Handbook of
Behavior Therapy
in the
Psychiatric Setting

CRITICAL ISSUES IN PSYCHIATRY
An Educational Series for Residents and Clinicians

Series Editor: Sherwyn M. Woods, M.D., Ph.D.
University of Southern California School of Medicine
Los Angeles, California

Recent volumes in the series:

CASE STUDIES IN INSOMNIA
Edited by Peter J. Hauri, Ph.D.

CHILD AND ADULT DEVELOPMENT: A Psychoanalytic Introduction
for Clinicians
Calvin A. Colarusso, M.D.

CLINICAL DISORDERS OF MEMORY
Aman U. Khan, M.D.

CONTEMPORARY PERSPECTIVES ON PSYCHOTHERAPY WITH
LESBIANS AND GAY MEN
Edited by Terry S. Stein, M.D., and Carol J. Cohen, M.D.

DECIPHERING MOTIVATION IN PSYCHOTHERAPY
David M. Allen, M.D.

DIAGNOSTIC AND LABORATORY TESTING IN PSYCHIATRY
Edited by Mark S. Gold, M.D., and A. L. C. Pottash, M.D.

DRUG AND ALCOHOL ABUSE: A Clinical Guide to Diagnosis and Treatment, Third Edition
Marc A. Schuckit, M.D.

EVALUATION OF THE PSYCHIATRIC PATIENT: A Primer
Seymour L. Halleck, M.D.

THE FREEDOM OF THE SELF: The Bio-Existential Therapy
of Character Problems
Eugene M. Abroms, M.D.

HANDBOOK OF BEHAVIOR THERAPY IN THE PSYCHIATRIC SETTING
Edited by Alan S. Bellack, Ph.D., and Michel Hersen, Ph.D.

NEUROPSYCHIATRIC FEATURES OF MENTAL DISORDERS
James W. Jefferson, M.D., and John R. Marshall, M.D.

RESEARCH IN PSYCHIATRY: Issues, Strategies, and Methods
Edited by L. K. George Hsu, M.D., and Michel Hersen, Ph.D.

SEXUAL LIFE: A Clinician's Guide
Stephen B. Levine, M.D.

STATES OF MIND: Configurational Analysis of Individual Psychology, Second Edition
Mardi J. Horowitz, M.D.

A Continuation Order Plan is available for this series. A continuation order will bring delivery of each new volume immediately upon publication. Volumes are billed only upon actual shipment. For further information please contact the publisher.

Handbook of Behavior Therapy in the Psychiatric Setting

Edited by
ALAN S. BELLACK, Ph.D.

Medical College of Pennsylvania at EPPI
Philadelphia, Pennsylvania

and

MICHEL HERSEN, Ph.D.

School of Psychology, Nova University
Fort Lauderdale, Florida

Plenum Press ● **New York and London**

Library of Congress Cataloging-in-Publication Data

Handbook of behavior therapy in the psychiatric setting / edited by
  Alan S. Bellack and Michel Hersen.
      p.   cm. -- (Critical issues in psychiatry)
    Includes bibliographical references and index.
    ISBN 0-306-44275-2
    1. Behavior therapy--Handbooks, manuals, etc.   I. Bellack, Alan
  S. II. Hersen, Michel. III. Series.
    [DNLM: 1. Behavior Therapy--methods.   WM 425 H23565]
  RC489.B4H344   1993
  616.89'142--dc20
  DNLM/DLC
  for Library of Congress   92-48877
                                                                   CIP

ISBN 0-306-44275-2

©1993 Plenum Press, New York
A Division of Plenum Publishing Corporation
233 Spring Street, New York, N.Y. 10013

Printed in the United States of America

To
Barbara, Jon, and Adam
and
Victoria, Jonathan, and Nathaniel

Contributors

Robert T. Ammerman • Western Pennsylvania School for Blind Children, Pittsburgh, Pennsylvania 15213

Marc S. Atkins • University of Pennsylvania School of Medicine and Department of Pediatric Psychology, Children's Hospital of Philadelphia and Children's Seashore House, Philadelphia, Pennsylvania 19104

Donald H. Baucom • Department of Psychology, University of North Carolina at Chapel Hill, Chapel Hill, North Carolina 27599

Alan S. Bellack • Medical College of Pennsylvania at EPPI, Philadelphia, Pennsylvania 19129

A. Lynn Bradshaw • Department of Psychology, Western Michigan University, Kalamazoo, Michigan 49008

Oscar G. Bukstein • Department of Psychiatry, University of Pittsburgh School of Medicine, Pittsburgh, Pennsylvania 15213

John V. Campo • Department of Psychiatry, Allegheny General Hospital and Medical College of Pennsylvania, Pittsburgh, Pennsylvania 15212

Mario Cappelli • Chedoke-McMaster Hospitals and Department of Psychiatry, McMaster University, Hamilton, Ontario L8N 3Z5, Canada

Laura L. Carstensen • Department of Psychology, Stanford University, Stanford, California 94305

David Celiberti • Rutgers, The State University of New Jersey, New Brunswick, New Jersey 08903

John A. Christopher • Department of Educational Psychology, University of Texas at Austin, Austin, Texas 78712

Paul Cinciripini • Department of Psychiatry and Behavioral Sciences, University of Texas Medical Branch at Galveston, Galveston, Texas 77555-0249

Michelle G. Craske • Department of Psychology, University of California—Los Angeles, Los Angeles, California 90024-1563

Charles E. Cunningham • Chedoke-McMaster Hospitals and Department of Psychiatry, McMaster University, Hamilton, Ontario L8N 3Z5, Canada

Margaret Dempsey • Department of Educational Psychology, University of Texas at Austin, Austin, Texas 78712

Faith B. Dickerson • The Sheppard and Enoch Pratt Hospital, 6501 North Charles Street, Baltimore, Maryland 21204

Michael G. Dow • Department of Community Mental Health, Florida Mental Health Institute, University of South Florida, Tampa, Florida 33612-3899

Ian R. H. Falloon • Department of Psychiatry and Behavioral Science, University of Auckland, New Zealand

Annette M. Farris • Department of Psychology, University of Houston, Houston, Texas 77204-5341

Jane E. Fisher • Department of Psychology, Northern Illinois University, DeKalb, Illinois 60115-2892

David M. Garner • Department of Psychiatry, Michigan State University, East Lansing, Michigan 48824-1316

David S. Glosser • Department of Neurology, Graduate Hospital, Philadelphia, Pennsylvania 19146

Guila Glosser • Department of Neurology, Graduate Hospital, Philadelphia, Pennsylvania 19146

Alan M. Gross • Department of Psychology, University of Mississippi, University, Mississippi 38677

Francis Harris • University of Pittsburgh, Pittsburgh, Pennsylvania 15213

Sandra L. Harris • Rutgers, The State University of New Jersey, New Brunswick, New Jersey 08903

Stephen N. Haynes • Department of Psychology, University of Hawaii, Honolulu, Hawaii 96822

Michel Hersen • School of Psychology, Nova University, 3301 College Avenue, Fort Lauderdale, Florida 33314

Diane Holder • Department of Psychiatry, University of Pittsburgh, 3811 O'Hara Street, Pittsburgh, Pennsylvania 15213

Ernest N. Jouriles • Department of Psychology, University of Houston, Houston, Texas 77204-5341

Erica Lilleleht • Rutgers, The State University of New Jersey, New Brunswick, New Jersey 08903

Marsha M. Linehan • Department of Psychology, University of Washington, Seattle, Washington 98195

Martin J. Lubetsky • Western Psychiatric Institute and Clinic, University of Pittsburgh School of Medicine, Pittsburgh, Pennsylvania 15213

Stephen A. Maisto • VA Medical Center, Brockton, Massachusetts 02401 and Brown University Medical School

Stephen C. Messer • University of Pittsburgh School of Medicine, Western Psychiatric Institute and Clinic, Pittsburgh, Pennsylvania 15213

J. Scott Mizes • Department of Psychiatry, MetroHealth Medical Center, Case Western Reserve University, School of Medicine, Cleveland, Ohio 44109

Tracy L. Morris • Department of Psychiatry and Behavioral Sciences, Medical University of South Carolina, Charleston, South Carolina 29425

Randall L. Morrison • William, Lynde, and Williams, Inc., Chagrin Falls, Ohio 44022

Kim T. Mueser • Medical College of Pennsylvania at EPPI, Philadelphia, Pennsylvania 19129

James P. Noll • Department of Psychology, Northern Illinois University, DeKalb, Illinois 60115-2892

Michael O'Boyle • Department of Psychiatry and Behavioral Sciences, University of Texas Medical Branch at Galveston, Galveston, Texas 77555-0429

William H. O'Brien • Department of Psychology, Bowling Green State University, Bowling Green, Ohio 43403

Timothy J. O'Farrell • VA Medical Center, Brockton, Massachusetts 02401 and Harvard Medical School

Mary L. Osborne • University of Pennsylvania School of Medicine and Department of Pediatric Psychology, Children's Hospital of Philadelphia and Children's Seashore House, Philadelphia, Pennsylvania 19104

Alan Poling • Department of Psychology, Western Michigan University, Kalamazoo, Michigan 49008

Lynn Rankin • Department of Psychology, University of North Carolina at Chapel Hill, Chapel Hill, North Carolina 27599

Robert C. Rinaldi • Division of Health Science, American Medical Association, Chicago, Illinois 60610

Alexander H. Sackeyfio • Eating Disorder Program, Beaumont Hospital, Royal Oak, Michigan 48073

Steven L. Sayers • Medical College of Pennsylvania at EPPI, Philadelphia, Pennsylvania 19129

Leslie J. Shapiro • School of Social Work, Boston University, Boston, Massachusetts 02215

Lori A. Sisson • Western Pennsylvania School for Blind Children, Pittsburgh, Pennsylvania 15213

Kevin D. Stark • Department of Educational Psychology, University of Texas at Austin, Austin, Texas 78712

Gail Steketee • School of Social Work, Boston University, Boston, Massachusetts 02215

Jill C. Taylor • Institute for Clinical Training and Research, The Devereux Foundation, Devon, Pennsylvania 19333

Susan E. Turk • Department of Psychology, Stanford University, Stanford, California 94305

Vincent B. Van Hasselt • School of Psychology, Nova University, Fort Lauderdale, Florida 33314

Eric F. Wagner • Emma Pendleton Bradley Hospital, Department of Psychiatry and Human Behavior, Brown University School of Medicine, East Providence, Rhode Island 02915

Kimberly Walitzer • VA Medical Center, Brockton, Massachusetts 02401

Elizabeth J. Wasson • Department of Psychology, University of Washington, Seattle, Washington 98195

Mark Worthen • VA Medical Center, Brockton, Massachusetts 02401

John T. Wixted • Department of Psychology, University of California—San Diego, La Jolla, California 92093

Preface

The Association for Advancement of Behavior Therapy, the primary professional organization for behavior therapists in North America, recently celebrated its 25th anniversary. The festivities surrounding this milestone highlighted the phenomenal growth of the field since the early 1960s. One of the most gratifying aspects of the celebration for those of us who have identified ourselves as "behavior therapists" over this period is the extent to which the behavioral approach has become part of the standard repertoire of psychiatric treatment approaches.

With a few notable exceptions, such as Joseph Wolpe, Stewart Agras, Robert Liberman, Mickey Stunkard, and John Paul Brady, behavior therapy was developed by psychologists. Its earliest acceptance was in university departments of psychology, schools, and specialized programs for retarded citizens. For many years, it was either ignored or discounted by much of psychiatry and many psychiatric facilities. That situation has now changed. Behavior therapy programs are now commonly found in medical school departments of psychiatry and in teaching hospitals. Behavior therapy training is a standard part of residency curricula, and questions on the approach are included on psychiatry board examinations. The topic is also found in an increasing number of medical school curricula.

The transition from university-based programs to the psychiatric setting is not simply a matter of acceptance of the scientific evidence that documents the efficacy of behavioral strategies. There are important differences in the types of patients seen in the two settings, in the way treatment is conducted, and in the context in which treatment is carried out. The medical tradition requires attention to issues that are not as germane in the psychology clinic (e.g., personal and family medical history), places increased emphasis on the role of medication as an alternate or ancillary treatment, and even applies a somewhat different set of ethical standards and practices.

The purpose of this book is to provide a manual for the practice of behavior therapy in the psychiatric setting. Particular emphasis has been placed on the special demands imposed by the difficult cases that present to the psychiatric clinic or the teaching hospital, rather than to university-based clinics, where most behavioral strategies were developed and validated. The book is divided into four parts. Part I, General Issues, is an introduction to the psychiatric setting. It covers practical and substantive issues that the clinician must attend to in this environment, including hospital practices, psychopharmacology, common medical complications, and neuropsychiatric complications. This book is intended for psychiatrists, as well as psychologists and social workers. Some of the material in this section (e.g., "Hospital Structure and Professional Roles") may be somewhat redundant for physicians and osteopaths, but the bulk of this section puts the subsequent sections in context and provides a general background for the practice of behavior therapy.

Parts II and III deal with the treatment of adults and of children and adolescents, respectively. Part IV covers family problems. Each chapter in these three sections includes a description of prototypical assessment and treatment strategies, followed by a discussion of "actual" or typical procedures. The prototypes represent the way in which techniques are often described in textbooks and journal articles, and the way in which they are designed to be carried out in research protocols. As will become apparent, patients in the real world rarely afford us the opportunity to use these prototypes. The authors have each described the types of problems that frequently arise and the solutions they have used. The reader who has no prior background in behavior therapy may wish to read original sources or textbooks for a more extended description of the prototype strategies, but the material in these three sections provides an excellent primer for clinical applications.

A book of this size and complexity requires the efforts of many individuals. Most of the credit belongs to our contributors, who shared their technical expertise and clinical knowledge in creative ways. We also appreciate their willingness to admit to the limitations of the techniques that they themselves have developed. As always, we are indebted to our secretarial staffs, without whom the book could never have been put together: Joan Gill and Peggy Mahon in Philadelphia, and Mary Newell and Mary Anne Fredrick in Pittsburgh. Finally, we thank our long-time friend and editor at Plenum, Eliot Werner; it is always a pleasure to be able to work with him.

ALAN S. BELLACK
MICHEL HERSEN

Contents

I
GENERAL ISSUES

1

Clinical Behavior Therapy with Adults

ALAN S. BELLACK and MICHEL HERSEN

INTRODUCTION

The history of behavior therapy can be roughly divided into three partially overlapping phases or eras: development, scientific documentation, and dissemination. The development phase comprises the first 10 or so years, in which Wolpe, Skinner, Lazarus, Cautela, Ayllon, Azrin, and others invented an entirely new repertoire of clinical techniques: systematic desensitization, contingency management, the token economy, thought stopping, and so on (Kazdin, 1978). The second phase, which comprised 10–15 years, established the efficacy of behavioral techniques. Stimulated by a series of seminal group-comparison studies by Paul, Lang, Davison, and others and by single-case designs by Hersen, Barlow, Leitenberg, Agras, and others, a new generation of clinical scientists conducted dozens of controlled trials that documented the superiority of the behavioral approach to other psychosocial strategies and our ability to modify behavior that had previously been thought to be intractable (Bellack, Hersen, & Kazdin, 1990).

Scientific "evidence," like beauty, is often only in the eye of the beholder. Although legions of behavior therapists were convinced of the value of the behavioral approach, the broader psychological/psychiatric community remained skeptical. Some of the reluctance to accept behavioral claims stemmed from the threat that such claims posed to traditional practices and theoretical beliefs. However, a good deal of the skepticism resulted from the well-founded contention that much of the research had questionable relevance to the clinical arena (Bellack & Hersen, 1985). As is by now well known, the creativity that led to the development of novel treatment strategies was matched by the development of innovative techniques for evaluating behavioral change and new designs for conducting outcome research. The *modus operandi* was the analogue study, as exemplified by the voluminous literature using college students with small-animal phobias as subjects and the Behavioral Approach Test as the primary criterion of outcome (Borkovec & Rachman, 1979; Matthews, 1978).

ALAN S. BELLACK • Medical College of Pennsylvania at EPPI, Philadelphia, Pennsylvania 19129.
MICHEL HERSEN • School of Psychology, Nova University, 3301 College Avenue, Fort Lauderdale, Florida 33314.

Handbook of Behavior Therapy in the Psychiatric Setting, edited by Alan S. Bellack and Michel Hersen. Plenum Press, New York, 1993.

Curiously, in the developmental phase, early behavior therapists worked with the most severely impaired clients, such as autistic and profoundly retarded children, chronic schizophrenics, and obsessive-compulsives and phobics unresponsive to conventional treatment. But in an effort to ensure scientific rigor, behavioral scientists substantially abandoned these difficult-to-study populations for much of the subsequent documentation era. The original intent of analogue studies was to provide a parallel to the clinical arena which afforded greater ability to objectify and standardize procedures. The legacy of this approach, including manualization of treatment protocols and behavioral observation, has been a profound influence on clinical practice and treatment outcome research (Kazdin, 1991). However, for an extended period, the analogue approach became reified in the behavioral literature, and the links to clinical practice were lost. Rather than being viewed as imperfect representations of the actual clinical environment, analogue protocols were frequently perceived as being equivalent. The conclusions about psychopathology and clinical practice derived from this mistaken assumption ranged from overly optimistic to inaccurate and, occasionally, naive (e.g., diagnosis is simply an overgeneralization and is superfluous; behavioral treatment is always brief and effective; if treatment is not effective, the fault lies in a faulty functional analysis). Of course, exaggerated claims and overstatements were partially a reaction to the cynicism and criticism that emanated from the mental health establishment. For much of the first 20 years, behavior therapists were something of a voice in the wilderness, needing to shout in order to be heard.

Fortunately, the field has continued to evolve and has moved from documentation and rhetoric to the current dissemination phase. The behavioral perspective has become more clinically realistic, techniques are more sophisticated, and claims are more tempered. Behavior therapy is increasingly becoming part of the mainstream of clinical practice. It is used in more diverse settings, including the psychiatric hospital and clinic. In many leading departments of psychiatry, it is seen as a partner to pharmacotherapy—the treatment of choice for some conditions and a reasonable alternative for others. Training in behavior therapy has also become a standard component of residency training curricula. Yet, the transition from research protocol and university clinic to the psychiatric environment is not complete. There are cultural, conceptual, and procedural differences that have yet to be resolved. In addition, further education is necessary both for behavior therapists making the translation to the psychiatric setting and for their nonbehavioral colleagues. The purpose of this book is to help bridge the gap. This initial chapter is intended to highlight some of the differences and issues that must be considered in the application of behavioral techniques in the psychiatric setting. We will briefly consider the nature of the clinical environment in such settings and the implications for assessment, implementation of treatment strategies, and issues related to the use of psychoactive medication.

THE CLINICAL ENVIRONMENT

The public and private mental-health establishment in most Anglo-European countries is based on a medical tradition. Whether or not a physician is in charge, this tradition has a powerful influence on clinical and administrative practices. It is reflected in the professional language, as well as in ways of thinking about cases; for example, the use of terms such as *patient* (vs. *client*), *diagnosis* (vs. *behavioral analysis*), and *medical record* or *chart* (vs. *behavioral observations*). It also affects the types of information needed to communicate about cases; for example, mental status, review of coexisting physical disorders and concurrent treatment, personal and family medical history, and blood work and toxicology screen. In contrast to the case in most psychology-oriented settings, treatment cannot begin in many psychiatric settings unless the individual has recently had a complete physical examination. In many cases, records must be signed by physicians even if the information is gathered or service is provided by a non-

M.D. This procedure is partly a function of tradition and is partly due to legal requirements or mandates by accreditation agencies. Even ethical practices differ in psychological and psychiatric settings. For example, psychologists generally will not communicate any information about a client without a written authorization, yet it is accepted practice in psychiatric settings to share information with referral sources and other colleagues who may be treating the individual.

Our intention is not to provide an encyclopedic listing of all of the special characteristics of the psychiatric setting. Rather, we simply wish to highlight the fact that the behavior therapist, who has traditionally been a psychologist trained with a university-based set of values and beliefs, must be attuned to the expectations of psychiatric colleagues and the requirements imposed on practice by a medically dominated system (e.g., hospital accreditation agencies, legal requirements, and restrictions on third-party reimbursement). These issues vary from state to state, country to country, and agency to agency. In many cases, they are arbitrary and antiquated (e.g., discriminatory reimbursement practices), and in other cases, they are reasonable, given the differences in areas of expertise (e.g., review and physician sign-off on concurrent medical condition). Moreover, the medical context does not necessarily preclude or impede the implementation of behavioral techniques; rather, it simply places the implementation in a different context and requires some additional considerations.

One aspect of the psychiatric setting that does appear to make a difference is the patient population. Psychiatric hospitals and clinics serve a more seriously ill population, including psychotic and suicidal patients, than psychology clinics. Moreover, this difference often appears to be the case *within* diagnostic categories as well as in the types of diagnoses that are served by the two different types of facilities. Clinical settings gradually develop a reputation among their primary referral sources and the local community that influences the types of patients that come for treatment. Whether it is true or not, psychiatric hospitals and clinics are often viewed as being appropriate or necessary for more difficult cases. In addition, the majority of individuals with psychological problems first seek help from family physicians, who tend to refer difficult cases to their psychiatric colleagues.

The term *difficult cases* in this context has two implications: the severity of the symptoms and the existence of concurrent conditions (e.g., dual diagnoses). Current diagnostic nomenclature (e.g., the revised third edition of the *Diagnostic and Statistical Manual*, or DSM-III-R; American Psychiatric Association, 1987) emphasizes the presence or absence of symptoms, rather than their severity. Yet patients at opposite ends of the severity spectrum are sometimes more different than patients with different diagnoses. For example, those with major depression range from individuals who can continue to work and maintain adequate social relationships to psychotic patients who cannot perform the activities of daily living (e.g., feeding and grooming themselves) and require inpatient care. Severely ill patients can have more symptoms and different symptoms (e.g., psychosis), as well as more severe symptoms. These differences often affect the type of treatment that is required, as well as how the treatment is implemented.

The Treatment of Depression Collaborative Research Program of the National Institute of Mental Health (NIMH) provides an example of the interaction of treatment type and severity. This multisite study found that cognitive behavior therapy was as effective as pharmacotherapy for moderately ill patients, but that the severely ill responded better to tricylic antidepressants (Elkin, Shea, Watkins *et al.*, 1989). These data are consistent with the general clinical wisdom that pharmacotherapy is indicated in the presence of psychosis or high suicidal risk, regardless of the documented effectiveness of behavior therapy for treating depression *per se*. The treatment of panic disorder provides another type of example. Behavior therapy has been shown to be a highly effective treatment for panic disorder (see Chapter 12 in this book), but it takes somewhat longer than pharmacotherapy to begin providing relief. Patients in acute distress due to severe or frequent attacks often require pharmacological intervention as an intermediary step or they will discontinue treatment. Behavior therapy has also proved to be an effective treatment for obsessive-compulsive disorder, even in the presence of depression (see Chapter 11 in this book).

However, severe depression can reduce energy and motivation to the point where the patient cannot participate in exposure and response prevention. Antidepressants are then indicated.

As illustrated by these examples, both empirical data and clinical necessity may dictate the use of pharmacotherapy as an adjunct or alternative to behavioral treatment. But the use of pharmacological treatment in severe cases does not preclude a role for behavior therapy. It is useful in maintaining gains (Frank, Kupfer, Perel, Cornes, Jarrett, Mallinger, Thase, McEochran, & Crochocinski, 1990) or remediating aspects of the disorder that are not effectively treated by medication (e.g., agoraphobic avoidance in panic disorder).

Few, if any, psychiatric disorders are mutually exclusive. Epidemiological data document that a large proportion of individuals with one disorder are apt to have a second (or third) disorder concurrently or at some time in the future (Robins, Helzer, Weissman, Orvaschel, Gruenberg, Burke, & Regies, 1984). Serious psychiatric disturbance also tends to have profound effects on social relationships and the ability to fulfill social roles (e.g., work and parenting). Consequently, few patients in psychiatric treatment settings are as "pure" as patients who participate in controlled treatment trials. There is an extensive literature on the difference between solicited volunteers (for experimental trials) and typical clinic referrals (Krupnick, Shea, & Elkin, 1986). Moreover, most trials have a rigorous set of exclusion criteria to avoid "messy" or unclear cases, which tend to obfuscate the results.

The clinician in the psychiatric setting does not have the luxury of referring out confusing or difficult cases. Rather, treatment must be accommodated to the difficulties presented by such patients. Treatment invariably takes longer than it does in protocols, often stretching to months or even years. Long-term treatment is especially common in the case of Axis 2 disorders, such as borderline personality (see Chapter 17 in this book). Negative life events, many of which are precipitated by social-role problems, interrupt the course of treatment. Patients miss sessions or insist that the focus shift to a current crisis or a new source of anguish. They self-medicate with alcohol, street drugs, or prescription medications (particularly benzodiazepines) secured from nonpsychiatric physicians. They are noncompliant with homework and inadvertently sabotage behavioral strategies. Family members resist the patient's efforts to change, or they increase the patient's stress because of their own psychiatric problems (e.g., physical abuse and alcoholism).

Another factor that distinguishes protocol cases from clinical cases is that the presenting problem is often an "acceptable" complaint that masks a more significant source of anxiety and distress, or a faulty assumption on the patient's part about what is really happening. It is not unusual for the focus of treatment to shift dramatically after a relationship is established and the patient feels comfortable admitting to all sources of concern. The clinician in the psychiatric setting must also accommodate to the unhappy fact that many problems cannot be alleviated with the current repertoire of behavior (or pharmacological) techniques, and that many patients are not amenable to the hard work of treatment at particular points in their lives. Complex cases may also require partial solutions or preclude any solutions.

BEHAVIORAL ASSESSMENT

The true hallmark of behavior therapy has always been its insistence on the precise selection and description of targets slated for modification. Although behavior therapists have traditionally been concerned with physiological responses and the patient's self-report (see Hersen, 1978), their most outstanding contribution to the general realm of assessment has been with respect to the measurement of motoric behavior (Tryon, 1991). As can be seen from the entries in the *Dictionary of Behavioral Assessment Techniques* (Hersen & Bellack, 1988a), both on-the-spot schemes to study a given patient's presenting behavioral difficulties and more formal and complex behavioral observation systems (e.g., the Marital Interaction Coding System; Tennenbaum, 1988) have been developed.

Behavioral assessment in the psychiatric setting certainly poses some unique challenges (Hersen, 1979), but it offers equally unique opportunities for innovative application within a medically oriented setting (cf. Hersen, 1988; Hersen & Bellack, 1988b; Hersen & Last, 1989; Hersen & Turner, 1988). We will not detail all of these issues here, as O'Brien and Haynes very ably discuss the specifics in Chapter 3 of this book; however, we will briefly highlight what we consider the most salient concerns. The first, of course (intuitively obvious), is that in the psychiatric arena, assessment is carried out under the umbrella system of the DSM-III (American Psychiatric Association, 1980) or DSM-III-R (APA, 1987), and, in the very near future, the forthcoming DSM-IV. Although the problems with overall psychiatric classification schemes are very well known and have received considerable critical attention for both adults (Hersen & Turner, 1988) and children (Hersen & Last, 1989), the reality of the situation is that these nosological systems are here to stay and have political ramifications with respect to medical control and reimbursement from third-party payers. Perhaps the overriding issue, however, is that classification is at the heart of every scientific endeavor, and that the alternative behavioral schemes that periodically appeared simply have not taken hold (see Hersen & Turner, 1988). Furthermore, in progression from the DSM-I (APA, 1952), the DSM-II (APA, 1968), the DSM-III (APA, 1980), the DSM-III-R (APA, 1987), and hopefully through the DSM-IV, both the reliability and the validity of the categories have improved considerably. The introduction of the multiaxial system also has yielded a more comprehensive picture, and in the DSM-III and the DSM-III-R, childhood and adolescent disorders were finally accorded an identity independent from adult diagnoses.

Unfortunately, despite increased diagnostic sophistication, the application of a particular label to the individual patient does not necessarily or specifically indicate which pharmacological or behavioral treatment should be used. Indeed, patients with identical symptomatic presentation and ensuing DSM-III-R diagnosis could (and often do) have totally different etiologies, requiring different therapeutic approaches. It is in this realm that an integration of behavioral assessment and psychiatric diagnosis is highly desirable from a clinical standpoint. Writing about children and adolescents, although these arguments are equally applicable to adults, Hersen and Last (1989) detailed the complementarity of psychiatric diagnosis and behavioral assessment as follows:

> In this conceptualization behavioral assessment is the *idiographic* approach and the DSM-III-R represents the *nomothetic approach*. That is, once a particular diagnosis has been established following DSM-III-R criteria, a behavioral analysis is carried out to determine the specific targets for either behavioral or pharmacological intervention. In so doing we have the advantage of the summary statement of diagnosis and the precision of relating specific targets to specific treatments in single-case strategies. (p. 525)

Useful versus Textbook Assessment

In a subsequent section of this chapter, "Pharmacotherapy and Behavior Therapy," we present highly sophisticated behavioral assessment schemes carried out over extensive periods of time by trained research technicians and evaluated in single-case research designs. Moreover, as motoric behavior was the primary target, and the assessments took place in the context of clinical research, adequate interrater agreement in each baseline and treatment phase was documented. Furthermore, in one case involving severe obsessive-compulsive psychopathology, the patient was observed for almost a three-month period on a 24-hour-a-day basis. Obviously, in the more typical clinical situation in the psychiatric setting, the therapist will have to forgo such experimental finesse. Indeed, there may be more reliance on the observation (albeit probably less reliable and valid) of nursing personnel. And when individuals are seen in outpatient settings (Hersen, 1983) for treatment, there may be a greater reliance on the therapist's own observations of behavior seen in the consulting room coupled with the patient's self-report (see Hersen, 1978).

In addition, in the clinical (versus the research) setting, it is unlikely that very expensive and sophisticated physiological equipment will be available, so the textbook tripartite assessment (motoric, cognitive, and physiological) is precluded. In spite of these limitations, however, the well-trained behavioral clinician can obtain sufficiently unbiased data to carry out the appropriate assessments during baseline, treatment, maintenance, and follow-up.

Increased Scope of Behavioral Assessment

Probably as a function of working in the context of a larger system (i.e., the psychiatric setting), behavior therapists have been exposed to a wide divergence of viewpoints and many different professionals. It should not be surprising, then, that this exposure has influenced how such clinicians perform their daily duties as behavioral assessors. As opposed to our earlier behavioral colleagues from the 1960s and 1970s, current behavior therapists have an increased scope in their practice of behavioral assessment (cf. Hersen, 1988):

1. As already noted, there is a concern with psychiatric diagnosis and how behavioral assessment can be integrated into the process.
2. Behavioral assessors now focus on neuropsychological findings and brain-behavior relationships.
3. There is a greater emphasis on developmental factors in psychopathology at all age levels.
4. There is an increased interest in the causative factors in particular diagnostic entities, especially insofar as different etiological considerations lead to identical symptomatic pictures across patients. Most definitely, the functional-analytic approach to assessment can contribute significantly to our understanding of both etiology and treatment.
5. Given the highly sensitive and sophisticated strategies developed by our more biologically oriented medical colleagues, contemporary behavioral assessors in psychiatric settings would be remiss if they ignored the biological substratum of observed behavior.

In short, behavioral assessment has become a much more comprehensive and inclusive endeavor that uses many tools previously not available to behavioral assessors (e.g., the plethora of structured and semistructured interview schedules).

CLINICAL STRATEGIES

Our charge to contributors to this volume was to describe "prototypical" treatment strategies, and then to discuss "actual" treatment practices. The following general principles are distilled from their recommendations and our own experience in conducting behavior therapy in the psychiatric setting:

1. Behavioral therapy is supposed to be based on a careful and systematic pretreatment assessment. In clinical practice, assessment must never end. The clinical behavior therapist must be attuned to new information that may alter how treatment is being implemented—or the entire conceptualization of the case. For example, a patient may not be compliant with homework because it is too difficult or is not relevant to the person's real concerns, or because she or he does not share the therapist's goals or approach to treatment, or a life crisis or recurrence of another disorder (e.g., depression) may make the initial presenting problem temporarily less relevant. Even decisions about termination must be based on an ongoing evaluation of residual symptomatology and the likelihood of further gains, rather than a predetermined decision about the number and focus of the sessions.

2. The therapist must be flexible. As implied by the discussion above, ongoing assessment frequently mandates a change in the form or direction of treatment. In some cases, the modifications involve relatively subtle changes in technique or additional attention to issues

covered in earlier sessions. However, it is not uncommon for the entire focus to change over time because of changes in the case formulation or the emergence of new problems. Rigid adherence to a protocol is a blueprint for failure with complex cases. Flexibility is essential in dealing with the ever-present problems in compliance. Most patients come to treatment expecting to talk and be semipassive recipients of the therapist's magic. They do not expect to keep diaries, do homework, or role-play during sessions. Although practice is essential in behavior therapy, we are aware of no data that explicitly document the necessity of self-monitoring or specific homework tasks (with the exception of exposure). The therapist must be creative in finding ways to induce the patient to comply with assignments but cannot insist on specific tasks. Such intransigence invariably leads to fruitless debate and derails sessions; it may also precipitate premature termination.

3. Patience is an essential virtue in the psychiatric setting. As previously indicated, progress with seriously ill patients characteristically is slow. Patients are afraid to make changes, and well-established habits are difficult to extinguish. Therapeutic progress is often characterized by the euphemism "two steps forward followed by one step backward." Frequently, treatment is temporarily interrupted by life crises, illness, decreases in motivation, or such prosaic issues as lapses in insurance coverage or changes in work schedules. In addition, gains are often modest. Success is reflected in symptom reduction and subtle improvements in quality of life, rather than in full symptom remission and recovery. Relapse and recurrence are also common. A therapist expecting a "quick fix" or "cure" is apt to lose many patients and experience frequent frustration.

4. Finally, the behavior therapist must be willing to consult with colleagues and consider referral of patients who are not progressing. Behavior therapy is the treatment of choice for several diagnostic categories and is demonstrably effective for many others. But it is not effective for *every* patient in any category. Consultation with both behavioral and nonbehavioral colleagues can provide a vital perspective on a case and may uncover reasons for roadblocks. Willingness to refer patients for alternative or ancillary treatment when needed is an ethical and legal mandate. It should not be avoided on purely theoretical grounds or for petty guild issues.

Pharmacotherapy and Behavior Therapy

By its very nature, the psychiatric-medical milieu sets the occasion for implementation of the combined pharmacotherapeutic and behavioral approach to difficult treatment cases. This integration, of course, is highlighted in the inpatient setting (Hersen, 1985c), but it is also representative of the outpatient setting (Hersen, 1983), although to a lesser extent. In inpatient psychiatry, the administrative control of biologically oriented psychiatrists is such that a behavioral treatment is unlikely to be applied by itself in the absence of any concurrent pharmacological strategy. However, the important issue is not who controls or dictates that treatment, but which treatment or combination serves the best interest of the particular patient.

As has been noted elsewhere, although both pharmacotherapy and behavior therapy have empirical bases (Hersen, 1985b), it was not until the middle 1970s and the decade of the 1980s that representatives of the pharmacological and behavioral disciplines began to contrast strategies and also consider their integration. More recently, the "combined effects of pharmacologic and behavioral treatment" have been heralded as "the wave of the future" (Hersen, 1985a, p. 10). This notion has been supported by the National Institute of Mental Health in the form of large grant awards to clinical researchers looking at the individual and possible synergistic effects of behavior therapy and pharmacotherapy in specified disorders (e.g., major depression: Hersen, Bellack, Himmelhoch, & Thase, 1984; Murphy, Simons, Wetzel, & Lustman, 1984; agoraphobia: Mavissakalian & Michelson, 1986; schizophrenia: Schooler, Keith, Bellack *et al.*, 1988).

Perhaps most representative of the interplay between pharmacotherapy and behavior therapy are the numerous single-case research designs that have appeared in the literature since the early 1970s in which either the drug has been kept consistent over time and a behavioral strategy has been added, or in which a behavioral strategy has been applied consistently over time and a pharmacological strategy has been added. Such combined strategies have been used in the treatment of schizophrenia (Agras, 1975; Hersen & Bellack, 1976), spasmodic torticollis (Turner, Hersen, & Alford, 1974), psychomotor seizures (Wells, Turner, Bellack, & Hersen, 1978), and obsessive-compulsive disorder (Turner, Hersen, Bellack, Andrasik, & Capparell, 1980). Although the large-scale clinical trials examining the separate and combined effects of pharmacotherapy and behavior therapy are specifically designed to provide confirmatory evidence of the possible synergistic effects (see Elkin, Pilkonis, Docherty, & Sotsky, 1988a, b; Hollon, Shelton, & Loosen, 1991; Kendall & Lipman, 1991; Marshall & Segal, 1990), they obviously cannot reflect the day-to-day nuances seen in clinical practice, as these are lost in the large-group parametric statistical analyses. Therefore, at this point, we will focus on drugs and behavior analysis and will identify some of the permutations of their combined use (cf. Liberman & Davis, 1975), illustrated by published single-case experimental designs.

In a seminal article on drugs and behavior analysis, Liberman and Davis (1975) categorized the interaction of pharmacotherapy and behavior therapy into four divisions:

1. Drugs used as adjuncts to facilitate behavior therapy.
2. Behavioral principles used to motivate medication use in chronic psychiatric patients.
3. Drug effects evaluated in single-case designs using behavioral measurement systems.
4. Drugs used as agents of punishment reinforcement, and of extinction.

In a chapter written a decade later, Hersen (1985a) reflected how the field looked at that time (and still does) and outlined the major categories of drug-behavior interactions. Two of the categories have the most relevance to current behavioral practice in psychiatric settings, and they are illustrated below: (1) drugs used to facilitate behavioral treatment and (2) the experimental analysis of pharmacological treatments using a behavioral indicant. A third use of the single-case strategy has involved the additive effects of drugs over behavior therapy; this use is also documented here.

Drugs Used to Facilitate Behavioral Treatment

We have already pointed out that the majority of inpatients treated behaviorally in psychiatric settings are medicated with psychotropic drugs. This certainly has been the case in the wardwide token economies frequently described in the 1970s (cf. Hersen, Eisler, Smith, & Agras, 1972; Kazdin, 1977). For example, Hersen et al. (1972) established a token economy unit for acutely disturbed male veterans whose psychiatric symptomatology was controlled pharmacologically, but whose work performance on the unit was managed behaviorally. When the token economy was artificially inflated and deflated (i.e., by a systematic increase or decrease in the point cost of privileges), the controlling effects of each economic contingency were clearly documented for the veterans' on-ward work performance. In a subsequent paper, Hersen, Turner, Edelstein, and Pinkston (1975) outlined the combined pharmacological and social skills treatment of a 27-year-old African-American patient (diagnosed schizophrenic, catatonic type, withdrawn), who participated in the token economy program originally described by Hersen et al. (1972). In this multifaceted treatment approach, an adjustment in phenothiazine levels enabled the patient to become more amenable to behavioral treatment. The token economy then led to an improvement in the patient's hygiene skills, whereas application of social skills training to identified behavioral targets led to improved interpersonal functioning to the extent that he was able to return to his home environment and obtain job retraining at Goodwill Industries. However, it is critical to underscore here that, in the absence of pharmacological control of psychotic symptoms, the amelioration of interpersonal deficits via social skills treatment would not have been possible.

Yet another example of the use of drugs to facilitate behavior therapy was reported by Hersen and Bellack (1976). In their multiple-baseline analysis of social skills training in chronic schizophrenics, two patients in a partial hospitalization program were first medicated in order to control psychotic symptomatology. In the first case, a 19-year-old single white male with a diagnosis of schizophrenia (catatonic type, with paranoid ideation) was administered Trilafon (32 mg, h.s.) and Cogentin (2 mg, h.s.). In the second case, a 27-year-old single white male, with a diagnosis of schizophrenia (chronic undifferentiated type) was administered Trilafon (16 mg, h.s.; 2 mg, q.i.d.) and Cogentin (2 mg, b.i.d.). In both cases, after medication was maximally effective, social skills training was directed to specific behavioral targets in sequence, leading to improved interpersonal functioning. However, in the absence of pharmacological remission of psychotic symptoms, behavioral treatment could not have been applied with success. Put more simply, the patients would not have learned the interpersonal skills while still psychotic.

At times, a drug proven to be only partially effective, and behavioral treatment is added for symptomatic relief after a reasonable period of pharmacotherapy. This is what took place in the case of a 22-year-old single female functioning in the "borderline" range of intelligence, whose psychomotor seizures were under only partial control with 1000 mg of Tegretol per day, Clonopin (2 mg, t.i.d.), and Prolixin (2.5 mg, t.i.d.) (Wells *et al.*, 1978). Indeed, seizures were still reported to occur at a rate of up to two to eight per day. As the patient reported a clear aura before each seizure, including anticipatory anxiety, a cue-controlled relaxation procedure was introduced, consisting of relaxation training paired with the cue word *relax*. The patient practiced this strategy while seizure-free and was then instructed to apply it when she experienced the aura. Cue-controlled relaxation procedures were evaluated in a single-case design during which medication was kept at a consistent level throughout each phase (Tegretol, 200 mg, t.i.d.). The results of this experimental analysis appear in Figure 1. Two target measures were examined:

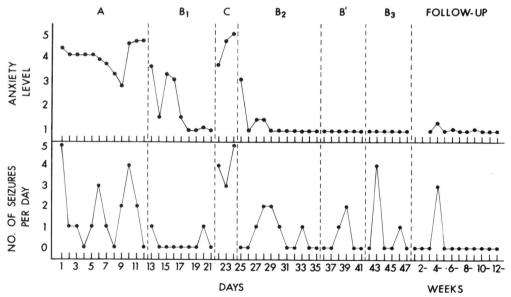

Figure 1. Frequency of seizure activity and ratings of anxiety level across experimental phases: A = Baseline; B$_1$ = cue-controlled relaxation; C = attention-placebo; B$_2$ = cue-controlled relaxation; B′ = cue-controlled relaxation with a novel therapist; B$_3$ = cue-controlled relaxation. From Wells *et al.* (1978, Figure 1). Reproduced with permission.

ALAN S. BELLACK and
MICHEL HERSEN

(1) the patient's self-reported anxiety level on a 1 to 5 point scale and (2) the number of seizures per day.

As can be seen in Figure 1, in Phase A (baseline), the anxiety level was higher, as was the seizure activity. In Phase B_1 (cue-controlled relaxation), the anxiety level decreased, as did the seizure activity. In Phase C (therapeutic attention in the absence of cue-controlled relaxation), the anxiety level rose considerably, as did the seizure activity. In Phase B_2 (cue-controlled relaxation), the anxiety level decreased again, as did the seizure activity. In Phase B' (cue-controlled relaxation with a novel therapist), the anxiety level and the seizure activity remained at the same level. In Phase B_3 (cue-controlled relaxation with the original therapist), the anxiety level was reported to be low, although the seizure activity increased, especially on Day 43. The patient was then discharged and followed up for 12 weeks. Except for Week 4, which was tension-filled for the patient, cue-controlled relaxation exercises were able to keep her anxiety level and the seizure activity under good control. In summary, the case documents the addition of a behavioral strategy to enhance the partial effects of pharmacotherapy.

Experimental Analysis of Pharmacological Treatments

According to Liberman and Davis (1975):

> The criteria for assessment of drug effects in clinical populations using single case designs should include: (a) continuous direct and reliable observations of behavior with enough observations to establish a clear trend within any condition; (b) controlled experimental designs, such as ABAB, BAB, or multiple baseline; and (c) double blind administration of the drug(s) and placebo. (p. 313)

The inpatient psychiatric setting, of course, is ideal for such evaluation, as it is able to provide the controls required by the particular design. Moreover, this type of experimental analysis provides the unique blend of pharmacotherapeutic intervention, behavioral observation, and a behavioral research strategy. Its importance is highlighted by the repeated measures used, which permit enough measurement points to document the controlling effects of the drug in question, as well as the possible variability over time.

Let us consider an illustration of the experimental analysis of Stelazine in a withdrawn 21-year-old male inpatient diagnosed schizophrenic, whose behavior had worsened over three years (Liberman, Davis, Moon, & Moore, 1973). On the inpatient unit, this patient was exceptionally socially isolated. Therefore, during the five phases of the experimental analysis, the mean number of his asocial responses (refusals to partake in brief conversations) served as the dependent measure. Figure 2 shows that, during the no-drug phase, his asocial responses increased dramatically. In the second phase (placebo), there was some initial improvement, but the patient's asocial responses again increased. The introduction of Stelazine (60 mg per day) in the third phase led to a marked reversal of his arousal responses. However, in the fourth phase, when placebo was reinstated, he once again was asocial. Finally, in the last phase, where Stelazine (60 mg per day) was reinstituted, his asocial responding dropped markedly.

Not only does the experimental analysis of drugs provide the investigator with documentation of their controlling effects on the targeted behavioral measure, but the analysis can also yield information about the most efficacious dosage level. Indeed, when different drug dosages are evaluated, the experimental analysis is capable of dictating the choice of the lowest possible discharge dosage that appears to be effective. This choice, of course, is a critical feature, which is permitted by the precision of the behavioral targets used to measure the success of the particular treatment.

Additive Effects of Drugs over Behavior Therapy

Our next illustration of the combined use of behavior therapy and pharmacotherapy involves the case of a 51-year-old severe obsessive-compulsive male who was underweight (Turner,

Hersen, Bellack, & Wells, 1979). In a long inpatient stay, response prevention and flooding had a marked positive effect on this patient's obsessive-compulsive symptomatology (which consisted of hand washing; hair combing; handling doorknobs and personal items with tissue paper; washing sinks, combs, and other personal items; food aversions; fear of constipation; general indecisiveness; and an inability to perform simple acts). However, the patient's inadequate sleep (hyposomnia) and low weight did not improve sufficiently until tricyclic antidepressants were added in the final phase of treatment. Throughout all phases of treatment, the patient was under constant observation, so we were provided with a wealth of data.

As can be seen in Figure 3, in Phase A (baseline) the percentage of rituals attempted was high, the patient's mean sleep duration was 4.5 hours, and his weight began to rise slightly (mean = 88.2 pounds). In Phase B (response prevention), the percentage of rituals attempted decreased (mean = 9%) sharply, mean sleep duration remained at 4.5 hours, and weight continued to rise (mean = 92.3 pounds). In the succeeding A phase, the percentage of rituals attempted increased (mean = 15%), sleep was unchanged (mean = 4.? hours), and weight continued to increase (mean = 97.0 pounds). In the next B phase (response prevention), the percentage of rituals attempted once again decreased (mean = 6%), sleep was essentially unchanged (mean = 4.6 hours), and weight stabilized (mean = 97.0 pounds). In Figure 4, with the addition of flooding to response prevention in Phase BC, the percentage of rituals attempted rose slightly (mean = 8%), sleep increased slightly (mean = 4.8 hours), and weight improved slightly (mean = 99.2 pounds). In the next A phase, baseline conditions were reinstated to test the generality of the treatment. There was a slight increase in percentage rituals attempted (mean = 11%), a slight increase in sleep (mean = 5.0 hours), and continued weight stabilization (mean = 99.2 pounds).

Given that the patient was still underweight and had remained virtually hypersomnic, a tricyclic antidepressant (imipramine) was introduced on Day 80 of treatment in Phase D (numeral 1). However, as this medication caused him to have extensive urinary retention, medication was changed to another tricyclic antidepressant (doxepin hydrochloride) on Day 84 (numerals 2–7 refer to dosage changes, increased gradually to 300 mg per day). In Phase D, there

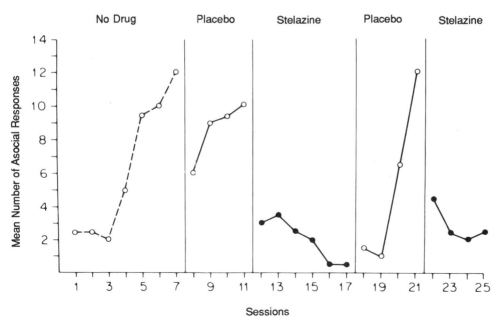

Figure 2. Average number of refusals to engage in a brief conversation. From Liberman *et al.* (1973, Figure 2). Reproduced with permission.

was a minimal increase in the percentage of rituals attempted (12%), the largest improvement in sleep (mean = 5.7 hours), and a more substantial weight gain (mean = 105.8 pounds).

In summary, it is clear that response prevention yielded marked decreases in ritualizing and that the addition of flooding had a minimal effect. The patient's sleep appeared essentially unaffected by behavioral treatment. His weight increased gradually during behavioral treatment, but this increase was undoubtedly due to the patient's inpatient stay and improved nutrition. Antidepressant medication had no effect on the rituals but did improve sleep to some extent and yielded the largest increase in body weight. Indeed, in the less structured combined use of behavioral therapy and pharmacotherapy in individual cases, it is not uncommon for behavioral treatment to be most efficacious with behavioral targets, whereas antidepressants and other forms of psychotropic medication tend to work fastest on vegetative symptoms.

Large-Scale Clinical Trials

Despite the apparent day-to-day utility of carrying out drug-behavioral-therapy interactions in clinical practice, the superiority of such dual conditions over drugs alone or behavioral treatments alone has not emerged consistently in the case of either major depression (Hersen *et al.*, 1984; Hollon *et al.*, 1991; Murphy, Simons, Wetzel, & Lastman, 1984; Simons, Murphy, Levine, & Wetzel, 1986) or the anxiety-based disorders (Marshall & Segal, 1990; Michelson & Marchione, 1991) when evaluated in large-scale clinical trials. Even when there has been some superiority in favor of the combined behavioral-pharmacological approach has been shown, this superiority has been reflected in nonsignificant trends. An exception is a recently published study by Agras, Rossiter, Arnow, Schneider, Telch, Raeburn, Bruce, Perl, and Koran (1992) showing

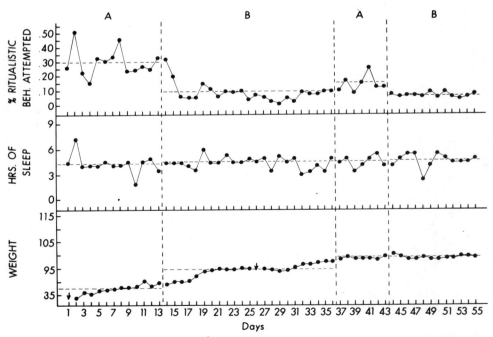

Figure 3. Percentage of time (observation periods) ritualizing, hours of sleep, and weight during initial baseline, initial response prevention, withdrawal, and second response prevention. From Turner *et al.* (1979, Figure 3A). Reproduced with permission.

the superiority of a combined cognitive-behavioral and desipramine condition in the treatment of bulimia nervosa. Also, in many instances, the outcome studies have been plagued by methodological problems (see Kendall & Lipman, 1991, for review). Among the many confounds are inadequate sample size, drug-alone subjects carrying out behavioral strategies on their own initiative, problems in treatment compliance, and superiority of the particular strategy *favored* by the research team. Also, in some instances, the addition of the pharmacological approach to behavior therapy has resulted in increased dropout from the study.

Despite these comments, we do not believe that the final verdict is in. Only a handful of outcome studies with adequate methodology have been carried out on relatively few disorders. Moreover, the heterogeneity of some of the samples does not allow the clinical researcher to pinpoint which subgroup of patients will benefit most from either the behavioral, the pharmacological, or the combined approach. Until such data are forthcoming, it is likely that the combined use of drugs and behavior therapy will continue in the psychiatric setting on a case-by-case basis.

SUMMARY

In this chapter, we have set the stage for the remainder of the book by identifying the unique role of behavior therapy in the psychiatric setting. In so doing, we have outlined both the benefits and the problems of carrying out behavioral strategies in this environment. In looking at the uniqueness of the psychiatric setting, we have examined the differences between private practice and university clinics and inpatient settings in terms of the severity of cases seen, the reality of dual diagnoses, and the overall medical atmosphere.

We then discussed behavioral assessment within the psychiatric setting, with a special

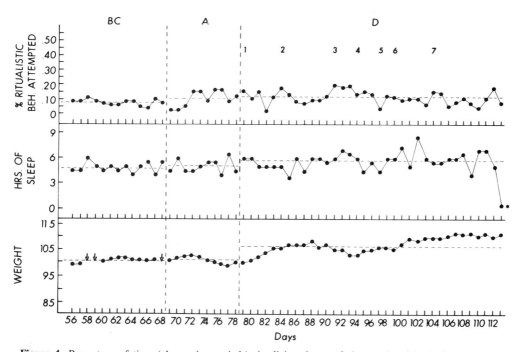

Figure 4. Percentage of time (observation periods) ritualizing, hours of sleep and weight during response prevention plus flooding, withdrawal and psychotropic medication. From Turner *et al.* (1979, Figure 3B). Reproduced with permission.

emphasis on its relationship to the umbrella of DSM diagnostic categories. We have also noted the increased scope of behavioral assessment, which probably is a direct function of the interaction of behavior therapists with colleagues harboring different theoretical positions within the medical environment. Apparently, this interaction has resulted in a fruitful collaboration and consequent yield. We then evaluated clinical strategies in the context of compliance, crises, and impediments to implementing behavioral protocols. Finally, in the section on pharmacotherapy and behavior therapy, we considered the concurrent application of the two treatment modalities from the clinical and research perspectives. However, to date, the large-scale clinical trials evaluating the separate and combined effects of pharmacotherapy and behavior therapy have not fully borne out the theoretical promise of synergistic effects.

What now follows are 30 chapters by colleagues who have carefully delineated the practice of behavior therapy in the psychiatric setting from many perspectives and with child, adolescent, and adult populations.

REFERENCES

Agras, W. S. (1975). Behavioral modification in the general hospital psychiatric unit. In H. Leitenberg (Ed.), *Handbook of behavior modification* (pp. 547–565). Englewood Cliffs, NJ: Prentice-Hall.

Agras, W. S., Rossiter, E. M., Arnow, B., Schneider, J. A., Telch, C. F., Raeburn, S. D., Bruce, B., Perl, M., & Koran, L. M. (1992). Pharmacologic and cognitive-behavioral treatment for bulimia nervosa: A controlled comparison. *American Journal of Psychiatry, 149*, 82–87.

American Psychiatric Association. (1952). *Diagnostic and statistical manual of mental disorders* (DSM-I). Washington, DC: Author.

American Psychiatric Association. (1968). *Diagnostic and statistical manual of mental disorders* (2nd ed.) (DSM-II). Washington, DC: Author.

American Psychiatric Association. (1980). *Diagnostic and statistical manual of mental disorders* (3rd ed.) (DSM-III). Washington, DC: Author.

American Psychiatric Association. (1987). *Diagnostic and statistical manual of mental disorders* (3rd ed., rev.) (DSM-III-R). Washington, DC: Author.

Bellack, A. S., & Hersen, M. (1985). General considerations. In M. Hersen & A. S. Bellack (Eds.), *Handbook of clinical behavior therapy with adults*. New York: Plenum Press.

Bellack, A. S., Hersen, M., & Kardin, A. E. (Eds.). (1990). *International handbook of behavior modification and therapy*. New York: Plenum Press.

Borkovec, T., & Rachman, S. (1979). The utility of analogue research. *Behaviour Research and Therapy, 17*, 253–262.

Elkin, I., Pilkonis, P. A., Docherty, J. P., & Sotsky, S. M. (1988a). Conceptual and methodological issues in comparative studies of psychotherapy and pharmacotherapy: 1. Active Ingredients and mechanisms of change. *American Journal of Psychiatry, 145*, 909–917.

Elkin, I., Pilkonis, P. A., Docherty, J. P., & Sotsky, S. M. (1988b). Conceptual and methodological issues in comparative studies of psychotherapy and pharmacotherapy: 2. Nature and timing of treatment effects. *American Journal of Psychiatry, 145*, 1070–1076.

Elkin, I., Shea, M. T., Watkins, J. T., *et al.* (1989). National Institute of Mental Health Treatment of Depression Collaborative Research Program: General effectiveness of treatments. *Archives of General Psychiatry, 46*, 971–982.

Frank, E., Kupfer, D. J., Perel, J. M., *et al.* (1990). *Three-year outcomes for maintenance therapies in recurrent depression. Archives of General Psychiatry, 47*, 1093–1099.

Hersen, M. (1978). Do behavior therapists use self-reports as major criteria? *Behavioral Analysis and Modification, 2*, 328–334.

Hersen, M. (Ed.). (1983). *Outpatient behavior therapy: A clinical guide*. New York: Grune & Stratton.

Hersen, M. (1985a). Historical issues. In M. Hersen (Ed.), *Pharmacological and behavioral treatment: An integrative approach*. New York: Wiley.

Hersen, M. (Ed.). (1985b). *Pharmacological and behavior treatment: An integrative approach* (pp. 5–14). New York: Wiley.

Hersen, M. (Ed.). (1985c). *Practice of inpatient behavior therapy: A clinical guide*. New York: Grune & Stratton.

Hersen, M. (1988). Behavioral assessment and psychiatric diagnosis. *Behavioral Assessment, 10*, 107–121.

Hersen, M., & Bellack, A. S. (1976). A multiple-baseline analysis of social-skills training in chronic schizophrenics. *Journal of Applied Behavior Analysis, 9*, 239–245.

Hersen, M., & Bellack, A. S. (Eds.) (1988a). *Dictionary of behavioral assessment techniques.* New York: Pergamon Press.

Hersen, M., & Bellack, A. S. (1988b). DSM-III and behavioral assessment. In M. Hersen & A. S. Bellack (Eds.), *Behavioral assessment: A practical handbook* (3rd ed.). New York: Pergamon Press.

Hersen, M., & Last, C. G. (1989). Psychiatric diagnosis and behavioral assessment in children. In C. G. Last & M. Hersen (Eds.), *Child psychiatric diagnosis* (pp. 517–528). New York: Wiley.

Hersen, M., & Turner, S. M. (1988). DSM-III, DSM-III-R, and behavior therapy. In A. S. Bellack & M. Hersen (Eds.), *Behavioral assessment: A practical handbook* (pp. 463–481). New York: Pergamon Press.

Hersen, M., Eisler, R. M., Smith, B. S., & Agras, W. S. (1972). A token reinforcement ward for young psychiatric patients. *American Journal of Psychiatry, 129,* 228–233.

Hersen, M., Turner, S. M., Edelstein, B. A , & Pinkston, S. G. (1975). Effects of phenothiazines and social skills training in a withdrawn schizophrenic. *Journal of Clinical Psychology, 31,* 588–594.

Hersen, M., Bellack, A. S., Himmelhoch, J. M., & Thase, M. E. (1984). Effects of social skill training, amitriptyline, and psychotherapy in unipolar depressed women. *Behavior Therapy, 15,* 21–40.

Hollon, S. D., Shelton, R. C., & Loosen, P. T. (1991). Cognitive therapy and pharmacotherapy for depression. *Journal of Consulting and Clinical Psychology, 59,* 88–99.

Kazdin, A. E. (1977). *The token economy.* New York: Plenum Press.

Kazdin, A. E. (1978). *History of behavior modification: Experimental foundations of contemporary research.* Baltimore: University Park Press.

Kazdin, A. E. (1991). Treatment research: The investigation and evaluation of psychotherapy. In M. Hersen, A. E. Kazdin, & A. S. Bellack (Eds.). *The clinical psychology handbook* (2nd ed.). New York: Pergamon Press.

Kendall, P. C., & Lipman, A. J. (1991). Psychological and pharmacological therapy: Methods and modes for comparative outcome research. *Journal of Consulting and Clinical Psychology, 39,* 78–87.

Krupnick, J., Shea, T., & Elkin, I. (1986). Generalizability of treatment studies utilizing solicited patients. *Journal of Consulting and Clinical Psychology, 54,* 68–78.

Liberman, R. P., & Davis, J. (1975). Drugs and behavior analysis. In M. Hersen, R. M. Eisler, & P. M. Miller (Eds.), *Progress in behavior modification* (Vol. 1, pp. 307–330). New York: Academic Press.

Liberman, R. P., Davis, J., Moon, W., & Moore, J. (1973). Research design for analyzing drug-environment-behavior interactions. *Journal of Nervous and Mental Disease, 156,* 432–439.

Marshall, W. L., & Segal, Z. V. (1990). Drugs combined with behavioral psychotherapy., In A. S. Bellack, M. Hersen, & A. E. Kazdin (Eds.), *International handbook of behavior modification and therapy* (pp. 267–279). New York: Plenum Press.

Matthews, A. (1978). Fear-reduction research and clinical phobias. *Psychological Bulletin, 85,* 390–404.

Mavissakalian, M., & Michelson, L. (1986). Agoraphobia: Relative and combined effectiveness of therapist-assisted in vivo exposure and imipramine. *Journal of Clinical Psychiatry, 47,* 117–122.

Michelson, L. K., & Marchione, K. (1991). Behavioral, cognitive, and pharmacological treatments of panic disorder with agoraphobia: Critique and synthesis. *Journal of Consulting and Clinical Psychology, 59,* 100–114.

Murphy, G. E., Simons, A. D., Wetzel, R. D., & Lustman, P. J. (1984). Cognitive therapy and pharmacotherapy. *Archives of General Psychiatry, 41,* 33–41.

Robins, L. M., Helzer, J. E., Weissman, M. M., Orvaschel, H,. Gruenberg, E., Burke, J. D., & Regies, D. A. (1984). Lifetime prevalence of specific psychiatric disorders in three sites. *Archives of General Psychiatry, 41,* 949–958.

Schooler, N. R., Keith, S. J., Bellack, A. S., *et al.* (1988, December). *Acute treatment response and short term outcome in schizophrenia.* Paper presented at the Annual Meeting of the American College of Neuropsychopharmacology, San Juan, PR.

Simons, A. D., Murphy, G. E., Levine, J. L., & Wetzel, R. D. (1986). Cognitive therapy and pharmacotherapy for depression. *Archives of General Psychiatry, 43,* 43–48.

Tennenbaum, D. L. (1988). Marital interaction coding system. In M. Hersen & A. S. Bellack (Eds.), *Dictionary of behavioral assessment techniques* (pp. 291–293). New York: Pergamon Press.

Tryon, W. W. (1991). *Activity measurement in psychology and medicine.* New York: Plenum Press.

Turner, A. M., Hersen, M., Bellack, A. S., Andrasik, F., & Capparell, H. V. (1980). Behavioral and pharmacological treatment of obsessive-compulsive disorders. *Journal of Nervous and Mental Disease, 168,* 651–657.

Turner, S. M., Hersen, M., & Alford, H. (1974). Effects of massed practice and meprobamate on spasmodic torticollis: An experimental analysis. *Behaviour Research and Therapy, 12,* 259–260.

Turner, S. M., Hersen, M., Bellack, A. S., & Wells, K. C. (1979). Behavioral treatment of obsessive-compulsive neurosis. *Behaviour Research and Therapy, 17,* 95–106.

Wells, K. C., Turner, S. M., Bellack, A. S., & Hersen, M. (1978). Effects of cue-controlled relaxation on psychomotor seizures: An experimental analysis. *Behaviour Research and Therapy, 16,* 51–53.

2

Clinical Behavior Therapy with Children

STEPHEN C. MESSER, TRACY L. MORRIS,
and ALAN M. GROSS

INTRODUCTION

The extent of childhood behavioral and psychological problems in need of services is enormous. At least 12% (about 7.5 million) of children under age 18 suffer from one or more psychological disorders (Gould, Wunsch-Hitzig, & Dohrenwend, 1981). Of these 7.5 million, nearly half are considered severely impaired by their condition (Office of Technology Assessment, 1986). Evidence also suggests that some of these childhood problems persist into late adolescence and possibly adulthood (e.g., Kazdin, 1989; Kovacs et al., 1984). Moreover the economic costs of the direct treatment of the behavior problems of children (under age 14) are estimated at a conservative $1.5 billion (Rice, Kelman, & Dunmeyer, in progress, cited in Institute of Medicine, 1989). Clearly, child behavior problems represent a significant social problem in search of potential solutions.

Many diverse disciplines, including clinical child psychology and psychiatry, pediatrics, and social work are called on to deliver effective services for these many children, their teachers, and their families. Treatments for children include a tremendous variety of approaches with interventions designed to reduce maladaptive behavior and increase social functioning (Johnson, Rasbury, & Siegel, 1986; Mash & Barkley, 1988). Only relatively recently have rigorous scientific methods been applied to the area of childhood psychopathology. At the forefront of clinical research and service is the field of child behavior therapy. Despite its short history, child behavior therapy has made substantial progress in the development of effective interventions for the treatment needed by a large number of children and their families.

The purpose of this chapter is to provide a broad overview of contemporary child behavior

STEPHEN C. MESSER • University of Pittsburgh School of Medicine, Western Psychiatric Institute and Clinic, Pittsburgh, Pennsylvania 15213.   TRACY L. MORRIS • Department of Psychiatry and Behavioral Sciences, Medical University of South Carolina, Charleston, South Carolina 29425. ALAN M. GROSS • Department of Psychology, University of Mississippi, University, Mississippi 38677.

Handbook of Behavior Therapy in the Psychiatric Setting, edited by Alan S. Bellack and Michel Hersen. Plenum Press, New York, 1993.

19

therapy. Following an attempt to put the field into perspective by providing some history and defining characteristics, our attention turns to a cornerstone of behavior therapy, the process of behavioral assessment. A brief and selective review of basic therapeutic paradigms and procedures follows. We conclude by highlighting some developmental and ethical issues. If we are able to provide the reader with an appreciation of the complexity and potential of a broad-based child behavioral-systems approach to the alleviation of children's suffering, we will have been successful.

HISTORICAL OVERVIEW

Attempts to modify the behavior of children date to antiquity, yet systematic behavioral applications to the treatment of childhood disorders were not evident until the early 1900s. Jones (1924) used conditioning principles to treat a 3-year-old boy's generalized fear of furry objects. Similarly, Mowrer and Mowrer (1938) successfully applied conditioning techniques to the treatment of enuresis. Despite such early efforts, applications of behavior therapy were generally limited to adult populations, and only occasional reports of behavior therapy with children occurred before the late 1950s.

During the 1950s and 1960s, many professionals grew discontented with the then-prevailing psychodynamic model. Many populations (e.g., those who were autistic and mentally retarded) were underserved. Reactions against the psychoanalytic establishments helped fuel the rise of applied behaviorism. The work of Skinner (1953), Eysenck (1957, 1960), Wolpe (1958), and Bandura (1961) addressed the utility of applying laboratory-derived methods to the modification of psychological disorders, and thus a firm foundation for the emerging field of behavior therapy was formed.

In the 1960s, operant conditioning principles came to be widely used in the treatment of child behavior problems. These techniques had demonstrated their efficacy in the laboratory, and it was believed that they could be easily adapted for use in "real life" settings. The transition from the laboratory, however, was not so smooth. Much of the work was done by researchers with little or no clinical experience. The focus was on demonstrating the efficacy of relatively simple operant procedures, and little was done to address developmental factors, cognitive variables, or the social network in which the behavior problems presented.

DEFINING CHILD BEHAVIOR THERAPY

Defining *behavior therapy*, whether for child or adult, is a difficult task. Different authors emphasize different features. Ollendick (1986) noted that

> some define behavior therapy by the techniques employed (e.g., London); others define behavior therapy by its allegiance to learning principles (e.g., Wolpe); still others define it by its methodological approach to behavior change (e.g., Yates). (p. 526)

Similarly, Emmelkamp (1986) identified four "schools" of behavior therapy: those stressing learning theory; those relying heavily on mediational concepts; the technical eclecticists, or multimodal behavior-therapy group; and those who emphasize an "experimental-clinical" or empirical-methodological approach. We can find no better working definition of child behavior therapy than that espoused by Ross (quoted by Ollendick, 1986):

> Like behavior therapy, in general, [it] is best defined as an empirical approach to psychological problems. It entails continuous evaluation of therapeutic interventions and thus calls for objectively defined terms and measurable procedures. It can thus be said that child behavior therapy is the application of psychology to the alleviation of the psychological distress of children. As such, it is an open-minded, self-correcting, and constantly changing field of endeavor. (p. 527)

One approach to characterizing child behavior therapy is to emphasize the methods of behavioral assessment. And one way to distinguish child behavioral assessment is to compare its assumptions, methods, and purposes with those of traditional psychological assessment. Several excellent reviews comparing the conceptual foundations of traditional and behavioral assessment can be found elsewhere (e.g., Barrios & Hartmann, 1986; Goldfried & Kent, 1972; Kanfer & Saslow, 1969). Ollendick and Hersen (1984) briefly summarized two major distinctions: 1) The traditional approach emphasizes psychological traits or dispositions that are assumed to underlie and produce behavioral consistency, whereas the behavioral approach focuses more on the behavior itself, while emphasizing situational influences upon behavior, and (2) traditional assessment interprets the child's response as a "sign" or indirect measure of some underlying personality trait, whereas behavioral assessment takes a "sample" approach, viewing the response as a sample of the target behavior to be assessed, relying on little inference. Though the process of contrasting behavioral assessment with "traditional" approaches has instructive and heuristic value, we agree with Mash and Terdal (1988), who emphasized the potential problems inherent in such a comparison. Such contrasts obscure a number of important and subtle distinctions, perpetuate the view of the field as reactionary, and foster dichotomous, either-or thinking (e.g., traits versus situations).

In the history of child behavioral assessment, two primary themes characterized early developments in the field (Ollendick & Hersen, 1984). Early child behavioral work evidenced a strong commitment to an operant perspective, emphasizing observable events, contemporaneous behavior and situational influences, and within-subject comparisons. In addition, little attention was directed to developmental issues and processes, including the utility of normative comparisons. The early adherence to the operant approach, while restricting and limiting the domain of inquiry, nevertheless provided the foundation for an empirical approach to the assessment of child behavioral disorders.

Several basic objectives of behavioral assessment can be identified (e.g., Barlow, Hayes, & Nelson, 1984; Bornstein, Bornstein, & Dawson, 1984; Gross & Wixted, 1988; Mash & Terdal, 1988; Ollendick & Hersen, 1984):

1. The identification of the problem behaviors and their controlling variables (see Mash & Terdal, 1988, for a discussion of target behavior versus disorder assessment).
2. The systematic, repeated measurement of those behaviors that assesses the change resulting from the treatment interaction.
3. An evaluation of the durability of the treatment gains after the intervention program has concluded.

Such objectives stimulate the behavioral assessor to ask such questions as

1. What is the child's current behavioral repertoire, including the maladaptive responses that brought him or her to the clinician?
2. What is the frequency, intensity, rate, and duration of the maladaptive responses?
3. Under what circumstances (antecedents and consequences) are the maladaptive responses emitted?
4. What environmental conditions in the child's life lend themselves to therapeutic manipulation? (Ross, 1974)

Current behavioral assessment approaches are attempting a fuller integration of the developmental, social, cognitive, and affective dimensions, representing a convergence on ecologically oriented systems models (e.g., Belsky, Lerner, & Spanier, 1984; Evans, 1985; Mash & Terdal, 1988). According to Ollendick and Hersen (1984), "recent developments expand the scope of child behavioral assessment to include broader and richer contexts in which ecological, social, cultural, and developmental influences on behavior can be examined more productively" (p. 6). These newer developments include a greater appreciation of developmental factors, such as the cognitive level and temperamental style of the child (e.g., Achenbach & Edelbrock, 1984); distal events, such as interactions with neighbors (e.g., Wahler, 1980); molar events, such as external stressors (e.g., Patterson, DeBarsyshe, & Ramsey, 1989); the wider social context (Bronfenbrenner, 1986); cognitions, such as parental expectations and attributions (e.g., Foster & Robin, 1989); and normative data (e.g., Achenbach & Edelbrock, 1984). The nature of behavioral assessment is changing from simple target behavior assessment to a more general, problem-solving analysis of system variables (e.g., Evans, 1985; Kanfer & Schefft, 1988; Mash & Terdal, 1988). In sum, the methods of assessment, but not the basic objectives, continue to change and evolve (Ollendick & Hersen, 1984).

Of course, the child behavior therapist requires specific procedures to actualize behavioral assessment objectives. Several criteria can be used to direct the selection of procedures (Ollendick & Hersen, 1984). First, a multimethod approach is useful in addressing the various contextual and behavioral dimensions evidenced by the child. The range of procedures and assessment strategies includes the clinical interview, self-monitoring, direct observation, psychophysiological recordings, standardized testing, ratings, and self-report (see Chapter 3 of this book or Mash & Terdal, 1988, for more extensive information). These various methods are assumed to provide incremental, unique information not derivable from one source in isolation (e.g., Mash, 1979). Second, empirically based and validated procedures should be given priority. Though the application of conventional psychometrics to behavioral measures is still somewhat controversial (e.g., Mash & Terdal, 1981), a number of sophisticated behavioral researchers acknowledge the importance of developing standardized and validated measures of child behavior (e.g., Cone, 1977; Ollendick & Hersen, 1984; Patterson, 1982). Finally, behavioral procedures should be chosen that demonstrate sensitivity to normal developmental processes (Ciminero & Drabman, 1977; Achenbach & Edelbrock, 1984; Mash & Terdal, 1988). Age-related constraints on assessment are notable and require further specification. For example, self-monitoring procedures appear to cause problems for preschool children (Ollendick & Cerny, 1981).

In addition, the child behavioral assessor must remain sensitive to several considerations unique to the process of child evaluation. First, children rarely refer themselves for treatment. Instead, the presenting complaint represents a complex series of judgments made by significant individuals in the child's environment (Mash & Terdal, 1988). Therefore, an examination of the referral process is essential. In particular, the therapist must assess the possible existence of problems originating elsewhere within the family system, such as marital discord, parental psychopathology, and social disadvantage. These issues may color parental perceptions and expectations, and such problems may supersede direct intervention targeting the child. Moreover, some evidence suggests that parent-referred children do not always differ from nonreferred siblings (Patterson, 1980) or from unrelated controls (Lobitz & Johnson, 1975). Second, an appreciation of the rapid and fluctuating developmental changes cutting across several dimensions of functioning is essential. Needless to say, it is important to know whether the desired behaviors are typically exhibited by children in the age group in question. The behaviors that constitute a problem for children of one age may not be a problem for children of another. One potential benefit of the incorporation of developmental data into behavioral assessment is the use of normative group comparisons to guide target selection and treatment (see later section on developmental issues).

Now, although behavioral assessment is a hallmark of behavior therapy characterized by an idiographic approach to the explication of behavior problems, some debate has arisen over the nomothetic application of such assessment data. In particular, the publication of the third edition of the *Diagnostic and Statistical Manual* (DSM-III; American Psychiatric Association, 1980) sparked some controversy (e.g., Haynes & O'Brien, 1988). Much of the controversy revolves around the issue of the classification of behavior.

CLASSIFICATION ISSUES

The revised third edition of the *Diagnostic and Statistical Manual of Mental Disorders* (DSM-III-R; American Psychiatric Association, 1987) has been put forth as the official diagnostic classification system for mental health professionals. The DSM-III and the DSM-III-R represent a significant advance over previous editions of the manual because they (1) take a descriptive, atheoretical approach; (2) provide explicit operational diagnostic criteria; (3) conducted basic reliability analyses during field trials; (4) provide increased attention to the problems of childhood and adolescence; and (5) incorporate a multiaxial approach to classification. Five major categories of "disorders first evident in infancy, childhood, or adolescence" have been identified: Disruptive Behavior Disorders (e.g., attention-deficit–hyperactivity disorder), Emotional Disorders (e.g., separation anxiety disorder), Habit and Eating Disorders (e.g., enuresis and anorexia), Developmental Disorders (e.g., mental retardation and dyslexia), and Gender Identity Disorders (e.g., transsexualism).

As noted, the DSM-III-R uses a multiaxial system of diagnosis. Specific classes of information are coded on each of the five axes as follows:

Axis I: Clinical Syndromes
Axis II: Personality and Developmental Disorders
Axis III: Physical Disorders and Conditions
Axis IV: Severity of Psychosocial Stressors
Axis V: Global Assessment of Functioning

In an attempt to provide a more broad-based classification, the multiaxial approach allows for recognition of the roles that physical condition and environmental circumstance play in the course and treatment of psychiatric dysfunction. Millon (1983) noted that

> the standard classification directs the clinician to address not the "disease entity," but an entire panorama of contextual dimensions, notably the person's overall style of psychological functioning, the qualities of the person's current situational environment, and his or her strengths and potentials for constructive and healthy coping. (p. 810)

Many behavior therapists have been reluctant to embrace the classification system presented in the DSM-III-R. This reluctance is largely based on a concern about the reliability and validity of the diagnostic categories and partly on the issue of classification itself. Concerning classification, some behavior therapists (usually operant) argue that a classification system like the DSM-III-R is antithetical to the idiographic behavior-analytic approach. In this approach, target behaviors are identified and classified functionally, based on the notion of response classes (i.e., responses are similar if they have the same controlling consequence). For the more typical, methodological behaviorist, concern about the DSM-III-R focuses on more traditional measurement issues, stimulating such questions as: How are the diagnostic criteria derived (empirically or intuitively)? How accurate is a diagnosis that is based on a single assessment measure (e.g., an informal interview)? Does information about diagnosis aid in the selection of a treatment strategy? Despite the need to address such questions in the development and refinement of any diagnostic scheme, the potential value of classification is evident. For example, a diagnostic classification system can serve an important function as a communication facilitator. A comprehensive diagnostic system provides a standard way of describing clinical populations. In addition, once a common communication system is empirically derived and in place, information can be compiled on the efficacy of specific treatments for specific disorders.

Another approach to the classification of child behavior problems that is receiving increasing attention and acceptance among behavior therapists, largely because of its empirical focus, is the multivariate approach. For several decades, multivariate statistical studies of childhood psychopathology have labored to identify reliable and coherent clusters of behavior problems (see Achenbach, 1985, and Quay, 1986, for reviews). Achenbach and Edelbrock's extensive investigations (1981), which are representative of the multivariate model (see also Quay, 1986), have identified two "broad-band" (or higher order) dimensions, labeled *internalizing* and *externalizing problems*. Subsumed within the internalizing dimension are more "narrow-band" (or first-order) behavioral clusters, such as social withdrawal and depressed, and within the externalizing dimension, aggressive and hyperactive (e.g., Achenbach & Edelbrock, 1984). The multivariate approach is generally atheoretical, except for its strong commitment to the underlying statistical assumptions and their implications, and is therefore compatible with a broad behavioral orientation. Notably, such classification systems may prompt behavioral therapists to examine the full set of potentially covarying behaviors, while furthering our understanding of response-response relationships that may otherwise be missed (Ollendick, 1986).

Unfortunately, the child behavior therapy literature has lacked uniformity in its classification. As Kazdin (1983) admonished,

> Failure to recognize or actively use DSM-III may make it difficult to integrate findings from child behavior therapy into clinical work in psychiatry, where the potential impact could and perhaps should be the greatest. (p. 94)

Behavioral assessment does not necessarily preclude the application of a diagnostic classification system. For example, behavioral assessment is conceptualized by Hersen and Bellack (1988) as an "idiographic approach within the broader nomothetic system" (p. 78). Consistent with this theme,

> Behavioral assessment can play at least three significant roles within the confines of DSM-III-R. First behavioral assessment can be used to determine if a person belongs within one of the diagnostic categories. Second, behavioral assessment can be used to enrich traditional diagnoses by illuminating the interpersonal components that maintain the behaviors upon which the diagnosis is based. Third, behavioral assessment can be used to track clinical change in response to treatment with the end product hopefully being that the diagnostic label no longer applies. (Tryon, 1989, p. 53)

Child behavioral assessment and classification have as their ultimate purpose the development and implementation of effective interventions that will assist children and their families. The section that follows provides a whirlwind and select review of behavioral procedures. An exhaustive exposition, considering the wide range of techniques and child problems, is clearly beyond the scope of this chapter (see Mash & Barkley, 1989). For the purpose of review, the internalizing-externalizing classification system will be used. This is not to claim that such an approach is the most empirically sound or comprehensive (cf. Achenbach, 1985; Rutter, Tuma, & Lann, 1988); but it does offer a useful framework for organizing some of the child behavior-therapy literature around the many problems involving children, adolescents, and their families.

TREATMENT FROM A BEHAVIORAL PERSPECTIVE: A BRIEF AND SELECTIVE REVIEW

Historically, behavior therapy has looked to the laboratory and experimental psychology for a grounding of its therapeutic procedures in the principles of learning. Such basic learning procedures include respondent conditioning, operant conditioning, and observational learning. Over the last several decades, basic behavioral research has expanded its borders to include "cognitive science" and the study of information processing. The following overview of child behavior-therapy methods is organized around basic learning paradigms, not because of a single one-to-one correspondence, but as a heuristic device to facilitate an understanding of the behavioral approach to intervention.

The Respondent Conditioning Paradigm and Internalizing Problems

The behavioral treatment of fear, anxiety, and avoidant or withdrawn behavior in children dates back to the classic work of Jones (1924) and the treatment of "Peter." The child appeared fearful of rabbits, fur coats, and similar objects. The treatment consisted of the progressive exposure of the child to a rabbit while he was engaged in a pleasurable activity (i.e., eating). The fear of the rabbit dissipated, as well as the fear of the related stimuli. This early case study is typically presented as an example of the application of classical or respondent conditioning principles to the amelioration of fear responses. Generally, the interpretation of the data has been that the child was gradually "deconditioned" to the fear stimuli.

Building on this early work, Wolpe (1958) developed a method he called "systematic desensitization" and presented adult case-study data supporting its effectiveness. The logic behind this approach rests on the assumption that fearful behavior can be reduced via "counter-conditioning" with anxiety-incompatible stimuli and responses. In practice, the fear- or anxiety-arousing stimuli are systematically and gradually paired (imaginally or *in vivo*) with competing stimuli, such as food, praise, imagery, or cues generated by muscular relaxation.

Early work with systematic desensitization used the predominantly imaginal presentation of the fearful stimuli. Systematic desensitization with children consists of three basic steps: (1) training in deep-muscle relaxation; (2) the rank ordering of fearful situations from lowest to highest; and (3) fear stimulus presentation via imagery while the subject is in a relaxed state (see Morris & Kratochwill, 1983, for a review). Such procedures appear to work well with older children and adolescents (see Barrios & O'Dell, 1989, for a review). However, younger children seem to have difficulty with both the imaginal presentation of fear stimuli and the acquisition of the incompatible muscular-relaxation response typically used (Ollendick & Cerny, 1981). Therefore, the constraints of development suggest that *in vivo* desensitization may be more effective with younger children (e.g., Hatzenbeuhler & Schroeder, 1978; Ultee, Griffiaen, & Schellekens, 1982).

According to the original formulation (Watson & Morgan, 1917), fear and anxieties are acquired via respondent conditioning. Demonstrations of fear induction through respondent conditioning are numerous, but criticisms abound regarding a strict respondent-conditioning theory of fear (see Barrios & O'Dell, 1989). Likewise, several alternative interpretations (other than counterconditioning) of behavior change following systematic desensitization have been proposed (e.g., Masters, Burish, Hollon, & Rimm, 1987). For example, the process of extinction, in which the fear-evoking stimuli are presented repeatedly while the nonoccurrence of the unconditioned (or other aversive) stimuli is ensured, may account for the observed fear reduction. Operant shaping, modeling, and self-instruction have been offered as explanations, as well as nonspecific factors such as positive expectancy and demand characteristics (Kazdin & Wilcoxon, 1976). At present, the relative influence of these various mechanisms on anxiety reduction in children is unknown.

Additional interventions for internalizing problems, largely based on a respondent conditioning paradigm, include flooding, implosion, and graduated exposure. To facilitate anxiety reduction, these procedures require the child to be exposed to the anxiety-eliciting stimuli for the extinction of the conditioned responses to occur (see Morris & Kratochwill, 1983). Flooding is characterized by prolonged *in vivo* exposure to the anxiety-arousing situation; implosion is similar but is conducted imaginally. Graduated exposure is the process of progressive *in vivo* exposure to the fearful stimuli. Numerous case reports and experiments support the efficacy of these approaches (Barrios & O'Dell, 1989). Though they are listed as distinct procedures, a comparison of the parameters related to these four methods reveals basic similarities. They do differ, however, along at least three dimensions: *in vivo* versus imaginal stimulus presentation, progressive versus prolonged presentations, and the presence or absence of programmed incompatible responses. Of course, the various procedures can be combined and tailored to the clinical situation, as when imaginal and *in vivo* desensitization are used concurrently (e.g., Phillips & Wolpe, 1981).

With respect to the relative effectiveness of respondent-conditioning-based methods, Ollendick (1986) concluded as follows:

> In summary, systematic desensitization, emotive imagery, flooding, and implosion all represent reasonably effective procedures for anxiety-based disorders in children. While several questions remain, they represent viable options and are welcome additions to the behaviorally-oriented clinicians armamentarium. (p. 533)

The Operant Conditioning Paradigm and Externalizing Problems

The operant-based approach to interventions, relying on the basic concepts of reinforcement, punishment, and stimulus control, and elaborated into more applied procedures such as the token economy, contingency contracting, time-out, and positive attention, enjoys increasing popularity in a variety of settings. Problem behaviors such as noncompliance, tantrums, and aggression can be influenced by altering the consequences of the behavior. Social or tangible rewards can be delivered for appropriate behavior to increase such behavior and withheld to suppress inappropriate behavior.

For example, token economies are reinforcement programs in which individuals earn tokens or points for certain behaviors (Ayllon & Azrin, 1968). The tokens can then be exchanged for a variety of tangible primary reinforcers or additional privileges. Often these programs include a "response cost" provision, in which previously earned tokens or points are deducted for inappropriate behavior. Token economies have been used successfully in many settings, such as in classrooms (Stumpf & Holman, 1985), in psychiatric wards (Ayllon & Azrin, 1968), as a component of parent training programs (Kazdin, 1977b; Patterson, Reid, Jones, & Conger, 1975), and in residential treatment programs (Phillips, Phillips, Fixsen, & Wolf, 1971).

One of the most noted residential treatment programs using the token economy is Achievement Place (Phillips, 1968). Originally established in 1967, the Achievement Place approach was developed for conduct-disordered adolescents and is now termed the Teaching-Family Model (TFM; Willner, Braukmann, Kirigin, & Wolf, 1978). The goal of the TFM is to teach prosocial behaviors. In each home, a family setting is established with a married couple (professionally trained to serve as teaching parents) and six to eight court-referred adolescents. The teaching parents model, role-play, and reinforce the use of appropriate social skills. There are currently more than 215 group homes using the TFM. Kirigin, Braukmann, Atwater, and Wolf (1982) examined police and court records in an evaluation of the effectiveness of the TFM and found significant reductions in the recorded offenses of adolescents in 13 TFM programs compared with those of adolescents from 9 "traditional" community-based residential programs, for the period during which the adolescents were in treatment. However, no differences were found between the groups in reported offenses for the one-year period following treatment. The initial success of the program and the subsequent decline in treatment gains at follow-up suggest the need for intervention with the family to which the adolescent is returned after treatment. The incorporation of "transition and maintenance" care is likely to enhance the long-term effectiveness of the program.

Contingency management methods are used routinely and "naturally" by many in our society, including day care centers, schools, and parents. The efficacy of more programmed contingency management procedures, often with parents acting as behavior modifiers and cotherapists, is well supported for children evidencing problems of the externalizing type (e.g., Barkley, 1989; Devany & Nelson, 1986; Kazdin, 1987; McMahon & Wells, 1989; O'Dell, 1974;

Ollendick, 1986; Wells & Forehand, 1981), especially younger children (Weisz, Weiss, Alicke, & Klotz, 1987). Such an approach to intervention is typically referred to as behavioral parent training (BPT). BPT focuses on teaching parents new ways to interact with their children, with the goal of changing the child's problem behavior in the natural environment. Parents are trained to be more effective in providing age-appropriate, consistent, and immediate consequences for both good and problem behavior. Successful programs train parents to give contingent praise for appropriate behaviors, to ignore annoying behaviors, to decrease criticism and nattering, and to use time-out for aggressive and noncompliant behavior (e.g., Barkley, 1987; Forehand & McMahon, 1981; Patterson & Chamberlain, 1988).

BPT programs are on the cutting edge of child behavior therapy. Consistent with the contemporary behavioral systems approach (e.g., Mash, 1989), BPT incorporates multiple procedures into a comprehensive, compound treatment package. Recent applications attempt to address developmental considerations (e.g., Eyberg, 1987), bidirectional influences (e.g., Patterson, 1982), and factors in the wider social environment (e.g., Dumas, 1986). Attempts are being made to promote generalization across settings (e.g., Sanders & Christensen, 1985) and to incorporate the educational components of normal development (e.g., Campbell, 1990). Programs are also being expanded to incorporate a systems view of family and school functioning, thereby focusing on more general social interactional processes that may influence the parents' successful participation in therapy (e.g., Dadds, Schwartz, & Sanders, 1987; Eyberg, 1987). Programs with the most general and long-term efficacy go beyond the strict operant approach, use other learning-based procedures such as modeling and instruction, and address broader family functioning (Eyberg, 1987). As Ollendick (1986) observed, the trend is away from "parent training" and toward "behavioral family therapy."

Campbell (1990) summarized a number of the preceding points nicely:

> Broad-based parent training approaches that take into account other aspects of family relationships and also involve direct observations of parent-child interaction or at least include role-playing, coaching, and feedback have the most obvious impact on the child and family and are most likely to lead to changes that are maintained at follow-up. In addition, it appears that families living under more stressful conditions or parents who feel less supported socially and emotionally may be either less able to follow through with the treatment initially or less able to maintain gains once treatment is over. (p. 191)

Observational Learning Paradigm and Internalizing Problems

The notion that persons can learn many different forms of behavior through "imitation" is not new, dating back to at least the days of Plato and Aristotle. Empirical research addressed this phenomenon in the work of Miller and Dollard (1941) and Bandura (1969; Bandura & Walters, 1963). Such work was stimulated by findings suggesting that learning occurs in situations not easily predicted by traditional conditioning theory. Through the process of observational learning (or modeling), one may acquire behavioral dispositions simply by viewing and cognitively processing the actions of another individual (Benson, Messer, & Gross, 1992). The process does not require an individual to actively perform the behavior; therefore, trial-and-error learning, along with its potential hazards, is not essential.

An observational learning approach to fear and anxiety acquisition has been explicitly addressed by a number of theorists and clinicians, including Rachman (1977) and Bandura (1986). For Rachman, modeling is one route, along with respondent conditioning and verbal instruction, for the acquisition of fears. Bandura also proposed that fear, avoidance, and withdrawal may be acquired through vicarious experience and are mediated by perceptions of self-efficacy in the face of threat.

Though exposure to a model is sufficient to promote observational learning, behavioral performance is influenced by reinforcement contingencies. Modeled behavior that is reinforced (or punished) is likely to increase (or decrease) the probability of the observer's behavior through the process of vicarious conditioning. Therefore, modeled behavior typically reflects the joint contributions of observational learning, operant conditioning, and probably respondent conditioning as well. Through observational learning and its associated mechanisms, behaviors may be increased in frequency through acquisition, disinhibition, and facilitation; they may be decreased in frequency through inhibitory and incompatible behavior effects (Bandura, 1986). Such learning has been demonstrated in a variety of children's behaviors, such as speech (Lovaas & Newsom, 1976), gender-role behaviors (Perry & Bussey, 1979), prosocial behavior (Bandura, 1977), and aggression (Bandura, Ross, & Ross, 1963), to list just a few.

The application of modeling procedures to fearful and avoidant behavior has proved effective (Barrios & O'Dell, 1989). Therapeutic modeling in this case involves the demonstration of nonfearful behavior as well as the exhibition of appropriate coping behavior. Following the demonstration, the child is prompted to imitate the model's performance, while feedback, coaching, and reinforcement are provided during repeated rehearsals (see Morris & Kratochwill, 1983). Moreover, modeling can be accomplished via filmed, live (*in vivo*), or participant approaches. Ollendick (1979) provided data suggesting the relative efficacy of participant modeling, at least for children with mild to moderate fears. Through this process, anxiety is reduced and coping skills are also acquired (Ollendick, 1986).

Modeling procedures have been used successfully to increase interaction among socially withdrawn children (Evers & Schwartz, 1973; Keller & Carlson, 1974; Ollendick, 1981) and to reduce childhood fears of snakes (Meichenbaum, 1971), the dark (Klingman, 1988), dental procedures (Melamed, Weinstein, Hawes, & Katin-Borland, 1975), and surgery and anesthesia (Melamed & Siegel, 1975). Though such procedures have yielded some success, many of the studies have used nonclinical populations. In addition, more studies are necessary to delineate the influence of particular parameters, such as the model's similarity, likability, and status; the use of multiple models; and the utility of active versus passive coping models (Graziano, DeGiovanni, & Garcia, 1979). Lastly, modeling techniques have proved versatile as adjunctive components in the compound treatment packages common in clinical practice (Barrios & O'Dell, 1989). Such compound treatments are consistent with the behavioral systems perspective.

The Cognitive Paradigm and Externalizing Problems

The last several decades have evidenced a tremendous upsurge of interest, research, and practice in cognitively based interventions. Associated with the cognitive paradigm are a number of creative and varied therapeutic approaches typically developed initially for adults, such as Ellis's rational-emotive therapy (1970), Beck's cognitive therapy (1976), Goldfried, Decenteceo, and Weinstein's systematic rational restructuring (1974), Lazarus's cognitive restructuring (1974), Meichenbaum's self-instructional training (1977), and Spivack and Shure's problem-solving approach (1974). Such cognitively based procedures often incorporate more traditional behavioral approaches, assuming that behavioral change be induced through direct, vicarious, and symbolically represented experience. The hallmark of the cognitive perspective is an explicit recognition of the influential role that cognitive processes play in mediating and regulating overt behavior. Foster, Kendall, and Guevremont (1988) noted that, "regardless of the procedures producing change, though, the mechanisms assumed to be responsible for the change lie in the cognitive events or processes producing behavior" (p. 79). These contemporary cognitively based procedures owe a major intellectual debt to the cognitive social learning theory developed and tested by Bandura and his colleagues (e.g., Bandura, 1969, 1986; Bandura & Walters, 1963), in which major emphasis is placed on information processing, reciprocal determinism, and self-regulation.

A cognitive approach to understanding and treating externalizing problems is based on the assumption that cognitive deficiencies are partly responsible for the unwanted behavior (e.g., Foster *et al.*, 1988). One primary deficiency proposed is the absence of self-guided private speech, which is hypothesized to promote self-regulation through covert self-instruction. Such a general framework has guided a number of therapeutic approaches to externalizing problems. For example, Camp, Blom, Herbert, and von Doornenck (1977) developed the "Think Aloud" program, of which self-instruction training was a major component, relying on the rehearsal of such self-statements as "What is my plan?" "Am I using the plan?" and "How did I do?" as well as the correction of faulty self-statements (Ollendick, 1986). In addition, social problem-solving training was conducted using games devised by Shure and Spivack (1978). Gains in classroom prosocial behavior and improved performance on various cognitive tests were noted, but nonsignificant reductions in aggressions were evidenced (Camp *et al.*, 1977). Similar findings have been reported by Kendall and Finch (1978) and Lochman, Nelson, and Sims (1981) for impulsive and aggressive children. More positive results were obtained among a sample of "delinquent" adolescents reported by Snyder and White (1979). Substantial improvements were demonstrated in the performance of daily activities as well as a reduction of impulsive behaviors maintained at the two-month follow-up.

Nevertheless, even when such studies suggest short-term improvements, many questions remain regarding the maintenance and generalization of the trained skills and the comparative efficacy of the cognitive and the traditional approaches, especially among clinically disturbed samples (Ollendick, 1986). In addition, further advances are necessary in cognitive assessment and the study of its implications for intervention strategies.

Regarding externalizing problems, increasing evidence suggests that a cognitive "deficiency" approach may tell only part of the story. Dodge (1980; Dodge & Frame, 1982) proposed and provided support for a cognitive "distortion" model of aggressive behavior. Aggressive children tend to misattribute neutral circumstances as reflecting peer hostility and to act accordingly. Conceptualization of the behavior problems as deficiency- or distortion-generated is likely to influence the selection and implementation of the treatment approach, and the behavioral component of the cognitive-behavioral conjunction must not be overlooked (Foster *et al.*, 1988). Last, more information is needed about the interaction of developmental factors with cognitive assessments and treatments (e.g., Cole & Kazdin, 1980; Kendall, 1984). Age-related differences in cognitive and conceptual abilities suggest that intervention targets and methods require tailoring to the child's developmental level.

DEVELOPMENTAL ISSUES

In general, theory and nomenclature relating to child psychopathology have reflected downward extensions from adult work. Age-related changes in behavioral manifestations have not been explicitly addressed. As Campbell (1990) noted:

> Although it is obvious to any student of child development that behavior, whether "normal" or "abnormal," must be examined within a developmental context, it is only recently that child psychiatry and clinical child psychology have paid more than lip service to this notion. (p. 5)

Likewise, traditional behavioral work has largely neglected the explicit recognition of developmental factors; probably partly because of the strong assumption that learning principles are universal across organisms and ages (Mash, 1989). Also, developmentalists (e.g., Piaget, 1969) have long espoused philosophical and theoretical positions that run counter to classical behavioral theory.

The developmental and behavioral positions are not necessarily incompatible, however. For example, Achenbach & Edelbrock (1984) argued that, if the two approaches are integrated, the assessment process is enriched. The nomothetic approach characterizing much of developmental psychology can provide normative baseline data. By use of these norms, individual patterns of behavior at the idiographic level can be compared with those of an appropriate reference group. As might be expected, numerous age differences were found in Achenbach & Edelbrock's inventory of problem behaviors (1983). According to Achenbach & Edelbrock (1983), such norms can be useful (1) in the establishment of the incidence and prevalence rates of child behavior problems; (2) as guides in the selection of appropriate target behaviors; (3) to assess the validity of informants' judgments of children's behavior; (4) in longitudinal epidemiological evaluations of behavioral stability; and (5) in the evaluation and "social validation" (Kazdin, 1977a) of treatment interventions (see Achenbach & Edelbrock, 1983, for such norms).

Developmental, or age-related, factors have implications for behavioral treatment as well. Take, for example, the notion of age-by-treatment interactions. A common clinical assumption is that treatments tend to be more efficacious for younger (versus older) children. Apparently, this assumption is based on the logic that younger are more malleable and their habits are less well established (Mash, 1989). A recent meta-analysis provides indirect support for such a proposition (Weisz *et al.*, 1987). The mean treatment-effect size was .92 for children aged 4–12 and was .58 for 13- 18-year-olds. Some evidence suggests that the effects of operant procedures are a function of age-related factors (e.g., Johnson & McGillicuddy-Delisi, 1983). For example, rewards that provide information regarding competence are more efficacious for older children (Schultz, Butkowsky, Pearce, and Shanfield, 1975). In addition, older children require a longer time-out period for the implementation of behavior change (White, Nielsen, & Johnson, 1972).

The preceding findings support the differential effectiveness of certain behavioral procedures as a function of age or developmental level. However, Mash (1989) emphasized the importance of identifying specific age-related developmental capacities and incorporating them into treatment. For example, cognitive and language-related capacities very likely interact with both the child's developmental level and her or his responses to environmental contingencies (Robinson, 1985). Age differences have been reported for the efficacy of cognitive self-instructional training across a range of problems (Hobbs, Moguin, Tyroler, & Lahey, 1980). Similarly, mental imagery capacities appear to be age-related. Nine-year-olds can effectively use mental imagery in recall conditions, whereas five- and six-year-olds cannot (Purkel & Bornstein, 1980).

Child behavior therapy may ultimately benefit from the recent emergence of a new subdiscipline, developmental psychopathology. The field represents "the study of the origins and course of individual patterns of behavioral maladaptation" (Sroufe & Rutter, 1984, p. 241). Developmental psychopathology holds great promise for the elucidation of the complex interactive processes that characterize both "normal" and "abnormal" behavioral development (Messer, 1990). The hallmark of the approach is a transactional or ecological view that assumes a coherence and predictability in development, despite changes and transformations (Sroufe, 1979).

Such a perspective is generally consistent with contemporary broad behavioral-systems approaches. Consequently, child behavior therapy appears to be more open to developmental issues. Such openness seems wise because the child therapy field is complicated by a host of factors influencing problem definition, treatment, course, and outcome, such as chronological age, level of cognitive and social development, family background, and sociocultural factors (Campbell, 1990).

Foster *et al.* (1988) listed several developmental considerations potentially relevant to an understanding of children's behavior: (1) the influence of age-graded tasks, situations, and transitions (Mize & Ladd, 1990); (2) qualitative changes in the developing child's attentional, perceptual, and memorial processes (Cohen & Schleser, 1984); (3) children's increasing utilization of symbolic activity, problem solving, and self-regulation (Bernard, 1984); (4) age-related differences in the efficacy of rewards and punishments (Robinson, 1985); and (5) age-related differences in the conceptual abilities necessary to generalize acquired skills. Looking to the future, Mash (1989) stated:

> At a more complex level, a developmental emphasis would require the incorporation of developmental principles and findings into our conceptualizations of child and family psychopathology, such that treatments are sensitive not only to a child's age and sex but also to ongoing developmental *processes* as they unfold and interact with and within one or more dynamic and changing social systems. (p. 9)

Such a tall order could be filled only by: (1) an extensive study of age/gender-by-treatment interactions; (2) an accumulation of normative data providing guidelines concerning "normal" development; (3) prognostic data enlightening us regarding the course and the long-term sequelae of problem behavior; and (4) an explication of developmental principles and processes (e.g., security of attachment and temperamental style). Once such knowledge was obtained, treatments could intervene and influence such processes.

ETHICAL CONSIDERATIONS

In closing, we would be remiss if we did not briefly address a few key ethical issues. First, children are not capable of granting legal (competent, voluntary, and informed) consent to treatment. Consent is provided on behalf of the child by a parent or a legal guardian. Likewise, children are not free to terminate treatment at their own discretion. This perceived lack of control by the child may result in refusal to cooperate with the therapist. It is wise to allow the child to play as active a role as possible in the selection of treatment strategies.

Second, children rarely refer themselves for treatment. Thus, the central issue is raised of whether the child is in need of treatment. Simply put, does the behavior noted in the presenting complaint warrant intervention? Stated otherwise, what is the appropriate treatment focus? As mentioned previously, an awareness of developmental factors and context is essential in making normative judgments. Is the parent knowledgeable about age-appropriate behavior? Unreasonable parent expectations and their consequences may serve only to frustrate the parent and the child alike and perhaps should be the treatment focus. Because the therapist relies to some degree on the parents' reports for assessment information, he or she needs to ascertain whether the parent is capable of providing an accurate report of the child's behavior. Panaccione and Wahler (1986) found that depressed mothers displayed a distorted perception of their children, reporting that their child's behavior was more negative than noted by objective observers. This finding further emphasizes the importance of conducting a thorough assessment that includes multiagent information from and about the parents, the siblings, and any significant others in the child's environment. Moreover, children are often referred by outside agencies (schools or courts) for problem behavior that may otherwise be adaptive in the child's home environment. In such cases, the most effective intervention is likely to be with the family as a unit rather than simply with the individual child. It should be clear, then, that the behavioral-systems approach stressed throughout this chapter facilitates an appreciation of the complex factors involved in the referral process.

Third, selecting the target behavior is more complicated when one is dealing with a child than when one is dealing with an adult. Who determines what behaviors are to be modified—the child, the parent, or the therapist? When the objectives of the child differ from those of the parent, which are given more weight? A widely held assumption is that parents know what is "best" for their child. For example, what about the child who presents with gender-identity disorder? One may question whether the modification of the child's sex-role behavior is in the interest of the child or of the parent (see Winkler, 1977).

Fourth, therapists have an ethical responsibility to provide the most effective treatment available. Related to this responsibility is accountability. The empirical approach of behavior therapy has long demonstrated an awareness of the need for accountability. As Harris (1983) pointed out, "the ability to specify goals and to measure change is one of the strong points in favor of a behavioral approach" (p. 437). Increased insurance benefits for psychiatric treatment and the proliferation of private psychiatric facilities will only fuel accountability demands.

Fifth, an often neglected ethical issue is the lack of treatment of children who need it. It has been estimated that only 20%–30% of children with clinically significant disturbances actually receive treatment (Knitzer, 1982). Exacerbating this problem is the fact that many children have not yet developed the communicative capacity to adequately express their subjective distress. Other children are unwilling to discuss their problems with their parents, for very obvious reasons, such as when the problem involves their parents (as in the case of child abuse). What is our obligation to these "invisible" clients? We take the position that child behavior therapists must educate those who work with children (e.g., teachers and day care workers) to make efforts to recognize behavioral problems and must provide adequate referral sources. In addition, there is a pressing need to provide behaviorally informed screening services for the identification of children at risk, as well as to develop prevention and early-intervention programs within communities.

SUMMARY

For many years the practice of behavior therapy with children was characterized by the downward extension of adult models. Recently, child behavior therapy has evolved into an independent discipline in which the application of clinical behavioral methods reflects a greater awareness of social, cognitive, and developmental variables.

This chapter has presented an overview of the current state of child behavior therapy from a behavioral-systems perspective. Following a brief survey of the nature of behavior therapy, we discussed the principles and procedures of child behavioral assessment. We also addressed some pertinent issues in the classification of child behavior disorders. In particular, we highlighted the strengths and weaknesses of examining children's behavioral difficulties from both the traditional DSM perspective and an empirical multivariate approach.

We also selectively reviewed child behavior-therapy treatments, including the basic respondent, operant, observational learning, and cognitive-behavioral paradigms, along with their application in treating the internalizing and externalizing disorders. The chapter concluded with a discussion of developmental and ethical issues in child behavior therapy. Interventions targeting the amelioration and prevention of childhood behavioral problems will benefit from further conceptual and methodological work, in the pursuit of comprehensive, empirically based approaches to child behavior therapy.

REFERENCES

Achenbach, T. M. (1985). *Assessment and taxonomy of child and adolescent psychopathology*. Beverly Hills, CA: Sage.

Achenbach, T. M., & Edelbrock, C. S. (1981). Behavioral problems and competencies reported by parents of normal and disturbed children aged 4 through 16. *Monographs of the Society for Research in Child Development, 46* (1, Serial No. 188).

Achenbach, T. M., & Edelbrock, C. S. (1983). *Manual for the Child Behavior Checklist and Revised Child Behavior Profile*. Burlington, VT: University Associates in Psychiatry.

Achenbach, T. M., & Edelbrock, C. S. (1984). Psychopathology of childhood. *Annual Review of Psychology, 35*, 227–256.

American Psychiatric Association. (1980). *Diagnostic and statistical manual of mental disorders* (3rd ed.; DSM-III). Washington, DC: Author.

American Psychiatric Association. (1987). *Diagnostic and statistical manual of mental disorders* (3rd ed., rev.; DSM-III-R). Washington, DC: Author.

Ayllon, T., & Azrin, N. H. (1968). *The token economy: Motivational system for therapy and rehabilitation.* New York: Appleton-Century-Crofts.

Bandura, A. (1961). Psychotherapy as a learning process. *Psychological Bulletin, 58*, 143–159.

Bandura, A. (1969). Social learning theory of identificatory processes. In D. A. Goslin (Ed.), *Handbook of socialization theory and research.* Chicago: Rand McNally.

Bandura, A. (1977). *Social learning theory.* Englewood Cliffs, NJ: Prentice-Hall.

Bandura, A. (1986). *Social foundations of thought and action: A social cognitive theory.* Englewood Cliffs, NJ: Prentice-Hall.

Bandura, A., & Walters, R. H. (1963). *Social learning and personality development.* New York: Holt, Reinhart, & Winston.

Bandura, A., Ross, D., & Ross, S. A. (1963). Imitation of film mediated aggressive models. *Journal of Abnormal and Social Psychology, 66*, 3–11.

Barkley, R. A. (1987). *Defiant children: A clinician's manual for parent training.* New York: Guilford Press.

Barkley, R. A. (1989). Attention deficit-hyperactivity disorder. In E. J. Mash & Barkley, R. A. (Eds.), *Treatment of childhood disorders* (pp. 39–72). New York: Guilford Press.

Barlow, D. H., Hayes, S. C., & Nelson, R. O. (1984). *The scientist practitioner.* New York: Pergamon Press.

Barrios, B., & Hartmann, D. P. (1986). The contributions of traditional assessment: Concepts, issues, and methodologies. In R. O. Nelson & S. C. Hayes, *Conceptual foundations of behavioral assessment* (pp. 81–110). New York: Guilford Press.

Barrios, B., & O'Dell, S. (1989). Fears and anxieties. In E. J. Mash & R. A. Barkley (Eds.), *Treatment of childhood disorders* (pp. 167–221). New York: Guilford Press.

Beck, A. T. (1976). *Cognitive therapy and the emotional disorders.* New York: International Universities Press.

Belsky, J., Lerner, R. M., & Spanier, G. B. (1984). *The child in the family.* New York: Random House.

Benson, B. A., Messer, S. C., & Gross, A. M. (1992). Learning theories of social development. In V. B. Van Hasselt & M. Hersen (Eds.), *Handbook of social development: A lifespan perspective* (pp. 81–111). New York: Plenum Press.

Bernard, M. E. (1984). Childhood emotion and cognitive behavior therapy: A Rational-emotive perspective. In P. C. Kendall (Ed.), *Advances in cognitive-behavioral research and therapy* (Vol. 3). New York: Academic Press.

Bornstein, P. H., Bornstein, M. T., & Dawson, B. (1984). Integrated assessment and treatment. In T. H. Ollendick & M. Hersen (Eds.), *Child behavioral assessment: Principles and procedures* (pp. 223–243). New York: Pergamon Press.

Bronfenbrenner, U. (1986). Ecology of the family as a context for human development: Research perspectives. *Developmental Psychopathology, 22*, 723–742.

Camp, B., Blom, G., Herbert, F., & Van Doornenck, W. (1977). "Think aloud": A program for developing self-control in young aggressive boys. *Journal of Abnormal Child Psychology, 5*, 157–169.

Campbell, S. B. (1990). *Behavior problems in preschool children: Clinical and developmental issues.* New York: Guilford Press.

Ciminero, A. R., & Drabman, R. S. (1977). Current developments in the behavioral assessment of children. In B. B. Lahey & A. E. Kazdin (Eds.), *Advances in clinical child psychology* (Vol. 1). New York: Plenum Press.

Cohen, R., & Schleser, R. (1984). Cognitive development and clinical interventions. In A. W. Myers & W. E. Craighead (Eds.), *Cognitive behavior therapy with children.* New York: Plenum Press.

Cole, P. M., & Kazdin, A. E. (1980). Critical issues in self-instructional training with children. *Child Behavior Therapy, 2*, 1–21.

Cone, J. D. (1977). The relevance of reliability and validity for behavioral assessment. *Behavior Therapy, 8*, 411–426.

Dadds, M. R., Schwartz, S., & Sanders, M. R. (1987). Marital discord and treatment outcome in behavioral treatment of child behavior problems. *Journal of Consulting and Clinical Psychology, 55*, 396–403.

Devaney, J., & Nelson, R. O. (1986). Behavioral approaches to treatment. In H. C. Quay & J. S. Werry (Eds.), *Psychopathological disorders of childhood* (3rd ed.). New York: Wiley.

Dodge, K. A. (1980). Social cognition and children's aggressive behavior. *Child Development, 51*, 162–170.

Dodge, K. A., & Frame, C. M. (1982). Social cognitive biases and deficits in aggressive boys. *Child Development, 53*, 622–635.

Dumas, J. E. (1986). Indirect influence of maternal social contacts on mother-child interactions: A setting events analysis. *Journal of Abnormal Child Psychology, 14*, 205–216.

Ellis, A. (1970). *The essence of rational psychotherapy: A comprehensive approach to treatment.* New York: Institute for Rational Living.

Emmelkamp, P. M. G. (1986). Behavior therapy with adults. In S. L. Garfield & A. Bergin (Eds.), *Handbook of psychotherapy and behavior change* (pp. 385–442). New York: Wiley.

Evans, I. M. (1985). Building systems models as a strategy for target behavior selection in child assessment. *Behavioral Assessment, 7,* 21–32.

Evers, W. L., & Schwartz, J. C. (1973). Modifying social effects in preschoolers: The effects of filmed modeling and teacher praise. *Journal of Abnormal Child Psychology, 1,* 248–256.

Eyberg, S. M. (1987, August). *Assessing therapy outcomes with preschool children: Progress and problems.* Presidential Address to the Section on Clinical Child Psychology of the American Psychological Association, New York.

Eysenck, H. S. (1957). *The dynamics of anxiety and hysteria.* New York: Praeger.

Eysenck, H. S. (Ed.). (1960). *Behavior therapy and the neuroses.* New York: Pergamon Press.

Forehand, R., & McMahon, R. (1981). *Helping the noncompliant child: A clinician's guide to parent training.* New York: Guilford Press.

Foster, S. L., Kendall, P. C., & Guevremont, D. C. (1988). Cognitive and social learning theories. In J. L. Matson (Ed.), *Handbook of treatment approaches in childhood psychopathology* (pp. 79–118). New York: Plenum Press.

Foster, S. L., & Robin, A. (1989). Parent-adolescent conflict. In E. J. Mash & R. A. Barkley (Eds.), *Treatment of childhood disorders* (pp. 493–528). New York: Guilford Press.

Goldfried, M. R., & Kent, R. N. (1972). Traditional versus behavioral personality assessment: A comparison of methodological and theoretical assumptions. *Psychological Bulletin, 77,* 409–420.

Goldfried, M. R., Decenteceo, E. T., & Weinstein, L. (1974). Systematic rational restructuring as a self-control technique. *Behavior Therapy, 5,* 247–254.

Gould, J., Wunsch-Witzig, R., & Dohrenwend, B. P. (1981). Estimating the prevalence of childhood psychopathology. *Journal of the American Academy of Child Psychiatry, 20,* 462–476.

Graziano, A. M., DeGiovanni, I. S., & Garcia, K. A. (1979). Behavioral treatment of children's fears: A review. *Psychological Bulletin, 86,* 804–830.

Gross, A. M., & Wixted, J. T. (1988). Assessment of child behavior problems. In A. S. Bellack & M. Hersen (Eds.), *Behavioral assessment: A practical handbook* (3rd ed., pp. 578–608). New York: Pergamon Press.

Harris, S. L. (1983). Behavior therapy with children. In A. E. Kazdin & A. S. Bellack (Eds.), *The clinical psychological handbook.* Elmsford, NY: Pergamon Press.

Hatzenbeuhler, L. C., & Schroeder, H. E. (1978). Desensitization procedures in the treatment of childhood disorders. *Psychological Bulletin, 85,* 831–844.

Haynes, S. N., & O'Brien, W. H. (1988). The Gordian knot of DSM-III-R use: Integrating principles of behavior classification and complex causal models. *Behavioral Assessment, 10,* 95–105.

Hersen, M., & Bellack, A. S. (1988). DSM-III and behavioral assessment. In A. S. Bellack & M. Hersen (Eds.), *Behavioral assessment: A practical handbook* (3rd ed.). New York: Pergamon Press.

Hobbs, S. A. Moguin, L. E., Tyroler, M., & Lahey, B. B. (1980). Cognitive behavior therapy with children: Has clinical utility been demonstrated? *Psychological Bulletin, 87,* 147–165.

Institute of Medicine. (1989). *Research on children and adolescents with mental, behavioral and developmental disorders.* Washington, DC: U.S. Department of Health and Human Services.

Johnson, J. E., & McGillicuddy-Delisi, D. A. (1983). Family environment factors and children's knowledge of rules and conventions. *Child Development, 54,* 218–226.

Johnson, J. H., Rasbury, W. C., & Siegel, L. J. (1986). *Approaches to child treatment: Introduction to theory, research, and practice.* New York: Pergamon Press.

Jones, M. C. (1924). The elimination of children's fears. *Journal of Experimental Psychology, 7,* 382–390.

Kanfer, F. H., & Saslow, G. (1969). Behavioral diagnosis. In C. M. Franks (Ed.), *Behavior therapy: Appraisal and status.* New York: McGraw-Hill.

Kanfer, F. H., & Schefft, B. K. (1988). *Guiding the process of therapeutic change.* Champaign, IL: Research Press.

Kazdin, A. E. (1977a). Artifact, bias, and complexity of assessment: The ABC's of reliability. *Journal of Applied Behavior Analysis, 10,* 141–150.

Kazdin, A. E. (1977b). *The token economy.* New York: Plenum Press.

Kazdin, A. E. (1983). Psychiatric diagnosis, dimensions of dysfunction, and child behavior therapy. *Behavior Therapy, 14,* 73–99.

Kazdin, A. E. (1987). Treatment of antisocial behavior in children: Current status and future directions. *Psychological Bulletin, 102,* 187–203.

Kazdin, A. E. (1989). Developmental psychopathology: Current research, issues, and directions. *American Psychologist, 44,* 180–187.

Kazdin, A. E., & Wilcoxon, L. A. (1976). Systematic desensitization and nonspecific treatment effects: A methodological evaluation. *Psychological Bulletin, 83*, 729–758.

Keller, M. F., & Carlson, P. M. (1974). The use of symbolic modeling to promote social skills in preschool children with low levels of social responsiveness. *Child Development, 45*, 912–919.

Kendall, P. C. (1984). Social cognition and problem-solving: A developmental and child-clinical interface. In B. Gholson & T. L. Rosenthal (Eds.), *Applications of cognitive-developmental theory*. New York: Pergamon Press.

Kendall, P. C., & Finch, A. J. (1978). A cognitive-behavioral treatment for impulsivity: A group comparison study. *Journal of Consulting and Clinical Psychology, 46*, 110–118.

Kirigin, K. A., Braukmann, C. J., Atwater, J. D., & Wolf, M. M. (1982). An evaluation of Teaching Family (Achievement Place) group homes for juvenile offenders. *Journal of Applied Behavior Analysis, 15*, 1–16.

Knitzer, J. (1982). *Unclaimed children: The failure of public responsibility to children and adolescents in need of mental health services*. Washington, DC: Children's Defense Fund.

Kovacs, M., Feinberg, T. L., Crouse-Novak, M., Paulaskas, S. L., Pollock, M., & Finkelstein, R. (1984). Depressive disorders in childhood. II. A longitudinal study of the risk of a subsequent major depression. *Archives of General Psychiatry, 41*, 643–649.

Lazarus, A. A. (1974). Desensitization and cognitive restructuring. *Psychotherapy Theory, Research, and Practice, 11*, 98–102.

Lobitz, W. C., & Johnson, S. M. (1975). Parental manipulation of the behavior of normal and deviant children. *Child Development, 46*, 719–726.

Lochman, J. E., & Nelson, W. M. (1981). A cognitive behavioral program for use with aggressive children. *Journal of Clinical Child Psychology, 10*, 146–148.

Lovaas, O. I., & Newsom, C. D. (1976). Behavior modification with psychotic children. In H. Leitenberg (Ed.), *Handbook of behavior modification and behavior therapy*. Englewood Cliffs, NJ: Prentice-Hall.

Mash, E. J. (1979). What is behavioral assessment? *Behavioral Assessment, 1*, 23–29.

Mash, E. J. (1989). Treatment of child and family disturbance: A behavioral-systems perspective. In E. J. Mash & R. A. Barkley (Eds.), *Treatment of childhood disorders* (pp. 3–38). New York: Guilford Press.

Mash, E. J., & Barkley, R. A. (Eds.). (1989). *Treatment of childhood disorders*. New York: Guilford Press.

Mash, E. J., & Terdal, L. G. (1981). Behavioral assessment of childhood disturbances. In E. J. Mash & L. G. Terdal (Eds.), *Behavioral assessment of childhood disorders* (pp. 3–76). New York: Guilford Press.

Mash, E. J., & Terdal, L. G. (1988). Behavioral assessment of child and family disturbance. In E. J. Mash & L. G. Terdal (Eds.), *Behavioral assessment of childhood disorders* (2nd ed., pp. 3–68). New York: Guilford Press.

Masters, J. C., Burish, T. G., Hollon, S. D., & Rimm, D. C. (1987). *Behavior therapy: Techniques and empirical findings* (3rd ed.). San Diego: Harcourt Brace Jovanovich.

McMahon, R. J., & Wells, K. C. (1989). Conduct disorders. In E. J. Mash & R. A. Barkley (Eds.), *Treatment of childhood disorders* (pp. 73–134). New York: Guilford Press.

Meichenbaum, D. H. (1971). Examination of model characteristics in reducing avoidance behavior. *Journal of Personality and Social Psychology, 17*, 298–307.

Meichenbaum, D. H. (1977). *Cognitive-behavior modification*. New York: Plenum Press.

Melamed, B. G., & Siegel, L. J. (1975). Reduction of anxiety in children facing hospitalization and surgery by use of filmed modeling. *Journal of Consulting and Clinical Psychology, 43*, 511–521.

Melamed, B. G., Weinstein, D., Hawes, R., & Katin-Borland, M. (1975). Reduction of fear related dental management problems with use of filmed modeling. *Journal of the American Dental Association, 90*, 822–826.

Messer, S. C. (1990, August). *Developmental psychopathology and psychotherapy: An integrative approach*. Paper presented at the American Psychological Association convention, Boston.

Miller, N., & Dollard, J. (1941). *Social learning and imitation*. New Haven, CT: Yale University Press.

Millon, T. (1983). The DSM-III: An insider's perspective. *Amerivan Psychologist, 38*, 804–813.

Mize, J., & Ladd, G. W. (1990). Toward the development of successful social skills training for preschool children. In S. R. Asher & J. D. Cole (Eds.), *Peer rejection in childhood* (pp. 338–364). New York: Cambridge University Press.

Morris, R. J., & Kratochwill, T. R. (1983). Childhood fears and phobias. In R. J. Morris & T. R. Kratochwill (Eds.), *The practice of child therapy* (pp. 53–86). New York: Pergamon Press.

Mowrer, O. H., & Mowrer, W. M. (1938). Enuresis—A method for its study and treatment. *American Journal of Orthopsychiatry, 8*, 436–459.

O'Dell, S. (1974). Training parents in behavior modification: A review. *Psychological Bulletin, 81*, 418–433.

Office of Technology Assessment. (1986). *Children's mental health: Problems and services—A background paper* (Publication No. OTA-BP-H-33). Washington, DC: U.S. Government Printing Office.

Ollendick, T. H. (1979). Fear reduction techniques with children. In M. Hersen, R. M. Eisler, & P. M. Miller (Eds.), *Progress in behavior modification* (Vol. 8). New York: Academic Press.

Ollendick, T. H. (1981). Assessment of social interaction skills in school children. *Behavioral Counseling Quarterly*, *1*, 227–243.

Ollendick, T. H. (1986). Behavior therapy with children and adolescents. In S. L. Garfield & A. E. Bergin (Eds.), *Handbook of psychotherapy and behavior change* (3rd ed., pp. 565–624). New York: Wiley.

Ollendick, T. H., & Cerny, J. A. (1981). *Clinical behavior therapy with children*. New York: Plenum Press.

Ollendick, T. H., & Hersen, M. (1984). An overview of child behavioral assessment. In T. H. Ollendick & M. Hersen (Eds.), *Child behavioral assessment: Principles and procedures* (pp. 3–19). New York: Pergamon Press.

Panaccione, V. F., & Wahler, R. G. (1986). Child behavior, maternal depression, and social coercion as factors in the quality of child care. *Journal of Abnormal Child Psychology*, *14*, 263–278.

Patterson, G. R. (1980). Mothers: The unacknowledged victims. *Monographs of the Society for Research in Child Development*, *45* (Serial No. 186).

Patterson, G. R. (1982). *Coercive family process*. Eugene, OR: Castalia.

Patterson, G. R., & Chamberlain, P. (1988). Treatment process: A problem at three levels. In L. C. Wynne (Ed.), *The state of the art in family therapy research: Controversies and recommendations* (pp. 189–223). New York: Family Process Press.

Patterson, G. R., Reid, J. B., Jones, R. R., & Conger, R. E. (1975). *A social learning theory approach to family intervention: Vol. 1. Families with aggressive children*. Eugene, OR: Castalia.

Patterson, G. R., DeBarsyshe, B. D., & Ramsey, E. (1989). A developmental perspective on antisocial behavior. *American Psychologist*, *44*, 329–335.

Perry, D. G., & Bussey, K. (1979). The social learning theory of sex differences: Imitation is alive and well. *Journal of Personality and Social Psychology*, *37*, 1699–1712.

Phillips, D., & Wolpe, S. (1981). Multiple behavioral techniques in severe separation anxiety of a twelve-year-old. *Journal of Behavior Therapy and Experimental Psychiatry*, *12*, 329–332.

Phillips, E. L. (1968). Achievement Place: Token reinforcement procedure in a home style rehabilitation setting for predelinquent boys. *Journal of Applied Behavior Analysis*, *1*, 213–223.

Phillips, E. L., Phillips, E. A., Fixsen, D. L., & Wolf, M. M. (1971). Achievement Place: Modification of the behaviors of the pre-delinquent boys within a token economy. *Journal of Applied Behavior Analysis*, *4*, 45–59.

Piaget, J. (1969). *Genetic epistemology*. New York: Columbia University Press.

Purkel, W., & Bornstein, M. H. (1980). Pictures and imagery both enhance children's short-term and long-term recall. *Developmental Psychology*, *16*, 153–154.

Quay, H. C. (1986). Classification. In H. C. Quay & J. S. Werry (Eds.), *Psychopathological disorders of childhood* (3rd ed.). New York: Wiley.

Rachman, S. J. (1977). The conditioning theory of fear-acquisition: A critical examination. *Behaviour Research and Therapy*, *15*, 375–387.

Rice, D. P., Kelman, S., & Dunmeyer, S. (in progress). *The economic costs of alcohol and drug abuse and mental illness: 1985*. Report to the Office of Financing and Coverage Policy (Alcohol, Drug Abuse, and Mental Health Administration, U.S. Department of Health and Human Services). San Francisco: University of California.

Robinson, E. A. (1985). Coercion theory revisited: Toward a new theoretical perspective on the etiology of conduct disorders. *Clinical Psychology Review*, *5*, 597–625.

Ross, A. O. (1974). *Psychological disorders of children: A behavioral approach to theory, research, and therapy*. New York: McGraw-Hill.

Rutter, M., Tuma, A. H., & Lann, I. S. (1988). *Assessment and diagnosis in child psychopathology*. New York: Guilford Press.

Sanders, M. R., & Christensen, A. P. (1985). A comparison of the effects of child management and planned activities training in five parenting environments. *Journal of Abnormal Child Psychology*, *13*, 101–117.

Schultz, T. R., Butkowsky, J., Pearce, J. W., & Shanfield, H. (1975). Development of schemes for the attribution of multiple psychological causes. *Developmental Psychology*, *11*, 502–510.

Shure, M. B., & Spivack, G. (1978). *Problem-solving techniques in childrearing*. San Francisco: Jossey-Bass.

Skinner, B. F. (1953). *Science and human behavior*. New York: Macmillan.

Snyder, J. J., & White, M. J. (1979). The use of cognitive self-instruction in the treatment of behaviorally-disturbed adolescents. *Behavior Therapy*, *17*, 7–16.

Spivack, G., & Shure, M. B. (1974). *Social adjustment of young children*. San Francisco: Jossey-Bass.

Sroufe, L. A. (1979). The coherence of individual development. *American Psychologist*, *34*, 834–841.

Sroufe, L. A., & Rutter, M. (1984). The domain of developmental psychopathology. *Child Development, 55,* 17–24.

Stumpf, J., & Holman, J. (1985). Promoting generalization of appropriate classroom behaviour: A comparison of two strategies. *Behavioural Psychotherapy, 13,* 29–42.

Tryon, W. W. (1989). Behavioral assessment and psychiatric diagnosis. In M. Hersen (Ed.), *Innovations in child behavior therapy* (pp. 35–56). New York: Springer.

Ultee, C. A., Griffiaen, D., & Schellekens, J. (1982). The reduction of anxiety in children: A comparison of the effects of systematic desensitization in vitro and systematic desensitization in vivo. *Behaviour Research and Therapy, 20,* 61–67.

Wahler, R. G. (1980). The insular mother: Her problems in parent-child treatment. *Journal of Applied Behavior Analysis, 13,* 207–219.

Watson, J. B., & Morgan, J. J. B. (1917). Emotional reactions and psychological experimentation. *American Journal of Psychology, 28,* 163–174.

Weisz, J. R., Weiss, B., Alicke, M. D., & Klotz, M. L. (1987). Effectiveness of psychotherapy with children and adolescents: A meta-analysis for clinicians. *Journal of Consulting and Clinical Psychology, 55,* 542–549.

Wells, K. C., & Forehand, R. (1981). Childhood behavior problems in the home. In S. M. Turner, K. S. Calhoun, & H. E. Adams (Eds.), *Handbook of clinical behavior therapy.* New York: Wiley.

White, G. D., Nielsen, G., & Johnson, S. M. (1972). Time out duration and the suppression of deviant behavior in children. *Journal of Applied Behavior Analysis, 5,* 111–120.

Willner, A. G., Braukmann, C. J., Kirigin, K. A., & Wolf, M. M. (1978). Achievement Place: A community model for youths in trouble. In D. Marholin (Ed.), *Child behavior therapy* (pp. 239–273). New York: Gardner.

Winkler, R. C. (1977). What types of sex-role behavior should behavior modifiers promote? *Journal of Applied Behavior Analysis, 10,* 549–552.

Wolpe, J. (1958). *Psychotherapy by reciprocal inhibition.* Stanford, CA: Stanford University Press.

3

Behavioral Assessment in the Psychiatric Setting

WILLIAM H. O'BRIEN and STEPHEN N. HAYNES

INTRODUCTION

Behavioral assessment, with its empirical and pragmatic emphasis on identifying important causal functional relationships[1] between setting events and biobehavioral responses, is the most appropriate and responsible means of meeting the specialized assessment demands of contemporary inpatient psychiatry. These specialized demands require that a comprehensive assessment be conducted to identify the components of disordered and/or adaptive behaviors and the variables that control them. The assessment information can then be used to (1) design interventions that bring about a modification of patient behavior and (2) monitor treatment effectiveness. Importantly, these assessment tasks must be accomplished rapidly, as most patients are discharged and become outpatients within two to three weeks of admission (Commission on Professional and Hospital Activities, 1988).

Although behavioral assessment and treatment methods are well suited to addressing the specialized demands of contemporary psychiatric settings, they are only infrequently incorporated into public and private inpatient treatment units (Boudewyns, Fry, & Nightengale, 1986; Dickerson, 1989). Bellack (1986) argued that the limited use of behavioral assessment and treatment procedures with severely disordered psychiatric patients (those diagnosed as schizophrenic) may be associated with an erroneous set of beliefs among behavior therapists that these disorders are (1) completely determined by biological processes; (2) adequately treated by pharmacological interventions alone, and (3) minimally influenced by behavioral treatments.

---

[1] The term *functional relationship* is often used in the behavioral assessment and treatment literature to indicate that two or more variables have a shared variance. Some functional relationships are causal, and others are not. When conducting assessments in clinical settings, the behavior analyst is usually most interested in identifying and evaluating functional relationships that have a causal impact on the problem behavior. Hence, the term *causal functional relationship* denotes the subset of functional relationships that are most relevant to clinical applications of behavioral assessment.

WILLIAM H. O'BRIEN • Department of Psychology, Bowling Green State University, Bowling Green, Ohio 43403.   **STEPHEN N. HAYNES** • Department of Psychology, University of Hawaii, Honolulu, Hawaii 96822.

Handbook of Behavior Therapy in the Psychiatric Setting, edited by Alan S. Bellack and Michel Hersen. Plenum Press, New York, 1993.

It is interesting that such faulty beliefs persist despite the voluminous research in the fields of behavioral medicine and health psychology (e.g., Haynes & Gannon, 1981; Keefe & Blumenthal, 1982; Taylor, 1991; Turpin, 1989; see also the special series on clinical applications of psychophysiological assessment in *Psychological Assessment: A Journal of Consulting and Clinical Psychology*, 1992) that has documented the importance of situational and behavioral variables in the course of many illnesses that were historically conceptualized as being determined by biological factors alone (e.g., cancer, cardiovascular heart disease, and diabetes). Indeed, these fields have rejected the traditional medical model in favor of a biobehavioral approach to illness (Schwartz, 1983). Consequently, the question of biological versus behavioral causation has been rendered meaningless, and interactive assessment questions (e.g., How do situational events and behavior influence the biological aspects of an illness?) have been put forward in their stead.

An empirically based biobehavioral perspective is also appropriate for assessing psychiatric illnesses and severe behavior disorders. For example, although the primary medical criteria for admission to an inpatient psychiatric setting are presumably related to the severity or dangerousness of the "symptomatic" behavior and the consequent need for specialized inpatient care (e.g., Goldman, 1988), a significant proportion of the variance in admission decisions can also be accounted for by a variety of sociocultural and situational determinants (Elliot, Hammer, Gitlin, Brown, & Jamison, 1990; Freeman, 1989; Kryter, 1990; Morrisey, 1988; Neale, Oltmans, & Winters, 1983), which are most adequately understood from a behavioral perspective. Similarly, the efficacy of pharmacological treatments can be enhanced or diminished as a result of situational and behavioral factors (e.g., Carlton, 1983; Falloon, Boyd, McGill, Williamson, Razani, Moss, Gilderman, & Simpson, 1985; Falloon, McGill, Boyd, & Pederson, 1987; Poling & Cleary, 1986; Tarrier, Barrowclough, Vaughn, Bamrah, Porceddu, & Freeman, 1989).

This chapter presents an overview of the basic assumptions of behavioral assessment and the major factors to be considered in the design of an individualized assessment battery. A review of the different behavioral assessment methods commonly used in inpatient psychiatric settings follows. Finally, functional analytic causal modeling, one specialized application of behavioral assessment, is presented as a heuristic for conceptualizing complex interactions between setting events and diverse biobehavioral responses for the purposes of intervention designs for and the evaluation of psychiatric inpatients.

BASIC ASSUMPTIONS OF BEHAVIORAL ASSESSMENT

Behavioral assessment is based on several assumptions about behavior. The first assumption is that behavior is lawfully *determined* by the confluence of interrelationships between setting events and individual responses (e.g., Barrios, 1988; Hawkins, 1986; Haynes, 1978, 1979, 1990; Haynes & Wilson, 1979; Nelson & Hayes, 1986; Skinner, 1974; Strosahl & Linehan, 1986). Failures in the prediction or control of behavior are presumed to stem from inadequate articulation (identification and measurement) of the causal functional relationships between setting and response factors (e.g., Haynes & O'Brien, 1990; Russo & Budd, 1987; Skinner, 1988). The second assumption is that the lawful interrelationships between settings and responses can be identified most effectively through the use of *minimally inferential empirical* methodologies (e.g., Barlow & Hersen, 1984; Cone, 1988; Hay, 1982; Krasner, 1988). The third assumption is that setting and response interrelationships can be systematically *modified* to foster improved functioning in patients with a wide range of behavior disorders (e.g., Eysenck, 1988; Kazdin, 1984).

Augmenting these fundamental assumptions about behavior and its determinants is an additional tenet that has been advanced more recently to accommodate empirical findings reported in the behavioral assessment and treatment literature. This tenet specifies that *dynamic* (i.e., time-limited and continuously changing), *nonlinear, multivariate* models of setting and response interrelationships are more capable of explaining behavior than the static univariate models that often characterized early behavioral conceptualizations (Evans, 1985; Haynes, 1991; Kanfer, 1985; Mash & Hunsley, 1990; Nelson & Hayes, 1986; Russo, 1990).

Behavior disorders are thus presumed to be the manifestation of complex setting × response interactions that may have transitory and/or lasting effects. Further, each factor in the setting × response interaction may subsume distinct components, levels, and parameters (Cone, 1988; Delprato & McGlynn, 1988; Haynes, 1988, 1991; Schwartz, 1986). For example, within the response factor alone, there are overt-motor, cognitive, and affective-physiological *components* (Hollandsworth, 1986) that can be examined at many *levels* of reduction (e.g., physiological responses can be measured at molecular, individual-organ, or systemic levels). Responses can also be defined along a number of quantitative and qualitative *parameters*, such as rate, magnitude, duration, and function. Similarly, setting events include many components, levels of reduction, and dimensions.

A fully interactive, dynamic, and multivariate model of behavior is reflected in the evolution and advancement of behavioral explanations of many disorders since the early 1970s. One advancement, arising from the recognition of distinctiveness across persons in learning history and genotype, is that the magnitude and form of effects of environmental events are influenced by individual differences (Haynes, 1979; Russo, 1990; Russo & Budd, 1987). A vulnerability-stress model of schizophrenia (Nuechterlein, Goldstein, Ventura, Dawson, & Doane, 1989; Olbrich, 1989) and sensitive periods in the acquisition of complex social behaviors (Morrison, 1990; Scott, Stewart, & DeGhett, 1974) are two examples of how genetically coded maturational sequences can mediate the effects of environmental variables.

A second advancement is the acknowledgment that cognitive and affective-physiological responses often account for a significant proportion of the variance in the onset, maintenance, or termination of dysfunctional behavioral repertoires (e.g., Beck, Rush, Shaw, & Emery, 1979; Lee, 1987; Lowe & Chadwick, 1990; Parks & Hollon, 1988; Sturgis & Gramling, 1988; Zahn, 1986). This incorporation of cognitive and affective-physiological responses into behavioral research, assessment, and treatment methodologies has constituted a major broadening of behavioral thinking, which traditionally eschewed the use of unobservable phenomena.

A third advancement, consistent with general systems theory (von Bertalanffy, 1968), is the recognition that complex *bidirectional causal functional relationships* between and within different responses, settings, and persons are commonly found in behavior disorders (Bandura, 1981; Evans, 1985; Haynes, 1991; Haynes & O'Brien, 1990; Schwartz, 1983, 1986; Voeltz & Evans, 1982). For example, symptom exacerbation among schizophrenic patients may be causally related to heightened physiological arousal and frequent interactions with family members who are rated high in negative expressed emotion (EE; Tarrier, 1989; Tarrier & Barrowclough, 1990). In this case, specific situational factors (i.e., frequent negative interactions with high-EE family members) are presumed to evoke elevated levels of physiological arousal, which, in turn, may lead to symptom exacerbation. Up to this point, a unidirectional model of causality has been presented (frequent negative interactions with high-EE family members → elevated arousal → symptom exacerbation). There may also be a reciprocal direction of causality, so that symptom exacerbation provokes an increase in negative interactions with high-EE family members, which, in turn, increases physiological arousal even further (symptom exacerbation → increased frequency of negative interactions with high-EE family members → elevated arousal). The model has thus become a bidirectional causal system. The relationships between depressive behavior and social reinforcement, fear and avoidance, and binging and self-induced vomiting are other examples of bidirectional causal relationships.

In summary, the basic foundations of behavioral assessment, which include environmental determinism, empiricism, and modifiability of behavior, have broadened to include an additional assumption that dynamic multivariate models of setting and response interactions are required to maximize the explanation, prediction, and control of behavior. As a result, it is now more frequently accepted that the causal functional relationships between environmental variables and severe behavior disorders are often (1) time-limited; (2) constrained by individual differences in learning history and biological makeup; (3) significantly influenced by cognitive and physiological responses; and (4) bidirectional.

The increased complexity of behavioral conceptualizations of disordered behavior requires that a wide range of environmental events and behaviors be carefully evaluated in any reasonably complete behavioral assessment of psychiatric patients. One task faced by the behavior analyst is to decide which combination of behavioral assessment methods will best "capture" the unique configuration of setting–behavior interactions that characterizes the disordered behavior of each psychiatric patient. The following section presents the major considerations involved in this decision.

GENERAL CONSIDERATIONS IN THE BEHAVIORAL ASSESSMENT OF PSYCHIATRIC PATIENTS

Behavioral assessment methods are designed to systematically sample relevant environmental events and behaviors out of a "stream" or universe of continuously changing environment–behavior interactions (Mudford, Beale, & Singh, 1990; Paul, 1986a,b; Schoenfeld & Farmer, 1970). Many behavioral assessment methods can be used to quantify these complex environment–behavior interactions. Some behavioral assessment methods use visual observation techniques (e.g., trained observers who systematically watch and code patient behavior). Other assessment methods, such as behavioral interviews and questionnaires, rely on self-report. Self-monitoring, a process in which the patient self-observes and self-reports his or her own behavior, combines observational and self-report methodologies. A final behavioral assessment methodology, product-of-behavior measurement, can be thought of as gathering circumstantial evidence (e.g., blood alcohol levels and weight fluctuations associated with food consumption) that indicates that a particular behavior has occurred.

No explicit formulas declare which method or combination of methods is most appropriate for patients with specific psychiatric diagnoses or target behaviors. Instead, the behavior analyst must identify the relevant situational and response variables, organize these variables into a meaningful model of setting–behavior interactions, and design an assessment battery that will efficiently and accurately quantify the most important setting–behavior interactions on an ongoing basis. To accomplish these tasks, the behavior analyst must first consider (1) how the target behavior will be defined; (2) where the target behavior will be assessed; and (3) how the target behavior will be sampled (Foster, Bell-Dolan, & Burge, 1988; Foster & Cone, 1986; Hartmann, 1984; Haynes, 1978, 1990; Haynes & Wilson, 1979; Mash & Hunsley, 1990; Paul, 1986a,b).

Factors to Consider in Defining the Target Behavior: Topography, Social Significance, and Functional Properties

A behavior must be precisely defined before it can be measured. An adequate definition of a target behavior should include information about (1) its form and content; (2) the extent to which it "deviates" from normality or impairs social functioning; and (3) the factors that control it. These three areas are referred to, respectively, as the topography, social significance, and functional properties of the target behavior (Nelson & Hayes, 1986).

Topography. A preliminary step in defining a target behavior involves describing its topography. Important topographical features to consider include (1) temporal characteristics, such as rate, duration, interresponse time, and latency (i.e., time that elapses between a causal event and onset of the target behavior); (2) the magnitude of the response; (3) the content or complexity of the behavior; and (4) the stability of the behavior. For example, depression may be evaluated in terms of its temporal characteristics (e.g., how often the patient experiences depressive episodes, how long they last, and whether they are cyclical), its magnitude (e.g., the extent to which the patient is dysphoric or suicidal), its content (e.g., what the patient's specific depressive symptoms are), and its stability (e.g., whether the depressive behavior is emitted at a constant rate or varies).

Social Significance. Psychiatric patients often present with many dysfunctional behaviors. Social significance information can be used to prioritize these behaviors. That is, the most "deviant," socially maladaptive, or dangerous behaviors should be targeted for assessment first.

Estimating social significance involves comparing some topographical aspect (e.g., the frequency or the magnitude) of the target behavior with a "normal" standard of performance. A number of authors (Foster & Cone, 1986; Foster *et al.*, 1988; Hartmann, 1984; Haynes, 1978, 1990; Haynes & Wilson, 1979; Kazdin, 1984, 1985) have suggested that several aspects of social significance be routinely examined before target selection: (1) the degree of danger of the behavior to the self or others; (2) the extent to which the behavior deviates from that observed in a nondisordered population; and (3) the extent to which the behavior impairs the patient's personal, occupational, or social functioning. Clinical cutoff scores on standardized measures of psycho-pathology and reports from the patient's family are two means of estimating the social significance of a target behavior.

Functional Properties. Changes in the target behavior are brought about by specific situational, cognitive, physiological, and behavioral events that precede, co-occur with, and/or follow it. These causal functional relationships between the target behavior and controlling events can be roughly depicted as elevated conditional probabilities (e.g., $P[A][B] > P[A]$ or $P[A][BC] > P[A]$, where P = probability; A = target behavior change; B = change in Controlling Event 1; and C = change in Controlling Event 2) that indicate that the probability of observing a change in the target behavior, given that some controlling event occurs (i.e., its conditional probability), is greater than the probability of observing a change in the target behavior without the occurrence of the controlling event (i.e., its base rate or unconditional probability; Haynes & O'Brien, 1990). For example, the suicidal verbalizations of a depressed patient may be more, or less, frequent when particular staff members are nearby. Or a patient may exhibit more aggressive behavior during active recreational activities (e.g., basketball) than during passive recreational activities (e.g., watching a movie).

A complete definition of any target behavior should include information about its functional properties because a topographical analysis (e.g., identifying the symptoms and making a diagnosis) does not always convey information about causation (Haynes & O'Brien, 1988). Indeed, the topography of certain behaviors may differ even though they are functionally related to a common causal event, or behaviors with similar topographies may be functionally related to different causal events (Evans, 1985; Voeltz & Evans, 1982; Wahler & Fox, 1981). For example, a patient's idiosyncratic facial expressions, inappropriate verbalizations, and unusual posturing are topographically dissimilar behaviors that may have causal functional relationships with a common controlling event such as paranoid ideation (Haynes, 1986). Alternatively, a single behavior, such as sexual arousal, may have causal functional relationships with maladaptive controlling events on some occasions (e.g., pedophilic stimuli) and adaptive controlling events (e.g., age-appropriate stimuli) on other occasions (Earls & Castonguay, 1989).

Failure to provide information about the functional properties of the target behavior will result in an incomplete and, perhaps, invalid definition. This is especially true when target behaviors are dysfunctional not because of topography, but because they have causal functional relationships with atypical events. For example, anxiety may be appropriate when it is causally related to an impending, uncontrollable stressor of significant magnitude (e.g., a job interview). It is maladaptive, however, when the frequency, magnitude, or duration of the anxiety is caused by events that do not typically provoke such a response (e.g., leaving the house or engaging in a conversation). When behaviors are targeted because of their functional properties, each occurrence of the behavior is not considered an occurrence of the target behavior. Instead, only those instances in which the performance of the behavior is functionally related to inappropriate controlling events qualify as an occurrence of the target behavior.

The identification of causal functional relationships between target behaviors and controlling events is a sophisticated, but infrequently studied, decisional process (Bellack & Hersen, 1978; Felton & Nelson, 1984; Groden, 1989; Hay, Hay, Angle, & Nelson, 1979; Haynes & O'Brien, 1990; Persons, 1991). Procedurally, however, the behavior analyst should observe the behavior of the patient in a wide range of settings, gather verbal reports from the patient and persons with whom he or she regularly interacts, and peruse the empirical literature. An observation of consistent relationships between the targeted behaviors and particular antecedent, coincident, or consequent events, along with a plausible causal explanation (often derived from the empirical literature), is a minimal requirement for inferring the function of a behavior. Groden (1989) and Touchette, MacDonald, and Langer (1985) have developed convenient observational systems that can assist in the identification of causal functional relationships. Evans (1985) and Haynes (1988) have presented methods that can be used to depict the relationships between multiple targeted behaviors and probable causal events.

In summary, details about the topography of behavior facilitate the development of precise descriptions. Social significance data assist in the prioritization of potential target behaviors. Information about the functional properties of the target behavior allow explanation. Consideration of the topography, social significance, and function of behavior, taken together, increases the likelihood that the subset of responses that are ultimately selected for ongoing assessment and treatment will be quantifiable, important, and valid. Thus, the time devoted to defining the target behavior is highly important. A behavioral assessment battery that quantifies a poorly defined behavior will not yield useful clinical data.

Factors to Consider in Selecting an Assessment Setting

A fundamental tenet of behavioral construct systems is that setting events account for a significant proportion of variance in behavior. This situational dependence of behavior is often observed among psychiatric patients. For example, Tarrier, Vaughn, Lader, and Leff (1979) examined differences in the level and variability of skin conductance (a measure of sympathetic arousal) among schizophrenic patients while they were conversing with high- and low-EE relatives. Three assessments were conducted in the patients' homes, and one assessment was conducted in a psychophysiological laboratory. The presence of the high-EE relative reliably evoked increased variability in skin conductance in two specific settings: (1) the first assessment occasion conducted in the patients' homes and (2) the assessment occasions that closely followed a stressful life event. The authors concluded that the sympathetic arousal associated with the novelty of the assessment situation and/or recent life events magnified the physiological effects of exposure to the high-EE relative. This observation and interpretation of the situational specificity of sympathetic arousal led to a number of follow-up studies that have furthered our understanding of how stressful events and particular family interaction patterns may provoke symptom exacerbation and eventual rehospitalization of schizophrenic patients (e.g., Falloon et al., 1985, 1987; Goldstein, Miklowitz, Strachan, Doan, Nuechterlein, & Feingold, 1989; Nuechterlein et al., 1989; Tarrier, 1989; Tarrier & Barrowclough, 1990).

Because of the importance of situational control over behavior, assessment should be conducted across diverse settings (Bellack & Hersen, 1978; Delprato & McGlynn, 1988; Foster *et al.*, 1988; Groden, 1989; Hersen & Bellack, 1978; Paul, 1986a; Touchette *et al.*, 1985). Assessment in *naturalistic settings* is a strategy by which patient behavior is sampled in everyday social, occupational, or domestic settings. This approach maximizes the ecological validity of the assessment data. The primary disadvantages associated with assessment in naturalistic settings are the cost (if observational procedures are used) and the difficulty of obtaining accurate measurements.

Because naturalistic assessments are difficult to conduct, many behavioral assessments of psychiatric patients take place in *analogue settings*, which range from highly controlled laboratory situations and classrooms to "quasi-naturalistic" hospital settings, such as the psychiatric unit, the hospital cafeteria, or the therapist's office (e.g., Boudewyns & Hyer, 1990; Curran, Faraone, & Dow, 1985; Douglas & Mueser, 1990; Falloon *et al.*, 1985; Hansen, St. Lawrence, & Christoff, 1989; Paul, 1986a,b,c). Analogue settings are designed to increase the probability that particular target behaviors will occur. For example, a patient whose social skills have been targeted for assessment may be placed in an analogue setting in which he or she is asked to initiate a conversation with another person. The target behaviors are much more likely to occur in this analogue setting than in a naturalistic setting, where the patient may avoid social encounters. Role-playing exercises, laboratory tasks, and planned social interactions are examples of analogue assessment situations that have been extensively used in psychiatric settings (Boudewyns & Hyer, 1990; Curran, Faraone, & Dow, 1985; Hahlweg, Hemmati-Webber, Heusser, Lober, Winkler, Muller, Feinstein, & Dose, 1990; Mueser, Bellack, Morrison, & Wixted, 1990).

The primary advantages of analogue assessment are associated with convenience, efficiency (e.g., infrequent target behaviors can be reliably evoked), and measurement precision (e.g., Foster *et al.*, 1988; Hartmann, 1984; Hartmann & Wood, 1990). Most analogue settings, however, contain only a small percentage of the important cues found in the patient's natural environment. Consequently, the assessor must carefully consider what stimuli should be present in the analogue setting in order to increase the probability that the assessment data obtained in these settings are ecologically valid.

To summarize, target behaviors are functionally related to specific controlling events. Naturalistic settings contain the full range of these controlling events, whereas analogue settings typically contain only a fraction of them. In many cases, the naturalistic assessment of psychiatric patients may be unfeasible (especially if observational assessment methods are used). Consequently, the behavior analyst must carefully determine which of many potential analogue and "quasi-naturalistic" settings will maximize the ecological validity of the assessment data.

Factors to Consider in Specifying a Method for Sampling Behavior

Thus far we have noted that target behaviors have unique topographical features, degrees of social significance, and functions. These different aspects of target behaviors are also presumed to vary across different settings. The behavior analyst must also consider what type of sampling strategies are appropriate for the assessment of such complex setting–behavior interactions. The imposition of a sampling strategy will undoubtedly result in the loss of some information, as every aspect of the target behavior and the settings within which it occurs cannot be realistically sampled. Thus, as Hartmann (1984) observed, the essential concern is to develop a sampling methodology that will "minimize costs and maximize representativeness, sensitivity, and reliability of data and the output per unit of time" (p. 114).

Sampling systems often segment behavior or setting–response interactions according to time units that range from a few milliseconds to years. The sampling intervals may also be contiguous (e.g., every hour) or discontiguous (e.g., every other hour). A number of time-sampling strategies that use different temporal sampling frames have been discussed in many textbooks and chapters on behavioral assessment (cf. Bellack & Hersen, 1988; Ciminero, Calhoun, & Adams, 1986; Foster & Cone, 1986; Hartmann, 1984; Hartmann & Wood, 1990; Haynes, 1978, 1990; Haynes & Wilson, 1979; Nelson & Hayes, 1986). Five major temporal sampling strategies are described below: event sampling, duration sampling, interval sampling, real-time sampling, and momentary-time sampling.

Event sampling is a procedure in which the occurrence of a behavior is noted and recorded. A frequency measure is then calculated by summing the number of occurrences across an appropriate time interval, such as minutes, hours, days, or weeks. Event samples can be obtained by direct observation or verbal report. For example, smoking behavior can be (1) observed directly; (2) self-monitored; or (3) verbally reported by the patient or the nursing staff during an interview.

Duration sampling involves measuring the amount of time that elapses between the onset and the cessation of a target behavior or a setting–behavior interaction. For example, the time that elapses between the presentation of a food tray and the onset of eating, or the time that elapses between the onset of eating and the cessation of eating for an anorectic patient may be assessed by duration sampling. Duration sampling can also be accomplished by direct observation and verbal report. In the anorectic example, the duration of eating behavior could be observed by nursing staff, self-monitored by the patient, or estimated from retrospective self-reports by the patient or by the nursing staff.

Duration sampling can provide important information about the target behavior that is not contained in frequency data. For example, a patient with obsessive-compulsive disorder may report that he or she infrequently engages in compulsive rituals. The problem may therefore seem to be under adequate control. However, if each compulsive ritual is several hours long, the problem may be quite serious.

Interval sampling segments time into discrete assessment intervals (e.g., 5 seconds, 5 minutes, or 60 minutes). The number of intervals during which the targeted response reaches some prespecified criterion level of rate, intensity, or quality are then recorded. Like event and duration sampling, interval sampling can be accomplished through direct observation or verbal report.

Interval sampling is most useful when the target behavior occurs frequently, or when the onset and termination of the target behavior are difficult to determine. For example, a patient may almost constantly engage in audible self-talk. With high-frequency behavior such as this, it is very difficult to determine when one response begins or ends. Consequently, event and duration sampling are not viable. An interval-sampling procedure may be devised, however, in which the day is divided into discrete 5-minute intervals. Whenever audible self-talk is observed, the entire interval is recorded as an occurrence of the target behavior. If self-talk is not observed for an entire interval, a nonoccurrence is recorded.

With interval-sampling methods, a marked occurrence may indicate one brief occurrence, one long occurrence, several brief occurrences, or a combination of brief and long occurrences. Therefore, one can determine only the number of intervals in which the target behavior has occurred. One cannot derive accurate frequency or duration estimates.

Real-time sampling combines event, duration, and interval sampling by recording the real time at the onset and cessation of a particular target behavior or setting–behavior interaction. Frequency information is derived by counting the number of times the behavior occurs across some period of time (e.g., seconds, minutes, hours, or days). Duration is derived by subtracting the time of onset from the time of cessation. To yield interval information, the day is divided into real-time intervals (e.g., 8 A.M.–9 A.M.). The number of times the behavior occurred within each interval is then counted.

Real-time sampling requires that the assessor record the onset and the termination of every occurrence of the target behavior. This requirement significantly limits the applicability of this methodology. Like event and duration sampling, it is not a viable method for high-frequency behaviors or behaviors with unclear beginning and end points. Additionally, real-time sampling usually cannot be done by means of verbal reports because most patients are not able to accurately recall and/or self-monitor the exact times when a target behavior began and ended. Consequently, this sampling strategy is used almost exclusively with observational assessment.

Momentary-time sampling is the fifth major sampling strategy. In momentary-time sampling, assessments are made during brief sampling intervals on a continuously rotating basis. This strategy can be likened to taking a "snapshot" of behavior at different times (Paul, 1986a). For example, Paul (1986c) developed an observational system of momentary-time sampling (The Time Sample Behavior Checklist) by which measurements can be obtained on up to 20 inpatients. Observers record each patient's behavior during successive 2-second sampling intervals. After completing one "round" of observations, the observers return to the first patient and run through the observational sequence again. A less elaborate time-sampling strategy was reported by Andrewes (1989), in which patient behavior was sampled for 15 minutes at the beginning of each shift on an inpatient psychiatric unit.

Momentary-time sampling is the most complex of all sampling strategies. It combines elements of interval sampling and real-time sampling. The intervals are extremely brief, discontiguous, and sequenced according to real-time units. Momentary-time sampling also has the limitations associated with interval and real-time sampling. As in interval sampling, information regarding the frequency and duration of the target behaviors may be suspect. Like real-time sampling, this methodology is largely restricted to direct observation because of its complexity.

In summary, event, duration, interval, real-time, and momentary-time sampling segment continuously occurring setting–behavior transactions in different ways. They also differ in their complexity and their labor demands. Event sampling, duration sampling, and interval sampling are less labor-intensive and can be easily taught to patients, nonprofessionals, and paraprofessionals. Consequently, these sampling methods can be used in direct observation, self-monitoring, and self-reports. Real-time sampling and momentary-time sampling are more complex and labor-intensive. For these reasons, they are almost exclusively used in direct observation in specialized psychiatric settings that are staffed by paid or volunteer assessment technicians.

Summary of General Considerations in the Behavioral Assessment of Psychiatric Patients

Many factors must be considered in the design of a behavioral assessment battery. To derive an adequate definition of the target behavior, the topography, the functional properties, and the social significance of the behavior must be examined. Once the target behaviors are defined, the behavior analyst must decide where ongoing assessment of the patient will occur. Assessment settings can range from highly controlled analogue situations to the natural environment. Each setting confers different advantages in measurement precision, cost, convenience, and ecological validity. In general, as the assessment setting moves from controlled analogue situations to naturalistic situations, measurement precision and convenience decline while cost and ecological validity increase. A number of sampling methodologies are available for segmenting continuous setting–behavior transactions into discrete elements. Event sampling, duration sampling, and interval sampling can be used for many clinical problems because patients and nonprofessionals can be taught to use the procedures to collect data. Real-time sampling and momentary-time sampling are more complicated approaches that are feasible only when assessment technicians are available to the behavior analyst.

Behavioral Assessment Methods Commonly Used in Psychiatric Settings

Many different behavioral assessment methods can be used in psychiatric settings. Table 1 lists patient diagnosis, target behaviors, assessment methods, and settings for assessment that were reported in the leading behavior assessment and treatment journals (*Behavioral Assessment*, *Behavior Modification*, *Behaviour Research and Therapy*, *Behavior Therapy*, *Journal of Applied Behavior Analysis*, and *Journal of Behavior Therapy and Experimental Psychiatry*) from 1988 through 1990.

A total of 679 individual or group assessment and intervention studies were examined for content. Eighteen (3%) explicitly described the behavioral assessment of adult patients in an inpatient psychiatric setting, a day-treatment center, or a residential psychiatric facility. Thirty-six target behaviors were assessed across the 18 studies. Fifty percent of the studies used more than one behavioral assessment method. The most commonly reported assessment methods were participant observation (42%), self-report inventories (28%), structured interviews (11%), nonparticipant observation (8%), product-of-behavior quantification (8%), behavioral assessment interviewing (3%), and archival data collection (3%). These assessment methods are described in the sections that follow.

Behavioral Assessment Interviewing

Behavioral assessment interviews can be differentiated from nonbehavioral (e.g., psychodynamic) assessment interviews in terms of structure, focus, interpretation of behavior, and purpose. Nonbehavioral interviews are relatively unstructured because nondirective questioning is used. In contrast, behavioral interviews are deliberately structured so that patient responses that provide important information about the topography, social significance, and function of the target behaviors are selectively reinforced (Turkat, 1986). For example, a behavioral interviewer usually questions the patient or informant about situational events, cognitions, behaviors, and physiological states that precede, coincide with, or follow the target behavior. A typical question for a patient presenting with major depression might be "Please tell me about the things you say to yourself, or do, when you are feeling particularly depressed?" The patient may initially provide an imprecise response, such as "I don't do anything; nothing can be done; I guess I just try to hang in there." The behavioral interviewer may then seek to improve the precision of the patient's response by restructuring the question as follows: "If I could tape-record your thoughts or follow you around with a movie camera, what would I hear and see?" At a maximal level of structure, the interviewer may used closed-ended questions (e.g., "When you are most depressed, do you say negative things to yourself?"). Closed-ended questions are usually required only for the most disordered patients.

In terms of focus, nonbehavioral assessment interviews concentrate largely on the semantic content of verbal responses (i.e., the words spoken and the meaning of those words). Behavioral assessment interviews, however, sample a much broader range of patient responses. Linguistic behavior (e.g., semantics, syntax, and phonetics), paralinguistic behavior (e.g., voice volume, rate of speech, and facial expressions), and nonverbal behavior (e.g., eye contact and posture) are all typically evaluated during behavioral interviews.

Patient responses are also interpreted quite differently in nonbehavioral and behavioral assessment interviews. From a nonbehavioral perspective, the main determinants of behavior are presumed to be internal, stable, and unobservable. Hence, the patient's responses are presumed to be a manifestation of these internal causal factors. In contrast, behavioral assessment interviews use an empirical perspective in which patient responses are treated as (1) markers of functional relationships that may be present in the patient's natural environment (e.g., a patient's report that his or her obsessive ruminations are most intense when he or she is at home) or (2) exemplars of the target behavior that are under the control of events that occur during the interview itself (e.g., depressive affect improves when a patient is asked to describe his or her positive attributes).

The broad empirical focus of behavioral assessment interviews is very useful in psychiatric settings. Patients who may have severely disordered interpersonal behavior or who have language impairments can still be assessed by an informal observation of paralinguistic and nonverbal responses during the interview (Bellack & Hersen, 1978; Mandal, Srivastava, & Singh, 1990). For example, a patient may respond to interview questions with nonsensical speech, and the semantic content of the speech may not provide useful information about the events that control the patient's behavior. However, the behavioral interviewer may observe that the patient consistently responds more appropriately when questions are highly structured, a result leading to the hypothesis that the patient's inappropriate speech is reduced when explicit cues are provided regarding socially appropriate responses. The interviewer may also observe that the patient is "taking turns" in the verbal interaction and is maintaining appropriate eye contact and adequate voice volume. These observations suggest that the factors controlling the semantic component of the patient's verbal responses may be independent of the factors that control the paralinguistic components. This example demonstrates how behavioral interviews may shift from *verbal correspondence encoding*, in which the semantic contents of verbal responses are presumed to be informative markers of naturalistic causal functional relationships, to *verbal performance encoding*, in which the verbal responses are treated as target behaviors that are causally related to events occurring within the interview itself (Paul, 1986a).

A final way in which behavioral assessment interviews differ from nonbehavioral assessment interviews is their purpose. The fundamental purpose of the nonbehavioral interview is to infer subjectively what internal pathological processes are causing the disordered behavior (Goldfried & Kent, 1972; Hartmann, Roper, & Bradford, 1979). The primary purpose of the behavioral interview is to define the topography, the social significance, and the functional properties of the target behavior. This approach, in turn, allows the behavior analyst to (1) develop a preliminary model of the patient's disorder that outlines the hypothesized interrelationships between important target behaviors and the relevant controlling factors; (2) select the settings and sampling methodologies for subsequent assessment; (3) make initial decisions regarding the design of an individualized treatment; (4) select the variables for treatment evaluation; (5) assess the subjective responses to behavioral interventions (e.g., the acceptability of the treatment); (6) assess compliance with the treatment recommendations; and (7) evaluate the patient's knowledge of behavioral principles (Haynes, 1988, 1990; McAndrew, 1989; Morganstern, 1988; Turkat, 1986).

To summarize, nonbehavioral assessment interviews tend to rely on the semantic content of speech and to assume that the patient's responses will provide information about the internal determinants of the patient's behavior. This approach reduces the utility of nonbehavioral assessment interviewing for patients who have severely disordered interpersonal behaviors or language processes. In contrast, behavioral assessment interviewing concentrates on a much broader range of patient responses and assumes that the responses are valid markers of causal functional relationships between social-environmental events and changes in the target behavior. At one level of analysis, the behavior analyst interprets verbal responses as valid markers of causal functional relationships that control the patient's behavior in naturalistic settings. At another level of analysis, the behavior analyst presumes that the patient's responses are functionally related to causal events that occur during the interview. This unique aspect of

WILLIAM H. O'BRIEN
and STEPHEN N.
HAYNES

Table 1. Representative Sample of Recently Published Studies Involving the Behavioral Assessment of Psychiatric Inpatients

Reference	Patient diagnosis	Target behavior	Method of assessment	Setting
Andrewes (1989)	Organic mental disorder	Screaming	Participant observation (discontinuous interval sampling: 15-minute interval at beginning of each shift by nursing staff)	Inpatient psychiatric ward
Belcher (1988)	Schizophrenia	Hallucinatory verbalizations	Participant observation (event recording by nursing staff)	Any location within nursing home
Blake *et al.* (1990)	Mixed diagnoses	(1) Therapeutic group attendance (2) Transitional living-unit satisfaction	(1) Participant observation (event recording by group facilitator) (2) Self-report questionnaire	(1,2) Postacute psychiatric ward
Boudewyns & Hyer (1990)	Posttraumatic stress disorder (PTSD)	(1) Behaviors associated with PTSD (2) Alcohol consumption (3) Physiological arousal (4) Quality of life	(1) Structured interview (2) Behavior by-product (breathylizer test) (3) Psychophysiological observation (muscle tension, heart rate, skin conductance) (4) Self-report questionnaire	(1,2) Inpatient psychiatric ward (3) Psychophysiological laboratory (4) Inpatient psychiatric ward
Bowen *et al.* (1990)	Schizophrenia	Excessive fluid consumption	Participant observation and behavior by-product (weight gain associated with fluid consumption)	Inpatient behavioral treatment unit
Carey *et al.* (1990)	Mixed diagnoses	(1) Intellectual functioning (2) Perceived stress (3) Problem-solving behavior	(1) Structured interview (2) Self-report questionnaire (3) Nonparticipant observation (ratings of audiotaped responses)	(1,2) Day treatment clinic (3) Analogue/role play situations
Douglas & Mueser (1990)	Mixed diagnoses	Social skills	Nonparticipant observation (ratings of audiotaped responses)	Analogue/role play situations
Earls & Castonuay (1989)	Pedophilia	(1) Situational precursors to pedophilic behavior (2) Inappropriate sexual arousal in the presence of pedophilic stimuli	(1) Behavioral interview and archival data collection (clinic records) (2) Psychophysiological observation	(1) Forensic psychiatric facility (2) Psychophysiological laboratory

Study	Diagnosis	Target behavior	Assessment method	Setting
Foxx et al. (1988)	Schizophrenia	(1) Delusional speech (2) Appropriate speech	(1) Participant observation (event recording by therapist) and nonparticipant observation (event recording of videotaped behavior) (2) Participant observation and nonparticipant observation (as described above)	(2) Social skills training room in psychiatric unit (2) Multiple noninstitutional settings
Harris (1989)	Mixed diagnoses	(1) Undesirable behavior (assaultiveness, hoarding medications, nuisance behavior) (2) Desirable behavior (self-care, positive mood, work attendance, appropriate social interactions)	(1) Participant observation (behavioral ratings by nursing staff) (2) Participant observation (behavioral ratings by nursing staff)	(1,2) Inpatient psychiatric ward
Lane et al. (1989)	Organic mental disorder	Hoarding edible and nonedible items	Participant observation (interval sampling by nursing staff)	Residential treatment unit
Miller et al. (1989)	Depressive disorder	Depressive behavior	Structured interview and self-report questionnaire	Inpatient psychiatric ward
Papworth (1989)	Organic mental disorder	(1) Nocturnal enuresis (2) Obsessive toileting	(1) Behavior by-product (checking sheets and underwear for dryness) (2) Participant observation	(1,2) Inpatient psychiatric ward
Peniston (1988)	Schizophrenia	(1) Disruptive behavior (2) Nonattendance at assignments (3) Grooming skills (4) Alcohol consumption	(1–3) Participant observation (discontinuous interval sampling by nursing aides) (4) Participant observation (event recording by nursing aides)	(1–4) Inpatient psychiatric ward
Sievert et al. (1988)	Mixed diagnoses	(1) Knowledge of legal rights (2) Use of appropriate behaviors to "redress legal rights violations"	(1) Structured interview (2) Participant observation (event recording by therapist)	(1) Legal rights training sessions (2) Analogue/role plays in several different settings (classroom and community)
Van Den Hout et al. (1988)	Obsessive-compulsive disorder	Obsessive-compulsive behavior	Self-report questionnaires	Inpatient psychiatric ward and outpatient clinic
Williamson et al. (1989)	Bulimia nervosa	(1) Bulimic behavior (2) Eating attitudes (3) Depression (4) General psychiatric symptoms	(1) Self-report questionnaire (2) Self-report questionnaire (3) Self-report questionnaire (4) Self-report questionnaire	(1–4) Inpatient psychiatric ward and outpatient clinic
Wong & Woolsey (1989)	Schizophrenia	Conversational behavior	Participant observation (event recording by therapist unit)	Simulated social interactions on an inpatient behavioral rehabilitation ward

behavioral interviewing is especially helpful in psychiatric settings, where many patients cannot be interviewed by the use of traditional approaches.

Sources for Behavioral Assessment Interviews.   In addition to the patient, a variety of informants who are familiar with the patient should be given behavioral assessment interviews (Bellack & Hersen, 1978). Direct-care staff (e.g., nurses and paraprofessionals) are a major source of information. These persons can provide information that is particularly useful in determining what situational, cognitive, or behavioral events may be causally related to the target behaviors in various "quasi-naturalistic" settings (e.g., the psychiatric unit or the day-treatment center). The validity and utility of staff observations, however, are significantly affected by the extent to which the interviewee attends to, and reliably reports objective information about, the targeted behavior and the impact on it of different controlling variables. Through structured questioning, paraphrasing, and selective reinforcement, the behavioral interviewer can encourage the interviewees to report their observations precisely, objectively, and noninferentially.

Nonprofessionals are another important source of information for behavioral assessment interviewers. Included in this category are members of the patient's family, friends of the patient, workmates, or fellow psychiatric inpatients. Interviews with these persons may also yield valuable information regarding the patient's social environment and the natural contingencies associated with both dysfunctional and adaptive behavior. As with direct-care staff, however, the interviewer must carefully design interview questions so that they encourage the interviewee to look for important causal functional relationships and to report his or her observations using behavioral terminology. Finally, it is extremely important that interviews conducted with nonprofessionals be conducted only after the patient or the legal guardian has consented.

The Reliability and Validity of Behavioral Assessment Interviews.   In a recent survey of the membership of the Association for Advancement of Behavior Therapy (AABT), 91% of those who responded to the survey ($n = 988$) said that they routinely used behavioral interviewing as an assessment method (Guevremont & Spiegler, 1990). In our survey of the published literature describing behavioral assessment in psychiatric settings (Table 1), however, only 3% of the studies explicitly referred to the use of behavioral interviewing. One may conclude that either (1) behavioral interviews are not routinely used in psychiatric settings or (2) behavioral interviews are underreported in the published literature. The latter conclusion seems most plausible, as it is hard to envision a behavior analyst instituting any other type of assessment strategy without interviewing *someone* about the patient's behavior beforehand. The behavioral interview may therefore be the most frequently used behavioral assessment method, although the extent of its use and the ways in which behavior analysts quantify and interpret the interview information are largely unknown.

There is also a paucity of empirical information available regarding the reliability and validity of the behavioral interview. Haynes and Wilson (1979) and Jensen and Haynes (1986) conducted reviews of the behavioral assessment and treatment literature and reported that the reliability of behavioral interviewing was largely unexplored. The extent to which interview-derived assessment data were correlated with noninterview assessment data was also undetermined. Hay *et al.* (1979) and Felton and Nelson (1984) examined the extent to which different assessors agreed on the classification of patient self-reported variables into antecedent, response, and consequence categories by using behavioral interviews conducted in analogue settings. The results of these studies indicated moderate levels of agreement, but there was significant variability in the results due to differences in interviewer behavior and the method of categorizing the data. Thus, although over a decade has elapsed since the issue of the reliability and validity of behavioral interviewing was raised (Haynes & Wilson, 1979), few empirical data have been generated, and the need for a psychometric evaluation of the behavioral interview remains a prominent concern.

In summary, the behavioral assessment interview is a frequently used assessment strategy that can be carried out effectively with even the most disordered psychiatric patients. Behavioral assessment interviews have the unique quality of treating verbal responses as both informational marker variables and target variables. The primary purpose of the behavioral interview is to gather preliminary information about the characteristics of the target behavior and its functional properties that allows the behavior analyst to create a preliminary model of the disordered behavior and to make decisions about the settings and sampling methods that will be used in subsequent assessment.

Despite the probable widespread use of the behavioral interview in psychiatric settings, very few studies have explicitly reported whether it was used as an assessment method. Additionally, few studies have examined the reliability and validity of behavioral interviewing. Further research is needed to improve our understanding of this frequently used assessment method.

Behavioral Observation

If numbers of book chapters and published journal articles are a valid index of research attention and sophistication, behavioral observation is the most extensively developed and frequently used behavioral assessment method (e.g., Alevizos, DeRisi, Liberman, Eckman, & Callahan, 1978; Foster & Cone, 1986; Foster et al., 1988; Hartmann & Wood, 1990; Haynes, 1978; Haynes & Wilson, 1979; Paul, 1986a,b,c; Paul & Lenz, 1977). The extensive research attention given to behavioral observation stems from its congruence with an empirical-behavioral perspective, in which observable, minimally inferential measures are preferred to nonobservable, indirect, or more inferential measures of behavior (Hartmann, 1984; Jacobson, 1985a,b). In this section, the observation methodologies most commonly used in psychiatric settings are described.

Nonparticipant Observation. Nonparticipant observation systems use observers whose sole function is to code behavior. Aside from this activity, they typically do not have any other patient care responsibilities. Paid observational technicians, university students, volunteer raters, and peer judges have been effectively used as nonparticipant observers in psychiatric settings (e.g., Douglas & Mueser, 1990; Paul, 1986a).

Because nonparticipant observers are not responsible for carrying out multiple caregiving activities (e.g., assisting patients with activities of daily living or dispensing medications), they can sample diverse and complex behaviors with a high degree of precision (Paul, 1986a). In psychiatric settings, nonparticipant observation has been frequently used to assess the many components of social skills (e.g., conversational skills, paralinguistic behavior, conflict resolution, and social problem solving) in analogue settings (Bellack & Mueser, 1990; Carey, Carey, & Meisler, 1990; Curran et al., 1985; Douglas & Mueser, 1990; Hahlweg et al., 1990; Halford, Hayes, & Varghese, 1990). Nonparticipant observation has also been used to assess inappropriate and bizarre behavior (e.g., Glynn, Bowen, Rose, Marshall, & Liberman, 1990; Paul & Lenz, 1977), the effect of pharmacological treatments on behavioral functioning (Munford, Tarlow, & Gerner, 1984), expressed emotion in the families of schizophrenic patients (Falloon et al., 1987; Tarrier, 1989), and therapist delivery of behavioral family therapy techniques during treatment sessions (Hahlweg et al., 1990).

The training of nonparticipant observers is often accomplished by having expert behavior analysts provide didactic instruction. Observers have also been successfully trained with written manuals and computer guidance (Bass, 1987; Miltenberger & Fuqua, 1985). Although nonparticipant observation could conceivably be conducted anywhere, it is most often used to assess patient behavior in analogue settings (e.g., social-skills-training sessions) and "quasi-

WILLIAM H. O'BRIEN
and STEPHEN N.
HAYNES

naturalistic'' settings (e.g., the psychiatric unit) because of the difficulties associated with conducting naturalistic observations.

The design of a nonparticipant observation method often follows a particular sequence. First, the behavior analyst must thoroughly define the target behaviors so that they can be reliably distinguished from other behaviors. These target behavior definitions are derived from informal observation and behavioral assessment interviews with the patient, the staff, and family members. Next, a decision must be made about where the observations will be conducted. If the behavior appears to be functionally related to controlling events that commonly occur in the hospital or treatment institution, a quasi-naturalistic observation setting (e.g., the ward, the cafeteria, or the day-treatment setting) is most appropriate. Alternatively, an analogue setting may be preferred if the target behaviors are controlled by events that occur infrequently in quasi-naturalistic or naturalistic settings. Finally, after the target and observation settings are defined, a sampling strategy must be selected. Any of the five sampling strategies (event, duration, interval, real-time, or momentary-time) can be used by nonparticipant observers.

Nonparticipant observation in psychiatric settings is limited in two significant ways. First, nonparticipant observation has been largely restricted to the assessment of overt motor behavior because cognitions and affective-physiological states are not easily distinguished by sight. Second, the costs of recruiting and training nonparticipant observers may be prohibitive. The first limitation may be partially remedied by the use of observational procedures that have been developed to assess the affective "tone" of marital interactions (e.g., Gottman, 1980; Gottman & Levenson, 1986; Julien, Markman, & Lindahl, 1989). The second limitation, the high cost per unit of observation, may be lessened by having observers code multiple targets and patients (Paul, 1986a,c).

In addition to these two limitations, three main sources of error are associated with nonparticipant observation: (1) error associated with the inadequate specification of the target behavior, the setting for observation, or the sampling procedures; (2) error associated with observer drift, observer fatigue, and observer expectancies; and (3) the reactive effects of observation on patient behavior (Foster *et al.*, 1988; Foster & Cone, 1986; Hartmann & Wood, 1990; Haynes, 1978; Jacobson, 1985a,b; Paul, 1986a,c). These sources of error can be reduced by (1) carefully detailing and revising (when problems are detected) a written procedure manual that explicitly specifies the target behavior, setting, and sampling procedures; (2) conducting intermittent and unannounced accuracy checks of observer data, scheduling rest periods within observation sessions, and consistently reinforcing accurate observations; and (3) minimizing the obtrusiveness of observation and scheduling an adaptation period that allows the patient to become accustomed to the presence of the observer (Delprato & McGlynn, 1988; Hartmann, 1984; Paul, 1986a,c).

In summary, nonparticipant observation can assess overt motor behavior with a good deal of precision. The costs of obtaining this information, however, may be quite high. Therefore, nonparticipant observation is most appropriate to research applications, where the investigator is interested in obtaining precise estimates of behavior and has the resources for procuring and training observational technicians. Nonparticipant observation is generally unsuitable for many idiographic clinical applications because of the limitations in the range of behaviors that can be assessed and because of the cost. Consequently, most clinicians in psychiatric settings will probably need to use alternative observational methodologies, which are described below.

Participant Observation. Participant observers have regular and ongoing interactions with the patient, independent of their responsibilities as behavioral coders. Participant observers are usually recruited from a patient's therapeutic (e.g., hospital, day-treatment center, or outpatient clinic), occupational, social, or domestic environment, are trained in observational methodology, and are then assigned to observe and record the patient's behavior in particular settings (Paul, 1986a). The participant observers available in psychiatric settings may include behavior therapists, psychiatrists, psychiatric nurses, paraprofessional staff workers, hospital roommates, other inpatients, work supervisors, co-workers, friends, and family members (cf. Alford, 1986; Elliot *et al.*, 1990; Fisher, Piazza, & Page, 1989; Hersen, 1985; Hersen & Bellack, 1978; Moyes, Tennent, & Bedford, 1985; O'Farrell, Goodenough, & Cutter, 1981).

Participant observation has been used to assess a very wide range of target behaviors in psychiatric settings, such as verbal abuse (Peniston, 1988), screaming (Andrewes, 1989), psychotic or bizarre verbalizations (Alford, 1986; Alford, Fleece, & Rothblum, 1982; Foxx, McMorrow, Davis, & Bittle, 1988), assaultive behavior (Harris, 1989; Moyes *et al.*, 1985; Peniston, 1988), suicidal behavior (O'Farrell *et al.*, 1981), self-care and grooming (Harris, 1989), property destruction (Foxx, McMorrow, Bittle, & Bechtel, 1986), obsessive toileting behavior (Papworth, 1989), and the expressed emotion of the patient's family members (e.g., Magana, Goldstein, Karno, Miklowitz, Jenkins, & Falloon, 1986). In most cases, these target behaviors have been observed and codified by nursing staff.

Designing a participant observation system involves a series of steps similar to those used in the design of nonparticipant observation. That is, the behavior analyst must carefully define the target behavior, specify the setting for the observations, select a sampling procedure, train the observers, and detect errors, and make corrections. Because participant observers have other responsibilities, it is also usually necessary to minimize the complexity of the observation system. Complexity can be reduced in a number of ways. First, the target behavior can be defined more broadly so that the observer does not have to make subtle discriminations of patient behavior. Second, the number or size of observation settings can be reduced. Third, sampling strategies that require less vigilance can be selected (e.g., event sampling or interval sampling with rest periods between each interval).

Two main advantages are associated with participant observation. First, it has a clear potential for enhanced ecological validity because (1) it is often less reactive, and (2) observers can be deployed across a wide range of quasi-naturalistic and naturalistic settings (Foster *et al.*, 1988; Foster & Cone, 1986; Hartmann, 1984; Haynes, 1978, 1990; Hersen & Bellack, 1978). Second, the costs associated with procuring observers are significantly lessened as they are already present in the patient's daily environment and may have some stake in bringing about improved behavioral functioning.

Several limitations must also be considered in the design of participant observation. Like nonparticipant observation, it has largely been restricted to the codification of overt motor behavior. Because participant observers may be less well trained than nonparticipant observers, there may also be an increased probability of observer error, especially if the coding scheme is complicated. Alternatively, some participant observers may want to influence the disposition of the patient (e.g., promote a rapid discharge), a desire that may impair the objectivity of their observations. Compliance may be a problem if the observers are required to conduct frequent or lengthy observations of patient behavior. Finally, a number of individual difference variables (e.g., age and motor skills) may influence the quality of the observational data (Hartmann, 1984; Hersen & Bellack, 1978).

A number of steps can be taken to counter these limitations. First, as noted earlier, the observational system should not be overly complex or require excessive time commitments. Obtaining feedback from the participant observers and monitoring compliance are two of the best ways to determine whether the observational system is excessively demanding. One can also use preestablished observational systems that have been designed for participant observers (Groden, 1989; Touchette *et al.*, 1985). To improve the accuracy of their observation, the participant observers should be given detailed training in (1) the basic assumptions of behavioral assessment and (2) the use of the particular observation system. Such initial training should be supplemented by frequent accuracy checks and consistent reinforcement for compliance (Foster *et al.*, 1988).

In summary, participant observers have been used to assess many different overt motor target behaviors in psychiatric settings. The data acquired from participant observation may be less precise than those obtained from nonparticipant observation because a simpler coding system is typically required. The economy of participant observation and the potential for gathering data across a wide range of naturalistic settings are two of the most important attributes of this assessment method. Participant observation is, therefore, a very useful means of obtaining behavioral assessment data in psychiatric settings.

Self-Monitoring.   In self-monitoring, the patient is the primary coder of his or her own behavior. Self-monitoring has been used in psychiatric settings to assess obsessive ruminations (Bornstein, Hamilton, & Bornstein, 1986), compulsive checking behavior (Turner, Holzman, & Jacob, 1983), the frequency of delusional thoughts and the strength of belief associated with those thoughts (Alford, 1986; Alford et al., 1982), and the frequency and duration of auditory hallucinations (Allen, Halperin, & Friend, 1985; Gloister, 1985; Hersen & Bellack, 1978; Turner, Hersen, & Bellack, 1977).

The content of auditory hallucinations and the affective consequences of the hallucinations can also be assessed by self-monitoring. For example, a behavioral consultation request was received by the first author about a patient who had been repeatedly hospitalized for suicidal gestures that were reportedly prompted by hallucinated voices commanding the patient to harm herself. A self-monitoring procedure was instituted in which the patient recorded the occurrence of hallucinations, the content of the hallucinated messages, the amount of distress experienced as a result of the hallucinations (on a 0–10 interval scale), her location and activity during the hallucinations, and "coping responses" she emitted to alleviate her distress. Results of this assessment indicated that her hallucinations occurred most often in the afternoon and early evening while the patient was sitting alone in her room or in the unit hallway. In response to the hallucinations, the patient typically reported her distress to the nursing staff, who consistently provided a tranquilizer and consolation (social reinforcement?) for her distress. An intervention was designed that used self-statements designed to counter the content of the hallucinations. The dosage level of the tranquilizer was also rapidly tapered, and the nursing staff were instructed to reinforce the patient for *not* reporting hallucinations and the attendant distress. As the intervention progressed, a reduction in the frequency of hallucinations, the levels of distress, and the requests for tranquilizers was observed.

In self-monitoring, as in all observational methods, the target behavior must be carefully defined so that the patient can reliably note and record its occurrence. The patient must also be carefully trained and reinforced for self-monitoring his or her behavior. Self-monitoring can be conducted in all therapeutic, occupational, social, and domestic environments. The full range of sampling procedures can also be used with self-observation, although event and interval recording are most often used because they are convenient and are less difficult to use than duration, real-time, and momentary-time sampling.

Many important benefits are associated with self-monitoring. First, it can be designed to sample cognitions and affective-physiological responses that cannot be seen by outside observers. This feature of multimodal target coverage distinguishes self-monitoring from nonparticipant and participant observation, which are largely restricted to the codification of overt motor responses (Bornstein et al., 1986). Second, infrequently occurring, clandestine, and private behavior (e.g., illicit drug use, masturbation, and sexual intercourse) can be recorded by self-monitoring (Hartmann, 1984). Third, training subjects to carefully observe their own behavior in relation to various antecedent and consequent events promotes the acquisition of "behavioral insight" (i.e., an improved understanding of the situational and behavioral factors that control their behavior) and may thus facilitate treatment generalization. Finally, self-monitoring may have reactive effects that directly promotes adaptive behavior change (Gloister, 1985; Kazdin, 1974; Willis & Nelson, 1982).

The limitations of self-monitoring stem primarily from questions about the accuracy of psychiatric patients' self-observation and recording. For example, depressed patients may underestimate the frequency of positively valenced events or behaviors and overestimate negative events, whereas nondepressed patients may do the opposite (Beck *et al.*, 1979; Bornstein *et al.*, 1986; Carson, 1986). Similarly, patients in acute psychotic states may not be able to monitor themselves accurately. Several studies, however, have shown that even severely disordered patients can be taught self-monitoring procedures (Alford, 1986; Allen *et al.*, 1985; Bornstein *et al.*, 1986; Gloister, 1985). Additional research designed to examine the accuracy of self-monitoring among different psychiatric patients is clearly needed.

In summary, self-monitoring procedures can be used to assess a wide range of unobservable, covert, and overt behaviors among psychiatric patients. Improvements in behavior and enhanced behavioral insight are two adaptive side effects of self-monitoring. The accuracy of observation among psychiatric inpatients is an area requiring additional research.

Self-Report Inventories

Self-report inventories are frequently used by behavior therapists in psychiatric settings (see Table 1). Many different target behaviors have been assessed with questionnaires: anxiety (Speilberger, Gorsuch, & Lushene, 1970), anxiety associated with delusional thoughts (Lowe & Chadwick, 1990), bulimic behavior and eating attitudes (Garner & Olmstead, 1984; Williamson, Prather, Bennet, Davis, Watkins, & Grenier, 1989), depression (Miller, Norman, Keitner, Bishop, & Dow, 1989), general psychiatric symptoms (Derogatis, 1983), hopelessness and suicide risk (Beck, Steer, Kovacs, & Garrison, 1985), knowledge of behavioral principles among nursing staff (Kolko, McCanna, & Donaldson, 1989; McKeegan & Donat, 1988), obsessive-compulsive behavior (Van Den Hout, Emmelkamp, & Griez, 1988), perceived control over negative life events (Jackson & Tessler, 1984), problem-solving ability (Carey *et al.*, 1990), quality of life (Boudewyns & Hyer, 1990; Frisch, Villanueva, Cornell, & Retzlaff, 1990), social skills (Curran, Corriveau, Monti, & Hagerman, 1980), and stressful life events (Elliot *et al.*, 1990).

The widespread use of self-report inventories is due, in large part, to their convenience. Self-report inventories are inexpensive and easily administered. There are also droves of self-report inventories that purport to measure the severity of many behaviors and the components of those behaviors.

A second reason for the popularity of self-report inventories is their clinical utility. Self-report inventories can be used for a variety of purposes, including the screening of patients, diagnosis, estimation of the social significance of a behavior, and treatment evaluation (Jensen & Haynes, 1986). A growing number of self-report inventories have been designed that are consistent with an empirical-behavioral perspective (Hersen & Bellack, 1988, compiled descriptions of many behavioral self-report inventories in the *Dictionary of Behavioral Assessment Techniques*). In this subset of self-report inventories, questions about the situational, cognitive, behavioral, or affective-physiological determinants of behavior are typically included so that causal-functional relationships can be tentatively identified.

Self-report inventories have a number of significant limitations. One problem is related to standardization. Unlike the previously described behavioral assessment methods that quantify individual behaviors within specific contexts, self-report inventories evaluate patient behavior by using predefined items and response formats. As a result, some of the questionnaire items are irrelevant and/or invalid for particular patients.

A second problem with self-report inventories is that the wording of items and the derivation of the scores may violate basic behavioral principles. For example, many questionnaires do not address the situational specificity of behavior but instead ask the patient to provide an estimate of "typical behavior" across settings. Analogously, questionnaire scores are often summaries of heterogeneous setting–response interactions or complex behavioral sequences.

A third problem is that the validity of many self-report inventories is unknown or, at best, only partially determined because of insufficient psychometric evaluation of the instrument using inpatient psychiatric samples. Validity problems may also be associated with the self-reports of psychiatric patients, or with the construction of the instrument (Baker & Brandon, 1990; Rankin, 1990). For example, information provided by a patient may be inaccurate because of reactive effects, purposeful distortions, recall errors, reading problems, disordered thinking, and/or lack of knowledge about the target behavior and its determinants. Alternatively, the questions contained in the inventory may be inappropriately worded, excessively limited in scope, or designed with an improper or insensitive response format (e.g., true/false versus Likert scale).

In sum, questionnaire administration is a popular assessment method among behavior therapists in psychiatric settings. Much of this popularity is associated with the convenience and the broad clinical utility of self-report inventories. Additionally, an increasing number of behaviorally oriented questionnaires are becoming available. Violations of basic behavioral principles and potential validity problems often limit the utility of questionnaire data. Behavior therapists in psychiatric settings should therefore use self-report inventories in conjunction with other, idiographic, behavioral assessment methods, such as behavioral interviewing, participant observation, nonparticipant observation, and self-monitoring.

Structured Interviews and Rating Scales

Structured interviews can best be thought of as verbalized questionnaires that present specific questions about disordered behavior to the patient. Unlike questionnaires, however, structured interviews are more flexible, as they often permit the interviewer to omit irrelevant items or slightly modify the wording of questions to improve the accuracy of the interviewee's self-reports. Rating scales are observational instruments that sample a restricted range of behaviors that are often associated with particular psychiatric disorders. In a sense, rating scales are like "visualized questionnaires" because the topography of predefined behavior is rated by an observer using nominal, ordinal, or interval response formats (e.g., a Likert scale that ranges from "not present" to "extremely severe"). Quite often, structured interviews contain rating-scale items and rating scales contain structured-interview items.

Structured interviews and rating scales are generally used to (1) assign diagnostic labels to psychiatric patients or (2) assess the severity of specific behaviors (symptoms) associated with diagnostic categories (Hasin & Skodol, 1989; Manchanda, Hirsch, & Barnes, 1989; Morrison, 1988; Thompson, 1989). Some of the more intensively researched structured interviews and rating scales that are used to assign diagnostic labels include the Schedule for Affective Disorders and Schizophrenia (SADS; Endicott & Spitzer, 1978), the Diagnostic Interview Schedule (DIS; Robins, Helzer, Croughan, & Ratcliff, 1981), the Structured Clinical Interview for the DSM-III-R (SCID; Spitzer & Williams, 1985), and the Anxiety Disorders Interview Schedule—Revised (ADIS; DiNardo, O'Brien, Barlow, Waddel, & Blanchard, 1985). Structured interviews and rating scales that are frequently used to assess the severity of symptomatic behavior include the Present State Exam (PSE; Wing, Cooper, & Sartorius, 1974), the Brief Psychiatric Rating Scale (BPRS; Overall & Gorham, 1962), the Global Adjustment Scale (GAS; Endicott, Spitzer, Fleiss, & Cohen, 1976), the Schedule for Assessing Negative Symptoms (SANS; Andreason, 1981), the Schedule for Assessing Positive Symptoms (SAPS; Andreason, 1984), and the Hamilton Rating Scale for Depression (HRSD; Hamilton, 1960, 1982).

The merits of structured interviews and rating scales are similar to those of self-report inventories: They are inexpensive, readily available, and relatively easy to administer. Further, modest flexibility in administration procedures allows the assessor to obtain information that is more idiographic than questionnaire data.

The limitations of structured interviews and rating scales are also similar to those of self-report inventories. First, topographical analyses of behavior do not always provide information about important causal functional relationships. This limitation may be intensified when the structured interview or rating scale measures the topography of a very restricted number of behaviors that are derived from, or are closely associated with, particular diagnostic categories. Although the merits of psychiatric diagnosis continue to be debated in the behavioral assessment literature (see the miniseries on the revised third edition of the *Diagnostic and Statistical Manual* [DSM-III-R; American Psychiatric Association, 1987] in *Behavioral Assessment*, Volume 10, 1988), there is consensus that diagnosis alone is often insufficient for treatment formulation (Haynes & O'Brien, 1988; Persons, 1991). Thus, the information derived from structured interviews and rating scales that concentrate on behaviors related to the DSM-III-R is most useful for descriptive purposes (i.e., defining the topography or social significance of the target behavior). Second, structured interviews and rating scales often violate basic behavioral principles by adding distinct behaviors together to form a global measure of pathology. Third, the validity of many structured interviews and rating scales has not been adequately addressed. In most cases, the focus of psychometric investigations has been on determining the extent to which structured interviews or rating scales correlate with assessments made by experienced psychiatrists or others using structured interviews and rating scales. Neither of these two psychometric strategies, however, assesses the validity of psychiatric diagnosis.

In summary, structured interviews and rating scales share many of the properties of self-report inventories; however, flexibility in administration procedures allows the assessor to take a more idiographic approach. Most often, structured interviews and rating scales are designed to evaluate the topography of target behaviors. As a result, they are less useful for identifying and/or evaluating causal functional relationships.

Product-of-Behavior Measurements and Archival Data

Product-of-behavior measures are convenient, lasting indexes of targeted responses or setting-response interactions (Hartmann, 1984; Haynes, 1978; Haynes & Wilson, 1979). Some examples of product-of-behavior measures are the metabolites in the urine associated with drug use, bruises and cuts associated with self-abuse, weight fluctuations that indicate overeating and purging, the amount of food left on a tray as an index of calorie consumption, and the number of cigarettes found in ashtrays as an index of smoking behavior.

Product-of-behavior measures have the advantage of forming a lasting record of the behavior that significantly reduces the complexity of the observation system. The validity of the measure, however, may be a problem. For example, the amount of food left on a tray may reflect (1) the amount of food the targeted patient ate; (2) the amount of food the patient gave to another patient; or (3) a combination of (1) and (2).

A final, and highly important, source of assessment information in inpatient psychiatric settings is archival data, which may include medical records, therapy records (e.g., case notes and treatment summaries), psychological test reports, military service records, and employment records. The medical record is usually the most important archival data source, as a broad range of physiological, behavioral, and self-reported data is sampled and recorded on an ongoing (usually daily) basis. Further, medical records often contain descriptions of previous therapy, military service, employment, and prior psychological assessments.

There are a number of advantages in using medical record information to assist in behavioral assessments. First, the information is provided by professionals and paraprofessionals from diverse disciplines (e.g., psychiatry, psychology, nursing, occupational therapy, social work, nutrition, and physical therapy). Consequently, many different components of patient functioning are evaluated and recorded. Second, medical record information is routinely recorded, so that minimal cost is involved in the data collection. Third, because staff observations are recorded frequently, important information about the situational specificity of behavior can be obtained (e.g., comparing the patient's behavior during the day shift and the evening shift).

A major problem with medical record information is the variation in the behavioral specificity of the reports of the various writers, their knowledge of behavioral principles, and their ability to articulate this information. For example, behavioral observations are often accompanied by an interpretation of what caused the patient to act in a particular way. These causal inferences rarely speculate on the situational antecedents and consequences of the behavior. Instead, unobservable psychological states are often cited as the probable cause (e.g., "the patient wanted attention"). Nonetheless, the behavior analyst can use the information as a starting point in a behavioral assessment by conducting behavioral interviews with the various persons who have recorded their observations in the medical record.

Summary of Methods Used in Psychiatric Settings

Many different behavioral assessment methods are available for obtaining data on target behaviors and causal functional relationships. The relative strengths and limitations of each assessment method can be evaluated in terms of (1) the component of the target behavior under investigation (overt motor, cognitive, or affective- physiological); (2) the settings within which the assessment occurs; (3) the sampling strategy desired; and (4) patient and staff resources.

Behavioral interviewing, self-monitoring, self-report inventories, structured interviews, and rating scales can be used to assess the overt motor, cognitive, and affective-physiological components of target behaviors. As well, product-of-behavior and archival records can be used as indirect indices of these three components of target behavior. Nonparticipant observation and participant observation have a restricted range of target coverage, as they are largely limited to the codification of overt motor responses.

Self-monitoring and participant observation are the only two methods that can easily be conducted in the patient's everyday domestic, occupational, or social environment. Consequently, these methods have the potential for providing direct information about the topography and function of the target behavior in naturalistic settings. All of the remaining assessment methods are usually conducted within a therapeutic setting. Thus, the ecological validity of the measurements cannot be assumed.

Event, duration, and interval samples can be readily obtained through self-monitoring and participant observation. Such information can also be estimated via self-reports, product-of-behavior measurements, and archival records. Because of their complexity, real-time and momentary-time samples are usually obtained through nonparticipant observation.

Each assessment method has a different personnel requirement and cost. Nonparticipant observation is the most labor-intensive and costly because it requires the acquisition and training of either paid technicians or volunteers. In many cases, nonparticipant observation is feasible only in psychiatric settings that are affiliated with a major university, where there is a steady supply of student observers. Participant observation uses observers who are already present in the patient's environment. It is often the most economical way to obtain observational data in psychiatric settings. Self-monitoring is useful when the patient is able to conduct regular self-observation and self-recording of behavior. An added advantage of this method is that it often promotes adaptive behavior change; hence, it can be used as both an assessment method and an intervention. The remaining assessment methods (behavioral interviewing, self-report questionnaires, structured interviews, and rating scales) do not generally require a significant investment of personnel.

A major purpose of behavioral assessment is to map out the complex causal functional relationships between target behaviors and the various factors that control them (e.g., Evans, 1985; Haynes, 1978; Haynes & O'Brien, 1990; Nelson & Hayes, 1986; Russo, 1990; Voeltz & Evans, 1982). Such information can be used in the design of interventions that modify the variables that control the target behavior.

Inferring that a causal functional relationship exists between two variables requires (1) "cues to causality," such as elevated conditional probabilities or reliable correlation (Einhorn, 1988); (2) a temporal ordering of variables so that the presumed causal variable precedes the dependent variable (James, Mulaik, & Brett, 1982); and (3) the exclusion of plausible alternative explanations for the observed relationship (Cook & Campbell, 1979). Many behavioral assessment methods can be used to evaluate empirically whether causal functional relationships exist between various controlling events (i.e., the independent variable) and target behaviors (i.e., the dependent variable). Time series analysis and experimental manipulations (e.g., A-B-A-B designs) can be used to measure the strength and reliability of causal functional relationships (Barlow, Hayes, & Nelson, 1985; Barlow & Hersen, 1984), but they also require a significant time investment and can evaluate the interactions between only a few independent and dependent variables.

The simultaneous administration of different behavioral assessment instruments can also yield information about causal functional relationships, but the resultant inferences must be held tentatively. For example, a patient may report increased levels of depression and endorse many items on a questionnaire assessing recent stressful life events. However, a causal functional relationship between the stressful life events and the heightened depression cannot be confidently inferred because a third unmeasured variable (marital distress) could be causing both the depression and the stressful life events.

The use of empirically validated marker variables is a third way to identify causal functional relationships (Haynes & O'Brien, 1988, 1990). For example, laboratory observation of heightened physiological arousal in the presence of a family member identified as high in expressed emotion is often interpreted as a marker of a causal functional relationship between sympathetic activation and naturalistic stressors (Olbrich, 1989; Tarrier, 1989). This inference, however, can be made only if it has been empirically established that laboratory-based causal relationships generalize to the natural environment. To summarize, establishing the presence of causal functional relationships by using rigorous statistical and empirical approaches is a formidable task for behavior analysts in psychiatric settings.

Functional analytic causal modeling has been proposed as an assessment method that attempts to bridge the gap between empirical rigor and clinical pragmatism in relation to causal inference and the modeling of complex environment–behavior interactions. Functional analytic causal models are vector diagrams that depict the important causal relationships between the target behavior and the controlling situational, cognitive, behavioral, and affective-physiological events (Haynes & O'Brien, 1990). Causal functional relationships are tentatively inferred when changes in the target behavior are accompanied by changes in one or more of the controlling events. These inferred relationships can be directly observed, self-monitored, or verbally reported by the patient, his or her family and friends, or professional staff. The strength of causal inference can be strengthened by (1) an observation (or report) of consistent temporal ordering of variables so that the presumed causal variable precedes the presumed effect and (2) empirical findings (either published or idiographically obtained) that support a hypothesis of causation. Thus, extensive empirical validation of the hypothesized causal relationships is not required, although the behavior analyst must seek to find converging evidence from different sources.

WILLIAM H. O'BRIEN
and STEPHEN N.
HAYNES

Figure 1 contains a model of a 39-year-old female patient who was admitted to a psychiatric hospital because of depression and severe weight loss (the patient weighed 87.2 lb, which was 79% of her ideal weight) resulting from food refusal. The patient received an admitting DSM-III-R Axis I diagnosis of Major Depression combined with an Atypical Eating Disorder. After one week of general inpatient treatment, the patient's weight had dropped an additional 8 lb to 72% of her ideal weight. The patient was subsequently placed on nasogastric (NG) tube feeding to slow her weight loss.

A behavior therapy consultation regarding this patient was received after the first week of inpatient treatment. Behavioral interviews were initially conducted with the patient's primary nurse, staff workers, and the attending psychiatrist. These informants reported that the patient frequently requested special meals and then stated that she was "not hungry" or was feeling "too upset to eat" when her specially ordered meal arrived. Informal observation and a careful reading of the medical record supported the verbal reports of the interviewed staff. However, it was also observed that staff members consistently tried to cajole the patient into eating or listened sympathetically to her various complaints during meals. Thus, it was hypothesized that a bidirectional causal functional relationship existed between staff-delivered social reinforcement and two target behaviors: food refusal and verbal complaints (e.g., food refusal increased the probability of receiving social reinforcement, and social reinforcement increased the probability of more food refusal).

Behavioral assessment interviews were conducted with the patient on several occasions. Three classes of target behavior were identified during these interviews: food refusal, frequent verbal complaints of distress, and depressed affect. A number of potential causal functional relationships between the controlling events and the target behaviors were also identified. First, the patient reported that she was experiencing a lack of hunger sensations, a chronic feeling of having a "pit" in her stomach, and uncomfortable "bloating sensations" whenever she ate even minute amounts of food. The patient also reported that she had "always" been depressed and did not know what different emotions should "feel like." These variables were subsumed under a more global term (*dysfunctional interoception*) in the functional analytic causal model

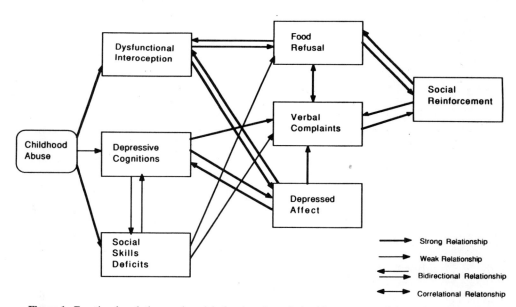

Figure 1. Functional analytic causal model of an inpatient admitted for treatment of depression and an atypical eating disorder.

(i.e., it was hypothesized that the patient was mislabeling interoceptive cues and/or failing to produce the appropriate interoceptive cues that are normally associated with variation in hunger states and affective states). In turn, the patient's dysfunctional interoception was presumed to be bidirectionally related to food refusal and depressed affect. Second, the patient reported that she continuously experienced depressive, helpless, and hopeless thoughts. These cognitive variables were presumed to be functionally related to verbal reports of distress and depressed affect. Third, the patient exhibited a very limited ability to assert herself and frequently mislabeled the intentions of persons with whom she interacted. These limitations in social skills were tentatively linked with food refusal, verbal complaints (i.e., the patient appeared to be using food refusal and/or complaints of distress rather than appropriate verbal assertion skills to influence the behavior of nursing staff and family members), and depressive (e.g., helpless) thoughts. Fourth, the patient reported that she had suffered an extensive amount of physical and psychological abuse as a child. The effect of this remote causal event on her current behavior was believed to be mediated by current interoception deficits, depressive thinking, and social skills deficits.

To obtain convergent evidence for the hypothesized functional relationships described above, a behavioral assessment battery was designed and implemented. The patient was instructed to self-monitor her eating behavior (what she ate and how much), her depressed affect, her feelings of hunger, and her cognitions by using an interval sampling methodology. A participant observation method was initially devised in which the nursing staff estimated the number of calories the patient had consumed during each meal. It was noted that the nursing staff members were only marginally compliant with this observational methodology because it was too difficult for them to estimate the patient's calorie consumption. Consequently, a simplified observation method was designed in which the staff merely recorded whether the patient had eaten one quarter, one half, three quarters, or all of her meal. To get an accurate calorie estimate, the nutritionist was instructed to send an equal amount of calories per meal (regardless of what the patient ordered). Several self-report inventories were also used to evaluate the severity of the patient's depression, negative cognitions, and social skills deficits.

The model presented in Figure 1 suggests that this patient's problem had multiple interacting components that were controlled by several variables acting alone and in combination. As presented in Figure 1, it was hypothesized that poor interoception and social reinforcement were the controlling variables that exerted the most impact on her food refusal. Hence, the functional relationships between these variables were targeted for change. To remove inappropriate social reinforcement, the patient was placed on a contract in which she agreed to consume a fixed number of calories at every meal. She was allowed 45 minutes to complete the meal, and the staff were instructed *not* to interact with her during this time. At the end of the 45-minute period, the staff recorded the amount of food consumed and removed her tray. If the patient had consumed all of the food, the staff were instructed to provide the patient with social reinforcement. If the patient failed to consume all of her food, she was matter-of-factly given a high-calorie liquid supplement that could be ingested by NG tube or by mouth. Further, if the patient ingested all of her prescribed calories by mouth for nine consecutive meals, the NG tube would be removed. To promote improved interoception, the patient was instructed to record differences in stomach sensations before and after each meal. She was also provided with an extensive list of words that she could use to describe different physiological and affective states. After 6 days of this intervention, the patient had gained 10 pounds and the NG tube was removed. Her self-monitoring records also began to show variation in hunger and depression levels. The remaining problem behaviors were subsequently targeted for change using the functional analytic causal model as a heuristic for intervention design.

There are several advantages in using functional analytic causal modeling. First, it systematizes the clinical decision-making process and thus forces the clinician to attend to the complexity of the case, to the functional properties of the target behaviors, and to whether the controlling factors have been adequately identified. Second, it encourages greater integration of assessment data with treatment design. Third, functional causal models can facilitate the identification of additional causal relationships which may be affecting the target behaviors. Fourth, functional causal models can provide a parsimonious behavior explanation of patient behavior that can be recorded in the medical record and presented to other professionals in psychiatric settings without lengthy verbal explanations.

SUMMARY

We have suggested that behavioral assessment is the most appropriate methodology for case conceptualization, treatment formulation, and treatment evaluation in contemporary psychiatric settings. Nonetheless, behavioral methodologies have been underused in psychiatric settings. This underuse may be associated with beliefs among behavior therapists that behavioral principles are not applicable to psychiatric disorders because they may have significant biological underpinnings.

The results of many empirical investigations that have examined relationships between severe psychopathology and situational or behavioral change have indicated that many components of these disorders can be modified by the use of behavioral technologies. Additionally, behavioral models of psychopathology and severe behavior disorders are becoming increasingly complex as empirical findings continue to refine our understanding of the interrelationships between settings events and target behaviors.

Because behavioral construct systems have significantly expanded since the early 1970s, behavior analysts in psychiatric settings must consider many different factors in the design of an assessment methodology. In order to adequately operationalize the target behavior, its topography, social significance, and functional properties must be evaluated. The behavior analyst also must decide where the target behavior will be assessed and how it will be sampled.

A number of behavioral assessment procedures have been used in psychiatric settings. Behavioral assessment interviewing is probably the most frequently used assessment method. Unfortunately, little is known about the reliability and validity of this method. Behavioral observation, self-report questionnaire administration, structured interviewing, rating-scale administration, and product-of-behavior measurement are other frequently used behavioral assessment methods. Each has strengths and weaknesses in its ability to measure overt motor, cognitive, and affective-physiological responses. The selection of a particular assessment method rests on a consideration of its ability to quantify particular components of the target response, the setting in which the assessment will occur, the sampling method to be used, and the resources available to the behavior analyst.

The output from behavioral assessment methods is often complex. Functional analytic causal modeling is offered as one strategy that can simplify the task of organizing behavioral assessment data so that causal functional relationships can be identified and evaluated.

Future research needs to be directed at strengthening our understanding of how behavior analysts derive causal inferences from assessment data and make decisions regarding treatment selection and evaluation. Empirical investigations of behavioral interviewing and functional analytic causal modeling would help in this endeavor. In addition, the extent to which functional analytic causal modeling facilitates the design of treatments that produce greater or more durable behavioral changes needs to be empirically evaluated.

REFERENCES

Alevizos, P. N., DeRisi, W., Liberman, R., Eckman, T., & Callahan, E. (1978). The behavior observation instrument: A method of direct observation for program evaluation. *Journal of Applied Behavior Analysis, 11,* 243–257.

Alford, B. A. (1986). Behavioral treatment of schizophrenic delusions: A single case experimental analysis. *Behavior Therapy, 17*, 637–644.

Alford, G. S., Fleece, L., & Rothblum, E. (1982). Hallucinatory-delusional verbalizations: Modification in a chronic schizophrenic by self-control and cognitive restructuring. *Behavior Modification, 6*, 421–435.

Allen, H., Halperin, J., & Friend, R. (1985). Removal and diversion tactics and the control of auditory hallucinations. *Behavior Research and Therapy, 23*, 601–605.

American Psychiatric Association. (1987). *Diagnostic and statistical manual of mental disorders* (3rd ed., rev.; DSM-III-R). Washington, DC: Author.

Andreason, N. C. (1981). *Scale for the assessment of negative symptoms (SANS)*. Iowa City: Department of Psychiatry, University of Iowa College of Medicine.

Andreason, N. C. (1984). *Scale for the assessment of positive symptoms (SAPS)*. Iowa City: Department of Psychiatry, University of Iowa College of Medicine.

Andrewes, D. (1989). Management of disruptive behavior in the brain-damaged patient using selective reinforcement. *Journal of Behavior Therapy and Experimental Psychiatry, 20*, 261–264.

Baker, T. B., & Brandon, T. H. (1990). Validity of self-reports in basic research. *Behavioral Assessment, 12*, 33–51.

Bandura, A. (1981). In search of pure unidirectional determinants. *Behavior Therapy, 12*, 30–40.

Barlow, D. H., & Hersen, M. (1984). *Single case experimental designs Strategies for studying behavior change* (2nd ed.). New York: Pergamon Press.

Barlow, D. H., Hayes, S. C., & Nelson, R. O. (1984). *The scientist practitioner: Research and accountability in clinical and educational settings*. New York: Pergamon Press.

Barrios, B. A. (1988). On the changing nature of behavioral assessment. In A. S. Bellack & M. Hersen (Eds.), *Behavioral assessment: A practical handbook* (3rd ed., pp. 3–41). Elmsford, NY: Pergamon Press.

Bass, R. F. (1987). Computer-assisted observer training. *Journal of Applied Behavior Analysis, 20*, 83–88.

Beck, A. T., Ward, C. H., Mendelsohn, M., Mock, J., & Erbaugh, J. (1961). An inventory for measuring depression. *Archives of General Psychiatry, 4*, 561–571.

Beck, A. T., Rush, A. J., Shaw, B. F., & Emery, G. (1979). *Cognitive therapy of depression*. New York: Guilford Press.

Beck. A. T., Steer, R. A., Kovacs, M., & Garrison, B. (1985). Hopelessness and eventual suicide: A 10 year prospective study of patients hospitalized with suicidal ideation. *American Journal of Psychiatry,145*, 559–563.

Belcher, T. (1988). Behavioral reduction of overt hallucinatory behavior in a chronic schizophrenic. *Journal of Behavior Therapy and Experimental Psychiatry, 19*, 69–71.

Bellack, A. S. (1986). Schizophrenia: Behavior therapy's forgotten child. *Behavior Therapy, 17*, 199–214.

Bellack, A. S., & Hersen, M. (1978). Assessment and single-case research. In M. Hersen & A. S. Bellack (Eds.), *Behavior therapy in the psychiatric setting* (pp. 3–39). Baltimore: Williams & Wilkins.

Bellack, A. S., & Hersen, M. (Eds.). (1988). *Behavioral assessment: A practical handbook* (3rd ed.). Elmsford, NY: Pergamon Press.

Bellack, A. S., & Mueser, K. T. (1990). Schizophrenia. In A. S. Bellack, M. Hersen, A. E. Kazdin (Eds.), *International handbook of behavior modification and therapy* (2nd ed., pp. 353–366). New York: Plenum Press.

Blake, D. D., Owens, M. D., & Keane, T. M. (1990). Increasing group attendance on a psychiatric unit: An alternating treatments design. *Journal of Behavior Therapy and Experimental Psychiatry, 21*, 15–20.

Bornstein, P. H., Hamilton, S. B., & Bornstein, M. T. (1986). Self-monitoring procedures. In A. R. Ciminero, C. S. Calhoun, & H. E. Adams (Eds.), *Handbook of behavioral assessment* (2nd ed., pp. 176–222). New York: Wiley.

Boudewyns, P. A., & Hyer, L. (1990). Physiological response to combat memories and preliminary treatment outcome in vietnam veteran PTSD patients treated with direct therapeutic exposure. *Behavior Therapy, 21*, 63–87.

Boudewyns, P. A., Fry, T. J., & Nightengale, E. (1986). Token economy programs in VA medical centers: Where are they today? *The Behavior Therapist, 6*, 126–127.

Bowen, L., Glynn, S. M., Marshall, B. D., Kurth, C. L., & Hayden, J. L. (1990). Successful behavioral treatment of polydipsia in a schizophrenic patient. *Journal of Behavior Therapy and Experimental Psychiatry, 21*, 53–61.

Carey, M. P., Carey, K. B., & Meisler, A. W. (1990). Training mentally ill chemical abusers in social problem solving. *Behavior Therapy, 21*, 511–518.

Carlton, P. L. (1983). *A primer of behavioral pharmacology: Concepts and principles in the behavioral analysis of drug action*. New York: W. H. Freeman.

Carson, T. P. (1986). Assessment of depression. In A. R. Ciminero, C. S. Calhoun, & H. E. Adams (Eds.), *Handbook of behavioral assessment* (2nd ed., pp. 404–445). New York: Wiley.

Ciminero, A. R., Calhoun, K. S., & Adams, H. E. (1986). *Handbook of behavioral assessment* (2nd ed.). New York: Wiley.

Commission on Professional and Hospital Activities. (1988). *Psychiatric length of stay by diagnosis, United States, 1987.* Ann Arbor, MI: CPHA Publications.

Cone, J. D. (1988). Psychometric considerations and multiple models of behavioral assessment. In A. S. Bellack & M. Hersen (Eds.), *Behavioral assessment: A practical handbook* (3rd ed., pp. 42–66). Elmsford, NY: Pergamon Press.

Cook, T. D., & Campbell, D. T. (1979). *Quasi-experimentation: Design and analysis issues for field settings.* Boston: Houghton Mifflin.

Curran, J. P., Corriveau, D. P., Monti, P. M., & Hagerman, S. B. (1980). Social skill and social anxiety. *Behavior Modification, 4,* 493–512.

Curran, J. P., Faraone, S. V., & Dow, M. G. (1985). Schizophrenia and other psychotic disorders. In M. Hersen (Ed.), *Practice of inpatient behavior therapy: A clinical guide.* Orlando, FL: Grune & Stratton.

Delprato, D. J., & McGlynn, F. D. (1988). Interactions of response patterns and their implications for behavior therapy. *Journal of Behavior Therapy and Experimental Psychiatry, 19,* 199–205.

Derogatis, L. R. (1983). *Description and bibliography for the SCL-90-R and other instruments of the psychopathology rating scale series.* Baltimore: Johns Hopkins University School of Medicine.

Dickerson, F. (1989). Behavior therapy in private hospitals: A national survey. *The Behavior Therapist, 12,* 7.

DiNardo, P. A., O'Brien, G. T., Barlow, D. H., Waddel, M. T., & Blanchard, E. B. (1985). *The anxiety disorders interview schedule.* Albany, NY: Center for Stress and Anxiety Disorders.

Douglas, M. S., & Mueser, K. T. (1990). Teaching conflict resolution skills to the chronically mentally ill: Brief social training groups for briefly hospitalized patients. *Behavior Modification, 14,* 519–547.

Earls, C. M., & Castonguay, L. G. (1989). The evaluation of olfactory aversion for a bisexual pedophile with a single-case multiple baseline design. *Behavior Therapy, 20,* 137–146.

Einhorn, H. J. (1988). Diagnosis and causality in clinical and statistical prediction. In D. C. Turk & P. Salovey (Eds.), *Reasoning, inference, and judgment in clinical psychology* (pp. 51–70). New York: Free Press.

Elliot, A., Hammer, C., Gitlin, M., Brown, G., & Jamison, K. (1990). Life events and the course of bipolar disorder. *American Journal of Psychiatry, 147*(9), 1194–1198.

Endicott, J., & Spitzer, R. L. (1978). A diagnostic interview: The schedule for affective disorders and schizophrenia. *Archives of General Psychiatry, 35,* 837–844.

Endicott, J., Spitzer, R. L., Fleiss, J. L., & Cohen, J. (1976). The global adjustment scale: A procedure for measuring the overall severity of psychiatric disturbance. *Archives of General Psychiatry, 33,* 766–771.

Evans, I. M. (1985). Building systems models as a strategy for target behavior selection in clinical assessment. *Behavioral Assessment, 7,* 21–32.

Eysenck, H. J. (1988). Psychotherapy to behavior therapy: A paradigm shift. In D. B. Fishman, F. Rotgers, C. M. Franks (Eds.), *Paradigms in behavior therapy: Present and promise.* New York: Springer.

Falloon, I. R. H., Boyd, J. L., McGill, C. W., Williamson, M., Razani, J., Moss, H. B., Gilderman, A. M., & Simpson, G. M. (1985). Family management in the prevention of morbidity of schizophrenia: 1. Clinical outcome of a longitudinal study. *Archives of General Psychiatry, 42,* 887–896.

Falloon, I. R. H., McGill, C. W., Boyd, J. L., & Pederson, J. (1987). Family management in the prevention of morbidity of schizophrenia: Social outcome of a two-year longitudinal study. *Psychological Medicine, 17,* 59–66.

Felton, J. L., & Nelson, R. O. (1984). Inter-assessor agreement on hypothesized controlling variables and treatment proposals. *Behavioral Assessment, 6,* 199–208.

Fisher, W., Piazza, C. C., & Page, T. J. (1989). Assessing independent and interactive effects of behavioral and pharmacological interventions for a client with dual diagnoses. *Journal of Behavior Therapy and Experimental Psychiatry, 20,* 241–250.

Foster, S. L., & Cone, J. D. (1986). Design and use of direct observation systems. In A. R. Ciminero, C. S. Calhoun, & H. E. Adams (Eds.), *Handbook of behavioral assessment* (2nd ed., pp. 253–324). New York: Wiley.

Foster, S. L., Bell-Dolan, D. J., & Burge, D. A. (1988). Behavioral observation. In A. S. Bellack & M. Hersen (Eds.), *Behavioral assessment: A practical handbook* (3rd ed., pp. 119–160). Elmsford, NY: Pergamon Press.

Foxx, R. M., McMorrow, M. J., Bittle, R. G., & Bechtel, D. R. (1986). The successful treatment of a dually diagnosed deal man's aggression with a program that included contingent electrical shock. *Behavior Therapy, 17,* 170–186.

Foxx, R. M., McMorrow, M. J., Davis, L. A., & Bittle, R. G. (1988). Replacing a chronic schizophrenic man's delusional speech with stimulus appropriate responses. *Journal of Behavior Therapy and Experimental Psychiatry*, *19*, 43–50.

Freeman, H. (1989). Relationship of schizophrenia to the environment. *British Journal of Psychiatry*, *155* (Suppl. 5), 90–99.

Frisch, M. B., Villaneuva, M., Cornell, J., & Retzlaff, P. J. (1990, November). *Clinical validation of the quality of life inventory: A measure of life satisfaction for use in treatment planning and outcome assessment.* Paper presented at the 24th Annual Convention of the Association for Advancement of Behavior Therapy, San Francisco.

Garner, D. M., & Olmstead, M. P. (1984). *Eating disorder inventory manual.* Odessa, FL: Psychological Assessment Resources.

Gloister, B. (1985). A case of auditory hallucination treatment by satiation. *Behavior Research and Therapy*, *23*, 213–215.

Glynn, S. M., Bowen, L., Rose, G., Marshall, B. D., & Liberman, R. P. (1990, November). *Behavioral correlates of negative symptoms in schizophrenia.* Paper presented at the 24th Annual Convention of the Association for Advancement of Behavior Therapy, San Francisco.

Goldfried, M. R., & Kent, R. N. (1972). Traditional versus behavioral assessment: A comparison of methodological and theoretical assumptions. *Psychological Bulletin*, *77*, 409–420.

Goldman, H. H. (1988). *Review of general psychiatry* (2nd ed.). Norwalk, CN: Appleton-Lange.

Goldstein, M. J., Miklowitz, D. J., Strachan, A. M., Doan, J. A., Nuechterlein, K. H., & Feingold, D. (1989). Patterns of expressed emotion and patient coping styles that characterize the families of recent onset schizophrenics. *British Journal of Psychiatry*, *155*, (Suppl. 5), 107–111.

Gottman, J. M. (1980). Consistency of nonverbal affect and affect reciprocity in marital interaction. *Journal of Consulting and Clinical Psychology*, *48*, 711–717.

Gottman, J. M., & Levenson, R. W. (1986). Assessing the role of emotion in marriage. *Behavioral Assessment*, *8*, 31–48.

Groden, G. (1989). A guide for conducting a comprehensive behavioral analysis of a target behavior. *Journal of Behavior Therapy and Experimental Psychiatry*, *20*, 163–169.

Guevremont, D. C., & Spiegler, M. D. (1990, November). *What do behavior therapists really do? A survey of the clinical practice of AABT members.* Paper presented at the 24th Annual Convention of the Association for Advancement of Behavior Therapy, San Francisco.

Hahlweg, K., Hemmati-Weber, M., Heusser, A., Lober, H., Winkler, H., Muller, U., Feinstein, E., & Dose, M. (1990). Process analysis in behavioral family therapy. *Behavior Modification*, *14*, 441–456.

Halford, W. K., Hayes, R. L., & Varghese, F. N. (1990, November). *Do social skills matter? The relationship between social skill, social functioning, and quality of life in schizophrenic patients.* Paper presented at the 24th Annual Convention of the Association for Advancement of Behavior Therapy, San Francisco.

Hamilton, M. (1960). A rating scale for depression. *Journal of Neurology, Neurosurgery, and Psychiatry*, *23*, 56–62.

Hamilton, M. (1982). Symptoms and assessment of depression. In E. S. Paykel (Ed.), *Handbook of affective disorders*. New York: Guilford Press.

Hansen, D. J., St. Lawrence, J. S., & Christoff, K. A. (1989). Group conversational skills training with inpatient children and adolescents. *Behavior Modification*, *13*, 4–31.

Harris, G. T. (1989). The relationship between neuroleptic drug dose and the performance of psychiatric patients in a maximum security token economy system. *Journal of Behavior Therapy and Experimental Psychiatry*, *20*, 56–67.

Hartmann, D. P. (1984). Assessment strategies. In D. H. Barlow & M. Hersen (Eds.), *Single case experimental designs: Strategies for studying behavior change* (pp. 107–139). New York: Pergamon Press.

Hartmann, D. P., & Wood, D. D. (1990). Observational methods. In A. S. Bellack, M. Hersen, & A. E. Kazdin (Eds.), *International handbook of behavior modification and therapy* (2nd ed., pp. 107–138). New York: Plenum Press.

Hartmann, D. P., Roper, B. L., & Bradford, D. C. (1979). Some relationships between behavioral and traditional assessment. *Behavioral Assessment*, *1*, 3–21.

Hasin, D. S., & Skodol, A. E. (1989). Standardized diagnostic interviews for psychiatric research. In C. Thompson (Ed.), *The instruments of psychiatric research* (pp. 19–58). New York: Wiley.

Hawkins, R. P. (1986). Selection of target behaviors. In R. O. Nelson, & S. C. Hayes (Eds.), *Conceptual foundations of behavioral assessment* (pp. 331–383). New York: Guilford Press.

Hay, L. R. (1982). Teaching behavioral assessment to clinical psychology students. *Behavioral Assessment*, *4*, 35–40.

Hay, W. M., Hay, L. R., Angle, H. V., & Nelson, R. O. (1979). The reliability of problem identification in the behavioral interview. *Behavioral Assessment*, *1*, 107–118.

Haynes, S. N. (1978). *Principles of behavioral assessment.* New York: Gardner Press.

Haynes, S. N. (1979). Behavioral variance, individual differences and trait theory in a behavioral construct system: A reappraisal. *Behavioral Assessment, 1*, 41–49.

Haynes, S. N. (1986). A behavioral model of paranoid behaviors. *Behavior Therapy, 17*, 266–287.

Haynes, S. N. (1988). Causal models and the assessment-treatment relationship in behavior therapy. *Journal of Psychopathology and Behavioral Assessment, 10*, 171–183.

Haynes, S. N. (1990). Behavioral assessment of adults. In G. Goldstein & M. Hersen (Eds.), *Handbook of Psychological Assessment* (2nd ed., pp. 423–463). New York: Pergamon Press.

Haynes, S. N. (1991). *Models of causality in psychopathology: Toward dynamic, synthetic, and nonlinear models of behavior disorders*. New York: Pergamon Press.

Haynes, S. N., & Gannon, L. R. (1981). *Psychosomatic disorders: A psychophysiological approach to etiology and treatment*. New York: Praeger.

Haynes, S. N., & O'Brien, W. H. (1988). The Gordian Knot of DSM-III-R use: Integrating principles of behavior classification and complex causal models. *Behavioral Assessment, 10*, 95–105.

Haynes, S. N., & O'Brien, W. H. (1990). Functional analysis in behavior therapy. *Clinical Psychology Review, 10*, 649–668.

Haynes, S. N., & Wilson, C. C. (1979). *Behavioral assessment*. San Francisco: Jossey-Bass.

Hersen, M. (1985). *Practice of inpatient behavior therapy: A clinical guide*. New York: Grune & Stratton.

Hersen, M., & Bellack, A. S. (1978). Chronic psychiatric patients: Individual behavioral approaches. In M. Hersen & A. S. Bellack (Eds.), *Behavior therapy in the psychiatric setting* (pp. 128–168). Baltimore: Williams & Wilkins.

Hersen, M., & Bellack, A. S. (Eds.). (1988). *Dictionary of behavioral assessment techniques*. New York: Pergamon Press.

Hollandsworth, J. G. (1986). *Physiology and behavior therapy: Conceptual guidelines for the clinician*. New York: Plenum Press.

Jackson, M., & Tessler, R. (1984). Perceived lack of control over life events: Antecedents and consequences in a discharged patient sample. *Social Science Research, 13*, 287–301.

Jacobson, N. S. (1985a). The role of observational measures in behavior therapy outcome research. *Behavioral Assessment, 7*, 297–308.

Jacobson, N. S. (1985b). Uses versus abuses of observational measures. *Behavioral Assessment, 7*, 323–330.

James, L. R., Mulaik, S. A., & Brett, J. M. (1982). *Causal analysis: Assumptions, models, and data*. Beverly Hills, CA: Sage.

Jensen, B. J., & Haynes, S. N. (1986). Self-report questionnaires. In A. R. Ciminero, C. S. Calhoun, & H. E. Adams (Eds.), *Handbook of behavioral assessment* (2nd ed., pp. 150–175). New York: Wiley.

Julien, D., Markman, H. J., & Lindahl, K. M. (1989). A comparison of a global and microanalytic coding system: Implications for future trends in studying interactions. *Behavioral Assessment, 11*, 81–100.

Kanfer, F. H. (1985). Target selection for clinical change programs. *Behavioral Assessment, 7*, 7–20.

Kazdin, A. E. (1974). Self-monitoring and behavior change. In M. J. Mahoney & C. E. Thorensen (Eds.), *Self-control: Power to the person* (pp. 218–246). Monterey, CA: Brooks-Cole.

Kazdin, A. E. (1984). *Behavior modification in applied settings* (3rd ed.). Homewood, IL: Dorsey Press.

Kazdin, A. E. (1985). Selection of target behaviors: The relationship of the treatment focus to clinical dysfunction. *Behavioral Assessment, 7*, 33–47.

Keefe, F. J., & Blumenthal, J. A. (1982). *Assessment strategies in behavioral medicine*. New York: Grune & Stratton.

Kolko, D. J., McCanna, M. W., & Donaldson, L. (1989). Sequential assessment of staff administration of contingency management procedures on a child psychiatry unit. *Behavior Modification, 13*, 216–244.

Krasner, L. (1988). Paradigm lost: On a historical/sociological/economic perspective. In D. B. Fishman, F. Rotgers, C. M. Franks (Eds.), *Paradigms in behavior therapy: Present and promise*. New York: Springer.

Kryter, K. D. (1990). Aircraft noise and social factors in psychiatric hospital admission rates: A re-examination of some data. *Psychological Medicine, 20*, 395–411.

Lane, I. M., Weslowski, M. D., & Burke, W. H. (1989). Teaching socially appropriate behavior to eliminate hoarding in a brain injured adult. *Journal of Behavior Therapy and Experimental Psychiatry, 20*, 79–82.

Lee, C. (1987). Affective behavior modification: A case for empirical investigation. *Journal of Behavior Therapy and Experimental Psychiatry, 18*, 203–213.

Lowe, C. F., & Chadwick, P. D. J. (1990). Verbal control of delusions. *Behavior Therapy, 21*, 461–480.

Matson, J. L., & Stephens, R. M. (1977). Overcorrection of aggressive behavior in a chronic psychiatric patient. *Behavior Modification, 1*, 559–564.

Magana, A. B., Goldstein, M. J., Karno, M., Miklowitz, D. J., Jenkins, J., & Falloon, I. R. H. (1986). A brief method for assessing expressed emotion in relatives of psychiatric patients. *Psychiatry Research, 17*, 203–212.

Manchanda, R., Hirsh, S. R., & Barnes, T. R. E. (1989). A review of rating scales for measuring symptom changes in schizophrenia research. In C. Thompson (Ed.), *The instruments of psychiatric research* (pp. 59–85). New York: Wiley.

Mandal, M. K., Srivastava, P., & Singh, S. K. (1990). Paralinguistic characteristics of speech in schizophrenics and depressives. *Journal of Psychiatric Research, 24,* 191–196.

Mash, E. J., & Hunsley, J. (1990). Behavioral assessment: A contemporary approach. In A. S. Bellack, M. Hersen, & A. E. Kazdin (Eds.), *International handbook of behavior modification and therapy* (2nd ed., pp. 87–106). New York: Plenum Press.

McAndrew, J. F. (1989). Obsessive-compulsive disorder: A behavioral case formulation. *Journal of Behavior Therapy and Experimental Psychiatry, 20,* 311–318.

McKeegan, G. F., & Donat, D. C. (1988). An inventory to measure knowledge of behavioral methods with inpatient adults. *Journal of Behavior Therapy and Experimental Psychiatry, 19,* 229–236.

Miller, I. W., Norman, W. H., Keitner, G. I., Bishop, S. B. & Dow, M. G. (1989). Cognitive-behavioral treatment of depressed inpatients. *Behavior Therapy, 20,* 25–47.

Miltenberger, R. G., & Fuqua, R. W. (1985). Evaluation of a training method for the acquisition of behavioral assessment interviewing skills. *Journal of Applied Behavior Analysis, 18,* 323–328.

Morganstern, K. P. (1988). Behavioral interviewing. In A. S. Bellack & M. Hersen (Eds.), *Behavioral assessment: A practical handbook* (3rd ed., pp. 86–118). Elmsford, NY: Pergamon Press.

Morrisey, J. P. (1988). Social psychiatry. In H. H. Goldman (Ed.), *Review of general psychiatry* (2nd ed., pp. 157–166). Norwalk, CT: Appleton & Lange.

Morrison, R. L. (1988). Structured interviews and rating scales. In A. S. Bellack & M. Hersen (Eds.), *Behavioral assessment: A practical handbook* (3rd ed., pp. 252–277). Elmsford, NY: Pergamon Press.

Morrison, R. L. (1990). Interpersonal dysfunction. In A. S. Bellack, M. Hersen, & A. E. Kazdin (Eds.), *International handbook of behavior modification and therapy* (2nd ed., pp. 503–522). New York: Plenum Press.

Moyes, T., Tennent, T. G., & Bedford, A. P. (1985). Long-term follow-up study of a ward-based behaviour modification programme for adolescents with acting-out and conduct problems. *British Journal of Psychiatry, 147,* 300–305.

Mudford, O. C., Beale, I. L., & Singh, N. N. (1990). The representativeness of observational samples of different durations. *Journal of Applied Behavior Analysis, 23,* 323–331.

Mueser, K. T., Bellack, A. S., Morrison, R. L., & Wixted, J. T. (1990). Social competence in schizophrenia: Premorbid adjustment, social skill, and domains of functioning. *Journal of Psychiatric Research, 24,* 51–63.

Munford, P. R., Tarlow, G., & Gerner, R. (1984). An experimental analysis of the interaction of chemotherapy and behavior therapy in anorexia nervosa. *Journal of Nervous and Mental Disease, 172,* 228–231.

Neale, J. M., Oltmans, T. F., & Winters, K. C. (1983). Recent developments in the assessment and conceptualization of schizophrenia. *Behavioral Assessment, 5,* 33–54.

Nelson, R. O., & Hayes, S. C. (1986). The nature of behavioral assessment. In R. O. Nelson & S. C. Hayes (Eds.), *Conceptual foundations of behavioral assessment* (pp. 3–41). New York: Guilford Press.

Nuechterlein, K. H., Goldstein, M. J., Ventura, J., Dawson, M. E., & Doane, J. A. (1989). Patient-environment relationships in schizophrenia: Information processing, communication deviance, autonomic arousal, and stressful life events. *British Journal of Psychiatry, 155* (Suppl. 5), 84–89.

O'Farrell, T. J., Goodenough, D. S., & Cutter, H. S. (1981). Behavioral contracting for repeated suicide attempts: Issues in the treatment of a hospitalized schizophrenic male. *Behavior Modification, 5,* 255–272.

Olbrich, R. (1989). Electrodermal activity and its relevance to vulnerability research in schizophrenics. *British Journal of Psychiatry, 155* (Suppl. 5), 40–45.

Overall, J. E., & Gorham, D. R. (1962). The brief psychiatric rating scale. *Psychological reports, 10,* 799–812.

Papworth, M. A. (1989). The behavioral treatment of nocturnal enuresis in a severely brain-damaged patient. *Journal of Behavior Therapy and Experimental Psychiatry, 20,* 265–268.

Parks, C. W., & Hollon, S. D. (1988). Cognitive assessment. In A. S. Bellack & M. Hersen (Eds.), *Behavioral assessment: A practical handbook* (3rd ed., pp. 161–212). Elmsford, NY: Pergamon Press.

Paul, G. L. (1986a). *Assessment in residential settings: Principles and methods to support cost-effective quality operations.* Champaign, IL: Research Press.

Paul, G. L. (1986b). *The staff-resident interaction chronograph: Observational assessment instrumentation for service and research.* Champaign, IL: Research Press.

Paul, G. L. (1986c). *The time sample behavioral checklist: Observational assessment instrumentation for service and research.* Champaign, IL: Research Press.

Paul, G. L., & Lenz, R. J. (1977). *Psychosocial treatment of chronic mental patients: Milieu versus social learning programs.* Cambridge: Harvard University Press.

Peniston, E. G. (1988). Evaluation of long-term therapeutic efficacy of a behavior modification program with chronic male psychiatric patients. *Journal of Behavior Therapy and Experimental Psychiatry, 19*, 95–110.

Persons, J. B. (1991). Psychotherapy outcome studies do not accurately represent current models of psychotherapy: A proposed remedy. *American Psychologist, 46*, 99–106.

Poling, A., & Cleary, J. (1986). The role of applied behavior analysis in evaluating medication effects. In A. Poling & R. W. Fuqua (Eds.), *Research methods in applied behavior analysis: Issues and advances* (pp. 299–311). New York: Plenum Press.

Rankin, H. (1990). Validity of self-reports in clinical settings. *Behavioral Assessment, 12*, 107–116.

Robins, L. N., Helzer, J. E., Croughan, J., & Ratcliff, K. S. (1981). National Institute of Mental Health diagnostic interview schedule: Its history, characteristics, and validity. *Archives of General Psychiatry, 38*, 381–389.

Russo, D. C. (1990). A requiem for the passing of the three-term contingency. *Behavior Therapy, 21*, 153–165.

Russo, D. C., & Budd, K. S. (1987). Limitations of operant practice in the study of disease. *Behavior Modification, 11*, 264–285.

Schoenfeld, W. N., & Farmer, J. (1970). Reinforcement schedules and the "behavior stream." In W. N. Schoenfeld (Ed.), *The theory of reinforcement schedules* (pp. 215–245). New York: Appleton-Century.

Schwartz, G. E. (1983). Social psychophysiology and behavioral medicine: A systems perspective. In J. T. Caccioppo & R. E. Petty (Eds.), *Social psychophysiology*. New York: Guilford Press.

Schwartz, G. E. (1986). Emotion and psychophysiological organization: A systems approach. In M. G. H. Coles, E. Donchin, S. W. Porges (Eds.), *Psychophysiology: Systems, processes, and applications* (pp. 354–377). New York: Guilford Press.

Scott, J. P., Stewart, J. M., & DeGhett, V. J. (1974). Critical periods in the organization of systems. *Developmental Psychobiology, 7*, 489–513.

Sievert, A. L., Cuvo, A. J., & Davis, P. K. (1988). Training self-advocacy skills to adults with mild handicaps. *Journal of Applied Behavior Analysis, 21*, 299–309.

Skinner, B. F. (1974). *About behaviorism*. New York: Knopf.

Skinner, B. F. (1988). The operant side of behavior therapy. *Journal of Behavior Therapy and Experimental Psychiatry, 19*, 171–179.

Spielberger, C. D., Gorsuch, R. L., & Lushene, R. D. (1970). *Manual for the state-trait anxiety inventory*. Palo Alto, CA: Consulting Psychologists Press.

Spitzer, R. L., & Williams, J. B. (1985). *Instruction manual for the structured clinical interview for DSM-III*. New York: Biometrics Research Department, New York State Psychiatric Institute.

Strosahl, K. D., & Linehan, M. M. (1986). Basic issues in behavioral assessment. In A. R. Ciminero, K. S. Calhoun, & H. E. Adams (Eds.), *Handbook of behavioral assessment* (2nd ed., pp. 12–46). New York: Wiley.

Sturgis, E. T., & Gramling, S. (1988). Psychophysiological assessment. In A. S. Bellack & M. Hersen (Eds.), *Behavioral assessment: A practical handbook* (3rd ed., pp. 213–251). Elmsford, NY: Pergamon Press.

Tarrier, N. (1989). Electrodermal activity, expressed emotion and outcome in schizophrenia. *British Journal of Psychiatry, 155* (Suppl. 5), 51–56.

Tarrier, N., & Barrowclough, C. (1990). Family interventions in schizophrenia. *Behavior Modification, 14*, 408–440.

Tarrier, N., Vaughn, C., Lader, M. H., & Leff, J. P. (1979). Bodily reactions to people and events in schizophrenics. *Archives of General Psychiatry, 36*, 311–315.

Tarrier, N., Barrowclough, C., Vaughn, C., Bamrah, J. S., Porceddu, K., & Freeman, H. (1989). Community management of schizophrenia: A two-year follow-up of a behavioral intervention with families. *British Journal of Psychiatry, 154*, 625–628.

Taylor, S. E. (1991). *Health psychology* (2nd ed.). New York: McGraw-Hill.

Thompson, C. (1989). Introduction. In C. Thompson (Ed), *The instruments of psychiatric research* (pp. 1–17). New York: Wiley.

Touchette, P. E., MacDonald, R. F., & Langer, S. N. (1985). A scatter plot for identifying stimulus control of problem behavior. *Journal of Applied Behavior Analysis, 18*, 343–351.

Turkat, I. D. (1986). The behavioral interview. In A. Ciminero, K. S. Calhoun, & H. E. Adams (Eds.), *Handbook of behavioral assessment* (2nd ed., pp. 109–149). New York: Wiley.

Turner, S. M., Hersen, M., & Bellack, A. S. (1977). Effects of stimulus interference and aversive conditioning on auditory hallucinations. *Behavior Modification, 1*, 249–258.

Turner, S. M., Holzman, A., & Jacob, R. C. (1983). Treatment of compulsive looking be imaginal thought stopping. *Behavior Modification, 7*, 576–582.

Turpin, G. (1989). *Handbook of clinical psychophysiology*. London: Wiley.

Van Den Hout, M., Emmelkamp, H., & Griez, E. (1988). Behavioral treatment of obsessive-compulsives: Inpatient versus outpatient. *Behaviour Research and Therapy, 26*, 331–332.

Voeltz, L. M., & Evans, I. M. (1982). The assessment of behavioral interrelationships in child behavior therapy. *Behavioral Assessment, 4*, 131–165.

von Bertalannfy, L. (1968). *General systems theory*. New York: Braziller.

Wahler, R. G., & Fox, J. J. (1981). Setting events in applied behavior analysis: Toward a conceptual and methodological expansion. *Journal of Applied Behavior Analysis, 14*, 327–338.

Williamson, D. A., Prather, R. C., Bennet, S. M., Davis, C. J., Watkins, P. C., & Grenier, C. E. (1989). An uncontrolled evaluation of inpatient and outpatient cognitive-behavior therapy for bulimia nervosa. *Behavior Modification, 13*, 340–360.

Willis, S. E., & Nelson, R. O. (1982). The effects and nature of target behavior on the accuracy and reactivity of self-monitoring. *Behavioral Assessment, 4*, 401–412.

Wing, J. K., Cooper, J. E., & Sartorius, N. (1974). *The measurement and classification of psychiatric symptoms*. New York: Cambridge University Press.

Wong, S. E., & Woolsey, J. E. (1989). Re-establishing conversational skills in overtly psychotic, chronic schizophrenic patients: Discrete trials training on the psychiatric ward. *Behavior Modification, 13*, 415–430.

Zahn, T. P. (1986). Psychophysiological approaches to psychopathology. In M. G. H. Coles, E. Donchin, & S. W. Porges (Eds.), *Psychophysiology: Systems, processes, and applications* (pp. 508–610). New York: Guilford Press.

4

Psychiatric Assessment and Diagnosis

Adults

JOHN T. WIXTED, RANDALL L. MORRISON,
and ROBERT C. RINALDI

INTRODUCTION

In psychiatry, as in any helping profession, effective clinical intervention depends on a comprehensive evaluation of the individual seeking treatment. The interrelated fields of psychiatric diagnosis and assessment constitute a wide and ever-expanding range of strategies designed to serve that purpose. Although an exhaustive survey of these methods would be impractical, this chapter details some of the more important and useful assessment techniques available to the practicing clinician. Our discussion of these techniques is divided into three main sections. The first concerns diagnosis and classification, including the use of structured diagnostic interviews. The second describes the growing use of convenient indirect measures of symptomatology, namely, self-report questionnaires and clinician rating scales. The third section reviews observation-based assessment techniques designed to measure abnormal behavior more directly in natural or in clinical or analogue settings. Because each of these methods has unique strengths and limitations, they are almost never used in isolation. Instead, the coordinated use of multiple assessment strategies, which allows for the identification of a consistent pattern of information, is generally the optimal approach.

JOHN T. WIXTED • Department of Psychology, University of California—San Diego, La Jolla, California 92093.   RANDALL L. MORRISON • William, Lynde, and Williams, Inc., Chagrin Falls, Ohio 44022.   ROBERT C. RINALDI • Division of Health Science, American Medical Association, Chicago, Illinois 60610.

Handbook of Behavior Therapy in the Psychiatric Setting, edited by Alan S. Bellack and Michel Hersen. Plenum Press, New York, 1993.

JOHN T. WIXTED *et al.*

The recent history of psychiatry has been characterized by wide variations in the general acceptance of efforts to classify psychopathology. Kraepelin's modest, but influential, nosology developed around the turn of the century, was largely overshadowed by subsequent developments in psychoanalytic and, later, behavioral theory. These schools of thought tended to eschew classification, preferring instead to interpret abnormal behavior solely in terms of theoretical models of unconscious conflict or empirical principles of conditioning. From either point of view, little was gained by the use of a conceptually vacuous verbal label that carried with it the veiled implication of biological dysfunction. Others, especially from the humanistic camp, emphasized the potential iatrogenic consequences of diagnostic labeling. According to this position, a diagnosis merely creates a distorting filter through which to perceive and interpret the behavior of the labeled individual.

Despite such opposition, efforts to create a workable psychiatric taxonomy never completely disappeared. Advocates of psychiatric classification envisioned a diagnostic system that would ultimately lead to important scientific advances, including improved communication among members of the research community, the possible identification of the etiological factors associated with individual disorders, and the eventual development of disorder-specific therapies. The first *Diagnostic and Statistical Manual* (DSM-I), published by the American Psychiatric Association (APA) in 1952, represented a major step forward in this regard. This manual, which listed 106 separate categories of psychopathology, was easily the most ambitious work of its kind. Its first revision, DSM-II (APA, 1968), listed 182 separate disorders.

Although impressive in scope, these initial systems did little to persuade the larger psychiatric community of the value of diagnosis. From a practical standpoint, their most important limitation was an embarrassingly low degree of interjudge reliability. If two trained clinicians using the same diagnostic manual are unable to agree on a patient's condition, the potential promise of psychiatric classification cannot possibly be realized. Most of the important developments in the field of psychiatric diagnosis occurring since the early 1970s, including the most recent revisions of the DSM, have addressed precisely this concern.

Diagnostic Reliability

The two principal factors contributing to a lack of diagnostic reliability are criterion variance and information variance. *Criterion variance* refers to differences in the inclusion and exclusion criteria that clinicians use to summarize patient data into psychiatric diagnoses (Endicott & Spitzer, 1978; Spitzer, Endicott, & Robins, 1978). Early diagnostic classification systems, including the first and second editions of the DSM, contained ambiguous clinical descriptions of each disorder rather than explicit, rule-governed diagnostic criteria. Deciding whether a patient matched one vague clinical summary better than another was a truly challenging task. Adding to this problem was *information variance*, which refers to differences in the quality and quantity of information obtained from patients during the course of a diagnostic interview. Throughout the successive reigns of the DSM-I and the DSM-II, few, if any, standardized procedures were developed to help guide the diagnostic interview process. Unfortunately, when assessment is left solely to the discretion of the individual clinician, some areas may not be probed in sufficient detail to permit a differential diagnosis, and other areas may be overlooked altogether.

In an effort to resolve problems such as these, several research groups began to develop their own explicit criteria and classification schemes. The first set of these, termed the Feighner criteria, represented the cumulative efforts of diagnostic research conducted at the Washington University School of Medicine over the course of several decades (Feighner, Robins, Guze, Woodruff, Winokur, & Monoz, 1972). Their system listed 16 psychiatric disorders along with specific behavioral and temporal criteria for each. The Feighner criteria were published in a book by Woodruff, Goodwin, and Guze (1974), and research conducted by Helzer, Robins, Taibleson, Woodson, Reich, and Wish (1977) demonstrated that they resulted in an immediate, dramatic improvement in clinician-clinician diagnostic reliability.

The Feighner criteria were later updated and enlarged to create the Research Diagnostic Criteria (RDC), published in 1978 (Spitzer *et al.*, 1978). *Exclusive* as well as *inclusive* criteria were included in the 25 psychiatric conditions listed in the RDC in an attempt to improve reliability still further. Thus, for example, a diagnosis of depression requires the presence of symptoms such as poor appetite, loss of energy, and feelings of guilt (inclusive criteria) as well as the absence of symptoms such as delusions of control, nonaffective hallucinations, and/or signs of formal thought disorder (exclusive criteria) that may imply the presence of schizophrenia.

In addition to developing explicit diagnostic criteria, these research groups also developed *structured diagnostic interviews* designed to reduce information variance. Helzer and colleagues at Washington University, for example, developed a standard interview based on the Feighner criteria called the Renard Diagnostic Interview (Helzer, Robins, Croughan, & Welner, 1981). This was soon modified and expanded to create the Diagnostic Interview Schedule (Robins, Helzer, Croughan, & Ratcliff, 1981). Similarly, concomitant with the development of the RDC, Endicott and Spitzer (1978) published the Schedule for Affective Disorders and Schizophrenia (SADS), a structured interview designed to elicit the information necessary for generating RDC diagnoses.

The demonstrable improvement in reliability occasioned by the use of objective criteria and structured interviews prompted a wholesale shift in the approach to diagnosis contained in the DSM series. Whereas the DSM-I and the DSM-II were basically clinical descriptions, the DSM-III (APA, 1980) and its recent revision, the DSM-III-R (APA, 1987), adopted the more objective criteria-based methodology of the RDC. Along with these developments, a number of structured interviews were created to facilitate diagnostic decisions based on the new DSM-III criteria. As might be expected, these developments have resulted in a considerable improvement in reliability compared to that of the DSM-I and the DSM-II (e.g., Matarazzo, 1983). Because of the enormous scientific progress that a reliable diagnostic system might be able to facilitate, earlier reservations about psychiatric classification have largely given way to widespread acceptance among psychiatrists and psychologists alike. The following section describes the current composition of the DSM-III and the DSM-III-R. Specific structured interviews designed to facilitate diagnoses based on the RDC and/or the DSM-III criteria are then reviewed in some detail.

DSM-III and DSM-III-R

Among the many changes introduced by the DSM-III is a multiaxial approach to diagnosis. Instead of a single diagnostic label, each patient is rated along five separate axes. Each axis is designed to provide information about the patient's psychiatric, psychosocial, or medical status. Axes I and II comprise all of the psychiatric conditions. The disorders coded on Axis I include most of the traditional clinical syndromes, such as mood disorders and schizophrenia, as well as a variety of nonmental disorders that may require psychiatric intervention (e.g., marital discord). Table 1 provides a comparison of the diagnostic descriptions for depression contained in the DSM-II and the DSM-III-R. Whereas the DSM-II lists a clinical description without explicit inclusion, exclusion, and temporal criteria, the DSM-III-R presents a much more precise description that contains all of these. Virtually every Axis I disorder contained in the DSM-III-R is characterized by inclusion and exclusion criteria described as objectively and athoeretically as possible.

Table 1. DSM-II versus DSM-III-R Descriptions of Major Depressive Episode

DSM-II clinical description[a]	DSM-III-R diagnostic criteria[b]
This disorder consists exclusively of depressive episodes. These episodes are characterized by severely depressed mood and by mental and motor retardation progressing occasionally to stupor. Uneasiness, apprehension, perplexity, and agitation may also be present. When illusions, hallucinations, and delusions (usually of guilt or of hypochondriacal or paranoid ideas) occur, they are attributable to the dominant mood disorder. Because it is a primary mood disorder, this psychosis differs from the *Psychotic depressive reaction*, which is more easily attributable to precipitating stress. Cases incompletely labelled as "psychotic depression" should be classified here rather than under *Psychotic depressive reaction* (pp. 36–37).	A. At least five of the following symptoms have been present during the same two-week period and represent a change from previous functioning: 1. depressed mood most of the day 2. markedly diminished interest and pleasure in all activities 3. significant weight loss or weight gain when not dieting 4. insomnia or hypersomnia nearly every day 5. psychomotor agitation or retardation nearly every day 6. fatigue or loss of energy nearly every day 7. feelings of woprthlessness or excessive guilt nearly every day 8. diminished ability to think or concentrate nearly every day 9. recurrent thoughts of death or suicidal ideation B. 1. It cannot be established that an organic factor initiated and maintained the disturbance 2. The disturbance is not a normal reaction to the death of a loved one (Uncomplicated Bereavement) C. At no time during the disturbance have there been delusions or hallucinations for as long as two weeks in the absence of prominent mood symptoms (i.e., before the mood symptoms developed or after they have remitted) D. Not superimposed on Schizophrenia, Schizophreniform Disorder, Delusional Disorder, or Psychotic Disorder NOS

[a]Adapted from American Psychiatric Association. (1968). *Diagnostic and Statistical Manual of Mental Disorders* (2nd ed.). Washington, DC: Author.
[b]Adapted from American Psychiatric Association. (1987). *Diagnostic and Statistical Manual of Mental Disorders* (3rd ed., rev.). Washington, DC: Author.

Axis II was included to encourage attention to more stable psychiatric conditions that are often overlooked when an Axis I disorder commands most of the initial attention. With regard to adults, the relevant Axis II disorders are the 11 personality disorders (the DSM-III-R also lists 3 experimental personality disorders coded on Axis II). These 11 disorders are grouped into three clusters: Cluster A includes the Odd/Eccentric disorders (Paranoid, Schizoid, and Schizotypal); Cluster B includes the Emotional/Erratic disorders (Histrionic, Narcissistic, Antisocial, and Borderline); and Cluster C includes the Anxious/Fearful disorders (Avoidant, Dependent, Compulsive, and Passive-Aggressive). With the exception of Antisocial Personality Disorder, the conditions coded on Axis II are described with less precision than those coded on Axis I. As a result, diagnostic reliability for the personality disorders is somewhat lower than that typically achieved for the more acute clinical syndromes (Matarazzo, 1983; Mellsop, Varghese, Joshua, & Hicks, 1982).

To complement the information provided by Axis I and/or Axis II diagnoses, the DSM-III includes a third axis on which physical disorders can be coded. This axis was included in the revision explicitly to encourage attention to known medical conditions that may be contributing to the psychological problem. In some instances, the physical disorder may be etiologically relevant to the mental disorder (e.g., a known neurological disorder may underlie dementia). In other cases, the physical condition may not be etiologically significant but may nevertheless serve to influence the treatment strategy. A major depressive episode occurring in the context of a life-threatening physical illness, for example, may have different treatment implications than one occurring in the context of a less serious physical disorder.

The two remaining axes, Axis IV and Axis V, were included for use by researchers and in special clinical settings, but one may assume that they are widely used in clinical practice as well. Ratings on Axis IV are designed to gauge the level of psychosocial stressors occurring over the past year that may have contributed to or perhaps exacerbated the psychiatric condition. The severity of a stressor is rated on a 6-point scale according to how stressful the event would be to an average person in similar circumstances. A rating of 1 indicates that no apparent stressors have occurred, whereas a rating of 6 indicates that the stressors have been catastrophic. Finally, Axis V is a global assessment of the patient's psychological, social, and occupational functioning over the last year. A rating in the range of 81–90 suggests minimal impairment, whereas a rating in the range of 1–10 implies very impaired functioning (e.g., inability to maintain minimal personal hygiene).

Sounding a recurrent theme of contemporary psychiatry, a number of research groups have argued that a multiaxial system offers potentially important etiological and prognostic information only to the extent that the axis ratings are reliable and valid. With regard to Axis IV ratings (psychosocial stressors), for example, some studies have reported moderately high levels of reliability (e.g., Schrader, Gordon, & Harcourt, 1986), whereas others have found reliability to be quite poor (Rey, Stewart, Plapp, Bashir, & Richards, 1988). Skodol and Shrout (1989) compared Axis IV ratings to an independent evaluation of psychosocial stress derived from a structured epidemiological research interview. Reasonably good agreement was found with regard to severe stressors, but many discrepancies were noted as well. The authors argued that the primary source of disagreement between the two measures was the DSM-III requirement that the clinician consider only stressors deemed to be important in the development or exacerbation of the disorder. If that requirement were dropped (so that severe stressors were coded regardless of their presumed etiological significance), more reliable ratings might be obtained. Future revisions of the DSM will probably need to incorporate suggestions such as these in order to strengthen the multiaxial approach to diagnosis.

Structured Diagnostic Interviews

Arriving at an Axis I and/or Axis II psychiatric diagnosis is now greatly facilitated by the use of standardized structured interviews. These interviews consist of a series of detailed questions, each addressing some aspect of the RDC or DSM-III-R nosology. For a given diagnostic category, a structured interview usually recommends a few broad questions (e.g., "Have you been sad or depressed lately?") and then suggests a series of more detailed inquiries to follow up a positive response. When the interview is completed, the patient's responses can be used to establish a diagnosis according to relatively clear rules and guidelines. The Schedule for Affective Disorders and Schizophrenia (SADS) developed by Endicott and Spitzer (1978) and the Diagnostic Interview Schedule (DIS) developed by Robins and her colleagues (e.g., Robins *et al.*, 1981) have seen widespread use since the early 1980s. More recently, a number of additional structured interviews designed to be used exclusively with the DSM-III-R (as opposed to the RDC or Feighner criteria) have also been developed.

The Schedule for Affective Disorders and Schizophrenia. There are actually three versions of the SADS: the regular version (SADS), the lifetime version (SADS-L), and the version for measuring change (SADS-C). The SADS is organized into two parts. Part 1 is designed to obtain a detailed description of the current episode and of the patient's functioning during the week before the interview. Part 2 focuses on information regarding psychiatric disturbance before the current episode. In general, the SADS-L is similar to Part 2 of the SADS. Thus, whereas the SADS is suitable for interviewing patients during a current episode of illness, the SADS-L is more appropriate for use with persons who are not experiencing a current episode (e.g., relatives of patients) (Endicott & Spitzer, 1978).

In completing the SADS, the interviewer is to use all available sources of information (including chart notes and information from significant others) and as many general or specific questions as needed to score the items accurately. The questions suggested by the SADS typically refer to the duration, course, or severity of specific symptoms. Several questions are suggested for each item in order to guide the interviewer in probing for additional information. For scoring, each question is rated on a Likert scale with anchor points that define discrete levels of symptom severity. More than 20 diagnostic categories are encompassed by the SADS, some of which contain subcategories or specific subsyndromes. A summary of these categories is presented in Table 2. Table 3 presents a small section of the SADS designed to elicit information relevant to the diagnosis of a manic episode.

The interview typically takes 1½ to 2 hours depending on the degree of pathology exhibited by the individual being interviewed. Endicott and Spitzer (1978) suggested that, because the interview requires decisions that involve knowledge of psychiatric concepts, it should be conducted only by psychiatrists, clinical psychologists, and psychiatric social workers.

With regard to the psychometric properties of the SADS, Endicott and Spitzer (1978) reported intraclass correlation coefficients of interrater reliability for the individually scaled items of the current section of the SADS and for summary scale scores. These coefficients were based on data from 210 newly admitted inpatients who were jointly evaluated by pairs of raters or who were independently interviewed twice within 72 hours. For all individual items and summary scale scores, with the exception of the Formal Thought Disorder Scale (FTDS) under the test-retest conditions, the reliabilities were quite high. Endicott and Spitzer (1978) examined the ratings of the FTDS and found that the low reliability was due to a lack of variability of ratings within this dimension (none of the subjects exhibited markedly disordered thought).

Spitzer *et al.* (1978) further examined joint-interview and test-retest reliability coefficients for specific subtypes of major depressive disorder identified in the RDC (see Table 2). Their findings indicate that, although these coefficients are smaller than those for the major diagnostic categories, "for the most part, they are quite satisfactory for research use, and much higher than generally reported" (p. 780). A subsequent study by Andreasen, Grove, Shapiro, Keller, Hirschfeld, and McDonald-Scott (1981) found that the lifetime version of the SADS generally had good reliability as well, although the coefficients for the 10 specific items that operationally define the global diagnosis of anxiety disorder were smaller than those for other disorders.

The SADS is currently the structured diagnostic interview most widely used in clinical research investigations. It is, of course, used most frequently in studies pertaining to schizophrenic and depressed patients, but it has been used in investigations of other disorders, including alcoholism (Jacob, Dunn, & Leonard, 1983). Although it was specifically developed in relation to the RDC criteria, it can be used to systematically gather information about symptoms that can then be applied to other diagnostic classification systems, such as the DSM-III. However, with the publication of the DSM-III-R (and the soon-to-be-released DSM-IV), the SADS is becoming increasingly dated. Indeed, as described later, the development of new interviews based primarily on the DSM-III and DSM-III-R criteria will undoubtedly reduce the use of the SADS in the coming years (Spitzer & Williams, 1985).

The Diagnostic Interview Schedule. The Diagnostic Interview Schedule (DIS) (Robins *et al.*, 1981) was specifically designed for administration by a lay interviewer. The exact wording to be used in all questions and probes is specified verbatim, as is the progression or sequence within the interview from one question to the next. The DIS, which was developed at

Table 2.   Research Diagnostic Criteria Covered by
the Schedule for Affective Disorders and Schizophrenia[a]

Schizophrenia	
Acute-chronic	Catatonic
Paranoid	Mixed (undifferentiated)
Disorganized	Residual
Schizoaffective disorder—manic	
Acute-chronic	Mainly affective
Mainly schizophrenic	
Schizoaffective disorder—depressed	
Acute-chronic	Mainly affective
Mainly schizophrenic	
Depressive syndrome superimposed on residual schizophrenia	
Manic disorder	
Hypomanic disorder	
Bipolar with mania (bipolar I)[b]	
Bipolar with hypomania (bipolar II)[b]	
Major depressive disorder	
Primary	Agitated
Secondary	Retarded
Recurrent unipolar[b]	Situational
Psychotic	Simple
Incapacitating	Predominant mood
Endogenous	
Minor depressive disorder with significant anxiety	
Intermittent depressive disorder[b]	
Panic disorder	
Generalized anxiety disorder with significant depression	
Cyclothymic personality[b]	
Labile personality[b]	
Briquet's disorder (somatization disorder)[b]	
Antisocial personality	
Alcoholism	
Drug use disorder	
Obsessive-compulsive disorder	
Phobic disorder	
Unspecified functional disorder	
Other psychiatric disorder	
Schizotypal features[b]	
Currently not mentally ill	
Never mentally ill	

[a]Adapted from J. Endicott and R. L. Spitzer. 1978. A Diagnostic Interview: The
  Schedule for Affective Disorders and Schizophrenia. *Archives of General Psychiatry*,
  35, 838. Copyright 1981 by the American Medical Association.
[b]These conditions are diagnosed on a longitudinal or lifetime basis. All other conditions
  are diagnosed on the basis of current or past episodes of psychopathology.

the request of the Division of Biometry and Epidemiology of the National Institute of Mental Health for use in a series of epidemiological studies, can provide diagnoses based on the DSM-III, RDC, or Feighner criteria. Diagnoses are first made on a lifetime basis, and then the interviewer inquires how recently the last symptom was experienced (Robins *et al.*, 1981). Disorders classified as "current" are further subdivided into those occurring within the past 2 weeks within the past month, within the past 6 months, or within the past year. The pattern of probes used to determine the clinical significance of a patient's endorsement of a symptom is specified and is the same for each item. Thus, the amount of discretion that the interviewer is to

Table 3. Screening Items for Manic Syndrome[a]

The next 5 items are screening items to determine the presence of manic-like behavior. If any of the items are judged present, inquire in a general way to determine how the patient was behaving at that time with such questions as: *"When you were this way, what kinds of things were you doing? How did you spend your time?"* Do not include behavior which is clearly explainable by alcohol or drug intoxication.

If the subject has only described dysphoric mood, the following questions regarding the manic syndrome should be introduced with a statement such as: *"I know you have been feeling (depressed). However, many people have other feelings mixed in or at different times, so it is important that I ask you about those feelings also."*

Elevated mood and/or optimistic attitude toward the future which lasted at least several hours and was out of proportion to the circumstances. *Have (there there been times when) you felt very good or too cheerful or high—not just your normal self?* If unclear: *When you felt on top of the world as if there was nothing you couldn't do?* *(Have you felt that everything would work out just the way you wanted?)* *If people saw you would they think you were just in a good mood or something more than that?* *(What about during the past week?)*	0. No information 1. Not at all: normal or depressed 2. Slight: e.g., good spirits, more cheerful than most people in these circumstances, but of only possible clinical significance 3. Mild: e.g., definitely elevated mood and optimistic outlook that is somewhat out of proportion to circumstances 4. Moderate: e.g., mood and outlook are clearly out of proportion to circumstances 5. Severe: e.g., quality of euphoric mood 6. Extreme: e.g., clearly elated, exalted expression and says, "Everything is beautiful, I feel so good" PAST WEEK 0 1 2 3 4 5 6
Less need for sleep than usual to feel rested (average for several days when needed less sleep). *Have you needed less sleep than usual to feel rested? (How much sleep do you ordinarily need?)(How much when you were/are high?)* *(What about during the past week?)*	0. No information 1. No change or more sleep needed 2. Up to 1 hour less than usual 3. Up to 2 hours less than usual 4. Up to 3 hours less than usual 5. Up to 4 hours less than usual 6. 4 or more hours less than usual PAST WEEK 0 1 2 3 4 5 6
Unusually energetic, more active than usual level without expected fatigue. *Have you had more energy than usual to do things? (More than just a return to normal or usual level?)(Did it seem like too much energy?)* *(What about during the past week?)*	0. No information 1. No different than usual or less energetic 2. Slightly more energetic but of questionable significance 3. Little change in activity level but less fatigued than usual 4. Somewhat more active than usual with little or no fatigue 5. Much more active than usual with little or no fatigue 6. Unusually active all day long with little or no fatigue PAST WEEK 0 1 2 3 4 5 6

[a]Adapted from J. Endicott and R. L. Spitzer. (1978). A Diagnostic Interview: The Schedule for Affective Disorders and Schizophrenia. *Archives of General Psychiatry*, *35*, 839. Copyright 1981 by the American Medical Association.

exercise, either in wording questions or in determining when to probe, is reduced to a minimum. Training for interviewers typically requires about one week. The actual diagnosis based on the interview can be derived by computer with a scoring program developed for the DIS. As noted above, diagnoses can be made for all three diagnostic systems. For most patients, the DIS can be completed within 60–75 minutes.

The psychometric properties of the DIS have been evaluated in a series of studies by Robins and her colleagues. Robins *et al.* (1981) presented data regarding the concordance of lay interviewers' and psychiatrists' diagnoses, as well as the sensitivity (percentage of cases correctly identified) and specificity (percentage of noncases correctly identified) of the lay interviewers' diagnoses, using the psychiatrists' interviews as a yardstick. The subjects were 118 psychiatric inpatients, 39 psychiatric outpatients, 24 nonpatient control, 10 members of Gamblers Anonymous, and 26 ex-patients. The subjects were interviewed by use of the DIS twice, once by a lay interviewer and once by a psychiatrist. The order in which the two interviews were conducted was randomized. For DSM-III diagnoses, the mean kappa value was .69. The mean sensitivity was 75% and the mean specificity was 94%. A more detailed examination of the DIS interview with the same 216 patients was provided by Robins, Helzer, Ratcliff, and Seyfried (1982). Their data indicate that disorders in remission or borderline conditions are diagnosed less accurately than current and severe disorders. However, this finding presumably would be true of any interview measure.

Finally, a study by Helzer, Robins, McEvoy, Spitznagel, Stolzman, Farmer, and Brockington (1985) examined the level of agreement between lay interviewers using the DIS and clinical diagnoses made by psychiatrists as part of a general population survey. The overall agreement between the lay DIS and the clinical impression of psychiatrists ranged from 79% to 96%. The chance-corrected concordance between lay DIS and psychiatrists' clinical diagnoses was .60 or greater for 8 of the 11 diagnostic categories. The specificity was 90% or better for each diagnostic category. Although sensitivity was lower, lay interview results indicated a bias for only two diagnoses. Major depression was significantly underdiagnosed by lay interviewers, and obsessive-compulsive disorder was overdiagnosed.

In general, the results of lay DIS interviews appear to agree with psychiatrists' judgments in most diagnostic categories. Thus, its use by lay interviewers would appear to be appropriate in those situations in which a psychiatrist or psychologist or other professionally trained diagnostician is unavailable. Robins and her colleagues are continuing to refine the DIS and to make additions to it that deal with a broader range of DSM-III diagnoses. For example, whereas earlier versions of the DIS did not include questions pertaining to social phobia (DiNardo, O'Brien, Barlow, Waddel, & Blanchard, 1983), this category is included in the most recent version (Helzer *et al.*, 1985).

The Structured Clinical Interview for the DSM-III-R. The Structured Clinical Interview for the DSM-III-R (SCID) is a structured diagnostic interview to be administered by a clinically trained interviewer in order to derive DSM-III-R diagnoses (Spitzer, Williams, & Gibbon, 1987). The SCID has been under development by Spitzer and his colleagues with input from numerous consultants, and it continues to be revised and expanded. Originally, sections of the SCID were introduced dealing with the diagnoses of schizophrenia and mood disorders based on the DSM-III criteria. These sections were revised with the publication of the DSM-III-R criteria, and other sections were added so that the SCID now provides screening for the following disorders: mood disorders, psychotic disorders, somatoform disorders, eating disorders, adjustment disorders, and all of the Axis II personality disorders. Future revisions may include sections pertaining to organic brain syndromes and a module for evaluating Axis IV and V and for noting Axis III conditions (Spitzer & Williams, 1988).

The SCID has been used most frequently in investigations of mood and psychotic disorders, although the SADS and the DIS are still more commonly used for that purpose. Because the SCID is still under development and revision, it is difficult to derive definitive information regarding its current psychometric status. However, the initial work on its development appears promising (e.g., Riskind, Beck, Berchick, Brown, & Steer, 1987), and it seems likely that the SCID will increase in popularity as further data regarding its efficacy are reported.

Other Structured Diagnostic Interviews for Adults. A number of additional structured interviews have been developed that focus on specific diagnostic categories. DiNardo *et al.* (1983), for example, developed the Anxiety Disorders Interview Schedule (ADIS) in order to (1) permit differential diagnosis among the DSM-III anxiety disorder categories and (2) provide sufficient information to rule out psychosis, substance abuse, and major affective disorders. The average time for administration is approximately 90 minutes. The ADIS is not intended as a general diagnostic instrument and is perhaps best suited for use with patients in whom there is reason to suspect an anxiety disorder (although it does evaluate depressive symptoms as well). Further, because some clinical judgment is required on the part of the interviewer, the ADIS should be administered only by clinicians with experience in interviewing and familiarity with the DSM-III. DiNardo *et al.* (1983) reported psychometric findings from test-retest interviews by two different interviewers on 60 consecutive outpatients at an anxiety disorders clinic. The findings indicate good agreement for anxiety, affective, and adjustment disorders as well as for the specific anxiety disorder categories of agoraphobia, panic, social phobia, and obsessive-compulsive disorder. However, agreement for generalized anxiety disorder failed to reach acceptable levels.

Other interviews have been developed that focus specifically on Axis II diagnoses. Of these, the Diagnostic Interview for Borderline Patients (DIBP) has been the most widely used (Gunderson, Kolb, & Austin, 1981). Acceptable test-retest reliability, sensitivity, and specificity have been reported in a series of studies with the DIBP (Frances, Clarkin, Gilmore, Hurt, & Brown, 1984; Gunderson *et al.*, 1981; Hurt, Hyler, Frances, Clarkin, & Brent, 1984). A similar instrument, the Schedule for Schizotypal Personalities (SSP), was developed by Baron, Asnis, and Gruen (1981) to facilitate the diagnosis of schizotypal personality disorder Test-retest interrater reliabilities of the SSP have generally been high, although agreement for individual items has often been far less than that for scaled scores or overall diagnoses (Baron *et al.*, 1981; Perry, O'Connell, & Drake, 1984). Sensitivity and specificity data revealed marked variations depending on which cutoff scores were used to declare an item positive or significant. When standard cutoff scores were used, false positives involving depressed patients and patients with other personality disorders were common. Higher cutoff scores, however, resulted in much better performance.

Finally, Stangl, Pfohl, Zimmerman, Bowers, and Corenthal (1985) undertook the ambitious task of developing the Structured Interview for DSM-III Personality Disorders (SIDP), an instrument intended to improve the reliability of Axis II diagnoses in general. Instructions to the patient emphasize that the questions pertain to their "usual" behavior and not to the acute symptomatology that they may be experiencing. In addition, a subset of the interview is routinely given to a knowledgeable informant in order to strengthen the quality of the clinical information obtained. Reliability data were collected on 63 subjects who were independently rated by two interviewers using the SIDP. Coefficients for interrater agreement were .70 or higher for histrionic, borderline, and dependent personalities, whereas coefficients for other disorders were lower. These findings suggest that some refinement of the instrument is needed before it can function efficiently in clinical settings.

A final issue regarding each of these measures (and the DSM-III-R itself) is the validity of the diagnostic information that is derived from them. Enhanced reliability, although critical to the success of any diagnostic system, does not in and of itself establish validity. More precisely, the reality of a psychiatric disorder is not established by the mere fact that clinicians have learned to agree on a diagnosis. The question of validity is especially problematic for the DSM-III Axis II disorders. For example, there is little evidence that borderline personality patients differ from histrionic personality patients with respect to phenomenology (Pope, Jonas, Hudson, Cohen, & Gunderson, 1983), etiology, family history, treatment response, or other parameters (Stangl *et al.*, 1985).

The difficulty in validating any diagnostic system for psychiatric illnesses involves finding an appropriate "gold standard" against which to compare the results. Unfortunately, no universally accepted criterion for psychiatric disorders can be identified. Spitzer (1983) argued that newly constructed diagnostic strategies should be validated against the opinion of mental health experts who have access to all of the information available on a particular patient. However, this strategy is far from perfect, especially when expert agreement is not very high (e.g., for Axis II disorders). Nevertheless, many of the instruments to be considered in later sections were validated in precisely this manner. During the next several years, as the DSM-III-R evolves into the DSM-IV, it seems likely that diagnostic categories will be expected to meet the more stringent requirements of predictive, descriptive, etiological, and construct validity (Widiger, Frances, Pincus, & Davis, 1990). Until that time, however, the validity of many psychiatric diagnoses, especially those coded on Axis II, remains uncertain.

INDIRECT ASSESSMENT TECHNIQUES

Although the rapid embrace of diagnostic activity correlated with publication of the DSM-III is remarkable, it has not served to invalidate concerns regarding the extent to which a diagnostic label captures the essential qualities of an individual patient. On the positive side, a valid diagnostic label is suggestive of the kinds of symptoms likely to be seen, the treatment strategies likely to be successful, and the natural course that the disorder may follow. On the negative side, the label offers no idiographic information relevant to the unique characteristics of the patient. The DSM-III and the DSM-III-R partially address this issue by means of the multiaxial system described earlier. However, additional assessment strategies are almost always needed in order to tailor treatment intervention to the needs of an individual patient. Some important functions not served by diagnosis alone include obtaining a quantitative picture of the pattern and severity of a patient's symptomatology, establishing an initial baseline measure of functioning, and providing ongoing measures to monitor treatment progress.

Two of the primary tools designed to serve these purposes are *self-report measures* and *clinician rating scales*. Both represent indirect assessments of patient functioning in that the information they provide is based on what the patient says rather than on what he or she actually does. In many respects, the general acceptance of these techniques paralleled the acceptance of psychiatric diagnosis and for similar reasons. Such measures were initially viewed with skepticism because the extent to which they were compromised by subjective factors was simply unknown. In recent years, these concerns have been addressed by exposing many of these instruments to a rigorous psychometric analysis.

Self-Report Measures

Asking a patient to complete a questionnaire covering a wide range of symptoms can be an extraordinarily efficient means of gathering clinically relevant information. Many such instruments now exist specifically for measuring depression (Beck, Ward, Mendelson, Mock, & Erbaugh, 1961), eating disorders (Garner & Garfinkel, 1979), assertiveness (Wolpe & Lazarus, 1966), anxiety (Spielberger, Gorsuch, & Lushene, 1970), marital satisfaction (Locke & Wallace, 1959; Spanier, 1976), and obsessions and compulsions (Rachman & Hodgson, 1980), to name a few. The popularity of these instruments derives from the fact that they can be quickly and efficiently completed by the patient before, during, and after a course of therapy in order to gauge treatment effectiveness. Moreover, in most cases, they provide a quick overview of specific problem areas that may warrant special consideration (e.g., suicidal ideation) within a broader domain.

A number of popular self-report instruments sample from a wide range of psychopathology and are thus especially useful for general psychiatric screening and initial patient evaluation. Although some of these instruments are intended to offer diagnostic information, they are perhaps more appropriately used to gather information of a *dimensional* rather than a categorical nature. Thus, for example, elevated scale scores on a self-report instrument may suggest that the patient exhibits paranoid tendencies, but other methods (e.g., a structured interview) would probably be necessary to determine whether or not the patient actually satisfies the DSM-III-R criteria for Paranoid Personality Disorder. In this section, we consider several of these instruments, each of which is currently in widespread use. The first measure to be considered is the Symptom Checklist-90 (SCL-90), an instrument designed to gauge acute symptom severity on nine clinical scales. Two additional self-report measures provide clinical information, in varying degrees, about both acute symptomatology and stable personality traits. These are the widely used Minnesota Multiphasic Personality Inventory (MMPI) and the Millon Clinical Multiaxial Inventory (MCMI). Finally, we consider an increasingly popular self-report measure designed specifically to provide information relevant to Axis II symptomatology, the Personality Diagnostic Questionnaire.

Symptom Checklist-90. The SCL-90—and its more recent successor, the SCL-90-R—is designed to serve both as a general screening device and as a clinical outcome measure (Derogatis, 1977, 1983). The instrument consists of 90 items, each briefly describing the experience of having a particular psychiatric symptom (e.g., "Feeling easily annoyed or irritated"). Patients rate each item on a 5-point scale, ranging from "Not at all" to "Extremely," to indicate the degree to which they have been bothered by that symptom over a specified period of time (usually the past week or the past month). The items are grouped into nine clinical scales: Somatization, Obsessive-Compulsive, Interpersonal Sensitivity, Depression, Anxiety, Hostility, Phobic Anxiety, Paranoid Ideation, and Psychoticism. In addition to these clinical scales, three summary scales can also be scored: the Positive Symptom Total (based on the total number of symptoms endorsed), the Positive Symptom Distress Index (based on the average intensity of the reported symptoms), and the General Severity Index (composed of both the number and the intensity of the symptoms). The questionnaire requires only about 20 minutes to complete, and normative information for nonpatients, psychiatric inpatients, and psychiatric outpatients has been published (Derogatis, 1983).

The SCL-90-R has adequate psychometric properties, with average test-retest and internal consistency coefficients exceeding .80 (Derogatis, 1983). However, in recent years, the instrument has been subjected to a thorough empirical analysis in an effort to evaluate the validity of its nine symptom dimensions. In this regard, recent research has been somewhat mixed. On the positive side, a number of studies have found that the SCL-90-R agrees quite well with alternative measures of symptomatology based on more intensive standardized clinical interviews (e.g., Peveler & Fairburn, 1990; Wilson, Taylor, & Robertson, 1985) and the much more time-intensive MMPI (Derogatis, Rickels, & Rock, 1976). On the negative side, researchers using factor-analytic techniques have often failed to reproduce the symptom dimensions of the SCL-90-R (e.g., Cyr, McKenna-Foley, & Peacock, 1985). Moreover, several studies have found that a single factor accounts for most of the total variance, which suggests that the instrument essentially provides an index of global distress rather than a detailed breakdown of symptomatology (e.g., Brophy, Norvell, & Kiluk, 1988). In practice, a patient's profile of scale elevations on the SCL-90-R should probably be regarded as tentative, subject to further inquiry using other methods of assessment.

Minnesota Multiphasic Personality Inventory. The MMPI was developed by Hathaway and McKinley in 1941 and is easily the most widely used and researched self-report inventory, with well over 9,000 books and articles devoted to it. The instrument consists of 566 true-false items that constitute 10 basic clinical scales, 4 validity scales, and a very large number of empirically derived subscales. The recently updated version (MMPI-2) is structurally similar, but some objectionable and outmoded items have been reworded or replaced altogether (Butcher, Dahlstrom, Graham, Tellegen, & Kaemmer, 1989). The 10 clinical scales are Hypochondriasis (Hs), Depression (D), Hysteria (Hy), Psychopathic Deviate (Pd), Masculinity/Femininity (MF), Paranoia (Pa), Psychasthenia (Pt), Schizophrenia (Sc), Hypomania (Ma), and Social Introversion (Si). The four validity scales are designed to measure the number of items not answered (the Cannot Say, or ? scale), the willingness of the individual to admit to even minor flaws (the L scale), the degree to which the individual responds in a deviant manner (the F scale), and test-taking "defensiveness" (the K scale). Hunsley, Hanson, and Parker (1988) provided a review of the voluminous research concerned with the psychometric properties of these scales. They concluded that, in general, all of the clinical and validity scales have adequate to impressive internal consistency (ranging from .71 to .84) and test-retest reliability (ranging from .63 to .86).

Like the SCL-90, the MMPI has often been used to obtain a dimensional analysis of acute symptomatology. Based on normative data, raw scale scores are converted to t scores with a mean of 50 and a standard deviation of 10. As a general rule, a t score two standard deviations above the mean is considered clinically significant. Thus, for example, a quick review of a patient's MMPI profile may suggest an abnormally high level of depression if the D scale exceeds 70 (65 if the MMPI-2 is used). The D scale in particular has often been used as a baseline and outcome measure in studies concerned with the treatment of depression.

A slightly different approach to profile interpretation emphasizes the *pattern* of scale elevations. In this regard, substantial clinical research has been directed at identifying patient characteristics associated with "two-point" codes (i.e., elevations on two clinical scales). For example, significant elevations on Scales 3 and 4 (Hysteria and Psychopathic Deviate) have been correlated with intense anger and aggressive impulses. Individuals with elevations on Scales 3 and 6 (Hysteria and Paranoia) have often been found to be defiant, uncooperative, and suspicious. Graham (1977) provided a particularly detailed and readable summary of patient characteristics that have been found to correlate with a variety of two-point code types.

In addition to the 10 clinical scales listed above, researchers have also developed a large number of empirically derived subscales for the purpose of identifying patients suffering from or at risk for various disorders. For example, the MacAndrew Alcoholism Scale was developed specifically to identify those at risk for alcohol abuse (MacAndrew, 1965, 1981). Hanvik (1951) developed the Lb scale to differentiate between the functional and organic etiology of low back pain. More recently, Morey and her colleagues created 11 new MMPI scales intended to correspond directly to the 11 DSM-III personality disorders (Morey, Waugh, & Blashfield, 1985). These scales have been shown to have a high degree of internal consistency (Morey *et al.*, 1985) and test-retest reliability (Hurt, Clarkin, & Morey, 1990). Moreover, factor analysis of these items yields three components that appear to closely match the three DSM-III-R Axis II clusters. Thus, these new MMPI scales provide an especially convenient way to gauge the extent to which a patient exhibits characteristics of the various personality disorders.

Although the MMPI is most often used to provide a dimensional analysis of psychopathology, a considerable amount of research is now under way to determine whether elevations based on the standard clinical scales (relevant to Axis I) and/or the supplementary personality scales (relevant to Axis II) can be used to make categorical diagnostic decisions (e.g., Dubro & Wetzler, 1989; Patrick, 1988). Although the initial results are somewhat promising in this regard, the use of the MMPI to establish a DSM-III-R diagnosis is probably inappropriate at this time. Until more research is available on its ability to classify individual patients correctly, the most important function of the MMPI is to provide detailed clinical information of a dimensional nature that is not captured by a single diagnostic label.

Millon Clinical Multiaxial Inventory. The MCMI is a self-report instrument designed specifically for the assessment of psychiatric patients rather than as a general screening instrument. Its most recent revision (the MCMI-II) consists of 175 true-false items, and it is designed for patients over age 17 (Millon, 1983, 1987). One advantage of this test over the MMPI is that it can generally be completed in about 30 minutes. The MCMI measures a wide range of psychopathology, including stable personality disorders as well as acute clinical syndromes. More specifically, the test yields scores on eight basic personality dimensions (Schizoid-Antisocial, Avoidant, Dependent-Submissive, Histrionic-Gregarious, Narcissistic, Antisocial-Aggressive, Compulsive-Conforming, and Passive-Aggressive-Negativistic), three pathological personality dimensions (Schizotypal-Schizoid, Borderline-Cycloid, and Paranoid), and nine clinical syndrome dimensions (Anxiety, Somatoform, Hypomanic, Dysthymic, Alcohol Abuse,

Drug Abuse, Psychotic Thinking, Psychotic Depression, and Psychotic Delusion). By design, each scale has a direct DSM-III Axis I or Axis II counterpart.

The psychometric properties of the MCMI are generally impressive: One-week test-retest reliabilities range from .78 to .91, and internal consistency values for the various scales average .88 (Millon, 1983). Not surprisingly, the more stable personality scales exhibit greater test-retest reliability during treatment than the acute syndrome scales, which tend to improve more readily (e.g., McMahon, Flynn, & Davidson, 1985). Factor-analytic studies generally find three dimensions roughly corresponding to the three pathological personality disorder scales (e.g., Wetzler, 1990). Like the personality scales of the MMPI, these three dimensions bear some similarity to the three personality disorder clusters listed in the DSM-III, although they clearly do not overlap.

One apparent problem with the MCMI is that intercorrelations between the various clinical scales are necessarily very high because of considerable item overlap (i.e., the same items appear in several scales). For example, the Dysthymic and Borderline-Cycloid scales share 65% of their items, primarily because Millon's personality theory regards these disorders as inter-related (Wetzler, 1990). Thus, the ability of the instrument to discriminate dysthymia from borderline personality disorder is obviously compromised. To address this problem, Millon (1987) reduced item overlap in the MCMI-2 and introduced different weightings for items that still appear on multiple scales.

As with the MMPI, some debate exists over whether the MCMI should be used for dimensional analyses or categorical diagnostic decisions. The MCMI was actually designed with the purpose of DSM-III diagnosis in mind, and Millon (1985) argued that the instrument performs very well in this regard. However, several studies investigating the agreement of MCMI scale scores with independently diagnosed inpatients have not entirely supported this claim. Wetzler (1990) provided a thorough review of the empirical research on this issue to date. With regard to Axis I disorders, the MCMI does not perform very well in most cases, although the Dysthymic scale seems to provide a reasonable measure of major depression. With regard to Axis II diagnoses, the performance of the MCMI has on several occasions been compared to DSM-III diagnoses based on structured clinical interviews. The results suggest that the MCMI is quite sensitive to the nonspecific presence of a personality disorder and fairly specific with regard to the proper DSM-III cluster. With regard to diagnosing individual personality disorders, however, the performance of the MCMI is still an open question.

The safest conclusion about the appropriate clinical use of the MCMI is similar to that reached for the MMPI. Specifically, the MCMI is clearly useful in answering questions of a dimensional nature (e.g., "To what extent does this patient exhibit characteristics typical of borderline personality disorder?"). Answering questions of diagnosis (e.g., "Does this patient satisfy the DSM-III-R criteria for borderline personality disorder?") is obviously a far more difficult challenge for self-report measures. An extensive body of research is likely to accumulate in the near future in an attempt to settle the debate over the utility of self-report measures in making diagnostic decisions. At present, however, neither the MCMI nor any other self-report measure should be used as the sole criterion for a diagnostic decision (cf. Widiger, Williams, Spitzer, & Frances, 1985).

Personality Diagnostic Questionnaire (PDQ). The PDQ-R is a 152-item, self-administered, true-false questionnaire designed specifically to yield information on personality functioning in terms consistent with the DSM-III-R (Hyler & Rieder, 1987). Indeed, most (137) of the items are derived directly from Axis II criteria. In that regard, the PDQ-R differs from the personality scales of both the MMPI and the MCMI. The remaining items attempt to evaluate a social desirability response set and malingering. The instructions encourage respondents to answer on the basis of their typical feelings, thoughts, and actions over the past several years.

The PDQ-R is still a relatively new instrument that is undergoing active research. Hyler, Lyons, Rieder, Young, Williams, and Spitzer (1990) conducted a factor analysis on the PDQ-R that yielded 11 components. Unfortunately, these 11 components did not correlate in any direct way with clinician ratings of specific personality disorders. On the other hand, the individual factors did tend to correlate specifically with only one of the DSM-III clusters. Thus, on a less specific level of analysis, the instrument performs quite well.

Hyler, Skodol, Kellman, Oldham, and Rosnick (1990) compared inpatient PDQ-R scores with clinician ratings based on a structured diagnostic interview. They found that the PDQ-R tended to overestimate the prevalence of personality disorder (a finding common to most self-report instruments) and that the correspondence between self-report and clinician ratings was acceptable for some disorders (e.g., avoidant and dependent personality disorder) but not for others (e.g., schizoid and histrionic). The authors prudently suggested that the PDQ-R is not a substitute for a structured interview assessment of Axis II disorders. Instead, the instrument may be used effectively as a screening device to select those for whom further inquiry is warranted and, more specifically, to direct attention to those personality attributes that appear to be deviant.

Clinician Rating Scales

Another common indirect method patient evaluation involves the use of clinician rating scales. These instruments contain many of the advantages of self-report scales (e.g., cost efficiency), but the information is acquired during a semistructured clinical interview rather than from paper-and-pencil tests. Like self-report measures, some of these scales are designed to sample from a broad range of psychopathology, such as the Brief Psychiatric Rating Scale (Overall & Gorham, 1962), whereas others provide a detailed analysis of a particular syndrome, such as the Hamilton Rating Scale for Depression (Hamilton, 1960). Because these scales are completed based on information obtained during an interview, they permit some degree of flexibility on the part of the therapist, who may wish to probe for details that the patient may neglect when completing a self-report measure. Like self-report scales, however, psychiatric rating scales provide a quantitative measure of the pattern and severity of the disturbance. As a result, these scales are often used to establish a baseline measure of the patient's symptomatology and to track progress during the course of therapy. In what follows, we consider rating scales of general psychiatric adjustment that are scored on the basis of a structured or semistructured interview.

Brief Psychiatric Rating Scale. The Brief Psychiatric Rating Scale (BPRS) was developed by Overall and Gorham (1962) as an easily administered interview measure of psychiatric symptoms. It was originally intended to be used to evaluate change in symptomatology over time. The BPRS was derived from a factor-analytic evaluation of two earlier scales: the Lorr Multidimensional Scale for Rating Psychiatric Patients (Lorr, Jenkins, & Holsopple, 1953) and the Lorr Inpatient Multidimensional Psychiatric Scale (Lorr, McNair, Klett, & Lasky, 1960). Eighteen symptom areas are rated on 7-point scales following a brief, unstructured interview. The symptom areas are Somatic Concern, Anxiety, Emotional Withdrawal, Conceptual Disorganization, Guilt Feelings, Tension, Mannerisms and Posturing, Grandiosity, Depressive Mood, Hostility, Suspiciousness, Hallucinatory Behavior, Motor Retardation, Uncooperativeness, Unusual Thought Content, Blunted Affect, Excitement, and Disorientation. The BPRS is intended for use by a trained clinician who makes ratings based on observations of the patient and the patient's verbal report. The 18 ratings of distinct symptom areas are summed to yield a "total pathology" score. Four composite "syndrome factor" scores can also be derived: Thought Disturbance, Withdrawal-Retardation, Hostility-Suspiciousness, and Anxiety-Depression (Overall & Klett, 1972). Brief descriptions of each symptom are provided on the BPRS rating form, and more detailed definitions are available in the original publication by Overall and Gorham (1962). Since its original development, the BPRS has undergone a number of revisions. Earlier versions contained 14 and 16 items.

The reliability of the BPRS is generally quite good. Overall and Gorham (1962), for example, reported interrater reliability coefficients ranging from .56 to .87, with an average of .78. The validity of the BPRS has been tested in several ways. In a study with 149 psychiatric patients by Zimmerman, Vestre, and Hunter (1975), the 16-item BPRS showed a canonical correlation of .65 with the Katz Adjustment Scales, .71 with the MMPI scales, .54 with global ratings of pathology by nurses, .61 with ratings by psychiatric residents, and .51 with patients' self-ratings. The BPRS has also been shown to be sensitive to clinical change. In a pharmacological outcome study with newly admitted schizophrenic patients, Hollister, Overall, Bennett, Kimbell, and Shelton (1965) reported significant treatment effects on 13 of the scales on the 16-item version of the BPRS and on all four syndrome factors. Also, the mean improvement of 28 points on the total pathology score reported by these authors represented "highly significant change" in the functioning of their patient sample.

Katz Adjustment Scale-Relative Form.   Although the use of trained, blind raters to obtain observations of patient or subject behavior is often recommended in order to maximize the objectivity of observational data, other methods of gathering independent ratings may sometimes be desirable. Significant others in the patient's life (e.g., husband, mother, or roommate) can often provide important observations that draw on their intimate knowledge of the patient's behavior. In this regard, the Katz Adjustment Scale-Relative Form (KAS-R) is a rating scale specifically designed to be completed by a knowledgeable informant (e.g., the parent of a schizophrenic patient) either independently or with the aid of a trained examiner (Katz & Lyerly, 1963). The instrument consists of 205 items covering a range of psychiatric symptomatology and social behavior. The informant rates the frequency and/or expected level of the patient's behavior on a 4-point scale for each. Eighteen separate scale scores are derived by summing the ratings of individual items. The 18 scales were identified through cluster analysis; they are Belligerence, Verbal Expansiveness, Negativism, Helplessness, Suspiciousness, Anxiety, Withdrawal and Retardation, General Psychopathology, Nervousness, Confusion, Bizarreness, Hyperactivity, Emotional Stability, Performance of Socially Expected Activities, Relative's Expectations of Performance, Performance of Free-Time Activities, Satisfaction with Free-Time Activities, and Satisfaction with Performance of Socially Expected Activities. The KAS-R is applicable to diverse ages, ranging from adolescents through geriatric patients. The time frame assessed is the past 3 weeks.

Crook, Hogarty, and Ulrich (1980) remarked that the KAS-R is the most widely used informant rating scale in mental health research. Nevertheless, data bearing on its psychometric properties are somewhat mixed. In one of the few studies concerned with the interrater reliability of the KAS-R, Parker and Johnston (1989) asked both parents of schizophrenic patients to complete the form at various periods. They found that agreement was extremely low when the patient was symptomatic but was more acceptable one month after discharge. On the other hand, Crook *et al.* (1980) reported generally good agreement between independent parent ratings of hospitalized schizophrenics.

With regard to validity information, an early study by Hogarty, Katz, and Lowery (1967) reported that all but 1 of the 18 KAS-R scales differentiated normal subjects from psychiatric day hospital patients. The results of several other studies found substantial agreement between KAS-R scores and postdischarge criterion measures such as relapse and probability of rehospitalization (Lyerly, 1973; Michaux, Katz, Kurland, & Gansereit, 1969). Still other studies reported significant changes in scale scores from pretreatment to follow-up, a finding suggesting that the measure is sensitive to clinical improvement (Lyerly, 1973; Michaux *et al.*, 1969). Finally, in a test of construct validity, Zimmerman *et al.* (1975) reported correlations between KAS-R scores and scores on the MMPI, the BPRS, the Psychotic Reaction Profile, and the Interpersonal Checklist (Family Form) that ranged between .53 and .87. However, KAS-R scores did not significantly correlate with global pathology ratings by nurses or psychiatry residents or with self-ratings by patients.

Unfortunately, there has been little effort to establish norms for particular patient groups, so the clinical significance of change scores may be difficult to determine. It is also unclear whether the results from self-report, relative informant, and interviewer-assisted administration are comparable. At the very least, however, the KAS-R provides important information regarding the family's attitudes toward the patient.

Global Adjustment Scale. The Global Adjustment Scale (GAS) is a 100-point rating scale of overall functioning (Endicott, Spitzer, Fleiss, & Cohen, 1976). Descriptive anchors are provided at 10-point intervals. The observer is to rate the subject's lowest level of functioning during the past week. Ratings may be based on direct observation, interview, or information provided by significant others. Outpatients typically attain scores between 31 and 70; inpatients typically score between 1 and 40. Scores above 70 are usually not obtained by persons who are receiving treatment (Endicott *et al.*, 1976). Endicott *et al.* reported interrater reliability coefficients ranging from .61 to .91 on interview ratings of inpatient and aftercare patients, and on ratings based on case notes. In a second study with a diagnostically heterogeneous inpatient sample, the interrater reliability coefficients ranged from .80 to .90 (Newman, 1980).

Evidence for the validity of GAS scores has also been reported. In their original article regarding the GAS, Endicott *et al.* (1976) reported moderate correlations between GAS scores and overall severity of illness scores from several other assessment measures, and between GAS scores and symptom dimensions on other measures. These correlations were typically higher at 6 months postadmission than at admission. Also, increases in GAS scores 3 months after the target admission were associated with decreasing readmission rates over the next 6 months. The GAS has been shown to be sensitive to treatment gains in schizophrenic (Meyer & King, 1980) and depressed patients (Van Putten & May, 1978).

The GAS is applicable to a wide range of patients and levels of functioning. However, only a portion of the scale is likely to be used by raters within any one study, or with any one type of patient. Within such a small range, the differentiation provided by the GAS may not be adequate for documenting differences between groups and/or changes over time. The GAS is simple for clinicians to use and results in easy data recording and statistical analysis.

DIRECT ASSESSMENT TECHNIQUES

The assessment strategies considered in the previous section are based on information provided by the patient. More direct *behavioral assessment* measures, based on observations of patient behavior, are also widely used. The field of behavioral assessment was originally developed as an alternative to the traditional diagnosis-based methods of psychiatric assessment. The purpose of behavioral assessment is not to diagnose clinical syndromes, but to identify the antecedents and consequences of maladaptive behavior. According to the behavioral philosophy on which this strategy is based, maladaptive behavior is generally maintained by the favorable consequences it produces (or the unfavorable consequences it avoids). For example, a patient's helpless and dependent interpersonal style may induce some family members to assume responsibility for tasks that the patient would prefer to avoid. Therefore, the patient is more likely to exhibit a greater degree of dependency in the presence of sympathetic relatives than in the presence of those who demand greater self-sufficiency. The most appropriate treatment intervention under these conditions would be directed not at changing characteristics of the patient *per se*, but at changing the environmental determinants of the problem behavior that have been identified through observational assessment.

In recent years, the once stark distinction between behavioral assessment and traditional diagnosis-based psychiatric assessment has become somewhat blurred. Originally, observational strategies were exclusively preferred in the behavioral assessment literature because they were, on the face of it, far more valid than alterative methods (such as self-report). However, an observational assessment necessarily records only a sample of behavior that may or may not be representative of the subject's behavior in general. Furthermore, different observers may not always agree about what they see. Thus, the reliability and validity of this approach, like those of any other assessment method, must be empirically documented (e.g., Hartmann, Roper, & Bradford, 1979).

Nelson (1988) observed that, for practical reasons, behavior therapists often follow a diagnostic strategy by default. For some problems, the same controlling variables are often identified through observational assessment (e.g., dependency maintained by the responses of significant others). For other problems, clinical outcome research reliably demonstrates the efficacy of a particular intervention (e.g., exposure therapy for the treatment of phobias). Under these conditions, the therapist may prefer to bypass the observational assessment phase designed to verify the hypothesized controlling variables and instead proceed directly to contingency management or exposure therapy once the "diagnosis" is made.

As a result of the shrinking gulf between behavioral and psychiatric assessment, the strategies derived from the two traditions are now commonly integrated. The addition of behavioral assessment strategies to the techniques considered earlier can provide an especially rich and detailed analysis of the patient's condition. As already indicated, the cornerstone of behavioral assessment is *observation*. Unlike self-report questionnaires and clinician rating scales (which gather data based on what the patient *says* about his or her performance), observational strategies attempt to measure what the patient actually does in different situations. The relevant observations of patient behavior may be taken in natural or in clinical analog settings.

Naturalistic Observation

Direct observation of a patient's behavior in his or her natural social environment is probably the method most closely identified with the field of behavioral assessment. It was one of the first techniques developed by behavior therapists, and it is well suited to both the precise measurement of maladaptive behavior and the elucidation of its possible environmental determinants. By directly observing the behavior of a depressed patient, for example, the therapist may be able to identify social skills deficits that lead to interpersonal conflict and rejection.

The technique of naturalistic observation is relatively simple in concept, but somewhat more difficult to apply. Foster, Bell-Dolan, and Burge (1988) provided a particularly detailed and comprehensive discussion of the advantages and disadvantages of this approach to assessment. The technique is generally more easily used on child populations, where observers have more ready access to natural social situations (e.g., the classroom). With regard to adults, this kind of access may be much more difficult. In the treatment of a sexual disorder, for example, many patients would be reluctant to agree to this method of assessment. Even if they did, the visible presence of trained observers may introduce *reactive* effects that invalidate otherwise accurate observations. Thus, for example, a couple may be much less likely to argue while an observer is present. For this reason, modified observational strategies are more often used to assess adult outpatients.

One innovative approach to dealing with the problems associated with naturalistic observation is the use of *participant observers*, that is, observers who are already part of the patient's social environment. To this end, couples have occasionally been trained to observe and record the clinically relevant behavior of their spouses (e.g., Floyd & Markman, 1983; Jacobson & Moore, 1981). Several spouse-observation instruments designed to facilitate this method of assessment have been shown to possess adequate psychometric properties (Margolin & Weiss, 1978; Markman, 1981). However, Floyd and Markman (1983) also showed that observations made by trained observers and spouses do not always coincide. Thus, although this approach to observational assessment provides a valuable "insider's" view of the dysfunctional system, it is clearly susceptible to subjective distortion. Therefore, participant observations should be only one component of a larger clinical assessment regimen.

Self-Observation and Self-Monitoring

A popular variant of participant observation is self-observation and self-monitoring. Indeed, because of its practical utility, asking patients to record their own behavior between sessions has become a standard component of behavioral assessment. In the study and treatment of agoraphobia, for example, patients are routinely asked to record their daily activities (e.g., where they traveled and how long they stayed) and to rate the intensity of any fear or panic attacks they have experienced (e.g., Arnow, Taylor, Agras, & Telch, 1985). Similarly, in the treatment of heterosocial anxiety and social phobia, therapists often ask patients to maintain a daily record of social behavior to monitor treatment progress (e.g., Heimberg, Madsen, Montgomery, & McNabb, 1980). The assumption underlying this procedure is that written records made when the targeted behavior occurs are considerably more accurate than in-session recall of the events occurring over the last week.

An important methodological concern often raised in the context of self-monitoring is, once again, the problem of *reactivity*, or the impact of self-monitoring on the measured behavior. An obese patient assigned the task of tracking food intake, for example, may start to eat less as soon as the measurements begin. Although such reactivity obviously complicates the acquisition of valid baseline measures, the direction of behavioral change is usually positive and several studies have attested to the therapeutic effect of this form of assessment (Stunkard, 1982). Because of the reliability and validity problems inherent in this approach, however, self-monitoring is almost never used alone. Two additional cost-effective observational strategies, one designed to measure the avoidance behavior associated with fear (the Behavioral Approach Test) and the other designed to evaluate the social deficits associated with a variety of psychiatric disorders (Behavioral Role Play), are often used to supplement self-monitoring.

Behavioral Approach Test

Developed in the early years of behavioral assessment, the Behavioral Approach Test (BAT) remains a standard tool for measuring the severity of a phobia. Although it has been used in various forms, this strategy basically involves a series of graded steps in which the patient and the feared object (e.g., a snake) are gradually moved closer together until the patient becomes uncomfortable. At that point, the test is terminated and the final distance between the patient and phobic object is recorded (e.g., Levis, 1969). The periodic use of this procedure provides an objective index of therapeutic gains, which should be reflected by a closer approach tolerance (i.e., decreased avoidance) as treatment progresses.

Strategies similar to the Behavioral Approach Test have been used with other anxiety patients, such as agoraphobics. The essential difference is that, instead of increasing her or his proximity to the feared object, the patient is instructed to proceed farther and farther away from a place of "safety." For example, Michelson, Mavissakalian, and Marchione (1985) routinely asked their agoraphobic patients to walk down the street away from the treatment clinic until they begin to experience anxiety. The distance the patient was able to walk provided the therapists with an initial baseline measure of phobic avoidance and, as treatment progresses, an index of the effects of intervention.

Mavissakalian and Hamann (1986) suggested that, contrary to earlier assumptions, the BAT may be less useful as a measure of avoidance *per se* and more useful as a means of obtaining *in vivo* measures of subjective anxiety and distress. In their study of female agoraphobics, they found that patients classified as "avoiders" or "nonavoiders" based on the BAT did not differ in their clinical characteristics or treatment responsiveness. One apparent reason for the lack of discriminant validity was that some patients avoided phobic situations entirely (experiencing minimal anxiety) and that others, perhaps because of intangible demand characteristics, tolerated the phobic situation despite intense apprehension and fear. A combined measure of both avoidance and subjective distress provided a more sensitive index of agoraphobic severity.

Behavioral Role Play

In the measurement of interpersonal behavior, a common alternative to naturalistic observation is role-play assessment, in which the patient and the therapist engage in a series of prearranged social interactions. In this way, the therapist gets an idea of the patient's performance in a range of social settings that would otherwise be impossible to obtain. In a typical test, a situation is described to the patient and the therapist (playing the role of another person in the scene) issues a verbal prompt. The patient is instructed to respond to the prompt as realistically as possible, and the therapist may then extend the interaction for one or two more exchanges. For example, the therapist might read the following scene description: "Imagine you are home watching television when your roommate walks in and changes the channel without asking. He says, 'Let's watch this channel for awhile.' " After the patient responds to this prompt, the therapist might continue; "You've been watching your shows all day. This one's better anyway." Again, the patient would respond as realistically as possible. These enactments can be videotaped and later scored for a variety of specific behavioral measures, including eye contact, voice quality, and gestures, or the therapist may simply gauge the patient's performance on a global basis after each scene is completed.

Role-play assessment has become a preferred method of evaluating the social performance of patients involved in social skills and assertiveness training. This method has also been used to evaluate the social competence of depressed patients, schizophrenics, and alcoholics, among others. A variety of standardized role-play tests have been devised for this purpose (e.g., St. Lawrence, 1987), beginning with the original Behavior Assertiveness Test (Eisler, Hersen, Miller, & Blanchard, 1975; Eisler, Miller, & Hersen, 1973). Typically, these tests consist of a series of specific scenes covering a range of social domains in which assertive behavior is appropriate (e.g., someone's cutting into the front of a line, or a waiter's presenting overcooked food).

One concern that has been raised about standardized role-play assessment is the extent to which performance under these conditions mirrors the patient's behavior under more natural conditions (Bellack, 1979, 1983). Indeed, initial empirical tests of this question were rather discouraging in that the concordance between role-play and *in vivo* performance was found to be low (e.g., Bellack, Hersen, & Turner, 1978). Improvements in the validity of this procedure have been obtained by using more extended role-play interactions and by personalizing role-play scenes to some degree rather than relying exclusively on standardized formats (Bellack, 1983). Ammerman and Hersen (1986) also found that manipulating subject *expectancies* may represent an important refinement of role-play assessment procedures. They found that a subject's social performance was strongly influenced by her or his expectation of the confederate's behavior (whose performance actually remained constant). When the confederate was expected to be "cold," the social performance of the subject declined. Although additional work of this kind may be needed to produce a truly sound procedure, role-play assessment in its current form often provides the practicing clinician with the only practical means of evaluating a patient's interpersonal behavior across a range of social situations.

The final observational strategy to be considered involves systematic observation of the patient during a diagnostic interview or therapy session. Although it is not widely practiced, several examples of this approach can be identified. Chamberlain, Patterson, Reid, Kavanagh, and Forgatch (1984) rated seven categories of resistant and cooperative responses made by patients during the course of therapy. They found that patients who eventually dropped out of therapy or who were referred to therapy by an external agency (as opposed to being self-referred) exhibited the highest levels of resistance. More recently, Bouhuys, Beersma, and Van den Hoofdakker (1987) coded six categories of patient behavior (e.g., head movements and gestures) during the administration of the Hamilton Depression Rating Scale. They found that the frequent occurrence of "relational" responses (e.g., looking, nodding, and gesturing) were predictive of subsequent treatment responsiveness, whereas "nonrelational" responses (e.g., random head movements) were predictive of minimal improvement. Although this approach is still in an early stage of development, the observation of responses found to be clinically significant can be readily integrated into existing clinician rating scales and standardized interviews. Indeed, some scales (e.g., the Motor Retardation subscale of the BPRS) already contain ratings based purely on observations of patient behavior.

SUMMARY

With the publication of the DSM-III-R just a few years ago and the publication of the DSM-IV just a few years away, the field of psychiatric assessment is in a state of rapid transition. Diagnostic categories introduced in the last edition may be modified or replaced altogether in the next. Indeed, some have argued that the official psychiatric taxonomy is changing faster than it can be empirically evaluated (e.g., Zimmerman, 1988). Nevertheless, the field's rapid evolution and increasing attention to empirical rigor may someday yield tests with the diagnostic accuracy of a laboratory blood assay. Until that time, we will be forced to rely on methods that are far less precise. Indeed, when exposed to the light of empirical scrutiny, none of the assessment techniques considered in this chapter emerges as a flawless measure of human nature. In view of the uncertainties associated with any single measure of psychopathology, the most reasonable solution is to use multiple assessment strategies whenever possible. Considering the field's current stage of development, the search for a consistent pattern of information across a variety of techniques represents the "state-of-the art."

REFERENCES

American Psychiatric Association. (1952). *Diagnostic and statistical manual of mental disorders* (1st ed.; DSM-I). Washington, DC: Author.

American Psychiatric Association. (1968). *Diagnostic and statistical manual of mental disorders* (2nd ed.; DSM-II). Washington, DC: Author.

American Psychiatric Association. (1980). *Diagnostic and statistical manual of mental disorders* (3rd ed.; DSM-III). Washington, DC: Author.

American Psychiatric Association. (1987). *Diagnostic and statistical manual of mental disorders* (3rd ed., rev.; DSM-III-R). Washington, DC: Author.

Ammerman, R. T., & Hersen, M. (1986). Effects of scene manipulation on role-play test behavior. *Journal of Psychopathology and Behavioral Assessment, 8,* 55–67.

Andreasen, N. C., Grove, W. M., Shapiro, R. W., Keller, M. B., Hirschfeld, R. M., & McDonald-Scott, P. (1981). Reliability of lifetime diagnosis. *Archives of General Psychiatry, 38,* 400–405.

Arnow, B. A., Taylor, C. B., Agras, W. S., & Telch, M. J. (1985). Enhancing agoraphobic treatment outcome by changing couple communication patterns. *Behavior Therapy, 16,* 452–467.

Baron, M., Asnis, L., & Gruen, R. (1981). The Schedule for Schizotypal Personalities (SSP): A diagnostic interview for schizotypal features. *Psychiatry Research, 4,* 213–228.

Beck, A. T., Ward, C. H., Mendelson, M., Mock, J. E., & Erbaugh, J. K. (1961). An inventory for measuring depression. *Archives of General Psychiatry, 4*, 561–571.

Bellack, A. S. (1979). A critical appraisal of strategies for assessing social skills. *Behavioral Assessment, 1*, 157–176.

Bellack, A. S. (1983). Recurrent problems in the behavioral assessment of social skills. *Behaviour Research and Therapy, 21*, 29–41.

Bellack, A. S., Hersen, M., & Turner, S. M. (1978). Role play tests for assessing social skill: Are they valid? *Behavior Therapy, 9*, 448–461.

Bouhuys, A. L., Beersma, D. G. M., & Van den Hoofdakker, R. H. (1987). Observed behaviors during clinical interviews predict improvement in depression. *Journal of Psychopathology and Behavioral Assessment, 9*, 13–33.

Brophy, C. J., Norvell, N. K., & Kiluk, D. J. (1988). An examination of the factor structure and convergent and discriminant validity of the SCL-90R in an outpatient population. *Journal of Personality Assessment, 52*, 334–340.

Butcher, J. N., Dahlstrom, W. G., Graham, J. R., Tellegen, A., & Kaemmer, B. (1989). *Manual for the restandarized Minnesota Multiphasic Personality Inventory: MMPI-2. An administrative and interpretive guide*. Minneapolis: University of Minnesota Press.

Chamberlain, P., Patterson, G., Reid, J. Kavanagh, K., & Forgatch, M. (1984). Observation of client resistance. *Behavior Therapy, 15*, 144–155.

Crook, J., Hogarty, G. E., & Ulrich, R. F. (1980). Interrater reliability of informant's ratings: Katz Adjustment Scale, R form. *Psychological Reports, 47*, 427–432.

Cyr, J. J., McKenna-Foley, M. M., & Peacock, E. (1985). Factor structure of the SCL-90R: Is there one? *Journal of Personality Assessment, 49*, 571–578.

Derogatis, L. R. (1977). *SCL-90 administration, scoring and procedures manual* (Vol. 1). Baltimore: Johns Hopkins University Press.

Derogatis, L. R. (1983). *SCL-90 administration, scoring and interpretation manual* (Vol. 2). Towson, MD: Clinical Psychometric Research.

Derogatis, L. R., Rickels, K., & Rock, A. F. (1976). The SCL-90 and the MMPI: A step in the validation of a new self-report scale. *British Journal of Psychiatry, 128*, 280–289.

DiNardo, P. A., O'Brien, G. T., Barlow, D. H., Waddel, M. T., & Blanchard, E. B. (1983). Reliability of DSM-III anxiety disorders using a new structured interview. *Archives of General Psychiatry, 40*, 1070–1074.

Dubro, A. F., & Wetzler, S. (1989). An external validity study of the MMPI personality disorder scales. *Journal of Clinical Psychology, 45*, 570–575.

Eisler, R. M., Miller, P., & Hersen, M. (1973). Components of assertive behavior. *Journal of Clinical Psychology, 29*, 295–288.,

Eisler, R. M., Hersen, M., Miller, P. M., & Blanchard, E. B. (1975). Situational determinants of assertive behavior; *Journal of Consulting and Clinical Psychology, 44*, 330–340.

Endicott, J., & Spitzer, R. L. (1978). A diagnostic interview: The Schedule for Affective Disorders and Schizophrenia. *Archives of General Psychiatry, 35*, 837–844.

Endicott, J., Spitzer, R. L., Fleiss, J. L., & Cohen, J. (1976). The Global Assessment Scale: A procedure for measuring overall severity of psychiatric disturbance. *Archives of General Psychiatry, 33*, 766–771.

Feighner, J. P., Robins, E., Guze, S. B. Woodruff, R. A., Winokur, G., & Monoz, R. (1972). Diagnostic criteria for use in psychiatric research. *Archives of General Psychiatry, 26*, 57–63.

Floyd, F. J., & Markman, H. J. (1983). Observational biases in spouse observation: Toward a cognitive/behavioral model of marriage. *Journal of Consulting and Clinical Psychology, 51*, 450–457.

Foster, S. L., Bell-Dolan, D. J., & Burge, D. A. (1988). Behavioral observation. In A. S. Bellack & M. Hersen (Eds.), *Behavioral assessment: A practical handbook* (3rd ed., pp. 119–160). New York: Pergamon Press.

Frances, A., Clarkin, J. F., Gilmore, M., Hurt, S. W., & Brown, R. (1984). Reliability of criteria for borderline personality disorder: A comparison of DSM-III and the Diagnostic Interview for Borderline Patients. *American Journal of Psychiatry, 141*, 1080–1083.

Garner, D. M., & Garfinkel, P. E. (1979). The Eating Attitudes Test: An index of the symptoms of anorexia nervosa. *Psychological Medicine, 9*, 273–279.

Graham, J. R. (1977). *The MMPI: A practical guide*. New York: Oxford University Press.

Gunderson, J. G., Kolb, J. E., & Austin, V. (1981). The Diagnostic Interview for Borderline Patients. *American Journal of Psychiatry, 138*, 896–903.

Hamilton, M. (1960). A rating scale for depression. *Journal of Neurology, Neurosurgery, and Psychiatry, 23*, 56–61.

Hanvik, L. J. (1951). MMPI profiles in patients with low back pain. *Journal of Consulting Psychology, 15*, 350–353.

Hartmann, D. P., Roper, B. L., & Bradford, D. C. (1979). Some relationships between behavioral and traditional assessment. *Journal of Behavioral Assessment, 1,* 3–19.

Hathaway, S. R., & McKinley, J. C. (1941). A multiphasic schedule (Minnesota): 1. Construction of the schedule. *Journal of Psychology, 10,* 249–254.

Heimberg, R.G., Madsen, C. H., Montgomery, D., & McNabb, C. E. (1980). Behavioral treatments for heterosocial problems: Effects on daily self-monitored and role-played interactions. *Behavior Modification, 4,* 147–172.

Helzer, J. E., Robins, L. N., Taibleson, M., Woodson, R. A., Reich, T., & Wish, E. D. (1977). Reliability of psychiatric diagnosis: 1. A methodological review. *Archives of General Psychiatry, 34,* 129–133.

Helzer, J. E., Robins, L. N., Croughan, J. L., & Welner, A. (1981). Renard Diagnostic Interview: Its reliability and procedural validity with physicians and lay interviewers. *Archives of General Psychiatry, 38,* 393–398.

Helzer, J. E., Robins, L. N., McEvoy, L. F., Spitznagel, E. L., Stolzman, R. K. Farmer, A., & Brockington, I. F. (1985). A comparison of clinical and Diagnostic Interview Schedule diagnoses: Physician reexamination of lay-interviewed cases in the general population. *Archives of General Psychiatry, 42,* 657–666.

Hogarty, G. E., Katz, M. M., & Lowery. H. A. (1967). Identifying candidates from a normal population for a community mental health program. In R. R. Monroe, G. D. Klee, & E. B. Brody (Eds.), *Psychiatric epidemiology and mental health planning.* Washington, DC: American Psychiatric Association.

Hollister, L. E., Overall, J. E., Bennett, J. L., Kimbell, I., & Shelton, J. (1965). Triperidol in newly admitted schizophrenics. *American Journal of Psychiatry, 122,* 96–98.

Hunsley, J., Hanson, R. K., & Parker, K. C. H. (1988). A summary of the reliability and stability of MMPI scales. *Journal of Clinical Psychology, 44,* 44–46.

Hurt, S. M., Hyler, S. E., Frances, A., Clarkin, J. F., & Brent, R. (1984). Assessing borderline personality disorder with self-report, clinical interview, or semistructured interview. *American Journal of Psychiatry, 141,* 1228–1231.

Hurt, S. W., Clarkin, J. F., & Morey, L. C. (1990). An examination of the stability of the MMPI personality disorder scales. *Journal of Personality Assessment, 54,* 16–23.

Hyler, S. E., & Rieder, R. O. (1987). *PDQ-R: Personality Diagnostic Questionnaire-Revised.* New York: New York State Psychiatric Institute.

Hyler, S. E., Lyons, M., Rieder, R. O., Young, L., Williams, J. B. W., & Spitzer, R. L. (1990). The factor structure of self-report DSM-III axis II symptoms and their relationship to clinicians' ratings. *American Journal of Psychiatry, 147,* 751–757.

Hyler, S. E., Skodol, A. E., Kellman, D., Oldham, J. M., & Rosnick, L. (1990). Validity of the Personality Diagnostic Questionnaire-Revised: Comparison with two structured interviews. *American Journal of Psychiatry, 147,* 1043–1048.

Jacob, T., Dunn, N. J., & Leonard, K. (1983). Patterns of alcohol abuse and family stability. *Alcoholism: Clinical and Experimental Research, 7,* 382–385.

Jacobson, N., & Moore, D. (1981). Spouses as observers of events in their relationship. *Journal of Consulting and Clinical Psychology, 49,* 269–277.

Katz, M. M., & Lyerly, S. B. (1963). Methods for measuring adjustment and social behavior in the community: 1. Rational, description, discriminative validity and scale development. *Psychological Reports, 13,* 503–535. (Monograph supplement 4-V13).

Levis, D. J. (1969). The phobic test apparatus: An objective measure of human avoidance behavior to small animals. *Behaviour Research and Therapy, 7,* 309–315.

Locke, H. J., & Wallace, K. M. (1959). Short-term marital adjustment and prediction tests: Their reliability and validity. *Journal of Marriage and Family Living, 21,* 251–255.

Lorr, M., Jenkins, R. L., & Holsopple, J. L. (1953). Multidimensional Scale for Rating Psychiatric Patients. *Veterans Administration Technical Bulletin, 10,* 507.

Lorr, M., McNair, D. M., Klett, C. J., & Lasky, J. J. (1960). A confirmation of nine postulated psychotic syndromes. *American Psychologist, 15,* 495.

Lyerly, S. B. (1973). *Handbook of psychiatric rating scales* (2nd ed.). Rockville, MD: National Institute of Mental Health.

MacAndrew, C. (1965). The differentiation of male alcoholic outpatients by means of the MMPI. *Quarterly Journal of Studies on Alcohol, 26,* 238–246.

MacAndrew, C. (1981). What the MAC scale tells us about alcoholics: An interpretive review. *Journal of Studies on Alcohol, 42,* 604–625.

Margolin, G., & Weiss, R. (1978). Comparative evaluation of the therapeutic components associated with behavioral marital treatments. *Journal of Consulting and Clinical Psychology, 46,* 1476–1486.

Markman, H. J. (1981). The prediction of marital distress: A five-year follow-up. *Journal of Consulting and Clinical Psychology, 49*, 760–762.

Matarazzo, J. D. (1983). The reliability of psychiatric and psychological diagnosis. *Clinical Psychology Review, 3*, 103–145.

Mavissakalian, M., & Hamann, M. S. (1986). Assessment and significance of behavioral avoidance in agoraphobia. *Journal of Psychopathology and Behavioral Assessment, 8*, 317–327.

McMahon, R., Flynn, P., & Davidson, R. (1985). Stability of the personality and symptom scales of the Millon Clinical Multiaxial Inventory. *Journal of Personality Assessment, 49*, 231–234.

Mellsop, G., Varghese, F., Joshua, S., & Hicks, A. (1982). The reliability of Axis II of DSM-III. *American Journal of Psychiatry, 139*, 1360–1361.

Meyer, J., & King, D. (1980, July). *Studying the reliability of clinician assessments of client mental health related problems.* Paper presented at the Region I Evaluation Conference, Durham, New Hampshire.

Michaux, W. W., Katz, M. M., Kurland, A. A., & Gansereit, K. H. (1969). *The first years out: Mental patients after hospitalization.* Baltimore: Johns Hopkins University Press.

Michelson, L., Mavissakalian, M., & Marchione, K. (1985). Cognitive-behavioral treatment of agoraphobia: Clinical, behavioral, and psychophysiological outcome. *Journal of Consulting and Clinical Psychology, 53*, 913–925.

Millon, T. (1983). *Millon Clinical Multiaxial Inventory manual* (3rd ed.). Minneapolis: National Computer Systems.

Millon, T. (1985). The MCMI provides a good assessment of DSM-III disorders: The MCMI-2 will prove even better. *Journal of Personality Assessment, 49*, 379–391.

Millon, T. (1987). *Manual for the Millon Clinical Multiaxial Inventory manual (MCMI-2).* Minneapolis: National Computer Systems.

Morey, L. C., Waugh, M. H., & Blashfield, R. K. (1985). MMPI scales for DSM-III personality disorders: Their derivation and correlates. *Journal of Personality Assessment, 49*, 245–251.

Nelson, R. O. (1988). Relationships between assessment and treatment within a behavioral perspective. *Journal of Psychopathology and Behavioral Assessment, 10*, 155–170.

Newman, F. L. (1980). Global scales: Strengths, uses and problems of global scales as an evaluation instrument. *Evaluation and Program Planning, 3*, 257–268.

Overall, J. E., & Gorham, D. R. (1962). The Brief Psychiatric Rating Scale. *Psychological Reports, 10*, 799–812.

Overall, J. E., & Klett, C. J. (1972). *Applied multivariate analysis.* New York: McGraw-Hill.

Parker, G., & Johnston, P. (1989). Reliability of parental reports using the Katz Adjustment Scales: Before and after hospital administration for schizophrenia. *Psychological Reports, 65*, 251–258.

Patrick, J. (1988). Concordance of the MCMI and the MMPI in the diagnosis of three DSM-III Axis I disorders. *Journal of Clinical Psychology, 44*, 186–190.

Perry, J. C., O'Connell, M. E., & Drake, R. (1984). An assessment of the Schedule for Schizotypal Personalities and the DSM-III criteria for diagnosing schizotypal personality disorder. *The Journal of Nervous and Mental Disease, 172*, 674–680.

Peveler, R. C., & Fairburn, C. G. (1990). Measurement of neurotic symptoms by self-report: Validity of the SCL-90R. *Psychological Medicine, 20*, 873–879.

Pope, H. G., Jonas, J. M., Hudson, J. L., Cohen, B. M., & Gunderson, J. G. (1983). The validity of DSM-III Borderline personality disorder. *Archives of General Psychiatry, 40*, 23–30.

Rachman, S., & Hodgson, R. (1980). *Obsessions and compulsions.* Englewood Cliffs, NJ: Prentice-Hall.

Rey, J. M., Stewart, G. W., Plapp, J. M., Bashir, M. R., & Richards, N. (1988). DSM-III Axis IV revisited. *American Journal of Psychiatry, 145*, 286–292.

Riskind, J. H., Beck, A. T., Berchick, R. J., Brown, G., & Steer, R. A. (1987). Reliability of DSM-III diagnoses for major depression and generalized anxiety disorder using the Structured Clinical Interview for DSM-III. *Archives of General Psychiatry, 44*, 817–820.

Robins, L. N., Helzer, J. E., Croughan, J., & Ratcliff, K. S. (1981). National Institute of Mental Health Diagnostic Interview Schedule: Its history, characteristics, and validity. *Archives of General Psychiatry, 38*, 381–389.

Robins, L. N., Helzer, J. E., Ratcliff, K. S., & Seyfried, W. (1982). Validity of the Diagnostic Interview Schedule, Version II: DSM-III diagnoses. *Psychological Medicine, 12*, 885–870.

St. Lawrence, J. S. (1987). Assessment of assertion. In M. Hersen, R. M. Eisler, & P. M. Miller (Eds.), *Progress in behavior modification* (Vol. 1, pp. 152–190). Newbury Park, CA: Sage.

Schrader, G., Gordon, M., & Harcourt, R. (1986). The usefulness of DSM-III Axis IV and Axis V assessments. *American Journal of Psychiatry, 143*, 904–907.

Skodol, A. E., & Shrout, P. E. (1989). Use of DSM-III Axis IV in clinical practice: Rating etiologically significant stressors. *American Journal of Psychiatry, 146,* 61–66.

Spanier, G. B. (1976). Measuring dyadic adjustment: New scales for assessing the quality of marriage and similar dyads. *Journal of Marriage and the Family, 38,* 15–28.

Spielberger, C., Gorsuch, A., & Lushene, R. (1970). *The State-Trait Anxiety Inventory.* Palo Alto, CA: Consulting Psychologists Press.

Spitzer, R. L. (1983). Psychiatric diagnosis: Are clinicians still necessary? *Comprehensive Psychiatry, 24,* 399–411.

Spitzer, R. L., & Williams, J. B. W. (1985). *Structured Clinical Interview for DSM-III—Psychotic Disorders Version.* New York: Biometrics Research Department, New York State Psychiatric Institute.

Spitzer, R. L., & Williams, J. B. W. (1988). Revised diagnostic criteria and a new structured interview for diagnosing anxiety disorders. *Journal of Psychiatric Research, 22,* 54–85.

Spitzer, R. L., Endicott, J., & Robins, E. (1978). Research diagnostic criteria. *Archives of General Psychiatry, 35,* 773–782.

Spitzer, R. L., Williams, J. B. W., & Gibbon, M. (1987). *Structured Clinical Interview for DSM-III-R (SCID).* New York: New York State Psychiatric Institute.

Stangl, D., Pfohl, B., Zimmerman, M., Bowers, W., & Corenthal, C. (1985). A structured interview for the DSM-III personality disorders. *Archives of General Psychiatry, 42,* 591–596.

Stunkard, A. J. (1982). Obesity. In A. S. Bellack, M. Hersen, & A. E. Kazdin (Eds.), *International handbook of behavior modification and therapy* (pp. 535–573). New York: Plenum Press.

Van Putten, T., & May, P. R. (1978). Subjective response as a predictor of outcome in psychotherapy: The consumer has a point. *Archives of General Psychiatry, 35,* 477–480.

Wetzler, S. (1990). The Millon Clinical Multiaxial Inventory (MCMI): A review. *Journal of Personality Assessment, 55,* 445–464.

Widiger, T. A., Williams, J. B. W., Spitzer, R. L., & Frances, A. J. (1985). The MCMI as a measure of DSM-III. *Journal of Personality Assessment, 49,* 366–378.

Widiger, T. A., Frances, A. J., Pincus, H. A., & Davis, W. W. (1990). DSM-IV literature reviews: Rationale, process, and limitations. *Journal of Psychopathology and Behavioral Assessment, 12,* 189–202.

Wilson, J. H., Taylor, P. J., & Robertson, G. (1985). The validity of the SCL-90 in a sample of British men remanded to prison for psychiatric reports. *British Journal of Psychiatry, 147,* 400–403.

Wolpe, J., & Lazarus, A. A. (1966). *Behavior therapy techniques.* New York: Pergamon Press.

Woodruff, R. A., Jr., Goodwin, D. W., & Guze, S. B. (1974). *Psychiatric diagnosis.* New York: Oxford University Press.

Zimmerman, M. (1988). Why are we rushing to publish DSM-IV? *Archives of General Psychiatry, 45,* 1135–1138.

Zimmerman, R. L., Vestre, N. D., & Hunter, S. H. (1975). Validity of family informants' ratings of psychiatric patients: General validity. *Psychological Reports, 37,* 619–630.

5

Psychiatric Assessment and Diagnosis

Children

MARTIN J. LUBETSKY

INTRODUCTION

It is only since the early 1970s that children and adolescents have been diagnosed with psychiatric disorders as described in the American Psychiatric Association's *Diagnostic and Statistical Manuals*. These diagnostic criteria have been expanded and revised four times to keep up with the progress in research in child and adolescent psychiatry. The expanding knowledge of child development, neurology, pharmacology, genetics, maternal and infant health, epidemiology, and adult disorders has led to a growth in the understanding of childhood disorders. In order to diagnose accurately, one must be able to assess the history, course, and presentation of symptoms, including the biological, medical, psychosocial, family, and school areas. Therefore, this chapter reviews a selection of the currently available methods for assessing behavioral and psychiatric problems in children and adolescents as they are commonly seen in a psychiatric setting. The major categorization of psychiatric disorders in children and adolescents is presented.

Historically, little child and adolescent psychopathology was covered in the psychiatric diagnostic literature before the Group for the Advancement of Psychiatry (GAP) publication in 1966. The GAP elaborated on deviations in childhood development and focused on psychopathology, including the categories of psychoneurotic, personality, and psychophysiological disorders. Preceding this document, the original *Diagnostic and Statistical Manual of Mental Disorders* (DSM-I) of the American Psychiatric Association (APA, 1952) reported only a few child or adolescent categories, such as adjustment reactions and schizophrenia. Following the GAP publication, the second edition of the *Diagnostic and Statistical Manual* (DSM-II; APA, 1968) included behavioral disorders of childhood and adolescence, adjustment reactions, and childhood schizophrenia. However, there were still few diagnostic groups and criteria on which

MARTIN J. LUBETSKY • Western Psychiatric Institute and Clinic, University of Pittsburgh School of Medicine, Pittsburgh, Pennsylvania 15213.

Handbook of Behavior Therapy in the Psychiatric Setting, edited by Alan S. Bellack and Michel Hersen. Plenum Press, New York, 1993.

to base decision making, and formulations were mostly theoretical. Then, in 1980, the third edition of the manual (DSM-III) provided a much improved framework of diagnostic criteria based on research findings. Included now were mental retardation, pervasive developmental disorders, and specific language and academic disorders; conduct disorders; oppositional disorder; attention deficit disorder; anxiety disorders; and eating disorders. In addition, the DSM-III provided an axis system for evaluating dysfunction. Axis I pertained to clinical psychiatric syndromes, Axis II dealt with developmental disorders and personality disorders, Axis III included the physical disorders and conditions, Axis IV was an index of the severity of psychosocial stressors, and Axis V listed the highest level of adaptive functioning in the past year.

In 1987, the APA published a revision (DSM-III-R) that incorporated research findings that allowed a reevaluation and expansion of diagnostic criteria. The purpose of this revision was to provide a better framework within which the clinician could assess symptoms, their duration, the course of the illness, and the family history, as well as a decision tree of alternative diagnoses. Some of the changes in DSM-III-R included moving all developmental disorders to Axis II (mental retardation, pervasive developmental disorders, specific language and academic disorders); combining infantile autism and pervasive developmental disorder (childhood onset) into autistic disorder; replacing atypical categories with "Not Otherwise Specified"; revising attention deficit disorder with or without hyperactivity to attention deficit-hyperactivity disorder; and altering subtypes of conduct disorders. Other revisions and clarifications in diagnoses are discussed later in this chapter.

PSYCHIATRIC ASSESSMENT AND DIAGNOSIS

Assessment is the process of gathering data in order to determine diagnoses and, consequently, treatment recommendations. This assessment process has undergone many changes over the years as a consequence of varying theoretical perspectives, diagnostic classification revisions, and research trials. The assessment should identify distinguishing characteristics that will allow a clustering of symptoms into operationalized categories in a reliable and valid manner. Thus, the process of evaluation involves many modalities of data gathering and presents the clinician with a vast and often confusing array of choices.

Assessment or evaluation of psychiatric/psychological/behavioral symptoms may take on different forms depending on the theoretical perspectives used (Achenbach & Edelbrock, 1989). A psychodynamic clinician considers personality development, the influence of damaging or confusing early experiences, defense mechanisms, and the patient's ability to develop an intimate and corrective therapeutic relationship (Bruch, 1974). This information is based on or inferred from extensive clinical interviews and, possibly, projective testing. A behaviorally oriented evaluator assesses specific behaviors, their antecedents, and their consequences by making direct observations, gathering specific behavioral data from the natural environment, and using behavioral rating scales. A family therapist explores the dynamics, structure, and development of the family to learn how the child's symptoms are symptomatic of disturbed family functioning. A physician uses the medical model, eliciting symptoms and signs through history taking, examination, and laboratory testing, to infer specific disease processes. A psychometrician thinks in quantitative terms and assesses with standardized tests. A clinician using a biopsychosocial model assesses aspects of many spheres: biological, medical, and genetic; psychiatric, psychological, and behavioral; interpersonal and family; and environmental, work, and school, as well as child development in all of these areas.

In following any of these aforementioned perspectives for assessing children and adolescents, one must consider the developmental process. Symptoms affect development, and developmental problems lead to symptoms (Cox & Rutter, 1985). For example, Rutter (1975, 1980) stated that children behave, think, and interact differently at different ages. Therefore, to assess a child adequately, it is necessary to know what is normal and abnormal for that child's age. In addition, the psychiatric disturbance may have interfered with the normal course of biopsychosocial development. The stresses inherent in each phase of development may produce normal or abnormal responses (Rutter, 1981). Thus, in order to assess a child's history and present symptoms, it is necessary to have a knowledge of the developmental process, its stresses, and its normal and abnormal variations.

Another requirement of assessing symptoms is an awareness of the child epidemiological and longitudinal study data that provide guidelines for evaluation (Rutter, 1982). Shepherd, Oppenheim, and Mitchell (1971) summarized findings that lead to better assessment, and therefore to the likelihood of identifying a psychiatric disorder. These elements include the number, frequency, duration, and severity of the symptoms; the abnormality of the behavior in relation to age and sex norms; and the circumstances in which the behavior occurs. Rutter, Tizard, and Whitmore (1970) showed that knowing which behaviors are better indicators of a disorder lead to a more competent evaluation. In addition, Rutter, Graham, Chadwick, and Yule (1976) reported that epidemiological findings have shown only moderate agreement among different informants about the same child. Moreover, there appears to be situation specificity for some behaviors. Therefore, information must be gathered from several sources in different settings; that is, at least from the child, the parents, and the school (Kazdin, 1983). Also, observation should be made with the child alone and with the other major caregivers, as well as in natural settings if possible (Young, Leven, Ludman, Kisnadwala, & O'Brien, 1990).

Categories of Assessment

The next consideration in assessment is choosing the type of interview. As previously described, this choice may be based on the clinician's theoretical perspective, and experience; epidemiological data; the situation; the client's age, cognitive functioning, and developmental level; the severity of the behavioral disturbance; the purpose or objective of the evaluation; and the type of information desired. As outlined by Young *et al.* (1990), the clinical interview is the primary source of the information used to determine the diagnosis and to guide treatment. One type of interview is the *unstructured* or *nondirective* approach used to explore conflicts, defenses, and conscious and unconscious components, in order to facilitate the treatment process (Goldblatt, 1972). A second style of interview is the directed method, in which the evaluator chooses specific topics and covers them within an assigned time period. The time limit requires persistent interruption and redirection to stay focused on the task in order to complete the necessary data base of information.

A third category of technique is the *structured* interview, in which the format, topics, and sequence are predetermined (Edelbrock & Costello, 1990). The questions are specified so that interviewer bias does not influence the outcome. The answers are limited to those choices listed, rather than being open-ended. One example of a highly structured interview is the Diagnostic Interview for Children and Adolescents (DICA) used in clinical and epidemiological research. The DICA was first developed in 1969 and was revised in 1981 (see Welner, Reich, Herjanic, Jung, & Amado, 1987, for a review). The DICA produces information on the presence or absence of more than 150 specific symptoms, as well as their severity, onset, duration, and associated impairments. There are child (DICA-C) and parent (DICA-P) versions. Another example of the structured interview is the Diagnostic Interview Schedule for Children (DISC) sponsored by the National Institute of Mental Health for epidemiological studies of child and adolescent psychopathology (see Costello, Edelbrock, Kalas, Kessler, & Klaric, 1982). Both child (DISC-C) and parent (DISC-P) versions have been developed. The DISC and the DICA are similar in purpose and structure in that each covers a broad range of symptoms and diagnoses and is suitable for use by professional and trained lay interviewers.

A fourth category of evaluation is the *semistructured* interview, which is similar to the structured interview but allows for individual differences (Edelbrock & Costello, 1990). The less structured areas allow the interviewer to start with specific topics or symptoms and to expand on them as necessary. One example of this kind of interview is the Kiddie-SADS or K-SADS (Schedule for Affective Disorders and Schizophrenia for School Age Children [6–18 years]; Puig-Antich & Chambers, 1978). The K-SADS is designed to assess current psychopathology focused on affective disorders, but it also includes conduct disorders, separation anxiety, phobias, attention deficits, and obsessions-compulsions. First, the parent is interviewed about the child; then the child is seen, and any discrepancies between parent and child reports are addressed. The interview begins with unstructured rapport building and an assessment of the presenting problems, continues with structured sections that cover specific symptoms by asking model questions, and then follows with unstructured questioning about symptoms to substantiate the ratings. The K-SADS-E is an epidemiological version for assessing lifetime psychopathology (Orvaschel, Puig-Antich, Chambers, Tabrizi, & Johnson, 1982).

Another example of a semistructured interview is the Interview Schedule for Children (ISC; Kovacs, 1982). It is for children aged 8–17 and their parents and focuses on current symptoms of depression. This instrument is available in two forms: one for initial clinical assessment and the other for follow-up. A third semistructured interview for children, aged 7–12, is the Child Assessment Schedule (CAS; Hodges, Kline, Stern, Cytryn, & McKnew, 1982). It has both a child and a parent version and was developed to facilitate the evaluation of a child and to aid in diagnostic formulation. It is a descriptive tool requiring clinical inference and did not originally incorporate the DSM criteria.

A fifth category of assessment is *formal* or *psychological* testing. Cronbach (1984) defined a test as a "systematic procedure for observing behavior and describing it with the aid of numerical scales or fixed categories" (p. 26). Psychometrics is the method of objectively administering, scoring, and interpreting tests. However, the person responsible for testing also assesses through interviewing, observing, and rating in combination with test results (Goldstein & Hersen, 1990).

One example of formal testing is *intelligence testing*. Intelligence tests not only give a numerical IQ score but allow the tester to examine cognitive processes, problem-solving skills, and language and nonverbal abilities (Goldstein & Hersen, 1990). The more commonly used intelligence tests for children are administered to identify special needs, to assist in school placement, and to act as an adjunct to clinical assessment (Perlman & Kaufman, 1990). A selection of tests is summarized in Perlman and Kaufman (1990), and in Achenbach and McConaughy (1987). The Wechsler Intelligence Scale for Children—Revised (WISC-R; Wechsler, 1974) is used for approximately ages 6–16 and yields three separate IQ scores, on the Verbal Scale, the Performance Scale, and the Full Scale. The Stanford-Binet, Fourth Edition (Thorndike, Hagen, & Sattler, 1986) is used for approximately ages 2 years to adults and yields scores on verbal reasoning, quantitative reasoning, abstract-visual reasoning, and short-term memory, as well as a composite score. The Kaufman Assessment Battery for Children (K-ABC; Kaufman & Kaufman, 1983) is used for ages 2½ to 12½. It yields four scales: two mental processing scales, a composite processing scale, and an achievement composite. The Bayley Scales of Infant Development (Bayley, 1969) are used for ages 2–30 months. It yields three scores: the Mental Developmental Index Standards score, the Psychomotor Developmental Index Standard score, and the Infant Behavioral Record. The McCarthy Scales of Children's Abilities (MSCA; McCarthy, 1972) are used for ages 2½ to 8½ years. They are 18 subtests grouped into six overlapping scales: Verbal, Quantitative, Perceptual-Performance, General Cognitive, Memory, and Motor. The Peabody Picture Vocabulary Test—Revised (PPVT-R; Dunn & Dunn, 1981) is used for ages 2½ years to adult and tests receptive language. The Slosson Intelligence Test (SIT; Slosson, 1983) is used for ages 2–18 years and, in 10–15 minutes, yield an estimate of intelligence on the basis of language production. The Vineland Adaptive Behavior Scales (Vineland; Sparrow, Balla, & Cicchetti, 1984) has eight categories of behavior related to

Social Competence. It is available in three forms, including the Survey and Expanded Forms for ages birth to 18 years 11 months, or the form for low-functioning adults, and the Classroom Edition for ages 3–12 years 11 months. The Wechsler Primary and Preschool Intelligence Scale (WPPSI; Wechsler, 1967) is used for ages 4–6½ years and yields a Verbal Comprehension Perceptual Organization factor.

Another example of formal evaluation is *achievement testing*. Such tests were developed to provide a standardized assessment are categorized as (1) group-administered; (2) individually administered; and (3) modality-specific (i.e., reading, math, etc.) (Katz & Slomka, 1990). Mitchell (1983) reported that over 2,672 standardized tests are in use. The testing approach today is based on the continuum of a learning model so that the assessment focuses on success rather than failure. The achievement test is used to obtain general academic skill competencies, individual performance in a specific area, and a measure of the "degree of learning" (Katz & Slomka, 1990). The screening battery or survey test allows a comparison of individual performances across diverse subjects and reflects both strengths and deficits. The content-focused diagnostic achievement tests are administered after an area of deficit is identified on a screening achievement test and examine more extensively that factors contributing to the academic dysfunction. In clinical use, these tests aid in assessing an individual's capacity to apply knowledge or native intelligence in practical problem-solving situations (Katz & Slomka, 1990).

Katz and Slomka (1990) provided a brief categorization of commonly used achievement tests. Group-administered achievement tests include the California Achievement Tests (CTB/ McGraw Hill, 1984), the Iowa Tests of Basic Skills (Hieronymus, Hoover, Lindquist *et al.*, 1978), the Metropolitan Achievement Tests (Balow, Farr, Hogan, & Prescott, 1978), the Stanford Achievement Test (Gardner, Rudman, Karlson, & Merwin, 1982), and the SRA Achievement Series (Naslynd, Thorpe, & Lefever, 1978). Individually administered achievement tests include Basic Achievement Skills Individual Screening (BASIS; Psychological Corporation, 1983), the Kaufman Test of Educational Achievement (Kaufman & Kaufman, 1985), the Peabody Individual Achievement Test—Revised (PIAT-R; Markwarat, 1989), the Wide Range Achievement Test (WRAT; Jastak & Wilkinson, 1984), and the Woodcock-Johnson Psychoeducational Battery (Woodcock, 1977). There are many modality-specific achievement tests: for reading the Classroom Reading Inventory (Silvaroli, 1986), the Durrell Analysis of Reading Difficulty (Durrell & Catterson, 1980), and others; for math the Enright Diagnostic Inventory of Basic Arithmetic Skills (Enright, 1983), the Key Math Diagnostic Arithmetic Test (Connolly, Nachtman, & Pritchett, 1971), and others. Thus, achievement tests can be used for (1) screening, to identify students potentially eligible for remedial programming; (2) classification and placement, to ascertain specific academic deficiencies; (3) prescriptive intervention, to make curriculum adjustments based on specific deficits; and (4) program evaluation, to evaluate the benefits of special programming (Katz & Slomka, 1990).

Another example of formal testing is a *neuropsychological assessment battery*. A neuropsychological test assesses performance change in cognitive, perceptual, and motor skills when brain function changes (Goldstein, 1990). Neuropsychological testing in children is appropriate if inherent cognitive problems contribute to a child's behavioral or psychiatric disturbance (Taylor & Fletcher, 1990). Taylor and Fletcher (1990) reviewed the "biobehavioral systems" approach to neuropsychological evaluation, in which a multifactorial framework is used to evaluate environmental, psychosocial, and developmental influences. Taylor and Fletcher emphasized that, rather than attempt a differential diagnosis of emotional and organic disorders, the biobehavioral systems approach focuses on an evaluation of the developing cognitive and behavioral skills associated with the disability in question.

The use of this neuropsychological assessment process with children involves, first, an analysis of the developmental disability through history, record review, checklist completion, parent and teacher interviews, and observations with specific testing (Rourke, Fisk, & Strang, 1986).

Second, the assessment includes cognitive testing of (1) intelligence; (2) language abilities; for example, the Peabody Picture Vocabulary Test (Dunn & Dunn, 1981), the Expressive One Word Picture Vocabulary Test (Gardner, 1979), and the Sequenced Inventory of Communication Development (Hedrick, Prather, & Tobin, 1975); (3) visual-spatial and constructional performance; for example, the Bender-Gestalt (Koppitz, 1964) and the Beery Test of Visual-Motor Integration (Beery, 1982); (4) somatosensory and motor functions; for example, the Bruininks-Oseretsky Test of Motor Proficiency (Bruininks, 1978); (5) attentional resources; for example, the Continuous Performance Test (Lindgren & Lyons, 1984); (6) memory and learning skills, for example, the Benton Visual Retention Test (Benton, 1974); and (7) problem solving and abstract reasoning, evaluated on subtests of several assessment batteries.

Third, the neuropsychological assessment model evaluates psychosocial functioning.

Fourth is the exploration of potential environmental influences, such as cultural values, language background, social and educational opportunities, parental attitudes, and family stressors.

Fifth is a review of evidence of any biological influence on the disability. This review encompasses a neurological and medical history, a physical examination, and laboratory and radiological testing. The child is still developing, and testing may change with development. Benton (1973) found that many children referred for neuropsychological examination do not have the definitive brain damage that may be found in adults.

The sixth part of this process, is the interpretation and management of the problems.

A final example of formal testing is *objective personality assessment*. This area has been controversial and has been better described in adults. One example is the Vineland Adaptive Behavior Scales (VABS; Sparrow *et al.*, 1984) used to assess adaptive and social abilities in a developmental context. Another instrument is the Personality Inventory for Children (PIC; Goldman, Stein, & Guerry, 1983).

A sixth category of assessment is the *behavioral evaluation*, in which an empirical approach "based on observations of experience" is conducted (Woolf, 1977). Such an empirically based behavioral assessment does not depend on any specific theory about the etiology of the behavior (Achenbach & Edelbrock, 1989). Ollendick and Hersen (1984) expanded on the definition of child behavioral assessment by describing it as, "an exploratory, hypothesis-testing process in which a range of specific procedures is used in order to understand a given child, group, or social ecology, and to formulate and evaluate specific intervention strategies" (p. 6). Ollendick and Greene (1990) concurred that child behavioral assessment must have a developmental, age-appropriate context; normative comparisons to ensure that change in behavior is related to treatment, not to normal developmental change; a knowledge of the context in which the child's behavior occurs and the function that it serves; and a multimethod assessment approach. In further defining behavioral assessment, Hersen (1973) referred to examining the triad of motoric, physiological, and self-report systems, when carrying out a fully comprehensive evaluation.

Many behavioral assessment schemes have been developed since the early 1960s. Kanfer and Grimm (1977) organized a review of patient symptoms into five categories: (1) behavioral deficiencies; (2) behavioral excesses; (3) inappropriate environmental stimulus control; (4) inappropriate self-generated stimulus control; and (5) reinforcement contingencies that cause problems. Lazarus (1973) proposed a comprehensive assessment scheme that incorporates seven elements: B = behavior; A = affect; S = sensation; I = imagery; C = cognition; I = interpersonal relationship; and D = drugs that are needed for pharmacological intervention. Wolpe (1977) documented the need to evaluate antecedents of behaviors in order to develop appropriate treatment strategies.

Achenbach and Edelbrock (1989) proposed the following rules for devising an empirically based behavioral assessment: (1) standardize procedures; (2) use multiple items to sample each aspect; (3) use items that provide quantitative scores for each aspect; (4) norm the scores for comparison; (5) take development or age into consideration when forming normative reference groups; and (6) use assessment procedures that are reliable, valid, and psychometrically sound. Following these principles, Achenbach and Edelbrock (1983) developed the Child Behavior Checklist (CBCL), comprising 20 social competence items and 118 behavior problems items, to assess child psychopathology. Parents of children aged 4–16 can complete this checklist in less than 20 minutes. This rating tool provides quantitative descriptions of behavioral problems and competencies through parental reports. Additional versions include Teacher Report and Youth Self-Report (ages 11–18). The CBCL is a useful instrument for assessing child psychopathology because it combines a behavioral perspective with DSM-III diagnostic categories and multiaxial information gathering.

Many other behavioral assessment instruments are available. For example, additional rating scales or checklists include the Behavior Problem Checklist—Revised (Quay & Peterson, 1983) and the Home Situations Questionnaire (HSQ; Barkley, 1981). Self-report instruments have been developed such as the Children's Depression Inventory (CDI; Kovacs, 1985). In addition, by self-monitoring, the child may observe and record the target behavior at the time it occurs. Finally, direct behavioral observation in the natural environment or in controlled simulated settings provides an informative accounting of the target behavior selected for modification.

Psychiatric Interview

The psychiatric interview combines many of the assessment styles or schemes already mentioned. An interview with a child has several special features. First, the child may not view herself or himself as having a problem at all; rather, she or he may see the parent or school as creating the problem. Second, the child may view the clinician in a mental health setting not as being in a helping role, but as being an ally of the parent or the school. Third, the agenda for the evaluation may not be specific and may be different for the parent, school, or mental agency. Fourth, the child's developmental, social, sexual, emotional, and intellectual level must be considered in the interview and evaluation.

A complete model for diagnostic interviews incorporates the child interview, the parent interview, and the family interview. Initially, the clinician may interview the parents, before the child or the family as a whole, in order to gather specific details that are sensitive or disturbing to the child or to the rest of the family. However, seeing the family first may provide much information about how the family interacts, how symptoms develop, how defensive strategies are used, and how family members react to stress. One clinician may see the child while another worker gathers history from the parents. Young children may be reassured by the presence of their parents during the initial interview. However, young children may fear disclosing certain information in front of their parents. It is common to interview adolescents alone and before their parents are interviewed, to reassure them that their opinion is taken seriously (Hill, 1985).

Sometimes, a physical examination is necessary in addition to the medical history. For example, a developmentally disabled child with mental retardation or autistic disorder, an anxious or depressed child with physical symptoms, or a highly somatic child should have a complete physical exam and laboratory work-up (if needed) in order to rule out any organic causes or contributions. For any child seen, it is necessary to clarify who is the primary medical caregiver and when the last physical exam occurred.

An Outline of Assessment and Diagnosis

It is helpful to follow an outline in working with a child client. The basic outline should include the *history* (usually from parents and records), the *mental status exam* (interviews with the child and the parents), a *family interview, additional information* (i.e., school reports and past psychiatric or medical records), a *diagnostic formulation* (the synthesis and integration of the information gathered), a *differential diagnosis* (using the five axes of the DSM-III-R), and a *treatment plan* (with recommendations).

History.   The following information is obtained through parental interviews, parental questionnaires, previous reports or records, and child interviews: (1) identifying information, such as age; (2) the chief complaint, the reason for referral, and the expectations of the assessment; (3) a history of the presenting problem, with specific details of duration, frequency, intensity, precipitant, consequences, coping or problem-solving skills, treatment attempts, disciplinary methods, and order of problem severity if there are several presenting problems; (4) a past psychiatric history, including previous treatment, psychotropic medication, and hospitalization; (5) strengths in the child as noted by the parents; (6) the child's psychodevelopmental history, including any perinatal problems (i.e., prenatal, birth, and postnatal), early infancy, milestones achieved at each developmental stage, and psychosocial stressors that may have influenced the developmental process; (7) school history from day care and preschool through grade levels, including any early intervention and academic achievements or failures; (8) a social history, including relationships with peers and adults (i.e., teachers, parents, and friends); drug, alcohol, and cigarette use; and sexual history; (9) a family history, including family members and their relationships with each other, family coping or problem-solving skills, family stressors, and a genetic history of any psychiatric or major medical illness; and (10) a medical history, including chronic illness, hospitalization, surgery, medications, medication reactions, and allergies.

Mental Status Exam.   Mental status information is obtained through child interview and observation, child self-reporting forms, previous reports or records, and parent interview. Portions of the information are similar to the information obtained in a review of symptoms or systems in a medical evaluation. The type of child interview is determined by the child's age, developmental level, language, social skills, and cooperation. A play interview is necessary for children younger than age 7, for children with developmental delay, or for older children who are not openly verbal about disturbing issues (Young *et al.*, 1990). Play is a child's work and "natural discourse" and, in revealing both content and process, provides useful information (Simmons, 1981). The interviewer is both an observer and a participant, eliciting the child's thoughts, feelings, fantasies, coping skills, and social skills. Hill's outline of the mental status exam (1985) includes the major topical areas of general appearance, parent-child interaction, emotion, thought content, social interaction, language, motor activity, and cognition. The format of the mental status exam is as follows:

1. Appearance
2. Attitude
3. Motor behavior
4. Speech and language
5. Reading and writing
6. Orientation
7. General information
8. Memory
9. Cognition and attention span
10. Abstracting ability
11. Intelligence (estimate)
12. Thought content and form
13. Hallucinations
14. Mood/affect
15. Symptom review (i.e., asking parents and child); one organized approach is to use the DSM-III-R categories:

a. Depression—sleep, appetite, energy, enjoyment, concentration, play, stressors, peer relationships, school
b. Mania—irritability, lability, hyperactivity, anger
c. Lethality—suicidality or homicidality: anger, hopelessness, helplessness, wish dead, wish not born, plan, attempts
d. Anxiety—fears, phobias, separation issues, peer relationships, obsessions, compulsions
e. Attention, distractibility, impulsivity, hyperactivity
f. Oppositionality, noncompliance, defiance, rule violation, legal involvement, destructiveness, aggressiveness
g. Image perception, eating patterns, weight changes
h. Communicative intent, quality of social interactions, symbolic play, stereotypies, self-injurious behavior
i. Tics, twitches (vocal and motor)
j. Abuse (physical, sexual, and neglect)
k. Insight and judgment

Family Evaluation. Observation of and interaction with the family are necessary if the clinician is to assess family structure, interactions, dynamics, and conflict resolution, as well as the role of the identified patient. The family process may be a vital link in resolving the identified problems or sustaining them. It is important to learn about family strengths, knowledge or understanding of the identified disorder, and willingness to participate in treatment. If the discussion is not productive or the children are too young to tolerate prolonged questioning, other creative means of assessment can be used. For example, the family puppet interview (Western Psychiatric Institute and Clinic, 1981), games, or storytelling (Gardner, 1986) can aid in facilitating a family interview or in assessing family interactions.

Additional Information. It is important to gather information from all available parts of a child's world in order to obtain as complete a picture as possible. School records and reports, the completion of rating scales, and documented observations provide a longitudinal view over a consistent period of time, with variations in stressors and in interactions with both peers and adults. The tasks in school require the child to display concentration, attention, self-control, and the ability to request assistance and to cooperate with teachers and peers. School also allows a comparison of the identified patient with classmates at similar developmental and intellectual levels.

In addition, the pediatrician, medical or other professional specialists, and medical records may provide helpful information about a child's life. The pediatrician may know the extended family and the community and may thus provide a broader background. Also, past psychiatrists, mental health clinicians, and records report valuable prior experience in dealing with the same or similar problems. Other community agencies in the child's or the family's life may be important sources for social service, legal (court, police, and child welfare), or religious involvement. YMCA, Girl or Boy Scouts, or athletic activities may provide a view of how a child deals with competition, rules, success or failure, delay of gratification, and social skills.

Diagnostic Formulation. A very difficult task is the synthesis and integration of all of the facts, observations, data, and inferences into a formulation that aids in diagnosis and treatment recommendations. It is helpful to summarize all of the interview categories and to review the major diagnostic groups in the DSM-III-R (APA, 1987) in order to assess the criteria for making a diagnosis. Throughout the assessment, the clinician should take a problem-solving approach to formulating hypotheses about the child and his or her family and exploring them during the interview and observation. This focused and purposeful appraisal should lead to a better understanding of the meaning and function of the specific aberrant behaviors exhibited. Also, the formulation provides a discussion of the biological or psychological mechanisms of the disorder, its underlying causes and precipitants, the factors perpetuating it, and the potential strengths of the client that may aid in treatment (Cox & Rutter, 1985).

The clinician should consider the impact of the specific diagnosis and the treatment recommendations before presenting them to the child and the family in order to be prepared to deal with their responses and level of understanding.

Differential Diagnosis. The DSM-III-R (APA, 1987) provides a multiaxial basis for forming a diagnosis. It clusters the symptoms found in an interview so that they may be used to form a diagnosis. The symptoms found may not meet all the criteria necessary for a specific diagnosis, and a differential diagnostic approach to alternatives may indicate areas that need further exploration. The multiaxial system of the DSM-III-R covers psychiatric syndromes, developmental disorders, personality disorders, physical disorders, psychosocial stressor severity, and global assessment of functioning.

The major child and adolescent diagnostic categories are briefly summarized here. Developmental disorders are coded on Axis II and include Mental Retardation (mild, moderate, severe, profound, and unspecified); Pervasive Developmental Disorders (Autistic Disorder or Pervasive Developmental Disorder Not Otherwise Specified); Specific Developmental Disorders such as Academic Skills Disorders (arithmetic, expressive writing, or reading); Language and Speech Disorders (articulation and expressive or receptive language); Motor Skills Disorder (coordination); and Not Otherwise Specified (NOS).

Axis I disorders include Disruptive Behavior Disorders such as Attention Deficit Hyperactivity Disorder, Conduct Disorder, and Oppositional Defiant Disorder; Anxiety Disorder of Childhood or Adolescence such as Separation Anxiety Disorder, Avoidant Disorder, and Overanxious Disorder; Eating Disorders such as Anorexia Nervosa, Bulimia Nervosa, Pica, Rumination Disorder of Infancy, and NOS; Gender Identity Disorders; Tic Disorders such as Tourette's Disorder, Chronic Motor or Vocal Tic Disorder, Transient Tic Disorder, and NOS; Elimination Disorders such as Functional Encopresis and Enuresis; and other disorders such Elective Mutism, Identity Disorder, Reactive Attachment Disorder of Infancy or Early Childhood, Stereotypy/Habit Disorder, Undifferentiated Attention-Deficit Disorder, Cluttering, and Stuttering. Still other Axis I diagnoses follow adult DSM-III-R criteria at the present time. The more common ones include Psychoactive Substance-Induced Organic Mental Disorders; Organic Mental Disorders with or without known etiology (Delirium, Dementia, etc.); Psychoactive Substance Use Disorders; Schizophrenia; Delusional (paranoid) Disorders; Other Psychotic Disorders (Brief Reactive Psychosis, Schizophreniform Disorder, Schizoaffective Disorder, and NOS); Mood Disorders such as Bipolar Disorder and Depressive Disorders; Anxiety Disorders (Panic, Phobias, Obsessive-Compulsive Disorder, Post-Traumatic Stress Disorder, etc.); Somatoform Disorders (Conversion, Hypochondriasis, Somatization, and Somatoform Pain); Dissociative Disorders; Sexual Disorders; Sleep Disorders such as dyssosomnias and parasomnias (Dream Anxiety—Nightmare, Sleep Terror, Sleepwalking, and NOS); Factitious Disorders; Impulse Control Disorders; and Adjustment Disorders.

Axis II disorders also include personality disorders. V- codes comprise conditions that are a focus of attention or treatment but that are not attributable to a mental disorder. Axis III allows physical disorders and conditions to be listed. Axis IV includes the psychosocial stressors affecting the child's functioning or psychopathology and its range of severity. Axis V allows a global assessment of the child's functioning on a hypothetical continuum of mental health to illness.

Summary Feedback Session

The summary feedback session should be conducted with the parents and without the child (By agreement, an adolescent client may be included.) This session is used to summarize all of the findings and recommendations, and to answer questions without the child's interrupting or being confused by the material. However, the interviewer should later meet with the child and her or his parents to explain the treatment plan and to answer questions simply and clearly. It is important to understand the "agenda" for this evaluation in order to present the feedback helpfully and constructively. It is often useful to give the parents paper on which to record aspects of the feedback sessions, and to repeat specific information that they find difficult to understand or anxiety-provoking. Organizing the feedback in categories and then pausing after each section will allow an opportunity for clarification before the parent becomes overwhelmed. For example, a feedback format may include a review of major concerns, medical findings, psychoeducational testing results, observational information, and the results of child, parent and family interviews, and then a diagnostic summary and the treatment recommendations. To be accepted and acted on, the treatment recommendations should consider the family's situation, such as the family's support system, its financial capability, the availability of transportation, and the availability of community services (e.g., psychiatrists, psychologists, therapists, special-education teachers, and speech therapists).

Asking parents how they feel about what they have heard will elicit their feedback and provide another chance to assist them in assimilating new and difficult or painful information, as well as to confirm accuracy or clarify misunderstandings. The interviewer should also offer to answer further questions by telephone, because many new ones will arise during the drive home or when the information is discussed with other family members. A follow-up phone call or visit may help to further clarify the information or facilitate the implementation of the treatment recommendations.

Summary

This chapter has provided a guide for approaches to the psychiatric assessment and diagnosis of children. A selection of theoretical perspectives and clinical and research methods has been presented. The DSM-III-R (APA, 1987) has been used as a model for diagnostic criteria. This chapter reviews the various approaches, assessment instrument, and rating tools to provide a framework for the clinician. Because children are constantly developing and growing, the interviewer is required to have a multidisciplinary knowledge base and approach to accurately assess and diagnose child psychopathology.

References

Achenbach, T. M., & Edelbrock, C. (1983). *Manual for the Child Behavior Checklist and Revised Child Behavior Profile*. Burlington: University of Vermont, Department of Psychiatry.

Achenbach, T. M., & Edelbrock, C. (1989). Diagnostic, taxonomic, and assessment issues. In T. H. Ollendick & M. Hersen (Eds.), *Handbook of child psychopathology* (2nd ed., pp. 53–69). New York: Plenum Press.

Achenbach, T. M., & McConaughy, S. H. (1987). *Empirically-based assessment of child and adolescent psychopathology: Practical applications*. Newbury Park, CA: Sage.

American Psychiatric Association. (1952). *Diagnostic and statistical manual of mental disorders* (DSM-I). Washington, DC: Author.

American Psychiatric Association. (1968). *Diagnostic and statistical manual of mental disorders* (2nd ed.; DSM-II). Washington, DC: Author.

American Psychiatric Association. (1980). *Diagnostic and statistical manual of mental disorders* (3rd ed.; DSM-III). Washington, DC: Author.

American Psychiatric Association. (1987). *Diagnostic and statistical manual of mental disorders* (3rd ed., rev.; DSM-III-R). Washington, DC: Author.

Balow, I. H., Farr, R., Hogan, T. P., & Prescott, G. A. (1978). *Metropolitan Achievement Tests* (5th ed.). Cleveland: Psychological Corporation.

Barkley, R. (1981). *Hyperactive children: A handbook for diagnosis and treatment*. New York: Guilford Press.

Bayley, N. (1969). *Bayley Scales of Infant Development: Birth to two years*. San Antonio: Psychological Corporation.

Beery, K. E. (1982). *Revised administration, scoring and teaching manual for the Developmental Test of Visual-Motor Integration*. Cleveland: Modern Curriculum Press.

Benton, A. L. (1973). Minimal brain dysfunction from the neuropsychological point of view. In F. F. de la Cruz, B. H. Fox, & R. H. Roberts (Eds.), *Minimal brain dysfunction*. New York: New York Academy of Sciences.

Benton, A. L. (1974). *Revised Visual Retention Test: Clinical and experimental application* (4th ed.). New York: Psychological Corporation.

Bruch, H. (1974). *Learning psychotherapy: Rationale and ground rules*. Cambridge: Harvard University Press.

Bruininks, R. H. (1978). *Bruininks-Osteretsky Test of Motor Proficiency examiner's manual*. Circle Pines, MN: American Guidance Service.

Connolly, A. J., Nachtmam, W., & Pritchett, E. M. (1971). *The Keymath Diagnostic Arithmetic Test*. Circle Pines, MN: American Guidance Service.

Costello, A. J., Edelbrock, C., Kalas, R., Kessler, M. D., & Klaric, S. H. (1982). *The NIMH Diagnostic Interview Schedule for Children (DISC)*. Unpublished interview schedule, Department of Psychiatry, University of Pittsburgh.

Cox, A., & Rutter, M. (1985). Diagnostic appraisal and interviewing. In M. Rutter & L. Hersov (Eds.), *Child and adolescent psychiatry: Modern approaches* (pp. 233–248). Boston: Blackwell Scientific.

Cronbach, L. J. (1984). *Essentials of psychological testing* (4th ed.). New York: Harper & Row.

CTB/McGraw Hill (1984). *California Achievement Tests*. Monterey, CA: Author.

Dunn, L. M., & Dunn, L. M. (1981). *Peabody Picture Vocabulary Test-Revised*. Circle Pines, MN: American Guidance Service.

Durrell, D. D., & Catterson, J. H. (1986). *Durrell Analysis of Reading Difficulty* (3rd ed.). Cleveland, OH: Psychological Corporation.

Edelbrock, C., & Costello, A. J. (1990). Structured interviews for children and adolescents. In G. Goldstein & M. Hersen (Eds.), *Handbook of psychological assessment* (2nd ed., pp. 308–323). New York: Pergamon Press.

Enright, F. E. (1983). *Enright Diagnostic Inventory of Basic Arithmetic Skills*. North Billerica, MA: Curriculum Associates.

Gardner, E. G., Rudman, H. C., Karlson, B., & Merwin, J. C. (1982). *Stanford Achievement Test*. Cleveland, OH: Psychological Corporation.

Gardner, M. F. (1979). *Expressive One-Word Picture Vocabulary Test*. Novato, CA: Academic Therapy Publications.

Gardner, R. A. (1986). *The psychotherapeutic techniques of Richard A. Gardner*. Cresskill, NJ: Creative Therapeutics.

Goldblatt, M. (1972). Psychoanalysis of the schoolchild. In B. B. Wolman (Ed.), *Handbook of child psychoanalysis*. New York: Van Nostrand Reinhold.

Goldman, J., Stein, C. L. E., & Guerry, S. (1983). *Psychological methods of child assessment*. New York: Brunner/Mazel.

Goldstein, G. (1990). Comprehensive neuropsychological assessment batteries. In G. Goldstein & M. Hersen (Eds.), *Handbook of psychological assessment* (2nd ed., pp. 197–227). New York: Pergamon Press.

Goldstein, G., & Hersen, M. (1990). Historical perspectives. In G. Goldstein & M. Hersen (Eds.), *Handbook of psychological assessment* (2nd ed., pp. 3–17). New York: Pergamon Press.

Group for the Advance of Psychiatry. (1966). *Psychopathological disorders in childhood: Theoretical considerations and a proposed classification* (Vol. 6, Report No. 62). New York: Author.

Hedrick, D. L., Prather, E. M., & Tobin, A. R. (1975). *Sequenced Inventory of Communication Development*. Seattle: University of Washington Press.

Hersen, M. (1973). Self-assessment and fears. *Behavior Therapy, 4*, 241–257.

Hieronymus, A. N., Hoover, D., Lindquist, E. F., Oberlen, K. R., Cantor, N. K., Burbick, O. O., Lewis, T. C., Hyde, E. C., & Rualls-Payne, A. C. (1978). *Iowa Test of Basic Skills*. Chicago: Riverside.

Hill, P. (1985). The diagnostic interview with the individual child. In M. Rutter & L. Hersov (Eds.), *Child and adolescent psychiatry: Modern approaches* (2nd ed., pp. 249–263). Boston: Blackwell Scientific.

Hodges, K., Kline, J., Stern, K., Cytryn, L., & McKnew, D. (1982). The development of a child assessment interview for research and clinical use. *Journal of Abnormal Child Psychology, 10*, 173–189.

Jastak, S., & Wilkinson, G. S. (1984). *Wide Range Achievement Test—Revised*. Wilmington, DE: Jastak Associates.

Kanfer, F. H., & Grimm, L. G. (1977). Behavior analysis: Selecting target behaviors in the interview. *Behavior Modification, 1*, 7–28.

Katz, L. J., & Slomka, G. T. (1990). Achievement testing. In G. Goldstein & M. Hersen (Eds.), *Handbook of psychological assessment* (2nd ed., pp. 123–147). New York: Pergamon Press.

Kaufman, A. S., & Kaufman, N. L. (1983). *Interpretive manual for the Kaufman Assessment Battery for Children.* Circle Pines, MN: American Guidance Service.

Kaufman, A. S., & Kaufman, N. G. (1985). *Kaufman Test of Individual Achievement.* Circle Pines, MN: American Guidance Service.

Kazdin, A. E. (1983). Psychiatric diagnosis, dimensions of dysfunction, and child behavior therapy. *Behavior Therapy, 14,* 73–99.

Koppitz, E. M. (1964). *The Bender Gestalt Test for Young Children.* New York: Grune & Stratton.

Kovacs, M. (1982). *The Interview Schedule for Children (ISC).* Unpublished interview schedule. Department of Psychiatry, University of Pittsburgh.

Kovacs, M. (1985). CDI (The Children's Depression Inventory). *Psychopharmacology Bulletin, 21,* 995–998.

Lazarus, A. A. (1973). Multimodal behavior therapy: Treating the "basic id." *Journal of Nervous and Mental Disease, 156,* 404–411.

Lindgren, S. D., & Lyons, D. A. (1984). *Pediatric Assessment of Cognitive Efficiency (PACE).* Iowa City: University of Iowa, Department of Pediatrics.

Markwarat, F. C. (1989). *Peabody Individual Achievement Test.* Circle Pines, MN: American Guidance Service.

McCarthy, D. A. (1972). *Manual for the McCarthy Scales of Children's Abilities.* San Antonio: Psychological Corporation.

Mitchell, T. V. (1983). *Tests in Print III.* Lincoln, Nebraska: The University of Nebraska Press.

Naslynd, R. A., Thorpe, L. P., & Lefever, D. W. (1978). *SRA Achievement Series.* Chicago: Science Research Associates.

Ollendick, T. H., & Greene, R. (1990). *Behavioral assessment of children.* In G. Goldstein & M. Hersen (Eds.), *Handbook of psychological assessment* (2nd ed., pp. 403–422). New York: Pergamon Press.

Ollendick, T. H., & Hersen, M. (Eds.), *Child behavioral assessment: Principles and procedures.* New York: Pergamon Press.

Orvaschel, H., Puig-Antich, J., Chambers, W., Tabrizi, M. A., & Johnson, R. (1982). Retrospective assessment of prepubertal major depression with the Kiddie-SADS-E. *Journal of the American Academy of Child Psychiatry, 21,* 392–397.

Perlman, M. D., & Kaufman, A. S. (1990). Assessment of child intelligence. In G. Goldstein & M. Hersen (Eds.), *Handbook of psychological assessment* (2nd ed., pp. 59–78). New York: Pergamon Press.

Psychological Corporation. (1983). *Basic Achievement Skills Individual Screener.* San Antonio: Author.

Puig-Antich, J., & Chambers, W. (1978). *The Schedule for Affective Disorders and Schizophrenia for School-aged Children.* Unpublished interview schedule, New York State Psychiatric Institute, New York.

Quay, H. C., & Peterson, D. H. (1983). *Manual for the Revised Behavior Problem Checklist.* Coral Gables, FL: Author.

Rourke, B. P., Fisk, J. L., & Strang, J. D. (1986). *Neuropsychological assessment of children: A treatment-oriented approach.* New York: Guilford Press.

Rutter, M. (1975). *Helping troubled children.* Harmondsworth, England: Penguin.

Rutter, M. (1980). Psychosexual development. In M. Rutter (Ed.), *Scientific foundations of developmental psychiatry* (pp. 322–339). London: Heinemann Medical.

Rutter, M. (1981). Stress, coping and development: Some issues and questions. *Journal of Child Psychology and Psychiatry, 22,* 323–356.

Rutter, M. (1982). Epidemiological-longitudinal approaches to the study of development. In W. A. Collins (Ed.), *The concept of development* (Vol. 15, pp. 105–144). Minnesota Symposia on Child Psychology. Hillsdale, NJ: Erlbaum.

Rutter, M., Tizard, J., & Whitmore, K. (Eds.) (1970). *Education, health and behaviour.* London: Longman. (Reprinted 1981, Huntington, NY: Krieger).

Rutter, M., Graham, P., Chadwick, O., & Yule, W. (1976). Adolescent turmoil: Fact or fiction? *Journal of Child Psychology and Psychiatry, 17,* 35–56.

Shepherd, M., Oppenheim, B., & Mitchell, S. (1971). *Childhood behaviour and mental health.* London: University of London Press.

Silvaroli, N. J. (1986). *Classroom Reading Inventory* (5th ed.). Dubuque, IA: Wm. C. Brown.

Simmons, J. E. (1981). *Psychiatric examination of children* (3rd ed.). Philadelphia: Lea & Febiger.

Slosson, R. L. (1983). *Slosson Intelligence Test (SIT) and Oral Reading Test (SORT) for children and adults.* East Aurora, NY: Slosson Educational Publications.

Sparrow, S. S., Balla, D. A., & Cicchetti, D. B. (1984). *The vineland Adaptive Behavior Scales: A revision of the Vineland Social Maturity Scale by E. A. Doll.* Circle Pines, MN: American Guidance Services.

Taylor, H. G., & Fletcher, J. M. (1990). Neuropsychological assessment of children. In G. Goldstein & M. Hersen (Eds.), *Handbook of psychological assessment* (2nd ed., pp. 228–255). New York: Pergamon Press.

Thorndike, R. L., Hagen, E. P., & Sattler, J. M. (1986). *Technical manual, Stanford-Binet Intelligence Scale: Fourth Edition*. Chicago: Riverside.

Wechsler, D. (1967). *Manual for the Wechsler Preschool and Primary Scale of Intelligence*. San Antonio: Psychological Corporation.

Wechsler, D. (1974). *Manual for the Wechsler Intelligence Scale for Children—Revised*. San Antonio: Psychological Corporation.

Welner, Z., Reich, W., Herjanic, B., Jung, K., & Amado, H. (1987). Reliability validity, and parent-child agreement studies of the Diagnostic Interview for Children and Adolescents (DICA). *Journal of the American Academy of Child Psychiatry*, 26, 649–653.

Western Psychiatric Institute and Clinic. (1981). *You can learn a lot from a lobster: The family puppet interview* (Videotape). Pittsburgh: Author.

Wolpe, J. (1977). Inadequate behavior analysis: The Achilles' heel of outcome research in behavior therapy. *Journal of Behavior Therapy and Experimental Psychiatry*, 8, 1–3.

Woodcock, R. W. (1977). *Woodcock Johnson Psychoeducational Battery: Technical Report*. Allen, TX: DLM Teaching Resources.

Woolf, H. B. (Ed.). (1977). *Webster's new collegiate dictionary*. Springfield, MA: Merriam.

Young, J. G., Leven, L., Ludman, W., Kisnadwala, H., & O'Brien, J. D. (1990). Interviewing children and adolescents. In B. D. Garfinkel, G. A. Carlson, & E. B. Weller (Eds.), *Psychiatric disorders in children and adolescents* (pp. 443–468). Philadelphia: W. B. Saunders.

6

Psychopharmacology

ALAN POLING and A. LYNN BRADSHAW

INTRODUCTION

This chapter considers how the use of psychotropic medications in hospital settings may influence the activities of behavior therapists in those settings. As the term is used here, psychotropic medications include all drugs that are prescribed with the intent of improving mood, thought processes, or overt behavior. Hospital settings are broadly defined as including all facilities that provide inpatient care for mentally ill, mentally retarded, and dually diagnosed people. Behavior therapists are practitioners who apply procedures based on the principles of experimental psychology to socially significant problems for the purpose of alleviating human suffering and enhancing human functioning (Brown, Wienckowski, & Stolz, 1975). These procedures usually involve operant or respondent conditioning, and their clinical efficacy is characteristically determined empirically, case by case. As the other chapters of this book indicate, the development of effective behavior therapy techniques has provided dramatic benefits for patients with a wide variety of behavior disorders. So, too, has the development of effective psychotropic medications, which have revolutionized psychiatry.

The psychopharmacological revolution in psychiatry began with the discovery of chlorpromazine (Thorazine), a compound that altered the history of the treatment of mentally ill people. Henri Laborit, the surgeon who in 1951 persuaded some of his colleagues in psychiatry to test this drug on psychotic patients, did not have a primary interest in the treatment of mentally ill people. Laborit was interested in drug-induced inhibition of the autonomic nervous system because of his belief that shock in surgical patients could be prevented through this mechanism. Chlorpromazine was one of the drugs that was synthesized and passed on to Laborit to be used for this purpose.

When Laborit administered chlorpromazine to patients being prepared for surgery, he observed that the drug calmed them without inducing obvious sedation. Although the patients were alert and aware of the forthcoming surgery, they seemed relatively unconcerned. As a result, Laborit rightly posited that chlorpromazine might be useful in the treatment of psychotic disorders. In marked contrast to the general depressant action produced by the sedative

ALAN POLING and A. LYNN BRADSHAW • Department of Psychology, Western Michigan University, Kalamazoo, Michigan 49008.

Handbook of Behavior Therapy in the Psychiatric Setting, edited by Alan S. Bellack and Michel Hersen. Plenum Press, New York, 1993.

113

114

ALAN POLING and
A. LYNN BRADSHAW

medications used early in this century to manage psychotic individuals, chlorpromazine produces a selective reduction in the signs and symptoms of schizophrenia and related disorders.

The availability of chlorpromazine revolutionized psychiatric practice because the drug reduced the undesirable behaviors of most psychotic patients. Many studies have shown that chlorpromazine and the related antipsychotic (neuroleptic) drugs introduced later are generally effective in managing schizophrenia and other psychoses. However, not all psychotic individuals benefit from these drugs, some improve in their absence, and all who receive them are at risk of developing motor dysfunctions and other adverse side effects (Baldessarini, 1985b; Berger, 1978; Kane, 1987).

Several antipsychotic drugs are now marketed in the United States (see Table 1). These medications have been prescribed for millions of people. For example, in 1985 in the United States alone, retail pharmacies dispensed 21 million prescriptions for antipsychotic drugs (Wysowski & Baum, 1989). In many cases, drug treatment sufficiently improves psychotic patients to allow them to leave hospitals and institutions. In fact, in the first half of the 20th century, the number of patients in U.S. mental hospitals (i.e., institutions) increased from approximately 150,000 to 500,000. In 1956, the first year in which chlorpromazine was widely used in this country, this trend reversed itself. By 1970, the number of hospitalized patients had fallen to fewer than 350,000 (Figure 1). The downward trend has continued to the present. Since the early 1960s, the number of beds in state psychiatric hospitals has been reduced by 75%. This reduction in the number of hospitalized patients has not resulted from a decrease in new admissions. Instead, effective psychotropic medication allows patients to leave the hospital after much briefer stays (Berger, 1978). Before the 1950s, patients with severe behavior disorders were commonly hospitalized for most of their lives.

Today, relatively few mentally ill people spend the majority of their lives in hospitals. Some do, however, and many others are hospitalized for periods of varying lengths. It is quite likely that these patients, whether mentally ill, mentally retarded, or dually diagnosed, will receive neuroleptic drug treatment. For example, Figure 2 shows that in 13 surveys of institutionalized (hospitalized) mentally retarded people in Canada (Tu, 1979), New Zealand (Pulman, Pook, & Singh, 1979; Sewell & Werry, 1976; White, 1983), the United Kingdom (Fischbacher, 1987; Spencer, 1974), and the United States (Briggs, Garrard, Hamad, & Wills, 1984; Cohen & Sprague, 1977; Hill, Balow, & Bruininks, 1985; Huessy & Ruoff, 1984; LaMendola, Zaharia, & Carver, 1980; Silva, 1979), the prevalence of neuroleptic drug use ranged from approximately 15% to 45%. Somewhat higher prevalence figures have characteristically been reported for neuroleptic use with institutionalized mentally ill people (Laska, Craig, Siegel, & Wanderling, 1981; Laska, Varga, Wanderling, Simpson, Logemann, & Shah, 1973; Prien, Haber, & Caffey, 1975; Prien, Klett, & Caffey, 1976; Sheppard, Collins, Fiorentino, Fracchia, & Merlis, 1969).

Neuroleptics are not, of course, the only kind of psychotropic medication prescribed for hospitalized patients. Psychotropic medications are conventionally divided into categories according to their primary effects and therapeutic applications (Usdin & Efron, 1972). In addition to antipsychotics, Table 1 lists selected stimulant, antianxiety (anxiolytic), antidepressant, and antimania drugs. *Many hospitalized patients with whom behavior therapists work receive one of these agents or some other psychotropic drug.* A sizable proportion of them continue to take psychotropic medication on leaving the hospital. Therefore, behavior therapists should have at least a rudimentary knowledge of psychopharmacology.

Space is not available here to summarize the characteristic uses, efficacy, and side effects of the drug classes in Table 1. This information is available in general overviews of the use of psychotropic medications (e.g., Poling, Gadow, & Cleary, 1991) and in reviews of the use of these medications with children (e.g., Gadow, 1986a,b; Werry, 1978), mentally ill people (e.g., Baldessarini, 1985a,b; Kane, 1987; Klein, Gittleman, Quitkin, & Rifkin, 1980), and mentally retarded people (Aman & Singh, 1988; Gadow & Poling, 1988). Useful information about the effects of particular medications is available in the *United States Pharmacopeia Dispensing*

Table 1. Selected Psychotropic Drugs

Generic (nonproprietary) name	Proprietary (trade) name	Generic (nonproprietary) name	Proprietary (trade) name
Neuroleptics		*Antidepressants*	
Phenothiazines		*Tricyclics*	
Aliphatic:		amitriptyline	Elavil, Endep
chlorpromazine	Thorazine	amoxapine	Asendin
triflupromazine	Vesprin	desipramine	Norpramin, Pertofrane
Piperidine:		doxepin	Adapin, Sinequan
mesoridazine	Serentil	imipramine	Janimine, Tofranil
piperacetazine	Quide	maprotiline	Ludiomil
thioridazine	Mellaril	nortriptyline	Aventyl, Pamelor
Piperazine:		protriptyline	Vivactil
acetophenazine	Tindal	trimipramine	Surmontil
fluphenazine	Prolixin, Permitil	*Monoamine oxidase inhibitors*	
perphenazine	Trilafon	isocarboxazid	Marplan
prochlorperazine	Compazine	phelelzine	Nardil
trifluoperazine	Stelazine	tranylcypromine	Parnate
Thioxanthenes		*Atypical*	
chlorprothixene	Taractan	bupropion	Wellbutrin
thiothixene	Navane	fluoxetine	Prozac
Butyrophenone		nomifensine	Merital
haloperidol	Haldol	trazodone	Desyrel
Dihydroindolone		*Antianxiety agents*	
molindone	Moban	*Propanediols*	
Dibenzoxazepines		meprobamate	Equanil
amoxapine	Asendin	*Diphenylmethane*	
loxapine	Loxitane	hydroxyzine	Atarax, Vistaril
Diphenylbutylpiperidine		*Benzodiazepines*	
pimozide	Orap	alprazolam	Xanax
Antimania agents		chlordiazepoxide	Librium
lithium carbonate	Eskalith, Lithane, Lithobid	clorazepate	Tranxene
		diazepam	Valium
Stimulants		flurazepam	Dalmane
amphetamine	Benzedrine	halazepam	Paxipam
deanol	Deaner	lorazepam	Ativan
dextroamphetamine	Dexedrine	oxazepam	Serax
methamphetamine	Desoxyn	prazepam	Centrax
methylphenidate	Ritalin	temazepam	Restoril
pemoline	Cylert	triazolam	Halcion

Information, the *American Hospital Formulary Service*, *AMA Drug Evaluations*, *The Medical Letter*, *Clin-Alert*, *Rational Drug Therapy*, *The United States Pharmacopeia*, and *The National Formulary*. *The Physicians' Desk Reference* (PDR) is a commonly used source of drug information, but not the best one. The manufacturers whose drugs are described in the PDR support the volume, and the material it contains is essentially identical to what appears in the drug package inserts.

SELECTION AND EVALUATION OF MEDICATION

Figure 3 shows the steps involved in the pharmacological treatment of a behavior disorder. On a descriptive level, behavior that creates a problem for patients can in most cases be divided into three general categories:

ALAN POLING and
A. LYNN BRADSHAW

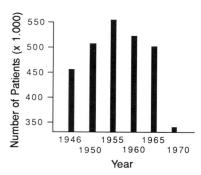

Figure 1. The number of resident patients in state and local mental hospitals in the United States in 1946, 1950, 1955, 1960, 1965, and 1970 as reported by Longo (1972). Chlorpromazine and other effective psychotropic medications were introduced in the mid-1950s. At that time, the number of resident patients, which had been steadily rising since the turn of the century, began to fall.

1. Behavior that is troublesome because of its topography (form). A patient's eating feces is an example; doing so is a problem whenever and wherever it occurs.
2. Behavior that is troublesome because of its rate or intensity. A second-grader's crying and asking to be hugged is an example. This is not a problem if it occurs occasionally, but most parents would be understandably vexed if the request were repeated every five

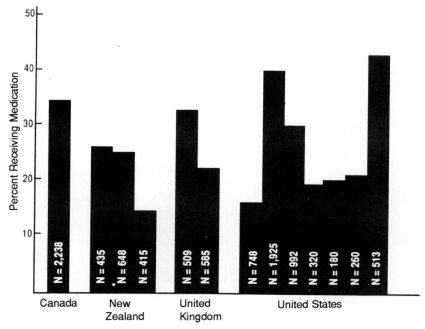

Figure 2. The prevalence of neuroleptic drug use in 13 institutions for mentally retarded as reported by Gadow and Poling (1988). From K. D. Gadow and A. Poling. (1988). *Pharmacotherapy and Mental Retardation* (p. 103). Copyright 1988 by Little, Brown and Company. Reproduced by permission.

minutes. Behavior that fails to occur or occurs rarely can also be a problem, as when a child consistently fails to comply with a parent's commands.

3. Behavior that is troublesome because it occurs in inappropriate circumstances. Masturbating is an example; it is not a problem in private, but it is undesirable in public.

When a person's behavior is sufficiently troublesome, help is sought from professionals in the hospital setting. At that point the behavior disorder constitutes an admitting problem. The problem may involve one or two discrete responses, as in nighttime bedwetting (enuresis) or self-injurious face slapping, or it may involve a broad range of signs and symptoms, as in schizophrenia.

Initial Assessment

Assessment, which involves collecting information about an individual, begins soon after a patient enters the hospital and continues until all treatment ends. One major function of

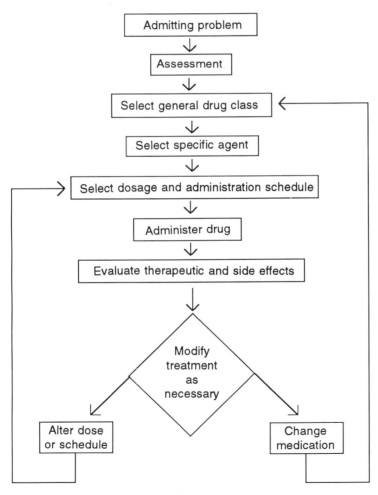

Figure 3. Simplified sequence of the steps involved in the pharmacological treatment of a behavior disorder.

ALAN POLING and
A. LYNN BRADSHAW

assessment is to identify individuals with certain characteristics, for example, those who are clinically depressed or anxious. A second is to guide caregivers in determining an individual's needs and developing interventions to meet these needs. A third is to ascertain whether the selected treatments are successful. Because of their skill in quantifying behavior problems, behavior therapists can play a valuable role throughout the assessment process.

When much, if not most, of an individual's behavior is troublesome, it is common to consider the specific behavior problems as symptoms of a clinical disorder. Psychiatric diagnosis involves categorizing people according to the troublesome things that they say and do. It is on this basis that the various forms of mental illness are distinguished.

In most cases, before receiving medication, a patient is assigned to a global diagnostic category. This assignment is frequently based on criteria described in the third revised edition of the *Diagnostic and Statistical Manual of Mental Disorders* (DSM-III-R) published by the American Psychiatric Association (1987). Appropriate psychiatric diagnosis is important, because the various classes of psychotherapeutic agents are fairly selective in their ability to modify the symptoms of mental illnesses (Baldessarini, 1985b, p. 388).

When the instruments used in psychiatric diagnosis do not clearly reflect the problem behaviors that treatment is intended to improve, direct and quantitative measures of those behaviors should be arranged before the initiation of pharmacotherapy. These direct measures of behavior provide a sound basis for treatment evaluation.

Selection of a Drug Class

After completing an initial assessment, the physician selects a treatment. In dealing with behavioral disorders, the first question to be answered concerning treatment is whether pharmacotherapy or an alternative, nonpharmacological intervention is appropriate. If a decision is made to medicate, further questions relating to the choice and administration of a specific agent must be addressed.

In a general way, how drugs are classified reflects empirical findings concerning their range of efficacy. The data indicate, for example, that neuroleptics are the drugs most likely to be useful in managing schizophrenia and other psychoses, anxiolytics in dealing with anxiety, antidepressants in treating unipolar depression, lithium in controlling bipolar affective disorders and mania, and stimulants in dealing with attention deficit disorder in children (Poling et al., 1991). Once a person is assigned to a diagnostic category, the initial choice of a drug class is usually simple and straightforward. If, for instance, the client is diagnosed as schizophrenic, a neuroleptic is indicated.

The selection of a drug class becomes complicated when prior findings have not indicated that any drug class is generally beneficial in treating the behavioral disorder at hand. This is the case, for instance, with self-injurious behavior in mentally retarded people, a problem for which no drug provides general and selective relief (Gadow & Poling, 1986). In such cases, the selection of a drug class is apt to rest on a clinician's personal experiences and on generalizations from reported drug effects in other kinds of patients. Suggestive but unreplicated research findings (e.g., case reports) may also guide the physician.

Behavior therapists characteristically play no direct role in the selection of a therapeutic drug class. They may, however, play an important role in suggesting alternatives to pharmacotherapy. For instance, it is widely acknowledged that stimulants are often of value in dealing with the short attention span, impulsiveness, restlessness, and aggression directed toward peers associated with attention-deficit hyperactivity disorder in children (e.g., Cantwell & Carlson, 1978; Gadow, 1986a; Ross & Ross, 1982). These drugs are also associated with several undesirable side effects, including diminished weight gain, increased heart rate, and insomnia. Because nonpharmacological treatments are often effective in managing hyperactivity, the decision to medicate a hyperactive child should be made with care, perhaps only after other kinds of interventions have proved ineffective (cf. O'Brien & Orbzut, 1986; O'Leary, 1980). Behavior therapists have a significant role to play in designing, implementing, and evaluating these interventions.

Although the variables involved in selecting and evaluating a nonpharmacological intervention are not considered here, it should be recognized that it is not uncommon for such an intervention to be given priority after initial assessment. In such cases, pharmacotherapy is begun only when the alternative is found to be ineffective. For the sake of simplicity, the selection and evaluation of nonpharmacological interventions is omitted from Figure 3.

In many cases, a decision is reached to use pharmacotherapy and another intervention concurrently. To derive maximum benefit, most patients with behavior disorders require more than drug therapy alone. As Baldessarini (1985b) pointed out:

> Despite the great success of the antipsychotic drugs, their use alone does not constitute optimal care of psychotic patients. The acute care, protection, and support of acutely psychotic patients, as well as mastery of techniques employed in their long-term care and habilitation continue to be important medical skills. (p. 409)

Behavior therapy is one of the techniques that are useful in the long-term treatment of psychotic patients (Bellack, 1986; Gomes-Schwartz, 1979). To best treat behavior disorders, integrated pharmacological and behavioral treatment are often required (see Hersen, 1986). Interestingly, some behavior therapists are unaware of the positive effects of psychotropic medications and are generally critical of their use in hospital settings. This attitude was pointed out by Hersen (1979):

> From my perspective as internship training director, I have seen many new behavioral trainees enter our program with a preconceived bias against the use of drugs with severely disturbed psychiatric patients. . . . Whatever the reason for such negative biases, the facts about the role and efficacy of psychotropic agents need to be faced squarely. In the treatment of schizophrenia, remission of major symptomatology (e.g., delusions, hallucinations, thinking disorders) is best accomplished with the antipsychotic agents (i.e., the phenothiazines and butyrophenones). Indeed, although we have not previously reported this finding in the literature, unless the medication of our schizophrenics is finely adjusted (i.e., correct dosage level), they simply do not show any evidence of learning in our social skills paradigm (consisting of instructions, modeling, feedback, behavioral rehearsal, social reinforcement). Other colleagues working in this area in different centers have corroborated our finding during the course of discussions. It is quite clear to us that with distracting hallucinatory stimuli, the schizophrenic is unable to fully attend. Therefore, it should not be surprising that under such conditions learning is minimized. (pp. 67–69)

An empirical demonstration of the positive interaction of behavioral and pharmacological interventions is evident in Figure 4, which shows data collected by Wallace, Donahoe, and Boone (1986). These data show the effects of haloperidol (10 mg/day) and a token reinforcement procedure (contingency), alone and in combination, on the number of seconds during a 2-minute period in which a 20-year-old schizophrenic patient read a newspaper aloud with appropriate volume. It appears that the reinforcement procedure was effective in the presence of the drug, but not in its absence.

Even when behavioral procedures are effective in the absence of medication, the combination of drug and behavior therapy may enhance therapeutic gains. For example, in considering the treatment of attention deficit disorder (ADD) and conduct disorder (CD), Pelham and Murphy (1986) concluded that

> There is considerable evidence that the combination of behavior therapy and psychostimulant medication is more effective short-term treatment than either alone for the average ADD child. This appears to be the case for children with a concurrent diagnosis of CD, as well as for those without CD, but more research directed at this dichotomy is needed. (pp. 137–138)

But they cautioned:

> No studies have systematically investigated the effects of combined interventions with CD children without concurrent ADD. No long-term studies of the combined treatments have been conducted. [Moreover,] there are large individual differences in response to combined treatments. For some children, who appear to respond only to one or the other treatment, the combined approach does not offer incremental benefit. Prediction of response to intervention is not possible given current knowledge, and functional analyses must be utilized to determine the most appropriate treatment for any one individual child. (p. 138)

Their final statement is true for all patients, regardless of age or behavior disorder.

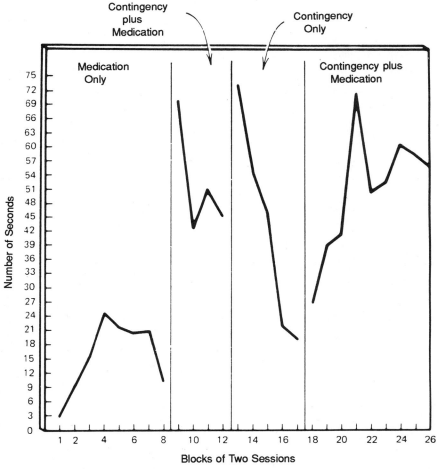

Figure 4. Effects of haloperidol and a behavioral contingency, alone and in combination, on the number of seconds during which speech exceeded the predetermined criterion level. From D. J. Wallace, C. P. Conahoe, Jr., and S. E. Boone. (1986). Schizophrenia. In M. Hersen (Ed.), *Pharmacological and Behavioral Treatment: An Integrative Approach* (pp. 357–381). New York: Wiley. Copyright 1986 by Wiley. Reproduced by permission.

Selection of a Specific Agent

Once a physician has decided to prescribe a drug from a particular therapeutic category, she or he is faced with the selection of a specific agent. In many cases, all members of a particular drug class are quite similar. For example, with respect to antipsychotic drugs:

> No one drug or combination of drugs has a selective effect on a particular symptom complex in groups of psychotic patients, although individual patients appear to do better with one agent than another; this can only be determined by trial and error. . . . Since the choice of a drug cannot be made on the basis of anticipated therapeutic effect, the *selection* of a particular medication for treatment often depends on side effects. If a patient has responded well to a drug in the past, it should probably be used again. (Baldessarini, 1985b, p. 415)

Although many drugs within a therapeutic category produce similar effects, it appears that a physician is well advised to become familiar with one or two well-studied members of each category and (unless there are clear contraindications) to use these drugs in preference to other, similar agents. The advantage of this strategy is that a clinician can more easily learn the pharmacological properties (e.g., indications, contraindications, side effects, usual dosage, appropriate schedule of administration, and interaction with other compounds) of a few drugs than of many. Being fully aware of a drug's pharmacological properties helps a clinician to optimize the treatment parameters and to avoid therapeutic errors.

Despite the advantages of regularly using a limited number of behavior-change medications, there are of course situations in which newly developed drugs merit application, or in which an unusual use of established drugs is warranted. Such situations are likely to be rare, limited to those instances in which conventional treatments have failed. They demand that a physician learn all that is possible about the agent under consideration, be cautious about its administration, and be absolutely certain to monitor its effects adequately. By providing accurate data about target behaviors and side effects, behavior therapists can provide valuable assistance in monitoring.

Selection of Dosage and Administration Schedule

Once a particular drug has been selected, an initial treatment schedule must be delineated. This involves specifying the route of administration, the time of administration, and the dose. Determining how a drug ought to be administered requires understanding its pharmacokinetics, "which deals with the absorption, distribution, biotransformation, and excretion of drugs. These factors, coupled with dosage, determine the concentration of drug at its sites of action and, hence, the intensity of its effects as a function of time" (Benet & Sheiner, 1985, p. 1). Behavior therapists generally play no direct role in deciding how a drug should be used. Nonetheless, they may be interested in what occurs once a drug enters the body, and for this reason, the process is summarized here. Many pharmacology books provide further coverage (e.g., Gilman, Goodman, Rall, & Murad, 1985; Goth, 1984).

The term *absorption* refers to a drug's entry into the bloodstream. A drug must enter the body before it can be absorbed, and the manner in which it does so is termed the *route of administration*. Although intravenous and intramuscular routes are occasionally used for special purposes (e.g., with extremely agitated individuals or with paranoid patients who refuse to swallow "poisons"), psychotropic drugs are usually given orally. This is a convenient and economical route of administration and is usually safer than other routes (e.g., intravenous). To be absorbed after ingestion, drugs in tablet or capsule form must dissolve in the fluids of the stomach or the intestine. They then pass through the cells that line the wall of the digestive tract and into the capillaries of the veins that lead from the stomach and the small intestine to the liver.

Drugs differ dramatically in how readily they are absorbed following ingestion. Moreover,

ALAN POLING and
A. LYNN BRADSHAW

individuals differ in their natural speed of absorption, which is also influenced by stomach and intestinal pH (acidity/alkalinity) and the presence of food or other drugs in the gut. Because food alters absorption, many medications are taken between meals. The usual exception is those agents that cause gastric upset if taken on an empty stomach.

The rate of absorption is determined, in part, by the form in which the drug is administered. Liquids are usually absorbed more readily than solids, although the two dosage forms are sometimes used interchangeably. Particulars of manufacture, such as the thickness of the pill coating, the type of filler substances, and the hardness of the tablet, also alter the rate of absorption. Therefore, different brands of the same drug may be absorbed at different rates. This difference may be of clinical significance because the amount of drug in the blood is related to the therapeutic response.

In some cases, manufacturers intentionally prepare drugs in a form that slows absorption. For example, CIBA Pharmaceuticals markets methylphenidate (Ritalin) in the form of regular and sustained-release (Ritalin SR) tablets. Drug molecules from the sustained-release tablets are more slowly absorbed, so that the duration of the drug effects is prolonged (Birhamer, Greenhill, Cooper, Fried, & Maminski, 1989). Because chewing sustained-release Ritalin tablets speeds absorption, patients are advised to swallow them whole.

Once in the bloodstream, drug molecules are distributed throughout the body, but they characteristically produce their effects at localized sites of action. Psychotropic drugs, for example, alter the functioning of cells located in the central nervous system (CNS). To reach these sites of action, molecules pass from the small arteries to the capillaries, then through the capillary walls to the extracellular fluid, where they diffuse and eventually contact neurons (nerve cells) in the brain. At a given time, only a tiny fraction of the drug molecules in the body is at the site of action.

The molecules of many drugs combine with large protein molecules in the blood in a process called *protein binding*. Protein-bound molecules are unable to pass out of the bloodstream and do not reach the site of action, but this process is not irreversible. As unbound molecules pass out of the bloodstream, bound molecules are released, so that the ratio of bound to unbound molecules in the blood remains roughly constant. Although the maximal effect of a drug is reduced by protein binding, the process prolongs the effect of the drug by creating a reservoir of bound drug molecules that are released over time (Briant, 1978). The concentration of drug molecules in fat or muscle cells (which occurs with some medications) has the same effect.

The passage of certain drugs out of the bloodstream and into the brain is impeded by the glial cells that closely surround the capillaries of the brain. The term *blood-brain barrier* is used to emphasize the difficulty with which drugs enter the brain, but the term has no precise structural referent. Most psychotropic drugs enter the brain with relative ease.

As they pass through the body, most drugs are changed into new compounds termed *metabolites*. This process is termed *biotransformation*. Substances within the cells of the liver called *enzymes* initiate and facilitate the chemical reactions that transform drugs into metabolites. In most cases, an active drug is metabolized into substances that are water-soluble and can be excreted through the kidneys. Some drugs, however, are not metabolized and pass from the body unchanged. Others are transformed into active metabolites.

Drugs and their metabolites are excreted from the body primarily by the actions of the kidneys. Although most drugs exit the body as water-soluble molecules dissolved in urine, significant quantities of certain drugs are excreted in feces or in exhaled air. Measurable amounts may also be present in sweat, saliva, tears, or the milk of nursing mothers. The rate of excretion of some drugs is affected by the pH of the urine. Drugs that are bases are generally excreted more rapidly when the urine is acidic, whereas acidic drugs are more rapidly excreted in basic urine. Many other variables influence the rate of the inactivation and elimination of drugs. Among them are genotype, age, drug history, and liver or kidney disease.

With the vast majority of psychotropic medications, a relationship clearly exists between the effects of the drug and its concentration in the body (e.g., in blood). When a drug is given on a single occasion (i.e., acutely), the level of drug in the blood and the effects it produces vary as a function of the time since administration. Each substance has a characteristic time course of action, which is the magnitude and direction of its physiological and behavioral actions as a function of time since administration. The time course of action for a given drug is determined by its physical properties, the dose administered, the route of administration, and the organismic variables (e.g., age, health, genotype, and drug history) that alter the body's response to the drug.

The rate of disappearance of drug molecules is described in terms of biological half-life, which is determined by measuring the amount of time required for a given blood level of the drug to decline by 50%. With many drugs, this value does not change significantly as a function of initial drug blood level or dosage, and these drugs are described as having linear (or first-order) kinetics. A constant fraction of such drugs is eliminated per unit of time.

Some drugs have nonlinear kinetics; that is, their eliminative mechanisms may become saturated. This saturation causes the relative rate of elimination to decrease (and the half-life to increase) with dosage and concentration. When this saturation occurs, there is a range of apparent half-lifes for any individual, each of which is affected by the dose and the initial concentration at which it is measured.

Even for drugs with linear kinetics, the rate of elimination varies across individuals as a function of genetics, physiological characteristics, and exposure to that drug and others (i.e., the person's drug history). Therefore, half-life values are expressed only within rather broad ranges. These values are, however, of therapeutic importance. For example, a medication should be administered approximately once per half-life to maintain stable blood levels. Because it takes approximately five half-lifes after the first administration to reach a stable blood level, evaluations of drug efficacy before that time will be inconclusive.

If a drug is taken in more rapidly than it can be inactivated, blood levels and overt effects increase over time. This phenomenon, known as *accumulation*, may be a clinically significant problem, especially with long-acting drugs with variable half-lifes.

As mentioned previously, psychotropic drugs produce their therapeutic effects by affecting the functioning of nerve cells in the brain, which is a wondrously complex organ. The human brain contains approximately 20 billion neurons, each of which may share up to 100,000 synapses (connections) with other neurons (Zimbardo, 1988). Learning how such a complex system works, and how it is affected by drugs, is a herculean task. Nonetheless, much has been learned in recent years. It is now known that the transmission of information in the CNS is an electrochemical process largely controlled by substances called *neurotransmitters*, which are produced in neurons. Information is passed along individual nerve cells by the movement of charged particles across the cell membrane into and out of cells, an action that produces a wave of electrical activity (termed the *neuronal impulse*) that moves down the length of the neuron. This activity can lead to the release of a neurotransmitter, a chemical produced and stored in the neuron. Neurotransmitter molecules cross the fluid-filled gap (synaptic cleft) between neurons and interact with receptors on the membrane of the next neuron. Receptors are parts of a cell (e.g., proteins, nucleic acids, or lipids of cell membranes) to which neurotransmitters bind chemically. Individual receptors are sensitive to specific neurotransmitters. Receptor–neurotransmitter interactions affect the probability that a neuronal impulse will be initiated. If the probability is increased, the effect is excitatory; if decreased, it is inhibitory. All neurons are affected by excitatory and inhibitory processes, and "the exquisite beauty of the nervous system is maintained by this delicate balance between excitation and inhibition" (Julien, 1985, p. 226).

Many substances are known to function as neurotransmitters, and the list grows each year. Among the best studied neurotransmitters are norepinephrine, serotonin, dopamine, acetylcholine, and gamma-aminobutyric acid (GABA). Drugs can affect neurotransmission in several ways, including the following:

1. By altering the synthesis (production in the body) of the neurotransmitter.
2. By interfering with the storage of the neurotransmitter.
3. By altering the release of the neurotransmitter.
4. By interfering with the inactivation of the neurotransmitter (by enzymes or reuptake).
5. By interacting with receptors.

The neuropharmacological actions of some psychotropic drugs are specifiable and relate to their clinical effectiveness. For instance, neuroleptics such as thioridazine (Mellaril) and chlorpromazine (Thorazine) appear to produce their antipsychotic effects by blocking receptors that respond to the neurotransmitter dopamine. A lock-and-key analogy is often used to explain this action: The receptor is envisioned as a lock, and molecules of dopamine and neuroleptics are envisioned as similar but not identical keys. The dopamine key matches the receptor lock perfectly and will unlock it, affecting the neuron on which the receptor is located. The neuroleptic key, in contrast, matches the receptor lock imperfectly: The key will enter the lock but will not unlock it. Therefore, when neuroleptic molecules combine with dopamine receptors, cellular activity is not directly affected. But just as ill-fitting keys prevent matching keys from entering and opening locks, neuroleptic molecules prevent dopamine molecules from combining with receptors and affecting the activity of the neuron. The result is a reduction in neuronal activity in parts of the brain where dopamine is the neurotransmitter.

Blocking dopaminergic activity with neuroleptic medication provides relief of symptoms in most patients diagnosed as schizophrenic. Moreover, prolonged exposure to drugs that increase dopaminergic activity (e.g., amphetamine) produces changes in behavior that resemble those characteristic of schizophrenia. These findings led to the speculation that schizophrenia results from metabolic errors leading to either (1) overproduction of dopamine in the limbic system or cortex of the brain or (2) production of an endogenous amphetaminelike compound. Such dopamine models of schizophrenia continue to be popular, but attempts to document metabolic differences in humans diagnosed as schizophrenic have yielded inconclusive results (Baldessarini, 1985a,b). Moreover, genetic studies have suggested that inheritance may account for only a portion of the causation of schizophrenia. In view of these considerations, biological models of schizophrenia based on inborn errors of metabolism that lead to an overproduction of dopamine or an amphetaminelike substance are not fully adequate. Nor, for that matter, are other models of the disorder.

With nearly all behavior-change medications, there is considerable variation in the range of doses commonly prescribed. Treatment is characteristically begun with a dosage described in the literature as low to moderate, administered at appropriate intervals. That dose is increased until the behavioral problem is adequately controlled, the side effects become intolerable, or the recommended maximum dose is reached. In dealing with extremely agitated clients, it is sometimes judicious to begin with a high dose, which is titrated downward once the problem behavior is initially controlled.

With neuroleptics, it is common practice to attempt to ascertain the minimum effective dose (MED), which is the least amount of medication that will produce the desired effect in a given patient. This dose is desirable because the frequency and severity of side effects are generally related directly to dosage. Figure 5 provides an example of the steps involved in determining the MED. By helping to ensure that a drug's effects will be adequately measured, behavior therapists can help to ensure that MEDs are accurately determined. By providing treatments that facilitate appropriate behavior, behavior therapists may also reduce the MED for individual patients. When that level is reached, even if it is zero (i.e., no drug), continued behavioral programming will be required to meet the needs of many, but not all, patients.

Of particular concern is providing adequate follow-up care for patients whose response to

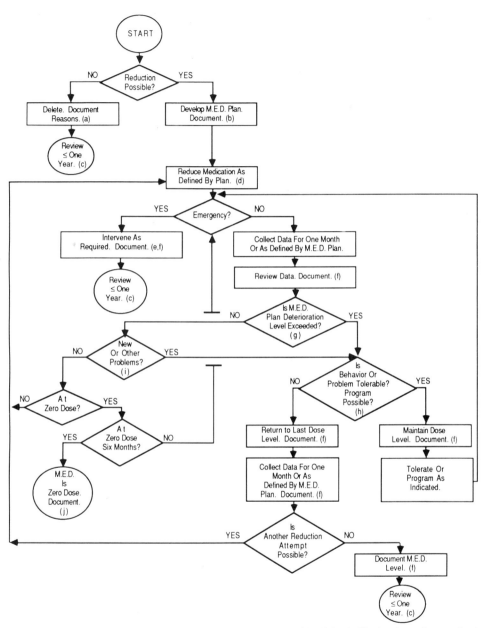

Figure 5. A flowchart describing the steps involved in ascertaining the minimal effective dose of a neuroleptic drug. From J. E. Kalachnik. (1988b). *Psychotropic Medication Monitoring Checklist and Manual for Rule 34 Facilities.* St. Paul: Minnesota Department of Human Services, Licensing Division. Reproduced by permission.

medication in the hospital setting is sufficient to allow them to return to the community. Recent findings indicate that many of these patients are readmitted to the hospital. For example, readmissions account for about 70% of all psychiatric hospital admissions, and the 2 million schizophrenics in the United States accumulate 500,000 admissions per year (Bellack, 1986). Developing programs for these people that improve the quality of their lives outside the institution while preventing the behavioral deterioration that leads to readmission is a worthy goal for behavior therapists. Gomez-Schwartz (1979) emphasized this goal and suggested a strategy:

> Few therapists, behavioral or otherwise, are content simply with improving hospital conditions and the patient's functioning within the hospital. An important goal is teaching patients new skills which will presumably permit them to function more appropriately in a nonhospital environment. . . . Thus, the behavior therapist who wishes to ensure that patients continue to perform a positive behavior once they have left the hospital must either design the treatment so that the patients learn to reinforce themselves or ensure that significant people on the outside, such as halfway house staff, family members, or employers are able to maintain the same contingencies which were in effect in the hospital. (pp. 459–460)

Drug Administration and Evaluation

Medications are unlikely to prove beneficial unless received by the patient at the dose and time intended by the physician. Nonetheless, data suggest that patients often fail to follow instructions for taking medications. Patient noncompliance may involve a full or partial omission of scheduled doses, the administration of inappropriate doses, a failure to take medication at the intended intervals, the addition of medications not prescribed, or the premature termination of drug therapy. A number of variables are known to influence the likelihood of noncompliance, among them the side effects of the medication, the treatment environment, the problem being treated, and the degree to which the importance of compliance is stressed by the physician. It is not possible to predict precisely which patients are at risk for noncompliance, but it appears that, unless very closely monitored, a sizable proportion of psychiatric patients fail to self-administer medications as intended by their physician. This result is shown in a study by Hare and Wilcox (1967), who examined noncompliance in a psychiatric hospital. They found that 19% of inpatients, 37% of day patients, and 48% of outpatients were noncompliant. An obvious goal for behavior therapists working in hospital settings is to develop programs to ensure patient compliance with dosing schedules.

Obviously, one can determine whether a patient benefits from a pharmacotherapeutic agent only if the medication is actually taken. Perhaps less obvious is the need to specify clearly the kinds of changes in behavior that constitute a benefit to a patient, and to determine beyond reasonable doubt whether a drug has produced such changes.

Sprague and Werry (1971) suggested that a small experiment is begun each time a drug is prescribed with the intent of improving behavior. In this experiment, the treatment team hypothesizes that drug administration will produce the desired alterations in the client's target behaviors without inducing intolerable side effects. Data that reflect target behaviors and side effects when the drug is and is not administered provide the only real means of testing this hypothesis. As in a formal research project, the data collected in clinical practice should be valid (i.e., should reflect the dimensions of concern), reliable (i.e., should yield constant scores if behavior does not change), and sensitive (i.e., should be capable of changing as a function of treatment).

Many different techniques can be used to assess behavior change along quantitative and qualitative dimensions. These include self-reports, global clinical evaluations, standardized tests, behavioral checklists and rating scales, and direct observation. The strengths and weakness of these techniques and their appropriateness for drug evaluation are considered elsewhere (e.g., Gadow & Poling, 1986; Poling *et al.*, 1991).

As a rule, the within-subject, direct-observation strategies that behavior therapists characteristically use to evaluate nonpharmacological interventions are well suited to clinical drug assessments. Consider, for example, a study conducted by Marholin, Touchette, and Stewart (1979), who used a withdrawal (B-A-B) design to examine how chlorpromazine affected four mentally retarded adults. (A fifth person was also studied in a similar but more complex withdrawal design; for simplicity, this subject is not considered here.) Several behaviors were carefully measured by direct observation in workshop and ward settings, among them compliance with verbal requests, the accuracy and rate of performance of workshop tasks, time on task, eye contact, talking to self, talking to others, standing, walking, being within 3 feet of others, being in bed, approaching others, and touching others. During the first 19 days of recording, chlorpromazine was administered. This period was followed by a 23-day drug-free (placebo) phase and a 25-day period in which drug treatment was reinstated.

Some of the data collected by Marholin *et al.* are shown in Figure 6. The effects of withdrawing the chlorpromazine differed appreciably across the subjects, but some desirable

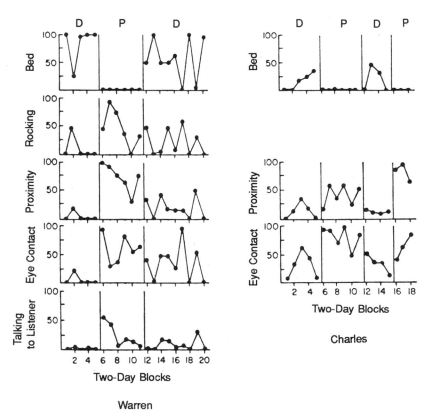

Warren

Charles

Figure 6. Percentage of intervals during which a variety of social behaviors occurred during chlorpromazine (D) and placebo (P) conditions. From D. Marholin, P. E. Touchette, and R. M. Stewart. (1979). Withdrawal of Chronic Chlorpromazine Medication: An Experimental Analysis. *Journal of Applied Behavior Analysis, 12,* 150–171. Copyright 1979 by the Society for the Experimental Analysis of Behavior. Reproduced by permission.

behaviors did emerge when the drug was withdrawn. Certainly the medication was not producing consistently beneficial effects: "Changes in the behavior of these severely retarded adults which we attributed to chlorpromazine were diverse and generally of no clear relevance to the patients' well being, access to the environment, or physical or psychological comfort" (Marholin *et al.*, 1979, p. 169). Because Marholin *et al.* provided a quantitative analysis of a range of behaviors under controlled conditions involving the alternate presence and absence of the drug, they were able to make such an assertion with relative confidence. Their study is an excellent example of how behavior therapists can assist in the accurate assessment of patients' responses to psychotropic medications.

In assessing these responses, it is important to ensure that side effects will be detected. Checklists and rating scales are often useful for this purpose. Table 2 lists a number of rating scales designed specifically to assess side effects. Several scales for rating tardive dyskinesias (involuntary motor activity produced by neuroleptic drugs) are listed in Table 3.

Although the evaluation of psychotropic medication is in principle no different from the evaluation of nonpharmacological interventions, unique characteristics of particular medications must be considered in evaluating the efficacy of these agents. For example, with antidepressants, therapeutic effects characteristically appear only after protracted exposure (e.g., of three to four weeks). With many neuroleptics, behaviorally active levels of the medication or its metabolites stay in the blood long after the medication is withdrawn. Moreover, in some patients, the abrupt withdrawal of neuroleptics precipitates a behavioral deterioration that is not evident with gradual withdrawal. An evaluation of a medication that does not take these features into consideration is unlikely to provide a fair assessment of its efficacy.

The same is true of evaluations that fail to arrange placebo control and double-blind conditions, the importance of which is covered fully by Gadow, White, and Ferguson (1986a,b).

Table 2.   Selected Side-Effect Rating Scales[a]

Scale	Source	Side effects evaluated
Abnormal Involuntary Movement Scale (AIMS)	Borison (1985)	Acute extrapyramidal side effects (akathisia, dystonia, pseudo-parkinsonism)
Dosage record and Treatment Emergent Symptom Scale (DOTES)	National Institute of Mental Health (1985b)	General side effects
Monitoring of Side-Effects System (MOSES)	Kalachnik (1988a)	General side effects
Neurological rating scale	Simpson & Angus (1970)	Acute extrapyramidal side effects
Parent's interval rating scales for side effects (also scales for physicians asking children)	Gofman (1972–1973)	General side effects
Scandinavian Society of Psychopharmacological Committee of Clinical Investigations Rating Scale	Scandinavian Society of Psychopharmacology (1987)	General side effects
Systematic Assessment for Treatment Emergent Effects (SAFTEE)	National Institute of Mental Health (1986)	General side effects
Subjective Treatment Emergent Symptoms Scale (STRESS)	National Institute of Mental Health (1985c)	General side effects
Systematic toxicity rating scale, neurotoxicity rating scale, seizure type and frequency rating	Cramer *et al.* (1983)	Antiepileptic effects and general side effects
Withdrawal Emergent Symptoms Checklist (WESC)	Engelhardt (1974)	General drug-withdrawal side effects

[a]From J. E. Kalachnik. (1988). Medication Monitoring Procedures. In K. D. Gadow and A. Poling (Eds.), *Pharmacotherapy and Mental Retardation* (p. 243). San Diego: College-Hill Press. Copyright 1988 by College-Hill Press. Reproduced by permission.

Table 3. Selected Tardive Dyskinesia Rating Scales

Scale name	Source
Abbreviated Dyskinesia Scale (ADS)	Simpson & Angus (1970)
Abnormal Involuntary Movement Scale (AIMS)	Guy (1976); National Institute of Mental Health (1985a)
Dyskinesia Identification System—Coldwater (DIS-Co)	Sprague, White, Ullmann, & Kalachnik (1984)
Dyskinesia Identification System: Condensed User Scale (DISCUS)	Sprague, Kalachnik, & White (1985)
Simpson Tardive Dyskinesia Rating Scale (TDRS)	Simpson, Lee, Zoubok, & Gardos (1979)
Smith-Texas Research Institute of Mental Sciences (TRIMS) dyskinesia scale	Smith, Allen, Gordon, & Wolff (1983)

In essence, to prevent nonspecific factors such as client or staff expectations and observer bias from confounding the drug effect, an inactive substance (placebo) similar to the drug being evaluated in size, shape, color, and taste should be administered during nondrug sessions. Further, to prevent bias and expectancy from confounding treatment effects, neither the clients nor the observers should be able to discriminate among the experimental conditions (i.e., conditions should be "double-blind"). In some instances, however, discriminable effects of the drug may break the double-blind. Patients can, for instance, probably ascertain whether they have received amphetamine or an inert placebo.

Although it may not always be possible to arrange placebo controls and double-blind conditions in everyday clinical drug evaluations, the failure to do so may render tentative any conclusions concerning efficacy. For example, Baldessarini (1989) noted that marked symptom suppression occurred in 65%–85% of adult patients with major depression who were treated with tricyclics, but 20%–40% also improved with placebo. Differentiating placebo responses from other beneficial effects of a medication is an important, but difficult, task.

SUMMARY

With few exceptions, behavior therapists do not prescribe psychotropic drugs. Nonetheless, as outlined in this chapter, the everyday activities of behavior therapists in hospital settings are much affected by the commonplace use of these agents to treat a wide variety of behavior disorders. Our discussion of this effect is by no means novel. For example, in a recent review of behavior therapy for schizophrenia, Bellack (1986) made several points similar to those emphasized here. He indicated that behavioral procedures are useful adjuncts to pharmacotherapy and are valuable in increasing patient compliance with drug treatments. Moreover, he noted, such procedures constitute an effective and humane alternative to other management procedures (e.g., restraint and seclusion) for those patients who do not respond to medication. Bellack also suggested that behavioral interventions may prove useful in reducing the neurological side effects associated with chronic neuroleptic treatment. This suggestion was not made in this chapter but is surely important.

REFERENCES

Aman, M. N., & Singh, N. N. (1988). *Psychopharmacology of the developmental disabilities*. New York: Springer-Verlag.

American Psychiatric Association. (1987). *Diagnostic and statistical manual of mental disorders* (3rd ed., rev.; DSM-III-R). Washington, DC: Author.

Baldessarini, R. J. (1985a). *Chemotherapy in psychiatry*. Cambridge: Harvard University Press.

Baldessarini, R. J. (1985b). Drugs and the treatment of psychiatric disorders. In A. G. Gilman, L. S. Goodman, T. W. Rall, & F. Murad (Eds.), *The pharmacological basis of therapeutics* (pp. 387–445). New York: Macmillan.

Baldessarini, R. J. (1989). Current status of antidepressants: Clinical pharmacology and therapy. *Journal of Clinical Psychiatry, 50,* 117–126.

Bellack, A. (1986). Schizophrenia: Behavior therapy's forgotten child. *Behavior Therapy, 17,* 199–214.

Benet, L,. Z., & Sheiner, L. W. (1985). Introduction. In A. G. Gilman, L. S. Goodman, T. W. Rall, & F. Murad (Eds.), *The pharmacological basis of therapeutics* (pp. 1–2). New York: Macmillan.

Berger, P. A. (1978). Medical treatment of mental illness. *Science, 200,* 974–981.

Birhamer, B., Greenhill, L. L., Cooper, T. B. Fried, J., & Maminski, B. (1989). Sustain released methylphenidate: Pharmacokinetic studies in ADDH males. *Journal of the American Academy of Child and Adolescent Psychiatry, 28,* 768–772.

Borison, R. (1985, May). *The recognition and management of drug-induced movement disorders (reversible type).* Paper presented at the annual meeting of the American Psychiatric Association, Dallas.

Briant, R. H. (1978). An introduction to clinical pharmacology. In J. S. Werry (Ed.), *The use of behavior modifying drugs with children* (pp. 3–28). New York: Brunner/Mazel.

Briggs, R., Garrard, S., Hamad, C., & Wills, F. (1984). A model for evaluating psychoactive medication use with mentally retarded persons. In J. A. Mulick & B. L. Mallory (Eds.), *Transitions in mental retardation: Advocacy, technology, and science* (pp. 229–248). Norwood, NJ: Ablex.

Brown, B. S., Wienckowski, L. A., & Stolz, S. B. (1975). *Behavior modification: Perspectives on a current issue.* Washington, DC: National Institutes of Mental Health.

Cantwell, D. P., & Carlson, G. A. (1978). Stimulants. In J. S. Werry (Ed.), *Pediatric psychopharmacology: The use of behavior modifying drugs with children* (pp. 253–301). New York: Brunner/Mazel.

Cohen, M. N., & Sprague, R. L. (1977, March). *Survey of drug usage in two midwestern institutions for the retarded.* Paper presented at the Gatlinburg Conference on Research in Mental Retardation, Gatlinburg, TN.

Cramer, J. A., Smith, D. B., Mattson, R. H., Excueta, A. V. D., Collins, J. F., & the VA Cooperative Study Group. (1983). A method of quantification for the evaluation of antiepileptic drug therapy. *Neurology, 33* (Suppl. 1), 26–27.

Engelhardt, D. M. (1974). *Withdrawal Emergent Symptoms (WES) Checklist.* (Available from author on request, Department of Psychiatry, Downstate Medical Center, State University of New York, 460 Clarkston Ave., Brooklyn, NY 11203.)

Fischbacher, E. (1987). Prescribing in a hospital for the mentally retarded. *Journal of Mental Deficiency Research, 31,* 17–29.

Gadow, K. D. (1986a). *Children on medication: Vol. 1. Hyperactivity, learning disabilities, and mental retardation.* San Diego: College-Hill Press.

Gadow, K. D. (1986b). *Children on medication: Vol. 2. Epilepsy, emotional disturbance, and adolescent disorders.* San Diego: College-Hill Press.

Gadow, K. D., & Poling, A. (1986). *Methodological issues in human psychopharmacology.* Greenwich, CT: JAI Press.

Gadow, K. D., & Poling, A. (1988). *Pharmacotherapy and mental retardation.* San Diego: College-Hill Press.

Gadow, K. D., White, L., & Ferguson, D. G. (1986a). Placebo controls and double-blind conditions: Part 1. In K. E. Gadow & A. Poling (Eds.), *Methodological issues in human psychopharmacology* (pp. 41–84). Greenwich, CT: JAI Press.

Gadow, K. D., White, L., & Ferguson, D. G. (1986b). Placebo controls and double-blind conditions: Part 2. In K. E. Gadow & A. Poling (Eds.), *Methodological issues in human psychopharmacology* (pp. 85–114). Greenwich, CT: JAI Press.

Gilman, A. G., Goodman, L. S., Rall, T. W., & Murad, F. (1985). *The pharmacological basis of therapeutics.* New York: Macmillan.

Gofman, H. (1972–1973). Interval and final rating sheets on side effects. *Psychopharmacology Bulletin (Special Issue), 8–9,* 182–187.

Gomes-Schwartz, B. (1979). The modification of schizophrenic behavior. *Behavior Modification, 3,* 439–468.

Goth, A. (1984). *Medical pharmacology.* St. Louis: Mosby.

Guy, W. (1976). *ECDEU assessment manual for psychopharmacology.* Washington, DC: U.S. Government Printing Office.

Hare, E. H., & Wilcox, D. R. C. (1967). Do psychiatric inpatients take their drugs? *British Journal of Psychiatry, 113,* 1435–1439.

Hersen, M. (1979). Limitations and problems in the clinical application of behavioral techniques in psychiatric settings. *Behavior Therapy, 10,* 65–80.

Hersen, M. (1986). *Pharmacological and behavioral treatment: An integrative approach.* New York: Wiley.

Hill, B. K., Balow, E. A., & Bruininks, R. H. (1985). A national study of prescribed drugs in institutions and community residential facilities for mentally retarded people. *Psychopharmacology Bulletin, 21,* 279–284.

Huessy, H. R., & Ruoff, P. A. (1984). Towards a rational drug usage in a state institution for retarded individuals. *Psychiatric Journal of the University of Ottawa, 9,* 56–59.

Julien, R. M. (1985). *A primer of drug action.* San Francisco: Freeman.

Kalachnik, J. E. (1988a). *Monitoring of side-effects scale (MOSES).* St. Paul: Minnesota Department of Human Services.

Kalachnik, J. E. (1988b). *Psychotropic medication monitoring checklist and manual for Rule 34 facilities.* St. Paul: Minnesota Department of Human Services, Licensing Division.

Kane, J. M. (1987). *Treatment of schizophrenia. Schizophrenia Bulletin, 13,* 133–151.

Klein, D. F., Gittelman, R., Quitkin, F., & Rifkin, A. (1980). *Diagnosis and drug treatment of psychiatric disorders: Adults and children.* Baltimore: Williams & Wilkins.

LaMendola, W., Zaharia, E., & Carver, M. (1980). Reducing psychotropic drug use in an institution for the retarded. *Hospital and Community Psychiatry, 31,* 272–272.

Laska, E., Varga, E., Wanderling, J., Simpson, G., Logemann, G. W., & Shah, B. K. (1973). Patterns of psychotropic drug use for schizophrenia. *Diseases of the Nervous System, 34,* 294–305.

Laska, E., Craig, T. J., Siegel, C., & Wanderling, J. (1981). Long-term monitoring of psychopharmacological treatment in hospitalized patients. In G. Tognoni, C., Belantuono, & M. Lader (Eds.), *Epidemiological impact of psychotropic drugs* (pp. 101–116). New York: Elsevier.

Longo, V. G. (1972). *Neuropharmacology and behavior.* San Francisco: Freeman.

Marholin, D., Touchette, P. E., & Stewart, R. M. (1979). Withdrawal of chronic chlorpromazine medication: An experimental analysis. *Journal of Applied Behavior Analysis, 12,* 150–171.

National Institute of Mental Health. (1985a). AIMS (Abnormal Involuntary Movement Scale). *Psychopharmacology Bulletin, 20,* 1077–1080.

National Institute of Mental Health. (1985b). DOTES (Dosage Record and Treatment Emergent Symptom Scale). *Psychopharmacology Bulletin, 20,* 1067–1068.

National Institute of Mental Health. (1985c). STRESS (Subjective Treatment Emergent Symptoms Scale). *Psychopharmacology Bulletin, 20,* 1073–1075.

National Institute of Mental Health. (1986). Systematic Assessment for Treatment Emergent Events (SAFTEE). *Psychopharmacology Bulletin, 22,* 347–381.

O'Brien, M., & Orbzut, J. (1986). Attention deficit disorder with hyperactivity: A review and implications for the classroom. *The Journal of Special Education, 20,* 281–297.

O'Leary, D. K. (1980). Pills or skills for hyperactive children? *Journal of Applied Behavior Analysis, 13,* 191–204.

Pelham, W. E., Jr., & Murpy, H. A. (1986). Attention deficit and conduct disorders. In M. Hersen (Ed.), *Pharmacological and behavioral treatment: An integrative approach* (pp. 108–148). New York: Wiley.

Poling, A., Gadow, K., & Cleary, J. (1991). *Drug therapy for behavior disorders: An introduction.* New York: Pergamon Press.

Prien, R. F., Haber, P. A., & Caffey, E. M. (1975). The use of psychoactive drugs in elderly patients with psychiatric disorders: Survey conducted in twelve Veterans Administration hospitals. *Journal of the American Geriatric Society, 23,* 104–112.

Prien, R. F., Klett, C. J., & Caffey, E. M. (1976). Polypharmacy in the psychiatric treatment of elderly hospitalized patients: A survey of 12 Veterans Administration hospitals. *Diseases of the Nervous System, 37,* 333–336.

Pulman, R. M., Pook, R. B., & Singh, N. N. (1979). Prevalence of drug therapy for institutionalized mentally retarded children. *Australian Journal of Mental Retardation, 5,* 212–214.

Ross, D. M., & Ross, S. A. (1982). *Hyperactivity: Current issues, research, and theory.* New York: Wiley.

Scandinavian Society of Psychopharmacology Committee of Clinical Investigations (UKU). (1987). The UKU side effects rating scale. *Acta Psychiatrica Scandinavica, 76* (entire supplement).

Sewell, J., & Werry, J. S. (1976). Some studies in an institution for the mentally retarded. *New Zealand Medical Journal, 84,* 317–319.

Sheppard, C., Collins, L., Fiorentino, D., Fracchia, J., & Merlis, S. (1969). Polypharmacy in psychiatric treatment: 1. Incidence at a state hospital. *Current Therapeutic Research, 11,* 765–774.

Silva, D. A. (1979). The use of medication in a residential institution for mentally retarded persons. *Mental Retardation, 17,* 285–288.

Simpson, G. M., & Angus, J. W. S. (1970). A rating scale for extrapyramidal side effects. *Acta Psychiatrica Scandinavica* (Suppl. 212), 11–19.

Simpson, G. M., Lee, J. H., Zoubok, B., & Gardos, G. (1979). A rating scale for tardive dyskinesia. *Psychopharmacology, 64,* 171–179.

Smith, R. C., Allen, R., Gordon, J., & Wolff, J. (1983). A rating scale for tardive dyskinesia and parkinsonian symptoms. *Psychopharmacology Bulletin*, *19*, 266–276.

Sneader, W. (1986). *Drug discovery: The evolution of modern medicines*. New York: Wiley.

Spencer, D. A. (1974). A survey of the medication in a hospital for the mentally handicapped. *British Journal of Psychiatry*, *124*, 507–508.

Sprague, R. L., & Werry, J. S. (1971). Methodology of psychopharmacological studies with the retarded. In N. R. Ellis (Ed.), *International review of research in mental retardation* (Vol. 5, pp. 147–219). Orlando, FL: Academic Press.

Sprague, R. L., White, D. M., Ullmann, R., & Kalachnik, J. E. (1984). Methods for selecting items in a tardive dyskinesia rating scale. *Psychopharmacology Bulletin*, *20*, 339–345.

Sprague, R. L., Kalachnik, J. E., & White, D. M. (1985). *Dyskinesia Identification System: Condensed User Scale (DISCUS)*. Champaign, IL: Institute for Child Behavior and Development.

Tu, J. B. (1979). A survey of psychotropic medication in mental retardation facilities. *Journal of Clinical Psychiatry*, *40*, 125–128.

Usdin, E., & Efron, D. H. (1972). *Psychotropic drugs and related compounds*. Washington, DC: U.S. Government Printing Office.

Wallace, C. J., Donahoe, C. P., Jr., & Boone, S. E. (1986). Schizophrenia. In M. Hersen (Ed.), *Pharmacological and behavioral treatment: An integrative approach* (pp. 357–381). New York: Wiley.

Werry, J. S. (1978). *Pediatric psychopharmacology: The use of behavior modifying drugs with children*. New York: Brunner/Mazel.

White, A. J. (1983). Changing patterns of psychoactive drug use with the mentally retarded. *New Zealand Medical Journal*, *96*, 686–688.

Wysowski, D. K., & Baum, C. (1989). Antipsychotic drug use in the United States, 1976–1985. *Archives of General Psychiatry*, *46*, 929–932.

Zimbardo, P. G. (1988). *Psychology and life*. Glenview, IL: Scott, Foresman.

Zimmermann, R. L., & Heistad, G. T. (1982). Studies of the long term efficacy of antipsychotic drugs in controlling the behavior of institutionalized retardates. *Journal of the American Academy of Child Psychiatry*, *21*, 136–143.

7

Hospital Structure and Professional Roles

FAITH B. DICKERSON

INTRODUCTION

Behavior therapy has made significant advances in the treatment of psychiatric patients since the mid-1960s. The opportunity to apply behavior therapy in psychiatric settings, however, depends on administrative factors within the settings. Because behavior therapy is a relative newcomer to hospital treatment, crosscuts usual professional boundaries, and contradicts aspects of the medical model, it does not readily "fit" in the psychiatric hospital structure. The collective experience of behavior therapists in psychiatric settings points to common organizational issues that may arise in the hospital practice of behavior therapy.

THE HOSPITAL SETTING

General Issues

Behavior therapists in psychiatric hospital settings find themselves in the midst of physician-dominated institutions, organized around the medical model of illness and treatment. The traditional hospital is a large bureaucracy with a rigid hierarchy of professional disciplines. Although each profession provides specific services for patients, frequent collaboration is necessary, and roles may overlap. Unlike the established medical professions, behavior therapy is typically outside the hospital power structure and lacks a specified place in the organization. As noted by Hersen (1979), there are enormous possibilities for conflict, dissent, and chaos in the psychiatric setting for behavior therapists.

Another prominent feature of hospital operations is a concern about costs. The hospital is a big business and is driven, at least in part, by economic considerations. Although the particular financial incentives vary by the type of hospital and the source of money, hospital efforts to increase revenues and reduce expenses are now universal. Even apart from issues of direct

---

FAITH B. DICKERSON • The Sheppard and Enoch Pratt Hospital, 6501 North Charles Street, Baltimore, Maryland 21204.

Handbook of Behavior Therapy in the Psychiatric Setting, edited by Alan S. Bellack and Michel Hersen. Plenum Press, New York, 1993.

patient care, behavior therapists may be influenced by economic contingencies operative within the hospital setting.

Behavior therapists in hospital settings not only are confronted by a complex, economically driven medical system but also espouse a model of treatment that is at odds with the psychiatric establishment. Psychiatry is currently dominated by biological and psychoanalytic models, with behavior therapy lying outside the psychiatric mainstream. Psychoanalysis is declining from its former dominance but still exerts some influence in most psychiatric settings and is usually part of the training of psychiatric residents. The biological model has overtaken psychoanalysis as psychiatry has become "remedicalized." In most psychiatric settings, there is now an increasing emphasis on the organic basis of psychiatric illnesses and treatment.

Behavior therapy challenges both the psychoanalytic and the biological ideologies, but it is more compatible with the biological model. The emergence of the biological model has permitted more collaboration with behavior therapy in psychiatric settings. Both the behavioral and the biological approaches are symptom- or problem-focused and take an objective, empirical stance toward treatment. Competition between the models still occurs. Conflict may emerge around the issue of which treatment to try first or around what caused clinical change ("It was the meds that made the patient better"; "No, the patient's improvement was due to the behavior program"). However, the models can complement and enrich each other and lead to an integrated treatment approach.

Types of Hospital Settings

Psychiatric hospital settings can be divided into those that are publicly funded and those that are in the private sector, either proprietary or not-for-profit. Psychiatric units within university hospitals constitute another group; they may combine features of both public and private settings and also provide training and research.

The public sector is composed primarily of state and veterans' (VA) hospitals. These settings tend to accumulate a population of chronically ill, geriatric, and indigent patients who have exhausted private health insurance benefits. The hospital settings themselves may lack professional and financial resources, a lack adding to the challenge for mental health professionals. For these reasons, there have been fewer competing models of care in public settings. Psychologists and behavior therapists have assumed broad roles in developing and carrying out treatment in these public facilities. In fact, it was in state hospitals that the early and pioneering behavioral work with psychiatric patients occurred (Ayllon & Azrin, 1968; Schaefer & Martin, 1966).

The current status of behavior therapy in public hospitals is highly variable. Given the relatively fewer numbers of professional staff in public than in private settings, psychologists and behavior therapists may have wide professional latitude and a wide range of responsibilities, enabling them to implement behavior therapy programs. On the other hand, public systems may be handicapped by limits in the funding and administrative support that are necessary for program development. Additionally, public hospital staff may be accustomed to providing custodial care and may resist the demands of active treatment such as behavior therapy. If public hospitals have a university affiliation, as many VA hospitals do, they are likely to have access to academic departments of psychology and trained behavior therapists, as well as greater overall professional resources.

Behavior therapy is underused in public, as well as in private, settings, despite its proven efficacy with severely disturbed psychiatric patients. A survey of VA hospitals in the mid-1980s (Boudewyns, Fry, & Nightingale, 1986) revealed that only 6.6% of all VA psychological services had social learning programs, and that only about 1% of all psychiatric patients in the VA system had access to this form of treatment. Survey respondents cited resistance to behavior therapy by their hospital administrations, as well as misconceptions of behavior therapy by nursing staff.

In the private psychiatric hospital as well, behavior therapy has only a limited presence and is by no means standard practice. A recent survey of private psychiatric hospitals (Dickerson, 1989) showed that fewer than one fifth have an inpatient program based on behavior therapy; the majority of these units treat children and adolescents. Behavior therapy consultation services are slightly more common, and about a quarter of hospitals provide these services.

As in the public sector, there are obstacles to the implementation of behavior therapy in private hospitals. Among the most prominent is that fact that private hospitals are often far removed from academic research settings, have their own established methods of operation, and may be slow to incorporate newer models of treatment. In the private setting, additionally, patient lengths of stay are typically short, and treating doctors are often private practitioners from the community rather than salaried hospital employees. Also, the patients are relatively high-functioning compared with the more severely and chronically ill patients in public hospitals. All of these factors conspire against the programmatic use of behavior therapy, particularly token economy programs.

There are indications, however, that behavior therapy has an increasing role in private hospitals. Contributing to this trend is the advent of contractual behavior therapy and more skill-based training with private hospitalized patients (Levendusky, Berglass, Dooley, & Landrau, 1983). These approaches have been found to be well suited to the range of psychiatric patients in the private hospital. Because these approaches are problem-focused, they also fare well in the increasingly competitive market of mental health care.

There is now intense financial competition in the private psychiatric sector. Contributing to this phenomenon is the recent and strenuous effort by third-party insurance companies to reduce costs by limiting benefits and overseeing treatment. Referred to as *managed care*, the practice involves a prospective and/or concurrent review of psychiatric treatment by the third-party payer, which then makes decisions about reimbursement. The third-party reviewer may also make recommendations about the types of treatment to be provided. Because the standards of mental health treatment are often ambiguous, decisions by third-party payers tend to be discretionary and rendered on a case-by-case basis.

Managed-care practices have been effective in reducing lengths of hospital stay in private settings. This reduction has affected all mental health professionals, including behavior therapists. In many ways, behavior therapy is well positioned to deal with managed-care reviews because behavior therapy tends to be clearly defined, empirically based, and cost-effective (Paul & Lentz, 1977). However, third-party reviewers may not always appreciate behavioral modalities. They may insist on a physician as the primary therapist, even when this is not the arrangement for a given patient. Also, they may promote more medical treatments, such as medication, on the assumption that they are less costly. Behavior therapists need to be ready and able to advocate for and justify behavioral treatment in this new era of cost containment.

INTERDISCIPLINARY COLLABORATION

Home Base within Psychology

Psychology has been the breeding ground for behavior therapy, and the ranks of behavior therapists are disproportionately filled by psychologists. Unlike professionals from other mental health disciplines, psychologists are routinely exposed to the principles of behavior therapy in the course of their training. This exposure leads to some background in and understanding of behavior approaches, even among psychologists who do not become behavior therapists.

In practicing behavior therapy in hospital settings, psychologists necessarily collaborate with a range of other professionals. The overlapping of responsibilities may promote professional sharing, but it may also lead to competition and turf battles, as well as ambiguity about professional roles.

FAITH B. DICKERSON

Psychiatry

Historically, psychiatrists have controlled the treatment of psychiatric inpatients. They continue to have the final authority and supervisory responsibility for hospitalized patients, and they usually assume the leadership roles in psychiatric hospital settings. In the administrative hierarchy, behavior therapists are usually housed within psychiatry or ultimately report to a psychiatrist administrator. However, only a minority of psychiatrists have been exposed to behavior therapy in their training. This fact contributes to the underuse of behavior therapy in psychiatric settings.

Psychiatrists tend not only to be uneducated about behavior therapy, but to have a view of psychiatric illness and treatment that is not fully consistent with a behavioral approach. The biological model, mentioned earlier, emphasizes psychiatric disorders as diseases with presumed organic etiologies. Differential diagnosis is central to the assessment process, which then leads to specific treatment (Kingsbury, 1987). The behavioral model assumes that psychological problems are often caused by multiple factors. Diagnosis *per se* is often less important than a behavioral inventory of the patient's skill deficits, cognitive distortions, and reinforcement contingencies.

Despite the potential differences between psychiatrists and behavior therapists, collaboration frequently can and does occur. Behavior therapy has gained wide respectability as the primary treatment for some disorders such as those in which anxiety is central. Conversely, medication may be a necessary first step in the treatment of other disorders. It is no longer a question of either/or strategies, but a question of how to best combine effective treatments. A good example is chronic schizophrenia, which usually requires both medication and skills training for a positive therapeutic outcome.

Nursing

As the front line of care in psychiatric hospitals, nursing staff are frequently called on to implement behavior therapy. More often than not, it is the nursing staff who actually carry out selective reinforcement, time-out, extinction, skills training, and so on. Nurses may also work one to one with patients in developing contracts and treatment plans. Because of their direct contact with patients, they are also best able to observe patients, assess problem areas, and recommend targets for behavioral interventions.

Even though they are well positioned to carry out behavior therapy, nurses may be subject to competing influences that conflict with their behavioral role. Like psychiatrists, nurses typically have had little formal exposure to behavioral techniques in the course of their training. Additionally, nurses are traditionally reinforced for their unconditional nurturance of patients and for their compliance with physician orders. By contrast, behavior therapy requires the use of selective rewards and independent judgment, which are contrary to the traditional nurse role.

Nurses are also accountable for their own routine of procedures and paperwork. These tasks usually have a high priority in nurses' day-to-day work. Unless a behavioral program is clearly defined as part of nursing's responsibility, it may not be consistently implemented.

Rehabilitation Therapies

The collaboration between behavior therapy and rehabilitation therapies can be a fruitful alliance in the hospital setting. Rehabilitation therapists such as occupational therapists and recreational therapists typically organize patient activities in psychiatric settings and serve as the leaders of rehabilitation groups for patients. Like behavior therapists, rehabilitation therapists tend to focus on practical behavioral skills, an objective assessment of functioning, and discrete skills training. Many of their therapeutic approaches are drawn directly from behavioral principles (e.g., Anthony, 1980).

Although the overlap is considerable between behavior and rehabilitation therapies, the latter tend to be less empirically based in both assessment and treatment methods. Also, in the psychiatric setting, rehabilitation therapies are typically focused on global adaptive functioning, whereas behavior therapy may be more strategic in its approach to the specific symptoms and problems of a particular patient. Rehabilitation therapists are often very receptive to behavioral colleagues, and the two groups can complement each other's work.

MODELS OF INPATIENT BEHAVIOR THERAPY

Behavior Therapy Programs

Behavior therapy programs that have been successfully established in psychiatric hospitals tend to display common organizational features that have been instrumental in their effectiveness. The consistency of these features is striking and occurs across a variety of hospital settings, both public and private (Merkel & Pollard, 1987; Morgan, Kremer, & Gaylor, 1979; Mosk, Kuehnel, Friedman, Collier, & Turley, 1988; Parker, Karol, & Doerfler, 1983). These behavior therapy programs tend to be the product of creative individuals who have established their credibility with the hospital administration. They have used personal power and diplomacy to persuade hospital authorities about the benefits of behavior therapy. This persuasion is necessary because institutions are generally opposed to change and need considerable pressure to establish new clinical programs. Sometimes, a foothold for behavior therapy has been established through the treatment of unusually difficult, so-called impossible patients, who have stumped their therapists and defied all conventional treatments. Behavior therapy may be called in as a last resort and may thus establish itself as a credible and potentially powerful approach.

A crucial ingredient in the development of behavioral programs is strong institutional support, both initial and ongoing. Support takes the form of underwriting start-up costs and also providing public endorsement of the program and its anticipated success. Autonomy from the hospital bureaucratic structure is also essential to enable the program to develop its own identity, to unburden the new program from unnecessary hospital policies and procedures, and to set the new program apart from traditional units.

The leadership on a behavioral unit is usually different from the typical arrangement of psychiatrists, who are responsible for individual patients and report to a physician service chief. On a behavioral unit, a psychologist/behavior therapist may be the clinical director or may share the leadership with a physician/psychiatrist. Whatever the arrangement, it is likely to be different from the usual power hierarchy of physician dominance and may threaten the existing order. As noted by Pollard *et al.* (1986), psychologists in such leadership roles may be "journeying into alien territory" and may elicit an unwelcome response.

The behavioral unit, with its clear boundaries, needs also to have the authority to choose both patients and staff. This is important if the unit is to maintain its autonomy from the hospital at large. Within the unit itself, the organization of roles is typically less hierarchical and more decentralized than in the traditional hospital unit. Professional roles are thus deemphasized, and clinicians from various disciplines are assigned to similar tasks and duties. For example, nursing staff may be patient coordinators or primary therapists, a psychologist and occupational therapist may colead a skills-training group, and a team of staff from various disciplines may work collaboratively to set patient goals and treatment plans. Decentralization is beneficial in promoting ongoing program development and facilitating a sense of group cohesion and shared purpose. Decentralization and role sharing also help to foster the skill development of front-line nursing staff, who carry out much of the behavioral treatment.

Consultation Services

Behavior therapists may also provide services to psychiatric patients in the role of consultants. In this situation, the behavior therapist responds to a referral from the patient's doctor or team for particular problems or issues in the patient's treatment. Typically, the clinical problems leading to a referral are behavioral management issues or focused clinical symptoms known to respond well to behavioral approaches. In some cases, the request for a behavioral consultation, as for any consultation, may be the product of team frustration or disagreement. The behavior therapist called in as a consultant may work directly with the patient or may direct the unit staff in behavioral strategies. The unit staff maintain primary control over the patient's treatment.

The behavior therapy consultation is fraught with potential pitfalls (see Chapter 8 in this book). One commonly noted problem is the lack of understanding of behavior therapy on the part of the inpatient staff, who have initiated the referral and remain the primary treaters. The behavioral consultant may not be sufficiently included in the patient's total treatment; other treatment decisions may be made without regard to their consistency with the behavioral plan. Unrealistic expectations of behavior therapy may lead to early frustrations by the team and, in the worst outcome, abandonment of the behavioral treatment.

Consultation with nonbehavioral colleagues is usually most effective when the consultant has personal credibility and some degree of authority. It is also helpful when the institution places value on behavioral approaches. As noted by behavior therapists who have developed successful consultation services (Malatesta, Aubuchon, Bloomgarden, & Kowitt, 1989; McGee, 1988), behavior therapy can be effectively combined with other treatments and can effectively complement the other aspects of the patient's primary treatment.

PROBLEMS AND TRENDS

Stigma and Misapplication of Behavior Therapy

Over the years, behavior therapy has often been stereotyped and misunderstood. Shortened to the pejorative term *b mod*, behavior modification has been perceived as a superficial, mechanistic approach that is dehumanizing and deterministic. Behavior therapy has been contrasted with the preferred methods of psychodynamic insight and emotional expressiveness. For reasons that remain mysterious, behavior therapy has also been erroneously linked with invasive medical procedures, such as electroshock and brain surgery.

Although some of the more gross distortions of behavior therapy have subsided somewhat, the term *behavior therapy* continues to be misapplied. In hospital settings, it may be used to describe harsh and arbitrary restrictive measures, such as locked-door seclusion, that appear to be more easily sanctioned if the term *behavior therapy* is applied. The term may also be used to describe crude reward or punishment schemes, devised off the cuff by front-line staff, again offering a professional sounding label to staff efforts to maintain order and control.

A related problem is the misconception that behavior therapy is easily performed by any clinician regardless of his or her training or expertise. Because of their extensive contact with psychiatric patients, mental health paraprofessionals may be considered behavioral specialists. Although, in fact, paraprofessional staff may be skilled in some behavioral techniques, a great deal of expertise is required to use behavior therapy well. Good behavioral treatment is very labor-intensive, requiring repeated and strategic interventions with patients. The kinds of settings that have limited professional resources and need quick and powerful management techniques may be ill equipped to carry out effective behavior therapy.

The acceptance and understanding of behavior therapy have also been reduced by the fact that behavior therapy was initially oversold. Early behavior therapists were expansive in claims that led to disappointment and disillusionment when the expectations of the new technology were not met. The idea that behavioral techniques could quickly and dramatically change behavior, regardless of the etiology and severity of the behavioral problems, was obviously bogus. Yet, even today in hospital settings, a behavioral plan may be prematurely set aside because it does not meet those unrealistically high expectations.

On the positive side, some aspects of behavior therapy have been so fully accepted that they have been incorporated into psychiatric programs as part of the mainstream of treatment. For example, concepts such as time-out, selective rewards, contingencies, and contracts may be used in programs without special designation as "behavior therapy." Although in some cases behavioral procedures may be borrowed and haphazardly applied, in other cases behavioral approaches have been well integrated and embedded in therapeutic programs.

Patients' Rights

The hospital treatment of psychiatric patients has been influenced and altered by the patients' rights movement and by landmark legal decisions that have set standards for aspects of hospital psychiatric care. The impetus to protect patients and to broaden their rights emerged from the powerless position of institutionalized patients. Many of these patients were, and are, highly impaired and have been institutionalized for extended periods, without their own advocates or the ability to defend themselves.

Pioneering behavior therapists developed and researched the token economy before the current era of sensitivity to patients' rights. They were able to draw on a full range of behavioral reinforcers and deprivations in their creation of the token economy approach. However, many of what were formerly potential reinforcers are now considered basic patient entitlements in a hospital setting. For example, food, comfortable living conditions, and, in some cases, cigarettes cannot be used as contingent rewards because they are givens in a patient's hospitalization. Similarly, patient work assignments, used as target behaviors in early token economy systems, are sharply limited legally. The historical reasons are clear; patients in the past were subject to potential abuse in hospitals that had little to offer in the way of effective treatment.

Although the legacy of patients' rights is understandable and even laudable, it has limited the potential of some kinds of behavioral programming. For example, it may be hard to gain enough control over the environment to institute an effective token economy program; patients' vocational training may be arbitrarily limited by hospital rules. But in a larger sense, the climate of expanded patients' rights has been a substantial gain for behavior therapy. Behavior therapy in hospital settings has shifted away from restrictive and operant approaches to skills training, education, and contractual models. Patients are now more directly encouraged to participate in their own treatment planning and to assume a more active, collaborative role with their treaters.

Behavior therapy in hospital settings is not without occasional and ongoing controversy. Aversive techniques, such as mild electroshock for severe self-injurious behavior, are the focus of current debate and generate conflict among mental health professionals (Gardner, 1989). Other restrictive strategies, such as time-out and overcorrection, are generally considered acceptable because they are carried out in a neutral, nonpunitive manner, are a direct response to focal patient problem behavior, and are typically offset by opportunities for positive reinforcement.

Advancement of Psychologists

No discussion of inpatient behavior therapy would be complete without a reference to the recent gains made by psychologists as health care providers (Youngstown, 1990a,b). Although these advancements have not been promoted exclusively by behavior therapists, their benefits are strongly felt by behaviorally oriented psychologists.

Within the past several years, psychologists have won inclusion in Medicare, the federal health insurance program for the elderly and the disabled. This gain not only gives psychologists more stature, in general, but also affords more real opportunities for psychologists to work with both geriatric and chronic mentally ill patients. Both of these groups are well suited for selective behavioral treatment and probably have been underserved by behavior therapists.

Within the hospital organization itself, psychologists have a stronger foothold in gaining hospital privileges to admit and treat inpatients. In the mid-1980s, the primary hospital accrediting body, the Joint Commission on Accreditation of Healthcare Organizations (JCAHO) changed its guidelines to allow psychologists membership on hospital medical staffs, if permitted by state law and hospital bylaws. The movement gained additional momentum with the 1990 *CAPP v. Rank* decision. The California Supreme Court decision upheld the rights of psychologists as independent health providers who are authorized by law to practice independently in hospitals. Although few other states permit psychologists full hospital admission and treatment privileges, the precedent has been set.

These gains for psychologists have occurred at some expense of the relationship between psychology and psychiatry, the latter assuming the main opposition to psychology's expanded role. Psychologists of all persuasions, and including behavior therapists, have been swept up in the parochial conflict (Freeman, 1990). Although the process is a difficult one, the outcome of the political tumult will further expand and solidify the role of behavior therapists as treatment providers in hospital settings.

SUMMARY

Behavior therapists in psychiatric settings are typically psychologists working in physician-dominated hospital environments that are organized around the medical model. Behavior therapy is not fully consistent with this model, though it can complement other treatment strategies used in the hospital setting. Behavior therapy has been underused in both private and public hospitals. The pattern of use and application varies widely among hospitals. Behavior therapy inpatient programs that have been successfully established tend to have strong administrative support, relative autonomy from the hospital organization, and a nonhierarchical use of program staff. Some stigma and misunderstanding of behavior therapy linger, in part because hospital professionals such as psychiatrists and nurses are not exposed to behavior therapy in the course of their training. The practice of behavior therapy is also influenced by legal guidelines for hospital treatment, by the current political climate of psychologists' push for hospital privileges, and by increased competition among mental health professionals for financial reimbursement.

ACKNOWLEDGMENTS.   The author acknowledges helpful comments from Dr. Patrick Boudewyns; Ms. Diane Gibson; Drs. Robert Heinssen, Arthur M. Horton, Richard Hunter, Philip Levendusky, James McGee, William Merkel, and John Moore; Mr. Mark Schade; and Dr. Robert Yolken in the preparation of this manuscript.

REFERENCES

Anthony, W. A. (1980). *The principles of psychiatric rehabilitation*. Baltimore: University Park Press.

Ayllon, T., & Azrin, N. (1968). *The token economy: A motivational system for therapy and rehabilitation*. New York: Appleton-Century-Crofts.

Boudewyns, P. A., Fry, T. J., & Nightingale, E. T. (1986). Token economy programs in VA medical centers: Where are they today? *The Behavior Therapist, 6*, 126–127.

Dickerson, F. B. (1989). Behavior therapy in private hospitals: Results of a national survey. *The Behavior Therapist, 12*, 157.

Freeman, A. (1990). The war continues. *The Behavior Therapist, 13*, 33, 45.

Gardener, W. I. (1989). But in the meantime: A client perspective of the debate over the use of aversive/intrusive therapy procedures. *The Behavior Therapist, 12*, 179–181.

Hersen, M. (1979). Limitations and problems in the clinical application of behavioral techniques in psychiatric settings. *Behavior Therapy, 10*, 65–80.

Kingsbury, S. J. (1987). Cognitive differences between clinical psychologists and psychiatrists. *American Psychologist, 42*, 152–156.

Levendusky, P. G., Berglas, S., Dooley, C. P., & Landrau, R. J. (1983). Therapeutic contract program: Preliminary report on a behavioral alternative to the token economy. *Behaviour Research and Therapy, 21*, 137–142.

Malatesta, V. J., Aubuchon, P. G., Bloomgarden, A., & Kowitt, M. P. (1989). Hospital-based behavior therapy services. *The Psychiatric Hospital, 20*, 119–123.

McGee, J. (1988). Inpatient cognitive behavioral therapy. In J. R. Lion, W. N. Adler, & W. L. Webb, Jr. (Eds.), *Modern hospital psychiatry* (pp. 136–168). New York: W. W. Norton.

Merkel, W. T., & Pollard, C. A. (1987). Applying modern management principles to clinical administration of a behavioral oriented inpatient unit. *Hospital and Community Psychiatry, 38*, 152–159.

Morgan, C. D., Kremer, E., & Gaylor, M. (1979). The behavioral medicine unit: A new facility. *Comprehensive Psychiatry, 20*, 79–89.

Mosk, M. D., Kuehnel, T., Friedman, D. S., Collier, R., & Turley, F. (1988). Behavior therapy in a state hospital: Overcoming obstacles to implementation. *The Behavior Therapist, 11*, 119–122.

Parker, J. C., Karol, R. C., & Doerfler, L. A. (1983). Pain unit director: Role issues for health psychologists. *Professional Psychology: Research and Practice, 14*, 232–239.

Paul, G. L., & Lentz, R. J. (1977). *Psychosocial treatment of chronic mental patients; Milieu versus social-learning programs.* Cambridge: Harvard University Press.

Pollard, C. A., Merkel, W. T., & Obermeir, H. J. (1986). Inpatient behavior therapy: The St. Louis model. *Behavior Therapy and Experimental Psychiatry, 17*, 233–243.

Schaefer, H. H., & Martin, P. L. (1966). Behavioral therapy for "apathy" of hospitalized schizophrenics. *Psychological Reports, 19*, 1147–1158.

Youngstown, N. (1990a, August). CAPP v. Rank is overturned: Ruling boosts hospital privileges. *The APA Monitor, 21*, 1, 17.

Youngstown, N. (1990b, June). On privilege issue, field is tilting to "yes." *The APA Monitor, 21*, 12, 13.

8

Staff Training and Consultation

MICHEL HERSEN, ALAN S. BELLACK, and FRANCIS HARRIS

INTRODUCTION

The precise implementation of behavioral programs in the psychiatric setting is dependent primarily on the technical expertise of a variety of paraprofessionals and professionals, such as nursing assistants, mental health workers (usually B.A. level personnel), psychiatric nurses, and social workers. Irrespective of the particular setting in which a behavioral program is introduced (i.e., a state hospital, a mental health center, a university hospital, a Veterans Administration Hospital, or a general hospital), the aforementioned staff have literally "life-and-death" powers over its success or failure. Many a naive behavior therapist, although well trained and certainly well intentioned, has failed in his or her attempts either to implement a behavioral program from scratch or to replace an existing program with one behaviorally oriented. In both cases, failure can usually be traced to poor administrative support and staff resistance. Staff resistance is undoubtedly a result of inadequate preparation, the contrasting (and often covert) goals of the staff and the program initiator, incomplete training of the staff, and ineffective staff consultation once the program has been established.

In this chapter, we examine the issue of staff training and consultation from a number of different perspectives.

First, we will examine the psychiatric setting (e.g., the inpatient ward) from the "political" vantage point. (The political issues are less critical in the outpatient setting, primarily because of the smaller staff numbers typically found in this setting and the relative independence or isolation of outpatient workers.) Thus, we will see how the introduction of a behavioral program on the psychiatric ward may or may not fit in with the existing political scheme and hierarchical structure. Indeed, it will become apparent that a behavioral program may very well upset the balance of power in the typical psychiatric unit.

Second, we will contrast how traditionally trained staff and behaviorally trained staff interact with their patients. Evaluation of the empirical findings to date will support the superiority of behavioral training.

MICHEL HERSEN • School of Psychology, Nova University, 3301 College Avenue, Fort Lauderdale, Florida 33314.   **FRANCIS HARRIS** • University of Pittsburgh, Pittsburgh, Pennsylvania 15213. **ALAN S. BELLACK** • Medical College of Pennsylvania at EPPI, Philadelphia, Pennsylvania 19129.

Handbook of Behavior Therapy in the Psychiatric Setting, edited by Alan S. Bellack and Michel Hersen. Plenum Press, New York, 1993.

Third, we will attempt to share with the reader some of our own experiences in developing and maintaining programs in several different psychiatric settings.

Fourth, we will evaluate the current research literature documenting the most efficacious methods for training staff in behavioral methodology. Also, we will examine those behavioral strategies that appear most promising for maintaining staff behaviors once initial instruction has been concluded.

Fifth, we will comment on the distinction between staff training and staff consultation.

Sixth, we will attempt to summarize all the findings reviewed and to present an outline for effecting maximum behavioral change in staff in the psychiatric setting.

In considering the above topics, it should be noted that, largely as a function of the specificity of the behavioral approach (see Bellack & Hersen, 1977, Chapter 1), it is possible to evaluate staff functioning empirically. That is, because of the behavior therapist's penchant for precision and measurement, many of the staff's interchanges with patients can be quantified. Along with definition and precision, it then becomes possible to establish a system of staff accountability. It will also become apparent that the notion of staff accountability, although a distinct advantage to the empirically minded behavior therapist, may become a political liability unless handled with consummate skill by the program initiator.

HOSPITAL POLITICS

In using the term *politics*, we are referring to the interpersonal forces, undercurrents, and informal networks that determine much of the day-to-day hospital operation, ranging from mores about the use of sick leave, to the degree of compliance required with directives, to which of two psychiatrists one approaches to get a medication change or pass for a patient. There can be no doubt that hospital politics are commonplace in the psychiatric setting, particularly with respect to the administration of inpatient units (see Hersen, 1976a,b; Kazdin, 1977; Patterson, 1975). In fact, we have often wondered whether the protagonists and antagonists on the "hospital battleground" frequently lose sight of their primary goal: patient care. (In our more facetious moments, we have argued that patient care is relegated to secondary or tertiary status and that politics assume primary status.) Therefore, when examined most dispassionately, such politics obviously are to be expected within the context of the hospital and ward hierarchy. The internal staff and administrative struggles found on the psychiatric unit long preceded the emergence of behavioral therapy. However, the introduction of a behavioral system (or, for that matter, any new system) on a given psychiatric ward can only intensify the struggles already found in the system. Consequently, the focus of the struggle will often shift, and the behavioral system will bear the brunt of existing conflicts.

Let us illustrate with the institution of a token economy ward in a psychiatric institution. In many instances, before the actual implementation of the behavioral program, the many virtues of token economics have been meticulously presented to the hospital administrator and to the staff of the designated unit. Frequently, the program has been portrayed with an overabundance of glowing terms and as a panacea for the many ills of the large psychiatric facility. Often, as a result of the young behavior therapist's (usually a psychologist) exposition of the program and accompanying enthusiasm, the hospital administrator will consent to implementing the program, promising administrative support. However, as previously articulated by Hersen (1976b):

> What the unsuspecting administration and staff frequently do not realize is how much *control* over patients they will lose once the token system if fully implemented (i.e., decisions about patient care now follow programmatic lines rather than being made more subjectively). We can not understand better why administrators in key hospital positions sometimes are reluctant to support fully token economy programs following their initiation. (p. 207)

As previously noted, the initiator of the large-scale behavioral program in the psychiatric setting is invariably a psychologist (see Hersen, 1976a; LeBow, 1973, 1976).[1] This creates problems because

1. The administrator of the psychiatric unit is typically a medical practitioner (i.e., a psychiatrist).
2. The "medical" or "disease" model of psychiatric disorder is generally followed.
3. The nursing staff has been trained to adhere to the dictates of the medical model, whereas the nursing assistants probably maintain a custodial orientation.
4. The psychologist instituting the behavioral program does not have administrative authority and therefore must rely on *staff cooperation* to implement his or her program.
5. The psychologist does not follow the medical model of psychiatric disorder but is more concerned with the socioenvironmental factors contributing to a given disorder (see Hersen, 1976a).

The above analysis strongly suggests that the seeds for conflictual staff relationships (psychologist versus psychiatrist, psychologist versus nurse, psychologist versus nursing assistant) are often present. When a *behavioral psychiatrist* such as Liberman (Liberman & Bryan, 1976) serves in the dual capacity of program initiator and administrator, many (but not all) of the "medical" problems can be obviated. Similarly, when a *behavioral psychologist*, such as Hersen (Hersen & Luber, 1977; Luber & Hersen, 1976), is clearly granted administrative control of his unit, many of the potential difficulties relating to authority are also avoided. Unfortunately, at this time, there are still relatively few behavioral psychiatrists and psychologists in such administrative positions:

> It is not surprising, then, that Watson (1975) concluded: It is very difficult to carry out regular client training in certain kinds of administrative models, particularly the custodial administrative model of the type usually found in the medical model residential institution. . . . Such a model is designed primarily to provide custodial treatment to patients. The two key administrative staff members, the superintendent and the director of nursing, are trained primarily to provide medical, psychiatric, and/or nursing treatment to patients. They typically subscribe to the "disease" orientation toward mental retardation and mental illness, and are not trained in psycho-educational procedures that are relevant to carrying out training programs with their residents or patients. Training usually is a low-priority item in this administrative system and usually is carried out only after all custodial obligations are satisfied. Their general orientation is basically incompatible with the behavior modification approach. (pp. 81–82)

An offshoot of this medical-behavioral dichotomy is the oft-seen conflict concerning the respective roles of pharmacology and behavioral intervention in the treatment of patients. This conflict is frequently manifested in useless debates and harangues by the partisans of both camps. These are particularly fruitless inasmuch as there is mounting evidence to support the complementary roles of drugs and behavioral analysis and therapy (see Hersen, 1986; Hersen & Bellack, 1976; Hersen, Turner, Edelstein, & Pinkston, 1975; Liberman & Davis, 1975; Liberman, Davis, Moon, & Moore, 1973; Turner, Hersen, & Alford, 1974). Unfortunately, the narrow proponents of each position fuel the fires, failing to recognize that both strategies can result in significant behavioral change in patients. (A thorough examination of drugs and behavior analysis appears in Chapter 6.)

---

[1] Similar problems are encountered by the behaviorist implementing *individual* treatment programs in the inpatient psychiatric setting. But, of course, the problems are less complex than those seen in the wardwide application of behavioral principles, as fewer and less diverse staff members tend to be involved in the primary care of the patient. On the other hand, on a well-functioning behavioral ward, it is relatively easy to carry out a novel behavioral manipulation (e.g., Hersen, Eisler, Alford, & Agras, 1973).

Behaviorists eager to implement wardwide programs are frequently insensitive to the historical role of the nursing profession in medicine in general and in psychiatry in particular. Throughout their training and during the course of clinical practice, nurses have been taught to obey medical dictums and reinforced for obeying them. In addition, nurses have been taught to respond positively to all patient communications, irrespective of whether reinforcement of these communications is ultimately of benefit to the patient. Of course, this approach is obviously contrary to the good practice of operant psychology and represents a source of frustration to behaviorists working in psychiatric settings. But no matter how skillfully and how politically it is introduced, the overall philosophy of the behavioral program is diametrically opposed to the traditional (although erroneous) conception of being the "good nurse." Moreover, with the introduction of a behavioral program (which is *infrequently* at the request of the nursing service), the nurse is being asked not only to perform in a manner alien to his or her training, but also to carry out duties as the *agent of the behavioral psychologist*. This requirement undoubtedly and understandably leads to considerable role conflict and may indeed account for much resistant behavior.

It should also be pointed out that the behavior modifier has spent years developing an intellectual and emotional commitment to behavioral techniques. This enthusiasm can blind him or her to the (natural) critical response of the nursing staff. It is sometimes difficult to remember that the ward staff has not been eagerly awaiting the behavioral revolution. If, as aptly suggested by LeBow (1976), the nurse were to become a *primary therapeutic agent* (i.e., a planner of treatment programs) as opposed to an ancillary agent of treatment, then cooperation, enthusiasm, and full participation would be likely to be ensured. However, until nursing schools become more familiar with what behavioral psychology has to offer them (e.g., LeBow, 1973), many of the role conflicts seen in day-to-day practice on behavioral treatment wards will remain.

Also related to the question of nursing resistance is the specific role of the head nurse in the behavioral format. Although many nursing functions are retained by the head nurse, usually as a direct result of the behavioral program (e.g., the token economy), decisions the nurse formerly may have made are now accomplished more automatically along programmatic lines. Thus, he or she has clearly lost some of the control associated with the position. In the absence of other compensating factors, cooperation with the spirit and the letter of the behavioral program is hardly a given (passive resistance is more likely). Indeed, the importance of the head nurse or nursing supervisor in ensuring the existence and implementation of the behavioral program cannot be sufficiently underscored, as clearly documented in the study conducted by Wallace *et al.* (1973). This study showed the powerful modeling influence (positive) of the nursing supervisor in carrying out the strictures of a specific behavioral program. (This study will be discussed in greater detail in a later section of the chapter.)

Still another aspect of the behavioral program that may be disturbing to some psychiatric personnel is the behavior therapist's interest in quantifying human behavior (i.e., that of the patients). Such quantification is done both for programmatic and research purposes. Despite the lectures given and the preparation of the staff for this feature of the program, frequent criticism and much staff discomfort tend to result once quantification is instituted. This phenomenon appears to be more prevalent in the larger and more isolated psychiatric settings, such as state hospitals. However, even in the university hospitals and their affiliates (where research activities are to be expected) with which we have been associated, we have sometimes found nursing staff concerned (and sometimes negativistic) about our clinical research efforts. We have found this to be true no matter what the level of the nurse's sophistication and even though our research efforts have *all* been directed toward improving patient functioning.

There are several reasons for this phenomenon:

1. Again, the nurse has been trained in the spirit of "caregiving" but not rigorous empiricism (naturally, exceptions to this rule are to be found).

2. Similarly, of all the medical disciplines, psychiatry (historically) appears to be the least

empirical and regrettably one of the most ridden with mythologies from the past that have no empirical basis. Thus, in many psychiatric settings, the notion of quantification and empiricism still is quite alien.

3. As noted in the introduction, there is an apprehension associated with quantification that may be properly labeled as *fear of accountability*. First, there is the possibility that individual competence (or lack of it) may be examined and exposed. Objective evaluation of patient progress necessarily implies some evaluation of staff performance. Second, quantification on the behavioral ward and the clinical decisions derived from it imply *change*. Of course, in many cases, change means that an entire philosophy of treatment and method of practice may have to undergo radical modification.

Thus, the empirical approach to the psychiatric management of patients undoubtedly represents an enormous challenge to the existing *procedures* and *way of life* of a preponderance of staff in most psychiatric units. Although the staff complaint may be articulated as "Measuring patient behavior is dehumanizing and degrading," the real concern is that long-standing practices will have to be discarded and/or modified, and that entirely new skills will have to be acquired and mastered. Most staff would obviously prefer the path of least resistance: no change in the system.

Although the preceding analysis may seem to discourage the behavioral clinician from implementing programs in the psychiatric setting, this is definitely not our intention. Rather, the goal was to document realistically the potential pitfalls faced by behavioral practitioners. Depending on the institution or even the specific unit within the institution, none, some, or all of these problems may be present.

Obviously, the question to be asked is: Can the situation be ameliorated? What can the behaviorist do to increase the probability of a program's succeeding and the staff's learning new techniques and carrying them out effectively? Fortunately, the precise techniques that behaviorists use so effectively to shape patient behavior (e.g., instructions, feedback, modeling, social reinforcement, and material reinforcement) can also be applied to shaping staff behavior (see Patterson, 1975). We will examine in some detail those procedures as they apply to staff training. However, let us first consider staff behavior (vis-à-vis psychiatric inpatients) in the absence of such training.

Unprogrammed Reinforcement on the Psychiatric Ward

There is ample evidence confirming the clinical impression that psychiatric staff on inpatient services often reinforce the specific deviant behaviors they ostensibly wish to eliminate (e.g., Ayllon & Azrin, 1968; Ayllon & Michael, 1959; Gelfand, Gelfand, & Dobson, 1967; Kazdin, 1977; Trudel, Boisvert, Maruca, & Leroux, 1974). Conversely, in the cited reports, there is equally good evidence that such psychiatric staff do not reinforce positive behaviors emitted by their patients.[1] In another publication (see Bellack & Hersen, 1977, Chapter 8), we have examined the status of patient-staff interactions within the context of chronic institutionalization and the extremely low staff-to-patient ratios found in large psychiatric hospitals. We noted that:

> Given this state of affairs it should be apparent that the chronic psychiatric patient receives little clinical attention and/or active psychotherapeutic treatment. In this system nursing assistants tend to have the greatest number of interactions with the chronic patient during the course of the typical hospital day. Ironically, the nursing assistant is, for the most part, the least well schooled, trained, or motivated to function in a therapeutic manner with the patient. It is little wonder, then, that nursing assistants tend to ignore positive behavior emitted by patients while systematically attending to their negative behaviors. Let us consider the following. The passive or "well-behaved"

[1] Clinical observation also suggests that nonbehaviorally oriented therapists in outpatient psychiatric settings do not optimize the reinforcement or extinction of behaviors of their patients.

chronic psychiatric patient who "goes about his business" without causing any disturbance on the unit is generally ignored, particularly for any *positive* initiatives that he may exhibit. By contrast, the "difficult" patient who causes disturbances on the ward frequently elicits an enormous amount of attention from doctors (when in evidence), nurses, nursing assistants, and other patients. The aforementioned, although prototypical, represents behavior modification in reverse. "Deviant" behavior receives attention, hence increasing the likelihood of its recurrence. "Positive" behavior is ignored, thus leading to its extinction. (p. 265)

Although the preceding analysis primarily reviewed practices conducted in the larger state psychiatric facilities for chronic patients, our own clinical experiences in a number of other settings (Veterans Administration hospitals and inpatient and partial hospitalization services in university hospitals) and those of others (cf. Gelfand *et al.*, 1967) suggest that staff (irrespective of staff-patient ratios or the chronicity of the patients) are very often ineffective and perhaps even detrimental in their interactions with patients. Let us examine this contention more specifically. Gelfand *et al.* (1967) planned a study in which the naturally occurring interactions between staff (i.e., psychiatrists, psychologists, social workers, nurses, and nursing assistants) and six severely psychotic chronic psychiatric patients were systematically observed on a well-staffed psychiatric inpatient unit at a Salt Lake City Veterans Administration Hospital. These six patients were selected for study because they were relatively active and because they evidenced both appropriate and inappropriate behavior. Throughout the study, these patients were observed for a total of 55 hours. In addition to staff-patient interactions, interactions between the six study patients and other patients on the ward were also monitored.

The study patients were closely observed by three graduate students as unobtrusively as possible. Patient behavior was rated on a 5-point scale: 1 for inappropriate behavior and 5 for appropriate behavior. For example, incoherent speech was rated 1, neutral behavior such as watching television was rated 3, and conducting a patient government meeting in a serious manner was rated 5. The interrater agreement between independent judges for 36 patient behavior units was 86%, yielding an r of .94. Staff and other patients' responses to the six study patients were put in three separate categories: (1) positive attention; (2) negative attention; and (3) ignoring. "Positive attention" was defined as "the other person reacts positively, praises, smiles, approves, continues to respond to the subject, instructs the subject, or asks for or gives information to the subject." "Negative attention" was defined as "reacts negatively, scolds, tells patient to shut up or go away, or refuses to comply." "Ignoring" was defined as "does not respond, looks away, walks away" (Gelfand *et al.*, 1967, p. 203). Independent raters were in 100% agreement on the environmental responses to patient behavior.

A summary of the results of this study is presented in Table 1.[1] In analyzing the results, let us keep in mind that the effective "behavioral engineer" is able to systematically reinforce instances of positive behavior while systematically ignoring instances of negative behavior. When such operant principles are followed, the emission of positive behavior should be maximized. In accord with these guidelines, the top part of the table indicates that nurses reinforced appropriate behavior 68% of the time, whereas nursing assistants did so only 48% of the time. Other patients on the ward fell inbetween, at 56%. On the other hand, with respect to inappropriate behavior, nurses rewarded it 39% of the time, nursing assistants 30%, and other patients 12%. Nursing assistants also ignored inappropriate behavior 64% of the time, whereas the patients did so 79% of the time. What then is the interpretation of these data? First and foremost, the data suggest that neither the nurses nor the nursing assistants were effective behavioral engineers. That is, the nurses tended to be indiscriminate in their responses in that they strongly rewarded *both* the positive and the negative initiatives of their patients. Obviously,

---

[1] The results are presented only for nurses, nursing assistants, and other patients, as psychiatrist, psychologist, and social worker interactions with the six study patients on the ward were too infrequent to be included for statistical purposes.

their ability to reinforce behavior was somewhat limited in the absence of specific training directed toward that end. (As previously noted, this limitation is likely to be the result of nurses' training to be warm and empathetic regardless of the communication emitted by the patient.) On the other hand, the nursing assistants generally were not very reinforcing of either positive or negative behavior. (This response was undoubtedly representative of their custodial attitude.)

Second, one of the most interesting findings of this study was that, on the whole, other patients were rather good natural "behavioral engineers." They were relatively reinforcing of appropriate behaviors (56% of the time) and most effective in ignoring inappropriate behavior (79% of the time). Indeed, other psychiatric patients on the ward reinforced inappropriate behavior only 12% of the time.

Third, the bottom part of the table shows that appropriate behavior received positive attention at a 61% rate; inappropriate behavior was given positive attention at a 26% rate. This latter finding is not at all encouraging, inasmuch as it is a well-known tenet of operant conditioning that partial reinforcement is most resistive to extinction. That is, if inappropriate behavior that is repeatedly presented is rewarded a small but noticeable proportion of the time, the likelihood of its becoming still more ingrained is significantly enhanced.

Gelfand *et al.* (1967) also examined the reinforcement contingencies operating with regard to the level of deviancy (psychoticism) of the six patients. This analysis indicated that there was a very high rank-order correlation (Kendall's tau = .73) between the inappropriateness of reinforcement contingencies and the severity of the patient's disturbance (i.e., the more severe the patient's disturbance, the more inappropriate the staff's responses to her or his behavior). This finding is very nicely illustrated in Table 2. Indeed, the data presented in Table 2 confirm "that the more severely psychotic the patient, the more likely it is that his prosocial behavior will be ignored and his bizarre behavior rewarded" (Gelfand *et al.*, 1967, p. 205).

Before examining the differences between staffs that have and have not had training in operant principles for patient management, let us present some of the conclusions that Gelfand *et al.* (1967) drew from their data:

> It would be most beneficial for the patients if hospital staff-members, and particularly the nursing assistants, could receive intensive training in reinforcement techniques.
>
> Since the nurses are the group most influential in the training and supervision of the nursing assistants, it is undoubtedly the nurses' attitudes and practices which are the most important to

Table 1.   Reinforcement Sequences[a]

Appropriate behavior	Reward (%)
Nurses	68
Nursing assistants	44
Other patients	56

Inappropriate behavior	Ignore %	Reward (%)
Nurses	Not indicated	39
Nursing assistants	64	30
Other patients	79	12

All observed instances	
Appropriate behavior	Positive attention (61%)
Inappropriate behavior	Positive attention (26%)

[a]Abstracted from Gelfand, Gelfand, & Dobson (1967).

change. In an attempt to increase their therapeutic effectiveness, psychiatric nurses have adopted a psychodynamic treatment approach which has led them to respond warmly to their patients regardless of the patient's behavior. However, these [sic] well-intended treatment interventions most probably serve to reinforce the very problem behavior they are attempting to alleviate. Because the nurses are not acquainted with reinforcement principles and therefore cannot visualize the role they might play in a behavioristic treatment program, many nurses view such procedures with considerable suspicion and unjustified alarm. Psychologists working in hospitals and in graduate schools of nursing can play a major role in instructing nurses in reinforcement principles and, more important, in training them in the actual use of behavior modification techniques. Once a nurse has had the highly gratifying experience of having produced dramatic improvements in her patients' behavior, it is likely that she will adopt with enthusiasm a treatment approach which allows her to play such a pivotal role in the lives of the people she is charged to help. (pp. 206–207)

Token Economy versus Control Ward

Does a staff, by virtue of its training and practice in token economics, respond differently to chronic psychiatric patients from a comparable staff (untrained in behavioral principles) on a control ward? This was the specific question posed by Trudel *et al.* (1974) in their comparison of unprogrammed reinforcement of patients' responses on wards with and without a token economy. In essence, this study represents a partial replication of the initial Gelfand *et al.* (1967) investigation.

The study was conducted on two similar wards. The control ward staff did not receive behavioral training; however, the treatment on that ward had been described as "active" by nursing personnel. On the token economy ward, behavioral training lasted for six months and involved classroom discussions of operant principles as well as viewing two films on the application of such principles. In addition, before the experiment was actually carried out, the token economy staff had accumulated two years of experience in behavioral technology. The characteristics of the two wards are presented in Table 3.

As in the Gelfand *et al.* study, Trudel *et al.* rated the patients behavior (on a scale of 1 to 5) on the basis of appropriateness; environmental responses were categorized as "positive attention," "negative attention," or "ignores." Interjudge reliability was very high (Spearman rho = .97). These ratings were based on nontoken economic exchanges between staff and patients (i.e., social reinforcement as opposed to simply giving the patient a token).

The results of this study are summarized in Table 4. These data indicates that the staff on the token ward reinforced appropriate behavior 6.53 times as frequently as comparable staff on the control ward. On the other hand, there did not appear to be any substantial differences between

Table 2. Percentage Reward, Punishment, and Ignoring Responses to Patient's Prosocial and Inappropriate Behavior[a]

	Reward (%)		Punishment (%)		Ignored (%)	
	Appropriate	Inappropriate	Appropriate	Inappropriate	Appropriate	Inappropriate
Patient A	44	53	9	4	47	43
Patient B	41	17	19	26	40	57
Patient C	64	50	0	6	36	44
Patient D	63	5	0	0	37	95
Patient E	66	32	4	13	30	55
Patient F	86	0	0	0	14	100
Group mean	61	26	5	8	34	66

[a]From Gelfand, Gelfand, & Dobson (1967).

Table 3.   Composition of Token and Control Wards[a]

	Aides	Mean length of service (aides)	Patients
Token ward	$N = 11$	8.27	$N = 49$
Control ward	$N = 9$	9.66	$N = 48$

[a]Abstracted from Trudel *et al.* (1974).

the two wards in the positive attention accorded inappropriate behavior. The results for negative attention (i.e., punishment) show very low levels across the two wards. However, with respect to behaviors ignored, ward staff on the control ward ignored positive behaviors 91.66% of the time; the percentage for the token economy staff was 45.58%. Inappropriate behaviors were ignored 80.76% of the time by token economy staff and 83.01% of the time by control ward staff.

What, then, are the conclusions that can be reached on the basis of this interesting study? First, it is apparent that training in specific behavioral methodology does make a difference. The token economy staff were definitely more socially reinforcing of appropriate behaviors than the control ward staff. Second, the staff on the control ward were much less effective in identifying and then reinforcing appropriate behavior. That is, they tended to ignore appropriate behavior more frequently (2:1 ratio) than the token economy staff. Third, despite behavioral training, the token economy ward staff continued to reinforce inappropriate behavior. Both the token economy and the control ward staff reinforced such behavior an equal proportion of the time (19.24 and 16.99%, respectively). Obviously, this area remained a problem, especially as "even rare reinforcements of unadaptive behaviors result in maintenance of these behaviors" (Trudel *et al.*, 1974, p. 149). Trudel *et al.* argued that more effective ways are needed to reinforce staff for correctly responding to patients. (In the next section, we will examine more specifically the empirical literature documenting how best to train staff and maintain their effective behavioral interactions once training is over.)

STAFF TRAINING

An extensive number of papers have been written that outline a variety of schemes for training psychiatric paraprofessionals and professionals in behavioral technology (cf. Bellack & Franks, 1975; Johnson, Katz, & Gelfand, 1972; Liberman, King, & Derisi, 1976; Patterson, Cooke, & Liberman, 1972; Wodarski, 1976). However, although these papers are useful to the behavior modifier working in several kinds of psychiatric settings, the data presented are at the clinical-descriptive level, and we cannot derive very firm conclusions about the efficacy of the techniques and strategies presented. In this discussion, rather than summarize the suggestions

**Table 4.   Unprogrammed Reactions of Staff to Behaviors of Patients
in Wards with and without a Token Economy**[a]

	Appropriate behaviors (%)		Inappropriate behaviors (%)	
	Ward with token economy	Ward without token economy	Ward with token economy	Ward without token economy
Positive attention	54.41	8.33	19.23	15.09
Negative attention	0.0	0.0	0.0	1.88
Behavior ignored	45.58	91.66	80.76	83.01

[a]Abstracted from Trudel *et al.* (1974).

offered in these papers, we will examine the empirical studies in which specific behavioral strategies have been evaluated (in single-subject or group comparison research) with respect to training staff in behavioral technology. We will clearly differentiate the initial training of the staff and the maintenance of staff behavior following the completion of training. This is an important distinction that has frequently been ignored in the behavioral literature. The reader should also be aware that the material must be interpreted in the context of the political issues discussed above, as well as in the context of general issues in human relations and effective management. It is naive to presume that even a perfect training program would be effective in a hostile political or interpersonal climate. In the same way that a positive therapeutic relationship is a necessary (but not sufficient) condition for effective outpatient interventions (Bellack & Hersen, 1977, Chapter 3), a positive staff environment and staff-director relationship is necessary for a behavioral unit to operate efficiently.

The Traditional Approach

The traditional approach to teaching psychiatric personnel new techniques has typically involved a series of lectures, classroom discussions coupled with reading assignments, films, and some on-the-job supervision. Generally, lectures and classroom discussions have preceded actual clinical practice, but the two have sometimes been carried out concurrently. However, until recently, relatively few evaluations of these teaching strategies have appeared in the literature. Thus, a number of important questions need to be raised and answered: (1) Does the typical in-service training offered result in improved learning and/or improved on-the-job performance? (2) What are the specific effects of academic (classroom) and on-the-job training? (3) How long are the effects of training maintained following the initial in-service experience? (4) What are the most effective techniques for maintaining staff performance following training?

Empirical Studies of Training

Before examining the relevant empirical literature on training psychiatric personnel, let us first summarize an investigation (McKeown, Adams, & Forehand, 1975) comparing several training strategies for training grade-school teachers in behavioral methods. Although the study concerns a different target population from the one in our discussion, the principles involved in training are quite similar. Moreover, the results of the study put into sharp focus some of the problems faced by the behavioral trainer.

In the McKeown *et al.* (1975) study, there were four groups of five teachers each. The first group was given a manual to read on behavior modification. In addition, the teachers participated in six, 1½-hour meetings (i.e., laboratory sessions) in which behavioral techniques were modeled and role-played. The second group was involved in laboratory sessions alone, and the third group only read the manual. The fourth group, a control, did not receive either of the "sources of information" (i.e., either the manual or the laboratory sessions). The effects of the training were evaluated by contrasting pre-post scores on two measures: (1) an observation of disruptive behavior in each teacher's classroom and (2) a 20-question multiple-choice examination on behavior modification.

The study indicated that the teachers who participated in the laboratory sessions evinced a significantly greater increase in knowledge (on the multiple-choice examination) than the teachers not exposed to the laboratory sessions. But more important, *only* the teachers who had participated in the laboratory sessions were able to effect a decrease in disruptive behavior in their classrooms. This latter finding suggests that if generalization from training to the actual educational or clinical situation is to occur, specific practice in behavioral management (even if only role-played) is required. As McKeown *et al.* argued, mere cognitive understanding of behavioral principles does not suffice. This makes sense in light of Hersen and Barlow's point (1976, Chapter 4) that the more closely the training situation (the laboratory in this case) approximates the natural environment (the classroom in this case), the more effective are the training results. Again, let us underscore the fact that the laboratory training on the McKeown *et al.* (1975) investigation was directly related to the specific problems that the teachers would face in their classrooms.

A parallel study comparing two instructional techniques (role playing and lecture) for training attendants in behavioral principles was earlier conducted by Gardner (1972). The study was carried out in a state institution for the mentally retarded and involved 20 female attendants enrolled in an in-service training program for new employees. The 20 attendants were matched in pairs and then randomly assigned first to role playing groups and then to lecture groups, or first to lecture groups and then role playing groups (crossover design). Matching was accomplished on a number of demographic variables (nursing skill knowledge, knowledge of mental retardation, attitude toward the retarded, and socioeconomic status). The role playing consisted of six 1-hour sessions in which shaping and reinforcement techniques were modeled and practiced, with attendants working in pairs alternating as trainer and trainee. Lectures consisted of eight 1-hour classroom sessions covering reinforcement, shaping techniques, and stimulus control.

The effects of the training were evaluated on the basis of two dependent measures: (1) The Training Proficiency Scale, a 30-item rating scale that assesses efficiency in applying behavioral techniques (e.g., speed of reinforcement), and (2) the Behavior Modification Test, a 229-item true-and-false examination covering the basic tenets of behavioral analysis and modification. The results of the study indicated that there was no order effect for the treatments. However, role playing resulted in a significantly improved ability to implement behavioral strategies, whereas the lectures effected increased gains in knowledge about behavior modification.

Gardner (1972) aptly presented the obvious conclusions to be drawn from his study:

> Perhaps the most parsimonious explanation is that performance skills are best taught within a teaching framework that emphasizes performance skills, while verbal skills are best taught in a framework emphasizing verbal skills. (p. 520)

As noted earlier, Gardner's results were fully concordant with those reported by McKeown *et al.* (1975), so that the results of training in behavioral methodology seem to be the same no matter what kind of group is being trained. Indeed, this principle is further supported by the results of the next two studies to be reviewed.

Paul and his associated (Paul & McInnis, 1974; Paul, McInnis, & Mariotto, 1973) examined two approaches to training paraprofessional mental health technicians in both milieu and social-learning programs. In one study (Paul & McInnis, 1974), two groups of 21 nonprofessional trainees hired from a high-unemployment area were exposed to two types of training. The first group initially received classroom instruction by professional staff and then on-the-job training (this was labeled the "sequential/professional" type of training). The second group received brief classroom instruction by professional staff concurrently with clinical assignments supervised by experienced technicians (this was labeled the "behavior-specific" type of training). Although the sequential/professional instruction led to better academic performance on a test of the content of the training, attitudinal changes (e.g,. results on the "Opinions about Mental Illness Scale) were related to the behavior-specific mode of training. Paul and McInnis noted:

> Trainee attitudes tended toward those of instructors, and attitudinal similarity was related to academic performance. Comparisons with attitudes of other occupational groups found current nonprofessional trainees to be unique but more similar to professionals than to nonprofessionals elsewhere. (p. 21)

In a second study, Paul *et al.* (1973) compared two groups of nonprofessional trainees. This time the sequential/professional mode of training was contrasted to an "integrated/technical approach" (i.e., brief academic instruction given concurrently with integrated clinical observation followed by on-the-job experience supervised by experienced workers). Both groups were trained in social-learning and milieu principles. The trainees were evaluated during a first six-week period while working independently on the ward. In this study, it was clear that the integrated/technical approach resulted in improved on-the-job performance, evaluated on the basis of 10-minute time samples observed by trained judges. (Parenthetically, performance on the social-learning unit was better irrespective of the mode of training followed.)

On the basis of their extensive work in this area and the work of others, Paul *et al.* (1973) reached the following conclusions concerning the initial training of psychiatric staff:

> In summary, the combined findings of the present study and those of the earlier report suggested that increased focus by professional staff in academic instruction results in greater *understanding* of principles and procedures. However, given basic understanding of principles and procedures, the integration of clinical observation with academic content, followed by practicum training by those who are performing the same functions results in more rapid acquisition and performance of duties. The relative importance of specific components of training must await studies designed to test those components. Meanwhile, the overall level of performance achieved by both groups of trainees in both treatment programs clearly supports previous recommendations in the literature to focus technician training on: (a) job-related behavior rather than general orientation, (b) concrete functions rather than abstract theory, (c) modeling and feedback rather than totally didactic presentation, and (d) specified programs and Staff Behavior × Resident Behavior × Setting interactions. (p. 531)

Since Paul *et al.*'s work, few staff-training studies have been conducted in psychiatric settings. One was conducted in a child psychiatric inpatient setting by Delamater, Conners, and Wells (1984). Single-case methodology was used to evaluate the effects of three procedures designed to train six staff members to use behavioral procedures in their work with children hospitalized for a wide range of acute psychiatric problems. The behavioral training procedures included (1) multimedia presentations and in-class exercises; (2) direct feedback to staff of appropriately and inappropriately attending to and rewarding child behavior during structured observation sessions; and (3) role playing with an experienced behavior therapist. Training was evaluated exclusively on the basis of direct observations of staff-child interactions during a free-play period. The ordering of the experimental conditions and the small number of subjects who participated in the role-playing condition make the results somewhat difficult to interpret. However, it does appear that the greatest gains in staff behavior occurred in conjunction with the role-playing condition. This result appears to confirm the notion of training hands-on skills through hands-on methods.

Several recent studies have been designed to evaluate various methods of training professional and paraprofessional staff to implement behavioral procedures with their developmentally disabled clients. These methods have included written instructions or a manual (Fitzgerald, Reid, Schepis, Faw, Welty, & Pyfer, 1984; Hundert, 1982), several types of verbal instruction (Ivancic, Reid, Iwata, Faw, & Page, 1981; Katz & Lutzker, 1980; Kissel, Whitman, & Reid, 1983; Stoddard, McIlvane, McDonagh, & Kledaras, 1986), and various combinations of modeling, behavior rehearsal, and performance feedback (Fitzgerald *et al.*, 1984; Kissel *et al.*, 1983; Mansdorf & Burstein, 1986; van den Pol, Reid, & Fuqua, 1983; Watson & Uzzell, 1980; Zlomke & Benjamin, 1983). Taken together, the results of the studies strongly support the previous conclusions reached by Gardner (1972), Paul and McInnis (1974), and Paul *et al.* (1973) that verbal skills are taught best by verbal means and performance skills are taught best by more interactive means, such as role playing and behavior rehearsal. A comprehensive review of the rapidly growing literature on developmental disabilities and staff-training literature is well beyond the scope of this chapter. However, excellent reviews have been written by Reid and Green (1990) and Reid, Parsons, and Green (1989).

On the basis of our foregoing review, it is eminently clear that a pragmatic approach involving practical training in combination with some lecture material is required to maximize both the behavioral and the cognitive skills of the neophyte behavioral technician. However, the question still remains how these skills, once acquired, are to be maintained in the clinical context. From our knowledge of operant psychology, we know very well that behavior in the absence of instructional control, feedback, reinforcement, or modeling invariably undergoes extinction, especially if the institutional system is not geared to promoting behavioral practice. Thus, in the following survey, we examine studies in which various behavioral techniques have been systematically applied to maintain staff performance.

In an early report concerned with application of operant principles to chronic psychiatric patients, Ayllon and Azrin (1964) pointed out that, despite repeated instructions to attendants about the appropriate use of verbal reinforcement, these instructions were not rigorously carried out. However, after direct verbal and audiotaped feedback were provided on a contingent basis, no further deviations from the prescribed procedures were noted. Unfortunately, no hard data were presented in this report to document the point.

The effects of systematic feedback were very nicely documented by Panyan, Boozer, and Morris (1970), using a multiple-baseline design across settings. Panyan *et al.* were interested in having attendants in a state institution for the retarded carry out operant techniques in their respective units (i.e., halls). Following a four-week course in operant strategies, attendants from each of the halls were asked to train their retarded residents in self-help skills (using operant shaping techniques) and to maintain performance records for each resident. During the baseline phase, the number of self-help training sessions conducted by hall personnel was tabulated. Figure 1 indicates that decreasing baselines were noted for Halls E, O, and C. During the feedback phase, the experimenters simply tabulated the number of sessions completed by each attendant on a feedback sheet and presented the sheet to the attendant. The graph shows that the effects of this feedback were marked and resulted in high levels of performance for each of the halls. Indeed, in Hall R, where feedback was given throughout the study, high levels of performance were consistently maintained.

Pomerleau, Bobrove, and Smith (1973) examined the effects of feedback, monetary reinforcement, consultation, and supervision on the performance of psychiatric aides working in a university-affiliated ward (run as a token economy) in a state hospital. There were 12 psychiatric aides, each of whom was randomly assigned one or two patients during his or her day-time tour of duty. None of the 12 psychiatric aides in the study was required to perform custodial duties of any sort. The dependent measure used to assess aid performance (i.e., indirectly) was the Ward Behavior Inventory. Pre-post changes per week were calculated for the assigned patients. Lowered scores on this inventory were related to improvements in the patient's behavior.

There were 11 separate phases in the study, each lasting 4 weeks: (1) B_1 = baseline; (2) NC = \$20 award to the "most cooperative aid" unrelated to improved patient behavior; (3) F = feedback to aides on the basis of patient improvement (the aides were ranked); (4) B_2 = baseline; (5) 10 = \$10 award to aide of the week based on ranked performance of assigned patients; (6) 20_1 = \$20 award to aide of the week based on ranked performance of assigned patients; (7) 30 = \$30 award to aide of the week based on ranked performance of assigned patients; (8) $20_2 = 20_1$; (9) C = aides were asked to consult with the second author about their patients, and the condition of 20_1 was also maintained; (10) S = aides were asked to consult with the second author about their patients, aides were supervised by the first author regarding reinforcement schedules, and condition 20_1 was also maintained; and (11) T = program terminated insofar as feedback, reinforcement schedules, consultation, and supervision were concerned.

MICHEL HERSEN
et al.

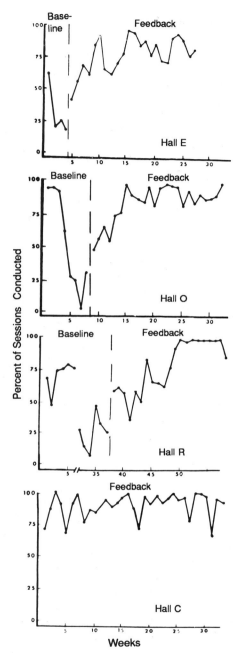

Figure 1. Percentage of requested training sessions conducted by the staff on Halls E, O, C, and R. Reprinted with permission from M. Panyan, H. Boozer, and N. Morris, *Journal of Applied Behavior Analysis*, *3*, 1–4, 1970.

The results of this study are presented in Figure 2, which suggests that the monetary reinforcement conditions (20₁ and 30) the feedback (F), and the consultation (C) resulted in the greatest behavioral change in the patients. As might be expected, condition 30 (the largest cash award) led to the greatest amount of behavioral change observed in patients. Although very clear conclusions are not permitted from the experimental design used by the investigators (e.g., different patients in different conditions), it is obvious that the application of contingent extrinsic reinforcement does lead to improved staff performance as evaluated indirectly via ratings of patient improvement.

Pommer and Streedbeck (1974) conducted a within-subject analysis to evaluate the effects of instructions and token reinforcement on motivating staff (child care workers) employed in a small residential facility for children. The behavioral disorders of the children included excessive activity, self-stimulatory behavior, temper tantrums, and aggressiveness. All staff members had received training in operant principles before the study. Staff performance was evaluated by counting the number of jobs and new procedures implemented within a one-week period. The instructions consisted of posting staff members' duties on a bulletin board (i.e., public notice). Token reinforcement consisted of filling out slips (equal to $1.00) contingent on staff's performing jobs and implementing procedures within the stated one-week time period.

The resulting data indicated that public notices led to an initial but short lived improvement in staff behavior. Token reinforcement in combination with public notices resulted in a renewed improvement. Public notices or token reinforcement alone did effect changes over baseline levels. However, the combination of the two strategies was most effective in starting and maintaining high levels of staff performance.

Loeber (1971) conducted an interesting study to determine the effects of monetary reinforcement and feedback about improvement in a patient's condition on the accuracy of nursing personnel's use of operant conditioning techniques. Twenty-eight nurses and attendants were assigned to four experimental conditions: (1) promise of reward ($4) contingent on accurate performance; (2) no promise of reward; (3) feedback about patient improvement; and (4) no feedback about patient improvement. Using a contrived laboratory task (pushing a lever that presumably dispensed tokens to a headbanger when he decreased this behavior), the investigator

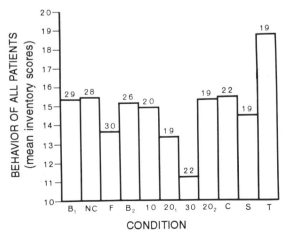

Figure 2. The mean Ward Behavior Inventory run for all patients as a function of the experimental condition; the number of patients in the program is shown for each condition. Reprinted with permission from O. F. Pomerleau, P. H. Bobrove, and R. H. Smith, *Journal of Applied Behavior Analysis, 6*, 383–390, 1973.

was able to record the accuracy with which the staff reinforced the patient. (It should be noted that deception was used in the experiment, in that the headbanging noises had actually been audiotaped; ostensibly, the nursing personnel were unaware of the deception.) The study showed that only the promise of reward led to improved accuracy in reinforcement on the part of the nurses and assistants. Again, as in several of the previous studies reviewed, it appears that monetary reinforcement, or the possibility of obtaining it, is a most potent reinforcer for maintaining accurate and consistent staff performance.

Hollander and Plutchik (1972) examined the effects of material reinforcement still more directly. Each of 13 psychiatric attendants was given 150 trading stamps contingently for each research task completed on an inpatient psychiatric unit. The results of this within-subject A-B-A analysis are presented in Figure 3. The data clearly indicate that, when the stamp contingency was in effect, the levels of staff performance were high. In the absence of the contingency, performance decreased. Also, as can be seen in Figure 4, the percentage of attendants who completed volunteer research tasks during the stamp contingency increased substantially. Finally, another by-product of the stamp contingency condition was that the attendants initiated more frequent contacts with their patients. As stated by Hollander and Plutchik (1972), "Prior to the program, the attendants avoided interactions with patients unless they acted out, or needed to be washed, fed, or clothed" (p. 300). Indeed, this was the case despite a prior six-week formal course in behavioral technology offered to the 13 attendants.

In yet another study, Hollander, Plutchik, and Horner (1973) found that the introduction and removal of the stamp contingency for attendants carrying out behavior modification tasks coincided with an increased and decreased percentage of patients doing work on the token economy ward. Again, the investigators pointed out that, during the stamp contingency, a marked increase in staff-patient interactions was noted, thus possibly enhancing the modeling value of the staff.

Katz, Johnson, and Gelfand (1972) systematically evaluated a number of strategies (instructions, verbal prompts, and monetary reinforcement) directed toward increasing the rate of reinforcement given to patients by psychiatric aides on a token economy unit. The baseline data indicated that aides gave low levels of reinforcement to their patients when appropriate behavior was exhibited. Although instructions did not result in improved performance, verbal prompts led to a moderate increase. Monetary reinforcement, on the other hand, yielded marked improvements in aide performance. Moreover, with increases in correct aide

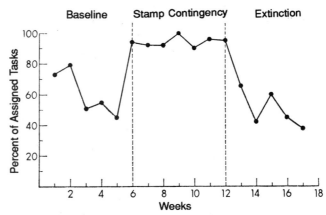

Figure 3. Percentage of assigned tasks completed by attendants during baseline, stamp contingency, and extinction conditions. Reprinted with permission from M. A. Hollander, and R. Plutchik, *Journal of Behavior Therapy and Experimental Psychiatry*, *3*, 297–300, 1972.

performance, improved functioning was recorded in two of the three patients selected for observation.

Recognizing that monetary reinforcement may not be available or possible in many settings (e.g., it may be contrary to administrative or union policies), Katz *et al.* (1972) offered the following suggestion:

> If it is not feasible to provide adequate reinforcers of psychiatric aides, it might be desirable to restructure the ward team. A new set of personnel could be added whose only assignment would be the implementation of the ward behavior modification program. These people could be directly responsible to the ward administrator and trained specifically in behavior modification theory and practice. It would not be necessary to have full-time personnel but it would be desirable to have them serve regularly for several hours each day. Those technicians could be undergraduates who are receiving independent study credit, or who are participating in a federally funded work-study program. (p. 587)

Although Katz *et al.*'s suggestion represents a possible solution (or alternative) to finding effective incentives for motivating psychiatric personnel, in our opinion it represents an avoidance of the issue (i.e., training and maintaining the behavior of existing psychiatric personnel found on the ward).

Over the past several years, the developmental disabilities literature has provided numerous evaluations of programs intended to improve the ongoing delivery of behavioral services (Reid *et al.*, 1989). Virtually all of these studies involve some type of performance feedback either alone or in conjunction with a positive reinforcement. Feedback has been delivered publicly and privately as well as verbally and in written form (Greene, Willis, Levy, & Bailey, 1978; Hutchison, Jarman, & Bailey, 1980; Parsons, Schepis, Reid, McCarn, & Green, 1987). Moreover, it has been provided in terms of staff behavior as well as in terms of client behavior. Money (Realon, Wheeler, Spring, & Springer, 1986), time away from the work setting (Seys & Duker, 1978), and preferred days off (Iwata, Bailey, Brown Foshee, & Alpern, 1976) have functioned as reinforcers for appropriate staff behavior. The results of these studies (in addition to those from the psychiatric setting) appear to provide clear evidence that well-designed and carefully implemented feedback and positive-reinforcement systems are likely to have a favorable impact on staff's implementation of behavioral procedures. However, for several reasons, we urge that program administrators proceed with caution in implementing such systems. First, such systems often present problems in settings where collective bargaining units exist. Second, costs

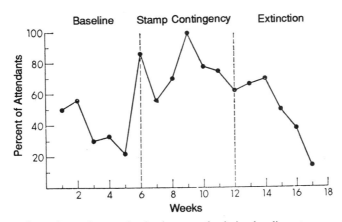

Figure 4. Percentage of attendants who completed volunteer tasks during baseline, stamp contingency, and extinction conditions. Reprinted with permission from M. A. Hollander, and R. Plutchik, *Journal of Behavior Therapy and Experimental Psychiatry*, *3*, 297–300, 1972.

in time as well as money are associated with the administration of reinforcement systems. Third, the novelty aspects of "new" rewards may wear off, so that a continuing investment of time may be required to update and maintain the program. Fourth, in some settings, it is difficult to design a program that precisely targets and rewards truly critical staff behaviors (Reid *et al.*, 1989). It is only after each of these issues is addressed that a contingency management program can be implemented. In the last study to be reviewed in this section, another, although much less costly, alternative for maintaining staff behavior is presented.

Wallace, Davis, Lieberman, and Baker (1973) conducted a within-subject analysis to determine the most effective means of increasing the frequency of interaction between nurses and technicians and their patients on a clinical research unit in a state hospital. There were eight separate phases in the study: (1) modeling by professional staff; (2) no modeling by professional staff; (3) no competing activities; (4) instructions; (5) no modeling by the nursing supervisor; (6) modeling by the nursing supervisor; (7) model absent at the appropriate time; and (8) follow-up. The results showed that neither an instructional set to interact nor the simple removal of competing activities effected substantial changes. The modeling of correct behaviors by both professional staff and the nursing supervisor proved to be the most effective strategy for increasing the target behavior. Wallace *et al.* (1973) rightly concluded that

> both nursing authority figures and professional staff members must be willing to do more than just administer treatment programs. The professional staff members are essential as models for the nursing authority figure who, in turn, is essential as a model for the nursing staff. (p. 425)

There can be no doubt that the behavioral program director cannot lead from behind if meaningful behavioral change is to occur in the staff. He or she must be visible, active, and involved.

STAFF CONSULTATION

A distinction needs to be made between staff training and maintenance and staff consultation. Whereas the former usually implies some type of commitment to establishing a behavioral program (unitwide or hospitalwide), the latter does not necessarily imply such a commitment. That is, because of interest, excess funds in the hospital budget, or an administrative intention of keeping up with the "latest fad," consultation (i.e., the consultant's time, effort, and presumed expertise) may be purchased by the unit or hospital administrator. This action most often taken without the staff's initial interest, recommendation, or approval. Thus, it should be little wonder that we behavioral consultants have experienced considerable frustration motivating staff to carry out the dictates of behavioral treatment. A game ensues. Consultants continue "to offer their wares" as they are reinforced (monetarily) for their efforts. The administration typically is happy because a "name" has been bought, giving the end-of-year report an aura of dignity and an academic flavor. On the other hand, the staff on whom the consultant has been foisted is unhappy and tends to resist most initiatives toward change.

Given this state of affairs, which typifies the consultant-consultee relationship, Bellack and Franks (1975) developed a four-stage model directed toward facilitating behavioral consultation in the community mental health center. The model is also applicable to other types of psychiatric settings.

To begin with, Bellack and Franks argued persuasively on behalf of a "soft-sell" program that minimizes the "real or presumed" theoretical differences that may distinguish the consultant from the consultee. If the consultee is less than enthusiastic about receiving consultation, he or she will certainly resist "seeing the behavioral light" and being disabused of current failings. The four-stage model is presented in the context of minimizing the threat by focusing on conservative and pragmatic goals.

The first consideration involves "The Goals of Consultation." Here, rather than teaching the consultee the theoretical underpinnings of the behavioral approach, the focus should initially be directed to applying techniques. Although most consultees are satisfied with the existing theoretical models, there is, characteristically, a need for and openness to effective techniques. Therefore, when the consultee begins to experience success in carrying out behavioral techniques, he or she may be more amenable to an in-depth evaluation of the basis for the technology being used.

The second consideration is labeled "The Format." Again, the pragmatic rather than the theoretical is stressed. Thus, the case conference method will be more "effective and efficient" than the didactic approach. This strategy avoids polemical lectures, while involving consultees at the locus of their own interests and concerns.

The third consideration is "The Consultant." To encourage the consultee to begin to conduct actual behavioral treatment, it is recommended that he or she serve as an active model (i.e., demonstrating techniques, relating clinical experience, and presenting taped sessions of treatment) rather than referring to the archival literature. This approach helps to counter the prevalent model of the "cold, totalitarian" behaviorist, as well as, again, focusing on the relevant clinical material.

The fourth consideration involves "The Consultee." Here, it is strongly recommended that the consultant avoid challenging the consultee's ideological position. Also, behavioral jargon should be minimized, even to the point of using the consultee's language system in describing behavioral technology. Bellack and Franks suggested that "The consultee can consider the presentation without threat if he believes that he can adopt less than the entire package and continue much of his customary activity" (p. 390).

This entire strategy requires the consultant to analyze the consulting environment in the same way that she or he analyzes a clinical situation. In both cases, the nature and timing of the intervention must be based on the specific characteristics of the target population, rather than on a predetermined or prepackaged blueprint.

Although the approach of Bellack and Franks has not been evaluated empirically, we have found these guidelines most helpful in our consulting efforts, particularly as they have markedly decreased consultee resistance. Of course, it would be interesting and useful to test empirically whether this approach is effective in changing the consultee's attitudes and actual behavior.

OUTLINE FOR INITIATING AND MAINTAINING A BEHAVIORAL PROGRAM

Consistent with our review of the relevant literature, we will now briefly outline the steps necessary to initiate, implement, and maintain a successful behavioral program in the psychiatric setting:

1. The hospital administration needs to be fully apprised of all of the consequences and implications of having a behavioral program either unitwide or hospitalwide. The issue of the unit director's losing some administrative power to the more automatically carried-out dictates of the behavioral program must not be overlooked or underemphasized.

2. The program director (unit administrator) should preferably be a behavior therapist himself or herself. If the behavior therapist attempting to institute a behavioral program is not accorded administrative authority (i.e., if she or he is not the unit director), then it is of utmost importance to ensure the full cooperation of the actual director and the head nurse. In the absence of such cooperation, the program is doomed to failure and will result only in a useless academic exercise.

3. Staff training should include both practical application and some theory. However, "on-the-spot" teaching of specific techniques should have precedence. Role playing in the classroom situation for staff should be promoted in order to maximize the transfer of skills to the on-ward clinical situation.

4. Behavioral techniques should be used systematically to promote the maintenance of staff performance. Where possible, advancement, raises, and extra monetary inducements should be arranged contingent on accurate staff performance (e.g., Iwata *et al.*, 1976; Patterson, Griffin, & Panyan, 1976). When these are not possible within the hospital's administrative structure, direct and public feedback, social reinforcement, and modeling techniques should be used to reinforce correct staff performance. Modeling of appropriate behavior by professional staff and supervising nursing personnel is critical. It is of the utmost importance to ensure that the head nurse model appropriate interactive behaviors with the patients.

5. It is also most apparent that the behavioral program director needs visibility on the unit in order to maximize the reinforcing and modeling power of his or her presence.

6. The political and interpersonal atmosphere should be examined before and during the implementation of any program. Although this step is not a characteristic and objective component of behavioral analysis, it is a critical aspect of effective programming.

SUMMARY

This chapter has dealt with the issues of staff training, the maintenance of staff performance, and staff consultation as they pertain to behavioral treatment programs in the psychiatric setting. Hospital politics, intrastaff power struggles, and the historical role of the nurse in the psychiatric setting were all examined vis-à-vis the implementation of behavioral programs. Empirically evaluated methods for teaching staff behavioral techniques were reviewed. The issue of behavioral consultation in psychiatric settings was also examined in light of the politics and the staff needs operating within them. Suggestions for improving the quality of consultation were outlined. Finally, a concise blueprint was presented for successfully initiating, effecting, and maintaining behavioral programs in the psychiatric setting.

REFERENCES

Ayllon, T., & Azrin, N. H. (1964). Reinforcement and instructions with mental patients. *Journal of Experimental Analysis of Behavior, 7*, 327–331.

Ayllon, T., & Azrin, N. H. (1968). *The token economy: A motivational system for therapy and rehabilitation.* New York: Appleton-Century-Crofts.

Ayllon, T., & Michael, J. (1959). The psychiatric nurse as a behavioral engineer. *Journal of Experimental Analysis of Behavior, 2*, 323–334.

Bellack, A. S., & Franks, C. M. (1975). Behavioral consultation in the community mental health center. *Behavior Therapy, 6*, 388–391.

Bellack, A. S., & Hersen, M. (1977). *Behavior modification: An introductory textbook.* Baltimore: Williams & Wilkins.

Delamater, A. M., Conners, C. K., & Wells, K. C. (1984). A comparison of staff training procedures: Behavioral applications in the child psychiatric inpatient setting. *Behavior Modification, 8*, 39–58.

Fitzgerald, J. R. Reid, D. H., Schepis, M. M., Faw, G. D., Welty, P. A., & Pyfer, L. M. (1984). A rapid training procedure for teaching manual sign language skills to multidisciplinary institutional staff. *Applied Research in Mental Retardation, 5*, 451–469.

Gardner, J. M. (1972). Teaching behavior modification to nonprofessionals. *Journal of Applied Behavior Analysis, 5*, 517–521.

Gelfand, D. M., Gelfand, S., & Dobson, W. R. (1967). Unprogrammed reinforcement of patients' behavior in a mental hospital. *Behaviour Research and Therapy, 5*, 201–207.

Greene, B. F., Willis, B. S., Levy, R., & Bailey, J. S. (1978). Measuring client gains from staff-implemented programs. *Journal of Applied Behavior Analysis, 11*, 395–412.

Hersen, M. (1976a). Historical perspectives in behavioral assessment. In M. Hersen & A. S. Bellack (Eds.), *Behavioral assessment: A practical handbook* (pp. 3–22). New York: Pergamon Press.

Hersen, M. (1976b). Token economies in institutional settings: Historical, political, ethical, and generalization issues. *Journal of Nervous and Mental Disease, 162*, 206–211.

Hersen, M. (Ed.). (1986). *Pharmacological and behavioral treatment: An integrative approach.* New York: Wiley.

Hersen, M., & Barlow, D. H. (1976). *Single case experimental design: Strategies for studying behavior change.* New York: Pergamon Press.

Hersen, M., & Bellack, A. S. (1976). A multiple-baseline analysis of social-skills training in chronic schizophrenics. *Journal of Applied Behavior Analysis, 9,* 239–245.

Hersen, M., & Luber, R. F. (1977). Use of group psychotherapy in a partial hospitalization service: The remediation of basic skill deficits. *International Journal of Group Psychotherapy, 27,* 361–376.

Hersen, M., Eisler, R. M., Alford, G. S., & Agras, W. S. (1973). Effects of token economy on neurotic depression: An experimental analysis. *Behavior Therapy, 4,* 392–397.

Hersen, M., Turner, S. M., Edelstein, B. A., & Pinkston, S. G. (1975). Effects of phenothiazines and social skills training in a withdrawn schizophrenic. *Journal of Clinical Psychology, 31,* 588–594.

Hollander, M. A., & Plutchik, R. (1972). A reinforcement program for psychiatric attendants. *Journal of Behavior Therapy and Experimental Psychiatry, 3,* 297–300.

Hollander, M., Plutchik, R., & Horner, V. C. (1973). Interaction of patient and attendant reinforcement programs: The "piggyback" effect. *Journal of Consulting and Clinical Psychiatry, 41,* 43–47.

Hutchison, J. M., Jarman, P. H., & Bailey, J. S. (1980). Public posting with a habilitation team: Effects on attendance and performance. *Behavior Modification, 4,* 57–70.

Ivancic, M. T., Reid, D. H., Iwata, B. A., Faw, G. D., & Page, T. J. (1981). Evaluating a supervision for developing and maintaining therapeutic staff-resident interactions during institutional care routines. *Journal of Applied Behavior Analysis, 14,* 95–107.

Iwata, B., Bailey, J. S., Brown, K. M., Foshee, T. J., & Alpern, M. (1976). A performance-based lottery to improve residential care and training by institutional staff. *Journal of Applied Behavior Analysis, 9,* 417–431.

Johnson, C. A., Katz, R. C., & Gelfand, S. (1972). Modifying the dispensing of reinforcers: Some implications for behavior modification with hospitalized patients. *Behavior Therapy, 3,* 589–592.

Katz, R. C., & Lutzker, J. R. (1980). A comparison of three methods for training timeout. *Behavior Research for Severe Developmental Disabilities, 1,* 123–130.

Katz, R. C., Johnson, C. A., & Gelfand, S. (1972). Modifying the dispensing of reinforcers: Some implications for behavior modification with hospitalized patients. *Behavior Therapy, 3,* 579–588.

Kazdin, A. E. (1977). *The token economy: A review and evaluation.* New York: Plenum Press.

Kissel, R. C., Whitman, T. L., & Reid, D. H. (1983). An institutional staff-training and self-management program for developing multiple self-care skills in severely/profoundly retarded individuals. *Journal of Applied Behavior Analysis, 16,* 395–415.

LeBow, M. D. (1973). *Behavior modification: A significant method in nursing practice.* Englewood Cliffs, NJ: Prentice-Hall.

LeBow, M. D. (1976). Applications of behavior modification in nursing practice. In M. Hersen, R. M. Eisler, & P. M. Miller (Eds.), *Progress in behavior modification* (Vol. 2, pp. 137–177). New York: Academic Press.

Liberman, R. P., & Bryan, E. (1976). A behavioral approach to community psychiatry. *Scandinavian Journal of Behavior Therapy, 5,* 57–73.

Liberman, R. P., & Davis, J. (1975). Drugs and behavior analysis. In M. Hersen, R. M. Eisler, & P. M. Miller (Eds.), *Progress in behavior modification* (Vol. 1, pp. 307–330). New York: Academic Press.

Liberman, R. P., Davis, J., Moon, W., & Moore, J. (1973). Research design for analyzing drug-environment behavior interactions. *Journal of Nervous and Mental Disease, 156,* 432–439.

Liberman, R. P., King, L. W., & DeRisi, W. J. (1976). Behavior analysis and therapy in community mental health. In H. Leitenberg (Ed.), *Handbook of behavior modification and behavior therapy* (pp. 566–603). Englewood Cliffs, NJ: Prentice-Hall.

Loeber, R. (1971). Engineering the behavioral engineer. *Journal of Applied Behavior Analysis, 4,* 321–326.

Luber, R. F., & Hersen, M. (1976). A systematic behavioral approach to partial hospitalization programming: Implications and applications. *Corrective and Social Psychiatry and Journal of Behavior Technology Methods and Therapy, 22,* 33–37.

Mansdorf, I. J., & Burstein, Y. (1986). Case manager: A clinical tool for training residential treatment staff. *Behavioral Residential Treatment, 1,* 155–167.

McKeown, D., Adams, H. E., & Forehand, R. (1975). Generalization to the classroom of principles of behavior modification taught to teachers. *Behaviour Research and Therapy, 13,* 85–92.

Panyan, M., Boozer, H., & Morris, N. (1970). Feedback to attendants as a reinforcer for applying operant techniques. *Journal of Applied Behavior Analysis, 3,* 1–4.

Parsons, M. B., Schepis, M. M., Reid, D. H., McCarn, J. E., & Green, C. W. (1987). Expanding the impact of behavioral staff management: A large-scale, long-term application in schools serving mentally handicapped students. *Journal of Applied Behavior Analysis, 20,* 139–150.

Patterson, E. T., Griffin, J. C., & Panyan, M. C. (1976). Incentive maintenance of self-help training programs for non-professional personnel. *Journal of Behavior Therapy and Experimental Psychiatry, 7*, 249–253.

Patterson, R., Cooke, C., & Liberman, R. P. (1972). Reinforcing the reinforcers: A method of supplying feedback to nursing personnel. *Behavior Therapy, 3*, 444–446.

Patterson, R. L. (Ed.). (1975). *Maintaining effective token economies.* Springfield, IL: Charles C Thomas.

Paul, G. L., & McInnis, T. L. (1974). Attitudinal changes associates with two approaches to training mental health technicians in milieu and social-learning programs. *Journal of Consulting and Clinical Psychology, 42*, 21–23.

Paul, G. L., McInnis, T. L., & Mariotto, M. J. (1973). Objective performance outcomes associated with two approaches to training mental health technicians in milieu and social-learning programs. *Journal of Abnormal Psychology, 82*, 523–532.

Pomerleau, O. F., Bobrove, P. H., & Smith, R. H. (1973). Rewarding psychiatric aides for the improvement of assigned patients. *Journal of Applied Behavior Analysis, 6*, 383–390.

Pommer, D. A., & Streedbeck, D. (1974). Motivating staff performance in an operant learning program for children. *Journal of Applied Behavior Analysis, 7*, 217–221.

Realon, R. E., Wheeler, A. J., Spring, B., & Springer, M. (1986). Evaluating the quality of training delivered by direct care staff in a state mental retardation center. *Behavioral Residential Treatment, 3*, 199–212.

Reid, D. H., & Green, C. W. (1990). Staff training. In J. L. Matson (Ed.), *Handbook of behavior modification with the mentally retarded* (pp. 71–90). New York: Plenum Press.

Reid, D. H., Parsons, M. B., & Green, C. W. (1989). *Staff management in human services.* Springfield, IL: Charles C Thomas.

Seys, D. M., & Duker, P. C. (1978). Improving residential care for the retarded by differential reinforcement of high rates of ward-staff behaviour. *Behavioural Analysis and Modification, 2*, 203–210.

Stoddard, L. T., McIlvane, W. J., McDonagh, E. C., & Kledaras, J. B. (1986). The use of picture programs in teaching direct staff. *Applied Research in Mental Retardation, 7*, 349–358.

Trudel, G., Boisvert, J. M., Maruca, F., & Leroux, P. A. (1974). Unprogrammed reinforcement of patients' behaviors in wards with and without token economy. *Journal of Behavior Therapy and Experimental Psychiatry, 5*, 147–149.

Turner, S. M., Hersen, M., & Alford, H. (1974). Effects of massed practice and meprobromate on spasmodic torticollis: An experimental analysis. *Behaviour Research and Therapy, 12*, 261–263.

van den Pol, R. A., Reid, D. H., & Fuqua, R. W. (1983). Peer training of safety-related skills to institutional staff: Benefits for trainers and trainees. *Journal of Applied Behavior Analysis, 16*, 139–156.

Wallace, C. J., Davis, J. R., Lieberman, R. P., & Baker, V. (1973). Modeling and staff behavior. *Journal of Consulting and Clinical Psychology, 41*, 422–425.

Watson, L. S. (1975). Shaping and maintaining behavior modification skills in staff using contingent reinforcement techniques. In R. L. Patterson (Ed.), *Maintaining effective token economies* (pp. 69–101). Springfield, IL: Charles C Thomas.

Watson, L. S., & Uzzell, R. (1980). A program for teaching behavior modification skills to institutional staff. *Applied Research in Mental Retardation, 1*, 41–53.

Wodarski, J. S. (1976). Procedural steps in the implementation of behavior modification programs in open settings. *Journal of Behavior Therapy and Experimental Psychiatry, 7*, 133–136.

Zlomke, L. C., & Benjamin, V. A. (1983). Staff in-service: Measuring effectiveness through client behavior change. *Education and Training of the Mentally Retarded, 18*, 125–130.

9

Medical Complications with Adults

MICHAEL O'BOYLE and PAUL CINCIRIPINI

INTRODUCTION

Many investigators have noted the high frequency of medical disorders among psychiatric patients, and the fact that medical disorders can mimic functional psychiatric illnesses (e.g., Marshall, 1949). An extensive literature documents failures to diagnose physical illness among psychiatric patients (Lazare, 1989). There are a number of reasons, which may be classified as patient-related, physician-related, or disease-related (Hoffman & Koran, 1984). For example, certain characteristics of the psychiatric patient may conspire to thwart an accurate medical diagnosis. Psychiatric patients may be unattractive (e.g., dirty, unkempt, malodorous, and hostile), may be uncooperative, or may have difficulty communicating clearly, and these factors may discourage accurate history taking or a thorough physical examination. Psychiatric patients may also be less likely to show evidence of physical pain, even in the face of acute, life-threatening medical illness (Talbott & Linn, 1978).

Physician-related reasons for misdiagnoses include inadequate assessments, overreliance on inadequate consultations, and uncritical acceptance of patients who have been "cleared medically," perhaps after a cursory examination. Patients with manifest psychiatric symptoms may be rejected by those in medical settings and referred to psychiatric facilities (Ananth, 1984). Referring physicians may use psychiatric facilities as primary-care sources for patients perceived as having psychiatric difficulties, perhaps doing so without completing an adequate evaluation for medical illness. It may be tempting to assume that a given problem or symptom has a psychiatric basis, especially in a patient with a psychiatric history, or in one with an obvious psychosocial stressor that "explains" the symptom. In some settings, such as emergency rooms, having a psychiatric history can inhibit a vigorous search for medical illness. The psychiatrist's skills in performing physical examinations may also erode (Patterson, 1978). A difficulty is that psychiatrists and other mental health professionals deal with illnesses that are characterized by mental symptoms, which potentially encompass all of medicine (Miller, 1967).

MICHAEL O'BOYLE and PAUL CINCIRIPINI • Department of Psychiatry and Behavioral Sciences, University of Texas Medical Branch at Galveston, Galveston, Texas 77555-0429.

Handbook of Behavior Therapy in the Psychiatric Setting, edited by Alan S. Bellack and Michel Hersen. Plenum Press, New York, 1993.

Psychiatric symptoms such as depression or anxiety are not pathognomonic for either physical or mental disorders. Subjective symptoms such as depression may herald physical disease and indeed precede objective signs of physical illness (Burke, 1972; Hoffman & Koran, 1984).

In this chapter, we summarize the literature on medical illnesses in psychiatric patients, outline common psychiatric presentations that may have medical causes, and suggest evaluation strategies for psychiatric patients. A high index of suspicion of physical illness, as well as an adequate history and physical examination, is required for all newly admitted psychiatric patients, regardless of how purely functional their psychiatric difficulties may appear to be.

PHYSICAL ILLNESS IN PSYCHIATRIC PATIENTS

Koranyi (1982) summarized a number of epidemiological studies describing rates of medical illness in psychiatric populations, indicating that the rate of physical illness was somewhat more than 50%. He noted that disorders of mood or behavior do not necessarily represent "first-rank" psychiatric illnesses, and he distinguished between primary and secondary psychiatric disorders, secondary disorders being caused by a medical illness or a toxic state. A number of possible relationships exist: The medical illness may cause or exacerbate the psychiatric syndrome; there may be no apparent relationship between the two entities; or the psychiatric syndrome may cause or exacerbate the medical illness (Maricle, Hoffman, Bloom, Faulkner, & Keepers, 1987). Lazare (1989) also summarized studies of medical illness in psychiatric populations, noting that from 34% to 84% of psychiatric inpatients were found to have physical disease. In 12%–40% of these patients, the physical illness was felt to have caused or contributed to the psychiatric symptoms. Although psychiatric symptoms are often non-specific, among psychiatric patients unrecognized medical illnesses are likely to present as organic mental states, acute psychosis, anxiety, or depression (Hall & Beresford, 1984). These presentations, as well as mania, are discussed below.

Organic Mental States

A common convention in psychiatry has been to separate disorders into organic and functional categories. This distinction cannot always be made reliably, and a number of functional disorders may eventually come to be understood in terms of brain dysfunction. However, confusion and other signs of cognitive impairment are often the hallmark of brain pathology.

Delirium. Confusion in psychiatric patients is common. Delirium may constitute a medical emergency and must always be considered in the differential diagnosis of any patient presenting with confusion. Delirium is common, causing substantial morbidity and mortality. Lipowski (1980) estimated that about 10% of hospitalized medical-surgical patients are delirious at any given time. The hallmark of delirium is a fluctuation in the ability to maintain and appropriately shift attention (American Psychiatric Association, 1987). The onset is usually acute and accompanied by disturbances in mood, perception, sleep-wake cycles, and psycho-motor activity (Lipowski, 1987).

Although an acute confusional state must be considered a delirium until proven otherwise, other diagnostic possibilities include dementia, psychosis, and dissociative states. Delirium should be suspected in all patients with a recent change in thinking, awareness, or behavior, especially if they have no psychiatric history. Delirium may have prodromal features such as anxiety or restlessness. The essential feature is fluctuation in the ability to concentrate or attend to the environment, so-called clouding of consciousness. This clouding can range from a slight impairment found only by explicit formal mental-status testing to sleepiness and disorientation, or paranoia, agitation and hypervigilance.

Perceptual disturbances, such as visual hallucinations (e.g., seeing insects) or illusions (e.g., the misidentification of people), are frequently observed. In addition, disorientation is frequently present, usually with respect first to time, then to place, and only rarely to person (if a patient in good physical health is disoriented only to person, one may suspect a psychiatric disorder such as a dissociative state as opposed to delirium).

Thinking disturbances are often present, and memory is usually impaired. Patients may become paranoid and delusional, feeling, for example, that they are being mistreated by staff members. Mood disturbance is the rule. Usually, patients are unhappy, with a labile affect, although delirious patients are occasionally euphoric.

In their psychomotor activity, patients are usually agitated, but one may also observe quiet deliriums. Autonomic dysfunction frequently occurs, its features depending on the etiology of the delirium (e.g., anticholinergic delirium is associated with dilated pupils).

Risk factors for delirium include older age, dementia, substance abuse, chronic disease, and surgery that involves general anesthesia. Mild cognitive impairment may be thought of as lowering an individual's threshold for developing a delirium. For this reason, simple mental-status screening-tests, such as the Mini-Mental Examination (Folstein, Folstein, & McHugh, 1975) are recommended for identifying patients at higher risk of delirium (Fields, MacKenzie, Charlson, & Sax, 1986), and for tracking a confusional state. Mild cognitive impairment or quiet deliriums may be missed if one relies only on casual conversation to screen for impairment. In a survey of patients over 65 admitted to a university general hospital, only 4 mental status examinations were recorded among 394 examinations (McCartney & Palmateer, 1985). Patients with clear cognitive deficits on admission were more likely to show acute confusional episodes later on, which would indicate the necessity of a thorough initial evaluation.

Although there may be a myriad causes of delirium, several etiological classes should always be considered when evaluating the disorder, although more than one cause may often be found:

1. *Toxic causes*. Intoxication by therapeutic as well as recreational drugs is not uncommon. Among the psychotropics, anticholinergic medications, including tricyclic antidepressants, are frequent offenders. A careful evaluation of the patient's current medications is essential because virtually all drugs in sufficient quantity may cause a delirium, especially in an elderly patient. A careful history may yield information regarding substance abuse or dependence, or exposure to poisons such as solvents or pesticides. Withdrawal from alcohol or sedative-hypnotic drugs is often a cause of delirium in patients of all ages.

2. *Systemic diseases*. Metabolic disturbances, systemic infections, cardiovascular disease, and collagen diseases are all potential causes of delirium. Metabolic causes include fluid and electrolyte imbalances. For example, among hypertensive patients, a delirium may be caused by hyponatremia precipitated by diuretics and a low-salt diet. Diabetes and nutritional deficiencies (e.g., vitamin deficiencies) may also cause delirium. Frequent infectious causes include pneumonia and urinary tract infections. A common cardiovascular cause is congestive heart failure.

3. *Primary brain disease*. Potential causes under this heading include brain trauma, such as subdural hematoma, and infections, such as meningitis; other cerebral insults include neoplasms or stroke.

It can be seen that delirium is a nonspecific syndrome that may have numerous, often multiple, causes. A high index of suspicion of delirium in anyone showing an acute onset of fluctuating cognitive and attentional deficits is crucial (Lipowski, 1987).

Dementia. Dementing illnesses are a significant cause of impairment among patients. *Dementia* refers to an acquired cognitive impairment, not seen exclusively during periods of delirium, of sufficient severity so as to interfere significantly with social or occupational functioning (American Psychiatric Association, 1987). Dementing illnesses may initially present with behavioral symptoms that overshadow the cognitive impairment. A common diagnostic mistake is the failure to recognize the cognitive impairment in the face of more prominent psychiatric symptoms such as depression, which may also be present in a person suffering from dementia (Moak, 1989).

Generally, one should be optimistic when evaluating a patient with a suspected dementing illness and should search for potentially treatable causes. The first task in an evaluation of dementia is to consider delirium, which is often reversible. In terms of functional disorders, depression sometimes mimics dementia. Depression and dementia are the two most common mental illnesses of old age. The interface between dementia and depression may be problematic. There may be an overlap in the clinical presentation of dementia, mood disorders, and physical disorders, leading to serious errors in diagnosis. Rabins (1983) reported that in from 10% to 33% of patients presenting with dementia, the cause of the dementia was potentially reversible; other patients were erroneously diagnosed as suffering from dementia. *Pseudodementia* is a syndrome of apparent organic deficit that is due to functional psychiatric illness (e.g., depression). It has been shown that a significant proportion of patients diagnosed as demented do not follow the expected downhill course of progressive dementia; their symptoms ameliorate, a finding suggesting that their dementia was the result of a psychiatric disorder (Wells, 1984). It has been suggested that a past history of depression, relatively acute onset, depressed mood, appetite disturbance, and self-blaming or somatic delusions are connected with dementia caused by depression (Rabins, Merchant, & Nestadt, 1984). Conversely, relatively more disorientation to time, greater difficulty finding one's way about, and impairment in dressing may suggest degenerative dementia (Reynolds, Hoch, Kupfer, Buysse, Houck, Stack, & Campbell, 1988).

However, although reversible dementias and depression-induced dementias (depressive pseudodementias) exist, we should realize that true progressive dementias are frequent as well. There may have been a tendency in recent years to overestimate the prevalence of reversible dementia, especially depression-induced dementia. Often, depression and dementia coexist, and although depressive symptoms may be reduced with treatment, cognition remains impaired (Reifler, 1986). Clarfield (1988) reviewed 32 studies that examined the prevalence of various causes of dementias, concentrating on potential and actual reversibility. In the 11 studies that gave follow-up information, it was found that 11% of the dementias resolved, 3% fully. The most common reversible dementias were those occurring secondary to drugs, depression, or metabolic disturbances. Clarfield felt that this 11% figure was probably an overestimate of the true community incidence of reversible dementias and argued for a conservative strategy in working up new cases of dementia. To this end, he cited Mulley (1986), who wrote that, "To deny demented patients comprehensive assessment is neglect; to subject them all to detailed investigation is unnecessary" (p. 1418).

There has been disagreement about how extensive the evaluation for suspected dementia should be. American authorities often recommend an elaborate work-up, whereas British and Canadian authorities tend to argue for a more restricted, clinically oriented evaluation (Clarfield, 1988). Generally, more extensive evaluations should be reserved for those patients in whom the dementing illness occurs earlier in life, for those in whom it occurs suddenly or for those who have had a particularly pernicious course. Dementing illnesses in which genetic patterns may be important (e.g., suspected Huntington's chorea) also warrant a more exhaustive evaluation (Popkin & Mackenzie, 1985).

Psychosis

Psychosis is a condition in which a patient's reality testing is grossly impaired, such impairment leading to the creation of a new reality (American Psychiatric Association, 1987). The term is quite nonspecific, and the condition may result from a number of physical or functional disorders. As with delirium, a complete listing of the medical conditions that can produce psychosis would encompass much of medicine. Major medical conditions that may cause psychosis include alcohol- or drug-related conditions and endocrine disturbances, especially thyroid disease (Sternberg, 1986). Because some medical conditions that cause psychosis are potentially fatal, one's first task in the evaluation of psychosis is to rule out a life-threatening physical cause. Anderson and Kuehnle (1974) listed eight potentially life-threatening conditions that may produce psychosis: cerebrovascular accident, drug withdrawal, hypertensive encephalopathy, hypoglycemia, hypoxic and hypoperfusion states, meningitis and encephalitis, poisoning, and Wernicke-Korsakoff syndrome. Once life-threatening diseases have been ruled out, one should look for disorders that, although not life-threatening, require medical attention (Sternberg & Pottash, 1986).

A high index of suspicion of medical illness is central to the evaluation of a psychotic patient. Factors reported to be suggestive of medical causes of psychosis include the onset of symptoms later in life and the acute onset and/or rapid progression of symptoms (Sternberg, 1986). Organicity should also be suspected in psychotic patients being treated for major medical illness, as a number of illnesses (e.g., Parkinson's disease) and the medications used to treat these illnesses may be associated with psychosis. A history of alcohol or drug abuse (including prescribed or over-the-counter medications) should also alert one to a possible organic psychosis. A family history of degenerative brain disease (e.g., Huntington's chorea or Wilson's disease) may be informative, as these disorders may present with psychotic symptoms. The presence of visual, olfactory, or tactile hallucinations should be considered medically caused until all medical causes are ruled out.

Anxiety

Symptoms of anxiety are seen in most psychiatric patients and have many causes. Because anxiety is observed at some time in virtually all psychiatric disorders, the correct diagnosis of anxiety symptoms may be difficult (Mackenzie & Popkin, 1983). Lawlor and Lazare (1989) classified conditions characterized by anxiety into four categories: (1) normal states; (2) psychiatric syndromes excluding anxiety disorders (such as schizophrenia); (3) anxiety disorders (panic disorders, phobias, etc.); and (4) organic anxiety syndrome. Organic anxiety syndrome must be ruled out before another diagnosis is made. The essential feature of organic anxiety syndrome is "prominent recurrent panic attacks or generalized anxiety caused by a specific organic factor" (American Psychiatric Association, 1987, p. 113).

As with delirium and psychosis, the number of potential medical causes of anxiety are myriad (e.g., see Lawlor & Lazare, 1989). The most common causes are endocrine disorders and drug use. Cardiovascular and/or pulmonary diseases (e.g., myocardial infarction and acute asthma) are also often associated with anxiety. The medical causes of panic attacks are similar to those that may cause generalized anxiety. In the case of panic disorder, one should recognize that patients may select only the most frightening symptom to report (e.g., chest pain). Katon (1986) found that 89% of 55 patients with panic disorder referred to psychiatrists by primary-care physicians had presented with just one or two somatic complaints. The most common complaints were cardiac, gastrointestinal (e.g., epigastric pain), and neurological (e.g., headache and dizziness). These selective presentations may lead to diagnostic confusion, and one should inquire about all possible panic symptoms should the diagnosis of panic disorder be suspected. Although many physical conditions are associated with anxiety and panic, some diagnoses are fairly uncomplicated (e.g., asthma attacks) and are not discussed here. A number of chronic illnesses, especially cardiovascular and/or pulmonary diseases (e.g., chronic obstructive pulmonary disease and heart failure) may also be associated with anxiety. Dealing with anxiety in such patients may be difficult, as they may have a coexisting panic disorder. Panic disorder should be considered if panic symptoms persist after optimal treatment of the chronic physical illness has been achieved.

One should next ask about drug use, both licit and illicit. Many medications (e.g., theophylline) and recreational drugs (e.g., cocaine), as well as commonly used drugs such as caffeine, may cause anxiety. Alcohol and drug withdrawal may also mimic panic.

Next, one should consider other medical conditions that may mimic panic disorder. Thyroid disorders may be associated with anxiety, and a high incidence of thyroid abnormalities has been reported among patients who self-refer for evaluation of panic attacks (Matuzas, Al-Sadir, Uhlenhuth, & Glass, 1987). For these reasons, thyroid function screening (T3, T4, and TSH) is suggested for all patients with a suspected panic disorder (Fyer & Sandberg, 1988; Lindemann, Zitrin, & Klein, 1984).

Although pheochromocytoma is another possible cause of panic, a work-up for it should be undertaken only if there is a positive family history; if panic attacks are associated with headache, flushing, and sweating; or if the physical exam yields findings consistent with such a diagnosis (e.g., abdominal mass) (Raj & Sheehan, 1987).

Temporal lobe seizures may be confused with panic attacks, but they are rare. Routine EEGs or neurological consultations are not recommended but should be considered for those whose panic attacks feature prominent feelings of depersonalization, derealization, or altered consciousness, or for those who have a history of seizures or head trauma (Fyer & Sandberg, 1988; Raj & Sheehan, 1987).

There is little evidence that hypoglycemia plays a role in panic attacks or generalized anxiety disorder. A work-up for hypoglycemia is not suggested unless the fasting blood sugar is quite low.

Last, mitral valve prolapse and panic disorder should be mentioned. Many studies have found that mitral valve prolapse is more common in patients with panic disorder (e.g., Liberthson, Sheehan, King, & Weyman, 1986). The exact nature of the relationship between the two remains to be elucidated, but it appears that the conditions may coexist. If the physical exam or EKG provide evidence suggestive of mitral valve prolapse, an echocardiogram should be considered. The medical evaluation, in addition to the physical examination, thyroid function testing, and EKG mentioned, should also include routine blood chemistries and a complete blood count. An EKG is recommended, as tricyclic antidepressants, suggested for treatment, may aggravate preexisting conduction defects (Glassman & Bigger, 1981).

Depression

Depressive symptoms often lead people to seek psychiatric help and, indeed, are ubiquitous among us. This ubiquity leads to difficulties in making the correct diagnosis of major depression, a syndrome of depressed mood or pervasive loss of interest and associated symptoms (i.e., sleep and/or appetite disturbance, psychomotor agitation or retardation, fatigue, difficulty in concentrating, and suicidal ideation) (American Psychiatric Association, 1987). As with psychotic disorders, organic causes of depression must be ruled out before a diagnosis of major depression can be made. This ruling out may be difficult, as major depression is also quite prevalent in those with chronic medical illness and may complicate the treatment of medical illnesses (Katon & Sullivan, 1990). The number of possible medical causes is immense, covering much of medicine. Classes of causes include (1) metabolic and endocrine disturbances, notably thyroid disorders; (2) drugs and toxic causes; (3) infections; (4) cancers; and (5) central nervous system degenerative disorders, such as Parkinson's disease (Sederer, 1986).

The most frequently occurring organic depressive states are due to drugs (Barreira, 1989), so a careful history that includes inquiry into all the medications (prescribed and over-the-counter) that a patient is taking is essential. A number of drugs have been associated with depressive symptomatology, most notably antihypertensives such as reserpine, clonidine, methyldopa, propranolol, and guanethidine (Goff & Jenike, 1986). Medications should be reviewed and simplified if possible. In addition, alcoholics and substance abusers may present a picture resembling a treatment-resistant depression. They can be identified only by obtaining an accurate estimate of the patient's alcohol or drug intake. Many of the medical conditions associated with depression can be detected with an evaluation that includes a detailed history and physical, routine blood tests (including a complete blood count, a thyroid panel, and automated chemistries), and a urinalysis. In the elderly, a pretreatment EKG is essential, as many of the drugs used to treat depression may affect the heart.

Mania

Although primary or functional manias are the rule, secondary manic syndromes, resulting from medical disorders, do occur. Krauthammer and Klerman (1978) reviewed the topic of secondary mania, reporting that drugs, metabolic disturbances, infection, neoplasm, and epilepsy have all been shown to cause mania. The authors defined secondary manias as manic syndromes occurring secondary to medical dysfunction. They excluded syndromes coexisting with confusional states (e.g., delirium and dementia), as well as manias occurring in a patient with a past history of mood disorder. Since their review, a number of reports have been made on secondary mania (for reviews, see Massion & Benjamin, 1989; Stasiek & Zetin, 1985). Again, the point is that all manic patients should be evaluated with the idea that their mania may result from an underlying medical or surgical condition. Particular attention should be given to those patients who have known medical illness or who are on medications. Those developing mania for the first time late in life are also quite likely to be suffering from a secondary mania.

EVALUATION STRATEGIES

The evaluation of a newly admitted psychiatric patient is a crucial task, for appropriate treatment follows from correct diagnoses. The most critical element may be an initial open-mindedness or benign skepticism, a stance in which previously gathered information or a referring diagnosis is not blindly accepted as fact. If other possible diagnoses are not at least somewhere on one's differential, they can easily be missed. An analogy may be made to the work done on bystander intervention in emergencies (Latané & Nida, 1981). Interest in this area was generated in large measure as a result of the Kitty Genovese case, in which a young woman was stalked and murdered in New York City in 1964 while numerous witnesses were present who did not intervene. One of the findings of this research, which may be overlooked because of its simplicity, is that a necessary prerequisite for acting on an emergency is perceiving one. Most of us feel that we will act appropriately in an emergency. However, a critical problem lies in correctly interpreting what constitutes an emergency. It is quite likely that true emergencies are missed because the situation is viewed as normal, or as to be expected. Overlooking a medical disorder in a psychiatric patient may well constitute an emergency that is missed. In addition, the fact that a given patient has been seen by a number of medical and/or mental health professionals during the evaluation process may lead to a diffusion of responsibility, also contributing to nonintervention (Latané & Nida, 1981). Thus, one should entertain the idea that a given psychiatric symptom may have a medical cause, even if that symptom may be explained as being due to functional psychiatric illness.

The first step in an evaluation includes a thorough history of the present illness, preferably from both the patient and knowledgeable others. The past psychiatric history must be outlined. A medical history, including medications, is also essential. Patients and informants should be questioned in detail about all medications taken (both prescribed and over-the-counter), as patients may not "count" non-prescribed medications or certain medications (such as birth control pills and vitamins) as medications unless they are explicitly asked. Patients may also neglect to mention medications they are taking that have been prescribed for others and are being shared. An accurate history of alcohol and recreational drug use should also be obtained. Inquiry should also be made into any history of toxic exposure (a case of mercury poisoning was clarified at our institution when family members reported that their children had been playing with a silvery liquid brought home by an acquaintance). At this time, documentation of prior hospitalizations should be obtained, as patients' accounts of hospitalizations may be vague or inaccurate. We advise formally requesting summaries of prior hospitalizations, including laboratory work and diagnostic tests. In addition to the medical history, a comprehensive review of systems may help to elicit symptoms that may not be spontaneously offered by a patient, but that may be helpful in pointing toward medical illnesses (e.g. heat intolerance associated with hyperthyroidism).

The family history, emphasizing inheritable disorders, both medical and psychiatric, may also provide crucial information. For example, a patient referred for an evaluation of a suspected psychiatric disorder reported that her father had died of "Parkinson's" disease at a relatively young age. Records obtained indicated that he had been diagnosed with Huntington's chorea. This information led to a tentative diagnosis of Huntington's chorea in the patient, who had presented with a number of complaints and had been ultimately referred to the psychiatry outpatient service after being seen by other specialists. The evaluation of each patient should include a comprehensive mental status examination. We recommend including a relatively brief standardized test of cognitive function, such as a Mini-Mental State Examination (Folstein *et al.*, 1975) or the Neurobehavioral cognitive status examination (NCSE; Mueller, Kiernan, & Langston, 1988).

In the physical examination, particular attention should be paid to vital signs. At times, rather obvious signs of illness (e.g., fever due to infection) may be overlooked because the patient has a psychiatric history. The physical examination should be thorough and, again, done in an open-minded way. Simply referring the patient for a screening physical, or to an internist for "medical clearance," may be unfair to the patient and to the consulting internist and may lead to a false sense of security (Hall, Gardner, Popkin, LeCann, & Stickney, 1981; Koranyi, 1979).

Laboratory Studies

As with the work-up for dementia, there is disagreement about what groups of tests constitutes an appropriate screening battery for psychiatric patients. Some recommend a comprehensive assessment, and others argue that a more selective battery is more cost-effective and efficient (Dolan & Mushlin, 1985). Laboratory tests are expensive and have the potential for morbidity. The cost of some tests commonly ordered for psychiatric patients is given in Table 1. The ordering of many tests increases the likelihood of obtaining a false-positive result, which may lead to more tests.

The argument against selective batteries is obviously that, without more extensive tests, treatable medical illnesses will not be detected (Rosse, Giese, Deutsch, & Morihisa, 1989). In addition, the cost of hospitalization is so high that a test that has the potential to shorten hospitalization may be cost-effective. Because drug toxicities, metabolic or endocrine disturbances, infections, and central nervous system disease are the most common medical causes of psychiatric illness, laboratory tests should be directed toward these entities. Test selection should always be guided by information gained from the history or physical; for individual patients, the tests may be more extensive. A complete blood count, an automated chemistry panel (e.g., electrolytes, glucose, liver and renal function tests), thyroid function tests (free T4 and TSH), a syphilis screen, and a urinalysis should be considered for all patients. B_{12} and folate levels, sedimentation rate, stool tests for occult blood, and skin testing for tuberculosis may also be helpful and are relatively inexpensive (Hoffman & Koran, 1984). We recommend a urinary drug screen despite its expense, as drug toxicity is a relatively common cause of

Table 1. Approximate Cost of Commonly Ordered Tests
for Psychiatric Patients[a]

Test	Cost ($)	Test	Cost ($)
Complete blood count[b]	19	HIV test	49
Blood chemistry panel[b]	90	Serum cortisol	41
Thyroid panel (free T4, TSH)[b]	153	Pregnancy test	35
Syphilis screen (e.g., VDRL)[b]	43	CT scan	442–513
Urinalysis[b]	21	MRI scan	763–1041
Urine drug screen[b]	150	EEG	200
Sedimentation rate	14	EKG	80
Blood alcohol level	43	Chest X ray	59
B_{12}, folate levels	82		

[a]Hospital charges only
[b]Recommended for all admissions

psychiatric presentations. The measurement of therapeutic drug levels is also reasonable. Such measurements may help in the detection of drug toxicity and also gauge a patient's compliance with prescribed medications (Estroff & Gold, 1986).

We recommend a head CT scan or MRI if an EEG has been abnormal, if focal findings are found on the neurological exam, if cognition is impaired, or if there is a history of seizure, head trauma, or alcoholism. Other possible indications include the first psychiatric episode or onset of psychiatric illness late in life (Rosse *et al.*, 1989). Although the tests recommended should help identify the majority of medical causes of psychiatric illness, we again emphasize that the most important elements in uncovering medically caused psychiatric presentations are a persistent open-mindedness and a willingness to search for medical causes. To explain symptoms as purely psychiatric in nature, without such an attitude, could be disastrous for the patient.

SUMMARY

Medical disorders are common among psychiatric patients and may cause or exacerbate psychiatric syndromes. Although medical illnesses may mimic virtually any psychiatric syndrome, they are more likely to present as organic mental states (e.g., delirium and dementia), acute psychosis, anxiety, or depression. As delirium may constitute a medical emergency, it should be suspected in anyone showing an acute onset of fluctuating cognitive deficits. Dementing illness may also be seen, and one should search for potentially treatable causes (e.g., depression and delirium) when evaluating a patient with a suspected dementing illness. Acute psychosis, anxiety states, and depression may also have medical causes.

Because the number of potential medical causes of these entities are myriad and encompass virtually all of medicine, a systematic evaluation strategy for psychiatric patients is crucial. Such an evaluation should include a thorough history of the present illness, from both the patient and informants. A medical history, including all medications, as well as a history of alcohol and drug use, must be obtained. A family psychiatric and medical history may also provide crucial information. A mental status examination, including a standardized test of cognitive function, is essential. In the physical examination, attention should be paid to the vital signs; the physical examination should not be a cursory screen. Selected laboratory tests (i.e., thyroid function tests, a drug screen, a chemistry panel, a complete blood count, a syphilis screen, and a urinalysis) are recommended for all patients. The most important element in such an evaluation is a willingness to search for medical causes of psychiatric symptoms, before viewing the symptoms as purely psychiatric in nature.

ACKNOWLEDGMENT. We thank Helen Cates for her help in preparing this manuscript.

174

MICHAEL O'BOYLE
and PAUL CINCIRIPINI

REFERENCES

American Psychiatric Association. (1987). *Diagnostic and statistical manual of mental disorders* (3rd ed., rev.; DSM-III-R). Washington, DC: Author.

Ananth, J. (1984). Physical illness and psychiatric disorders. *Comprehensive Psychiatry, 25*, 586–593.

Anderson, W. H., & Kuehnle, J. C. (1974). Strategies for the treatment of acute psychosis. *Journal of the American Medical Association, 229*, 1884–1889.

Barreira, P. (1989). Depression. In A. Lazare (Ed.), *Outpatient psychiatry: Diagnosis and treatment* (2nd ed., pp. 252–255). Baltimore: Williams & Wilkins.

Burke, A. W. (1972). Physical illness in psychiatric hospital patients in Jamaica. *British Journal of Psychiatry, 121*, 321–322.

Clarfield, A. M. (1988). The reversible dementias: Do they reverse? *Annals of Internal Medicine, 109*, 476–486.

Dolan, J. G., & Mushlin, A. I. (1985). Routine laboratory testing for medical disorders in psychiatric inpatients. *Archives of Internal Medicine, 145*, 2085–2088.

Estroff, T. W., & Gold, M. S. (1986). Medical evaluation of the psychiatric patient. In M. S. Gold & A. L. C. Pottash (Eds.), *Diagnostic and laboratory testing in psychiatry* (pp. 9–26). New York: Plenum Press.

Fields, S. D., MacKenzie, C. R., Charlson, M. E., & Sax, F. L. (1986). Cognitive Impairment—Can it predict the course of hospitalized patients? *Journal of the American Geriatric Society, 34*, 579–585.

Folstein, M. F., Folstein, S. E., & McHugh, P. R. (1975). "Mini-Mental State": A practical method for grading the cognitive state of patients for the clinician. *Journal of Psychiatric Research, 12*, 189–198.

Fyer, A. J., & Sandberg, D. (1988). Pharmacologic treatment of panic disorder. In A. J. Frances & R. E. Hales (Eds.), *American Psychiatric Press review of psychiatry, Vol. 7* (pp. 88–120). Washington, DC: American Psychiatric Press.

Glassman, A. H., & Bigger, J. I. (1981). Cardiovascular effects of therapeutic doses of tricyclic antidepressants: A review. *Archives of General Psychiatry, 38*, 815–820.

Goff, D. C., & Jenike, M. A. (1986). Treatment-resistant depression in the elderly. *Journal of the American Geriatric Society, 34*, 63–70.

Hall, R. C. W., & Beresford, T. P. (Eds.). (1984). *Handbook of psychiatric diagnostic procedures* (Vol. 1). New York: Spectrum.

Hall, R. C. W., Gardner, E. R., Popkin, M. K., LeCann, A. F., & Stickney, S. K. (1981). Unrecognized physical illness promoting psychiatric admission: A prospective study. *American Journal of Psychiatry, 138*, 629–635.

Hoffman, R. S., & Koran, L. M. (1984). Detecting physical illness in patients with mental disorders. *Psychosomatics, 25*, 654–660.

Katon, W. (1986). Panic disorder: Epidemiology, diagnosis, and treatment in primary care. *Journal of Clinical Psychiatry, 47*(10, Suppl.), 21–27.

Katon, W., & Sullivan, M. D. (1990). Depression and chronic medical illness. *Journal of Clinical Psychiatry, 51*(6, Suppl.), 3–11.

Koranyi, E. K. (1979). Morbidity and rate of undiagnosed physical illness in a psychiatric clinic population. *Archives of General Psychiatry, 36*, 414–419.

Koranyi, E. K. (1982). Undiagnosed physical illness in psychiatric patients. *Annual Review of Medicine, 33*, 309–316.

Krauthammer, C., & Klerman, G. L. (1978). Secondary mania: Manic syndromes associated with antecedent physical illness or drugs. *Archives of General Psychiatry, 35*, 1333–1339.

Latané, B., & Nida, S. (1981). Ten years of research on group size and helping. *Psychological Bulletin, 89*, 308–324.

Lawlor, T., & Lazare, A. (1989). Anxiety. In A. Lazare (Ed.), *Outpatient psychiatry: Diagnosis and treatment* (2nd ed., pp. 246–251). Baltimore: Williams and Wilkins.

Lazare, A. (1989). Medical disorders in psychiatric populations. In A. Lazare (Ed.), *Outpatient psychiatry: Diagnosis and treatment* (2nd ed., pp. 240–245). Baltimore: Williams and Wilkins.

Liberthson, R., Sheehan, D. V., King, M., & Weyman, A. (1986). The prevalence of mitral valve prolapse in patients with panic disorders. *American Journal of Psychiatry, 143*, 511–515.

Lindemann, C. G., Zitrin, C. M., & Klein, D. F. (1984). Thyroid dysfunction in phobic patients. *Psychosomatics, 25*, 603–606.

Lipowski, Z. J. (1980). *Delirium: Acute brain failure in man*. Springfield, IL: Charles C Thomas.

Lipowski, Z. J. (1987). Delirium (acute confusional states). *Journal of the American Medical Association, 258*, 1789–1792.

Mackenzie, T. B., & Popkin, M. K. (1983). Organic anxiety syndrome. *American Journal of Psychiatry, 140*, 342–344.

Maricle, R. A., Hoffman, W. F., Bloom, J. D., Faulkner, L. R., & Keepers, G. A. (1987). The prevalence and significance of medical illness among chronically mentally ill outpatients. *Community Mental Health Journal, 23*, 81–90.

Marshall, H. E. S. (1949). Incidence of physical disorders among psychiatric inpatients. *British Medical Journal, 2*, 468–470.

Massion, A. O., & Benjamin, S. (1989). Manic behavior. In A. Lazare (Ed.), *Outpatient psychiatry: Diagnosis and treatment* (2nd ed., pp. 256–266). Baltimore: Williams and Wilkins.

Matuzas, W., Al-Sadir, J., Uhlenhuth, E. H., & Glass, R. M. (1987). Mitral valve prolapse and thyroid abnormalities in patients with panic attacks. *American Journal of Psychiatry, 144*, 493–496.

McCartney, J. R., & Palmateer, L. M. (1985). Assessment of cognitive deficit in geriatric patients: A study of physician behavior. *Journal of the American Geriatric Society, 33*, 467–471.

Miller, H. (1967). Depression. *British Medical Journal, 1*, 257–262.

Moak, G. (1989). Disturbances of higher intellectual functioning. In A. Lazare (Ed.), *Outpatient psychiatry: Diagnosis and treatment* (2nd ed., pp. 280–291). Baltimore: Williams and Wilkins.

Mueller, J., Kiernan, R. J., & Langston, J.W. (1988). The mental status examination. In H. Goldman (Ed.), *Review of general psychiatry* (2nd ed., pp. 193–207). Norwalk, CT: Appleton & Lange.

Mulley, G. P. (1986). Differential diagnosis of dementia. *British Medical Journal Clinical Research, 292*, 1416–1418.

Patterson, C. W. (1978). Psychiatrists and physical examinations: A survey. *American Journal of Psychiatry, 135*, 967–968.

Popkin, M. K., & Mackenzie, T. B. (1985). The provisional diagnosis of dementia: Three phases of evaluation. In R. C. W. Hall & T. P. Beresford (Eds.), *Handbook of psychiatric diagnostic procedures* (Vol. 2, pp. 197–211). New York: Spectrum.

Rabins, P. V. (1983). Reversible dementia and the misdiagnosis of dementia: A review. *Hospital and Community Psychiatry, 34*, 830–835.

Rabins, P. V., Merchant, A., & Nestadt, G. (1984). Criteria for diagnosing reversible dementia caused by depression: Validation by 2-year follow-up. *British Journal of Psychiatry, 144*, 488–492.

Raj, A., & Sheehan, D. V. (1987). Medical evaluation of panic attacks. *Journal of Clinical Psychiatry, 48*, 309–313.

Reifler, B. V. (1986). Mixed cognitive-affective disturbances in the elderly: A new classification. *Journal of Clinical Psychiatry, 47*, 354–356.

Reynolds, C. F., Hoch, C. C., Kupfer, D. J., Buysse, D. J., Houck, P. R., Stack, J. A., & Campbell, D. W. (1988). Bedside differentiation of depressive pseudodementia from dementia. *American Journal of Psychiatry, 145*, 1099–1103.

Rosse, R. B., Giese, A. A., Deutsch, S. I., & Morihisa, J. M. (1989). *Concise guide to laboratory and diagnostic testing in psychiatry*. Washington, DC: American Psychiatric Press.

Sederer, L. (1986). Depression. In L. Sederer (Ed.), *Inpatient psychiatry: Diagnosis and treatment* (2nd ed., pp. 3–35). Baltimore: Williams and Wilkins.

Stasiek, C., & Zetin, M. (1985). Organic manic disorders. *Psychosomatics, 26*, 394–396, 399, 402.

Sternberg, D. E. (1986). Testing for physical illness in psychiatric patients. *Journal of Clinical Psychiatry, 47* (1, Suppl.), 3–9.

Sternberg, D. E., & Pottash, A. L. C. (1986). Evaluation of psychotic syndromes. In M. S. Gold & A. L. C. Pottash (Eds.), *Diagnostic and laboratory testing in psychiatry* (pp. 191–214). New York: Plenum Press.

Talbott, J. A., & Linn, L. (1978). Reactions of schizophrenics to life-threatening disease. *Psychiatric Quarterly, 50*, 218–227.

Wells, C. E. (1984). Diagnosis of dementia: A reassessment. *Psychosomatics, 25*, 183–187, 190.

10

Neuropsychiatry

A Multidimensional Approach

GUILA GLOSSER and DAVID S. GLOSSER

INTRODUCTION

Increased scientific interest in the neurobiological bases of behavioral disorders has brought about numerous changes in clinical practice within the psychiatric setting. One of the most conspicuous changes has been the renewed collaboration of behavioral neurologists and neuropsychologists with psychiatrists and behavioral psychologists in the assessment and treatment of patients. The term *neuropsychiatry* refers to an evolving multidimensional approach to a variety of well-recognized behavioral disorders. The neuropsychiatric approach assesses and develops interventions for the interactive biological and psychological aspects of behavioral disorders.

One significant consequence of the resurgent interest in the neuropsychiatric perspective has been that the dichotomous distinction between "functional" and "organic" disorders has been abandoned. Attempts to identify behavioral markers or tests that reliably distinguish between organic and functional disorders have failed (Heaton, Baade, & Johnson, 1978; Sillitti, 1982). There is wider recognition now that no core set of symptoms is common to all organic disorders, and that what previously had been termed the organic disorders encompasses a diverse group of neurobehavioral syndromes, each with its own identifiable set of unique symptoms, etiology, and/or pathology (Seltzer & Sherwin, 1978). Increasingly sophisticated neurodiagnostic procedures have revealed a variety of neurological changes among patients who were considered previously to have functional disorders without biological abnormalities (e.g., Nasrallah & Weinberger, 1986). Moreover, developments in the rehabilitation of patients with neurobehavioral disorders, such as those associated with closed-head injury and stroke, have reinforced the conclusion that many of the same behavioral interventions that are successful in the management of patients with certain psychiatric disorders can also successfully modify maladaptive behaviors of patients with known neurological illnesses (Wood, 1987). Thus, it has become untenable, both scientifically and clinically, to maintain a separation between the psychiatric and neurological disorders.

GUILA GLOSSER and DAVID S. GLOSSER • Department of Neurology, Graduate Hospital, Philadelphia, Pennsylvania 19146.

Handbook of Behavior Therapy in the Psychiatric Setting, edited by Alan S. Bellack and Michel Hersen. Plenum Press, New York, 1993.

GUILA GLOSSER and
DAVID S. GLOSSER

Neuropsychiatry is an evolving field integrating knowledge from psychiatry, clinical and neuro-psychology, neurology, and other neurosciences to assess and treat patients with behavioral disorders. The neuropsychiatric approach is not limited to certain patient groups, and thus, it is not possible to compile an exhaustive list of neuropsychiatric diseases or disorders for the purposes of a review. Perusal of current textbooks on clinical neuropsychiatry (e.g., Cummings, 1985) reveals discussion of disorders as diverse as apraxia, schizophrenia, narcolepsy, and obsessive-compulsive disorder. Rather than denoting specific illnesses or patient populations, the neuropsychiatric approach entails the application of a coherent set of principles of brain-behavior relationships to clinical problems.

The classificatory principles that guide neuropsychiatric diagnosis and treatment are different from those in traditional psychiatric practice. In fact, the subtypes of dysfunction that are revealed through neurobehavioral and neurodiagnostic assessments often are not coextensive with established psychiatric diagnoses (Goldstein & Shelly, 1987; Townes, Martin, Nelson, Prosser, Pepping, Maxwell, Peel, & Preston, 1985; Yozawitz, 1986). The relevant dimensions and principles that guide neuropsychiatric classification, assessment, and interventions are those that specify the relationships between various locations, patterns, and dynamics of neurological dysfunction and particular cognitive, emotional, and behavioral-adaptive capabilities. We describe these classificatory principles briefly, and then illustrate the application of these principles in a discussion of epilepsy and dementia.

CLASSIFICATION IN NEUROPSYCHIATRY

Neurological Variables

Three features of neurological dysfunction are most relevant to neuropsychiatric diagnosis and intervention:

1. The *location* of neurological dysfunction can be specified by anatomical criteria (e.g., the left temporal lobe), neurochemical criteria (e.g., the cholinergic system), and/or physiological criteria (e.g., the limbic system).

2. *Patterns* of neurological dysfunction are conceived of as gradients of activation versus deactivation within each of the aforementioned neurological loci. For example, during an epileptic seizure, there may be heightened activation in a particular anatomical region, while between seizures, there may be hypoactivation in the same brain area; or there may be chronic and progressive hypoactivation in a specific neurochemical system, such as the dopaminergic defect in Parkinson's disease.

3. The *dynamics* of neurological dysfunction include distinctions such as whether there is insult to a developing as opposed to a mature nervous system; whether the onset of the dysfunction is sudden or if it evolves gradually over time; and whether the subsequent temporal course of the dysfunction is stable, remitting or progressing. Dementia of the Alzheimer's type, for example, involves slowly evolving alterations in the adult nervous system that follow a progressively deteriorating course. A traumatic brain injury in an adult also involves an insult to a developed nervous system, but the neurological dysfunction in this case is of acute onset, and it subsequently tends to follow a remitting course with a decelerating rate of improvement over time. Tourette's syndrome, by contrast, begins insidiously in childhood, during a period of neural development and tends to evolve slowly over time. Subsequently, it follows a chronic progressive or a "waxing and waning" course.

Psychological Variables

A comprehensive discussion of all the psychological and behavioral symptoms that might be related to specific aspects of neurological dysfunction, and that constitute the focus of neuropsychiatric assessment and treatment, is beyond the scope of this chapter. However, the general categories of psychological and behavioral function relevant to neuropsychiatric practice are outlined below:

1. The cognitive domains that are traditionally assessed in the mental status examination (e.g., Strub & Black, 1977) and in standard neuropsychological evaluations (e.g., Lezak, 1983) consist of attention-concentration, language, visuospatial (constructional) abilities, learning and memory, and higher-order conceptual, reasoning and executive control abilities. More elementary motor and sensory functions along with specific symptoms of higher cortical dysfunction (e.g., apraxia and agnosia), are also commonly included in a comprehensive neuropsychological assessment. Such an assessment typically yields a detailed characterization of impaired and spared cognitive functions, as well as statements regarding relationships between the pattern of observed cognitive impairment(s) and the presumed underlying neurological dysfunction.

2. Alterations in mood, affect, and insight into one's disabilities, as well as symptoms such as delusions, illusions, and hallucinations, are also related in definable ways to specific aspects of neurological dysfunction. For example, depression is characteristic among non-fluent aphasics with lesions in anterior structures of the left cerebral hemisphere; while patients with posterior lesions and fluent aphasia of the Wernicke's type are more likely to present with paranoid delusions (Benson, 1973). As another example, the high incidence of depression among Parkinson's disease patients, who have dysfunction in the dopaminergic neural systems, contrasts sharply with the much lower incidence of depression among Alzheimer's Disease patients (see below), who are believed to have primary disruption in cholinergic neurochemical systems.

3. Particular forms of neurological dysfunction result in predictable behavioral syndromes, and these may be associated with certain patterns of adaptive functioning. For example, patients with damage in the right cerebral hemisphere are more often unaware of or indifferent to their physical and cognitive impairments (Weinstein & Kahn, 1955). Consequently, not being able to apprehend or appreciate the need for help, these patients are less likely to comply with rehabilitation efforts. Unlike many of the cognitive and emotional symptoms that remain as relatively stable dispositions of the neurologically impaired individual across situations, behavioral and adaptive patterns tend to be more variable, as they are determined by the interaction between the attributes of the impaired individual and attributes of particular environments. The distinction that is made in the field of rehabilitation between *impairment* and *disability* is relevant here. Neurological injuries and their consequent physical, cognitive and psychological impairments are considered to be properties of the individual. These impairments are measured and interpreted in comparison with fixed normative standards. Behavioral disabilities and adaptive abilities, on the other hand, can be specified only as a function of the interaction between the impaired person and the particular social and physical environment that must be addressed by that person. Disabilities of adaptive functioning are measured and interpreted in comparison to norms which are conditional or situationally determined and which vary according to changing environments.

EPILEPSY

The high comorbidity of epilepsy and frank psychopathology has been recognized for centuries. It has been estimated that 12% of the institutionalized mentally ill in the United States have epilepsy (Commission for the Control of Epilepsy and Its Consequences, 1978). Among patients with epilepsy, there is an increased incidence of psychotic disorders (Flor-Henry, 1969), nonpsychotic interictal personality disorders (Hermann & Whitman, 1984), and depression (Robertson & Trimble, 1983). Even in the absence of the most severe psychopathology, cognitive inefficiency, personality anomalies, and problems in social adjustment are ubiquitous in this population. Some epileptologists assert that psychosocial problems of varying magnitude are universal among patients with chronic seizure disorders (Rodin, 1977).

Epilepsy patients presenting in the psychiatric setting often display the full range of psychosocial adjustment problems, and in many cases, the specific sources of the various problems cannot be determined easily. As a rule, the problem behaviors are due to the interaction of variables in multiple domains. Neuropsychiatric assessment requires a consideration of neurological, neuropsychological, medical, and social factors.

Neurological Variables and Neuropsychiatric Complications of Psychiatry

The most obvious sources of some of the cognitive, behavioral, and affective symptoms in epilepsy are the periodic epileptiform discharges that disrupt normal brain function. Many of the most florid psychiatric symptoms seen in epilepsy patients are direct manifestations of seizures and are observed peri-ictally. Symptoms may occur in different modalities, dependent on the type and focus of the seizure (Bolwig, 1986). Most common are the changes in consciousness, confusion, and the psychomotor symptoms seen in complex partial seizures. Disturbances of thought characterized by delusions of familiarity (*déjà vu*) or strangeness (*jamais vu*) and the intrusion of complex alien ideas or remembrances are present as well. Strong affective symptoms, ranging from terror to depression, may also be part of the ictus. Sexual arousal or orgasm, though unusual, may be a feature of seizures as well (Lesser, Lueders, Dinner, & Morris, 1987). The phenomena most likely to create diagnostic confusion are hallucinations, which may occur in visual, auditory, or other sensory modalities. The hallmarks of most of the peri-ictal psychiatric symptoms are rapidity of onset, brevity of duration, and stereotypical similarity from seizure to seizure in a given patient. In certain patients, complex psychiatric symptoms evolve when seizures are repetitive and prolonged (Adebimpe, 1977; Penfield & Jasper, 1954).

All clinicians are aware that epilepsy patients emit unusual behaviors during the ictal phase of a seizure disorder. Clinicians are less cognizant generally of the relationships between behavioral symptoms and interictal electrophysiological abnormalities, some of which may be present for hours before and after seizures. Subclinical epileptiform or spike discharges as well as abnormal slowing of the electroencephalogram interictally are related to impaired information processing capacities and to disrupted behavior (Aarts, Binnie, Smit, & Wilkins, 1984; Shewmon & Erwin, 1988). When a patient with a known seizure disorder presents with a change in behavior, serious consideration should be given to the possibility that the new clinical symptoms are related to electroencephalographic (EEG) abnormalities.

Assessing the mere presence or absence of electroencephalographic (EEG) abnormalities is not sufficient; it is also important to consider variables such as the type, location, duration, and frequency of the epileptiform discharges. Certain types of seizure disorder, such as complex partial seizures of temporal lobe origin, are known to have higher associations with severe psychiatric disorders, than other types of seizure disorders, such as absence seizures of centrencephalic origin (Rodin, Katz, & Lennox, 1976). In terms of neuropsychological impairment, patients with epileptiform discharges confined to a focal brain area (partial seizures) tend to display a different pattern of cognitive impairment from that of patients with generalized discharge throughout the brain (Fedio & Mirsky, 1969; Wilkus & Dodrill, 1976). It is generally believed that the earlier the age of onset and the longer the duration of the seizures, the greater the likelihood of cognitive impairment (Dikmen, Matthews, & Harley, 1975; Saykin, Gur, Sussman, O'Connor, & Gur, 1989). Increased seizure frequency and severity are also related to increased cognitive and behavioral impairment, especially in more extreme cases where repeated and severe generalized tonic-clonic (*grand mal*) seizures result in prolonged periods of hypoxia

(Blumer & Benson, 1982). The greater availability of long-term EEG monitoring with concurrent behavioral videorecordings (Delgado-Escueta, 1979) has increased diagnostic accuracy and specificity in relating behavioral seizure morphologies to particular electroencephalographic abnormalities.

Increasingly sophisticated neurodiagnostic procedures have provided clearer evidence that the majority of patients with seizure disorders have identifiable structural brain lesions. More often than not, the location of the brain lesion corresponds to the location of the primary seizure focus. The actual extent of the areas of neuroanatomical and neurophysiological pathology, however, may be much wider than the circumscribed focus from which the seizures originate (Gur, 1985). Seizure disorders may occur in combination with or as a result of numerous types of neurological illnesses. Seizures may occur in conjunction with pervasive developmental disorders (e.g., cerebral palsy), following acute cerebral injury (e.g., stroke), as symptoms of metastatic disease, or as a result of diffuse encephalopathies (e.g., chronic seizure disorders often develop following an episode of febrile convulsions in childhood). The neuropsychiatric assessment of patients with known or suspected epilepsy requires consideration of the full extent of the neuropathology that results in disrupted brain function, even between actual seizure events. The underlying neuropathology may contribute significantly to abnormalities in mood, cognition, behavior, and adaptive function, and it is usually not treatable pharmacologically.

Neuropsychological Issues in Epilepsy

The cognitive and neuropsychological profiles associated with various types of seizure disorders have received extensive attention in both the clinical and the basic science literatures. Studies have ranged from examinations of global measures of cognitive functioning, such as the overall intelligence quotient in various epilepsy groups to detailed assessments of material-specific verbal and nonverbal memory problems that are differentially associated with dysfunction in the left or the right mesial temporal lobes (Milner, 1975). The preceding discussion of the neurobiological abnormalities associated with seizure disorders should lead the reader to anticipate that the cognitive and neuropsychological manifestations in epilepsy are also complex and variable. A complete neuropsychological evaluation should be considered for any patient presenting with a history of chronic seizure disorder. The reader is referred to Lezak (1983) for a comprehensive review of current practices in neuropsychological assessment.

In the neuropsychological assessment of patients with chronic seizure disorders some specific issues need emphasis: In the majority of clinical settings, the most common reason for referral to a neuropsychologist (including referrals of seizure disorder patients) is that either the patient or someone in the patient's environment notes "memory problems." The prevalence of complaints about memory is probably due to several factors. The capacity to encode and consolidate new information in a long-lasting representation entails a complex set of higher-order cognitive procedures that depend on the integrity of numerous lower-level cognitive and sensorimotor functions. It is rare to find a case where memory abilities are completely preserved in the face of significant impairments in primary sensory, attentional, linguistic, visuospatial or other basic cognitive functions. It is simply not possible to learn new information normally when basic perceptual, conceptual, and response systems are not functioning optimally. Memory disturbance, therefore, is found in association with a wide range of cognitive disturbances.

Complaints of "memory" dysfunction sometimes reflect impairment in another cognitive domain that is subserved by completely different neural systems. Patients often refer to a language disorder manifested by inconsistent retrieval of specific words or names as a memory problem (e.g., Mayeux, Brandt, Rosen, & Benson, 1980). Distinguishing between a true impairment in the processes necessary for the encoding, storage, and retrieval of new information in long-term memory and a selective word-finding disorder (anomia) is important for

GUILA GLOSSER and
DAVID S. GLOSSER

localizing the underlying neurological disturbance, for educating patients and caregivers regarding the disabilities, and for rehabilitation planning.

A distinction should also be made between memory complaints and actual memory performance. The former tend to correlate highly with variables such as depression, rather than with objective indices of memory functions among neurologically impaired populations (Bolla *et al.*, 1991; Kahn, Zarit, Hilbert, & Niederehe, 1975). In patients with chronic seizure disorders metamemory, or self-monitoring of memory functions, has been shown to be variably impaired (Prevey, Delaney, & Mattson, 1988). Like other groups, temporal lobe epilepsy patients' memory complaints do not reflect the adequacy of their actual memory performances, but rather seem to be determined by social-emotional factors and reflect the patients' sense of well-being (McGlone & Wands, 1991). A comprehensive neuropsychological assessment can distinguish among the various types of "memory" disorders and can often associate the pattern of memory/cognitive dysfunction with a particular neuropathological or psychiatric disorder.

Neuropsychological assessment of patients with chronic seizure disorders, unlike assessments of patients with strokes or brain tumors, often yield imperfect correlations between the domain of most serious cognitive impairment and the locus of maximal electroencephalographic abnormality. The neuropsychological assessment tends to highlight more stable regions of structural anatomical damage and of physiological underactivation, which do not always coincide with the primary focus of electrophysiological overactivation. Because the neurological dysfunction in epilepsy often begins at a time when the developing nervous system has the greatest potential for plasticity early in life, recovery or reorganization of neurological and neuropsychological function is often a consideration in localizing brain dysfunction. There is perhaps no better demonstration of the reorganization of function in the developing nervous system than the finding that, after excision of the damaged region of a temporal lobe for control of intractable seizures, there is sometimes *improvement* in memory and other cognitive functions that would otherwise have been expected to be subserved by the removed structure (Novelly, Augustine, Mattson, Glaser, Williamson, Spencer, & Spencer, 1984). Such sparing of neuropsychological function is characteristic of patients with an onset of seizures early in life (Powell, Polkey, & McMillan, 1985). Because of the developmental nature of the neurological disorder in many seizure disorder patients and because of the variability of the neuropathologies underlying epilepsy, special caution is required in applying conventional principles of brain-behavior relationships to localizing neurological dysfunction in epilepsy.

Although neuropsychological assessment may have limited utility in the absolute localization of the neurophysiological dysfunction in epilepsy, such an assessment can document a patient's profile of cognitive abilities and disabilities. This information is directly relevant to the educational and vocational planning problems of many epilepsy patients, who typically present with psychosocial adaptation complaints in their early adult years (Dodrill, Breyer, Diamond, Dubinsky, & Geary, 1984). Delineating perceptual and cognitive competencies is also important to understanding problems of interpersonal adjustment and behavior. Hermann (1981), among others, has demonstrated relationships between the severity of overall neuropsychological impairment and the severity of general psychopathology among people with epilepsy. Growing numbers of investigations have demonstrated relationships between particular patterns of lateralized neuropsychological dysfunction and specific patterns of social-emotional maladaptation in children and adults (Gainotti, 1978; Glosser & Koppell, 1987; Robinson, Kubos, Starr, Rao, & Price, 1984), and such relationships also apply to epilepsy patients.

Medications

Chronic anticonvulsant treatments must also be regarded as potential contributions to the cognitive-behavioral symptoms of epilepsy patients. Reynolds (1985) reviewed investigations documenting that, among healthy individuals, cognitive functioning is impaired following administration of various anticonvulsants at subtherapeutic doses; and among epilepsy patients, different anticonvulsants disrupt cognitive functioning and behavior even when administered at therapeutic, subtoxic, levels. Though a matter of debate, phenytoin and valproate have been described as having the worst impact on cognitive functioning, while carbamazepine is thought to be the least noxious (Trimble & Thompson, 1986). In maintaining therapeutic anticonvulsant levels, inadvertent toxicity is a common problem. Sometimes, anticonvulsant toxicity is indexed by a change in behavior. For example, in the case of gradually emerging depression and irritability as the main presenting symptoms, consideration should be given to the possibility that toxic levels of primidone or phenobarbital are responsible (Mattson & Cramer, 1989).

Most epileptologists regard the effects of uncontrolled recurrent seizures as more damaging cognitively and behaviorally than the side effects of anticonvulsants. Rather than setting therapeutic levels according to laboratory standards of serum drug concentrations, most epileptologists administer the maximum individually tolerable dose (usually of a single anticonvulsant) that is required to achieve substantially complete seizure control (Duncan, 1989). It should be noted that, although good seizure control generally produces improvement in the psychiatric complications of epilepsy, this is not always the case. Paradoxical exacerbation of emotional disturbances, particularly on the abolition of generalized absence seizures with ethosuximide and normalization of the EEG, has been reported and is termed *forced normalization* (Landolt, 1958). Wolf (1986) reported that this controversial phenomenon occurs in approximately 1% of epilepsy patients but may account for up to 15% of the psychotic illness in this population.

Pharmacological treatment of seizure patients' interictal behavior problems is complicated by the concurrent administration of anticonvulsants. For example, pharmacological treatment of depression, the most common psychiatric correlate of epilepsy, is constrained by the fact that tricyclic antidepressants may inadvertently lower the seizure threshold and thereby increase seizure frequency (Robertson, 1985). Certain antidepressants, maprotiline in particular, can produce seizures in vulnerable but non-epileptic individuals. The pharmacological management of psychiatric problems in epilepsy requires the same degree of specialized knowledge as is needed for the optimal psychopharmacological treatment of affective, schizophrenic and other major psychiatric disorders.

As in all medical conditions, medication compliance is a major issue in the behavioral management of patients with chronic seizure disorders. In a recent study medication compliance rates for 24 subjects followed for 3,428 days ranged from 87% to 39% (Cramer *et al.*, 1989). Failure to take prescribed anticonvulsant medication is the most common cause of subtherapeutic blood levels in epilepsy patients (Masland, 1982). Medication noncompliance not only increases risk of seizures but also increases the risk of peri-ictal psychiatric complications in epilepsy.

Social Learning Factors in Epilepsy

The contribution of the social environment to the problems of adjustment among epilepsy patients can not be overstated. The social environment can pose numerous barriers to adjustment. Patients with incompletely controlled seizures can not drive legally, or engage in many occupations because of potential safety risks and may be deprived of full participation in many other activities as well because of the prevalent stigma attached to epilepsy. Early in life, the person with epilepsy may encounter negative social responses within his/her family, and later in development, the individual may be confronted with negative reactions in school, at work, and sometimes even in the mental health setting. The individual's response and adjustment to his/her disability may be considered largely a function of the social environment, either through the current impact that other people have on the patient's behavior or through the cognitions and

GUILA GLOSSER and
DAVID S. GLOSSER

attributions concerning illness in general and epilepsy in particular that are learned socially by the patient.

The concept of stigma is central to understanding the social aspects of epilepsy. *Stigma* refers to the possession of a public attribute that is deeply discrediting and that causes the stigmatized person to be regarded as fundamentally different from, and globally inferior to, other people (Goffman, 1963). Historically, in the United States, epilepsy has been regarded as a negative personal attribute, as evidenced by the survival, until relatively recent times, of legal proscriptions against marriage and childbearing by people with epilepsy (Dell, 1986). The stigma of epilepsy has been regarded by many as more disruptive to normal function than the seizures themselves (Commission for the Control of Epilepsy and Its Consequences, 1978). In Collings's study (1990) of the correlates of subjective well-being among epilepsy patients, the importance of social identity and self-perception is well-demonstrated. In that survey, the best predictor of impaired global well-being was not the severity of the illness, but low self-image. Among epilepsy patients, the experience of stigmatization, impaired self-esteem, and feelings of helplessness have all been associated strongly with the development of anxiety and depression as well as with impaired life satisfaction (Arntson, Droge, Norton, & Murray, 1986).

The behavioral and cognitive adaptations by which an individual minimizes the impact of a defective public identity may be termed a *stigma management strategy*. The development of an effective strategy in epilepsy is rendered difficult by certain unique factors. Unlike conditions leaving a stable change in physical appearance, such as paraplegia or amputation, the discrediting public attribute in epilepsy ordinarily entails a defect not of physique, but of consciousness. The display of highly salient and embarrassing behaviors during seizures, such as incontinence or stereotypical automatisms, imposes a stigma burden similar to that encountered by the mentally ill. The unpredictable and intermittent nature of the expression of non-normative behaviors further complicates adoption of a stigma management strategy that is effective consistently.

A prime issue in stigma management for seizure patients is the question of disclosure versus secrecy. Unlike people with stable visible physical disabilities, people with epilepsy must repeatedly decide if it is wiser to preemptively make the disorder known to new social contacts, in the hope of preventing negative appraisal in the event of a seizure, or to conceal it and thereby not announce themselves as members of a stigmatized class. When seizures are well controlled, patients may elect not to disclose their epilepsy. Concealment relies on perfect seizure control, however, or on careful partitioning of one's social life so that the stigmatizing attribute does not become known. The secrecy strategy has many drawbacks. Threats to secrecy include the necessity to take medications frequently or to account for their side effects. There is an increasing possibility that a job-related urinalysis for drug abuse detection will reveal the presence of anticonvulsants. In addition to the long-term stress imposed by fears of discovery, secrecy may also serve as a barrier to the establishment of intimate relationships. Concealment of epilepsy is sometimes maintained by social avoidance when the patient has experienced or anticipates that he or she may have increased seizures. Episodic unexplained social withdrawal may yield negative consequences, which, in turn, may justify the patient's initial fear of rejection.

A less-often-appreciated, but equally important, source of behavioral dysfunction in epilepsy is the effect of disadvantageous conditioning processes. That seizures may be highly aversive events is understandable in light of the risk of injury imposed by many seizures. Patients often suffer lacerations, fractures, broken teeth, and burns during seizures, and drownings while swimming or bathing are unusually common. Even when injury does not occur, the adverse social consequences of seizures may be lastingly painful. An intense fear of seizures, including the fear of death, is common among seizure patients (Mittan, 1986). A more-or-less random schedule of potent aversive stimulation may foster the rapid development of avoidance behavior and anxiety. The most obvious and common adverse reaction is avoidance of situations that are recalled as being antecedent to seizures. When a seizure has occurred in association with a particularly discriminable antecedent event, a circumscribed phobia may be expected. When aversive seizures occur frequently and randomly, rapid generalization may result in avoidance of a wide range of situations and may produce a clinical picture similar to that of severe panic disorder with agoraphobia. The consequent loss of control over response contingent reinforcement and the inability to escape aversive events may partly account for the high prevalence of depression in epilepsy patients in much the same way as it does in other populations (Grosscup & Lewinsohn, 1980).

Many of the issues that have been raised in the discussion of the neuropsychiatric conceptualization of epilepsy also apply to a host of other neurodevelopmental disorders ranging from attention deficit disorder to schizophrenia. We have stressed the multifaceted aspects of the neurological dysfunction underlying the observed behavioral, cognitive, and emotional symptoms. The location of the neurological dysfunction in terms of its anatomy, physiology, and biochemistry; the fluctuating patterns of neurological disturbance; and the effects of psychopharmacological agents—all are relevant. The moderating effects of the age at which the neurological dysfunction occurred are also important. In many of the neurodevelopmental disorders, there is no exact correspondence between the location, severity, or pattern of the neurological dysfunction and the apparent cognitive, behavioral, and affective symptoms. Nonetheless, careful delineation of the pattern of spared and impaired neuropsychological functioning can lead to the development of rational behavioral rehabilitation programs. We have stressed the importance of the social environment in determining the public acceptability of people with neurological impairments. For many patients with epilepsy or with other neurodevelopmental disorders, all of the behavioral, cognitive, and affective symptoms will not be abolished by either psychopharmacological or psychological treatments. It is often necessary for the environment to be adapted to the patient's functional limitations, rather than to expect the patient to adapt to situations posing unattainable cognitive, social, or physical demands.

DEMENTIA OF THE ALZHEIMER'S TYPE

Dementia is defined as a decline from previously higher levels of functioning in two or more cognitive domains (usually including memory) and in personality. The declines in cognitive functioning must be evident in the absence of delirium and must significantly interfere with work and usual social relationships and activities (American Psychiatric Association, 1987; McKhann, Drachman, Folstein, Katzman, Price, & Stadlon, 1984).

Dementia refers to a constellation of mental and behavioral symptoms that may be associated with numerous diseases. There need not be a progression of symptoms, though in practice the overwhelming majority of dementing illnesses follow a progressively deteriorating course. Dementia is a symptom complex that is associated with certain psychiatric disorders such as chronic schizophrenia and what has been termed the *dementia of depression*, as well as with more than 50 other neuromedical conditions (Haase, 1977). Our discussion focuses on Alzheimer's disease (AD), as this is the most common dementing illness, but much of the presented material also applies to the other major classes of progressive dementing illnesses (e.g., multi-infarct dementia, Parkinson's disease, and Pick's disease).

Neuropsychological Evaluation

A determination of dementia must be made relative to an estimate of premorbid functional levels. The presence and the degree of cognitive impairment cannot be judged on an absolute scale; rather, dementia is defined as a change compared to premorbid performance levels that have a variable distribution in the normal population. There are numerous brief tests intended to screen for dementia, but they must be used cautiously in the psychiatric setting and should not be substituted for a more comprehensive mental status examination. Short screening tests typically do not correct for individual differences in premorbid characteristics, such as levels of education, that are known to affect cognitive test performances. Unacceptably high rates of both false-positive dementia classification (e.g., among illiterate or poorly educated individuals and among patients with primary language disorders) and false-negative dementia classification (e.g., among highly educated patients and those with mild diffuse encephalopathies or with nonlinguistic cognitive impairments) have been reported with these tests (Nelson, Fogel, & Faust, 1986). Formal neuropsychological assessment uses several methods to estimate premorbid levels of cognitive functioning that may be used as a basis of comparison with current levels of performance (e.g., Nelson & O'Connell, 1979; Wilson, Rosenbaum, & Brown, 1979). Also, many neuropsychological tests correct the obtained scores according to relevant demographic characteristics (e.g., age) of the patient. Because a comprehensive neuropsychological assessment obtains multiple measures of each cognitive domain, it yields estimates of current mental functioning that are more reliable, and more valid, than the results of simple screening procedures.

Dementia does *not* refer to an isolated impairment in memory functions; rather, impairment in multiple cognitive domains must be demonstrated. The initial presentation of a dementia, such as AD, more often than not entails changes in several cognitive domains and also in behavior, mood, and activity levels. Although memory impairment is usually one of the earliest presenting symptoms of dementia, it is not a sufficient and, according to some investigators (Cummings & Benson, 1983), not a necessary condition for the diagnosis of dementia. An assessment for dementia, therefore, requires a full evaluation of all facets of the mental status. Among the very elderly and patients with significant mood disorders, such an examination may require more specialized neuropsychological and behavioral assessment procedures than those done routinely in the psychiatric clinic. It is important to note also that the success of different tests in identifying dementia and in grading degree of cognitive impairment varies according to the severity of the dementia (Vitaliano, Breen, Albert, Russo, & Prinz, 1984).

Though there is variability in the clinical presentation of patients with AD, the following are some of the of the most commonly observed cognitive features:

1. Impairments of both immediate (primary) and long-term (secondary) memory functions are characteristic of patients with AD and differentiate them from patients with isolated amnestic disorders (Corkin, 1982). Memory dysfunction is one of the earliest manifestations of most, but not all, dementing disorders. The apparently disproportionate memory impairment in the early stages of AD has been linked to focal dysfunction in cerebral structures that are believed to be critical for the consolidation of new memories (Damasio & van Hoesen, 1986). As stated earlier in the discussion of memory dysfunction associated with epilepsy, adequate memory functioning depends on the integrity of many other basic cognitive processes. Hence, in patients with dementia, who have known impairments in multiple cognitive domains, memory is especially vulnerable. In addition to an impaired ability to form new memories and to acquire new information (anterograde amnesia), patients with AD also demonstrate significantly impaired recall and recognition of events that transpired before the onset of dementia (retrograde amnesia) (Wilson, Kaszniak, & Fox, 1981).

2. Some investigators consider a disturbance in language necessary for the diagnosis of AD (Obler & Albert, 1981). The language disorder in AD is different from that seen in aphasia (Glosser & Deser, 1991), and it appears to change somewhat over the course of the disease (Bayles & Kaszniak, 1987). In the earlier stages of dementia, when patients present for diagnosis, they usually manifest impairments in naming (lexical retrieval), in auditory and reading comprehension (particularly of conceptually more complex language), and in writing (especially in spontaneous descriptive writing). At least in the early to middle stages of the disease, AD patients show relatively preserved articulation and fluency, oral reading, writing

to dictation, and repetition, abilities that do not draw on their presumably impaired semantic processing (Schwartz, Marin, & Saffran, 1979). With advancing disease, patients manifest more diffusely impaired language skills, often progressing to mutism.

3. Impairments in visuospatial processing are seen in all stages of AD. The visuospatial processing disorders range from frank visual agnosia, to topographic disorientation, to more subtle impairments in visual perception, to almost universal visuoconstructional (e.g., drawing) deficits (Cummings & Benson, 1983).

4. Impairments in all aspects of attention, concentration, and immediate memory are also seen in AD and probably contribute to compromised performance on numerous tasks (Morris & Baddeley, 1988).

5. Finally, impaired reasoning, abstraction, problem solving, judgment, and higher level executive control functions are the hallmarks of all dementing disorders and appear quite early in the course of AD (Moss & Albert, 1988).

Assessing Behavioral Disturbances

Virtually all AD patients demonstrate a change in their usual activity levels. Such changes are manifested by either decreased activity (aspontaneity and apathy) or increased activity (restlessness) (Larson, 1963). A certain proportion of patients also demonstrate behaviors that resemble psychotic disorders. In the large series reported by Larson (1963), approximately one third of the AD patients exhibited psychotic or depressive symptoms. Cummings, Miller, Hill, and Neshkes (1987) conducted very detailed psychiatric examinations of 30 patients with the diagnosis of probable AD. These authors found that simple paranoid beliefs, usually concerning the fidelity of a spouse or the whereabouts of misplaced valuables, comprised the most common psychotic symptom among dementia patients and were documented in approximately 50% of both AD and multi-infarct dementia cases. In contrast to conventional clinical lore, hallucinations (both auditory and visual) were found to be *un*common among patients with the primary diagnosis of AD. Patients with suspected multi-infarct dementia who had significant visual sensory disturbances (specifically visual field constriction) were most likely to report visual hallucinations.

The incidence of depressive symptoms among Cummings *et al*.'s (1987) series of AD patients, and also in the series reported by Larson (1963), Kral (1983), and Reding, Haycox, and Blass (1985), has been approximately 20%. Cummings *et al.* (1987) made an important distinction between the presence of symptoms of depression and the presence of a major depression syndrome. These investigators reported that none of the dementia patients they examined exhibited the full symptom complex of major depression (but see Greenwald, Kramer-Ginsburg, Marin, Laitman, Hermann, Moks, & Davis, 1989), although many patients did exhibit isolated symptoms of depression. It is becoming increasingly recognized that elements of depression co-occur with dementia of the Alzheimer's type. Estimates of the absolute incidence of coexistent dementia and depression vary considerably, however, depending on the population from which study patients are drawn (i.e., either from psychiatry or neurology clinics), depending on the assessment procedures and criteria for the diagnosis of depression (e.g., self-report versus observational methods), and depending on the stage of dementia when patients are studied. Overall, the findings tend to suggest that depression is no more common among AD patients than in the general population of the elderly, and that the incidence of some forms of depression, in fact, may be lower in AD patients than in the general population of medically ill elderly (Cummings *et al.*, 1987; Reifler, Larson, & Hanley, 1982). In AD, the depressive symptoms are most likely to occur in the early and middle stages of dementia (Reifler *et al.*, 1982), and the predominant symptoms are behavioral (e.g., crying) and somatic (e.g., sleep and appetite disturbance), rather than cognitive (Cummings *et al.*, 1987). Most important, depressive symptoms in patients with AD respond as well to conventional pharmacotherapy as in patients without coexisting dementia (Kral, 1983; Greenwald *et al.*, 1989).

Specific relationships have been demonstrated between particular patterns of cognitive impairment and certain symptoms of disrupted behavior among patients with dementia. As reported above, it appears that patients with disproportionately severe impairments in visual sensation and perception may be more susceptible to experiencing visual illusions-hallucinations. If they also have significantly impaired reasoning and judgment, or if they lack insight about their illness, such patients are more likely to act inappropriately based on these misperceptions. The inverse relationship between dementia severity and the presence of symptoms of depression reported above may be explained by the fact that patients with more severe memory and executive control disorders are less likely to be able to sustain depressogenic cognitions (Merriam, Aronson Gaston, Wey, & Katz, 1988). Dementia patients with more severe auditory comprehension problems (like patients with severe Wernicke's aphasia) are at greater risk of developing paranoid delusions, which seem to be due, in large part, to the patient's misinterpretation of the linguistic communications of others.

In a comprehensive study of agitation over the course of progressively dementing illnesses, Cohen-Mansfield, Marx, and Rosenthal (1990) found that different levels of cognitive and functional abilities predicted different *types* of agitated behaviors. "Verbally agitated" behaviors (e.g., complaining and cursing) and "hoarding and hiding" behaviors were most prominent in the earlier stages of dementing illnesses, when language skills are least impaired and when patients still retain the ability to accomplish some activities of daily living. "Physically nonaggressive" behaviors (e.g., pacing and repetitive mannerisms), on the other hand, were manifested by more severely cognitively impaired patients who, though confused, still retained some physical and instrumental functional abilities. In the most advanced stages of dementing illnesses, the behavioral problems that require greatest attention are patients' impaired abilities to execute activities of daily living and self-care functions (e.g., problems of continence and feeding problems). Haley and Pardo (1989) also noted that the more disruptive kinds of behavior, such as wandering, yelling, and agitated pacing, decrease with more severe levels of cognitive impairments in the advanced stages of dementia. Careful individual behavioral assessment may reveal these and other types of associations between behavioral, affective, and cognitive symptoms in dementia. And these observations, in turn, can inform the treatment and management of some of the more disruptive behavioral symptoms of AD (Rabins, 1989).

Functional Assessment

In addition to assessing cognitive and behavioral symptoms, an assessment of functional abilities is also indicated in patients with suspected AD or another dementia. As noted above, current definitions of dementia require a change in the patients' performance of usual social roles to establish the diagnosis. This type of information is obtained from the history or by ratings on formal scales that have been developed to define the disabilities in various functional domains (Kane & Kane, 1981). Obtaining information about the functional abilities of dementia patients poses special problems. Because of their cognitive loss, even in the early stages of dementia, patients are not usually aware of the full extent of their cognitive and behavioral impairments, and they are not able to provide a reliable history of current symptoms or an accurate portrayal of their current functional abilities. Moreover, their cognitive impairments may interfere with their comprehension of and ability to respond to the simplest self-report scales. In patients suspected of having dementia, the history should *always* be confirmed by a reliable family member or another observer.

There is a moderate, but imperfect, correlation between the degree of impairment in functional adaptation and the degree of cognitive loss in dementia (Cohen-Mansfield *et al.*,

1990; Mayeux, Stern, & Spaton, 1985). Discrepancies between the severity of functional and cognitive impairments are due, in part, to the fact that patients may come from different environments that require functional capacities of varying degrees of complexity for adequate adaptation. Patients that are functioning in more demanding environments, such as those holding higher level administrative or professional positions, often present for diagnosis and treatment earlier in the course of the dementing illness. The cognitive impairments of these individuals impinge on their usual activities more quickly than for certain other retired individuals, who may engage in only limited activities outside the home. As noted in the introduction to this chapter, functional disability is determined not only by the severity of neurological dysfunction and concomitant cognitive impairments, but by an interaction between these person variables and environmental-social factors.

Several global rating scales for dementia severity are useful in initial diagnostic assessment as well as in monitoring changes over time and in predicting the progression of dementia (Berg, Hughes, Coben, Danziger, Martin, & Knesevich, 1982; Schneck, Reisberg, & Ferris, 1982). These rating scales generally identify three stages of dementia that are characteristic of AD:

1. The first stage consists of obvious, but mild, impairments in memory and other cognitive functions that affect the ability to carry out activities outside the home, such as work, travel, shopping, and managing finances. At this stage, the relatively mild cognitive impairments have a minimal effect on more routine activities at home (e.g., cooking and hobbies) and on self-care functions.

2. The second stage of dementia is characterized by severe memory and cognitive impairments usually sparing only the most overlearned and simple memories and skills. Self-care activities (e.g., dressing, toileting, and feeding) may be performed with minimal assistance or supervision, but the patient is no longer able to function independently either outside the home or, in most cases, within the home.

3. In the final stages of dementia, fragments of the patient's past knowledge, memories, and skills surface, but only infrequently. The patient depends on others for all activities, is often completely noncommunicative, and may be nonambulatory.

AD is a type of *progressive* dementia. In addition to the retrospective history of progressive decline, it is advisable to follow patients with suspected AD or another progressive dementia prospectively and to obtain serial assessments at a minimum of two points in time. Serial assessments are useful for confirming the suspected diagnosis and for projecting the future rate of progression. Dementia in AD patients progresses at different rates depending on a variety of factors, but in most cases, the rate of progression appears to be relatively constant for each individual (Mayeux *et al.*, 1985). Deviations from the typically steady rate of progression may be the result of a new, intercurrent illness or an abrupt change in the patient's environment. Once the acute problem is resolved, often a return to the more steady rate of functional decline may be expected.

Various factors have been suggested as contributing to differences in the base rate of progression of AD. The disease appears to follow a more rapidly progressing course in patients with a younger age at onset of symptoms, and in those with a strong family history of dementia, with accompanying extrapyramidal symptoms, or with disproportionately severe behavioral disturbances and psychotic symptoms earlier in the disease (Heston, Mastri, Anderson, & White, 1981; Seltzer & Sherwin, 1983; Stern, Mayeux, Sano, Hauser, & Bush, 1987). The rate of disease progression is a dynamic property of neurological dysfunction. In general, more rapidly evolving or abrupt onset of neurological dysfunction yields more severe behavioral symptoms. With more slowly progressing or serial CNS lesions, there is a greater possibility of restitution of function and of functional adaptation (Finger & Stein, 1982). The severity of the symptoms attributable to equal amounts of brain damage varies depending on the rate of progression of the damage. In AD, a more malignant presentation and more severe symptoms tend to be related to more rapidly progressing disease.

Diagnostic Issues

GUILA GLOSSER and
DAVID S. GLOSSER

The full debate about the differential diagnosis of dementia cannot be reviewed here. Controversy remains regarding how extensive a neuromedical evaluation should be performed, and how important it is to distinguish among etiologically different dementing illnesses in the clinical setting (Larson, Reifler, Featherstone, & English, 1984). Accuracy of the differential diagnosis of dementia is related to several factors: In neurological or medical clinics, when the initial presenting problem is cognitive change in an older individual, the accuracy rate for diagnosing the presence of a dementing illness and its etiology is greater than 80% (Sulkava, Haltia, Paetau, Wikstrom, & Palo, 1983; Wade, Mitsen, Hachinski, Fisman, Lau, & Merskey, 1987). Higher diagnostic error rates tend to prevail for patients presenting at a younger age, for those seen initially in a psychiatric setting where a behavioral disorder (such as depression) may be the primary presenting problem, and in patients who have a prior psychiatric treatment history. High rates of false-positive diagnoses of dementia tend to predominate in psychiatric settings (Nott & Fleminger, 1975; Ron, Toone, Garralda, & Lishman, 1979), whereas dementia clinics in nonpsychiatric settings tend to report higher rates of false-negative diagnoses (Reding, Haycox, & Blass, 1985).

It is generally agreed that the probability of finding a reversible cause of dementia is small among the geriatric population presenting with primary cognitive changes. The probability of finding a *coexisting* problem that contributes to, but does not cause, the dementia is quite high, however. It has been estimated that approximately 50% of patients with AD present initially with another co-occurring medical or psychiatric disorder (Reifler & Larson, 1989; Terry & Katzman, 1983). In such cases, the coexisting disease, or what has been termed the *excess disability*, may be treated successfully. And although such treatment will not reverse the dementing process, it certainly removes a factor that may otherwise accelerate the rate of progression and the severity of the primary degenerative disease.

In progressive dementias such as AD, the onset of dysfunction is usually insidious. Significant progression of the disease may occur before a patient is brought to medical attention. Often, disruptive behaviors, rather than cognitive changes, prompt the family to seek treatment, and commonly, social rather than medical factors determine when the patient will first be brought to medical attention. Arie (1973) and others have noted that patients' first contact with medical personnel often occurs at a time of crisis. The crisis may be in response to a sudden deterioration in behavior that is due to an acute change in the patient's physical or medical status (e.g., the occurrence of a new, intercurrent medical illness that itself may be benign) or to a recent change in the patient's environment (e.g., a move to a new home or the loss of a spouse). The crisis need not entail a change in the patient's behavior, but sometimes it is due to changes in the behavior of those around the patient with dementia. Medical attention may be sought in an emergent fashion because a family caregiver becomes ill suddenly and is unable to assist the patient, or a family member reaches a state of exhaustion from the considerable stress associated with caregiving, or a relative, who does not live with the patient, first notes cognitive-behavioral changes after a long absence from the patient and believes that the changes are of recent acute onset. During these periods of crisis, patients are more likely to present with confusion and disordered behavior that, in turn, increase the likelihood of emergency psychiatric hospitalization. Because of the pervasive cognitive impairments, medical problems are less likely to be noted by the patient and his or her family. The initial assessment of the dementia patient may reveal many coexisting medical and social-psychological problems that also require attention.

Dementia is a common disorder among the elderly, affecting approximately 15% of individuals over the age of 65 and as much as a third of the "old-old" population over the age of 80. Dementia in the elderly, or what used to be termed *organic brain syndrome*, is the major reason for long-term psychiatric hospitalization in the United States (Butler & Lewis, 1983). With increasing proportions of older adults in the general population, it can be expected that the demented elderly will make up a larger share of the patients in the psychiatric setting as well.

Although no therapeutic strategies are currently available to arrest or reverse the neurological impairments in AD, optimal management of the condition requires appreciation of its multiple dimensions. Overattribution of all behavioral-cognitive dysfunction in the elderly to progressive brain failure can produce an unwarranted attitude of therapeutic nihilism that may deprive patients of access to restorative treatments. Conversely, failure to appreciate the progressive neuropsychological impairments in AD deprives the patient and the family of the opportunity to make timely plans to adjust the environment to meet the patient's growing need for prosthesis.

The issues discussed in the neuropsychiatric conceptualization of Alzheimer's disease are not unique to the situation of elderly patients seeking psychiatric services. Rather, they are pertinent to many other groups of nonelderly patients with multifocal cerebral dysfunction (e.g., patients with metabolic-infectious disorders such as AIDS, patients with multiple sclerosis, and certain patients with traumatic brain injuries). In all these conditions, careful consideration of the relationships between neuropsychological, behavioral, functional, and neurological variables clarifies the nature of the psychiatric disturbance and leads to the development of rational interventions for the specific patient.

SUMMARY

The heterogeneity within the general class of neurobehavioral disorders is as great as that found within the general class of "psychiatric" disorders. There are as many differences between a child with a developmental language disorder and an elderly patient with Parkinson's disease as there are between a patient with bulimia nervosa and one with schizophrenia. Because patients with neurobehavioral disorders are so widely divergent etiologically, pathologically, and in terms of their clinical presentations, it is useful to integrate the facts in each case through the application of certain organizing principles. We have proposed a multidimensional neuropsychiatric approach in which characteristic cognitive, behavioral, and affective symptoms of various kinds of neurological dysfunction are related also to the individual's developmental history and social environment.

The discussions of epilepsy and Alzheimer's disease illustrate the application of a multidimensional approach to the behavioral assessment and treatment of two common clinical entities. The neuropsychiatric approach is not limited only to patients with defined neurological diseases; it may be applied to the full range of patient groups within the psychiatric setting.

REFERENCES

Aarts, J. H. P., Binnie, C. D., Smit, A. M., & Wilkins, A. J. (1984). Selective cognitive impairment during focal and generalized epileptiform EEG activity. *Brain, 107,* 293–308.

Adebimpe, V. R. (1977). Complex partial seizures simulating schizophrenia. *Journal of the American Medical Association, 237,* 1339–1341.

American Psychiatric Association. (1987). *Diagnostic and statistical manual of mental disorders* (3rd ed., rev.; DSM-III-R). Washington, DC: Author.

Arie, T. (1973). Dementia in the elderly: Diagnosis and assessment. *British Medical Journal, 4,* 540–543.

Arntson, P., Droge, D., Norton, R., & Murray, E. (1986). The perceived psychosocial consequences of having epilepsy. In S. Whitman & B. P. Hermann (Eds.), *Psychopathology in epilepsy: Social dimensions* (pp. 143–161). New York: Oxford University Press.

Bayles, K. A., & Kaszniak, A. W. (1987). *Communication and cognition in normal aging and dementia.* Boston: Little, Brown and Company.

Benson, D. F. (1973). Psychiatric aspects of aphasia. *British Journal of Psychiatry, 123,* 555–566.

Berg, L., Hughes, C. P., Coben, L. A., Danziger, W. L. Martin, R. L., & Knesevich, J. (1982). Mild senile dementia of Alzheimer type: Research diagnostic criteria, recruitment, and description of a study population. *Journal of Neurology, Neurosurgery and Psychiatry*, *45*, 962–968.

Blumer, D., & Benson, D. F. (1982). Psychiatric manifestations of epilepsy. In D. F. Benson & D. Blumer (Eds.), *Psychiatric aspects of neurologic disease* (Vol. 2, pp. 25–48). New York: Grune & Stratton.

Bolla, K. I., Lindgren, K. N., Bonaccorsy, C., & Bleecker, M. L. (1991). Memory complaints in older adults. Fact or fiction? *Archives of Neurology*, *48*, 61–64.

Bolwig, T. G. (1986). Classification of psychiatric disturbances in epilepsy. In M. R. Trimble & T. G. Bolwig (Eds.), *Aspects of epilepsy and psychiatry* (pp. 1–8). Chichester, England: Wiley.

Butler, R. N., & Lewis, M. I. (1983). *Aging and mental health*. New York: C. V. Mosby.

Cohen-Mansfield, J., Marx, M. S., & Rosenthal, A. S. (1990). Dementia and agitation in nursing home residents: How are they related. *Psychology and Aging*, *5*, 3–8.

Collings, J.A. (1990). Psychosocial well-being and epilepsy: An empirical study. *Epilepsia*, *31*, 418–426.

Commission for the Control of Epilepsy and Its Consequences. (1978). *Plan for Nationwide Action on Epilepsy*. DHEW Publication # NIH 78–276. Washington, DC: U.S. Government Printing Office.

Corkin, S. (1982). Some relationships between global amnesias and the memory impairments in Alzheimer's Disease. In S. Corkin, K. L. Davis, J. H. Growden, E. Usdin, & R. J. Wurtman (Eds.), *Alzheimer's disease: A report of progress in research* (pp. 149–164). New York: Raven Press.

Cramer, J. A., Mattson, R. H., Prevey, M. L., Schreyer, R. D., Valinda, L., & Oullette, R. N. (1989). How often is medication taken as prescribed? *Journal of the American Medical Association*, *261*, 3273–3277.

Cummings, J. L. (1985). *Clinical neuropsychiatry*. Orlando, FL: Grune & Stratton.

Cummings, J. L., & Benson, D. F. (1983). *Dementia: A clinical approach*. Boston: Butterworth.

Cummings, J. L., Miller, B., Hill, M. A., & Neshkes, R. (1987). Neuropsychiatric aspects of multi-infarct dementia and dementia of the Alzheimer type. *Archives of Neurology*, *44*, 389–393.

Damasio, A. R., & van Hoesen, G. W. (1986). Neuroanatomical correlates of amnesia in Alzheimer's Disease. In A. B. Scheibel, A. F. Wechsler, & M. A. Brazier (Eds.), *The biological substrates of Alzheimer's disease* (pp. 65–71). New York: Academic Press.

Delgado-Escueta, A. V. (1979). Epileptogenic paroxysms: Modern approaches and clinical correlations. *Neurology*, *29*, 1014–1022.

Dell, J. E. (1986). Social dimensions of epilepsy: Stigma and response. In S. Whitman & B. P. Hermann (Eds.), *Psychopathology in epilepsy: Social dimensions* (pp. 185–210). New York: Oxford University Press.

Dikmen, S., Matthews, C. G., & Harley, J.P. (1975). The effect of early versus late onset of major motor epilepsy upon cognitive intellectual function. *Epilepsia*, *16*, 73–81.

Dodrill, C. B., Breyer, D. N., Diamond, M. B., Dubinsky, B. L., & Geary, B. B. (1984). Psychosocial problems among adults with epilepsy. *Epilepsia*, *25*, 168–175.

Duncan, J. S. (1989). Strategies of antiepileptic drug treatment in patients with chronic epilepsy. In M. R. Trimble (Ed.), *Chronic epilepsy, its prognosis and management* (pp. 143–150). Chichester, England: Wiley.

Fedio, P., & Mirsky, A. F. (1969). Selective intellectual deficits in children with temporal lobe or centrencephalic epilepsy. *Neuropsychologia*, *7*, 287–300.

Finger, S., & Stein, D. G. (1982). *Brain damage and recovery*. New York: Academic Press.

Flor-Henry, P. (1969). Psychosis and temporal lobe epilepsy: A controlled investigation. *Epilepsia*, *10*, 363–395.

Gainotti, G. (1978). The relationship between emotions and cerebral dominance: A review of clinical and experimental evidence. In J. Gruzelier & P. Flor-Henry (Eds.), *Hemispheric asymmetries of function in psychopathology* (pp. 21–34). Elsevier/North Holland: Biomedical Press.

Glosser, G., & Deser, T. (1991). Patterns of discourse production among neurological patients with fluent language disorders. *Brain and Language*, *40*, 67–88.

Glosser, G., & Koppell, S. (1987). Emotional-behavioral patterns in children with learning disabilities: Lateralized hemispheric differences. *Journal of Learning Disabilities*, *20*, 365–368.

Goffman, E. (1963). *Stigma: Notes on the management of spoiled identity*. Englewood Cliffs, NJ: Prentice-Hall.

Goldstein, G., & Shelly, C. (1987). The classification of neuropsychological deficit. *Journal of Psychopathology and Behavioral Assessment*, *9*, 183–202.

Greenwald, B. S., Kramer-Ginsberg, E., Marin, D. B., Laitman, L. B., Hermann, C. K., Mohs, R. C., & Davis, K. L. (1989). Dementia with coexistent major depression. *American Journal of Psychiatry*, *146*, 1472–1478.

Grosscup, S. J., & Lewinsohn, P. M. (1980). Unpleasant and pleasant events and mood. *Journal of Clinical Psychology*, *36*, 252–259.

Gur, R. C. (1985). Imaging regional brain physiology in behavioral neurology. In M. M. Mesulam (Ed.), *Principles of behavioral neurology* (pp. 347–359). Philadelphia: F. A. Davis.

Haase, G. R. (1977). Diseases presenting as dementia. In C. E. Wells (Ed.), *Dementia* (pp. 27–67). Philadelphia: F. A. Davis.

Haley, W. E., & Pardo, K. M. (1989). Relationship of severity of dementia to caregiving stressors. *Psychology and Aging, 4*, 389–392.

Heaton, R. K., Baade, L. E., & Johnson, K. L. (1978). Neuropsychological test results associated with psychiatric disorder in adults. *Psychological Bulletin, 85*, 141–162.

Hermann, B. P. (1981). Deficits in neuropsychological functioning and psychopathology in epilepsy: A rejected hypothesis revisited. *Epilepsia, 22*, 161–167.

Hermann, B. P., & Whitman, S. (1984). Behavioral and personality correlates of epilepsy: A review, methodological critique and conceptual model. *Psychological Bulletin, 95*, 451–497.

Heston, L. L., Mastri, A. R., Anderson, V. E., & White, J. (1981). Dementia of the Alzheimer type: Clinical genetics, natural history and associated conditions. *Archives of General Psychiatry, 38*, 1085–1090.

Kahn, R. L., Zarit, S. H., Hilbert, N. M., & Niederehe, G. (1975). Memory complaint and impairment in the aged. *Archives of General Psychiatry, 32*, 1569–1573.

Kane, R. A., & Kane, R. L. (1981). *Assessing the elderly*. Lexington, MA: Lexington Books.

Kral, V. A. (1983). The relationship between senile dementia (Alzheimer type) and depression. *Canadian Journal of Psychiatry, 28*, 304–306.

Landolt, H. (1958). Serial electroencephalographic investigations during psychotic episodes in epileptic patients and during schizophrenic attacks. In A. M. Lorentz de Haas (Ed.), *Lectures on epilepsy* (pp. 91–133). Amsterdam: Elsevier.

Larson, E. B., Reifler, B. V., Featherstone, H. J., & English, D. R. (1984). Dementia in elderly outpatients: A prospective study. *Annals of Internal Medicine, 100*, 417–423.

Larson, T. (1963). Senile dementia. *Acta Psychiatrica Scandinavica* (Suppl. 167), *39*, 1–259.

Lesser, R. P., Lueders, H., Dinner, D. S., & Morris, H. H. (1987). Simple partial seizures. In H. Lueders & R. P. Lesser (Eds.), *Epilepsy: Electroclinical syndromes* (pp. 223–278). London: Springer-Verlag.

Lezak, M. D. (1983). *Neuropsychological assessment*. New York: Oxford University Press.

Masland, R. (1982). The nature of epilepsy. In H. Sands (Ed.), *Epilepsy: A Handbook for the Mental Health Professional* (pp. 5–57). New York: Brunner/Mazel.

Mattson, R. H., & Cramer, J. A. (1989). Phenobarbital toxicity. In R. Levy, R. Mattson, B. Meldrum, J. K. Penry, & F. B. Dreifuss (Eds.), *Antiepileptic drugs* (pp. 341–355). New York: Raven Press.

Mayeux, R., Brandt, J., Rosen, J., & Benson, F. (1980). Interictal memory and language in temporal lobe epilepsy. *Neurology, 30*, 120–125.

Mayeux, R., Stern, Y., & Spaton, S. (1985). Heterogeneity in dementia of the Alzheimer type: Evidence of subgroups. *Neurology, 36*, 453–461.

McGlone, J., & Wands, K. (1991). Self-report of memory function in patients with temporal lobe epilepsy and temporal lobectomy. *Cortex, 27*, 19–28.

McKhann, G., Drachman, D., Folstein, M., Katzman, R., Price, D., & Stadlon, E. M. (1984). Clinical diagnosis of Alzheimer's disease. *Neurology, 34*, 939–944.

Merriam, A. E., Aronson, M. K., Gaston, P., Wey, S. L., & Katz, I. (1988). The psychiatric symptoms of Alzheimer's disease. *Journal of the American Geriatric Society, 36*, 7–12.

Milner, B. (1975). Psychological aspects of epilepsy and its neurosurgical management. In D. P. Purpura, J. K. Penry, & R. D. Walter (Eds.), *Advances in neurology, Vol. 8* (pp. 299–321). New York: Raven Press.

Mittan, R. (1986). Fear of seizures. In S. Whitman & B. P. Hermann (Eds.), *Psychopathology in epilepsy: Social dimensions* (pp. 90–121). New York: Oxford University Press.

Morris, R. G., & Baddeley, A. D. (1988). Primary and working memory functioning in Alzheimer's-type dementia. *Journal of Clinical and Experimental Neuropsychology, 10*, 279–296.

Moss, M. B., & Albert, M. S. (1988). Alzheimer's disease and other dementing disorders. In M. S. Albert & M. B. Moss (Eds.), *Geriatric neuropsychology* (pp. 145–178). New York: Guilford Press.

Nasrallah, H. A., & Weinberger, D. R. (1986). *The neurology of schizophrenia*. Amsterdam: Elsevier.

Nelson, A., Fogel, B. S., & Faust, D. (1986). Bedside cognitive screening instruments. *Journal of Nervous and Mental Disease, 174*, 73–83.

Nelson, H. E., & O'Connell, A. (1979). Dementia: The estimation of premorbid intelligence levels using the New Adult Reading Test. *Cortex, 14*, 234–244.

Nott, P. N., & Fleminger, J. J. (1975). Presenile dementia: The difficulties of early diagnosis. *Acta Psychiatrica Scandinavica, 51*, 201–217.

Novelly, R., Augustine, E. A., Mattson, R. H., Glaser, G. H., Williamson, P. D., Spencer, D. D., & Spencer, S. S. (1984). Selective memory improvement and impairment in temporal lobectomy for epilepsy. *Annals of Neurology, 15*, 64–67.

Obler, L. K., & Albert, M. L. (1981). Language in the elderly aphasic and dementing patient. In M. Sarno (Ed.), *Acquired aphasia* (pp. 385–398). New York: Academic Press.

Penfield, W., & Jasper, H. (1954). Epilepsy and the functional anatomy of the human brain. Boston: Little, Brown.

Powell, G. E., Polkey, C. E., & McMillan, T. (1985). The new Maudsley series of temporal lobectomy. I: Short-term cognitive effects. *British Journal of Clinical Psychology, 24*, 109–124.

Prevey, M. L., DeLaney, R. C., & Mattson, R. H. (1988). Metamemory in temporal lobe epilepsy: Self-monitoring of memory functions. *Brain and Cognition, 7*, 298–311.

Rabins, P. V. (1989). Behavior problems in the demented. In E. Light & B. D. Lebowitz (Eds.), *Alzheimer's disease treatment and family stress: Directions for research* (pp. 322–339). Rockville, MD: National Institute of Mental Health.

Reding, M., Haycox, J., & Blass, J. (1985). Depression in patients referred to a dementia clinic. *Archives of Neurology, 42*, 894–896.

Reifler, B. V., & Larson, E. (1989). Excess disability in dementia of the Alzheimer's type. In E. Light & B. D. Lebowitz (Eds.), *Alzheimer's disease treatment and family stress: Directions for research* (pp. 363–382). Rockville, MD: National Institute of Mental Health.

Reifler, B. V., Larson, E., & Hanley, R. (1982). Coexistence of cognitive impairment and depression in geriatric outpatients. *American Journal of Psychiatry, 139*, 623–626.

Reynolds, E. H. (1985). Antiepileptic drugs and psychopathology. In M. R. Trimble (Ed.), *The psychopharmacology of epilepsy* (pp. 49–64). Chichester, England: Wiley.

Robertson, M. M. (1985). Depression in patients with epilepsy: An overview and clinical study. In M. R. Trimble (Ed.), *The psychopharmacology of epilepsy* (pp. 65–82). Chichester, England: Wiley.

Robertson, M. M., & Trimble, M. R. (1983). Depressive illness in patients with epilepsy: A review. *Epilepsia, 24*, 109–116.

Robinson, R. G., Kubos, K. L., Starr, L. B., Rao, K., & Price, T. R. (1984). Mood disorders in stroke patients. *Brain, 107*, 81–93.

Rodin, E. A. (1977). Psychosocial management of patients with seizure disorders. *Mclean Hospital Journal* (June), 74–84.

Rodin, E. A., Katz, M., & Lennox, K. (1976). Differences between patients with temporal lobe seizures and those with other forms of epileptic attacks. *Epilepsia, 17*, 313–320.

Ron, M. A., Toone, B. K., Garralda, M. E., & Lishman, W. A. (1979). Diagnostic accuracy in presenile dementia. *British Journal of Psychiatry, 134*, 161–168.

Saykin, A., Gur, R. C., Sussman, N. M., O'Connor, M. J., & Gur, R. E. (1989). Memory deficits before and after temporal lobectomy: Effects of laterality and age of onset. *Brain and Cognition, 9*, 191–200.

Schneck, M. K., Reisberg, B., & Ferris, S. H. (1982). An overview of current concepts of Alzheimer's disease. *American Journal of Psychiatry, 139*, 165–173.

Schwartz, M. F., Marin, O. S. M., & Saffran, E. M. (1979). Dissociations of language function in dementia: A case study. *Brain and Language, 7*, 277–306.

Seltzer, B., & Sherwin, I. (1978). "Organic brain syndromes": An empirical study and critical review. *American Journal of Psychiatry, 135*, 13–21.

Seltzer, B., & Sherwin, I. (1983). A comparison of clinical features in early- and late-onset primary degenerative dementia. *Archives of Neurology, 40*, 143–146.

Shewmon, D. A., & Erwin, R. J. (1988). The effect of focal interictal spikes on perception and reaction time: 2. Neuroanatomic specificity. *Electroencephalography and Clinical Neurophysiology, 69*, 338–352.

Sillitti, J. (1982). MMPI: Derived indicators of organic brain dysfunction. *Journal of Clinical Psychology, 38*, 601–605.

Stern, Y., Mayeux, R., Sano, M., Hauser, W. A., & Bush, T. (1987). Predictors of disease course in patients with probable Alzheimer's disease. *Neurology, 37*, 1649–1653.

Strub, R. L., & Black, F. W. (1977). *The Mental Status Examination in neurology*. Philadelphia: F. A. Davis.

Sulkava, R., Haltia, M., Paetau, A., Wikstrom, J., & Palo, J. (1983). Accuracy of clinical diagnosis in primary degenerative dementia: Correlation with neuropathological findings. *Journal of Neurology, Neurosurgery and Psychiatry, 46*, 9–13.

Terry, R. D., & Katzman, R. (1983). Senile dementia of the Alzheimer type. *Annals of Neurology, 14*, 497–506.

Townes, B. D., Martin, D. C., Nelson, D., Prosser, R., Pepping, M., Maxwell, J., Peel, J., & Preston, M. (1985). Neurobehavioral approach to classification of psychiatric patients using a competency model. *Journal of Consulting and Clinical Psychology, 53*, 33–42.

Trimble, M. R., & Thompson, P. J. (1986). Neuropsychological aspects of epilepsy. In I. Grant & K. M. Adams (Eds.), *Neuropsychological assessment of neuropsychiatric disorders* (pp. 321–346). New York: Oxford University Press.

Vitaliano, P. P., Breen, A. R., Albert, M. S., Russo, J., & Prinz, P. N. (1984). Memory, attention, and functional status in community residing Alzheimer type patients and optimally healthy aged individuals. *Journal of Gerontology, 39*, 58–64.

Wade, J. P. H., Mirsen, T. R., Hachinski, V. C., Fisman, M., Lau, C., & Merskey, H. (1987). The clinical diagnosis of Alzheimer's disease. *Archives of Neurology, 44*, 24–29.

Weinstein, E. A., & Kahn, R. L. (1955). *Denial of illness*. Springfield, IL: Charles C Thomas.

Wilkus, R. J., & Dodrill, C. B. (1976). Neuropsychological correlates of the electroencephalogram in epileptics: 1. Topographic distribution and average rate of epileptiform activity. *Epilepsia, 17*, 890–100.

Wilson, R. S., Rosenbaum, G., & Brown, G. (1979). The problem of premorbid intelligence in neuropsychological assessment. *Journal of Clinical Neuropsychology, 1*, 49–53.

Wilson, R. S., Kaszniak, A. W., & Fox, J. H. (1981). Remote memory in senile dementia. *Cortex, 17*, 41–48.

Wolf, P. (1986). Forced normalization. In M. R. Trimble & T. G. Bolwig (Eds.), *Aspects of epilepsy and psychiatry* (pp. 101–115). Chichester, England: Wiley.

Wood, R. L. (1987). *Brain injury rehabilitation: A neurobehavioral approach*. London: Croom Helm.

Yozawitz, A. (1986). Applied neuropsychology in a psychiatric center. In I. Grant & K. M. Adams (Eds.), *Neuropsychological assessment of neuropsychiatric disorders* (pp. 121–146). New York: Oxford University Press.

II

TREATMENT OF
ADULT DISORDERS

11

Obsessive-Compulsive Disorder

GAIL STEKETEE and LESLIE J. SHAPIRO

INTRODUCTION

Definition

According to the revised third edition of the *Diagnostic and Statistical Manual of Mental Disorders* (DSM-III-R; American Psychiatric Association, 1987), obsessions are "recurrent and persistent ideas, thoughts, impulses, or images that are experienced . . . as intrusive and senseless" (p. 245). The individual recognizes the obsessions as a product of his or her own mind and attempts to ignore, suppress, or neutralize them with some ritualistic thought or action. The content of clinical obsessions differs little from the intrusive thoughts exhibited by nonobsessionals, but the former provoke more anxiety and are less easily dismissed than the latter (Dent & Salkovskis, 1986; Rachman & De Silva, 1978; Salkovskis & Harrison, 1984). Compulsions are repetitive, stereotypical behaviors performed in response to an obsession. They are designed to reduce discomfort or prevent a feared event, although this intention may not always be apparent to an observer. Rituals are excessive and are recognized as unreasonable by the individual.

Prevalence

According to the Epidemiology Catchment Area (ECA) survey, the lifetime prevalence of obsessive-compulsive disorder (OCD) is 2.5% (1 in 40 people) so that it is the fourth most common psychiatric disorder (Karno, Golding, Sorenson, & Burnam, 1988). Other studies have reported similar figures, with a slight preponderance of women (e.g., Henderson & Pollard, 1988). Onset age in most studies is late adolescence to the early 20s, males exhibiting symptoms earlier than females (Rasmussen & Eisen, 1990; White, Steketee, & Julian, 1990). OCD runs in families: nearly one quarter of nuclear family members also met criteria for this disorder, and

GAIL STEKETEE and LESLIE J. SHAPIRO • School of Social Work, Boston University, Boston, Massachusetts 02215.

Handbook of Behavior Therapy in the Psychiatric Setting, edited by Alan S. Bellack and Michel Hersen. Plenum Press, New York, 1993.

an additional 17% reported obsessional traits (Swedo, Rapoport, Leonard, Lenane, & Cheslow, 1989).

Presentation

Most obsessive-compulsives are identified by the type of ritual(s) they exhibit, though patients may have more than one type. Washing rituals are designed to remove "contamination" from some specific source, such as germs or chemicals; typically, some specific disaster (e.g., illness) is feared. Checking is intended to prevent a particular catastrophe (for example, burglary, fire, harming someone, social embarrassment, or rejection). Repeating compulsions may be likened to superstitions: ordinary actions (such as crossing a threshold or touching something) are repeated to prevent some imagined harm from occurring (for example, a loved one's dying in an accident). Less common are ordinary rituals, in which objects must be arranged to produce a satisfying symmetry or balance, usually to alleviate a general feeling of discomfort. Although Greenberg (1987) differentiated "hoarders" (or collectors) from other obsessionals, in our view this is another subtype of OCD whose compulsions serve to prevent the loss of potentially important objects or information.

Subtypes based on the content of obsessions (e.g., religious or aggressive) have been proposed but not widely adopted (Akhtar, Wig, Verma, Pershad, & Verma, 1975; Capstick & Seldrup, 1973; Dowson, 1977). Efforts to identify subtypes of obsessions or compulsions have not been useful in predicting responses to treatments. By contrast, Foa and Tillmanns's categorization of OCD symptoms (1980) has direct clinical relevance. According to this model, obsessions are discomfort-evoking and may be prompted by environmental or internal cues (thoughts and images), as well as by fears of potential disasters. To relieve this discomfort, the individual avoids the feared situation passively or carries out mental or behavioral rituals to restore safety or prevent harm (Rachman, 1976a). This definition leads directly to the treatment interventions discussed later in this chapter.

Diagnosis

Several disorders have been likened to OCD. The somatic preoccupations and repeated requests for medical reassurance found in hypochondriasis appear to be very similar to the obsessive fears and compulsive rituals of OCD (Salkovskis & Warwick, 1986; Tynes, White, & Steketee, 1990). Similarly, the overconcern with fatness or fullness observed in anorexia nervosa and the vomiting and purging of bulimia have much in common with obsessions and compulsions. In fact, behavioral treatments similar to those found to be effective for OCD have also been successfully used for these disorders (e.g., Rosen & Leitenberg, 1982; Salkovskis, 1989).

Although body dysmorphic disorder (BDD) has recently drawn attention as an OCD-like syndrome (e.g., Brady, Austin, & Lydiard, 1990; Hollander, Liebowitz, Winchel, Klumker, & Klein, 1989), a noteworthy difference is the ego-syntonic nature of the ruminations of BDD patients. However, medications helpful for OCD have also been useful for BDD. Hollander *et al.* (1989), and Phillips (1990) concluded that there is a convincing association with OCD, at least in some cases. The same cannot be said of trichotillomania, which has been associated with OCD primarily because of the feeling of "compulsion" to pull hair and the response of trichotillomania patients to serotonergic drugs (Swedo, Lenane, Leonard, & Rapoport, 1990). However, this disorder lacks the characteristic obsessive thought, and hair pulling is typically experienced as pleasurable or satisfying (positively reinforcing), rather than only discomfort-reducing (negatively reinforcing) as in OCD. Instead, trichotillomania should be classed as a habit or impulse control disorder, much like nail biting or scab picking (Mansuedo & Goldfinger, 1990).

Personality Disorders. The personality disorders that most frequently co-occur with OCD are avoidant, dependent, and histrionic (Baer, Jenike, Ricciardi, Holland, Seymour, Minichiello, & Buttolph, 1990; Mavissakalian, Hamman, & Jones, 1990a; Steketee, 1990). Interestingly, although several traits of obsessive-compulsive personality disorder (OCPD; orderliness, rigidity, indecisiveness, and perfectionism) are commonly found in OCD patients, fewer than 10% actually qualify for a diagnosis of OCPD (Black, 1974; Mavissakalian *et al.*, 1990a; Steketee, 1990). Certain comorbid personality disorders, including borderline, schizotypal, and passive-aggressive, appear to adversely affect the outcome of pharmacological or behavioral treatment (Hermesh, Shahar, & Munitz, 1987; Jenike, Baer, Minichiello, Schwartz, & Carey, 1986; Steketee, 1990). However, Mavissakalian *et al.* (1990a) found that personality functioning improved with clomipramine and had no prognostic significance in the drug treatment of OCD patients.

Depression and Anxiety Disorders. Depression is undoubtedly the most common psychological concomitant of OCD. The ECA study found that 32% of OCD subjects met the diagnostic criteria for major depression (Karno *et al.*, 1988). It appears that depression most often develops secondary to OCD (Welner, Reich, Robins, Fishman, & Van Doren, 1976), probably because of increasing debilitation. The biological link between these two disorders has been widely debated, and the evidence has been interpreted both pro and con. Although some data have suggested that concomitant depression bodes ill for treatment outcome, this interpretation is disputed by other findings (Tynes, White, & Steketee, 1990). About one quarter of OCD patients report specific phobias, and slightly fewer have comorbid social phobia (18%) and panic disorder (14%) (Rasmussen & Tsuang, 1986). So far, evidence supporting any prognostic significance of such comorbid anxiety disorders is lacking.

Psychosis. Although some psychotic patients exhibit classic obsessions and compulsions concurrently with delusions and hallucinations (Rosen, 1957), treatments for these patients are appropriately focused on the latter symptoms. In 1878, K. Westphal noted the distinction between obsessive and psychotic thinking, describing OCD as "abortive insanity," much like French clinician J. Esquirol's term "insanity with insight." However, a small proportion of OCD patients evidence delusional or "overvalued" thinking with little insight into the unreasonable nature of their symptoms (Foa, 1979; Insel & Akiskal, 1986; McKenna, 1984; Perse, 1988). Suggestions for classification of these patients range from placing them in a separate diagnostic category somewhere between OCD and psychosis (Perse, 1988) to specifying their place along a continuum from typical OCD to "obsessive-compulsive psychosis" (Ballerini & Stanghellini, 1989; Insel & Akiskal, 1986). Such patients have failed to respond to behavior therapy (Foa, 1979) or to antidepressant medication (Perse, 1988), but they may respond to cognitive therapy directed at negative automatic thoughts (Salkovskis & Warwick, 1986).

Alcoholism. Recent studies suggest that OCD occurs in 6%–12% of alcohol-dependent patients, a rate substantially higher than would be expected from population prevalence rates (Eisen & Rasmussen, 1989; Riemann & McNally, 1990). However, OCD patients did not have higher than expected rates of alcoholism (Riemann & McNally, 1990). Nonetheless, identifying such dual-diagnosis patients is likely to assist in improving clinical outcome, as OCD symptoms may have been partly responsible for development of drinking patterns.

PROTOTYPICAL ASSESSMENT

Ideally, the assessment of patients with obsessive-compulsive disorder encompasses not only the obsessions and compulsions, but also related symptomatology and personality traits, as well as environmental factors that may affect treatment strategies. Interviews serve as the primary source of information; questionnaires and behavioral observations complement the patient's description of the problem. Psychophysiological recordings provide additional information regarding typical physical responses to feared situations.

Interview

To assess obsessions, the interviewer solicits information about the triggers for discomfort, including (1) external situations, such as seeing lights on and touching doorknobs; (2) internal thoughts, images, or impulses; and (3) ideas of the disastrous consequences that may ensue unless compulsions are performed. For those with more than one type of obsessive concern, such as fears of pesticides and fears of AIDS, questioning should be conducted separately for each category. Knowing which cues provoke discomfort (anxiety or guilt) also allows the interviewer to anticipate and inquire about situations that the patient unwittingly avoids. Inquiries about presymptomatic functioning may help solicit information about prior activities that are currently avoided. For example, one patient had given up parallel parking to avoid backing up, lest she run over a child. Very helpful in soliciting information about feared and avoided cues is the patient's description of a typical day in minute detail from the time he or she wakes up until he or she goes to sleep.

In addition to obsessions and avoidance behavior, the therapist should inquire about all behaviors or thoughts that the patient uses to reduce discomfort. Patients may have more than one ritual for a single source of obsessive fear, or they may use the same ritual to relieve discomfort caused by more than one obsessional theme. The interviewer should look particularly for abbreviated versions of more complex rituals, such as wiping or rinsing rather than washing with soap. In addition, many patients have developed cognitive compulsions that are not readily recognized unless information is specifically requested. A question such as "Do you ever try to reduce your discomfort by thinking particular thoughts?" may prompt the reporting of mental rituals. Because rituals serve to maintain obsessive fears, the identification of all discomfort-reducing compulsions is essential to the success of behavioral treatment. To assist in identifying any obsessions or rituals not mentioned by the patient, the Yale Brown Obsessive-Compulsive (YBOCS) Symptom Checklist is a very useful adjunct to the interview (Goodman, Price, Rasmussen, Mazure, Delgado, Heninger, & Charney, 1989b; Goodman, Price, Rasmussen, Mazure, Fleischman, Hill, Heninger, & Charney, 1989c). This checklist of 36 obsessive and 23 compulsive symptoms includes such categories as aggressive, contamination, sexual, hoarding/saving, religious, symmetry/exactness, somatic, and miscellaneous.

Ideally, the Structured Interview for DSM-III-R (SCID; Spitzer, Williams & Gibbon, 1987) is also conducted by a trained interviewer to identify comorbid problems that may require additional treatment strategies or modification of the planned behavioral treatment. For example, if alcohol is used to relieve discomfort, specific measures to reduce consumption may be needed so that, during exposure homework, obsessive discomfort can habituate without interference by chemical agents. The finding that a patient also suffers from a marked social phobia suggests that additional treatments aimed at this difficulty will be essential to return the patient to a reasonably functional lifestyle. An awareness of particular personality traits, such as perfectionism or rigid moral beliefs, may lead the therapist to include cognitive treatment strategies to alter dysfunctional beliefs and attitudes that may also underlie some of the obsessive fears.

Questionnaires

Both interviewer-rated and self-report measures of OCD allow an assessment of the severity and, in some cases, the identification of OCD symptoms not mentioned by the patient. Using the 10-item Yale-Brown Obsessive Compulsive Scale (YBOCS; Goodman, Price, Rasmussen, Mazure, Delgado, Heninger, & Charney, 1989) an interviewer rates obsessions and compulsions separately for time spent, interference, distress, resistance, and controllability. Used in conjunction with the symptom checklist discussed earlier, this measure has demonstrated good reliability and validity in assessing symptom severity and has rapidly become the industry standard for assessing the outcome in drug trials for OCD (Goodman *et al.*, 1989b,c). Likert-like scales adapted from phobia research have been used by independent assessors, patients, and therapists to measure the severity of the main obsessive fears, avoidance, and compulsions (for a review, see Kozak, Foa, & McCarthy, 1987). These instruments are particularly useful for rating change following treatment, as they assess the particular symptoms targeted during behavioral treatment.

Also used as both an assessor-rated and a self-report questionnaire is the Compulsive Activity Checklist (CAC) (Cottraux, Bouvard, Defayolle, & Messy, 1988), which assesses the severity of impairment in specific activities and thus allows the identification of problem situations not necessarily covered in an interview (Cottraux *et al.*, 1988; Freund, Steketee, & Foa, 1987; Steketee & Freund, 1990). The CAC has satisfactorily detected changes following treatment and meets acceptable validity, though not reliability, criteria. Commonly used in behavioral research applications has been the self-report Maudsley Obsessional Compulsive Inventory (MOCI), which contains 30 true-false questions and yields a total score and five subscale scores (checking, cleaning, slowness, doubting/conscientiousness, and ruminating) (Hodgson & Rachman, 1977). Adequate validity and reliability have been reported (Rachman & Hodgson, 1980; Sternberger & Burns, 1990a,b). The subscales of the MOCI render it useful in assessing changes in particular symptoms. Several other questionnaire measures are available for assessing OCD symptoms, but we have selected only the two that have been most commonly used in recent research studies.

Behavioral Measures

Two types of behavioral measures can be used with OCD patients; (1) the Behavioral Avoidance Test (BAT), which measures the degree of avoidance of feared situations and (2) monitoring of the amount of ritualizing. The number of steps completed in a hierarchy of feared situations and the amount of subjective anxiety experienced in each have been used in some research studies (e.g., Marks, Hodgson, & Rachman, 1975; Steketee & Foa, 1985). Behavioral measures of the frequency and duration of compulsions usually request the patient (or observer) to record the number of minutes spent on compulsive activity (Emmelkamp & van Kraanen, 1977; Foa, Steketee, & Milby, 1980a). Despite occasional problems with compliance, daily self-monitoring provides extremely useful clinical insight into the patient's typical routine. In special situations, observer monitoring by parents, spouses, nurses, and so on may be used.

Psychophysiological Measures

Physiological recordings, such as heart rate, skin conductance, and respiration, have been used to measure the intensity of anxiety (e.g., Lang, 1979). The concordance between subjective and psychophysiological recordings is far from perfect, but in most studies, elevations in one sphere in response to exposure to feared obsessive situations are accompanied by increases in the other. Interested readers are referred to Kozak *et al.* (1987) for further information regarding assessment of the physiology of fear. In addition to the above measures of physiology, some investigators have studied biochemical responses of OCD patients (e.g., DST (dexamethasone suppression test), cortisol, and cerebral blood flow), as well as neurological activity using magnetic resonance imaging (MRI) and positron emission tomography (PET) scan technology (for reviews, see Jenike, Baer, & Minichiello, 1990a). The implications of these assessments for obsessive discomfort and behavior are not yet clear. Physiological measures are expensive and inconvenient unless an existing laboratory facility or portable equipment is already available.

Even with ready equipment and expertise, such assessments are often not practical because few obsessive situations can be reproduced accurately in the laboratory. For these reasons, physiological measures are rarely used clinically and are not considered critical to successful assessment and treatment.

ACTUAL ASSESSMENT

Because it is rarely possible to use all the available assessment methods for OCD patients in clinic settings, the essential strategies are highlighted below.

Interview

Although the SCID is extremely useful in identifying comorbid problems that may affect treatment methodology, such information can be obtained more informally via several specific questions about social and familial relationships, drug or alcohol use, psychotic processes, and other sources of anxiety. Inquiries about family members' reactions to the patient's symptoms provide information about personality traits and functioning difficulties not otherwise reported. The interview process should leave the therapist with a clear understanding of the interrelationship between the rituals and the obsessions. If the information seems conflicting, the therapist should inquire further until the relationship between the two seems consistent and logical.

In addition to the general interview, we suggest the inclusion of the YBOCS Symptom Checklist and of the 10-item YBOCS scale to measure overall symptom severity and functional difficulty. At present, the latter is the only measure that assesses the severity of OCD in a standardized fashion without regard to the patient's particular types of obsessions or compulsions. Both measures together require 30 to 45 minutes.

Questionnaires

Although most symptoms can be identified by means of the YBOCS Symptom Checklist, the degree of difficulty with particular activities can be measured with the CAC and, to a limited extent, with the MOCI. However, neither measure is appropriate for patients whose obsessions or rituals are atypical or idiosyncratic.

Behavioral Measures

Observation of patients in situations where obsessions and rituals typically occur is invaluable in providing informative details about symptomatology. We strongly suggest that clinicians accompany the patient to two or more locations, especially the home, where difficulties occur to observe the extent of avoidance and discomfort and the rituals. For example, one patient's kitchen contents were clearly arranged in the "clean" and "dirty" dichotomy that her contamination fears provoked. In another case, the foot-deep pile of dirty underwear and towels covering the entire bedroom floor provided a new understanding of the severity of one man's symptoms and of his inability to invite others to his home. Observation of actual ritualistic behavior can help one identify problem behaviors that will require attention during response prevention. Because it is not always possible to observe compulsions (for example, one of our patient's worst compulsions occurred just before going to bed at night), self-monitoring is an essential source of information. We have also requested monitoring by significant others to supplement what we believed was questionable or incomplete information from the patient. In the case mentioned above, the patient's husband provided forgotten details about the bedtime ritual.

In this section, we provide some theoretical background for the selection of treatment methods, along with research findings that have guided the development of current clinical practice with OCD patients in outpatient and inpatient settings.

Theoretical Conceptualizations Underlying Behavioral Treatment

According to Mowrer's theory (1960), neutral events become associated with fear when they are paired with inherently aversive events. For OCD patients, concrete objects, as well as thoughts and images, acquire the ability to produce discomfort or anxiety; to reduce this discomfort, escape or avoidance responses are developed (Dollard & Miller, 1950). Because some behaviors cannot be avoided (for example, going to the bathroom), rituals are developed to reduce fear. Support for the fear acquisition stage of this model is inadequate, as many subjects report no early traumatic conditioning experience associated with onset (e.g., Rachman & Wilson, 1980). Several theoreticians have suggested additional sources of symptom acquisition, including early and recent stressful life events, as well as sensitization and heightened arousal processes (Boulougouris, 1977; Rachman, 1971; Teasdale, 1974; Watts, 1971). Regardless of the source of onset of OCD symptoms, there is sufficient evidence to suggest that obsessions provoke discomfort and compulsions reduce it (e.g., Rachman & Hodgson, 1980). Based on this formulation, behavioral treatment is designed to reduce obsessive anxiety or discomfort via exposure to the feared situations and to eliminate rituals by blocking them.

Early behavioral researchers failed to distinguish the functional difference between obsessions and compulsions, indiscriminately applying exposure (desensitization, flooding, satiation, and paradoxical intention) and blocking (thought stopping and aversion via shock) to either or both symptoms. Not surprisingly, none of these methods was strikingly effective (see Steketee & Cleere, 1990). By contrast, behavioral techniques developed from the theoretical model considerably improved the prognostic picture for OCD.

Treatment by Combined Exposure and Response Prevention

The two-pronged approach of using exposure for obsessions and using response prevention for compulsions was first administered by Meyer in 1966. Hospitalized patients were exposed to circumstances that normally evoked obsessive fears, while performance of rituals was prevented (see details below under "Actual Treatment"). Of 15 patients treated, all improved and only 2 had relapsed at follow-up (Meyer & Levy, 1973; Meyer, Levy, & Schnurer, 1974). These exceptional results sparked considerable interest in this treatment approach. Findings from over 20 research studies implementing exposure and response prevention are summarized in Table 1.

Most of these studies examined variants of exposure (e.g., imagined versus *in vivo* and self-controlled versus therapist-assisted). The sample sizes and data included in the table pertain only to the use of the *combination* of exposure and response prevention; information about comparison treatments has been omitted. We have included findings from standardized measures of OCD symptoms and from Likert-like scales assessing the target obsessions and compulsions; whenever possible, we have averaged scores across assessors (patient, therapist and/or independent assessor) and across symptoms (obsessions and compulsions) to yield a single score.

As is evident from the table, exposure and response prevention produced a significant improvement in most measures over time. Not surprisingly, the most positive results were evident in measures of the targeted obsessions and compulsions, where the average benefit ranged from 40% to 75%. On the MOCI and the CAC, the improvement rates were in the same range; two studies reported substantially lower numbers (Cottraux, Mollard, Bouvard, Marks, Sluys, Nury, Douge, & Cialdella, 1989; Emmelkamp, de Haan, & Hoogduin, 1990); LOI scores

**GAIL STEKETEE and
LESLIE J. SHAPIRO**

Table 1. Outcome of Behavior Therapy (BT) for OCT[a]

Study	No. of cases of BT	No. of wks.	No. of sessions	Design	General results	Mean % change posttest	#Ss improved[b] at posttest	Follow-up time	Mean % change at follow-up	# Ss improved by category[b] at follow-up
Meyer et al. (1974)	15	2–8	Daily	Open trial EX + RP	Sig. improv.	NA	20% vmi targ. Sx; 47% mi; 33% imp; 0% no chg	.5–6 yr	NA	17% vmi-targ. Sx; 50% mi; 17% imp; 17% no chg
Marks et al. (1975)	20	4–12	15	Mixed, gradual EX modeling	Sig. improv; EX > relax.; model = no model	57% targ. obs.; 35% LOI-Int	40% mi-targ. Sx; 35% imp; 25% no chg	2 yr.	64% targ. obs.	70% mi-targ. Sx; 5% imp; 25% no chg
Roper et al. (1975)	10	3	15	Passive vs. partic. modeling	Model > relax.; partic. > passive	52% targ. Sx; 52% LOI-Sx	50% mi-targ. Sx; 30% imp; 20% no chg	6 mo.	63% targ. Sx; 66% LOI	40% mi-targ. Sx; 40% imp; 20% no chg
Rabavilas et al. (1976)	12	NA	8+	Imag. vs. in vivo, short vs. long	Long > short (in vivo); long = short (imag.)	46% total obs.; 43% main obs.	50% mi-targ. Sx; 33% imp; 17% no chg	6 mo. (mean)	NA	50% mi-targ. Sx; 33% imp; 17% no chg
Boulougouris (1977)	15 (incl. 12 from above)	NA	11 (mean)	Open trial in vivo + imag. EX	Sig. improv.	43% total obs.; 41% main obs.; 39% LOI-Sx	87% imp-targ. Sx	2.8 yr. (mean) (2–5 yr)	52% main obs.; 55% total obs.; 41% LOI-Sx	60% vmi-targ. Sx
Boersma et al. (1976)	13	5–6	15	Grad. vs. rapid EX, model vs. no model	Sig. improv.	62% main obs.; 59% other obs.; 42% LOI-Sx	NA	3 mo.	Sig. improv.	54% vmi-targ. Sx; 23% imp; 23% no chg
Emmelkamp & van Kraanen (1977)	13	5–6	10	Ther. vs. self-cntrl.	Sig. improv.; therapist = self-control	65% targ. Sx; 70% other Sx; 38% LOI-Sx	NA	3.5 mo.	Sig. improv.	NA

Study										
Emmelkamp et al. (1980)	15	NA	10	SIT + EX vs. EX	Sig. improv.; SIT + EX = EX	54% main obs.; 69% other obs.; 41% LOI-Sx	NA	6 mo.	67% main obs.; 78% other obs.; 47% LOI-Sx	NA
Marks et al. (1978)	13	NA	14 (mean)	Open trial EX + RP	Sig. improv.	75% rituals; 75% CAC	NA	6 mo.	72% rituals; 78% CAC	NA
Foa & Goldstein (1978)	21	2–3	10–15	Open trial EX + RP	Sig. improv.	68% targ. Sx	71% vmi-targ. Sx; 10% mi; 14% imp; 5% no chg	1.5 yr. (mean) (.3–3 yr.)	70% targ. Sx	71% vmi-OC Sx; 3% mi; 13% imp; 13% no chg
Foa et al. (1980a)	15 (incl. 7 from above)	2–3	10	in vivo + imag. EX vs. in vivo	Sig. improv.; imag + vivo > vivo at follow-up	71% targ. SX	NA	1 yr. (.3–2.5 yr.)	61% targ. Sx	53% stable/impr.; 47% relapse
Foa et al. (1980b)	8	4	20	EX vs. RP	Sig. improv. 78% rituals; 83% BAT	NA	NA	NA	NA	NA
Foa et al. (1983)	50 (incl. 37 from other studies)	NA	10–20	Combined studies	Sig. improv.	NA	38% mi-targ. Sx; 38% imp; 4% no chg	1 yr. (.3–3 yr.)	NA	59% mi-targ. Sx; 17% imp; 24% no chg
Cobb et al. (1980)	11	NA	10	EX + RP vs. marital Tx	Sig. improv. EX > mar. Tx	40% targ. Sx; 35% CAC	NA	1.6 yr. (1–2 yr.)	Stable gains; 54% targ. Sx	NA
Julien et al. (1980)	18	9 (2–96)	x̄ = 20 (8–192)	Open trial EX + RP	NA	NA	67% vmi-targ. Sx; 27% mi; 6% no chg	1 yr. (.5–3 yr.)	NA	27% vmi-targ. Sx; 33% mi; 22% imp; 17% no chg
Emmelkamp & de Lange (1983)	12	5	10	Selfcntrl. vs. partner-assisted EX	Part. asst. > selfcntrl.	38% targ.Sx; 51% MOCI	NA	1 mo.	52% targ. Sx; 44% MOCI	NA
Emmelkamp et al. (1985)	42	NA	10 more Tx as needed	EX + RP	Sig. improv.	57% anxiety; 56% MOCI (N = 20)	38% vmi-anxiety; 43% imp; 19% no chg	3.5 yr. (2–6 yr.)	65% anxiety; 50% MOCI	57% vmi-anxiety; 24% imp; 19% no chg

(Continued)

GAIL STEKETEE and
LESLIE J. SHAPIRO

Table 1. (Continued)

Study	No. of cases of BT	No. of wks.	No. of sessions	Design	General results	Mean % change posttest	#Ss improved[b] at posttest	Follow-up time	Mean % change at follow-up	# Ss improved by category[b] at follow-up
Foa et al. (1984)	12	4	17	EX vs. RP vs. EX + RP	EX + RP > EX = RP	60% targ. Sx; 66% MOCI; 74% CAC	60% vmi-targ. rit.; 10% imp; 30% no chg	1 yr. (.3–2 yr.)	45% targ. Sx; 43% MOCI; 53% CAC	44% vmi-targ. rit.; 44% imp.; 12% no chg
Hoogduin & Hoogduin (1984)	25	NA	x̄ = 20 (8–80)	Open trial self-cntrl. EX + RP	Sig. improv.	NA	80% vmi-targ. Sx; 4% mi; 16% min	1.2 yr. (.3–2 yr.)	NA	80% vmi-targ. Sx; 4% mi; 16% min
Emmelkamp et al. (1988)	18	8	10	EX + RP vs. RET	Sig. improv.	51% anxiety; 19% MOCI	22% mi-anxiety; 67% imp; 11% no chg	6 mo.	56% anxiety; 27% MOCI	22% mi-anxiety; 78% imp; 0% no chg
Hoogduin & Duivenvoorden (1988)	60	20	10	Open trial EX + RP	Sig. improv.	NA	78% imp-targ. Sx; 22% no chg	NA	NA	NA
Emmelkamp et al. (1990)	50	5	8	Self EX + RP vs. spouse	Sig. improv.; self = spouse	37% anxiety; 18% MOCI	NA	1 mo.	20% MOCI; 41% anxiety	NA
Mehta (1990)	30	12	24	Self EX + RP vs. family-assisted	Sig. improv.; family > self	42% anxiety; 48% MOCI	NA	6 mo.	59% anxiety; 45% MOCI	NA

Study	N		Sessions	Comparison		Post results		Follow-up period	Follow-up results	
Marks et al. (1980)	20	3–6	15–30	EX vs. relax.	EX > relax	53% targ. Sx; 56% CAC	NA	1.2 yr. (mean)	Sig. improv.; 55% targ. Sx; 44% CAC	NA
Rachman et al. (1979)	10 (subset)	6	30	(CMI vs. PBO)		61% targ. Sx; 57% CAC	NA		NA	
Marks et al. (1988)	12 (PBO + EX)	23	x̄ = 10 (4–19)	EX + RP vs. CMI vs. combo	Sig. improv. w/EX homewk.; therapist EX added little	75% targ. Sx	NA	1 yr.	NA	50% mi-targ. Sx; 30% imp; 20% no chg
Cottraux et al. (1989)	15 (PBO + EX)	24	Up to 25	EX + RP vs. FLV vs. combo	All improv.; combo best at follow-up	32% targ. Sx; 18% CAC; 52% BAT	40% respond (target Sx)	1 yr.	45% targ. Sx; 23% CAC; 53% BAT	50% responded (targ. Sx)
Foa et al. (in press)	38	4	17 EX + RP 12 supprt	IMI vs. PBO all EX + RP	Sig. improv.; IMI + BT > IMI	64% targ. Sx; 47% MOCI; 73% CAC	45% vmi-targ Sx; 52% mi; 3% no chg	1.4 yr. (mean) (.8–2 yr.)	53% targ. Sx; 39% MOCI; 52% CAC	32% vmi-targ. Sx; 50% mi; 18% no chg
Emmelkamp et al. (1989)	14	2.5 or 5	10	Ther vs. self massed vs. spaced	Sig. improv. ther = self massed = spaced	68% targ. obs.; 57% MOCI	43% no Sx-targ. obs.; 14% mi; 29% imp; 14% nochg	1 mo.	61% targ. obs.; 45% MOCI	50% no Sx-targ. obs.; 7% mi; 21% imp; 21% no chg
Emmelkamp & Beens (1991)	11	17	12	Self EX + RP vs. RET	Sig. improv. EX + RP = RET	50% targ. obs.; 26% MOCI	NA	6 mo.	65% targ. obs.; 32% MOCI	NA

aAbbreviations: BAT = behavioral avoidance test; CAC = Compulsive Activity Checklist; CMI = clomipramine; EX = exposure; grad. = gradual; IMI = imipramine; imag. = imaginal; FLV = fluvoxamine; LOI = Leyton Obsessional Inventory; MOCI = Maudsley Obsessional Compulsive Inventory; NA = not available; obs. = obsessions; PBO = placebo; RET = rational emotive therapy; rit. = rituals; RP = response prevention; selfcntrl. = self-controlled treatment; sig. improv. = significant improvement; SIT = self-instructional training; Sx = symptoms; targ. = target; Tx = treatment.
bTarget symptoms were averaged across obsessions and compulsions and across assessors; vmi = very much improved; mi = much improved; imp = improved; no chg = no change/minimally improved.

had a somewhat lower range of 35%–52% average improvement across six studies. Overall, then, most measures indicated that OCD symptoms were improved by 50%–70%.

Next, we examined how many subjects were improved after behavioral treatment. Investigators often defined their categories of improvement quite differently, so that it was difficult to compare across studies. Thus, our summarization here is only approximate. Nearly all studies for which data were available indicated that approximately 85% of patients (range, 75%–100%) were at least "improved," and about 55% (range 40%–70%) fell into the "much" or "very much improved" categories, typically meaning target symptom gains of more than half. The extent of improvement and the consistency of these results across multiple treatment sites and countries are quite impressive.

At follow-up ranging from 3 months to 6 years, the findings also indicated significant benefits over time on various measures. The treatment gains were fairly stable, the average improvement rates being in the 45%–70% range for the target symptoms, only slightly below the posttest figures. Questionnaire measures showed slightly more decline: MOCI scores ranged from 40% to 50%, and CAC scores from 23% to 78%, most being in the 50% range. Scores from two studies using the LOI at follow-up were 41% and 66%. Again, the percentage of subjects who were at least "improved" was quite high, averaging about 75% (range, 50%–88%), and approximately 50% of patients (range, 40%–70%) were "much" or "very much" improved. Thus, the results were largely maintained, with some response evident and some patients needing additional therapy (e.g., Emmelkamp, Visser, & Hoekstra, 1988a; Foa & Goldstein, 1978).

Most of the data on treatment by exposure and response prevention are derived from group studies rather than single-case reports, so that the integrity and generalizability of these findings was substantiated. This treatment proved superior to relaxation, which was quite ineffective (e.g., Marks *et al.*, 1975), and to marital therapy, which improved marital problems but not OCD symptoms (Cobb, McDonald, Marks, & Stern, 1980). Exposure therapy has not been compared to combinations of other exposure and blocking treatments (e.g., desensitization or paradoxical intention and thought stopping or aversion therapy), but it is doubtful that these treatments could improve on the success rate of exposure therapy. Exposure and relapse prevention, then, can be considered the psychological treatment of choice for OCD.

Specific Effects of Exposure and Response Prevention

Exposure and response prevention have typically been used in tandem, so that the separate effects of each procedure have not been examined. Theoretically, prolonged exposure facilitates the habituation of obsessive fears, and response prevention affects urges to ritualize. Both case studies (Mills, Agras, Barlow, & Mills, 1973; Turner, Hersen, Bellack, Andrasik, & Capparell, 1980) and two between-subjects comparisons (Foa *et al.*, 1980a; Foa, Steketee, Grayson, Turner, & Latimer, 1984) have substantiated this differential effect. As hypothesized, exposure affected obsessive anxiety more than rituals, and response prevention reduced rituals more than obsessions. The greatest benefit was clearly produced by the combination.

Although exposure consistently reduced obsessions in ritualizers, it is puzzling that, in the form of satiation, it has yielded inferior results with "obsessionals" (e.g., Emmelkamp & Kwee, 1977; Stern, 1978). One explanation is that "pure" ruminators who have no overt behavioral rituals do have cognitive compulsions that remain undetected and therefore untreated by response prevention (Salkovskis & Westbrook, 1989; Steketee & Foa, 1985). That is, fearful thoughts are interspersed with cognitions or images that briefly reduce anxiety (mental rituals). Prolonged exposure to the entire chain may fail on two counts: (1) because they are repeatedly evoked, mental rituals are strengthened through their ability to reduce anxiety (negative reinforcement), and (2) frequent interruption of obsessions by cognitive rituals may prevent exposure that is long enough to allow the habituation of discomfort. In fact, Salkovskis and

Westbrook (1989) reported preliminary results demonstrating that following an obsessive thought with a "neutralizing" (compulsive) thought designed to reduce anxiety actually *increases* discomfort. For effective treatment, exposure should be applied to anxiety-provoking thoughts and blocking strategies to cognitive compulsions. Rachman (1976b) and Salkovskis and Westbrook (1989) have demonstrated the effectiveness of this approach in case studies.

Variations in Delivery of Exposure and Response Prevention

Imagined versus *In Vivo* Exposure.   Early trials of exposure treatment used both imagined "flooding" and *in vivo* or direct contact with feared situations. Combining both strategies (with blocking of rituals) led to very positive outcomes in several reports (e.g., Boulougouris & Bassiakos, 1973; Foa & Goldstein, 1978; Rabavilas, Boulougouris, & Stefanis, 1976). Not surprisingly, *in vivo* exposure appeared to be significantly more effective than exposure in fantasy (Rabavilas *et al.*, 1976). According to Lang's model of phobic anxiety (1977), exposure should closely replicate the content of the patient's own internal fear construct. For most patients, actual practice produces more direct exposure to all aspects of their obsessive fears. However, catastrophic thoughts (e.g., death, disease, burglary, accident, and fire) are a prominent feature of the obsessions of some patients. In such cases, these ideas can be confronted through imagined exposure. The usefulness of imagined exposure has been tested with checkers who had such fears of disastrous consequences (Foa, Steketee, Turner, & Fischer, 1980a). All responded equally at posttest either to *in vivo* exposure or to combined imagined and *in vivo* exposure, but at follow-up, the combined-exposure treatment had led to significantly better retention of the gains.

Number and Frequency of Sessions.   In most studies of behavioral therapy, 10–20 sessions produced very positive results. Controlled trials comparing different durations of treatment have not been conducted with OCD patients, but the findings in Table 1 indicate little difference in outcome between studies using more sessions and those using fewer. However, in the study by Rachman, Cobb, Grey, McDonald, Mawson, Sartory, & Stern (1979), 30 sessions appeared to produce somewhat greater gains on most measures of OCD symptoms than 15 sessions; no formal statistical comparison was made of treatment duration (see also Marks, Stern, Mawson, Cobb, & McDonald, 1980). In a similar vein, Emmelkamp *et al.* (1985) reported more improved at follow-up after further treatment was provided as needed. It appears that more than 20 sessions of direct exposure and response prevention may not be necessary for OCD symptoms, although a further treatment of other related problems may indeed be required in many cases.

With respect to frequency of sessions, Emmelkamp and colleagues found no differences between improvement produced by masses sessions (10 sessions in 2.5 weeks) and spaced sessions (10 sessions in 5 weeks) (Emmelkamp, van den Heuvell, Rüphan, Sanderman, 1989). Again, when the results of studies using daily treatments were compared with those of studies using more spaced sessions (Table 1), there was little difference in outcome, with a slight advantage for more frequent sessions. Individual data reported by Julien, Riviere, and Note (1980) allowed analysis of the degree of improvement in subjects receiving different frequencies of sessions (range, 1–5 per week). All five patients who received frequent sessions (4–5 per week) were at least 70% improved, whereas 8 of the 13 subjects (62%) treated once or twice weekly achieved this degree of benefit. When frequency and duration of treatment were examined as predictors of exposure treatment outcome, however, they did not predict outcome (Steketee, Foa, & Grayson, 1982). Ideally, daily sessions are provided, and they are usually feasible in inpatient settings, though impractical for many outpatient clinicians.

Duration and Speed of Exposure.   Studies of both animal and volunteer subjects indicate that prolonged exposure is more effective than brief exposure. For example, 80 minutes of continuous *in vivo* exposure led to better results than eight 10-minute segments (Rabavilas *et al.*, 1976). This difference was not evident for imagined exposure. With respect to the speed of exposure, desensitization is perhaps the most gradual method available but has yielded poor results in reducing obsessive anxiety. By contrast, prolonged and intense exposure has been highly effective. Hodgson, Rachman, and Marks (1972) observed that rapid exposure to more difficult hierarchy items did not produce better results than exposure to less difficult items. Both were equally effective, although patients reported greater comfort with the gradual approach.

Modeling. Comparisons between exposure *in vivo* with and without modeling have showed no differences between treatments according to two studies (Boersma, Den Hengst, Dekker, & Emmelkamp, 1976; Rachman, Marks, & Hodgson, 1973). As Marks *et al.* (1975) noted, this does not mean that certain individuals cannot benefit from modeling. Indeed, when asked to confront feared situations, patients commonly ask, "Would *you* do that?" Noncompulsive behavior modeled by the therapist seems to help some patients overcome their resistance and fear.

Distraction. In two studies of patients with washing rituals, distraction from contaminants produced less habituation of heart rate but more habituation of subjective fear than did focusing attention on the obsessive cues (Grayson, Foa, & Steketee, 1982; Grayson, Steketee, & Foa, 1986). As Baum (1987) noted in relation to the literature on both humans and animals, the role of distraction vis-à-vis fear reduction and avoidance is not yet well understood, and thus, it is difficult to provide treatment recommendations.

Therapist's Role. Informal observations led Marks *et al.* (1975) to propose that exposure and response-prevention treatment requires a good patient-therapist relationship and sometimes a sense of humor. Therapists who were respectful, understanding, interested, encouraging, challenging, and explicit produced more improvement than those who gratified dependency needs and were permissive and tolerant (Rabavilas, Boulougouris, & Perissaki, 1979). The prescription for the therapist's behavior during exposure treatment is apparent from these findings.

Although the personal style of the therapist seems to be important in the treatment relationship, his or her presence during exposure may not be crucial to a positive outcome. According to two studies (Emmelkamp, Van den Meuvell, Rüphan, & Sanderman, 1989; Emmelkamp & Kraanen, 1977), therapist-directed exposure has not improved on the outcome of self-controlled treatment. Further, patients who conducted their own exposures required fewer treatment sessions at follow-up, perhaps gaining greater skill by working *independently* on their fears (Emmelkamp & Kraanen, 1977). Marks and his colleagues concurred that adding therapist-aided exposure after 8 weeks of self-exposure instructions produced only temporary additional benefits, which were lost at Week 23 (Marks, Lelliott, Basoglu, Noshirvani, Monteiro, Cohen, & Kasvikis, 1988). These studies suggest not that therapists are dispensable, but that *in vivo* exposure may be successful without their immediate presence.

Well-trained nurse therapists have produced excellent results with OCD patients in hospital settings (Marks, Hallam, Connolly, & Philpott, 1977; see Table 1). Some inpatient behavioral programs in the United States have also used nurses as behavioral clinicians, though psychologists most often provide this service. Paraprofessionals (usually students) are another often overlooked resource for outpatient settings (Pruitt, Miller, & Smith, 1989). Both patients and paraprofessionals appear to benefit from the mutual learning that *in vivo* exposure provides.

Family members can also be trained as cotherapists to help facilitate exposure and response prevention at home. Emmelkamp and De Lange (1983) found a consistent trend for spouse-assisted exposure to yield better results than patient-alone treatment at posttest, though there were no differences at follow-up and a later study found no difference in outcome at any point (Emmelkamp *et al.*, 1990). Most spouses were enthusiastic assistants to the therapist. However, in one maritally distressed couple, the patient failed to improve until the spouse was no longer involved in therapy. As Emmelkamp and De Lange noted, spouse involvement may not always be wise, particularly when dependency is an issue between the partners. Steketee (1987) observed that relapse was more likely if close family members were critical or angry or believed the patients were not trying hard enough to control their symptoms. Nonanxious, firm, and *supportive* family members were effective in helping to reduce rituals (Mehta, 1990).

    Comment.   In view of the evident potency of exposure and response prevention in treating anxiety-based disorders, the failure to detect differences between most variants of exposure may be due to a ceiling effect. The number of subjects per cell in studies comparing methodological variations is small, permitting only dramatic effects to be detected. Additionally, response prevention was used simultaneously and may have further obscured differences among variants of exposure. Thus, the results cannot be interpreted to confirm that variables such as therapist presence and rapidity of presentation do not affect treatment outcome, but they do not appear to be decisive factors for most patients. The clinical implications of the above findings are discussed below.

    Response Prevention Variants.   The strictness of response prevention has varied widely across studies, ranging from continuous observation and direct interference with rituals (such as turning off water faucets) (e.g., Meyer *et al.*, 1974) to mere verbal instructions for home restrictions (e.g., Emmelkamp *et al.*, 1985) or requests that the ritual be delayed (Junginer & Turner, 1987). A study of five washers indicated that verbal instructions alone blocked some compulsions, whereas strict supervision completely eliminated rituals (Mills *et al.*, 1973). Rachman *et al.* (1973) and Marks *et al.* (1975) attributed most of their failures to patients' inadequate compliance with response prevention instructions. These few findings suggest that strict supervision is not crucial for most patients but may result in a more thorough elimination of rituals.

Concomitant Treatments

    Marital Therapy and Assertiveness Training.   It is generally recognized that obsessive-compulsive symptoms have a negative effect on the afflicted person's ability to fulfill marital, familial, social, and occupational roles. With respect to marital issues, Marks (1981) suggested that exposure therapy is indicated despite marital problems. His contention is supported by research showing that marital adjustment did not predict behavioral treatment outcome (Emmelkamp & De Lange, 1983; Emmelkamp *et al.*, 1990) and by findings that exposure treatment alleviated both OCD symptoms and marital problems (Cobb *et al.*, 1980). Concerning social relationships, patients who had obsessions about harming others improved with assertiveness training, although its efficacy relative to exposure was not tested (Emmelkamp & van der Heyden, 1980). Exposure combined with assertiveness training and marital therapy for patients with such difficulties may yield better treatment outcome (e.g., Queiroz, Motta, Madi, Sossai, & Boren, 1981), particularly at follow-up when relationship problems may lead to relapse.

    Cognitive Treatment.   While treating the behavioral symptoms, clinicians can readily observe the cognitive distortions evident in OCD patients. Common among these are overesti-mates of the risk of the negative consequences of many actions (Foa & Kozak, 1985), including exaggerations of ordinary concerns about health, safety, death, sex, morality, religious matters, and scrutiny by others (Carr, 1974). Other cognitive distortions include unrealistic expectations of competence in all endeavors; self-castigation for failure to fulfill perfectionistic ideas; beliefs that certain behaviors "magically" prevent catastrophes (McFall & Wollersheim, 1979); and beliefs that every situation has a "correct" solution (Guidano & Liotti, 1983). Beech and Liddell (1974) suggested that OCD patients have an excessive need for certainty.

    These apparent cognitive difficulties have led to efforts to relieve symptoms via cognitive therapy. Self-instructional training (SIT) added little to exposure treatment (Emmelkamp *et al.*, 1980) but may have failed because it did not directly address the cognitive deficits peculiar to

OCD. By contrast, rational emotive therapy (RET) was found to be as effective as self-controlled *in vivo* exposure for OCD symptoms and also decreased depression and irrational beliefs (Emmelkamp & Beens, 1991; Emmelkamp, Visser, & Hoekstra, 1988a). Kearney and Silverman (1990) reported that alternating between cognitive therapy and response prevention was effective in treating a suicidal adolescent with OCD for whom *in vivo* exposure was too distressing to tolerate. So far, there is inadequate evidence regarding the efficacy of cognitive treatments for OCD symptoms, and it is not routinely included in standard behavioral treatment programs.

Pharmacotherapy

Although this chapter is intended to assist clinicians using behavioral treatment for OCD, some knowledge of the effects of medications is essential. Patients invariably ask for such information or are already receiving drugs. The relative efficacy of drugs and behavior therapy for OCD is of important concern to many patients. The most effective drugs for OCD symptoms appear to be the serotonin reuptake inhibitors clomipramine (CMI, Anafranil), fluoxetine (FLX, Prozac) and fluvoxamine (FLV), which is not yet approved in the United States (for review see Jenike *et al.*, 1990a).

As Table 2 demonstrates, although all of these drugs have been shown to be significantly more effective than placebo, the average amount of improvement is consistently below that produced by behavior therapy (Greist, 1990). Studies of clomipramine show an average improvement rate ranging from 20% to 45% after 4 to 12 weeks; only 1 of 15 studies gives figures as high 65%. Seven investigations of fluoxetine and six of fluvoxamine showed average benefits of about 20%–40%, slightly below those of CMI. These figures contrast with substantially greater average improvement rates of 50%–70% following behavioral treatment, although it is somewhat difficult to compare across studies that used different measures of outcome. Still, comparisons of outcomes using identical measures (i.e., CAC and MOCI) showed greater mean benefits for exposure treatment. Unfortunately, no behavioral studies have yet used the YBOCS commonly used in recent drug studies.

With respect to the number of subjects who were improved, medication was again less effective than behavior therapy. On CMI, about 60% of subjects were considered "improved" or "responders"; on FLX, the figures were about 65%; and on FLV, 55%. By contrast, at least 75% were "improved" with behavior therapy. Very few studies allowed an examination of drug effects at follow-up, but it appears that gains were consistently maintained or increased. However, 89% of CMI responders relapsed when the drug was replaced by placebo in a double-blind design, even after 27 months of treatment (Pato, Zohar-Kadouch, Zohar, & Murphy, 1988). The duration of CMI treatment did not affect the relapse response.

To date, three studies have compared the effects of serotonergic drugs with exposure and response prevention and the combination (see Tables 1 and 2). Two by Marks and his colleagues used complicated research designs to compare CMI with placebo, and behavioral treatment with relaxation (Marks *et al.*, 1980) and with instructions not to expose (Marks *et al.*, 1988). In the first study, CMI improved mood and OCD symptoms; behavior therapy led to additional improvement on most OCD symptoms, but not on mood. Combined CMI plus exposure therapy had slight advantages over CMI alone at 10 weeks. At follow-up conducted two years later (Mawson, Marks, & Ramm, 1992) and six years later (O'Sullivan, Noshirvani, Marks, Monteiro, & Lelliott, 1991), gains in OCD symptoms were maintained, though anxiety had returned to pretreatment levels (moderate). At six years, 61% were taking medications, one-fourth of which were on clomipramine and the remainder on other tricyclic antidepressants or anxiolytics. The original CMI group was superior to the placebo group on only one of 16 measures. In the second study, CMI initially enhanced the effect of exposure, but this effect disappeared with continued exposure treatment and was not evident at follow-up. A third study compared FLV with FLV plus exposure and with placebo plus exposure (Cottraux *et al.*, 1989).

Table 2. Outcome of Drug Treatments for OCT[a]

Study	No. of cases	No. of wks.	Design	General results	Mean % change posttest	#Ss improved[b] at posttest	Follow-up time	Mean % change at follow-up	# Ss improved[b] by category at follow-up
Clomipramine (CMI)									
Marks et al. (1980)	20 (10 w/relax)	4 (7 w/ relax)	DB vs. PBO	CMI > PBO	16% targ. Sx; 14% CAC; (45% targ. Sx; 39% CAC)	NA	1.2 yr.	NA	NA
Montgomery (1980)	14 (nondep.)	4	DB crossover	CMI > PBO	NA	NA	NA	NA	NA
Thoren et al. (1980)	8	5	DB vs. NOR	CMI > PBO; NOR = PBO	33% obs. Sx; 42% CPRS-OC	50% respond	NA	NA	CMI continued; 55% responders
Ananth et al. (1981)	10	4	DB vs. AMI	CMI > DMI	31% OC Sx; 65% OC severity	2 normal-CGI; 4 mild ill; 2 mod. ill; 1 severe	NA	NA	NA
Insel et al. (1983)	12	6	DB crossover vs. PBO, CLG	CMI > PBO; CLG = PBO	21.5% OCRS; 30% NIMH-OC; 34% CPRS-OC; 31% CAC	NA	NA	NA	Relapse on drug w/drawal
Mavissakalian et al. (1985)	7 (low dep)	12	DB vs. PBO	CMI > PBO	35% OCNS	43% respond	NA	NA	NA
Volavka et al. (1985)	8	12	DB	CMI > IMI	32% SRONS (slight improv.)	75% mi-obs.; 25% imp	NA	NA	NA
Insel et al. (1985)	13	5	DB ZMD vs. DMI, then CMI	CMI > ZMD = DMI	21% CPRS-OC; NIMH-OC	NA	NA	NA	NA
Zohar & Insel (1987)	10 (nondep.)	6	DB crossover vs. DMI	CMI > DMI	20% CPRS-OC; 22% NIMH-OC	10% vmi-CPRS; 60% imp; 30% no chg	12 wk. cont'd	40–90% imp CPRS-OC	NA
Marks et al. (1988)	12	12–17	BT vs. CMI vs. combo	CMI > PBO	22% targ. Sx	25% respond	1 yr.	NA	22% mi targ. Sx; 17% imp; 67% no chg

(*Continued*)

Table 2. (*Continued*)[a]

Study	No. of cases	No. of wks.	Design	General results	Mean % change posttest	#Ss improved[b] at posttest	Follow-up time	Mean % change at follow-up	# Ss improved[b] by category at follow-up
DeVaugh-Geiss et al. (1990)	194 (nondep.)	10	DB vs. PBO	CMI > PBO	40–45% YBOCS; mod. improv. CGI	NA	NA	Further improv. w/CMI	NA
Greist et al. (1990)	13 (nondep.)	10	DB	CMI > PBO	35% YBOCS; 28% NIMH-OC	33% mi-YBOC; 40% imp; 27% no chg	NA	NA	NA
Katz et al. (1990)	134 (nondep.)	10	DB	CMI > PBO	38% NIMH-OC	61% respond on CGI	1 yr. (N = 101)	48% NIMH-OC	71% respond- CGI
Mavissakalian et al. (1990b)	33	10	DB and open trial	Sig. improv.	31% MOCI; 37% OCNS; 47% YBOCS; 36% NIMH-OC	35% mi-NIMH; 39% imp (47% subclin.)	NA	NA	NA
Jenike et al. (1989a)	13	10	DB vs. PO	CMI > PBO	37% YBOCS; 40% NIMH-OC	8% vmi YBOCS; 39% mi; 31% imp; 23% no chg	NA	NA	NA
Pato et al. (1988)	18	5–27	DB CMI, then PBO	Sig. loss	53% YBOCS; 46% CPRS-OC; 43% NIMH-OC	89% relapse	No effect of CMI duration on relapse at FU		
Fluoxetine (FLX)									
Fontaine & Chouinard (1985)	7	8	Open trial	Sig. improv.	59% CPRS-OC; 44% CGI; 17% HSCL-OC	71% respond	NA	NA	NA
Turner et al. (1985)	8	10	SB	Sig. improv.	37% CGI; 20% HSCL-OC; 10% MOCI; 22% targ. Sx	50% vmi; 13% imp; 25% min; 12% no chg	NA	NA	NA
Lipinski et al. (1988)	34	8–30	Open trial	Sig. improv.	23% NIMH-OC; 17% CGI	77% respond	7 mos	31% NIMH-OC; 23% CGI	NA

Study	N	Wk	Design	Result					
Modell et al. (1989)	5	8.5 (mean)	Open trial	No improv.	NA	100% no chg	NA	NA	NA
Jenike et al. (1989b)	61	12	Open trial	Sig. improv.	37% YBOCS; 17.5% MOCI	NA	NA	NA	NA
Markovitz et al. (1990)	11	7–48	Open trial	Sig. improv.	37% MOCI; 30% SCL-90-R	9% vmi; 18% mi; 55% imp; 18% n chg	NA	NA	NA
Fluvoxamine (FLV)									
Perse et al. (1987)	16	8	DB crossover vs. PBO	FLV > PBO	38% SCL-90-R; 15% MOCI; 21% CAC; 34% OC rating	56% imp; 25% sl. imp; 19% no chg	NA	NA	NA
Price et al. (1987)	10	4–8	SB	Sig. improv.	39% YBOCS; 23% MOCI	60% imp; 20% min. imp; 20% no chg	NA	NA	NA
Cottraux et al. (1989)	13	24	DB vs. FLV + BT vs. PBO + BT	FLV > PBO	49% targ. Sx; 34% CAC; 49% BAT	54% respond	48 wk.	43% targ. Sx; 24% CAC; 39% BAT	45% respond
Goodman et al. (1989a)	21	6–8	DB	FLV > PBO	22% YBOCS; 13% MOCI	43% mi/vmi YBOCS, CGI; 56% mi/vmi PGIS	6–8 wk.	NA	NA
Jenike et al. (1990b)	18	10	DB vs. PBO	FLV > PBO	17% YBOCS; 22% NIMH-OC; 15% CGI	NA	NA	NA	NA
Goodman et al. (1990)	21	8	DB vs. DES	FLV > DMI	29% YBOCS	52% mi/vmi YBOCS, CGIS	NA	NA	NA

[a] Abbreviations: BT = behavior therapy; CAC = Compulsive Activity Checklist; CGI = Clinical Global Improvement Scale; CLG = clorgyline; CMI = clomipramine; CPRS = Comprehensive Psychiatric Rating Scale; dep. = depressed; DB = double blind; DMI = desipramine; FLV = fluvoxamine; FLX = fluoxetine; HSCL = Hopkins Symptom Checklist; NIMH-OC = NIMH Obsessive Compulsive Scale; NOR = nortriptyline; OCNS = Obsessive-Compulsive Neurotic Scale; PBO = placebo; sig. improv. = significant improvement; SRONS = Self-Rating Obsessional Neurotic Scale; targ. Sx = target symptoms, YBOCS = Yale-Brown Obsessive Compulsive Scale; ZMD = zimelidine.

[b] Target symptoms were averaged across obsessions and compulsions and across assessors; vmi = very much improved; mi = much improved; imp = improved; no chg = no change/minimally improved.

All three groups improved, with a slight advantage for combined drug and behavioral treatment at six months.

A detailed examination of the results of these studies provides some information about the differences in effectiveness of medication and behavioral treatment. Two Marks *et al*. studies (1980 and 1988) indicated greater average improvement for exposure over CMI at posttest, the later study demonstrating that many more patients had improved from exposure than from CMI (75%–80% vs. 22%–33%). Combined treatment led to more subjects who were "much" improved after one year (73% vs. 50% for exposure alone), but not to more average improvement. Surprisingly, FLV alone showed better average improvement than exposure in two of three measures and produced more successes (54% vs. 40%) at posttest (Cottraux *et al*., 1989). However, after 11 months, the mean improvement was nearly equivalent across the treatments, and slightly more exposure patients were improved (50% vs. 45%). The combination treatment showed some potentiating effect at 6 months, but this effect was minimal at 11 months.

It appears, then, that clomipramine, fluoxetine, and fluvoxamine are effective antiobsessive drugs, but that they are less potent than exposure and response prevention in eliminating OCD symptoms. CMI appears to have a slight advantage over FLX and FLV. The side effects (much less with fluoxetine than CMI) and the tendency of patients to relapse on drug withdrawal (at least of CMI) suggest that medications are not the first treatment of choice. However, for patients who are very apprehensive about or not highly motivated for exposure treatment, and for those who experience high levels of arousal, beginning with drug treatment may enable engagement in exposure treatment.

ACTUAL TREATMENT

Above, we summarized the literature on effective treatments for OCD and on variations in treatment methodology that affect efficacy. That these research-based treatments are transferable to routine clinical practice is quite evident (Kirk, 1983), although modifications, such as reliance on homework assignments rather than accompanied *in vivo* practice, are often made. Issues pertaining to the practice of exposure and response prevention in clinic and hospital settings are presented below. More detailed information is available in Steketee and Foa (1985).

Clinical Application of Exposure and Ritual Prevention

Conducting Exposure Therapy. Most patients show good results with 15 sessions of treatment, but 20 or more sessions are often needed for those whose symptoms are severe or complex (that is, for those with several obsessions or rituals and/or comorbid psychiatric difficulties). Although a few clinical trials showed good results with weekly treatment, most trials used more frequent sessions. Based on our experience from an ongoing OCD treatment program, a minimum of at least two appointments a week is recommended. Following a thorough information-gathering and mutual treatment-planning phase of three to six hours, the practitioner begins exposing the patient for at least an hour to mild to moderately disturbing situations (wherever they are located) and then assigning specific structured exposure between sessions. Writing out homework assignments and providing a written format for recording practice and outcome (e.g., discomfort reduction and urges to ritualize) facilitate the patient's cooperation and accurate following of instructions. Only if the patient cannot carry out particular homework assignments should the therapist accompany him or her to that context.

Although gradual exposure is usually preferred by patients, it is not more effective, and some circumstances, especially unexpected ones, require more rapid confrontation. Modeling is useful in some situations to help assuage patients' fearful attitudes and enable them to carry out the exposure. A sense of humor is invaluable in helping patients over difficult situations.

After all, many practice exposure sessions put both patient and therapist in awkward and even ridiculous situations. Patients are encouraged to concentrate on, rather than distract their attention from, exposure situations. However, this does not mean they cannot discuss feelings, historical information about their fears, or other relevant issues during exposure sessions.

Constant supervision of rituals is rarely possible even in an inpatient setting, nor it is likely to be more beneficial than encouraging a self-controlled reduction of rituals. Therapists are urged to help patients monitor their rituals by requiring self-recording and to remind patients firmly of their commitment to overcome their OCD symptoms and the necessity of stopping even minor rituals. We recommend eliminating as many rituals as possible from the outset. Often, however, complete response prevention exposes patients too quickly to situations that are extremely discomfiting and that, for some patients, are too overwhelming. A modified version may be used in which patients immediately reduce rituals to near-normal levels (for example, with washers, one 10- to 15-minute shower per day and 5 to 10 handwashes) and gradually eliminate their remaining excessive behaviors as exposure progresses. Similar restrictions are placed on checking rituals, and repeating rituals are increasingly eliminated according to the exposure treatment schedule.

Mental Rituals. Applying exposure and response prevention appropriately requires a correct identification of the patient's obsessions and compulsions, particularly cognitive rituals which may be mistaken for obsessions. Blocking mental rituals may be difficult, as they are not directly observable by the therapist or the patient. We suggest enlisting the patient's aid in finding creative strategies. Strong distractions from the compulsive thought may be helpful, or mental rituals may be interrupted by immediately rethinking the obsessive thought that led to the ritual. For example, a patient who interpolated "good" thoughts to undo potential damage from thoughts or reminders of the devil was exposed to written and imagined "evil" words and asked to focus on these whenever she noticed herself engaging in "good" thoughts.

Imagined Flooding. Based on research findings, routine inclusion of *imagined* exposure is appropriate for any patient who reports obsessional fears of catastrophes. Many clinicians inexperienced in "flooding" feel uncomfortable using this treatment, as it requires the patient to give verbal and visual expression to his or her worst fears, which are invariably unpleasant. However, it is very clear that trying to *avoid* thinking about or imagining these unpleasant ideas has only led to their entrenchment as provocative cues for discomfort. A reasonable strategy for managing such ingrained cognitions is to stop avoiding and instead to allow oneself free thinking of unwanted thoughts. These may be tape-recorded and replayed regularly as homework.

Exposure in fantasy may also be indicated for patients whose severe avoidance and anxiety make the prospect of *in vivo* exposure seem unmanageable. For example, in two cases with "bowel obsessions," imagined exposure to fears of fecal incontinence, somatic sensations, distressing thoughts, and feared social consequences facilitated subsequent *in vivo* exposure (Beidel & Bulik, 1990). The extensive data supporting the efficacy of flooding certainly warrants its inclusion in treatment. See Steketee and Foa (1985) or Steketee and White (1990) for detailed information about conducting flooding.

Outpatient versus Inpatient Treatment. Although no differences in results for inpatient and outpatient treatment were found in one study (Van den Hout, Emmelkamp, Kraaykamp, & Griez, 1988), there are clinical advantages in both inpatient and outpatient settings. Hospital treatment may be indicated when (1) the symptoms are severe and patients have difficulty tolerating the discomfort provoked by exposure; (2) depression is severe; (3) functioning in everyday living situations is very poor; and (4) the patient lacks an adequate support network (Megens & Vandereycken, 1989). An inpatient setting also allows better monitoring of medications where it is needed. The disadvantages of inpatient treatment include its high cost, potential dependency on continual staff availability, and its being an inappropriate context for exposure treatment (e.g., patients with home-checking rituals may experience no urges to ritualize while in the hospital) (Megens & Vandereycken, 1989). Outpatient treatment is desirable whenever it is feasible.

Problems Encountered during Therapy

Compliance.   Failure to comply with either exposure or response prevention instructions is widely viewed as a clear signal of treatment failure (Foa *et al.*, 1984; Rachman & Hodgson, 1980). Similarly, we are convinced that arguments between therapist and patient are never productive. Assuming that the therapist has been sensitive to the patient's capacity to withstand discomfort and has prescribed exposure accordingly, such arguments can only signal a conviction that the obsessive fears are reasonable (overvalued ideation) or ambivalence about eliminating the OCD symptoms. We suggest that the therapist consider terminating treatment or, with the patient's agreement, redirecting it at issues other than OCD symptoms.

Generalization.   Particularly in inpatient settings, the generalization of symptom reduction from the treatment site to natural situations requires special planning and assignments. Treatments in which most exposure is self-conducted entail little difficulty with generalization. But patients treated in the hospital, especially in a distant city, will undoubtedly require a home visit or special arrangements with a "cotherapist," whether this is a family member or another therapist in the hometown. Difficulties in doing exposure without the therapist's reassuring presence may be minimized by increasingly requiring patients to self-expose and to prevent rituals during the last half of treatment.

Cognitive Issues.   Overvalued ideation or a conviction that the obsessive fears are correct has predictive of a poor outcome with behavioral treatment (e.g., Foa, 1979). Cognitive treatment involving a logical discussion of the actual probability of a negative outcome or of its potential impact (its valence) seems to produce little change in firmly held beliefs. Efforts to correct misconceptions may be useful in cases where there is genuine inaccuracy in assumptions, but this is not the problem in most instances. Instead, OCD patients have *exaggerated* the perceived danger of a potentially harmful situation. Beck's model (Beck, Emery, & Greenberg, 1985) recommends testing such automatic beliefs, which is precisely the problem: To test the belief requires direct exposure, which overvaluing patients either refuse to do or carry out convinced that the apparent absence of catastrophe can be explained by other circumstances (such as luck).

Cognitive treatments may have more validity for OCD patients if they are focused on basic assumptions about themselves, the world, and the future. Indeed, there is both research evidence and clinical conviction that OCD patients often hold unrealistic assumptions (e.g., "I must do everything perfect," "People will reject me if I make mistakes," "Taking even small risks is unnecessary and dangerous," "I am responsible for every action I take and will be held accountable"). However, apart from Emmelkamp *et al.*'s study of RET (1988), we have no empirical evidence that this strategy is effective for most patients. Further study on this issue is essential, as many failures and relapses appear to occur among those who hold such unchanging beliefs, particularly when guilt and excessive responsibility are involved.

Concomitant Pharmacotherapy.   Most patients are likely to be taking either clomipramine or fluoxetine when they seek behavioral treatment. It is advisable to stabilize medications for two to three months before beginning exposure sessions so that the patient is better enabled to distinguish the separate benefits of the two treatments. As evident from the Pato *et al.* (1988) study, patients who wish to discontinue drug therapy face a high risk of relapse. Behavioral treatment may protect against relapse, though this possibility has not yet been tested. As medications are withdrawn, the therapist is advised to carefully monitor the patient's symptoms, to consult regularly with the pharmacologist regarding dosage adjustment, and to use booster exposure sessions to consolidate gains in the nondrugged state.

SUMMARY

Obsessive-compulsive disorder is a complex anxiety disorder, characterized by multiple types of obsessions and compulsions. The variety of manifestations of OCD make diagnosis more difficult, particularly in the case of mental rituals, which often go unreported and are "invisible" to all but the patient. Complicating the picture are comorbid disorders, such as major depression, personality disorders, and other anxiety disorders, including panic and social phobia. Some disorders, including hypochondriasis, body dysmorphic disorder, and eating disorders, bear a strong resemblance to OCD and may respond to similar treatments. Several traits common to OCD that appear to play a role in symptomatology have been identified: perfectionism, difficulty in making decisions, excessive guilt and responsibility, and avoidance of risk taking.

The assessment of OCD requires a careful interview with the assistance of the YBOCS Symptom Checklist. Other questionnaires are available that allow a comparison of patients' scores with normative data and with the scores of other OCD subjects. An assessment of the change in symptoms can be accomplished by the YBOCS, which measures the severity of overall obsessions and compulsions, by target symptom ratings, or by the behavioral self-monitoring of obsessions and rituals.

The behavioral treatment of choice for OCD is exposure to obsessive fear situations and the prevention of rituals. This combination has proved highly effective, yielding an average improvement rate of 50%–70% on most measures and leaving about 85% of patients improved, with 55% very much improved. These results are fairly stable at follow-up, with some loss of gains. Variations in the delivery of exposure have made little difference in outcome, except for prolonged exposure and the addition of imagined exposure, which improved gains.

Drug treatments have also led to substantial improvement, but with lower response rates: average improvement ranged from 20% to 40%, and about 60% of patients were rated improved. Combined treatment was only slightly better than behavior therapy alone. Despite this finding, concurrent drug and behavior therapy is very common in clinical settings, particularly inpatient ones.

The ideal behavioral treatment is delivered at least twice a week by a therapist who is firm and supportive, who assigns regular homework, who travels with the patient to conduct exposure in actual feared situations, and who enlists the aid of supportive family members. Exposure should be prolonged and graduated in difficulty, and rituals should be strictly limited in concert with the pace of exposure. Imagined exposure can be added to exposure *in vivo* when catastrophic fears are a prominent part of obsessive ideation. Medication (clomipramine or fluoxetine) is included when high anxiety or low motivation prevents patients from adequately exposing themselves. Noncompliant patients are encouraged to postpone behavior therapy or to redirect its focus.

At present, there are several complications of OCD for which proved treatments are lacking. These include near-delusional beliefs (overvalued ideation) in the validity of obsessive fears and assumptions regarding the importance of perfectionism, risk avoidance, and personal responsibility or guilt. In addition, schizotypal, borderline, and passive-aggressive personality disorders appear to bias outcome negatively. It is hoped that specialized cognitive treatments may provide strategies for addressing these problems.

ACKNOWLEDGMENT.   Preparation of this chapter was supported in part by NIMH grant R01 MH44190 awarded to the first author.

GAIL STEKETEE and
LESLIE J. SHAPIRO

REFERENCES

Akhtar, S., Wig, N. A., Verma, V. K., Pershad, D., & Verma, S. K. (1975). A phenomenological analysis of symptoms in obsessive-compulsive neurosis. *British Journal of Psychiatry, 114*, 342–348.

American Psychiatric Association. (1987). *Diagnostic and statistical manual of mental disorders* (3rd ed., rev.; DMS-III-R). Washington, DC: Author.

Ananth, J., Pecknold, J. C., Van den Steen, N., & Englesmann, F. (1981). Double-blind comparative study of clomipramine and amitriptyline in obsessive neurosis. *Progress in Neuropsychopharmacology, 5*, 257–262.

Baer, L., Jenike, M. A., Ricciardi, J. N., Holland, A. D., Seymour, R. J., Minichiello, W. E., & Buttolph, M. L. (1990). Standardized assessment of personality disorders in obsessive-compulsive disorder. *Archives of General Psychiatry, 47*, 826–830.

Ballerini, A., & Stanghellini, G. (1989). Phenomenological question about obsession and delusion. *Psychopathology, 22*, 315–319.

Baum, M. (1987). Distraction during flooding (exposure): Concordance between results in animals and man. *Behaviour Research and Therapy, 25*, 227–228.

Beck, A. T., Emery, G., & Greenberg, R. L. (1985). *Anxiety disorders and phobias: A cognitive perspective*. New York: Basic Books.

Beech, H. R., & Liddell, A. (1974). Decision making, mood states, and ritualistic behavior among obsessional patients. In H. R. Beech (Ed.), *Obsessional states*. London: Methuen.

Beidel, D. C., & Bulik, C. M. (1990). Flooding and response prevention as a treatment for bowel obsessions. *Journal of Anxiety Disorders, 4*, 247–256.

Black, A. (1974). The natural history of obsessional neurosis. In H. R. Beech (Ed.), *Obsessional states*. London: Methuen.

Boersma, K., Den Hengst, S., Dekker, J., & Emmelkamp, P. M. G. (1976). Exposure and response prevention: A comparison with obsessive compulsive patients. *Behaviour Research and Therapy, 14*, 19–24.

Boulougouris, J. C. (1977). Variables affecting the behaviour modification of obsessive-compulsive patients treated by flooding. In J. C. Boulougouris & A. D. Rabavilas (Eds.), *The treatment of phobic and obsessive-compulsive disorders*. Oxford, England: Pergamon Press.

Boulougouris, J. C., & Bassiakos, L. (1973). Prolonged flooding in cases with obsessive-compulsive neurosis. *Behaviour Research and Therapy, 11*, 227–231.

Brady, K. T., Austin, L., & Lydiard, R. B. (1990). Body dysmorphic disorder: the relationship to obsessive-compulsive disorder. *Journal of Nervous and Mental Disease, 178*, 538–539.

Capstick, N., & Seldrup, J. (1973). Phenomenological aspects of obsessional patients treated with clomipramine. *British Journal of Psychiatry, 122*, 719–720.

Carr, A. I. (1974). Compulsive neurosis: A review of the literature. *Psychological Bulletin, 8*, 311–318.

Cobb, J., McDonald, R., Marks, I. M., & Stern, R. (1980). Marital versus exposure therapy: Psychological treatments of co-existing marital and phobic obsessive problems. *Behavioural Analysis and Modification, 4*, 3–16.

Cottraux, J., & Bouvard, M., Defayolle, M., & Messy, P. (1988). Validity and factorial structure study of the compulsive activity checklist. *Behavior Therapy, 19*, 45–53.

Cottraux, J., Mollard, E., Bouvard, M., Marks, I., Sluys, M., Nury, A. M., Douge, R., & Cialdella, P. (1989). A controlled study of fluvoxamine and exposure in obsessive compulsive disorder. *International Clinical Psychopharmacology, 5*, 1–14.

Dent, H. R., & Salkovskis, P. M. (1986). Clinical measures of depression, anxiety and obsessionality in non-clinical populations. *Behaviour Research and Therapy, 24*, 689–691.

DeVeaugh-Geiss, J., Landau, P., & Katz, R. (1990). Preliminary results from a multicenter trial of clomipramine in obsessive-compulsive disorder. *Psychopharmacology Bulletin, 25*, 36–40.

Dollard, J., & Miller, N. E. (1950). *Personality and psychotherapy: An analysis in terms of learning, thinking and culture*. New York: McGraw-Hill.

Dowson, H. H. (1977). The phenomenology of severe obsessive-compulsive neurosis. *British Journal of Psychiatry, 131*, 75–78.

Eisen, J. L., & Rasmussen, S. A. (1989). Coexisting obsessive compulsive disorder and alcoholism. *Journal of Clinical Psychiatry, 50*, 96–98.

Emmelkamp, P. M. G., & Beens, H. (1991). Cognitive therapy with obsessive-compulsive disorder: A comparative evaluation. *Behavior Research and Therapy, 29*, 293–300.

Emmelkamp, P. M. G., & De Lange, I. (1983). Spouse involvement in the treatment of obsessive-compulsive patients. *Behaviour Research and Therapy, 21*, 341–346.

Emmelkamp, P. M. G., & Kwee, K. G. (1977). Obsessional ruminations: A comparison between thought stopping and prolonged exposure in imagination. *Behaviour Research and Therapy, 15*, 441–444.

Emmelkamp, P. M. G., & van der Heyden, H. (1980). The treatment of harming obsessions. *Behavioural Analysis and Modification, 4,* 28–35.

Emmelkamp, P. M. G., & von Kraanen, J. (1977). Therapist-controlled exposure *in vivo*: A comparison with obsessive-compulsive patients. *Behaviour Research and Therapy, 15,* 491–495.

Emmelkamp, P. M. G., van der Helm, M., van Zanten, B. L., & Plochg, I. (1980). Contributions of self-instructional training to the effectiveness of exposure *in vivo*: A comparison with obsessive compulsive patients. *Behaviour Research and Therapy, 18,* 61–66.

Emmelkamp, P. M. G., Hoekstra, R. J., & Visser, S. (1985). The behavioral treatment of obsessive-compulsive disorder: Prediction of outcome at 3.5 years follow-up. In P. Pichot, P. Berner, R. Wolf, & K. Thau (Eds.), *Psychiatry: The state of the art* (Vol. 4). New York: Plenum Press.

Emmelkamp, P. M. G., Visser, S., & Hoekstra, R. J. (1988). Cognitive therapy vs. exposure *in vivo* in the treatment of obsessive-compulsives. *Cognitive Therapy and Research, 12,* 103–114.

Emmelkamp, P. M. G., van den Heuvell, C. V. L., Rüphan, M., & Sanderman, R. (1989). Home-based treatment of obsessive-compulsive patients: Intersession interval and therapist involvement. *Behavior Research and Therapy, 27,* 89–93.

Emmelkamp, P. M. G., de Haan, E., & Hoogduin, C. A. L. (1990). Marital adjustment and obsessive-compulsive disorder. *British Journal of Psychiatry, 156,* 55–60.

Esquirol, J. E. D. (1838). *Des maladies mentales (Vol. II).* Paris: Baillière.

Foa, E. B. (1979). Failure in treating obsessive-compulsives. *Behaviour Research and Therapy, 17,* 169–176.

Foa, E. B., & Goldstein, A. (1978). Continuous exposure and complete response prevention of obsessive-compulsive disorder. *Behavior Therapy, 9,* 821–829.

Foa, E. B., & Kozak, M. J. (1985). Treatment of anxiety disorders: Implications for psychopathology. In A. H. Tuma & J. Maser (Eds.), *Anxiety and the anxiety disorders.* Hillsdale, NJ: Erlbaum.

Foa, E. B., & Tillmanns, A. (1980). The treatment of obsessive compulsive neurosis. In A. Goldstein & E. B. Foa (Eds.), *Handbook of behavioral interventions: A clinical guide.* New York: Wiley.

Foa, E. B., Steketee, G. S., & Milby, J. B. (1980a). Differential effects of exposure and response prevention in obsessive compulsive washers. *Journal of Consulting and Clinical Psychology, 48,* 71–79.

Foa, E. B., Steketee, G. S., Turner, R. M., & Fischer, S. C. (1980b). Effects of imaginal exposure to feared disasters in obsessive compulsive checkers. *Behaviour Research and Therapy, 18,* 449–455.

Foa, E. B., Grayson, J. B., Steketee, G., Doppelt, H. G., Turner, R. M., & Latimer, P. R. (1983). Success and failure in the behavioral treatment of obsessive-compulsives. *Journal of Consulting and Clinical Psychology, 51,* 287–297.

Foa, E. B., Steketee, G. S., Grayson, J. B., Turner, R. M., & Latimer, P. R. (1984). Deliberate exposure and blocking of obsessive-compulsive rituals: Immediate and long term effects. *Behavior Therapy, 15,* 450–472.

Foa, E. B., Steketee, G. S., Kozak, M. J., & McCarthy, P. R. (in press). Imipramine and behavior therapy in the treatment of depressive and obsessive compulsive symptoms. *British Journal of Clinical Psychology.*

Fontaine, R., & Chouinard, G. (1985). Fluoxetine in the treatment of obsessive compulsive disorder. *Progress in Neuro-psychopharmacological Biological Psychiatry,9,* 605–608.

Freund, B., Steketee, G. S., & Foa, E. B. (1987). Compulsive activity checklist (CAC): Psychometric analysis with obsessive-compulsive disorder. *Behavioral Assessment, 9,* 67–79.

Goodman, W. K., Price, L. H., Rasmussen, S. A., Delgado, P. L., Heninger, G. R., & Charney, D. S. (1989a). Efficacy of fluvoxamine in obsessive-compulsive disorder. *Archives of General Psychiatry, 46,* 36–44.

Goodman, W. K., Price, L. H., Rasmussen, S. A., Mazure, C., Delgado, P., Heninger, G. R., & Charney, D. S. (1989b). The Yale-Brown Obsessive Compulsive Scale: 2. Validity. *Archives of General Psychiatry, 46,* 1012–1016.

Goodman, W. K., Price, L. H., Rasmussen, S. A., Mazure, C., Fleischman, R. L., Hill, C. L., Heninger, G. R., & Charney, D. S. (1989c). The Yale-Brown Obsessive Compulsive Scale: 1. Development, use, and reliability. *Archives of General Psychiatry, 46,* 1006–1011.

Goodman, W. K., Price, L. H., Delgado, P. L., Palumbo, J., Krystal, J. H., Nagy, L. M., Rasmussen, S. A., Heninger, G. R., & Charney, D. S. (1990). Specificity of serotonin reuptake inhibitors in the treatment of obsessive-compulsive disorder. *Archives of General Psychiatry,47,* 577–585.

Grayson, J. B., Foa, E. B., & Steketee, G. S. (1982). Habituation during exposure treatment: Distraction versus attention focusing. *Behaviour Therapy and Research, 20,* 323–328.

Grayson, J. B., Steketee, G. S., & Foa, E. B. (1986). Exposure *in vivo* of obsessive-compulsives under distracting and attention-focusing conditions: Replication and extension. *Behaviour Research and Therapy, 24,* 475–479.

Greenberg, D. (1987). Compulsive hoarding. *American Journal of Psychotherapy, 41,* 409–416.

Greist, J. H. (1990). Treatment of obsessive compulsive disorder: Psychotherapies, drugs, and other somatic treatment. *Journal of Clinical Psychiatry, 51* (8, Suppl.), 44–50.

Greist, J. H., Jefferson, J. W., Rosenfeld, R., Gutzman, L. D., March, J. S., & Barklage, N. E. (1990). Clomipramine and obsessive compulsive disorder: A placebo-controlled double-blind study of 32 patients. *Journal of Clinical Psychiatry, 51*, 292–297.

Guidano, V. L., & Liotti, G. (1983). *Cognitive processes and emotional disorders.* New York: Guilford Press.

Henderson, J. G., & Pollard, C. A. (1988). Three types of obsessive compulsive disorder in a community sample. *Journal of Clinical Psychology, 44*, 747–752.

Hermesh, H., Shahar, A., & Munitz, H. (1987, January). Obsessive-compulsive disorder and borderline personality disorder (letter to the editor). *American Journal of Psychiatry, 144*, 120–121.

Hodgson, R. J., & Rachman, S. (1977). Obsessional compulsive complaints. *Behaviour Research and Therapy, 15*, 389–395.

Hodgson, R. J., Rachman, S., & Marks, I. M. (1972). The treatment of chronic obsessive-compulsive neurosis: Follow-up and further findings. *Behaviour Research and Therapy, 10*, 181–189.

Hollander, E., Liebowitz, M. R., Winchel, R., Klumker, A., & Klein, D. F. (1989). Treatment of body-dysmorphic disorder. *American Journal of Psychiatry, 146*, 768–770.

Hoogduin, C. A. L., & Duivenvoorden, H. J. (1988). A decision model in the treatment of obsessive-compulsive neuroses. *British Journal of Psychiatry, 152*, 516–521.

Hoogduin, C. A. L., & Hoogduin, W. A. (1984). The outpatient treatment of patients with an obsessional-compulsive disorder. *Behaviour Research and Therapy, 22*, 455–459.

Insel, T. R., & Akiskal, H. S. (1986). Obsessive-compulsive disorder with psychotic features: A phenomenological analysis. *American Journal of Psychiatry, 143*, 1527–1533.

Insel, T. R., Murphy, D. L., Cohen, R. M., Alterman, I., Kilts, C., & Linnoila, M. (1983). Obsessive-compulsive disorder: A double-blind trial of clomipramine and clorgyline. *Archives of General Psychiatry, 40*, 605–612.

Insel, T. R., Mueller, E. A., Alterman, I., Linnoila, M., & Murphy, D. L. (1985). Obsessive-compulsive disorder and serotonin: Is there a connection? *Biological Psychiatry, 20*, 1174–1189.

Jenike, M. A., Baer, L., Minichiello, W. E., Schwartz, C. E., & Carey, R. J. (1986). Concomitant obsessive-compulsive disorder and schizotypal personality disorder. *American Journal of Psychiatry, 143*, 530–532.

Jenike, M. A., Baer, L., Summergrad, P., Weilburg, J. B., Holland, A., & Seymour, R. (1989a). Obsessive-compulsive disorder; A double-blind, placebo-controlled trial of clomipramine in 27 patients. *American Journal of Psychiatry, 146*, 1328–1329.

Jenike, M. A., Buttolph, L., Baer, L., Ricciardi, J., & Holland, A. (1989b). Open trial of fluoxetine in obsessive-compulsive disorder. *American Journal of Psychiatry, 146*, 909–911.

Jenike, M. A., Baer, L., & Minichiello, W. E. (1990a). *Obsessive compulsive disorders: Theory and management.* Chicago: Year Book Medical Publishers.

Jenike, M. A., Hyman, S., Baer, L., Holland, A., Minichello, W. E., Buttolph, L., Summergrad, P., Seymour, R., & Ricciardi, J. (1990b). A controlled trial of fluvoxamine in obsessive-compulsive disorder: Implications for a serotonergic theory. *American Journal of Psychiatry, 147*, 1209–1215.

Julien, R. A., Riviére, B., & Note, I. D. (1980). Traitement comportemental et cognitif des obsessions et compulsions resultats et discussion. *Séance du Lundi 27 Octobre*, 1123–1133.

Junginger, J., & Turner, S. M. (1987). Spontaneous exposure and "self-control" in the treatment of compulsive checking. *Journal of Behavioral Therapy and Experimental Psychiatry, 18*, 115–119.

Karno, M., Golding, J. M., Sorenson, S. B., & Burnam, M. A. (1988). The epidemiology of obsessive-compulsive disorder in five U.S. communities. *Archives of General Psychiatry, 45*, 1094–1099.

Katz, R. J., DeVeaugh-Geiss, J., & Landau, P. (1990). Clomipramine in obsessive-compulsive disorder. *Biological Psychiatry, 20*, 401–414.

Kearney, C. A., & Silverman, W. K. (1990). Treatment of an adolescent with obsessive-compulsive disorder by alternating response prevention and cognitive therapy: An empirical analysis. *Journal of Behavior Therapy and Experimental Psychiatry, 21*, 39–47.

Kirk, J. W. (1983). Behavioral treatment of obsessional-compulsive patients in routine clinical practice. *Behavior Research and Therapy, 21*, 57–62.

Kozak, M. J., Foa, E. B., & McCarthy, P. R. (1987). Assessment of obsessive-compulsive disorder. In C. Last & M. Hersen (Eds.), *Handbook of anxiety disorders.* New York: Pergamon Press.

Lang, P. J. (1977). Imagery in therapy: An information processing analysis of fears. *Behavior Therapy, 8*, 862–886.

Lang, P. J. (1979). A bio-informational theory of emotional imagery. *Psychophysiology, 16*, 495–512.

Lipinski, J., White, K., & Quay, S. (1988). *Antiobsessional effects of fluoxtine: An open trial.* Unpublished manuscript.

Mansuedo, C. S., & Goldfinger, R. I. (1990, November). *Group treatment of trichotillomania with multi-system habit-competition training*. Paper presented at the annual meeting of the Association for the Advancement of Behavior Therapy, San Francisco.

Markovitz, P. J., Stagno, S. J., & Calabrese, J. R. (1990). Buspirone augmentation of fluoxetine in obsessive-compulsive disorder. *American Journal of Psychiatry*, *147*, 798–800.

Marks, I. M. (1981). *Cure and care of the neuroses*. New York: Wiley.

Marks, I. M., Hodgson, R., & Rachman, S. J. (1975). Treatment of chronic obsessive-compulsive neurosis *in vivo* exposure: A 2 year follow-up and issues in treatment. *British Journal of Psychiatry*, *127*, 349–364.

Marks, I. M., Hallam, R. S., Connolly, J., & Philpott, R. (1977). *Nursing in behavioral psychotherapy*. London: Royal College of Nursing of the United Kingdom.

Marks, I. M., Bird, J., & Lindley, P. (1978). Behavioral nurse therapists. *Behavioural Psychotherapy*, *6*, 25–35.

Marks, I. M., Stern, R. S., Mawson, D., Cobb, J., & McDonald, R. (1980). Clomipramine and exposure for obsessive-compulsive rituals. *British Journal of Psychiatry*, *136*, 1–25.

Marks, I. M., Lelliott, P., Basoglu, M., Noshirvani, H., Monteiro, W., Cohen, D., & Kasvikis, Y. (1988). Clomipramine, self exposure and therapist-aided exposure for obsessive compulsive rituals. *British Journal of Psychiatry*, *152*, 522–534.

Mavissakalian, M., Turner, S. M., Michelson, L., & Jacob, R. (1985). Tricyclic antidepressants in obsessive-compulsive disorder: Anti-obsessional or antidepressant agents. *American Journal of Psychiatry*, *142*, 572–576.

Mavissakalian, M., Hamann, M. S., & Jones, B. (1990a). A comparison of DSM-III personality disorders in panic/agoraphobia and obsessive-compulsive disorder. *Comprehensive Psychiatry*, *31*, 238–244.

Mavissakalian, M. R., Jones, B., Olson, S., & Perel, J. M. (1990b). Chlomipramine in obsessive-compulsive disorder: Clinical response and plasma levels. *Journal of Clinical Psychopharmacology*, *10*, 261–268.

McFall, M. E., & Wollersheim, J. P. (1979). Obsessive-compulsive neurosis: A cognitive behavioral formulation and approach to treatment. *Cognitive Therapy and Research*, *3*, 333–348.

McKenna, P. J. (1984). Disorders with overvalued ideas. *British Journal of Psychiatry*, *45*, 579–585.

Megens, J., & Vandereycken, W. (1989). Hospitalization of obsessive-compulsive patients: The "forgotten" factor in the behavior therapy literature. *Comprehensive Psychiatry*, *30*, 161–169.

Mehta, M. (1990). A comparative study of family-based and patient-based behavioral management in obsessive-compulsive disorder. *British Journal of Psychiatry*, *157*, 133–135.

Meyer, V., & Levy, R. (1973). Modification of behavior in obsessive-compulsive disorders. In H. E. Adams & P. Unikel (Eds.), *Issues and trends in behavior therapy*. Springfield, IL: Charles C Thomas.

Meyer, V., Levy, R., & Schnurer, A. (1974). A behavioral treatment of obsessive-compulsive disorders. In H. R. Beech (Ed.), *Obsessional states*. London: Methuen.

Mills, H. L., Agras, W. S., Barlow, D. H., & Mills, J. R. (1973). Compulsive rituals treated by response prevention. *Archives of General Psychiatry*, *28*, 524–527.

Modell, J. G., Himle, J., Nesse, R. M., Mountz, J. M., & Schmaltz, S. (1989). Sequential trials of fluoxetine, phenelzine, and tranylcypromine in the treatment of obsessive-compulsive disorder. *Journal of Anxiety Disorders*, *3*, 287–294.

Montgomery, S. A. (1980). Clomipramine in obsessional neurosis: A placebo controlled trial. *Pharmaceutical Medicine*, *1*, 189–192.

Mowrer, O. H. (1960). *Learning theory and behavior*. New York: Wiley.

O'Sullivan, G., Noshirvani, H., Marks, I., Monteiro, W., & Lelliott, P. (1991). Six-year follow-up after exposure and clomipramine therapy for obsessive-compulsive disorder. *Journal of Clinical Psychiatry*, *52*, 150–155.

Pato, M. T., Zohar-Kadouch, R., Zohar, J., & Murphy, D. (1988). Return of symptoms after discontinuation of clomipramine in patients with obsessive-compulsive disorder. *American Journal of Psychiatry*, *145*, 1521–1527.

Perse, T. (1988). Obsessive-compulsive disorder: A treatment review. *Journal of Clinical Psychiatry*, *49*, 48–55.

Perse, T. L., Greist, J. H., Jefferson, J. W., Rosenfeld, R., & Dar, R. (1987). Fluvoxamine treatment of obsessive-compulsive disorder. *American Journal of Psychiatry*, *144*, 1543–1548.

Phillips, K. A. (1990, May). *Body dysmorphic disorder: The distress of imagined ugliness*. Paper presented at the American Psychiatric Association, New York.

Price, L. H., Goodman, W. K., Charney, D. S., Rasmussen, S. A., & Heninger, G. R. (1987). Treatment of severe obsessive-compulsive disorder with fluvoxamine. *American Journal of Psychiatry*, *144*, 1050–1061.

Pruitt, S. D., Miller, W. R., & Smith, J. E. (1989). Outpatient behavioral treatment of severe obsessive-compulsive disorder: Using paraprofessional resources. *Journal of Anxiety Disorders*, *3*, 179–186.

Queiroz, L. O. S., Motta, M. A., Madi, M. B. B. P., Sossai, D. L., & Boren, J. J. (1981). A functional analysis of obsessive-compulsive problems with related therapeutic procedures. *Behaviour Research and Therapy*, *19*, 377–388.

Rabavilas, A. D., Boulougouris, J. C., & Stefanis, C. (1976). Duration of flooding sessions in the treatment of obsessive-compulsive patients. *Behaviour Research and Therapy, 14*, 349–355.

Rabavilas, A. D., Boulougouris, J. C., & Perissaki, C. (1979). Therapist qualities related to outcome with exposure *in vivo* in neurotic patients. *Journal of Behavior Therapy and Experimental Psychiatry, 10*, 293–299.

Rachman, S. J. (1971). Obsessional ruminations. *Behaviour Research and Therapy, 9*, 229–235.

Rachman, S. J. (1976a). Obsessional-compulsive checking. *Behaviour Research and Therapy, 14*, 437–443.

Rachman, S. J. (1976b). Obsessional ruminations. *Behaviour Research and Therapy, 9*, 229–235.

Rachman, S. J., & De Silva, P. (1978). Abnormal and normal obsessions. *Behaviour Research and Therapy, 16*, 233–248.

Rachman, S. J., & Hodgson, R. (1980). *Obsessions and compulsions.* Englewood Cliffs, NJ: Prentice-Hall.

Rachman, S. J., & Wilson, G. T. (1980). *The effects of psychological therapy.* Oxford: Pergamon Press.

Rachman, S. J., Marks, I. M., & Hodgson, R. (1973). The treatment of obsessive-compulsive neurotics by modelling and flooding *in vivo. Behaviour Research and Therapy, 11*, 463–471.

Rachman, S. J., Cobb, J., Grey, S., McDonald, B., Mawson, D., Sartory, G., & Stern, R. (1979). The behavioral treatment of obsessional-compulsive disorders with and without chlomipramine. *Behavior Research and Therapy, 17*, 467–468.

Rasmussen, S. A., & Eisen, J. L. (1990). Epidemiology of obsessive compulsive disorder. *Journal of Clinical Psychiatry, 51*, 10–13.

Rasmussen, S. A., & Tsuang, M. T. (1986). Epidemiological and clinical findings of significance to the design of neuropharmacologic studies of obsessive-compulsive disorder. *Psychopharmacological Bulletin, 22*, 723–733.

Riemann, B. C., & McNally, R. J. (1990, November). *The comorbidity of obsessive-compulsive disorder and alcoholism.* Paper presented at the meeting of the Association for the Advancement of Behavior Therapy. San Francisco.

Roper, G., Rachman, S., & Marks, I. M. (1975). Passive and participant modelling in exposure treatment of obsessive-compulsive neurotics. *Behaviour Research and Therapy,13*, 271–279.

Rosen, I. (1957). The clinical significance of obsessions in schizophrenia. *Journal of Mental Science, 103*, 773–786.

Rosen, J. C., & Leitenberg, H. (1982). Bulimia nervosa: Treatment with exposure and response prevention. *Behavior Therapy, 13*, 117–124.

Salkovskis, P. M. (1989). Somatic problems. In K. Hawton, P. M. Salkovskis, J. Kirk, & D. M. Clark (Eds.), *Cognitive behaviour therapy for psychiatric problems.* Oxford, England: Oxford University Press.

Salkovskis, P. M., & Harrison, J. (1984). Abnormal and normal obsessions: A replication. *Behaviour Research and Therapy, 22*, 549–552.

Salkovskis, P. M., & Warwick, H. M. C. (1986). Morbid preoccupations, health anxiety and reassurance: A cognitive-behavioural approach to hypochondriasis. *Behaviour Research and Therapy, 24*, 597–602.

Salkovskis, P. M., & Westbrook, D. (1989). Behavior therapy and obsessional ruminations: Can failure be turned into success? *Behaviour Research and Therapy, 27*, 149–160.

Spitzer, R. L., Williams, J. B. W., & Gibbons, M. (1987). Structured Clinical Interview for DSM-III-R-Patient Version. Biometrics Research Department, New York State Psychiatric Institute, 722 W. 168th St., New York, New York 10032.

Steketee, G. S. (1987). *Predicting relapse following behavioral treatment for obsessive-compulsive disorder: The impact of social support.* Ann Arbor, Michigan: UMI Dissertation Information Service.

Steketee, G. (1990). Personality traits and disorders in obsessive-compulsives. *Journal of Anxiety Disorders, 4*, 351–364.

Steketee, G., & Cleere, L. (1990). Obsessive-compulsive disorders. In A. S. Bellack, M. Hersen, & A. E. Kazdin (Eds.), *International handbook of behavior modification and therapy.* New York: Plenum Press.

Steketee, G. S., & Foa, E. B. (1985). Obsessive-compulsive disorder. In D. H. Barlow (Ed.), *Clinical handbook of psychological disorders: A step-by-step treatment manual.* New York: Guilford Press.

Steketee, G., & Freund, B. (1990, November). *Psychometric properties of the Compulsive Activity Checklist.* Paper presented at the Association for Advancement of Behavior Therapy, San Francisco.

Steketee, G., & White, K. (1990). *When once is not enough.* Oakland, CA: New Harbinger.

Steketee, G. S., Foa, E. B., & Grayson, J. B. (1982). Recent advances in the behavioral treatment of obsessive-compulsives. *Archives of General Psychiatry, 39*, 1365–1371.

Stern, R. S. (1978). Obsessive thoughts: The problem of therapy. *British Journal of Psychiatry, 133*, 200–205.

Sternberger, L. G., & Burns, G. L. (1990a). Compulsive Activity checklist and the Maudsley Obsessional-Compulsive Inventory: Psychometric properties of two measures of obsessive-compulsive disorder. *Behavior Therapy, 21*, 117–127.

Sternberger, L. G., & Burns, G. L. (1990b). Maudsley Obsessional-Compulsive Inventory: Obsessions and compulsions in a nonclinical sample. *Behaviour Research and Therapy, 28,* 337–340.

Swedo, S. E., Rapoport, J. L., Leonard, H. L., Lenane, M. C., & Cheslow, D. L. (1989). Obsessive-compulsive disorder in children and adolescents. *Archives of General Psychiatry, 46,* 335–341.

Swedo, S. E., Lenane, M. C., Leonard, H. L., & Rapoport, J. L. (1990, November). *Drug treatment of trichotillomania: Two year follow-up.* Paper presented at the meeting of the Association for the Advancement of Behavior Therapy, San Francisco.

Teasdale, J. D. (1974). Learning models of obsessional compulsive disorder. In H. R. Beech (Ed.), *Obsessional states.* London: Methuen.

Thoren, P., Asberg, M., Cronholm, B., Jornstedt, L., & Traskman, L. (1980). Clomipramine treatment of obsessive-compulsive disorder: A controlled clinical trial. *Archives of General Psychiatry, 37,* 1281–1285.

Turner, S. M., Hersen, M., Bellack, A. S., Andrasik, F., & Capparell, H. V. (1980). Behavioral and pharmacological treatment of obsessive-compulsive disorders. *Journal of Nervous and Mental Disease, 168,* 651–657.

Turner, S. M., Jacob, R. G., Beidel, D. C., & Himmelhock, J. (1985). Fluoxetine treatment of obsessive-compulsive disorder. *Journal of Clinical Psychopharmacology, 5,* 207–212.

Tynes, L. L., White, K., & Steketee, G. (1990). Toward a new nosology of obsessive compulsive disorder. *Comprehensive Psychiatry, 31,* 465–480.

Van den Hout, M., Emmelkamp, P., Kraaykamp, H., & Griez, E. (1988). Behavioral treatment of obsessive-compulsives: Inpatient vs. outpatient. *Behavior Research and Therapy, 26,* 331–332.

Volavka, J., Neziroglu, F., & Yaryura Tobias, J. A. (1985). Clomipramine and imipramine in obsessive-compulsive disorder. *Psychiatry, 14,* 85–93.

Watts, E. N. (1971). *An investigation of imaginal desensitization as a habituation process.* Unpublished doctoral dissertation, University of London.

Welner, A., Reich, T., Robins, E., Fishman, R., & Van Doren, T. (1976). Obsessive-compulsive neurosis: Record, follow-up, and family studies. *Comprehensive Psychiatry, 17,* 527–539.

Westphal, K. (1878). Über Zwangsvorstellungen. *Archiv Psychiatric Nervenkrankheiten, 8,* 734–750.

White, K., Steketee, G., & Julian, J. (1990). *Course and comorbidity in OCD.* Unpublished manuscript.

12

Assessment and Treatment of Panic Disorder and Agoraphobia

MICHELLE G. CRASKE

INTRODUCTION

In a medical-psychiatric setting, panic disorder and agoraphobia (PDA) may be either a primary reason for admission or an additional feature of other medical or psychiatric difficulties. A psychiatric hospital has particular relevance to the assessment and treatment of PDA: Because PDA is characterized by a fear of specific bodily sensations and the avoidance of being alone or without help, the setting itself may inadvertently reinforce agoraphobic fear and avoidance behavior. That is, the medical setting is a particularly "safe" environment for the panicker and/or agoraphobic because of the availability of medical care and support personnel and the protectiveness of the environment. Consequently, the medical setting may be (although, not necessarily) counterproductive to the treatment goals of learning to be less fearful and more independent.

In this chapter, a description of the disorder is followed by a delineation of the reasons that PDA may present in a medical-psychiatric setting. The prototypical method of assessment for PDA is outlined, as well as the considerations relevant to assessment in a medical-psychiatric setting. Similarly, the prototypical cognitive-behavioral treatment for PDA is described, along with recommended modifications and considerations relevant to particular settings.

DESCRIPTION OF PANIC DISORDER AND AGORAPHOBIA

Features of the Clinical Syndrome

Definition of Panic Attack. In the most recent edition of the *Diagnostic and Statistical Manual of Mental Disorders* (DSM-III-R; American Psychiatric Association, 1987), panic attacks are defined as acute episodes of intense fear or discomfort, associated on at least one occasion with at least 4 of 13 physical and cognitive symptoms. The criteria for panic disorder (PD) specify that at least one attack must be "unexpected," and that the attacks must

MICHELLE G. CRASKE • Department of Psychology, University of California—Los Angeles, Los Angeles, California 90024-1563.

Handbook of Behavior Therapy in the Psychiatric Setting, edited by Alan S. Bellack and Michel Hersen. Plenum Press, New York, 1993.

have occurred at least four times in four weeks or must have been followed by at least one month of apprehension about their recurrence. Revisions of the criteria will appear in the publication of the DSM-IV projected in 1993. Nevertheless, the defining features will remain (1) the experience of sudden rushes of intense fear or discomfort for no apparent reason, which are distinct from gradually building anxious arousal and from phobic reactions to clearly discernible, circumscribed stimuli, and (2) apprehension about the attacks, even in the absence of identifiable triggers. The symptoms reported to occur most frequently during panic attacks include dizziness, unsteadiness or faintness, palpitations or tachycardia, trembling or shaking, parasthesias, sweating, and fears of going crazy and losing control (Barlow, Vermilyea, Blanchard, Vermilyea, DiNardo, & Cerny, 1985; Rapee, Craske, & Barlow, 1990a).

Conceptualization of Panic Attacks. The phenomenon of panic has been conceptualized from various perspectives, including cognitive (Beck, 1988; Clark, Salkovskis, & Chalkley, 1985), neurochemical (e.g., Charney, Heninger, & Breier, 1984; Gorman, Fyer, Goetz, Askanazi, Liebowitz, Fyer, Kinney, & Klein, 1988), and psychobiological or cognitive-behavioral (Barlow, 1988; Ehlers & Margraf, 1989). The psychobiological models are the most comprehensive and include the following types of factors: physiological predispositions, stressful life events, learned associations between certain bodily sensations and panic, and danger-laden beliefs about the symptoms of anxious arousal.

According to the psychobiological conceptualization presented by Barlow (1988), panic attacks are triggered by certain bodily sensations of which the individual has learned to be afraid (through earlier traumatic associations with panic attacks). A positive feedback loop is proposed to account for the acceleration into panic, because the stimulus that is feared (i.e., symptoms of arousal) intensifies as a function of the fear response. According to this model, panic attacks are not spontaneous but are triggered by subtle physiological changes of which the individual may not be fully aware. As a result, panic attacks may be triggered by subtle changes in breathing, or by activities that elicit sensations of arousal (such as ingesting caffeine, sexual arousal, aerobic activities, and hot, steamy showers). A full description of this formulation can be found in Barlow (1988).

Definition of Agoraphobia. Agoraphobia is specified in the DSM-III-R as avoidance, or endurance with distress, of situations from which escape may be difficult or in which help is unavailable in the event of a panic attack, or a fear of developing symptoms that may be incapacitating or embarrassing (e.g., loss of bowel control or vomiting). Typical agoraphobic situations include shopping malls, waiting lines, movie theaters, buses or cars, and crowded restaurants and stores, as well as being far from home and being alone. Three levels of avoidance are specified to reflect differing levels of restriction on mobility: mild, moderate, and severe, the last characterizing the truly "housebound" agoraphobic. As the degree of agoraphobia worsens, individuals typically become increasingly dependent on others. As a result, family roles and the assignment of daily responsibilities may alter dramatically.

The avoidance component extends beyond overt avoidance of agoraphobic-type situations. For example, it may include persistent attempts to "keep busy" in order to distract oneself from feared bodily sensations, an avoidance of activities that elicit sensations similar to panic attack symptoms (such as cardiovascular exercise or the ingestion of caffeine), or the maintenance of proximity to safety signals, such as medical facilities and telephones, in the event of a panic attack. In other words, avoidance behavior may be subtle or obvious.

Relationship between Panic and Agoraphobia. In most instances, agoraphobic avoidance develops following an initial, unexpected panic attack (Craske, Miller, Rotunda, & Barlow, 1990; Noyes, Crowe, Harris, Hamra, McChesney, & Chaudhry, 1986; Pollard, Bronson, & Kenney, 1989a; Swinson, 1986; Thyer, Himle, Curtis, Cameron, & Nesse, 1985). Therefore, agoraphobia is conceptualized as one means of coping with the threat of panicking (Craske & Barlow, 1988). This view is supported by the fact that panic disorder with agoraphobia and panic disorder without agoraphobia share many features, including age of onset, symptom profiles, fears of symptoms, and panic frequency (see Craske & Barlow, 1988, for a review).

As the degree of avoidance becomes more severe, the proportion of females increases (Reich, Noyes, & Troughton, 1987; Thyer *et al.*, 1985). On average, 57% of mild avoiders are female, in comparison to 80% of severe avoiders. The predominance of females has been attributed to sociocultural factors, as dependency and avoidance behaviors are more acceptable for females than for males. This conjecture is supported by the finding that the degree of agoraphobic avoidance is predicted more strongly by "femininity-masculinity" measures than by sex-gender measures (Chambless & Mason, 1986). In addition, it is believed that males are more likely to use alcohol and/or drugs (as opposed to avoidance) to alleviate panic and anxiety (Barlow, 1988).

Panic Apprehension. Of the general population, 6%–12% report having experienced a panic attack that occurred for no apparent reason in the previous year (Brown, Cash, & Deagle, 1988; Craske & Kreuger, 1990; Norton, Doward, & Cox, 1980; Salge, Beck, & Logan, 1988; Telch, Lucas, & Nelson, 1989). However, according to data from the Epidemiological Catchment Area (ECA) Study, only 2%–6% meet the criteria for PD or PDA (Weissman, Leaf, Blazer, Boyd, & Florio, 1986).

What differentiates infrequent panickers from those who go on to develop PD? The key variable may be chronic, anxious apprehension about the experience of panic (Barlow, 1988). Chronic apprehension is characterized by heightened chronic arousal, body vigilance or selectivity of attention to feared bodily sensations, and cognitive misappraisals of bodily sensations as being harmful. These features may result in a maintaining pattern of continuing panic and apprehension (Barlow, 1988). In support of Barlow's model (1988), PD/PDAs tend to misappraise bodily symptoms as more threatening (Chambless, Caputo, Bright, & Gallagher, 1984; Reiss, Peterson, Gursky, & McNally, 1986), to report more arousal symptomatology (Holt & Andrews, 1989), and to be more interoceptively aware (Ehlers & Margraf, 1989) than other anxiety disorder groups.

Familial Patterns. On average, anxiety disorders are observed in 15%–20% of first-degree relatives of PDA patients. This proportion is about five times higher than the rate observed in the general population (Carey & Gottesman, 1981; Weissman, Myers, Leckman, Harding, Pauls, & Prusoff, 1984b). Concordance ratios from twin studies are suggestive of familial transmission also, particularly in the case of agoraphobic avoidance (Crowe, Noyes, Pauls, & Slymen, 1983; Torgersen, 1983). PDA also tends to be predictive of familial depression and substance abuse (Harris, Noyes, Crowe, & Chaudhry, 1983; Weissman, Leckman, Merikangas, Gammon, & Prusoff, 1984a). These data suggest neither a simple recessive genetic transmission nor purely cultural transmission. Rather, a family history of panic or agoraphobia may reflect an inherited vulnerability to a cluster of emotional problems.

Clinical Presentation

The mean age of onset of PDA ranges from 23 to 29 years, and the mean age at which treatment is sought is 34 years (Breier, Charney, & Heninger, 1986; Craske *et al.*, 1990; Noyes *et al.*, 1986). The initial attack usually occurs in the context of stressful life events (Craske *et al.*, 1990; Faravelli & Pallanti, 1989; Pollard, Pollard, & Corn, 1989b; Rapee, Litwin, & Barlow, 1990b; Roy-Byrne, Geraci, & Uhde, 1986). Approximately one half report having experienced "panicky" feelings at some time before their first attack. Thus, the onset may be either insidious or acute (Craske *et al.*, 1990). In most cases, PDA is accompanied by additional diagnoses or diagnostic features. For example, Sanderson, DiNardo, Rapee, and Barlow (1990) found that of 55 principally diagnosed PD/PDAs, 22% had additional diagnostic features of social phobia; 13% the diagnostic features of generalized anxiety disorder; 40%, of specific phobias; and 2%, of obsessive-compulsive disorder.

Depressive Features. Depending on the particular study, from 7% to 35% of PD/PDAs meet the criteria for additional concurrent diagnoses of major depression or dysthymia (Moras, 1989). Furthermore, the lifetime incidence of depression in PDAs is in the range of 20%–90% (Cassano, Perugi, Musetti, & Akiskal, 1989). Chronological surveys indicate that anxiety precedes the onset of depression in most cases (Alloy, Kelly, Mineka, & Clements, 1989).

Personality Disorders. Depending on the method of personality assessment, from 27%–50% of PD/PDA patients meet the DSM-III or DSM-III-R criteria for an Axis II disorder (Reich, 1988; Reich & Noyes, 1987). The most predominant personality disorders are dependent and avoidant (Mavissakalian & Hamman, 1986; Reich, Noyes, & Troughton, 1987). Currently, it is unclear whether the personality features precede and/or predispose one to the development of PD/PDA or develop as a consequence of PD/PDA. In support of the latter supposition, Mavissakalian and Hamman (1987) found that dependent personality features improved following a successful combined drug-behavioral treatment for PDA. On the other hand, avoidant personality features did not change as a result of this treatment.

Alcohol and Drug Use. PDA is frequently associated with alcohol and drug use. Anthony, Tien, and Petronis (1989) found that panic attacks were associated with cocaine and heavy alcohol use in the ECA community sample. Cox, Norton, Swinson, and Endler (1990) found that approximately 10%–40% of alcoholics met the criteria for a panic-related anxiety disorder, and about 10%–20% of anxiety disorder patients abused alcohol or other drugs. The relationship between PDA and alcohol and drug use may take various forms. For example, a substantial minority of PDA patients relate the onset of their anxiety problem to drug use (Aronson & Craig, 1986; Craske *et al.*, 1990). In addition, panic attacks and symptoms are frequently experienced during withdrawal from drug use. Furthermore, alcohol and drugs are commonly used to alleviate anxiety, and at the same time, others report discontinuation of drugs for fear that continued drug use will exacerbate panic symptomatology.

Presentation in a Medical or Psychiatric Setting

PDA may present in a medical-psychiatric setting for one of two main reasons: as a direct function of the symptomatology of PDA or as a result of comorbid diagnoses. In the domain of direct symptomatology, three possibilities are presented here.

First, the acute physical symptomatology of PDA may serve as a major impetus to seek medical help, especially because the symptoms are commonly misappraised as being life-threatening. For example, Thompson, Burns, Barkto, Boyd, Taube, and Bourdon (1988) found agoraphobia to be the most common phobia leading to the use of health services, especially when accompanied by panic attacks. Similarly, Boyd (1986) reported that the presence of panic attacks in a diagnostic profile (of various emotional and psychotic disorders) was associated with a significantly increased use of medical services. Also, the urgency of obtaining medical assistance is reflected in the high frequency with which panickers attend emergency room facilities. Extreme fears for one's own physical or mental well-being may easily result in admission to a hospital.

A second reason why PDA might lead directly to hospitalization is the risk of suicide. Weissman, Klerman, Markowitz, and Ouellette (1989) reported a marked elevation in suicide attempts by PDs in comparison to other anxiety and mood disorder groups. It is noteworthy, however, that many PDAs fear harming themselves because of "loss of control" (e.g., fears of loss of control while driving leading to driving off the side of the road); this fear is very distinct from thoughts about wanting to end one's life. Therefore, care must be taken not to confuse fears of losing control and inadvertently harming oneself with suicidal ideation.

Third, the severity of agoraphobic avoidance and panic attacks may lead to hospitalization. In some instances, impairment in functioning is extreme, as fears of leaving the house, even if accompanied, may be extremely debilitating. The severity of the disorder may be compounded by lack of social support systems. Very severe presentations of PDA may be the result of an insidious development over the course of months or years. Alternatively, very severe presentations may be the result of acute withdrawal and rebound effects from the termination of anxiolytic medications.

Reasons for hospitalization that are not a direct function of PDA include additional psychiatric diagnoses, such as alcohol or drug abuse or dependence, severe depression, psychosis, or impairment in functioning due to personality disorders. The recently reported incidence of panic attacks in schizophrenic samples is one such example (Argyle, 1990; Kahn, Drusin, & Klein, 1987). Finally, medical conditions that exacerbate a PDA condition may cause hospitalization. Examples include heart disease, diabetes, or chronic obstructive lung disease, which may complicate behavioral and pharmacological treatment approaches.

Assessment of Panic Disorder and Agoraphobia

Prototypical Assessment

The prototypical method of assessing PDA includes diagnostic interview instruments, standardized self-report inventories, client ratings, self-monitoring, behavioral assessment, and medical evaluation. On average, the diagnosis of PDA is not particularly difficult, as evidenced by the generally high rates of agreement between two independent diagnosticians (e.g., DiNardo & Barlow, 1989; Mannuzza, Fyer, Martin, Gallops, Endicott, Gorman, Liebowitz, & Klein, 1990). The areas of most confusion and disagreement include the level of agoraphobia (i.e., mild, moderate, or severe), the differentiation of PDA with mild avoidance from specific phobias of certain "agoraphobia-type" situations (such as claustrophobic situations), and the differentiation of PDA and social phobia. These diagnostic boundary issues are being addressed by the DSM-IV Anxiety Disorders Task Force.

Interviews.   Several semistructured diagnostic interviews yield reliable diagnostic judgments for PDA. One is the Anxiety Disorders Interview Schedule—Revised (ADIS-R; DiNardo & Barlow, 1988; DiNardo & Barlow, 1989), which covers anxiety and depressive disorders, brief screens for other psychiatric disorders, and psychosocial history factors. The Hamilton Anxiety and Depression scales are also embedded in this interview. Two other structured interviews are also commonly used. The Structured Clinical Interview for DSM-III diagnoses (SCID; Spitzer, Williams, & Gibbons, 1985) and the Schedule for Affective Disorders and Schizophrenia-Lifetime Anxiety Version—Revised (SADS-LA; Fyer, Endicott, Mannuzza, & Klein, 1985) have been shown to yield reliable PDA diagnoses. The SCID and SADS-LA cover other psychiatric conditions in more detail and anxiety disorders in less detail than the ADIS-R. Clinicians in practice may not want to administer these interviews in their entirety, given their length (i.e., the complete ADIS-R may take two to three hours to complete). However, certain items may be particularly valuable aids in differential diagnosis.

Whether one is using a semistructured interview or an open clinical interview, it is important to obtain information regarding the frequency of panic, the panic symptoms and cognitions, worry or apprehension about the recurrence of panic, avoidance behavior, and associated features (such as depression, alcohol or drug abuse, and complicating medical conditions). Also, information about idiosyncratic safety signals, which are used as "protectors" against panicking, is important for treatment planning because they represent another form of avoidance. Typical safety signals include medication, food or drink, bags, bracelets, smelling salts and antacid, paper bags (to control hyperventilation), reading materials, alcohol, and relaxation tapes (Barlow, 1988).

Self-Report Inventories.   Several standardized and normatively based questionnaires take little time to complete yet provide valuable supplementary information. One is the Mobility

Inventory for gauging the degree of agoraphobic avoidance (Chambless Caputo, Jasin, Gracely, & Williams, 1985). This inventory is a 27-item checklist of situations that are rated in terms of the degree to which they are avoided when the patient is alone and when the patient is accompanied. The Marks and Mathews Fear Questionnaire includes a short subscale of five agoraphobia terms (Marks & Mathews, 1979); however, a more complete profile of the various situations that are avoided may be obtained from the Mobility Inventory.

Fear of panic symptoms may be measured with the Anxiety Sensitivity Index (Reiss *et al.*, 1986). This 16-item scale has good psychometric properties and measures the extent to which the physical symptoms of anxious arousal are viewed as harmful. The Agoraphobia Cognitions Questionnaire and the Body Sensations Questionnaire (Chambless *et al.*, 1984) also measure fear of panic symptoms. They correlate highly with the Anxiety Sensitivity Index. Because the measures developed by Chambless and colleagues are in the form of checklists, they are clinically useful in identifying the person's most feared sensations and most typical danger-laden cognitions.

All of these self-report measures are sensitive to change as a result of treatment. Hence, they can be used to gauge therapeutic progress.

Client Ratings. An alternative to the Mobility Inventory is an individualized hierarchy of situations that are feared and/or avoided (Barlow, 1988). The hierarchy may be generated with the help of the client, following the interview. The fear and avoidance hierarchy is useful for assessing progress because it reflects the areas of most functional relevance to the particular client. In addition, it may be used as a guide for conducting *in vivo* exposure practices because the list of situations is ordered by difficulty level.

Self-Monitoring. Years of research in behavioral assessment have demonstrated the value of self-monitoring of events as they occur in contrast to retrospective recall. The value of self-monitoring seems to be particularly strong for panic attacks because of the tendency to overestimate the number and severity of panic attacks experienced in the past (Margraf, Taylor, Ehlers, Roth, & Agras, 1987; Rapee *et al.*, 1990a). Inflationary recall biases may contribute to increased apprehension about future attacks. Therefore, self-monitoring provides more accurate information about progress, and therapeutically, it minimizes the negative influence of inflationary biases. In addition, a functional analysis of antecedents and consequences is obtainable through self-monitoring.

Self-monitoring procedures have been incorporated fully into the assessment and treatment of PDA (e.g., Barlow, Craske, Cerny, & Klosko, 1989). However, compliance with instructions for on-the-spot monitoring may create problems. Increased time spent with the client to emphasize the value of self-monitoring and to give corrective feedback about the self-monitoring procedures usually increases compliance rates (Barlow, 1988).

Three self-monitoring procedures for PDA have been developed and refined at the Center for Stress and Anxiety Disorders at the University at Albany, State University of New York (SUNY). The first is the Panic Attack Record (see Figure 1) for recording symptomatology, duration, presence of others, expectedness, and maximum level of anxiety.

The Weekly Record of Anxiety and Depression entails end-of-the-day ratings of background anxiety, depression, pleasantness, "fear" of panic attacks, and medication use (see Figure 2). Instructions for discriminating panic attacks from generalized anxiety are usually given. The discrimination is based primarily on the suddenness of onset and the immediacy of the sense on fear or danger, as opposed to a slowly building, anxious arousal in anticipation of future events.

Finally, the Daily Activity Record is useful for assessing agoraphobic avoidance (see Figure 3). This record is a behavioral checklist. At the end of the day, clients check which tasks they attempted or completed. For attempted or completed tasks, the level of anxiety and the presence of others are indicated. In addition to keeping track of progress, this form is useful for recording structured exposure-practice assignments.

Behavioral Assessment. Direct observation of clients in their own environment provides information about changes in approach behavior as a result of treatment, as well as subtle patterns of avoidance of which the individual may not be fully aware. Unfortunately, behavioral observation is time-consuming and not always practical. Nevertheless, the results of behavioral assessments do not always coincide with the results of self-report and interview assessments (Rachman & Hodgson, 1974). For example, clients may report that they are comfortably able to enter a shopping mall but show severe distress and escape behavior during behavioral testing. For this reason, a comprehensive and accurate assessment warrants the inclusion of behavioral assessment. In a research setting, the behavioral assessment is frequently supplemented with physiological measures of anticipatory and actual arousal while the subject confronts feared situations. In an individualized behavioral assessment, clients may be asked to attempt three to five items from their fear and avoidance hierarchy, to the best of their ability, while fear levels and behaviors are recorded (see Barlow, 1988, for a complete description).

Also, specific exercises that have been designed to elicit paniclike physical symptoms may be used in behavioral assessments of fear and avoidance of bodily sensations (Barlow *et al.*, 1989). These exercises include spinning in a swivel chair, overbreathing or hyperventilating, and forms of cardiovascular exercise. The exercises are described in more detail in the treatment section.

Medical Evaluation. Medical evaluation is important for at least two reasons. First, the presence of certain medical conditions may place limits on the types of treatment procedures used. For example, high-intensity exposure would be contraindicated for patients with high blood pressure or angina pectoris. Second, several medical conditions produce symptoms that mimic the symptoms of high anxiety or panic attacks (Taylor, 1987). Therefore, differential diagnosis is important.

The medical conditions that mimic panic attack symptomatology include hypoglycemia

---

Panic Attack Record

Name: ____________________

Date: ____________ Time: ________ Duration: ________ (mins.)

With Spouse ______ Friend ______ Stranger ______ Alone ______

Stressful situation: Yes/No Expected: Yes/No

Maximum anxiety (circle):

0——1——2——3——4——5——6——7——8

None Moderate Extreme

Sensations (check):

Pounding heart	___	Sweating	___	Hot/cold flash	___
Tight/painful chest	___	Choking	___	Fear of dying	___
Breathless	___	Nausea	___	Fear of going crazy	___
Dizzy	___	Unreality	___	Fear of losing	
Trembling	___	Numb/tingle	___	control	___

Figure 1. Panic Attack Record Form (Center for Stress and Anxiety Disorders, Albany, New York).

(low blood sugar levels), hyperthyroidism (hyperactive thyroid gland), hypoparathyroidism (deficiencies in secretion of the parathyroid hormone), Cushing's syndrome (increased circulating levels of cortisol), pheochromocytoma (tumor, usually on the adrenal glands), temporal lobe epilepsy, caffeine intoxication, and illicit drug use. A review of these conditions is found in Katon (1989). However, although these conditions may account completely for panic symptomatology, they may co-occur with panic and exacerbate panic disorder pathology.

Assessment in Medical-Psychiatric Settings

Differentiation from Medical Conditions. As noted above, identifying medical conditions that either mimic or exacerbate PDA symptomatology is a key issue. Differentiation of PDA from medical conditions is difficult because of the predominant somatic component of

---

WEEKLY RECORD OF ANXIETY AND DEPRESSION

Name _____ Date _____

Each evening before you go to bed, please rate your *average* level of anxiety (taking all things into consideration) throughout the day, the *maximum* level of anxiety which you experienced that day, your *average* level of depression throughout the day and your average feeling of pleasantness throughout the day. Use the scale below. Next, please list the dosages and amounts of any medication you took. Finally, please rate, using the scale below, how worried or frightened you were on average about the possibility of having a panic attack throughout the day.

Level of anxiety/depression/pleasant feelings

```
0———————1———————2———————3———————4———————5———————6———————7———————8
None         Slight        Moderate           A lot        As much
                                                            as you
                                                            can
                                                            imagine
```

Date	Average anxiety	Maximum anxiety	Average depression	Average pleasantness	Medication type, dose, number (mg)	Fear of panic

Figure 2. Weekly record of anxiety and depression (Center for Stress and Anxiety Disorders, Albany, New York).

Daily Activity Monitoring

Name _____ Date _____

Maximum and
average anxiety: 0————————2————————4————————6————————8
                    None   Mild   Moderate   Strong   Extreme

Activity	Check if done today	Mostly alone (75%)	Duration (mins.)	Maximum anxiety (0–8)	Average anxiety (0–8)
Work					
Shopping Mall					
Large store					
Small store					
Supermarket					
Corner store					
Bank					
Gas station					
Standing in line					
Driving Highway					
Other roads					
Bridge					
Passenger Highway					
Other roads					
Bridge					
Bus					
Taxi					

Figure 3. Excerpt from Daily Activity Monitoring form (Center for Stress and Anxiety Disorders, Albany, New York).

PDA. A balanced perspective is needed to prevent discounting medical factors, on the one hand, and excessive medical testing (in response to physical symptomatology), on the other hand.

Overreporting of symptoms is a characteristic feature of PDA because of oversensitivity to internal physical changes and fear of the symptoms of arousal (Barlow, 1988). Katon (1984) found that 89% of a group of 55 primary-care patients who were referred for psychiatric consultation (and received a diagnosis of PDA) had initially presented with one or more somatic symptoms. In addition, in some instances, misdiagnosis as a medical problem had continued for months or years. Overuse of medical testing was reported by Clancy and Noyes (1976); their group of PDA patients had undergone an average of 7.5 medical tests. In their sample, medical testing was particularly likely when cardiovascular symptoms were reported. Another example of symptom overreporting is the common report of hyperventilatory symptoms in the absence of physical evidence (i.e., low pCO_2 values) of hyperventilatory respiration patterns (Holt & Andrews, 1989).

The differentiation is even more difficult when physical conditions coexist with PDA or exacerbate PDA symptomatology. A fairly common example is mitral valve prolapse (MVP). With MVP symptoms, the panicker may be more likely to spiral into a full-blown panic attack than without them. Barlow (1988) wrote that "the ultimate test is whether the patient with a physical disorder stops panicking once the disorder is properly diagnosed and treated. If not, then it is probably time to deal with the panic disorder in its own right" (p. 372).

Differentiation from Somatoform Disorders. Another difficult differentiation likely to be encountered in the medical setting is between PDA and somatoform disorders. In general, somatoform disorders are more likely to be characterized by a disease conviction (as in hypochondriasis), or by symptoms that do not match the cluster of panic attack symptoms (as in somatization). Another differentiating factor is onset and course. Somatization usually begins in the late teens and is chronic, whereas PDA tends to occur in the mid to late 20s and shows a more fluctuating course. On the other hand, PDA patients tend to score high on illness attitude scales and measures of somatization (Katon, 1984; Salkovskis, Warwick, & Clark, 1990).

Timing of Assessment. The timing of the assessment of PDA is important, particularly when PDA is not the primary reason for hospitalization. An assessment of PDA is best conducted following the stabilization of physical and mental status, such as after withdrawal from abused substances or after the successful control of a complicating medical condition. Otherwise, the overlap in physical symptomatology of PDA and the coexisting conditions may prevent an accurate diagnosis. Furthermore, coexisting conditions may limit the physical and/or mental capacity necessary to complete the PDA assessments.

The recent initiation of a medication regime raises issues of assessment timing also. For example, the side effects of the medication may confound PDA assessment, as may the period of psychological adjustment to receiving a pharmacological substance. Consequently, an initial screen should be followed by a more complete assessment once a stabilization of medication has been achieved.

Compliance with Assessment Procedures. Compliance with assessment procedures requiring ongoing effort (such as self-monitoring) may be particularly poor as a result of the types of comorbid diagnoses most likely to present in a medical-psychiatric setting (such as severe depression, psychoses, or impairing personality traits). At the least, repeated prompting and corrective feedback may be necessary. Similarly, self-reporting of symptoms or distress levels may be overdramatized. This bias may be minimized by corrective training regarding the defining characteristics of panic attacks, or by the use of scales with behaviorally descriptive anchors. For example, anxiety levels may be tied to the number of times that verbal reassurances of safety are sought, or to the number of times that the heart rate is checked (for fear of heart attack). Despite the potential problems in self-monitoring, it is considered worthwhile, given the potentially therapeutic effect of learning to record anxiety and panic reactions objectively.

An alternative to self-monitoring is event sampling or time sampling of relevant PDA behaviors (such as panicking, help seeking, or approach-avoidance) by the staff of the medical-psychiatric facility. Recording by independent observers provides information regarding the antecedents and consequences of the PDA behaviors to be targeted for modification. For example, the number of times that patients request medication or verbal reassurances of their mental and/or physical safety (e.g., "Am I losing control?" "Am I going to die?" "Will I faint?") or remain close to walls or rails for physical support (to prevent collapsing) may be monitored.

Assessment of Generalization. Cognitive-behavioral treatment conducted in a hospital environment entails practice exposure to tasks within the constraints of that environment. Therefore, for effective treatment planning, the behavioral measures (i.e., daily activity monitoring, the fear and avoidance hierarchy, and behavioral assessments) should include items relevant to the hospital setting. After completion of the hospital-based treatment, an equally important assessment is of behavior in the home environment, which determines the degree to which gains made in the hospital environment have generalized to the home environment, as well as the need for further outpatient care. For this reason, daily activity forms of fear and avoidance hierarchies should also include items relevant to the home environment.

Behavioral Treatment of Panic and Agoraphobia

Behavioral treatments for agoraphobia began in the 1960s with systematic desensitization. The behavioral treatments for panic attacks did not begin until the 1970s, when "stress management" techniques were used, consistent with the conceptualization of panic attacks as nonspecific, free-floating anxiety. In the 1980s, significant advances were made in the behavioral treatments for PD, and refinements were made in the treatments for agoraphobia.

Prototypical Treatment of Agoraphobia

The treatment procedure of choice for agoraphobia is *in vivo* exposure, that is, repeated confrontation with or approach to situations that have been avoided. Outcome results can be summarized as follows. When dropouts are excluded, 60%–70% of agoraphobics who complete treatment show clinical improvement, which is maintained, on average four years or more (Burns, Thorpe, & Cavallaro, 1986; Cohen, Monteiro, & Marks, 1984; Hafner, 1976; Jansson, Jerremalm, & Ost, 1986; Jansson & Ost, 1982; Marks, 1971; Munby & Johnston, 1980). However, the median dropout rate is 12% (Barlow & Waddell, 1985), with a range as high as 25%–40% under certain conditions (Jansson & Ost, 1982; Zitrin, Klein, & Woerner, 1980). Also, 30%–40% who complete treatment fail to benefit, and of the remaining 60%–70%, a substantial proportion may not attain clinically meaningful levels of functioning. The percentage who are classified as high end-state (i.e., minimal or no symptoms) ranges from 15%–50%. Finally, as many as 50% who have benefitted clinically may relapse, although the relapse is usually transient and followed by a return of clinical gains (Munby & Johnston, 1980). Attempts to improve efficacy have continued through the examination of various procedural variations, which are described below.

Massed versus Spaced Exposure. At its most intensive, exposure therapy may be conducted three to four hours a day, five days a week (i.e., massed exposure). Spaced exposure entails lengthier intervals between exposure sessions. Long, continuous sessions are generally considered more effective than shorter or interrupted sessions (Chaplin & Levine, 1981; Marshall, 1985; Stern & Marks, 1973).

Originally, it was believed that, although massed sessions produced superior short-term effects (Foa, Jameson, Turner, & Payne, 1980), the long-term effects and consideration of treatment dropouts favored spaced exposure (see Barlow, 1988, for a review of this literature). Recently, comparable short- and long-term effects, including dropout rates, have been demonstrated for massed- and spaced-exposure treatments (Chambless, 1989). However, given the intensive nature of the treatment, massed exposure is not acceptable for everyone. Chambless (1989) concluded by suggesting that the choice of masses versus spaced exposure should be the decision of the therapist and the client.

Graduated versus Intense Exposure. *In vivo* exposure is typically conducted in a graduated format, progressing from the least to the most difficult hierarchy items. Higher level hierarchy items are targeted initially in the more intensive approaches. Feigenbaum (1988) reported very impressive short-term and long-term outcomes from intensive (and massed) exposure treatment conditions. At posttreatment and eight months later, graduated and intensive exposure conditions proved to be equally effective. However, intensive exposure was clearly superior at the five-year follow-up assessment, at which time 76% of the intensive group versus 35% of the graded group reported themselves to be completely free of symptoms. This dramatic set of results suggests that an intensive approach is most beneficial (at least, for massed exposures). Unfortunately, acceptance rates were not reported. It is possible that massed and intensive exposure are acceptable to fewer PDAs, but for those who do assent, the outcome is likely to be more effective than for spaced or graduated exposure. Therefore, the decision to use graduated or intense exposure may best be left to the individual client and therapist.

Self-Directed versus Therapist-Directed Exposure. Several manuals that outline self-directed exposure methods are available (Marks, 1978; Mathews, Gelder, & Johnston, 1981; Weeks, 1976). Ghosh and Marks (1987), Mathews *et al.* (1981), and Jannoun, Munby, Catalan, & Gelder (1980) have found that structured, manualized programs, with minimal therapist contact, are as effective as more intensive therapist contact. Similar success has been obtained with telephone-directed exposure (McNamee, O'Sullivan, Lelliot, & Mark, 1989). However, some evidence suggests that self-directed behavioral treatment is less effective for the more severe, housebound agoraphobics (Holden, O'Brien, Barlow, Stetson, & Infantino, 1983).

Another way of encouraging self-directed exposure practice is to include family members or significant others in the treatment process. The involvement of significant others in all aspects of assessment and treatment has been shown to produce results superior to the exclusion of significant others (Barlow, O'Brien, & Last, 1984), a finding that is particularly evident two years following treatment (Cerny, Barlow, Craske, & Himadi, 1987). In this type of treatment, couples participate in a group treatment and are instructed in methods of exposure practice. Spouses are taught to serve as coaches in the design and practice of exposure tasks, and in the application of anxiety-control strategies. The addition of communication training to exposure conducted in a couples format has also been found to enhance gains from exposure procedures (Arnow, Taylor, Agras, & Telch, 1985).

Cognitive and Somatic Coping Strategies. Various anxiety-control strategies have been used to reduce levels of anxiety during *in vivo* exposure. These include cognitive methods such as distraction, coping self-statements (e.g., instructing oneself to stay in the situation, accept the feelings, and discount unrealistic beliefs), and paradoxical intention (e.g., confronting and exaggerating fearful imagery). Physical coping strategies include relaxation and medication.

It is clear that the various coping strategies alone are not effective forms of treatment for agoraphobic avoidance (e.g., Emmelkamp, Kuipers, & Eggeraat, 1978). The combination of cognitive strategies with *in vivo* exposure has been shown to be effective (Vermilyea, Boice, & Barlow, 1984), although distraction strategies may have deleterious long-term effects (Craske, Street, & Barlow, 1989). However, the mechanisms by which cognitive strategies, as well as relaxation strategies, enhance the efficacy of *in vivo* exposure have been questioned (Emmelkamp & Mersch, 1982; Jansson *et al.*, 1986; Michelson, Mavissakalian, & Marchione, 1985;

Williams & Rappaport, 1983). On the other hand, attrition rates have been found to be as much as twice as high in exposure-alone conditions (Michelson *et al.*, 1985).

Currently, it is believed that the major value of coping strategies is their positive effect on dropout rates and compliance with exposure instructions. For example, Michelson, Mavissakalian, Marchione, Dancu, and Greenwald (1986) found that subjects who received relaxation training practiced exposure more frequently than did other subjects, both during treatment and at follow-up assessment. Practice has been shown to relate positively to degree of improvement (Barlow *et al.*, 1984; Craske *et al.*, 1989; Vermilyea *et al.*, 1984). Decreasing attrition and increasing compliance with exposure enhances the efficacy of exposure-based treatments. For these reasons, the addition of coping strategies to exposure procedures is generally recommended.

Prototypical Treatment for Panic

Recently developed behavioral treatments for panic can be divided into panic management approaches and interoceptive exposure approaches. The panic management approaches include somatic and cognitive techniques. The somatic techniques include breathing, retraining, applied relaxation, and vagal innervation techniques.

Somatic Strategies. One of the earliest, most dramatic, but uncontrolled, reports of the nonpharmacological treatment of panic attacks was by Clark *et al.* (1985). They developed a cognitive-behavioral treatment, emphasizing breathing retraining. Breathing retraining entails learning slow and sometimes diaphragmatic breathing. Breathing retraining has been used as a treatment procedure because of the similarity between hyperventilatory symptoms and panic attacks, at least in 50%–60% of persons with Panic Dirsorders (e.g., Kraft & Hoogduin, 1984; Rapee, 1985; Salkovskis, Warwick, Clark, & Wessels, 1986).

Unfortunately, the results of respiratory-control training programs are difficult to interpret. Recent research suggests that, despite symptom report, hyperventilation physiology may not play a major role for the majority of panickers (Holt & Andrews, 1989). Therefore, it is unclear whether the benefits of breathing retraining are directly attributable to changes in respiratory patterns. Also, subjects have typically been selected on the basis of exhibiting hyperventilatory symptoms, and therefore, it is unclear how far the findings generalize to patients who do not experience hyperventilatory symptoms. Finally, at least one study did not replicate the success of breathing-retraining treatments (de Ruiter, Rijken, Garssen, & Kraaimaat, 1989).

Another approach used to control physical symptomatology is vagal innervation (Sartory & Olajide, 1988). This procedure entails teaching control of the heart rate through various massage techniques, such as stimulating the vagal receptors through massaging the carotid artery or pressing on one eye during expiration. An initial study showed this procedure to be relatively effective (Sartory & Olajide, 1988).

A form of relaxation known as *applied relaxation* has also shown promising results as a treatment for panic attacks (Ost, 1988). Applied relaxation entails training in progressive muscle relaxation (PMR) until the patient becomes skilled in the use of cue-control procedures. At this point, the relaxation skill is applied to the practice of items from a hierarchy of anxiety-provoking tasks. In contrast to Ost's results (1988), Barlow *et al.* (1989) found that applied PMR was no more effective in the control of panic than a wait-list control condition (when dropouts were included in the outcome analysis). Ost (1988) included interoceptive tasks in the hierarchy of practices, whereas Barlow *et al.* (1989) limited the relaxation practices to situational tasks. As will be discussed below, interoceptive exposure seems to be very effective in the control of panic attacks.

Cognitive Restructuring. Cognitive treatments that focus on correcting misappraisals of bodily sensations as threatening began with Beck's extension (1985) of his cognitive model of depression to anxiety and panic. In this approach, cognitive therapy is conducted in conjunction with behavioral techniques, although the effective mechanism of change is assumed to lie in the cognitive realm. Most emphasis is placed on the tendency to overestimate the danger associated with panic symptoms (e.g., estimates of going crazy, dying, fainting, or doing something embarrassing). Beck (1988) reported an uncontrolled study in which 25 PD patients were treated with cognitive techniques in combination with interoceptive and *in vivo* exposure for an average of 17 individual sessions. At posttreatment and 12-month assessments, the panic response had been eliminated in the 17 patients who did not have additional diagnoses of personality disorder. However, it is difficult to attribute the outcome to cognitive procedures, given the inclusion of specific behavioral treatment procedures.

On the other hand, the preliminary reports of studies going on in Oxford (Clark, 1989) and Marburg (Margraf, 1989) have suggested that cognitive procedures conducted in isolation from exposure procedures are highly effective in controlling panic attacks. The full results of these studies may prove to be very important.

Interoceptive Exposure. The purpose of interoceptive exposure is to disrupt or weaken associations between specific bodily cues and panic reactions. The theoretical basis for the implementation of interoceptive exposure is fear extinction, given the conceptualization of panic attacks as "conditioned" or learned alarm reactions to salient bodily cues (Barlow, 1988). Interoceptive exposure is conducted through procedures that reliably induce panic-type sensations. Based on the promising results of earlier studies using repeated infusions of sodium lactate (Bonn, Harrison, & Rees, 1973; Haslam, 1974) and repeated carbon dioxide inhalations (Griez & van den Hout, 1986), a treatment package incorporating interoceptive exposure was developed and tested (Barlow *et al.*, 1989). Interoceptive exposure entails repeated exposures to exercises entailing forced hyperventilation, spinning, or cardiovascular effort. The "simulation" exercises are followed by practice with naturalistic activities that have been feared and/or avoided because of the physical sensations they elicit. Examples include sports, saunas, and drinking coffee. The treatment conditions entailing interoceptive exposure and cognitive restructuring were significantly superior to applied PMR and wait-list conditions in terms of panic frequency, producing freedom from panic in 87% of patients at posttreatment. These patterns were maintained up to 24 months following treatment completion (Craske, Brown, & Barlow, 1992). A prototypical treatment outline is given in Table 1.

Table 1. Prototypical Treatment of Panic and Agoraphobia

1. *Education* about the nature of panic attacks, including a description of the physiology of panic and a conceptual model of panic attacks emphasizing cognitive misappraisals, learned fear responses, hypervigilance to bodily symptoms, and chronic hyperarousal.
2. *Cognitive restructuring* to learn to correct tendencies to overestimate the danger of physical symptoms, and to catastrophize about panicking.
3. Training in a method of *symptom control*, such as cue-controlled progressive muscle relaxation, breathing retraining, or vagal innervation.
4. *Interoceptive exposure*, to teach patients to be less fearful of certain bodily sensations, using structured exercises (e.g., hyperventilating and cardiovascular exercises) and naturalistic activities (e.g., drinking coffee).
5. *Situational exposure*, to teach patients to be less fearful of certain anticipated situations, with the aid of cognitive and somatic strategies.

Interoceptive and situational exposure may be conducted in a graded or intense format, and in a massed or spaced format, depending on the choice of the patient and the therapist. In addition, self-directed or therapist-directed exposure may be conducted, depending on the severity of the fear and avoidance.

Treatment in Medical and Hospital Settings

The issues to consider with respect to implementing these treatment procedures in a medical hospital environment fall into three main areas: severity, comorbidity, and the setting itself.

Severity. The treatment implications of severe PDA include the pace at which treatment proceeds, the extent to which a therapist directly assists in the *in vivo* exposure practices, and the importance of maximizing generalization to the natural environment following discharge (see "Hospital Setting," below). For example, items in situational and/or interoceptive exposure hierarchies may be divided into smaller steps and may be practiced when accompanied before being practiced alone. On the other hand, a hospital environment is in some ways the best setting for conducting massed and intense exposure, given the environmental controls.

Comorbidity. A question that may arise for patients with additional psychiatric conditions is when to treat PDA. In most cases, the treatments outlined in Table 1 can be implemented in the presence of coexisting conditions, assuming that the coexisting conditions do not predominate (in terms of impairment in functioning or severity). For example, the co-occurrence of depression or personality disorders does not necessarily prohibit the behavioral treatment of PDA. It must be noted, however, that specific issues may arise in each case, such as the effect of depression on motivation for exposure practice. Similarly, compliance with instructions and trust in the therapist may need to be addressed when certain DSM-III-R Axis II conditions coexist. The results of an uncontrolled study reported by Beck (1988) suggested that a cognitive-behavioral treatment was effective for PDAs with additional personality disorder diagnoses but took considerably longer than when Axis II conditions were not present (32 weeks on average in comparison to 18 weeks).

On the other hand, suicidal ideation, florid psychotic states, manic episodes, active stages of substance abuse withdrawal, and so on prohibit a behavioral treatment for PDA. In those cases, the PDA treatments should follow the stabilization of physical and mental state.

A related issue is the need to modify exposure procedures when medical complications exist that may place the patient in danger if high levels of fear or stress are elicited. Situational and interoceptive exposure may be very provocative, particularly when carried out in an intense and massed format. When certain serious medical complications exist, a very graduated and spaced approach is warranted. In addition, the level of physical stress caused by exposure tasks may be continuously monitored, so that intensity levels can be gauged and controlled. For example, portable heart-rate or blood-pressure recorders may be used to ensure that responding will not exceed certain cutoff levels.

When complicating medical factors coexist, patients may benefit from learning to discriminate the physical symptomatology of the medical problem from the physical symptomatology of stress and anxiety. Examples include education about the symptoms of heart disease and education about the side effects of certain medications and their distinctiveness from panic symptoms. However, medical symptom information should be accompanied by education about the nature of panic, in order to minimize a fearful tendency to use the newly acquired information as a way of persistently and unadaptively checking the "dangerousness" of different symptoms.

Hospital Setting. Issues related to the medical-psychiatric setting include the potential for professional staff to directly or inadvertently reinforce excessive illness behavior, which has been identified as an important component of PDA (Salkovskis, 1988). For example, fears of fainting or collapsing may be reinforced by the provision of wheelchairs or the aid of another person when the patient moves around. Similarly, verbal reassurances of safety to allay fear and distress may interfere with the premise of behavioral treatment; that is, learning that panic symptoms are not dangerous in and of themselves, even if the patient is alone or without medical help. The same difficulty may arise if medication is given "as needed."

Another factor to consider in the hospital setting is the importance of coordinating the various treatment procedures and interactions with patients. An example of a potential area of conflict concerns the conceptualization of PDA. Traditionally, medical personnel have conceptualized the underlying basis of PDA as a neurochemical dysregulatory mechanism, possibly genetic in origin, that is most appropriately treated within a disease model. In contrast, the prototypical treatment described earlier is based on a psychobiological model. This model recognizes the role of physiological predisposition, but it also places a strong emphasis on learning and psychological factors. The presentation of contrasting conceptualizations by the medical personnel may interfere with the patient's progress. This problem is paramount when drug and behavioral treatments are combined. In the patient's best interests, all professional staff involved should fully understand each other's perspective and convey a cohesive formulation to the patient. For example, a cohesive rationale for drug and behavioral treatments recognizes both the value of medications in reducing or dampening physical symptomatology and the value of exposure practices in teaching the patient to be less afraid of the physical symptomatology. A cohesive rationale for the causes of PDA acknowledges the roles of both physiological predispositions and learned fear reactions.

The combination of drug and behavioral treatments is particularly likely in a medical-psychiatric setting because of either the clinical orientation of the professional staff or the severity of the presenting condition. Several arguments exist against the combination of drugs and behavioral treatments, including state-dependent learning (e.g., Overton, 1977). Furthermore, there is a possibility that patients will attribute their therapeutic gains to the drug rather than to their own personal efforts; this attribution is believed to increase the risk of relapse when the drugs are withdrawn. Indeed, relapse rates from medication treatments (particularly the benzodiazepines) tend to be high (Fyer, 1988). On the other hand, several studies have suggested that the combination of tricyclic antidepressants (e.g., imipramine) and behavioral treatment is more effective than either treatment alone (see Telch, 1988, for review), at least in the control of agoraphobic avoidance. The effectiveness of combination treatments in the control of panic attacks is currently being investigated in a large cross-site study (SUNY, Yale, Cornell, and Columbia). It is noteworthy that the cognitive-behavioral treatment is an effective means of helping patients withdraw from medications, particularly benzodiazepines (Bruce, Spiegel, Falkin, & Nuzzarello, 1992).

A final major issue concerns generalization from the hospital setting to the home environment. Generalization can be facilitated in several ways. First, while the patient is hospitalized, exposure practices can be designed to increase the distance from the hospital setting, accompanied and alone. Second, significant others who are willing to participate may be educated about the nature of PDA and encouraged to help the patient design and practice exposure tasks when he or she returns home. Third, practice tasks to be completed on leaving the hospital environment should be designed and rehearsed before the patient returns to the home environment. The rehearsals should take into consideration the types of difficulties likely to be encountered and the methods of controlling the fear and urges to escape or avoid. Finally, successful generalization may be facilitated if a therapist accompanies the patient home for a few hours and practices exposure tasks in the home. This strategy may be particularly valuable for patients without significant others. Follow-up phone contact and contact with an outpatient therapist may also be valuable, depending on the patient's level of distress.

SUMMARY

Panic disorder and agoraphobia may be very severe, debilitating conditions that may be seen in a psychiatric-medical setting because of the severity of the disorder or as an additional diagnostic feature of other medical or psychiatric conditions. In particular, PDA may present with coexisting depressive disorders, substance abuse or dependence, personality disorders, or psychoses. There are various ramifications of a medical setting for the assessment and treatment of PDA. The prototypical assessment of PDA includes diagnostic interviews; standardized self-report inventories; self-monitoring of panic, anxiety, and behavior; behavioral assessments, and medical evaluation. The assessment issues that arise in a medical setting include differential diagnosis from medical conditions that either mimic PDA symptomatology or exacerbate PDA symptomatology; differentiation from somatoform disorders; physical and mental status at the time of assessment; the confounding effects of recently initiated medications; compliance with assessment procedures (particularly self-monitoring); alternative methods of monitoring via independent-observer ratings; and the assessment of fear and avoidance outside the hospital setting.

The prototypical treatment of PDA includes education about panic and anxiety, cognitive restructuring to correct misappraisals of physical panic symptoms, somatic control strategies, interoceptive exposure, and situational exposure. The treatment issues that arise in a medical setting include the pace of the treatment due to the severity of the PDA condition; physical and mental status when initiating PDA treatments; modifications of PDA treatments due to coexisting psychiatric and medical conditions; the reinforcement of agoraphobic fear and avoidance as a result of the medical setting; the importance of a cohesive rationale and treatment for patients being treated by different professionals; and methods for enhancing generalization from the hospital to the home environment. Ultimately, although special considerations exist within a medical-psychiatric setting, the prototypical methods of assessment and treatment of PDA can be tailored to suit the patient and the setting.

ACKNOWLEDGMENT.   The author would like to express appreciation to Lori Zoellner for her helpful editing and comments on the chapter.

REFERENCES

Alloy, L. B., Kelly, K. A., Mineka, S., & Clements, C. M. (1989). Comorbidity of anxiety and depressive disorders: A helplessness-hopelessness perspective. In J. D. Maser & C. R. Cloninger (Eds.), *Comorbidity in anxiety and mood disorders*. Washington, DC: American Psychiatric Press.

American Psychiatric Association. (1987). *Diagnostic and statistical manual for mental disorders* (3rd ed., rev.; DSM-III-R). Washington, DC: American Psychiatric Press.

Anthony, J. C., Tien, A. Y., & Petronis, K. R. (1989). Epidemiological evidence on cocaine use and panic attacks. *American Journal of Epidemiology*, *129*, 543–549.

Argyle, N. (1990). Panic attacks in chronic schizophrenia. *British Journal of Psychiatry*, *157*, 430–433.

Arnow, B., Taylor, C. B., Agras, W. S., & Telch, M. J. (1985). Enhancing agoraphobia treatment outcome by changing couple communication patterns. *Behavior Therapy*, *16*, 452–467.

Aronson, T. A., & Craig, T. J. (1986). Cocaine precipitation of panic disorder. *American Journal of Psychiatry*, *143*, 643–645.

Barlow, D. H. (1988). *Anxiety and its disorders: The nature and treatment of anxiety and panic*. New York: Guilford Press.

Barlow, D. H., & Waddell, M. (1985). Agoraphobia. In D. H. Barlow (Ed.), *Clinical handbook of psychological disorders: A step-by-step treatment manual*. New York: Guilford Press.

Barlow, D. H., O'Brien, G. T., & Last, C. G. (1984). Couples treatment of agoraphobia. *Behavior Therapy*, *15*, 41–58.

Barlow, D. H., Vermilyea, J. A., Blanchard, E. B., Vermilyea, B. B., DiNardo, P. A., & Cerny, J. A. (1985). The phenomenon of panic. *Journal of Abnormal Psychology*, *94*, 320–328.

Barlow, D. H., Craske, M. G., Cerny, J. A., & Klosko, J. (1989). Behavioral treatment of panic disorder. *Behavior Therapy*, *20*, 261–282.

Beck, A. T. (1985). Theoretical perspectives on clinical anxiety. In A. H. Tuma & J. D. Maser (Eds.), *Anxiety and the anxiety disorders*. Hillsdale, NJ: Erlbaum.

Beck, A. T. (1988). Cognitive approaches to panic disorder: Theory and therapy. In S. Rachman & J. D. Maser (Eds.), *Panic: Psychological perspectives*. Hillsdale, NJ: Erlbaum.

Bonn, J. A., Harrison, J., & Rees, W. (1971). Lactate-induce anxiety: Therapeutic application. *British Journal of Psychiatry, 119*, 468–470.

Boyd, H. H. (1986). Use of mental health services for the treatment of panic attacks. *American Journal of Psychiatry, 143*, 1569–1574.

Breier, A., Charney, D. S., & Heninger, G. R. (1986). Agoraphobia with panic attacks. *Archives of General Psychiatry, 43*, 1029–1036.

Brown, T. A., Cash, T. F., & Deagle, E. A. (1988). *Prevalence and phenomenology of panic in nonclinical samples: Additional findings and methodological considerations.* Poster presented at 22nd Annual Association for the Advancement of Behavior Therapy, New York.

Bruce, T. J., Spiegel, D., Falkin, S., & Nuzzarello, A. (1992, March). *Does cognitive-behavioral therapy assist slow-taper alprazolam discontinuation in panic disorder?* Poster presented at the annual meeting of the Anxiety Disorders Association of America, Houston, Texas.

Burns, L. E., Thorpe, G. L., & Cavallaro, L. A. (1986). Agoraphobia eight years after behavioral treatment: A follow-up study with interview, self-report, and behavioral data. *Behavior Therapy, 17*, 580–591.

Carey, G., & Gottesman, I. (1981). Twin and family studies of anxiety, phobic, and obsessive disorders. In D. Klein & J. Rabkin (Eds.), *Anxiety: New research and changing concepts.* New York: Raven Press.

Cassano, G. B., Perugi, G., Musetti, L., & Akiskal, H. S. (1989). The nature of depression presenting concomitantly with panic disorder. *Comprehensive Psychiatry, 30*, 473–482.

Cerny, J. A., Barlow, D. H., Craske, M. G., Himadi, W. G. (1987). Couples treatment of agoraphobia: A two-year follow-up. *Behavior Therapy, 18*, 401–415.

Chambless, D. L. (1989, November). *Spacing of exposure sessions in the treatment of phobia.* Paper presented at the 22nd Annual Association for Advancement of Behavior Therapy, New York.

Chambless, D. L., & Mason, J. (1986). Sex, sex role stereotyping, and agoraphobia. *Behaviour Research and Therapy, 24*, 231–235.

Chambless, D. L., Caputo, G. C., Bright, P., & Gallagher, R. (1984). Assessment of fear in agoraphobics: The Body Sensations Questionnaire and the Agoraphobic Cognitions Questionnaire. *Journal of Consulting and Clinical Psychology, 52*, 1090–1097.

Chambless, D. L., Caputo, G. C., Jasin, S. E., Gracely, E. J., & Williams, C. (1985). The Mobility Inventory for Agoraphobia. *Behaviour Research and Therapy, 23*, 35–44.

Chaplin, E. W., & Levine, B. A. (1981). The effects of total exposure duration and interrupted versus continued exposure in flooding therapy. *Behavior Therapy, 12*, 360–368.

Charney, D. S., Heninger, G. R., & Breier, A. (1984). Noradrenergic function in panic anxiety: Effects of yohimbine in healthy subjects and patients with agoraphobia and panic disorder. *Archives of General Psychiatry, 41*, 751–763.

Clancy, J., & Noyes, R. (1976). Anxiety neurosis: A disease for the medical model. *Psychosomatics, 17*, 90–93.

Clark, D. (1989, June). *Cognitive treatment of panic disorders.* Paper presented at the annual meeting of the European Association of Behavior Therapy, Vienna.

Clark, D., Salkovskis, P., & Chalkley, A. (1985). Respiratory control as a treatment for panic attacks. *Journal of Behavior Therapy and Experimental Psychiatry, 16*, 23–30.

Cohen, S. D., Monteiro, W., & Marks, I. (1984). Two-year follow-up of agoraphobics after exposure and imipramine. *British Journal of Psychiatry, 144*, 276–381.

Cox, B. J., Norton, G. R., Swinson, R. P., & Endler, N. (1990). Substance abuse and panic-related anxiety: A critical review. *Behaviour Research and Therapy, 28*, 385–393.

Craske, M. G., & Barlow, D. H. (1988). A review of the relationship between panic and avoidance. *Clinical Psychology Review, 8*, 667–685.

Craske, M. G., & Kreuger, M. (1990). The prevalence of nocturnal panic in a college population. *Journal of Anxiety Disorders, 4*, 125–139.

Craske, M. G., Street, L., & Barlow, D. H. (1989). Instructions to focus upon or distract from internal cues during exposure treatment for agoraphobic avoidance. *Behaviour Research and Therapy, 27*, 663–672.

Craske, M. G., Miller, P., Rotunda, R., & Barlow, D. H. (1990). A descriptive report of features of initial unexpected panic attacks in minimal and extensive avoiders. *Behaviour Research and Therapy, 28*, 395–400.

Craske, M. G., Brown, T. A., & Barlow, D. H. (1991). Behavioral treatment of panic disorder: A two-year follow-up. *Behavior Therapy, 22*, 289–304.

Crowe, R., Noyes, R., Pauls, D., & Slymen, D. (1983). A family study of panic disorder. *Archives of General Psychiatry, 40*, 1065–1069.

de Ruiter, C., Rijken, H., Garssen, B., & Kraaimaat, F. (1989). Breathing retraining, exposure, and a combination of both, in the treatment of panic disorder with agoraphobia. *Behaviour Research and Therapy, 27*, 647–656.

DiNardo, P. A., & Barlow, D. H. (1988). *Anxiety Disorders Interview Schedule-Revised (ADIS-R)*. Albany, NY: Phobia and Anxiety Disorders Clinic, State University of New York at Albany.

DiNardo, P. A., & Barlow, D. H. (1989). *Reliability of DSM-III-R anxiety disorder categories using ADIS-R*. Unpublished manuscript.

Ehlers, A., & Margraf, J. (1989). The psychophysiological model of panic attacks. In P. M. G. Emmelkamp (Ed.), *Anxiety disorders: Annual series of European research in behavior therapy. Vol. 4*. Amsterdam: Swets.

Emmelkamp, P. M. G., & Mersch, P. P. (1982). Cognition and exposure in vivo in the treatment of agoraphobia: Short term and delayed effects. *Cognitive Therapy and Research, 6*, 77–88.

Emmelkamp, P. M. G., Kuipers, A., & Eggeraat, J. (1978). Cognitive modification versus prolonged exposure in vivo: A comparison with agoraphobics as subjects. *Behaviour Research and Therapy, 16*, 33–41.

Faravelli, C., & Pallanti, S. (1989). Recent life events and panic disorder. *American Journal of Psychiatry, 146*, 622–626.

Feigenbaum, W. (1988). Long-term efficacy of ungraded versus graded masses exposure in agoraphobics. In I. Hand & H. U. Wittchen (Eds.), *Panic and phobias* (Vol. 2). Berlin: Springer-Verlag.

Foa, E. B., James, J. S., Turner, R. M., & Payne, L. L. (1980). Massed vs. spaced exposure sessions in the treatment of agoraphobia. *Behaviour Research and Therapy, 18*, 333–338.

Fyer, A. (1988). Effects of discontinuation of antipanic medication. In I. Hand & H. U. Wittchen (Eds.), *Panic and phobias* (Vol. 2). Berlin: Springer-Verlag.

Fyer, A., Endicott, J., Mannuzza, S., & Klein, D. (1985). *Schedule for Affective Disorders and Schizophrenia: Lifetime Version* (modified for the study of anxiety disorders). New York: Anxiety Disorders Clinic, New York State Psychiatric Institute.

Ghosh, A., & Marks, I. M. (1987). Self-directed exposure for agoraphobia: A controlled trial. *Behavior Therapy, 18*, 3–16.

Gorman, J. M., Fyer, M. R., Goetz, R., Askanazi, J., Leibowitz, M. R., Fyer, A. J., Kinney, J., & Klein, D. F. (1988). Ventilatory physiology of patients with panic disorder. *Archives of General Psychiatry, 45*, 31–39.

Griez, E., & van den Hout, M. A. (1986). CO_2 inhalation in the treatment of panic attacks. *Behaviour Research and Therapy, 24*, 145–150.

Hafner, R. J. (1976). Fresh symptom emergence after intensive behavior therapy. *British Journal of Psychiatry, 129*, 145–150.

Harris, E., Noyes, R., Crowe, R., & Chaudhry, D. (1983). A family study of agoraphobia. *Archives of General Psychiatry, 40*, 1061–1064.

Haslam, M. T. (1974). The relationship between the effect of lactate infusion on anxiety states and their amelioration by carbon dioxide inhalation. *British Journal of Psychiatry, 125*, 88–90.

Holden, A., O'Brien, G., Barlow, D., Stetson, D., & Infantino, A. (1983). Self-help manual for agoraphobia: A preliminary report of effectiveness. *Behavior Therapy, 14*, 107–115.

Holt, P., & Andrews, G. (1989). Hyperventilation and anxiety in panic disorder, social phobia, GAD, and normal controls. *Behaviour Research and Therapy, 27*, 453–460.

Jannoun, L., Munby, M., Catalan, J., & Gelder, M. (1980). A home-based treatment program for agoraphobia: Replication and controlled evaluation. *Behavior Therapy, 11*, 294–305.

Jansson, L., & Ost, L-G. (1982). Behavioral treatments for agoraphobia: An evaluative review. *Clinical Psychology Review, 2*, 311–336.

Jansson, L., Jerremalm, A., & Ost, L-G. (1986). Follow-up of agoraphobic patients treated with exposure in vivo or applied relaxation. *British Journal of Psychiatry, 149*, 486–490.

Kahn, J. P., Drusin, R. E., & Klein, D. F. (1987). Schizophrenia, panic anxiety and alprazolam. *American Journal of Psychiatry, 144*, 527–528.

Katon, W. (1984). Panic disorder and somatization: A review of 55 cases. *American Journal of Medicine, 77*, 101–106.

Katon, W. (1989). *Panic disorder in the medical setting*. Washington, DC: National Institute of Mental Health.

Kraft, A. R., & Hoogduin, C. A. (1984). The hyperventilation syndrome: A pilot study of the effectiveness of treatment. *British Journal of Psychiatry, 145*, 538–542.

Mannuzza, S., Fyer, A., Martin, L., Gallops, M., Endicott, J., Gorman, J., Liebowitz, M., & Klein, D. (1990). Reliability of anxiety assessment: 1. Diagnostic agreement. *Archives of General Psychiatry, 46*, 1093–1101.

Margraf, J. (1989, June). *Comparative efficacy of cognitive, exposure, and combined treatments for panic disorder*. Paper presented at the annual meeting of the European Association of Behavior Therapy, Vienna.

Margraf, J., Taylor, C. B., Ehlers, A., Roth, W. T., & Agras, W. S. (1987). Panic attacks in the natural environment. *Journal of Nervous and Mental Disease, 175*, 558–565.

Marks, I. M. (1971). Phobic disorders four years after treatment: A prospective follow-up. *British Journal of Psychiatry, 118*, 683–686.

Marks, I. M. (1978). *Living with fear*. New York: McGraw-Hill.

Marks, I., & Mathews, A. M. (1979). Brief standard self-rating for phobic patients. *Behaviour Research and Therapy*, *17*, 263–267.

Marshall, W. L. (1985). The effects of variable exposure in flooding therapy. *Behavior Therapy*, *16*, 117–135.

Mathews, A. M., Gelder, M., & Johnston, D. W. (1981). *Agoraphobia: Nature and treatment*. New York: Guilford Press.

Mavissakalian, M. L., & Hamman, M. S. (1986). DSM-III personality disorders in agoraphobia. *Comprehensive Psychiatry*, *27*, 471–479.

Mavissakalian, M. L., & Hamman, M. (1987). DSM-III personality disorders in agoraphobia. II. Changes with treatment. *Comprehensive Psychiatry*, *28*, 356–361.

McNamee, G., O'Sullivan, G., Lelliot, P., & Marks, I. M. (1989). Telephone-guided treatment for housebound agoraphobics with panic disorder: Exposure vs relaxation. *Behavior Therapy*, *20*, 491–497.

Michelson, L., Mavissakalian, M., & Marchione, K. (1985). Cognitive and behavioral treatments for agoraphobia: Clinical, behavioral, and psychophysiological outcomes. *Journal of Consulting and Clinical Psychology*, *53*, 913–925.

Michelson, L., Mavissakalian, M., Marchione, K., Dancu, C., & Greenwald, M. (1986). The role of self-directed in vivo exposure practice in cognitive, behavioral, and psychophysiological treatments of agoraphobia. *Behavior Therapy*, *17*, 91–108.

Moras, K. (1989). *Diagnostic comorbidity in the DSM-III and DSM-III-R anxiety and mood disorders: Implications for the DSM-IV*. Unpublished manuscript.

Munby, J., & Johnston, D. W. (1980). Agoraphobia: The long-term follow-up of behavioral treatment. *British Journal of Psychiatry*, *137*, 418–427.

Norton, G. R., Doward, J., & Cox, B. J. (1980). Factors associated with panic attacks in nonclinical subjects. *Behavior Therapy*, *17*, 239–252.

Noyes, R., Crowe, R. R., Harris, E. L., Hamra, B. J., McChesney, C. M., & Chaudhry, D. R. (1986). Relationship between panic disorder and agoraphobia: A family study. *Archives of General Psychiatry*, *43*, 227–232.

Ost, L-G. (1988). Applied relaxation vs. progressive relaxation in the treatment of panic disorder. *Behaviour Research and Therapy*, *26*, 13–22.

Overton, D. A. (1977). Drug state-dependent learning. In M. E. Jarvik (Ed.), *Psychopharmacology in the practice of medicine*. New York: Appleton-Century-Crofts.

Pollard, C. A., Bronson, S. S., & Kenney, M. R. (1989a). Prevalence of agoraphobia without panic in clinical settings. *American Journal of Psychiatry*, *146*, 559.

Pollard, C. A., Pollard, H. J., & Corn, K. J. (1989b). Panic onset and major events in the lives of agoraphobics: A test of contiguity. *Journal of Abnormal Psychology*, *98*, 318–321.

Rapee, R. M. (1985). A case of panic disorder treated with breathing retraining. *Behavior Therapy and Experimental Psychiatry*, *16*, 63–65.

Rapee, R. M., Craske, M. G., & Barlow, D. H. (1990a). Subject described features of panic attacks using a new self-monitoring form. *Journal of Anxiety Disorders*, *4*, 171–181.

Rapee, R. M., Litwin, E. M., & Barlow, D. H. (1990b). Impact of life events on subjects with panic disorder and on comparison subjects. *American Journal of Psychiatry*, *147*, 640–644.

Reich, J. (1988). DSM-III personality disorders and family history of mental illness. *Journal of Nervous and Mental Disease*, *176*, 45–49.

Reich, J., & Noyes, R. (1987). A comparison of DSM-III personality disorders in acutely ill panic and depressed patients. *Journal of Anxiety Disorders*, *1*, 123–131.

Reich, J., Noyes, R., & Troughton, E. (1987). Dependent personality disorder associated with phobic avoidance in patients with panic disorder. *American Journal of Psychiatry*, *144*, 323–326.

Reiss, S., Peterson, R. A., Gursky, D. M., & McNally, R. J. (1986). Anxiety sensitivity, anxiety frequency, and the prediction of fearfulness. *Behaviour Research and Therapy*, *24*, 1–8.

Roy-Byrne, P. P., Geraci, B., & Uhde, T. (1986). Life events and the onset of panic disorder. *American Journal of Psychiatry*, *143*, 1424–1427.

Salge, R., Beck, G., & Logan, A. (1988). A community survey of panic. *Journal of Anxiety Disorders*, *2*, 157–167.

Salkovskis, P. (1988). Phenomenology, assessment and the cognitive model of panic. In S. Rachman & J. D. Maser (Eds.), *Panic: Psychological perspectives*. Hillsdale, NJ: Erlbaum.

Salkovskis, P., Warwick, H., Clark, D., & Wessels, D. (1986). A demonstration of acute hyperventilation during naturally occurring panic attacks. *Behaviour Research & Therapy*, *24*, 91–94.

Salkovskis, P., Warwick, H., & Clark, D. (1990). *Hypochondriasis, illness phobia, and other anxiety disorders*. Unpublished manuscript.

Sanderson, W. S., DiNardo, P. A., Rapee, R. M., & Barlow, D. H. (1990). Syndrome comorbidity in patients diagnosed with a DSM-III-Revised anxiety disorder. *Journal of Abnormal Psychology*, *99*, 308–312.

Sartory, G., & Olajide, D. (1988). Vagal innervation techniques in the treatment of panic disorder. *Behaviour Research and Therapy*, *26*, 243–266.

Spitzer, R., Williams, J., & Gibbons, M. (1985). *Instruction manual for the Structured Clinical Interview for DSM-III (SCID)*. New York: Biometrics Research Department, New York State Psychiatric Institute.

Stern, R. S., & Marks, I. M. (1973). Brief and prolonged flooding: A comparison of agoraphobic patients. *Archives of General Psychiatry*, *28*, 270–276.

Swinson, R. P. (1986). Reply to Kleiner. *The Behavior Therapist*, *9*, 110–128.

Taylor, M. (1987). DSM-III organic mental disorders. In G. L. Tischler (Ed.), *Diagnosis and classification in psychiatry: A critical appraisal of DSM-III*. Cambridge, England: Cambridge University Press.

Telch, M. J. (1988). Combined pharmacological and psychological treatments for panic sufferers. In S. Rachman & J. D. Maser (Eds.), *Panic: Psychological perspectives*. Hillsdale, NJ: Erlbaum.

Telch, M. J., Lucas, J. A., & Nelson, P. (1989). Nonclinical panic in college students: An investigation of prevalence and symptomatology. *Journal of Abnormal Psychology*, *98*, 300–306.

Thompson, J. W., Burns, B. J., Barkto, J., Boyd, J. H., Taube, C. A., & Bourdon, K. H. (1988). The use of ambulatory services by persons with and without phobia. *Medical Care*, *26*, 280–288.

Thyer, B. A., Himle, J., Curtis, G. C., Cameron, O. G., & Nesse, R. M. (1985). A comparison of panic disorder and agoraphobia with panic attacks. *Comprehensive Psychiatry*, *26*, 208–214.

Torgersen, S. (1983). Genetic factors in anxiety disorders. *Archives of General Psychiatry*, *40*, 1085–1089.

Vermilyea, J. A., Boice, & Barlow, D. H. (1984). Rachman and Hodgson (1974) a decade later: How do desynchronous response systems relate to the treatment of agoraphobia? *Behaviour Research & Therapy*, *22*, 615–621.

Weeks, C. (1976). *Simple, effective treatment of agoraphobia*. New York: Hawthorne.

Weissman, M. M., Leckman, J., Merikangas, K., Gammon, G., & Prusoff, B. (1984a). Depression and anxiety disorders in parents and children. *Archives of General Psychiatry*, *41*, 845–852.

Weissman, M. M., Myers, J., Leckman, J., Harding, P., Pauls, D., & Prusoff, B. (1984b). Anxiety disorders: Epidemiology and familial patterns. *Archives of General Psychiatry*, *41*, 845–852.

Weissman, M. M., Leaf, P. J., Blazer, D. G., Boyd, J. H., & Florio, L. (1986). The relationship between panic disorder and agoraphobia: An epidemiological perspective. *Psychopharmacology Bulletin*, *43*, 787–791.

Weissman, M. M., Klerman, G., Markowitz, J., & Ouellette, R. (1989). Suicidal ideation and suicide attempts in panic disorder and attacks. *New England Journal of Medicine*, *321*, 1209–1214.

Williams, S. L., & Rappaport, J. A. (1983). Cognitive treatment in the natural environment for agoraphobics. *Behavior Therapy*, *14*, 299–313.

Zitrin, C. M., Klein, D. F., & Woerner, M. G. (1980). Behavior therapy, supportive psychotherapy, imipramine, and phobias. *Archives of General Psychiatry*, *37*, 63–72.

13

Affective Disorders

MICHAEL G. DOW

INTRODUCTION

Diagnostic Criteria

The two primary categories of affective disorders (also called *mood disorders*) are major depression and bipolar disorder. The *Diagnostic and Statistical Manual* (third edition, revised) of the American Psychiatric Association (DSM-III-R; APA, 1987) is typically used in inpatient psychiatric settings to define and diagnosis these affective disorders. A major depressive episode requires the occurrence of at least five of nine symptoms listed in the manual: (1) depressed mood; (2) diminished interest or pleasure; (3) significant weight change (gain or loss); (4) difficulty sleeping or excessive sleeping; (5) psychomotor agitation or retardation; (6) fatigue or loss of energy; (7) feelings of worthlessness or guilt; (8) difficulty thinking or concentrating; and (9) suicidal ideation or behavior. A further requirement is that either Symptom 1 (depressed mood) or Symptom 2 (diminished interest or pleasure) must be present. Symptoms must be present most of the day, nearly every day for two weeks. These symptoms must also represent a change in functioning from prior behavior.

Individuals who experience a major depressive episode and are not also shown to have an organic disorder, uncomplicated bereavement, or a major psychotic disorder like schizophrenia, are typically diagnosed as experiencing major depression. Other individuals have one or more manic episodes in addition to the depressive episode and are therefore diagnosed as having a bipolar disorder. The criteria for a manic episode require a period of distinctly elevated, irritable, or expansive mood and at least three (or four, if the mood is only irritable) of the following: inflated self-esteem, reduced need for sleep, pressured speech, racing thoughts, distractibility, increased goal-oriented activity, and increased involvement in pleasurable activities that may have negative consequences. The mood disturbance must also be sufficiently severe to disrupt normal occupational or social functioning, or to require hospitalization.

The criteria for somewhat less acute versions of these disorders are provided by the DSM-III-R and are termed *dysthymia* (depressive neurosis) and *cyclothymia*. Although less severe,

MICHAEL G. DOW • Department of Community Mental Health, Florida Mental Health Institute, University of South Florida, Tampa, Florida 33612-3899.

Handbook of Behavior Therapy in the Psychiatric Setting, edited by Alan S. Bellack and Michel Hersen. Plenum Press, New York, 1993.

these disorders must be present for two years to warrant diagnosis and are therefore serious in their own right.

The DSM-III-R criteria are widely used in inpatient facilities. Even though behavioral psychologists traditionally have had some qualms about the medical model and the value of formal diagnosis, the DSM-III-R diagnostic structure is widely used by behavioral psychologists. Part of the reason is that insurance reimbursement in private settings is tied to diagnosis.

Prevalence

Depression is a very common disorder; about 10% of all men and 20% of all women experience a clinical level of depression at least once in their life (Weissman & Myers, 1978). Because of concern about suicide and the clear deterioration in social and occupational functioning that often occurs with depression, it is not unusual for severely depressed persons to be admitted to an inpatient setting at some time during their affective disturbance. Depression also tends to be somewhat episodic, and about one half of all depressed persons have more than one distinct episode of depression during their lifetime. Bipolar disorder is less common than major depression. Estimates indicate that between 0.4% to 1.2% of the population have had bipolar disorder (American Psychiatric Association, 1987). Thus, roughly only about 1 of every 15 depressed persons experiences bipolar disorder. However, in inpatient facilities, the ratio of bipolar disorder to major depression is much higher, and some facilities report almost equal numbers. Unlike major depression, bipolar disorder affects males and females at approximately the same rate.

The vast majority of research and writing on the behavioral treatment and assessment of affective disorders has emphasized unipolar depression, that is major depression and dysthymia. Much less emphasis has been placed on bipolar disorder. There may be several reasons. First, genetic evidence suggests that bipolar disorder is more clearly related to genetic transmission (Allen, 1976; Smith & Winokur, 1984) than major depression. Environmental factors appears less important in bipolar disorder. Second, the primary treatment for bipolar disorder is lithium. No widely supported cognitive-behavioral treatments have been developed specifically for bipolar disorder. Third, major depression is much more prevalent than bipolar disorder in outpatient settings—the primary settings for cognitive-behavioral clinicians. For all of these reasons, behavioral psychologists have tended to ignore bipolar disorder and have focused on major depression.

Cognitive-Behavioral Theories of Depression

Behavioral and cognitive-behavioral models of depression have been very influential since the late 1960s and have been discussed elsewhere in considerable detail (e.g., Abramson, Seligman, & Teasdale, 1978; Beck, 1967; Lewinsohn & Hoberman, 1982; Rehm, 1977).

Lewinsohn (1974), drawing on seminal work by Ferster (1966) introduced a behavioral approach to depression that emphasizes the role of reinforcement. It was theorized that response-contingent positive reinforcement received by the individual acts to maintain a positive mood state. When reinforcement is low, extinction of motor behavior tends to occur, further isolating the individual and reducing the level of reinforcement received. As part of this model, depressed people are often seen as having low social skill, which tends to minimize the amount of positive reinforcement received from the environment.

Cognitive tendencies were emphasized by Rehm (1977), who developed a self-control model of depression, emphasizing deficits in the depressed individual's self-monitoring, self-evaluation, and self-reinforcement.

Beck (1967) also developed a cognitive model of depression that emphasizes the depressed person's tendency to perceive events negatively. Because of cognitive biases or schemata, depressed persons are said to have a negative view of themselves, the world, and the future. These schemata result in cognitive errors of perception and attribution, such as arbitrary inference, selective attention, minimization of positive events, and magnification of negative events.

Seligman (1975) developed a "learned-helplessness" model of depression, drawing on animal research that showed that, when there is a lack of contingency between one's effort and its results (particularly for negative events), extinction of behavior occurs. This model was refined by Abramson *et al.* (1978) to underscore the importance of attributions about events. In particular, depressed persons are said to have an internal, stable, and global attribution for negative events.

Although they are sometimes viewed as competing, there appears to be substantial overlap among these models (Biglan & Dow, 1981; Craighead, 1980). All emphasize cognitive-behavioral factors in terms of etiology, assessment, and treatment.

PROTOTYPICAL ASSESSMENT

Cognitive-behavioral clinicians typically conceptualize psychological disturbances as having behavioral, cognitive-subjective, and physiological aspects. An appropriate assessment should involve an investigation of each of these areas.

Assessment Methods

Because depression is predominantly a disturbance of mood, it should be of no surprise that self-report assessment has been used most widely. Perhaps the two most widely used assessment inventories are the Beck Depression Inventory, a 21-item scale first published by Beck, Ward, Mendelson, Mock, and Erbaugh (1961), and revised by Beck (1978), and the Minnesota Multiphasic Personality Inventory D scale (MMPI; Hathaway, & McKinley, 1942), which has also been revised with the publication of the MMPI-2 (Butcher, Dahlstrom, Graham, Tellegen, & Krammer, 1989). These scales have well-established reliability and validity data. A number of other self-report assessments for depression were reviewed by Rehm (1988), but these tend not to be used as frequently, particularly in inpatient settings. As Rehm (1988) noted, the MMPI has frequently been used to discriminate depressed and nondepressed samples in research studies, at least partly because the test was originally developed by the use of an empirical construction approach that identified items based on their ability to distinguish depressed and nondepressed samples. The Beck Depression Inventory is unequaled in ease of use and has been used widely.

Although self-report assessments cover symptoms that include behavioral, cognitive-subjective, and physiological processes, the individual is ultimately asked to make evaluations of himself or herself using this format, so these assessments may be heavily influenced by one's cognitive-subjective state, even when being asked about a behavioral or physiological symptom. A related problem in the use of self-report depression inventories is that none of them provide subscales to determine the relative emphasis of various symptom domains, such as cognitive-subjective, physiological, and behavioral symptoms. Two patients, each with a score of 20 on the Beck Depression Inventory, may present very differently, with different symptom clusters, prognosis, and preferred approach to treatment.

Although a number of physiological or psychophysiological assessments have attempted to diagnosis depression, none is widely used except for the dexamethasone suppression test (DST). In the most widely used procedure for the DST, 1.0 mg of dexamethasone is taken at 11:00 P.M., which is typically the low point in the circadian rhythm of endogenous corticosteroid secretion. Dexamethasone normally suppresses the release of plasma cortisol for at least 24 hours. Blood samples are typically drawn at 8:00 A.M., 4:00 P.M., and 11:00 P.M. An elevated plasma concentration of cortisol in any blood sample obtained between 9 and 24 hours after the ingestion of dexamethasone indicates a failure in the normal suppression of cortisol (Glassman, Arana, Baldessarini, Brown, Carroll, Davis, Greenblatt, Klerman, Orsulak, Schildkraut, & Shader, 1987). Depressed individuals are more likely to be nonsuppressors of cortisol; thus, the test has been used to confirm the diagnosis of major depression and to predict responses to antidepressant medications. However, patients with other psychiatric conditions, such as anorexia nervosa and Alzheimer's disease without depression, have also been shown to have abnormal DST results (Starkman, 1987). Thus, the test has been criticized for lacking sufficient specificity, sensitivity, and predictive value (Coppen, Abou-Saleh, Milln, Metcalfe, Harwood, & Bailey, 1983; Insel & Goodwin, 1983).

Behavioral assessment procedures for recording types of behavior emitted on the unit by depressed inpatients were described by Williams, Barlow, and Agras (1972). Telemetric monitoring of motor behavior was described by Kupfer, Weiss, Foster, Detre, Delgado, and McPartland (1974). In addition, a number of research studies have used behavioral assessment procedures to examine social skills, and some of these studies have concerned the social skills of depressed persons. However, none of these behavioral assessments have been widely adopted for clinical use. The two primary types of assessments in the area of social skills have involved a brief social interaction task with a research assistant or confederate (Arkowitz, Lichtenstein, McGovern, & Hines, 1975; Dow & Craighead, 1987) or a taped role-play situations test (Rehm & Marston, 1968). There are some concerns, however, that the role-play test may not generalize well to a typical conversation (Bellack, Hersen, & Turner, 1979).

Lewinsohn has used self-reports to assess social behavior in developing the Pleasant Events Schedule (MacPhillamy & Lewinsohn, 1971) and the Interpersonal Events Schedule (Youngren & Lewinsohn, 1980). These assessments involve long lists of pleasant events and interpersonal events, respectively, in which the respondents record how often they have been involved in a specific event during the last 30 days (or other time period) and how much enjoyment they obtained. Because these assessments rely on a memory of past events, they may be influenced by subjective factors associated with depression.

Differential Diagnosis

Despite the tradition of functional analysis, which argues that all relevant problems should be addressed when one is treating individual patients, most published studies of the behavioral treatment of depression fail to present data on specific symptom configurations or additional problems outside the apparent monolith of depression.

Lewinsohn is one of the few behavioral researchers in the area of depression who has attempted to determine that the depressed subjects in his research studies do not experience other psychiatric disturbances. He has used a subject selection protocol in a number of research studies that uses MMPI clinical scale elevations, in conjunction with an interview-based symptom checklist, to identify depressed subjects, psychiatric nondepressed control subjects, and normal control subjects. The specific procedures were described by Lewinsohn and Lee (1981).

The advent of structured clinical interviews has seen other attempts to ensure subject purity. Miller, Norman, Keitner, Bishop, and Dow (1989) used the Diagnostic Interview Schedule (DIS; Robins, Helzer, Croughan, & Ratcliff, 1981) to determine that depressed inpatients did not also have other psychiatric diagnoses that would complicate interpretation of their results. The Structured Clinical Interview for the DSM-III-R (Spitzer, Williams, Gibbon, & First, 1990) and the Research Diagnostic Criteria (Spitzer, Endicott, & Robins, 1978) have also been used in various research studies.

The differential diagnosis of depression also requires that depression be differentiated from a variety of medical illnesses that may present with depressionlike symptoms. Endocrinological disorders may not be adequately considered or assessed in many clinical settings. Behavioral psychologists, by orientation and training, are not always fully aware of these possibilities. Thus, a brief review seems in order.

The first major type of endocrinological disorder that may mask as depression involves disorders of hypothalamic-pituitary-adrenocortical hyperactivity (HPAH). Cushing's syndrome is the classic example of this type of disorder. As described by Starkman (1987) in her excellent review of HPAH disorder as it relates to depression, some possible indicators of Cushing's syndrome include obesity, hirsutism (excess body hair), menstrual irregularities, hypertension, myopathy (muscle disease or damage), diabetes mellitus, irritability, decreased libido, skin and mucous membrane hyperpigmentation or ecchymoses (small blue or purplish patches on the skin), sleep disturbance, memory difficulties, an abnormal DST result (nonsuppression of cortisol), and depressed mood. Depressed mood is reported by 75% of patients with Cushing's disease. Although it is similar to the experience of major depression in many respects, irritability is more likely to be pronounced in Cushing's syndrome, and depressed affect is more likely to be intermittent, with episodes of one to three days occurring frequently. Patients with Cushing's syndrome may also feel their best in the morning, rather than at night (Starkman, 1987).

The treatment for Cushing's syndrome may involve surgery to remove a pituitary microadenoma tumor or an adrenal adenoma or carcinoma, if present. Alternatively, cobalt irradiation of the pituitary gland or controlling cortisol secretion by chemical agents such as metyrapone may be effective (Starkman, 1987).

A second major type of endocrine disorder that may mask as depression involves thyroid dysfunction, principally hypothyroidism, an underproduction of thyroid hormone. Certain symptoms may be common to depression and hypothyroidism, including depressed mood, loss of interest or pleasure, weight gain, appetite loss, sleep increase, constipation, decreased libido, fatigue, decreased concentration, and suicidal ideation (Sinaikin & Gold, 1987). Other symptoms may assist in differential diagnosis. Specifically, depression, but not hypothyroidism, may present with weight loss, appetite increase, or sleep decrease. On the other hand, hypothyroidism, but not depression, may produce goiter, cold intolerance, brittle hair, loss of eyebrow hair, dry skin, bradycardia (slow heart rate), and delayed reflexes (Sinaikin & Gold, 1987).

Specific laboratory tests are available that diagnosis hypothyroidism. Sinaikin and Gold (1987) indicated that a comprehensive evaluation of thyroid function is needed to differentiate hypothyroidism and depression. Specifically, they recommended T_4, T_3RIA, T_3RU, basal TSH, and TRH stimulation testing.

Of additional concern in psychiatric settings is the finding that lithium inhibits thyroid function. Thus, bipolar patients treated with lithium may develop hypothyroidism. In some cases, these individuals may appear to be cycling in a depressive period when, in fact, they are experiencing hypothyroidism. Sinaikin and Gold (1987) recommended that, before introducing antidepressant medication for depressed patients who are taking lithium, thyroid function should be assessed.

The incidence of hypothyroidism among 250 consecutively admitted depressed inpatients was found to be 8% in a study by Gold, Pottash, and Extein (1981). None of these individuals were referred for thyroid evaluation or received thyroid medication. Hypothyroidism is a serious, but not uncommon, condition that can be readily treated with thyroid replacement therapy. Therefore, it is crucial to distinguish this condition from major depression.

ACTUAL ASSESSMENT

Assessment Methods

Clinicians often consider major depression a fairly easy disorder to diagnose. The most frequent approach is probably the clinical interview, in which the patient is asked questions about depressive symptoms, the patient is observed for demonstrated affect, and an attempt is made to rule out other complicating diagnoses such as substance abuse, organicity, primary insomnia, obsessive-compulsive disorder, or schizoaffective disorder. Although psychologists are typically taught to ask open-ended questions and to do a specific functional analysis of individual problems, the reality in many applied inpatient settings is that many patients have so many problems of such different types that such a thorough assessment would take weeks of intense effort. Instead, applied clinicians tend to take on more of the medical-model style during a first interview, in which a wide variety of symptoms are assessed quickly by asking a series of close-ended questions, and then a few areas that appear most salient are emphasized. Such carving up of the clinical material is basically a triage process, in which specific goals are identified and decisions are made to meet certain goals in a specified time.

Bipolar Disorder is often considered more difficult to diagnose, unless the patient is currently in a manic episode at the time of the assessment.

As an adjunct to the clinical interview, various self-report assessments are often administered, the most common appearing to be the Beck Depression Inventory. If an MMPI-2 is administered, Scale 2 (D) or the New Depression Content scale (DEP; Butcher, Graham, Williams, & Ben-Porath, 1990) is typically used as a measure of depression. Scale 9 (Hypomania) may be helpful in identifying bipolar disorder.

A complete physical exam is typically part of the admission procedure in most inpatient settings and is required by the Joint Commission on Accreditation of Health Care Organizations (JCAHO). In addition to standard laboratory work on blood and urine samples, one of the most frequently conducted physiological assessments relevant to depression is the dexamethasone suppression test (Glassman et al., 1987). The test is conducted in a relatively standardized way and is conducted fairly often in many private facilities. Public facilities, which often have staffing patterns with fewer nurses, appear to conduct this test less frequently. What seems to distinguish the "prototypical" from the "actual" use of this test is how the test is presented to the patient and how the test is interpreted by some medical staff. As mentioned above, the prototypical use of this test acknowledges the high false-positive error rate. Thus, the test should not be used as a primary source of data, but it may reasonably be used in conjunction with other sources of data to confirm depression. Similarly, a normal test result does not rule out depression, but it may suggest a lack of depression if this seems reasonably consistent with other data. Unfortunately, I have talked to many depressed inpatients (who have had many different doctors) who indicated that their psychiatrist did a blood test that showed "that I have a biochemical imbalance in my brain." This tendency to overinterpret the test results may be meant, in part, to enhance compliance with medication or to enhance nonspecific placebo and demand effects.

As part of the physical examination in inpatient facilities, routine thyroid screening is typically conducted on serum thyroxine (T_4) and triiodothyronine (T_3), and possibly basal thyroid-stimulating hormone (TSH). However, differential diagnosis of depression and thyroid dysfunction requires a more comprehensive evaluation than is typically conducted.

Other than in published research studies, extensive behavioral assessment procedures are rarely used in inpatient facilities. However, many inpatient facilities do 15-minute or 30-minute checks, which involve having a staff member with a clipboard walk around the unit and identify the location of each patient and/or the behavior that each patient is engaged in. These checks constitute a form of behavioral assessment that may be used for diagnostic purposes or to evaluate treatment outcome. The form used in the adult inpatient unit at the Florida Mental Health Institute was described by Ward and Naster (1991). It has six major categories of activity: Bedroom, Meals, Therapeutic Activity, Unit Social Area, Off Unit, and Seclusion. Each of these categories is separated into finer subcategories. For example, the Unit Social Area codes are categorized as Not Interacting, Activity Alone, and Interacting. Bedroom codes include Inactive (asleep), Resting, and Active. During treatment team meetings, descriptive statistics are given on the codes of interest. For example, for a depressed person who is socially isolative, data may routinely be aggregated on the daily percentage of the checks during which the client was interacting with others, involved in a solitary activity, or not engaged in either activity.

Differential Diagnosis

As contrasted with published reports of outpatient cognitive-behavioral treatment for depression, inpatient treatment settings appear to emphasize the importance of differential diagnosis. In private inpatient settings, full work-ups of patients, including several hours of psychological tests, laboratory reports, and medical consultations, are fairly routine for seriously disturbed patients or patients with multiple problems. Public facilities also attempt to approximate these efforts, but staffing and resources are severely limited in most public facilities, so that it is more difficult to follow through on these attempts.

As an example of the difficulty in assessing real patients in an applied setting, I would like to briefly describe a patient who was assessed on a public-funded inpatient unit. The patient was a woman in her early 30s who was admitted with the diagnosis of schizoaffective disorder. She had had about 15 prior admissions to psychiatric facilities since her late teenage years, had made three significant suicide attempts, and experienced auditory self-critical hallucinations. She had experienced three visual hallucinations. She currently experienced a wide range of depression symptoms. In various settings, she had been treated with several antidepressants, several major tranquilizers, and lithium, all with minimal success. The chart indicated that she had recently been diagnosed with diabetes.

The assessment process began with an hour-long clinical interview, which involved reviewing the circumstances surrounding her admission to the hospital; a review of her social, occupational, physical health, and psychiatric history; questions about a wide variety of psychiatric symptoms; and a brief mental status exam. Observations of her physical appearance, dress, movement, verbal and nonverbal behavior, and gait were all relevant. The interview raised several salient diagnostic issues. First, in terms of appearance, it was noted that the woman had dark hair on her arms, was greatly overweight (about 270 lb), and appeared very tired. It was learned that the woman had started her menstrual periods at age 8, began to have emotional problems at this time, and had had intermittent and sometimes infrequent menstrual periods. Second, it was learned that her sleep was chronically disturbed, during periods of both psychiatric decompensation and relative well-being. All of her visual hallucinations and most of her auditory hallucinations had occurred at night or in the early morning during the sleep-wake transition. She also had a 10-year history of alcohol dependence, with abstinence during the previous year. The hallucinations had decreased in frequency during her period of abstinence but had not disappeared altogether. She denied ever having experienced seizures. She showed multiple elevations on the MMPI-2 scales, the overall profile most closely approximating a 2–7 profile, which suggests an anxious, ruminative type of depression. Her WAIS-R (Wechsler Adult Intelligence Scale—Revised; Wechsler, 1981) showed an average IQ with little subtest scatter and no significant Verbal-Performance difference.

These results suggested the need for an endocrinological consultation, given the menstrual irregularities, the patient's weight, and the hair on her arms. The possibility of Cushing's syndrome or some other type of endocrinological disorder was considered. A dietary consultation was also recommended. Given the normal WAIS-R, consistent with expectation, and no history of head injury or other likely causes of organic impairment except for 10 years of alcohol abuse, no referral for a neurological exam or additional neuropsychological testing was recommended. An extended sleep record on the unit was arranged, with a request that the staff pay particular attention to her breathing during room checks to see if there were periods of sleep apnea.

The picture of this woman that emerged was of someone who was probably experiencing major depression, recurrent, with mood-congruent psychotic features. A primary sleep disorder was strongly suggested, with difficulty in the sleep-wake transition period. The visual hallucinations and auditory hallucinations appeared to be related primarily to her sleep disturbance and prior alcohol abuse and appeared to reflect REM (rapid-eye-movement) rebound effects. No significant evidence of organicity or epilepsy was obtained. When taken off the major tranquilizers, she showed no increase in hallucinations or other psychotic symptoms. She did show greater energy and some improvement in mood. The issue of possible endocrinological disturbance was never clarified because the patient did not have any source of reimbursement for such a consultation and the treatment program had limited resources for such consultations. The patient was discharged after 30 days of inpatient treatment to a day treatment program in a community mental health center and was followed for medication management. The recommendation was communicated that this woman receive an endocrinological evaluation and further assessment of sleep disorder, but I do not know whether she ever received such an evaluation.

This example serves to communicate several points about the actual assessment of real patients in applied settings, particularly publicly funded programs. At times, there are so many diagnostic issues that should be investigated that patients leave the inpatient facility before their diagnostic picture is clear. At various times during her inpatient stay, some treatment staff felt that this woman might best be diagnosed as experiencing schizophrenia, alcohol dependence, major depression, organicity, schizoaffective disorder, borderline personality disorder, sleep disorder, or an endocrinological disorder. Consensus was reached among the treatment staff that she was not schizophrenic, currently dependent on alcohol, organic, or experiencing a borderline personality disorder. However, the range of diagnostic issues not fully clarified was wide, and could have had significant implications for treatment.

PROTOTYPICAL TREATMENT

The hallmark of behavior therapy is an individualized assessment of behavioral deficits, a treatment plan designed to remediate all relevant deficits, and continual assessment throughout the course of treatment. When interventions are not successful in modifying targeted behaviors, additional interventions are designed and implemented. This is a flexible, problem-specific approach, designed to capitalize on the individual difficulties of a specific client. Assessment is integral to the process of treatment in that it identifies and monitors the relevant target behaviors.

Despite the emphasis on an individualized, or idiographic, approach to treatment, essentially all large-scale outcome studies of the behavioral treatment of depression have used the group comparison format, in which patients are given a structured clinical program such as cognitive therapy, social skills training, assertiveness training, or interventions to increase pleasant activity. These treatments often use a treatment manual, employ relatively inexperienced therapists, and typically conduct the research study on outpatients. Relatively few behavioral-treatment outcome studies have been conducted on depressed inpatients.

Behavioral Treatment Components for Depression

Some of the major behavioral treatment components for depression are (1) increasing pleasant activities; (2) cognitive therapy; (3) social skills and assertiveness training; and (4) problem solving.

Increasing Pleasant Activities. Lewinsohn provided systematic procedures for increasing pleasant activities for outpatient depressives. Basically, his procedure involves the administration of the Pleasant Events Schedule (MacPhillamy & Lewinsohn, 1971) to determine the frequency of patients' engagement in pleasant activities during the past month and their subjective enjoyment of these events. A 160-item or 80-item activity schedule is then developed based on the items judged by the patient to be the most pleasant. The patient completes daily records of how many activities have been engaged in and rates her or his overall mood on a daily basis. The patient is encouraged to engage in more pleasant activities and is shown the relationship between rated mood and the number of positive events engaged in. Active discussion and problem solving of how the patient can engage in more activities is also undertaken.

Cognitive Therapy.   Procedures for cognitive therapy have been described in some detail by Beck, Rush, Shaw, and Emery (1979). The basic procedure involves helping the client to examine instances of negative thinking and to help the client challenge negative thoughts and avoid the negative distortion of information. A Socratic dialogue is used to bring the client into greater awareness of the thought patterns that predispose him or her to see things in a depressive way.

Research on depressed outpatients has generally found that cognitive therapy is as effective as antidepressant medication. Some research has actually suggested that cognitive therapy may be more effective than medication (Rush, Beck, Kovacs, & Hollon, 1977). Both types of treatment are more effective than control conditions. Moreover, some studies comparing the combination of antidepressant medication with cognitive therapy have shown that the combination is typically more effective than either treatment alone (Blackburn, Bishop, Glen, Whalley, & Christie, 1981; Teasdale, Fennell, Hibbert, & Amies, 1984).

Social Skills and Assertiveness Training.   In the organizational format provided by Twentyman and Zimering (1979), the major components of social skills training include behavioral rehearsal of desired responses, modeling, coaching, feedback, homework assignments, projected positive consequences (where the client is taught to imagine positive reactions to specific social behavior), and cognitive modifications. The types of behaviors that are often taught in these programs include asking questions, giving compliments, making positive statements, making eye contact, asking others for specific behavior change, speaking in a clear tone of voice, and avoiding fidgets and self-denigrations. Bellack, Hersen, and Himmelhoch (1981) presented data on female depressed outpatients that showed that social skills training improved social functioning and depressive symptomatology. Many other research studies have been conducted on outpatients and inpatients of varying diagnostic groups. Generally, although it seems clear that improvement in social functioning may occur as a result of social skills training, the extent of generalizability to the natural environment is less clear.

Problem Solving.   D'Zurilla and Goldfried (1971) and McLean (1976) have presented discussions of the steps necessary to solve personal problems. Both approaches include a specification of the problem, the generation of likely alternative approaches to the problem, an evaluation of these alternatives, and a reevaluation of the effects after attempts have been made. Such a structured approach to personal problems is often used clinically with depressed individuals as part of a comprehensive behavioral treatment of depression, such as was evaluated by McLean and Hakstian (1979). The rationale for these interventions is that depressed individuals are often overwhelmed by a multitude of specific problems and avoid decision making, thus further compounding their personal problems.

Actual Treatment

Extensive behavioral or cognitive-behavioral treatment for depression on inpatient units is still relatively rare. There are several barriers to this type of approach, such as the medicalization of the hospital environment; the extreme level of client distress, which often mandates pharmacological treatment; the difficulty of implementing behavioral techniques when the client is not in his or her natural environment; the relatively short length of inpatient stays, particularly in private facilities; and the difficulty of providing continuity of care.

Examples from Research Studies

Reisinger (1972) published one of the earliest examples of behavioral treatment for depression in an inpatient setting. In this single-case-study token-economy program, tokens were provided to the subject when she smiled and fines were applied when she cried. The results were that smiling and crying behavior could be readily manipulated by the token economy program. Although this study illustrates this approach, a wider range of target behaviors would seem to be desirable.

Miller, Bishop, Norman, and Keitner (1985) conducted a preliminary study with six chronically depressed, drug-refractory inpatients, in which three subjects who received cognitive therapy plus medication were compared with three subjects treated with social skills training plus medication. Two of three of these poor-prognosis patients improved in each group.

A subsequent controlled-treatment study by Miller *et al.* (1989) investigated the incremental effects of either cognitive therapy or social skills training in addition to standard unit programming (hospital milieu and pharmacotherapy) and psychiatric follow-up after discharge. The patients were randomly assigned to one of three treatment conditions: standard treatment, standard treatment plus cognitive therapy, and standard treatment plus social skills training. All treatments began on the inpatient unit and continued for four months on an outpatient basis after discharge. The patients in all treatment conditions showed significant improvement at discharge and at the end of the outpatient treatment period. Although there was no difference among the three conditions at discharge from the inpatient unit, the subjects assigned to either the cognitive therapy condition or the social skills condition showed reduced symptomatology at the end of treatment compared with patients who received the standard treatment.

Bowers (1988) conducted a study on depressed inpatients in which 10 patients received medication (nortriptyline) only, 10 patients received relaxation plus medication, and 10 patients received cognitive therapy plus medication. Although all groups improved over the course of the study, the cognitive therapy and relaxation subjects reported fewer depressive symptoms and fewer negative cognitions at discharge. Also, fewer subjects in the cognitive therapy group were judged to be depressed at discharge, compared with the other groups.

Clinical Applications in the Psychiatric Setting

The effort to increase pleasant activities is often difficult within an inpatient setting, as relatively few opportunities exist of the type described by MacPhillamy and Lewinsohn (1971). I have used copies of their Pleasant Events Schedule (MacPhillamy & Lewinsohn, 1971) or a shortened version that I have adapted, as a technique to help depressed individuals become more aware of opportunities for pleasant events. For example, in a group format, I have passed out copies of a list of pleasant events and asked the group members to check off how many of these events they were involved in during the last three months before admission. A brief discussion would ensue, in which, typically, at least some clients exclaimed that they had forgotten all about going bowling or to the beach and so on, even though such experiences had been pleasurable in the past. Sometimes, clients remark that they had not realized how isolated they have become. Using the principle of behavioral contracting, I typically ask each person in the group to commit verbally to doing several positive things during the first two weeks after discharge. I also attempt to get a commitment from group members to attempt to do some positive things together on the unit during the rest of the day or the next day. Clients also take home their list of positive events after discharge.

On more than one occasion, the attempt to increase pleasant activities has made clear to me that an individual I was treating for depression was really bipolar. For example, during the assessment process, it may become clear that an individual has been involved in an incredibly broad range of activity before admission, or the attempt to increase pleasant events may be met with a general increase in activity, pressured speech, and a flight of ideas. Obviously, for bipolar individuals, it is not desirable to encourage greater activity.

Social skills programs seem relatively common in publicly funded inpatient programs, or in day treatment programs for the severely mentally ill. Such programs do not seem to be as common in private psychiatric hospitals that deal with a somewhat higher functioning group of patients. An exception that I observed was a group social-skills-training program at Butler Hospital in Providence, Rhode Island. The psychologist in charge of the group conducted a series of rotating topics involving assertiveness, problem solving, increasing social activities, and so on. The attending psychiatrists were able to refer interested patients to this group, and specific fees were billed for group psychotherapy. The group was very popular and was essentially a clinical service—not part of a research effort. Two nurses assisted the group leader with this group.

Cognitive therapy, in its classic form, is still relatively rare on inpatient units. On these relatively short-stay units, the emphasis is typically to start medication, stabilize the patients, provide support, and after ensuring that the patients will not be a danger to themselves or others, discharge them to a less restrictive form of outpatient treatment. In the private setting, some "managed-care" insurance plans allow for as little as six days of reimbursement for major depressive disorder. The modal length of stay in private settings for major depressive disorder is probably approximately two weeks.

Concerns have been raised about the applicability of cognitive therapy in inpatient settings. Cognitive therapy is a somewhat intellectually demanding form of treatment, requiring the patient to make fine distinctions between thoughts, beliefs, ideas, and feelings. Some inpatients may lack the cognitive capacity to make these distinctions either because of severe depression or because of low intelligence. The concept of thoughts as specific events (talking to oneself) and the impact that this talking to oneself can have on one's emotional state is fairly abstract. I have used a somewhat simplified form of cognitive therapy with a large number of depressed inpatients whom I have treated, using several worksheets. One of the worksheets lists the following four items, with space after each item in which the client can write responses.

1. Describe a specific situation that happened today or yesterday that brought out your feelings of depression.
2. List your negative self-statements (thoughts) that made the depression feel worse.
3. Argue against those negative self-statements.
4. List some positive self-statements.

I have found it helpful to introduce this worksheet as follows:

> I want to work with you on a strategy for getting rid of depressing thoughts. It's true that big problems usually cause depression (like the things that happened to you before going into the hospital), but what do you think keeps that depression going? It's really the day-to-day problems and hassles—little things—and the way you think about those problems that feed the depression and keep it going weeks and months after all the bad things happened to you. Most people who get depressed think they need to keep thinking about their big problems and try to make sense of what has happened. And although you do need to spend some time thinking about those things, you've spent enough time thinking about them right now. You need a break from those problems. Besides, you're also finding it hard to deal with the smaller problems in your life right now. Let's work on those problems right now. Let's take today, for example. When did you feel your most depressed today? At what time? What happened to you that brought out those feelings of depression?

After I work with the client to get a specific "trigger," he or she writes it down in the first space. If nothing can be identified for today, I try yesterday. I resist going back much further, as the here-and-now perspective is important if the client is ever to implement this strategy as new problems develop. An example of a response to the answer to the first item is

> Good example: You felt your most depressed today when the nurse came in and told you that you would have to change rooms. Now, I want you to try to remember what specific thoughts popped into your head when you were told that. What did you say to yourself in your mind?

At this point, many inpatients have a lot of trouble being specific or identifying their thoughts. Instead, they start talking about some tangential issue, such as why they didn't want to change rooms. This may be helpful information for the therapist, but it is important to steer the conversation back to specific thoughts. I often tell patients that thoughts are "words that you say in your head." Ultimately, the patient will settle on a few thoughts like "My new roommate won't like me. This hospital moves people around like cattle—they don't really care about me. I never should have come into this hospital, anyway. I'll never get better here." I try to be fairly inclusive at this point and list several thoughts that the person had. It is only by seeing the depressive spiral of negative thoughts—the snowballing that occurs—that the patients can distance themselves for a moment from what has happened in order to take more rational perspective:

> Now I want you to start with the thought you mentioned: "My new roommate won't like me." If someone else told you that he or she had that thought, how could you argue against it? What could you tell that person about the way he or she was looking at things?

After a while, the client may come up with some examples like: "Hold it, I'm jumping the gun. I'm not going to assume this person won't like me. Some people have liked me in the past. Besides, I'm here to get help just as this person is. I need to concentrate on getting better. It doesn't mater that much what this person thinks of me. Sure, it's an inconvenience having a new roommate, but I can handle that." Then, I say:

> As a last step, it sometimes helps to think some positive thoughts related to this type of experience. Try to wash out those negative feelings. Tell me something positive about yourself.

Here the client may say that she or he can be a good friend, or is trustworthy, or that people like her or him once they become acquainted, and so on.

My experience is that most depressed inpatients can use this simplified format, but some patients absolutely cannot grasp the concept of a thought or may be so preoccupied with the big events that brought on the depression that they do not cooperate. Other patients cannot read or write, may not speak English very well, or may be very hard of hearing. Some patients refuse to cooperate, saying that they can't be helped. When this occurs, I try to take that thought as an example and try to work with it. When patients are preoccupied with the big events, I point out to them that they seem preoccupied with what happened in the past and that they need to take a break from those thoughts right now. I tell them that, generally, one's thoughts can concern only the past, the present, or the future: "Right now, I want you to think about the present, today, only things that happened today."

Complications in Multiple Diagnoses or Multiple Problem Areas

A significant number of inpatients may qualify for more than one diagnostic category or may otherwise have significant problems not directly related to their primary psychiatric condition. For example, a depressed person may have a significant marital problem, obesity, a drinking problem, borderline intellectual functioning or mild mental retardation, obsessive-compulsive disorder, or a primary sleeping disorder. The cognitive-behavioral approach to treatment emphasizes the importance of assessing all problem areas and developing interventions for all significant problems. Thus, for a depressed person who is experiencing obesity and is complaining about a lack of significant relationships, interventions may be developed that deal with depression, social relationships, and obesity. Inherent in the comprehensive, problem-specific nature of cognitive-behavioral treatment is the role of case management, in addition to treatment. The behavior therapist need not provide all necessary interventions in the team approach to treatment that occurs in inpatient settings. Medications, dietary programs, adjunctive marital therapy, vocational assessment and consultation, and other interventions may be available from other professional staff.

Although it is not possible to discuss treatments for all problems that may coincide with depression, substance abuse and marital discord are two relatively common complicating conditions in the treatment of depression found in the inpatient setting.

Substance Abuse: Dual-Diagnosis Issues.   An area of growing national attention in clinical research concerns dually diagnosed individuals, that is, those who present with a clinical disorder such as schizophrenia or depression and also abuse drugs or alcohol. There appears to be much more evidence on the association of depression and alcohol abuse than on the association of depression and drug abuse (Mayfield, 1985). Also, individuals with bipolar disorder are more likely to have substance abuse problems than individuals with unipolar depression.

It has become increasingly clear that depressed individuals who also abuse alcohol should have focused treatment for the alcohol abuse, in addition to treatment for depression. Schuckit (1986) concluded that 5%–10% of patients with affective disorder increase their drinking when depressed to the point where a secondary diagnosis becomes warranted. Although depression may bring on alcohol abuse in some individuals, it is also clear that alcohol abuse can worsen or maintain depression. On a basic level, alcohol is a depressant drug, which reduces motor behavior. It also brings on the associated stress of family, social, and occupational problems that may come with alcohol abuse. Research by Woodruff, Guze, Clayton, and Carr (1973) found that dually diagnosed patients were more similar to alcoholics than to depressed persons. This type of research seems to support current clinical lore, which argues that alcohol abuse must be treated concurrently with depression. The behavioral model of functional analysis argues that all deficits should be targeted in a comprehensive treatment plan. It is unwise to assume that remediating one deficit will necessarily remediate another type of deficit.

Marital Problems.   Marital discord is quite frequent among married depressed persons and may have etiological significance for some couples (Jacobson, Holtzworth-Munroe, & Schmaling, 1989). In the inpatient setting, social workers are often assigned the task of conducting a family assessment and beginning marital or family therapy during the inpatient stay, if necessary. However, little or no research has been conducted on the effect of cognitive-behavioral marital therapy on depressed inpatients. However, cognitive-behavioral marital therapy has been shown to alleviate depression among married depressed outpatients (O'Leary & Beach, 1990). Thus, this area needs more investigation.

Implementation Issues within Private "Medical-Model" Facilities

During the 1980s, there was a tremendous increase in the number of private, for-profit treatment facilities. Major corporations such as Charter Hospital Corporation and Hospital Corporation of America built new facilities and bought existing private nonprofit treatment facilities. Some of these hospitals advertise on television and in the newspapers, refer to their clients as "customers," and sometimes provide staff incentives of various kinds for admitting patients. Many academic psychologists and public-mental-health staff view this trend with increasing concern. These programs generally endorse a medical-model approach to treatment, with a high proportion of nursing staff, low staff-to-client ratios, and an admitting psychiatrist who is clearly in charge of the treatment team. It may come as a surprise, therefore, that some of these corporations are fairly open to structured cognitive-behavioral interventions for the treatment of depression.

Part of the reason this opportunity exists is that these corporations often use a marketing approach that emphasizes patient tracks such as affective disorders programs, women's programs, eating-disorders programs, and chemical dependency programs. These corporations have found that patients are very interested in the types of group treatments and individual therapy approaches that are offered. The business maxim that "the customer is always right" seems to hold sway, even when it is in conflict with the views of the medical staff. Second, some of these corporations have become aware of the large number of psychologists and "allied mental-health professionals" in clinical practice, compared to the number of psychiatrists. To position their hospitals for inpatient referrals, some of these hospitals are allowing professional staff membership and granting more inclusive privileges for psychologists and other allied mental-health professionals. The American Psychological Association has also fought for more inclusive treatment opportunities for psychologists and has published a book entitled *A Hospital Practice Primer for Psychologists* (1985).

While they are working to improve funding opportunities and to improve the less restrictive forms of care in the community, particularly for the severely mentally ill, it can be argued that cognitive-behavioral psychologists should not ignore the clear national trend toward privatization and should participate in establishing cognitive-behavioral treatments for the inpatients in these private hospitals. Dorwart, Schlesinger, Davidson, Epstein, and Hoover (1991), using 1988 data, reported that 18.2% of the patients in public psychiatric hospitals were depressed; 34.0% of the patients in private nonprofit hospitals were depressed; and 34.7% of the patients in private for-profit hospitals were depressed. Thus, private psychiatric hospitals, both nonprofit and for-profit, tend to emphasize the treatment of depressed inpatients. If cognitive-behavioral interventions are to occur with depressed inpatients, they must occur in the types of settings that emphasize the treatment of depression.

I was a consultant and therapist for 3 1/2 years at a private, for-profit hospital and developed and implemented a depression group program that involved three one-hour group therapy sessions per week on an inpatient unit. The patients were admitted to the affective disorders program, stayed an average of three to four weeks, and were almost all treated with antidepressant medication. The group had a rotating series of eight topics: negative thinking, problem solving, cognitive therapy, increasing social activities, irrational beliefs and expectations, assertiveness training, positive self-statement training, and improving sleep patterns. The group size varied from 5 to 18 patients, about 12 patients being the norm. On any one day, there might be two or three new admissions and two or three discharges.

The group was designed to help patients learn various coping techniques to overcome depression, as well as to provide information about the psychiatric problem of depression. Only one topic was discussed in a particular session. These topics were designed to cover the major problems that depressed people often experience. The topics were general enough so that most patients were able to identify some difficulties, concerns, and goals for behavior change within each topic.

I began a typical group session by introducing myself and any new members of the group and giving the name of the group and a brief description of it. I then identified and discussed the topic for the day, explaining the relevance of that topic to depression. I elicited input from the patients to help determine the relevance and importance of the topic for each individual. I then encouraged the patients to discuss the real-life problems they were having that were related to the topic being discussed, and we worked on a variety of therapeutic exercises, including role playing, written exercises, written practice, group feedback, and homework exercises, in the effort to help the patients improve their coping responses or to develop more effective skills in dealing with problem situations. I used interpretation, direct questioning, reflecting feelings, emotional support, catharsis, and other therapeutic techniques, as well as the specific psycho-educational practices that were being discussed.

The specific patient goals were to

1. Learn basic information about the prevalence of depression, its symptoms, the expected course of the disorder, the types of treatment, and the causes of depression.
2. Identify repetitive negative thought patterns, challenge those thoughts, and reduce depressive thinking.
3. Become more aware of positive experiences and interactions, learning to monitor positive activities and increasing participation in social activities.
4. Learn several approaches for improving and strengthening positive sleep patterns and sleep habits.
5. Become more assertive in expressing requests and dealing with problems before they build up into resentment and depression.
6. Identify positive coping thoughts that help to improve negative moods, learning how thoughts often precede mood states and learning to gain better control over moods.
7. Become more aware of the basic beliefs that influence one's behavior and lifestyle, reevaluating one's basic beliefs and lifestyle to consider whether irrational expectations are adding unnecessary stress.
8. Become more adept at problem solving, learn to quickly identify when problems are becoming overwhelming and learn to evaluate problems rationally, one at a time.

There was no opportunity to collect research data on the effectiveness of this program, although prior research and anecdotal data would suggest that these types of procedures should improve treatment effectiveness, compared with unit "milieu" treatment.

SUMMARY

At this point, a number of studies have established the efficacy of cognitive-behavioral treatments for depressed outpatients. Much less research has been conducted on inpatients. The initial emphasis on outpatient research was appropriate, in that this is the setting where most psychological interventions for depression occur. However, the relative dearth of funding available in public mental-health programs, among other reasons (cf. Knox, 1988), has tended to demedicalize public programs and offers opportunities for psychosocial, behavioral, and cognitive-behavioral interventions. Community mental-health centers, public crisis-stabilization units, and state hospitals are relatively open to cognitive-behavioral interventions. Recent changes in private hospitals, with more hospitals adopting specialized programs for affective disorder patients, and a greater push to include psychologists as allied mental-health practitioners provide opportunities for focused cognitive-behavioral interventions.

Thus, in this environment, it is important to research further the effectiveness of cognitive-behavioral interventions for depressed inpatients. However, it may be necessary to adapt these interventions to the needs of these patients.

Several issues should also be raised concerning the training of psychologists. Some graduate students in clinical psychology go into internship with little clinical experience in working with severe psychopathology, or without sufficient background in neuropsychology, basic endocrinology, pharmacology, or medical terminology. Although behaviorally oriented graduate programs may eschew aspects of the medical model, they should not ignore it. Graduate programs can do more to provide students with information about medical issues. A graduate course that includes medical abbreviations and describes common medical laboratory tests and medical procedures would be very helpful.

There is currently an opportunity for behavioral psychologists to make a real impact on clinical treatment, research, and administration in publicly funded mental-health programs because of the shortage of physicians willing to take these positions. Changes in the private sector may also open doors for psychologists. But to function in these applied settings, a cognitive-behavioral clinician must be willing to expand his or her knowledge base in medical procedures, terminology, and ways of thinking. Only then can we reduce the gap between the prototype of behavioral treatment and the realities in applied settings.

REFERENCES

Abramson, L. Y., Seligman, M. E. P., & Teasdale, J. D. (1978). Learned helplessness in humans: Critique and reformulation. *Journal of Abnormal Psychology*, *87*, 49–74.

Allen, M. (1976). Twin studies of affective illness. *Archives of General Psychiatry*, *33*, 1476–1478.

American Psychiatric Association. (1987). *Diagnostic and statistical manual of mental disorders* (3rd ed., rev.; DSM-III-R). Washington, DC: Author.

American Psychological Association. (1985). *A hospital practice primer for psychologists*. Washington, DC: Author.

Arkowitz, H., Lichtenstein, E., McGovern, K., & Hines, P. (1975). The behavioral assessment of social competence in males. *Behavior Therapy*, *6*, 3–13.

Beck, A. T. (1967). *Depression: Causes and treatment*. Philadelphia: University of Pennsylvania Press.

Beck, A. T. (1978). *Beck Depression Inventory*. New York: Psychological Corporation, Harcourt Brace Jovanovich.

Beck, A. T., Ward, C. H., Mendelson, M., Mock, J., & Erbaugh, J. (1961). An inventory for measuring depression. *Archives of General Psychiatry*, *4*, 561–571.

Beck, A. T., Rush, A. J., Shaw, B. F., & Emery, G. (1979). *Cognitive therapy of depression*. New York: Guilford Press.

Bellack, A. S., Hersen, M., & Turner, S. M. (1979). Relationship of role-playing and knowledge of appropriate behavior to assertion in the natural environment. *Journal of Consulting and Clinical Psychology*, *47*, 670–678.

Bellack, A. S., Hersen, M., & Himmelhoch, J. (1981). Social skills training compared with pharmacotherapy and psychotherapy in the treatment of unipolar depression. *American Journal of Psychiatry*, *138*, 1562–1567.

Biglan, A., & Dow, M. G. (1981). Toward a second generation model: A problem-specific approach. In L. Rehm (Ed.), *Behavior therapy for depression*. New York: Academic Press.

Blackburn, I. M., Bishop, S., Glen, A. I. M., Whalley, L. J., & Christie, J. E. (1981). The efficacy of cognitive therapy in depression: A treatment trial using cognitive therapy and pharmacotherapy, each alone and in combination. *British Journal of Psychiatry*, *139*, 181–189.

Bowers, W. A. (1988). *Treatment of depressed inpatients: Cognitive therapy plus medication, relaxation plus medication, and medication alone*. Paper presented at the annual meeting of the American Psychological Association, Atlanta.

Butcher, J. N., Dahlstrom, W. G., Graham, J. R., Tellegen, A., & Krammer, B. (1989). *MMPI-2 manual for administration and scoring*. Minneapolis: University of Minnesota Press.

Butcher, J. N., Graham, J. R., Williams, C. L., & Ben-Porath, Y. S. (1990). *Development and use of the MMPI-2 content scales*. Minneapolis: University of Minnesota Press.

Coppen, A., Abou-Saleh, M., Milln, P., Metcalfe, M., Harwood, J., & Bailey, J. (1983). Dexamethasone suppression test in depression and other psychiatric illness. *British Journal of Psychiatry*, *142*, 498–504.

Craighead, W. E. (1980). Away from a unitary model of depression. *Behavior Therapy*, *11*, 122–128.

Dorwart, R. A., Schlesinger, M., Davidson, H., Epstein, S., & Hoover, C. (1991). A national study of psychiatric hospital care. *American Journal of Psychiatry*, *148*, 204–210.

Dow, M. G., & Craighead, W. E. (1987). Social inadequacy and depression: Overt behavior and self-evaluation processes. *Journal of Social and Clinical Psychology*, *5*, 99–113.

D'Zurilla, T. J., & Goldfried, M. R. (1971). Problem-solving and behavior modification. *Journal of Abnormal Psychology*, *78*, 107–126.

Ferster, C. B. (1966). Animal behavior and mental illness. *Psychological Record*, *16*, 345–356.

Glassman, A. H., Arana, G. W., Baldessarini, R. J., Brown, W. A., Carroll, B. J., Davis, J. M., Greenblatt, D. J., Klerman, G. L., Orsulak, P., Schildkraut, J. J., & Shader, R. I. (1987). The Dexamethasone Suppression Test: An overview of its current status in psychiatry. *American Journal of Psychiatry*, *144*, 1253–1262.

Gold, M. S., Pottash, A. L. C., & Extein, I. (1981). Hypothyroidism and depression, evidence from complete thyroid function evaluation. *Journal of the American Medical Association*, *245*, 1919–1922.

Hathaway, S. R., & McKinley, J. C. (1942). *Minnesota Multiphasic Personality Inventory*. Minneapolis: University of Minnesota Press.

Insel, T. R., & Goodwin, F. K. (1983). Promises and problems of diagnostic laboratory tests in psychiatry. *Hospital and Community Psychiatry*, *34*, 1131–1138.

Jacobson, N. S., Holtzworth-Munroe, A., & Schmaling, K. B. (1989). Marital therapy and spouse involvement in the treatment of depression, agoraphobia, and alcoholism. *Journal of Consulting and Clinical Psychology*, *57*, 5–10.

Knox, M. D. (1988). Factors affecting psychiatrists' availability to serve in public programs. *Psychiatric Quarterly*, *59*, 113–120.

Kupfer, D. J., Weiss, B. L., Foster, F. G., Detre, T. P., Delgado, J., & McPartland, R. (1974). Psychomotor activity in affective state. *Archives of General Psychiatry*, *30*, 765–768.

Lewinsohn, P. M. (1974). Clinical and theoretical aspects of depression. In K. S. Calhoun, H. W. Adams, & K. M. Mitchell (Eds.), *Innovative treatment methods in psychopathology* (pp. 63–120). New York: Wiley.

Lewinsohn, P. M., & Hoberman, H. M. (1982). Behavioural and cognitive approaches. In E. S. Paykel (Ed.), *Handbook of affective disorders*. New York: Guilford Press.

Lewinsohn, P. M., & Lee, W. M. L. (1981). Assessment of affective disorders. In D. Barlow (Ed.), *Behavioral assessment of adult disorders* (pp. 129–179). New York: Guilford Press.

MacPhillamy, D. J., & Lewinsohn, P. M. (1971). *A scale for the measurement of positive reinforcement*. Unpublished mimeo, University of Oregon.

Mayfield, D. (1985). Substance abuse in the affective disorders. In A. I. Alterman (Ed.), *Substance abuse and psychopathology* (pp. 69–90). New York: Plenum Press.

McLean, P. (1976). Therapeutic decision-making in the behavioral treatment of depression. In P. O. Davidson (Ed.), *Behavioral management of anxiety, depression, and pain* (pp. 54–90). New York: Brunner/Mazel.

McLean, P., & Hakstian, L. (1979). Clinical depression: Comparative efficacy of outpatient treatments. *Journal of Consulting and Clinical Psychology*, *47*, 818–836.

Miller, I. W., Bishop, S., Norman, W. H., & Keitner, G. I. (1985). Cognitive-behavioral therapy and pharmacotherapy with chronic, drug-refractory depressed inpatients: A note of optimism. *Behavioral Psychotherapy*, *13*, 320–327.

Miller, I. W., Norman, W. H., Keitner, G. I., Bishop, S. B., & Dow, M. G. (1989). Cognitive-behavioral treatment of depressed inpatients. *Behavior Therapy*, *20*, 25–47.

O'Leary, K. D., & Beach, S. R. H. (1990). Marital therapy: A viable treatment for depression and marital discord. *American Journal of Psychiatry*, *147*, 183–186.

Rehm, L. P. (1977). A self-control model of depression. *Behavior Therapy*, *8*, 787–804.

Rehm, L. P. (1988). Assessment of depression. In A. S. Bellack & M. Hersen (Eds.), *Behavioral assessment: A practical handbook*. New York: Pergamon Press.

Rehm, L. P., & Marston, A. R. (1968). Reduction of social anxiety through modification of self-reinforcement: An instigation therapy technique. *Journal of Consulting and Clinical Psychology*, *32*, 565–574.

Reisinger, J. J. (1972). The treatment of "anxiety-depression" via positive reinforcement and response cost. *Journal of Applied Behavior Analysis*, *5*, 125–130.

Robins, L., Helzer, J. E., Croughan, J., & Ratcliff, K. S. (1981). National Institute of Mental Health Diagnostic Interview Schedule. *Archives of General Psychiatry*, *38*, 381–389.

Rush, A. J., Beck, A. T., Kovacs, M., & Hollon, S. (1977). Comparative efficacy of cognitive and pharmacotherapy in the treatment of depressed outpatients. *Cognitive Therapy and Research*, *1*, 17–37.

Schuckit, M. A. (1986). Genetic and clinical implications of alcoholism and affective disorder. *American Journal of Psychiatry*, *143*, 140–147.

Seligman, M. E. P. (1975). *Helplessness: On depression, development, and death*. San Francisco: Freedman.

Sinaikin, P., & Gold, M. S., (1987). Endocrinology and depression: 2. Thyroid function, In O. G. Cameron (Ed.), *Presentations of depression: Depression in medical and other psychiatric disorders* (pp. 275–290). New York: Wiley.

Smith, R. E., & Winokur, G. (1984). Affective disorders—Bipolar. In S. M. Turner & M. Hersen (Eds.), *Adult psychopathology and diagnosis* (pp. 245–262). New York: Wiley.

Spitzer, R. L., Endicott, J., & Robins, E. (1978). Research diagnostic criteria: Rationale and reliability. *Archives of General Psychiatry*, *35*, 773–782.

Spitzer, R. L., Williams, J. B. W., Gibbon, M., & First, M. B. (1990). *Structured clinical interview for DSM-III-R*. Washington, DC: American Psychiatric Press.

Starkman, M. N. (1987). Endocrinology and depression: 1. Hypothalamic-pituitary-adrenocortical hyperactivity and depression. In O. G. Cameron (Ed.), *Presentations of depression: Depression in medical and other psychiatric disorders* (pp. 251–273). New York: Wiley.

Teasdale, J. D., Fennell, M. J., Hibbert, G. A., & Amies, P. L. (1984). Cognitive therapy for major depressive disorder in primary care. *British Journal of Psychiatry*, *144*, 400–406.

Twentyman, C. T., & Zimering, R. T. (1979). Behavioral training of social skills: A critical review. In M. Hersen, R. M. Eisler, & P. M. Miller (Eds.), *Progress in behavior modification* (Vol. 7). New York: Academic Press.

Ward, J. C., & Naster, B. J. (1991). Reliability of an observational system used to monitor behavior on a mental health residential treatment unit. *Journal of Mental Health Administration, 18,* 64–68.

Wechsler, D. (1981). *Wechsler Adult Intelligence Scale—Revised.* New York: Psychological Corporation.

Weissman, M. M., & Myers, J. K. (1978). Affective disorders in a U.S. urban community. *Archives of General Psychiatry, 35,* 1304–1310.

Williams, J. G., Barlow, D. H., & Agras, W. S. (1972). Behavioral measurement of severe depression. *Archives of General Psychiatry, 27,* 330–333.

Woodruff, R. A., Guze, S. B., Clayton, P. J., & Carr, D. (1973). Alcoholism and depression. *Archives of General Psychiatry, 28,* 97–100.

Youngren, M. A., & Lewinsohn, P. M. (1980). The functional relation between depression and problematic interpersonal behavior. *Journal of Abnormal Psychology, 89,* 333–341.

14

Schizophrenia

KIM T. MUESER

INTRODUCTION

Schizophrenia is a chronic, debilitating illness that afflicts approximately 1% of the adult population. Before the discovery of antipsychotic medications, effective treatments for schizophrenia were not known, and most patients were destined to spend their lives languishing in state hospitals with little hope of returning to the community. Between 1950 and 1965, the widespread use of antipsychotic medications, coupled with the spiraling costs of long-term inpatient treatment for mental illness, led to the "deinstitutionalization" movement, the locus of most psychiatric treatment shifting from the hospital to the community (Johnson, 1990). The change in treatment locus is reflected in the reduction of hospital beds in the United States occupied by patients with psychiatric illness, from 560,000 in 1955 to under 140,000 in the mid-1970s (Meyer, 1976) and the drop in average length of hospital stay from six months to three weeks (Sharfstein, 1984).

As the inpatient population of schizophrenics declined, new problems emerged when it became clear that antipsychotic medications were not a panacea and that most patients remained chronically symptomatic, although in the community. The influx of patients into the community made the pervasive social deficits of schizophrenia more apparent to the general public, who often responded with fear and rejection. The dismal quality of life experienced by discharged schizophrenic patients and the social impoverishment of many residential and treatment settings in the community (Levitt, Hogan, & Bucosky, 1990) suggest that the term *transinstitutionalization* better describes the trend toward outpatient treatment than *deinstitutionalization* (Bellack & Mueser, 1986). Furthermore, most schizophrenics experience symptom relapses requiring brief inpatient treatment; cumulative relapse rates exceed 65% over 2 years and 90% over 10 years postdischarge (Hogarty, Anderson, & Reiss, 1987; Vaillant, 1978). Thus, the psychiatric hospital continues to play a pivotal role in the management of schizophrenia, and most patients return periodically to the hospital for the treatment of acute symptoms although they reside in the community. In many cases, the hospital continues to coordinate pharmacological and psychosocial outpatient treatment for patients living in the community.

KIM T. MUESER • Medical College of Pennsylvania at EPPI, Philadelphia, Pennsylvania 19129.

Handbook of Behavior Therapy in the Psychiatric Setting, edited by Alan S. Bellack and Michel Hersen. Plenum Press, New York, 1993.

Behavior therapy has evolved since the early 1960s as the most promising psychosocial treatment approach to improving the outcome of schizophrenia. Early behavioral treatments based on the token economy showed that even severely impaired, chronically ill schizophrenics were capable of learning new social behaviors in an inpatient setting (Ayllon & Azrin, 1968; Paul & Lentz, 1977). Later developments in social skills training and behavioral family therapy have demonstrated the importance of these interventions in improving the adjustment of patients living in the community (Liberman & Mueser, 1989). The discovery of novel antipsychotic medications for treatment-resistant schizophrenia (e.g., clozapine) is likely to further increase the number of patients living in the community who are amenable to behavioral interventions (Stephens, 1990). Although behavior therapy for schizophrenia is an emerging technology, research and clinical experience suggests that combining behavioral treatment with pharmacological treatment and case management reduces symptom relapses and optimizes social functioning.

DESCRIPTION OF DISORDER

Schizophrenia is a biological illness that can be precipitated or made worse by environmental stress. Family studies of schizophrenia indicate that vulnerability to the illness may be transmitted genetically, although other factors may also play a role. The concordance ratio for schizophrenia among monozygotic twins is between 25% and 50%, indicating that environment or nongenetic biological factors play a role in the etiology of schizophrenia (Holtzman & Matthysse, 1990). The pathogenesis of schizophrenia is not known at the present. Major theories hypothesize that an imbalance in brain neurotransmitters (e.g., dopamine), structural abnormalities in the brain (e.g., enlarged ventricles), and altered blood flow and activation of specific brain structures (e.g., the prefrontal cortex, the limbic system, and the basal ganglia) are involved in the pathophysiology of the disorder (Buchsbaum, 1990; Crow, 1990).

The Course of Schizophrenia

The onset of schizophrenia usually occurs in late adolescence or early adulthood, in most cases between the ages of 16 and 30 years. The disorder rarely develops after the age of 35, although it occasionally occurs later in life (Grahame, 1984). The onset often follows a period of time ranging from three months to over one year in which the person experiences a deterioration in social functioning accompanied by *prodromal* symptoms. The symptoms of the prodrome overlap with the symptoms of schizophrenia but are not identical, and they refer mainly to social withdrawal, odd ideas or form of speech, or perceptual aberrations.

The longitudinal course of schizophrenia is episodic, and the intensity of the symptoms varies over time. Often, during severe relapses, when the symptoms worsen dramatically, the patient must be hospitalized in order to minimize the risk of self-harm or injury to others. Persons with poor premorbid sexual and social competence are more likely to develop schizophrenia (Walker & Lewine, 1990), have a more severe course of the illness (Zigler & Glick, 1986), and have greater impairments in social skill (Mueser, Bellack, Morrison, & Wixted, 1990). Once schizophrenia has developed, the course of the illness is usually chronic across the adult life span; few patients return to their premorbid social or vocational levels of functioning between symptom relapses. However, symptom severity decreases over long periods of time, and a significant number of patients have symptom remissions later in life (Ciompi, 1985; Harding, Brooks, Ashikaga, Strauss, & Breier, 1987). Females tend to have a later onset of illness and a more benign course—including fewer hospitalizations and better social functioning—than males (Angermeyer & Kuhn, 1988; Mueser, Bellack, Morrison, & Wade, 1990a).

Diagnosis and Characteristic Symptoms

Impairment in social and/or vocational functioning is the most fundamental symptom of schizophrenia, and without this symptom, the illness cannot be diagnosed according to the criteria of the revised third edition of the *Diagnostic and Statistical Manual* (DSM-III- R; American Psychiatric Association, 1987). The DSM-III-R criteria require the continuous presence of symptoms over a minimum of six months for the diagnosis of schizophrenia. If symptoms have been present for more than one week and less than six months, the person meets the criteria for *schizophreniform disorder*, which often develops into schizophrenia over time.

The symptoms of schizophrenia can be divided into three broad categories: negative symptoms, positive symptoms, and mood disturbances. *Negative symptoms* are defined by the absence or paucity of behaviors, mood states, or cognitions ordinarily present in healthy individuals. The most common symptoms include *blunted or flattened affect* (diminished facial and vocal expressiveness), *emotional withdrawal*, *alogia* (low amount of speech or poverty of content), *anhedonia* (diminished hedonic capacity), *asociality* (lack of social drive and libido), *apathy*, *lack of curiosity*, *social withdrawal*, *poor attention*, and *motor and psychomotor retardation*. These symptoms are relatively stable over time and exist independent of depression. There is a strong association between severity of negative symptoms and impairment in social functioning (Bellack, Morrison, Wixted, & Mueser, 1990b).

In contrast to negative symptoms, positive symptoms are defined as the presence or excess of behaviors, cognitions, or mood states that are ordinarily absent in healthy persons. The most common positive symptoms are *hallucinations* (experiencing perceptions in the absence of sensory stimulation) and *delusions* (beliefs that are not culturally bound and that others recognize as clearly false or impossible). About 80% of schizophrenic patients experience hallucinations, auditory hallucinations being the most common, followed by visual hallucinations, and then other types of hallucinations (Mueser, Bellack, & Brady, 1990). The most common types of delusions are *perscutory delusions*, *delusions of control* (e.g., thought insertion or thought withdrawal), *delusions of reference* (e.g., the television is talking to the patient), and *delusions of grandeur*. Positive symptoms that are disorders of communication and motor behavior include *word salad* (disordered syntax), *loose associations*, *stereotypical behaviors*, *mannerisms*, and *posturing*. These symptoms are comparatively rare and usually occur only briefly during florid psychotic episodes. Positive symptoms tend to be less stable over time than negative symptoms and, because of their subjective quality, are more difficult to assess reliably (Lewine, 1990; Mueser, Douglas, Bellack, & Morrison, 1991).

Mood disturbances such as *depression*, *anxiety*, *anger*, and *hostility* are common in schizophrenia and often appear secondary to chronic positive symptoms. Paranoid delusions are often accompanied by anger and hostility. Persistent auditory hallucinations or delusions frequently cause anxiety and depression as patients become aware of a loss of control over their own subjective experiences. Most schizophrenics experience depression, approximately 50% attempt suicide at some time in their lives, and 10% die from suicide (Roy, 1986).

Subtypes of Schizophrenia

There have been many attempts to subtype schizophrenia over the past 100 years. The DSM-III-R retains the vestiges of subtypes originally described by Emil Kraepelin: paranoid, undifferentiated, disorganized, and catatonic schizophrenia. Other subtypes that have been the focus of previous research include acute/chronic, reactive/process, and approach/withdrawn schizophrenia. These subtypes have not been found to be consistently useful, either clinically or prognostically. Since the early 1980s, extensive research has been conducted on the positive/ negative symptom subtypes of schizophrenia (Andreasen, 1982; Crow, 1980). The theory postulates that the positive/negative symptom distinction reflects two distinct disease processes. Prominent positive symptoms are hypothesized to be the consequence of hyperdopaminergic transmission in the limbic system and are associated with good premorbid social functioning, a rapid onset of symptoms, favorable response to antipsychotic medications, and a fair prognosis. Prominent negative symptoms, on the other hand, are thought to result from neuronal loss and atrophy and are associated with poor premorbid social functioning, an insidious onset of symptoms, poor response to medication, and a poor prognosis. Although the positive/negative distinction continues to be a focus of research (Greden & Tandon, 1991), the validity of the subtype has been challenged. Patients with solely negative or positive symptoms are rare (Andreasen, Flaum, Swayze, Tyrrell, & Arndt, 1990), and stable high levels of negative symptoms are correlated with worse positive symptoms (Mueser, Douglas, Bellack, & Morrison, 1991). In addition, research has not supported the predicted differences between the positive and negative subgroups in response to antipsychotic medications nor in structural brain anomalies (Meltzer, 1985). At the present, evidence does not support the clinical utility of any schizophrenia subtypes.

Schizoaffective disorder is categorized in the DSM-III-R as a separate Axis I disorder, although it overlaps considerably with schizophrenia. The diagnostic criteria for schizoaffective disorder require the presence of a depressive or manic syndrome (see Chapter 13) for at least two weeks, irrespective of concomitant schizophrenic symptoms, and the presence of schizophrenic symptoms for at least two weeks when an affective syndrome is *not* present. Studies of the course of schizoaffective disorder indicate that the outcome falls between that for schizophrenia and that for the major affective disorders (Marneros & Tsuang, 1986). Research on the treatment of schizoaffective disorder suggests that it is responsive to antipsychotic medications and behavioral interventions similar to those to which schizophrenia is responsive.

PROTOTYPICAL ASSESSMENT

The behavioral assessment of schizophrenia requires a consideration of two broad areas related to the severity and the outcome of the illness: (1) characteristic impairments of the illness, including symptomatology and social adjustment; and (2) factors that can influence the severity of the illness and the vulnerability to symptom relapses, such as environmental stress, social skills, and substance abuse. The different assessment areas, methods of assessment, and instruments are summarized in Table 1.

Symptomatology and Social Adjustment

The diagnosis of schizophrenia should be established with a structured clinical interview. Symptom severity is best assessed through semistructured interviews that yield information based on both patient verbal reports and behavioral observations conducted in the interview. Patient self-report instruments are also useful, particularly in the assessment of mood. Self-reported negative mood states have been found to be more predictive of later thought disorder, relapse, and suicide than interview-based ratings (Blanchard, Mueser, & Bellack, in press; Cohen, Test, & Brown, 1990; Hogarty, Schooler, Ulrich, Mussare, Ferro, & Herron, 1979). Measures of social adjustment provide information about role functioning (e.g., social relationships and independent-living skills) and subjective quality of life. Information about social functioning can be obtained through standardized interviews with the patient and significant others, self-report instruments, and behavioral observation. Overt behavioral observations are useful for the assessment of social adjustment in the hospital, particularly self-care skills and ability to conduct basic social interactions.

Schizophrenia is a biological illness, but its course can be influenced by a myriad of biological, environmental, and patient variables. The stress-vulnerability-coping-skills model can guide the assessment of factors related to symptomatology, relapses, and social functioning in schizophrenia (Liberman & Mueser, 1989; Zubin & Spring, 1977). According to the model,

Table 1. Assessment Areas, Methods, and Instruments for Schizophrenia

Area	Methods	Instruments
Diagnosis	Structured interviews	Present state examination (Wing, Cooper, & Sartorius, 1974)
		Schedule for Affective Disorders and Schizophrenia (Endicott & Spitzer, 1978)
		Structured Clinical Interview for DSM-III-R (Spitzer & Williams, 1985)
Symptomatology	Semistructured interviews	Brief Psychiatric Rating Scale (Overall & Gorham, 1962)
		Positive and Negative Symptom Scale (Kay, Fiszbein, & Opler, 1987)
		Scale for the Assessment of Negative Symptoms (Andreasen & Olsen, 1982)
	Self-report	Symptom Checklist (Derogatis, 1977)
Social adjustment	Semistructured interviews: patient	Quality of Life Interview (Lehman, 1988)
		Quality of Life Scale (Heinrichs, Hanlon, & Carpenter, 1984)
		Social Adjustment Scale II—Patient Version (Schooler, Hogarty, & Weissman, 1979)
	Semistructured interviews: Relative and significant other	Social Adjustment Scale II—Family Version (Schooler, Hogarty, & Weissman, 1979)
		Social Performance Schedule (Wykes & Sturt, 1986)
	Self-report	Life Satisfaction Scale (Test, Knoedler, & Allness, 1985)
Biological vulnerability		
Medical noncompliance	Pill counts	
	Interviews with patient and significant others	
	Plasma	
Substance abuse	Interviews with patient and significant others	Case Manager Rating Scale (Drake, Osher, Noordsy, Hurlbut, Teague, & Beaudett, 1990)
	Toxicology screens	
Environmental stress and support		
Life events	Interviews with patient	Life Events Interview (Ventura, Nuechterlein, Lukoff, & Hardesty, 1989)
Expressed emotion	Interviews with patient	Camberwell Family Interview (Brown, Birley, & Wing, 1972)
Social support	Interviews with patient	Social Network Inventory (Escobar & Randolf, 1981)
Coping skills		
Social skills	Role-play tests	The Role-Play Test (Bellack, Morrison, Mueser, Wade, & Sayers, 1990a)
Coping with symptoms	Interview with patient	

social functioning, symptom severity, and sensitivity to symptom relapses are determined by three dynamic, interactive factors: biological vulnerability, environmental stress, and coping skills.

Vulnerability is assumed to be caused by genetic and early biological influences (e.g., birth complications) and is reflected by measures such as genetic loading, cognitive and attentional deficits, and schizotypal personality disorder. Biological vulnerability is necessary for the development of schizophrenia, but it is unclear whether it is sufficient for the illness to develop, or if environmental stress is a necessary trigger. *Stress* impinges on vulnerability to worsen social functioning and to cause symptom relapses. Stress can be defined as either discrete events or environmental contingencies that require the person to adapt in order to minimize negative effects. The negative impact of stress on vulnerability is mediated by the patient's *coping skills* (e.g., social skills). These skills are defined as abilities that enable the person to eliminate or reduce the source of stress, or to lessen its unpleasant effects. Coping skills are ordinarily acquired during childhood and adolescence through social learning, but they may be lost after the onset of the illness through disuse, lack of motivation, or reinforcement of the "sick" role.

The stress-vulnerability model points to possible avenues of behavioral intervention in schizophrenia. The model suggests that symptom relapses can be precipitated by changes in either vulnerability or stress that overwhelm the individual's coping skills. These areas must be assessed if future symptom relapses are to be reduced and the quality of social functioning is to be improved.

Changes in patients' biological vulnerability often cause symptom relapses in schizophrenia. Noncompliance with antipsychotic medications is common in over 25% of persons with schizophrenia, and it must be rectified if the illness is to be effectively managed (Corrigan, Liberman, & Engle, 1990; Kane, 1985). The assessment of compliance with oral medication can be conducted through direct questioning of the patient, significant others, or staff members, through pill counts, or through blood plasma levels. The use of more than one assessment method increases the reliability of the evaluation.

Another common way in which changes in vulnerability trigger relapses is substance abuse, particularly the abuse of stimulants, such as cocaine or amphetamines (Turner & Tsuang, 1990). The incidence of substance abuse in schizophrenia and schizoaffective disorder ranges between 15% and 50% (Mueser, Yarnold, Levinson, Singh, Bellack, Kee, Morrison, & Yadalam, 1990c). Patients may abuse drugs or alcohol in an attempt to self-medicate negative mood states or because the drugs are available from peers. Like the assessment of medication noncompliance, detecting substance abuse requires multiple sources of information, including the reports of patients, significant others, and mental health workers familiar with the patient (Drake, Osher, Noordsy, Hurlbut, Teague, & Beaudett, 1990). Toxicology screens are also useful in identifying covert substance abuse, which may be denied by patients who fear losing basic services if their abuse is detected.

Several different types of stress may increase patients' vulnerability to relapses. Life events, such as the loss of a significant other, are potent stressors that may trigger symptom relapses. Semistructured interviews can be used to assess recent life events and their perceived impact (Ventura, Nuechterlein, Lukoff, & Hardesty, 1989). Another important stressor is the presence of high levels of negative ambient emotion in the patient's family, "expressed emotion" (EE), which is predictive of relapses following a recent hospitalization (Parker & Hadzi-Pavlovic, 1990). Further information on the assessment of EE is included in Chapter 29. Other types of stress associated with increased symptomatology and relapse rates include lack of environmental structure (Rosen, Sussman, Mueser, Lyons, & Davis, 1981; Wong, Massel, Mosk, & Liberman, 1986) and treatment programs that expect rapid change and high patient turnover (Linn, Caffey, Klett, Hogarty, & Lamb, 1979).

Just as the environment in which the patient lives may be a source of stress to the patient, it may also buffer the noxious effects of stress. Social support and network size may both reduce stress on the patient. Social contacts are a strong predictor of outcome (Strauss & Carpenter, 1977), and reduced network size is common in schizophrenia (Cohen & Kochanowicz, 1989). Interviews with patients and significant others may be used to ascertain the availability of social support for the patient.

Two broad types of coping skill mediate the effects of stress: (1) self-regulation strategies for coping with chronic symptoms and (2) social skills for achieving socially oriented goals. Schizophrenic patients frequently develop methods for coping with persistent, distressful symptoms, such as auditory hallucinations and delusions of reference (Carr, 1988). Most effective coping methods involve shifting one's focus of attention, changing one's activity level, or modifying the intensity of sensory input. The use of multiple coping strategies is associated with improved coping effectiveness (Falloon & Talbot, 1981). However, not all patients report significant distress from chronic symptoms or use strategies to cope with these symptoms. Table 2 summarizes common strategies for coping with psychotic symptoms.

Social Skills Assessment

The assessment of social skills forms an important cornerstone in the behavioral treatment of schizophrenia. The remediation of skill deficits through social skills training serves two primary goals. First, there is compelling evidence that an adequate repertoire of social skills is necessary to achieve a good quality of life and to meet social role expectations. Second, the

Table 2. Adaptive Strategies for Coping with Chronic Symptoms

Modality	Strategies	Examples
Behavior	1. Increasing nonsocial activity	a. Walking
		b. Engaging in nonsocial leisure activity (e.g., doing puzzles, reading, or pursuing a hobby)
	2. Increasing interpersonal contact	a. Initiating conversation
		b. Doing a leisure activity with someone else
	3. Reality testing	a. Seeking opinions from others
Cognition	1. Shifting attention	a. Thinking about something different (e.g., something pleasant or plans)
		b. Passive diversion (e.g., watching TV)
		c. Blocking all thoughts
	2. Fighting back	a. Telling voices to "stop" (e.g., thought stopping)
	3. Self-instruction	a. Telling oneself to "be responsible," "take it easy," or "You can handle it"
		b. Problem solving (e.g., asking oneself "What is the problem?" "What can I do about it?" "What else can I do?" etc.)
	4. Ignoring symptom	
	5. Attending calmly	a. Listening or thinking about symptom
		b. Reflecting back content
		c. Accepting symptom
	6. Prayer	
Sensation and physiology	1. Decreasing arousal and sensory input	a. Relaxation, deep breathing
		b. Blocking ears, closing eyes
	2. Increasing arousal and sensory input	a. Physical exercise
		b. Listening to loud, stimulating music
	3. Aversive conditioning	a. Snapping a rubber band against the wrist (combining symptom with aversive stimulus)
		b. Conjuring up an image

stress-vulnerability model of schizophrenia posits that social skills mitigate the negative effects of environmental stress, thereby lowering vulnerability to relapses. Research on social skills training for schizophrenia provides support for both of these assumptions (Donahoe & Dreisenga, 1988).

Social skills are defined as abilities that enable an individual to achieve instrumental or affiliative goals. *Social competence* is the actual attainment of social goals. Different types of social skills are required for effective communication, including perceptual, cognitive, and behavioral skills. Social interactions first require perceptual skills that identify situational and affective parameters that may constrain the range of appropriate behaviors (e.g., affect recognition, public vs. private setting). Schizophrenics have pronounced deficits in social perception, particularly in the recognition of negative facial affect (Morrison, Bellack, & Mueser, 1988), which limits their ability to effectively handle conflict situations.

After perceptual skills have been used to size up the situation, cognitive skills are needed to generate possible responses, to evaluate these options, and to choose the best course of action for achieving the specific goal. Choosing the best response is critical to social success. The pervasive cognitive impairments characteristic of schizophrenia often result in poor problem-solving skills, which lead to a range of social impairments (Bellack, Morrison, & Mueser, 1989). The poor fund of social knowledge possessed by schizophrenics contributes further to difficulties in evaluating the consequences of their social behaviors and in choosing the most effective response (Cutting & Murphy, 1990).

When a response has been selected, behavioral skills are needed to enact the plan. A range of different behaviors is required for effective social interactions. *Speech content* refers to what is actually said, including both topic and word choice. Poverty of speech, a common negative symptom, severely impairs social performance. *Paralinguistic elements* are the vocal characteristics that qualify and give meaning to the verbal content, such as voice tone and loudness. Flattened voice tone is frequently present in schizophrenia, and it can be improved through training in expressive tonality. *Nonverbal behaviors* are the bodily positions and movements that also convey meaning during an interaction. Some impairments in nonverbal behavior that are typical in schizophrenia include blunted facial expression, minimal eye contact, and a paucity of gestures. The final type of behavioral skill is *interactive balance*, which includes latency of response, timing of turn taking, and social reinforcement (e.g., head nodding, occasional smiles, and saying, "Uh-huh"). Schizophrenics frequently exhibit inappropriately long response latencies and do not appear to grasp the give and take of verbal interactions, so that their conversational partners feel uncomfortable.

Effective social behavior is assumed to be the consequence of a smooth integration of the specific components constituting social skill into complex behavioral repertoires. Examples of complex repertoires that constitute skillful interpersonal behavior include conversational skill, friendship and dating skills, assertiveness, conflict resolution, medication management, job interviewing, and vocational skills. Schizophrenics may be impaired in any or all of these areas, and all have been the target of social-skills training-programs. For assessment and training purposes, each complex repertoire can be broken down into skills, each skill consisting of specific component behaviors. Table 3 illustrates the skills involved in conflict resolution and the component behaviors required for each of these skills (Douglas & Mueser, 1990).

Determining whether problems in social functioning are related to social skill deficits requires an examination of the nonskill factors that may influence social functioning. A socially impoverished environment may result in poor social adjustment because there is a lack of social opportunities, rather than of interpersonal skills. Mood states, such as depression, anger, or hostility, may interfere with social functioning in patients with adequate skill repertoires. Similarly, negative symptoms such as anhedonia, asociality, and apathy may limit the social performance of patients who are socially withdrawn and not motivated to use their social skills. Delusions and hallucinations may also worsen social functioning independent of social skill deficits, particularly during an acute exacerbation. Antipsychotic medication side effects, such as *akathisia* (subjective and behavioral restlessness) and *akinesia* (diminution of body and facial movement and vocal inflection), may mimic nonverbal and paralinguistic skill deficits, but they are responsive to medication reduction or to side-effect medications. In summary, patients' social skills should be evaluated within the context of associated factors that may affect their social performance.

Ideally, social skill should be assessed through direct observation in the natural environment. Behavioral observation may be possible in some situations, but not in others, and it is impractical in most hospital settings. Interviews with the patient, significant others, and clinical staff may provide valuable insights into the patient's social dysfunction. The limitations of direct observation and the lack of specific behavioral information from verbal reports have led to the development of role-play tests as an analogue measure of social skill.

A role-play test is a brief simulated social encounter, conducted in a standardized fashion, in which the patient is instructed to respond as if the situation were actually occurring. In a typical test, the situation is described to the patient, and the therapist, playing the role of another person in the scene, begins the interaction with a verbal prompt. The conversation continues for several exchanges and is then ended. For example, a scene description might be as follows: "Imagine that you and a friend want to go out to eat together, but you disagree about where to eat. Your friend wants to eat hamburgers, but you prefer pizza. How would you deal with this situation?" The therapist would then initiate the interaction: "How would you like to go out for burgers tonight?" Following the patient's statement of a preference for pizza, the therapist might continue, "The last time I ate pizza I got sick. How about burgers?" Once again, the patient would respond to the therapist's prompt. The interaction can be recorded and later rated for the behavioral components of social skill. The validity of role-play tests as a measure of social skill and social role performance in schizophrenia has been empirically supported (Bellack, Morrison, Mueser, Wade, & Sayers, 1990).

ACTUAL ASSESSMENT

An axiom of behavior therapy is that assessment is an ongoing process throughout therapy. Assessment and treatment of schizophrenia need to be integrated because of time limitations, as well as the cognitive and social impairments characteristic of the illness. The comprehensive

Table 3. Specific Skills and Component Skills for Conflict Resolution

Conflict resolution skills
1. Expressing negative feelings
2. Compromising and negotiating

Component skills in expressing negative feelings
1. Looking at the other person with a serious facial expression; speaking firmly
2. Telling the other person what she or he did that upset you
3. Telling her or him how it made you feel
4. Suggesting how this situation can be prevented in the future

Component skills on compromise and negotiation
1. Stating your point of view
2. Listening to the other person's point of view
3. Repeating back what you heard
4. Suggesting a compromise

assessment previously outlined must be conducted over an extended period of time when treatment is also provided. With some patients, the therapist gains important information (e.g., about substance abuse, subjective distress from symptoms, and aspects of social functioning) only after the therapeutic relationship has been firmly established. In addition, pressing clinical issues (e.g., an acute symptom exacerbation) may dominate the focus of early treatment, delaying a more detailed assessment of other areas.

The general strategy is to perform a cursory assessment of the patient's social and clinical functioning so that interventions occur in the order of greatest need. The initial assessment may be divided into two tiers corresponding to level of importance. The first tier, which is of primary importance, requires the assessment of current clinical functioning and factors that have an immediate impact on such functioning. The following questions are pertinent during the first tier of assessment:

Have the patient's symptoms been pharmacologically stabilized?
Is the patient actively suicidal?
Is the patient a threat to others' safety?
Does the patient comply with his or her antipsychotic medication regimen?
Does the patient abuse psychoactive drugs?

Symptom Stabilization

The psychosocial treatment of patients whose symptoms are not yet stabilized is notoriously difficult. Patients who have experienced a recent relapse usually require two to four weeks of treatment before their symptoms are adequately stabilized, after which their symptoms gradually decline over a period of months. It is preferable to initiate behavioral assessment and treatment after symptoms have been stabilized. However, 15%–30% of schizophrenics get little or no benefit from antipsychotic medications (Schulz, Conley, Kahn, & Alexander, 1989). If a patient's symptoms have not abated after several weeks of treatment, behavioral assessment and intervention may need to be started, despite persistent symptomatology.

Suicide and Violence

The assessment of suicidal ideation may often be accomplished by direct questioning of the patient. Most schizophrenics who attempt suicide have one of two overlapping symptom profiles: (1) severe unremitting dysphoria, including hopelessness, depression, and anxiety, which leads to a suicide attempt, or (2) positive symptoms that precipitate self-destructive behavior (e.g., a delusion that the person can fly, or auditory hallucinations that command the person to hurt herself or himself). Suicide attempts are usually impulsive, but in most cases, the patient has mentioned the possibility to others. Young males with severe symptoms and relatively high-functioning peers are especially vulnerable to suicide (Caldwell & Gottesman, 1990).

Assessing whether a patient presents a danger to others is necessary with a small subsample of severely ill schizophrenics, most of whom are chronic inpatients. A history of violent behavior is the most important predictor of future violence. Fixed paranoid delusions and command hallucinations to commit violent acts have also been related to violence, although only a small proportion of patients act on these symptoms (Volavka & Krakowski, 1989).

Medication Noncompliance and Substance Abuse

Medication noncompliance and substance abuse pose the greatest threat to stable clinical functioning in patients living in the community, although these problems also exist in a small proportion of hospitalized schizophrenics (Alterman, Erdlen, Laporte, & Erdlen, 1982). As discussed in the section on prototypical assessment, identifying substance abuse or medication noncompliance is difficult and requires multiple sources of information (e.g., significant others and laboratory assays). Often, the most important clue to these problems is provided when a patient exhibits a symptom exacerbation and/or a clear deterioration in social adjustment in the absence of identifiable life stressors or of high levels of negative familial affect. The therapist who notes such a change in clinical functioning and suspects either substance abuse or medication noncompliance can discuss this with the patient and pursue other sources of information. There is some evidence that medication noncompliance may be *negatively* corre-lated with substance abuse. Patients with a history of substance abuse tend to report higher satisfaction with their antipsychotic medications than nonabusers (Selzer, Lavelle, Frechen, Goldstein, & Lauve, 1990).

Social Adjustment

The second tier of assessment pertains to the patient's social functioning, subjective distress, and motivation to participate in treatment, as reflected by the following questions:

Does the patient lack social contacts?
Does the patient make others feel uncomfortable during social interactions?
Does the patient engage in few recreational activities, have poor personal hygiene, or report an unsatisfactory quality of life?
Does the patient have social skill deficits?
Is the patient disturbed by persistent symptoms?
Is the patient unmotivated to participate in treatment?
Does the patient reject attempts to help him or her and/or deny the illness?

The assessment of social functioning involves pinpointing specific problem areas in order to conduct a more thorough behavioral analysis. Standardized interview instruments for patients and significant others require extensive interviewer training, are time-consuming and are not feasible in many applied settings. Frequently, significant others are unavailable to comment on patients' social functioning, although mental health workers (e.g., board-and-care operators and caseworkers at community mental health centers) may be valuable informants.

Another practical consideration when assessing social adjustment is determining what constitutes "adequate" social functioning for the schizophrenic person. The adequacy of a patient's ability to meet society-based role demands is generally accepted as a measure of his or her social adjustment, regardless of his or her level of subjective distress or ability to sus-tain social roles without increased risk of relapse. For example, for some schizophrenics, working part time or on a volunteer job results in a better quality of life and fewer relapses than working full time, although an "objective" measure of social adjustment suggests that working full time reflects better adjustment. The assessment of social adjustment takes into account both accepted social norms and the individual patient's perception of his or her adjustment.

Social Skills

According to the social skills model, impairments in social functioning are often related to social skills deficits, but they may also be influenced by nonskill factors (e.g., medication side effects or apathy). Virtually all schizophrenics have impairments in the social skills needed to deal with at least some social situations. Approximately 50% of schizophrenics have clear, stable deficits in the basic social skills of conversation initiation, positive assertion, and negative assertion (Mueser, Bellack, Douglas, & Morrison, 1991). Even more patients lack the skills to cope with difficult situations, such as problem solving and resolving interpersonal conflicts (Bellack, Mueser, Wade, & Sayers, 1992).

Because social skill deficits are widespread in schizophrenia, most patients are good candidates for skills training. Videotaped or audiotaped role-play tests may be used to assess specific skills before one engages the patient in treatment, but they are not essential for identifying target behaviors for modification. In many clinical settings, the resources are not available to conduct rigorous pretreatment evaluations, and skills are assessed in role plays conducted during treatment sessions as the first step toward remediation. Frequently, deficits in social skills and specific problem areas are identified during the course of treatment as information about patients' social functioning gradually emerges.

Motivation for Treatment

Poor motivation for treatment is a common problem in schizophrenia. Negative symptoms result in poor motivation to change, which can be further worsened by depression and a personal sense of hopelessness and futility. If one is to engage patients in treatment, they must be motivated to change by identifying goals that are important to them. Usually, the goals need to be established over several meetings with the patient. Assessment and goal setting may be interspersed with the provision of basic information about schizophrenia (e.g., characteristic symptoms, medication and side effects, and early warning signs of relapse) during the first two to five sessions. This strategy permits ample time to develop specific treatment goals while laying a foundation for the patient's understanding of his or her illness and the methods used to treat it. For many patients, the motivation to participate in treatment is highest following recovery from a symptom exacerbation and hospitalization. Schizophrenic patients living in the community usually prefer to remain out of the psychiatric hospital and to live as independently as possible. The goals of preventing rehospitalization and improving the quality of social relationships are common to all patients. These goals, coupled with more specific personal goals, can help to galvanize the patient's motivation to participate in treatment.

PROTOTYPICAL TREATMENT

Behavioral treatments for schizophrenia are effective only when provided with a range of other services necessary for the comprehensive management of the illness. Bellack and Mueser (1986) suggested that the comprehensive treatment of schizophrenia requires the integration of four types of service: treatment (e.g., medication, social skills training, and medical care), rehabilitation (e.g., self-maintenance skills and job training), social services (e.g., income and housing), and continuity of care. Often the primary therapist bears the responsibility of identifying specific service needs and coordinating the delivery of these services.

The stress-vulnerability model points to specific areas for behavioral intervention to improve the outcome of schizophrenia. The generic goals of treatment are to (1) decrease biological vulnerability (e.g., by reducing substance abuse and promoting medication compliance); (2) decrease exposure to ambient stress; (3) improve social skills and the ability to manage stress; and (4) improve the ability to cope with persistent, disturbing symptoms. These goals can be accomplished either through the modification of the patient's immediate environment or by enhancing the individual's social and coping skills.

Environmental Modification

Two general strategies can be used to modify the patient's environment. The first is behavioral family therapy for patients with high contact with their families in order to reduce stressful conflict in the family and improve family members' understanding of schizophrenia

(Mueser, 1989; also see Chapter 29). This approach can also be used to reduce stress in nonfamily environments, such as community rehabilitation residences, board-and-care homes, and foster homes. Second, a token economy can be used to harness the principles of operant conditioning in order to reinforce prosocial behaviors and extinguish inappropriate ones (Glynn & Mueser, 1986). Token economy procedures were among the first behavioral interventions to be studied for the treatment of chronic schizophrenic inpatients, and the early results supported its efficacy (Ayllon & Azrin, 1968). In a landmark study of the effects of the token economy on chronic state-hospital psychiatric patients, Paul & Lentz (1977) demonstrated that the token economy program was more effective than an equally intensive milieu therapy or standard hospital treatment in improving adaptive behavior, decreasing the need for medication, discharging patients into the community, and maintaining patients in the community.

Although the token economy continues to be the treatment of choice for many severely ill schizophrenics, the impressive results of Paul and Lentz's study have never been replicated, and relatively few token economy programs currently exist. Glynn (1990) identified a range of different factors that have contributed to the low acceptance of token economy programs, including false assumptions by mental health professionals about the mechanistic nature of behavior therapy, the reduced length of hospital stays, the emphasis on community-based treatment, economic issues (e.g., costs of hiring and training additional staff), and legal and ethical issues (e.g., the use of food as a primary reinforcer). Other operant treatment approaches have also been applied successfully to schizophrenic patients, such as contingency contracting (Liberman, Wallace, Teigen, & Davis, 1974), overcorrection (Sumner, Mueser, Hsu, & Morales, 1974), and aversive conditioning (Turner, Hersen, & Bellack, 1977). However, relatively few of these interventions have been systematically studied and replicated, and their impact on domains of the illness such as relapse rates, social adjustment, and quality of life is unknown. For these reasons, the token economy and other operant treatments are not discussed further here.

Training Strategies for Coping with Chronic Symptoms

It has long been recognized that schizophrenics spontaneously develop strategies for coping with chronic symptoms. Numerous case reports have suggested that some schizophrenic patients are capable of learning more effective methods of managing symptoms (Piatkowska & Farnill, in press). Only recently have efforts been made to develop systematic, replicable techniques for enhancing the coping of patients. Tarrier (in press) and Liberman (Liberman & Corrigan, in press) have developed methods for improving the ability of patients to cope with disturbing symptoms. Although these methods are still in the experimental phase of development and validation, preliminary data support their feasibility (e.g., Tarrier, in press).

The behavioral approach to training in coping methods uses the following sequence: (1) *assessment* (identifying the antecedents and consequences of the symptom and determining the currently used coping strategies and their effectiveness); (2) *providing a rationale for learning new coping strategies* (establishing motivation to improve coping skills); (3) *selecting and teaching a new coping strategy* (strategies are taught by modeling, role playing, guided rehearsal, and covert rehearsal; see Table 2 for a list of possible coping strategies); (4) *implementing the strategy through homework assignments* (giving assignments to practice the strategy in specific situations and to monitor its effects); and (5) *evaluating, modifying, and teaching new coping strategies* (teaching at least two new coping skills for each problem symptom).

Social Skills Training

Social skills training is now one of the interventions most widely used in the treatment of schizophrenia and other chronic psychiatric disorders (Taylor & Dowell, 1986). The primary goal of skills training is to increase the ability of patients to interact effectively with others, both to improve their social adjustment and to increase their resilience from stress.

Format.   Social skills training is usually conducted in small groups, although individual treatment is a viable alternative. Some of the advantages of group training are that it is more economical than individual treatment, it provides patients with an opportunity to learn from others and to help others, and it gives patients a chance to relax for brief periods during the session. Sessions are highly structured, using preplanned agendas based on curriculum designed to teach an array of skills related to an area of social behavior (e.g., assertiveness, conversational skill, friendship, and dating). The training is conducted in more of a classroom setting than traditional psychotherapy, with a liberal use of instructional aids such as posters, blackboards, and handouts displaying the different steps in the skill.

The best group size is 5–10 patients. Sessions last 1 to 1½ hours and are conducted two to five times per week. Frequent training sessions are essential to the acquisition of the targeted skills because overlearning is thought to facilitate the generalization of skills to patients' natural environment. It is preferable for treatment sessions to be conducted by two cotherapists. These therapists alternate responsibility for segments of each session, use one another as models of appropriate behavior, and split up the group in order to provide individualized training for patients who are either more or less advanced in a particular skill area. The training can be conducted by staff with degrees at the bachelor's or master's level, by nurses, and by nurses' aides. The requirements for therapists include experience working with severely ill patients, an understanding of the structured behavioral approach (i.e., not feeling obliged to develop insight or discuss patients' problems at length), and the ability to be socially reinforcing, especially in the face of slow progress.

The preferred method of assigning patients to treatment groups is to match them on the basis of deficits in similar areas of social skill. However, this matching is not always feasible. Patients with different levels of social skill can be managed in the same group by the use of the more skillful patients as role models, and by providing training to the relatively skilled patients in more difficult social situations.

Training Methods.   The main strategy of social skills training is to choose individual motor behaviors based on what the patient can most easily learn, to ensure continuing success throughout the treatment. Skills training follows a sequence derived from social learning theory: (1) instructions; (2) modeling by therapists; (3) behavior rehearsal by patients; (4) feedback and social reinforcement; (5) additional rehearsal and feedback; and (6) homework to practice the skill.

The first step in teaching a new skill is to provide a rationale for its use. The rationale may be elicited from patients by asking open-ended questions about the value of a particular skill. For example, as an introduction to teaching the skill of "expressing negative feelings," the therapist may ask group members questions such as "Why is it important to be able to express negative feelings?" "What happens when you have a negative feeling and you don't express it?" and "How can expressing negative feelings improve a problem situation?" Group members' responses are written down on a blackboard or chart, and therapists supplement these reasons with additional ones. When the rationale has been established, the specific components of the skill are reviewed, and each is briefly discussed. For example, when addressing the common problem of low voice volume, the therapist might say, "If you want people to hear you and take you seriously, you need to speak loudly and with a firm tone of voice."

Following the provision of instructions, the therapists model (i.e., demonstrate) the skill in a brief, preplanned role play. The situation depicted in the role play should be plausible so that patients can see the relevance of learning the skill. Immediately before the role play, the therapist draws the patients' attention to important components of the skill. When the role play has been completed, the therapist asks the patients to describe the different steps of the skill they have observed. Some patients require additional modeling with focused instructions to observe specific components of the skill.

After the skill has been modeled, a patient is selected to rehearse it with the therapist in a role play of the same situation. To ensure that the patient understands the role play, the description of the scenario is repeated, and the patient is requested to state his or her goal in the interaction. Role playing is the heart of social skills training, and all patients participate in numerous rehearsals throughout the course of treatment. Following the role play the patient is given feedback by the therapist and the group members about how to improve her or his performance, and depending on her or his level of skill, the role play is repeated two to four times. Each patients rehearses the skill at least twice, because the first time often involves mimicking the therapist, and additional rehearsal gives the patients the opportunity to practice the skill using their own words and personal style.

The nature of the feedback given to the patient after each role play is the key to successful training. Feedback must be specific, positive, and brief (e.g., "I liked the way you spoke loudly and firmly in that role play. I'd like you to try it once more and this time remember to look at the other person while you speak"). Behaviorally specific feedback helps the patient to focus on particular components of the skill that either were done well or need to be improved. Feedback always focuses first on the positive qualities of the patient's behavior, even if the overall performance was poor. Rather than criticizing the patient, areas in need of improvement are identified, and constructive suggestions are made for changes in the next role play. When negative feedback is avoided, patients' efforts are reinforced, and social embarrassment during role play is minimized. Corrective feedback focuses on modifying one component skill per role play so that patients' limited attentional capacity is not overwhelmed. Positive and corrective feedback is given by both the therapist and the group members (e.g., "What did you like about the way Fred expressed his negative feeling just then?"). Although noticeable improvements in social skill may occur after just several role plays, most significant gains occur over weeks and months of training, with gradual improvements shaped by abundant, specific social reinforcement.

When one patient has completed several role plays, the focus shifts to the next patient, who rehearses the skill using the same scenario. The remaining patients use the same sequence of role plays, followed by positive and corrective feedback. To vary the role-play scene, a new scenario can be substituted for the initial one after several patients have completed their role plays. At the end of the session, homework is assigned to practice the skill. Homework assignments are designed to program the generalization of the skill from training session into patients' natural social environment. In order for generalization to be successful, the assignment must be clear, relevant to the patients' goals, and within their capability.

Subsequent training sessions begin with a review of the homework assignment, which is used to set up role-play situations based on the patients' actual experiences in trying to use the skill. As the patients become more adept in the targeted skill, the role-play scenarios are tailored to the needs of each patient, such as rehearsing the skill in a situation that the patient had difficulty managing or expects to encounter in the near future. In addition, as the patients improve their skills in role plays, the training shifts from focusing exclusively on behavioral skills to the remediation of perceptual and cognitive skills. This focus is accomplished by asking the patients questions before and after each role play and correcting their responses (or rerunning the role play) as necessary. Questions for assessing perceptual skills include "What emotion was the other person feeling?" and "What was the other person's point of view?" Questions for assessing cognitive (problem-solving) skills include "What is your goal in this situation?" "What could you do if this strategy didn't work?" "What do you think the other person would do if you did that?" and "Would that strategy achieve your goal?"

Efficacy of Social Skills Training. Numerous studies have been conducted since the early 1970s on the effects of skills training on chronic psychiatric patients (Benton & Schroeder, 1990). Unfortunately, many of the studies are methodologically flawed, limited by the absence of control groups, diagnostic heterogeneity or the failure to use standardized diagnostic instruments, lack of attention to the possible confounds of psychotropic medication, or the failure to examine important dimensions of outcome in schizophrenia (e.g., relapse and rehospitalization rate, social adjustment, and quality of life).

Despite these limitations, early research on social skills training produced several convergent results. First, there is compelling evidence that schizophrenics can be taught a wide range of different social skills, such as skills for conflict resolution (Douglas & Mueser, 1990), initiating and maintaining conversations (Urey, Laughlin, & Kelly, 1979), problem solving (Foxx & Faw, 1990), assertiveness (Bellack, Hersen, & Turner, 1976), and medication management (Dow, Verdi, & Sacco, 1991). Second, moderate generalization of skills to patients' natural environment can be expected, the extent of generalization being limited by the complexity of the targeted skill and the severity of patients' cognitive deficits (Bellack *et al.*, 1976; Mueser, Bellack, Douglas, & Wade, 1991). Third, skills training results in reductions in the anxiety experienced by patients during social interactions (Monti, Curran, Corriveau, DeLancey, & Hagerman, 1980).

Three controlled studies with a random assignment of patients to treatment and control groups have provided further support for the efficacy of social skills training for schizophrenics. Bellack, Turner, Hersen, and Luber (1984) compared the effects of a 12-week (3 sessions/week) group social-skills training-program plus day treatment with day treatment only for chronic schizophrenics recently discharged from the hospital after treatment for an acute exacerbation. They found that the two groups showed similar improvements in a range of different measures at the three-month posttreatment assessment, but at the six-month follow-up, only the group that had received skills training had maintained their gains. There were no differences in relapse rate one year after the end of treatment, however.

Liberman, Mueser, and Wallace (1986) found that intensive (12 hours/week) group skills training with schizophrenic inpatients over a two month period resulted in a broad range of improvements in social adjustment and in symptoms at two years posttreatment compared to equally intensive "holistic health" treatment. The cumulative relapse rates over the two years also differed between the social-skills and holistic-health groups (50% vs. 78%), although this difference was not statistically significant.

Hogarty and colleagues (Hogarty *et al.*, 1987; Hogarty, Anderson, Reiss, Kornblith, Greenwald, Javna, & Madonia, 1986) compared four different treatments for schizophrenia over a two-year period: individual social skills training (weekly sessions for the first year and biweekly sessions for the second year), psychoeducational family therapy, skills training plus family therapy, and medication only. In the first year of treatment, social skills training and family therapy were equally effective in reducing relapse rates (20% and 19%) compared to medication only (41%), and the combined treatment (0%) was even more effective. At the end of the second year, the social skills treatment continued to result in lower relapse rates than in the medication-only group (42% vs. 66%), but the difference was no longer statistically significant. Thus, skills training has shown modest effects in improving domains of functioning in schizophrenia. The chronic nature of schizophrenia probably requires intensive and/or extensive social skills training for significant clinical effects to accrue.

ACTUAL TREATMENT

The actual engagement of schizophrenics in social skills training involves managing a variety of different problems related to patient characteristics and the generalization of targeted social skills to real-life situations. Because skills training is most frequently conducted in groups, the problems encountered with this format are the main focus of attention here. In general, patients who are lower functioning and more symptomatic are more difficult to work with and learn at a slower rate. The question of whether a patient is in enough control to be able to attend a skills training group and be nondisruptive is the primary criterion for including patients.

Patients need not be asymptomatic to learn social skills and to benefit from skills training. It is common for patients to occasionally drift off or hallucinate during a session and still be able to participate if they are "there" most of the time. Some patients with prominent positive symptoms are often preoccupied with these symptoms and may benefit from some individual work with a therapist to develop strategies for coping with the symptoms. These symptomatic patients can often participate in group skills training after some individual sessions, whereas other patients require individualized social skills training.

Low Functioning Patients

A number of different steps can be taken to address the problems in training lower functioning patients in social skills. Lowering the patient-therapist ratio by reducing the number of patients per group permits more attention to be paid to each patient. Shortening the interval between each patient's turn to rehearse the targeted skill and increasing the frequency of skills training sessions afford more behavioral rehearsal, the main ingredient in social skills training. Two strategies can be used to handle disruptive patients during a group session. First, placing one of the therapists next to the difficult patient enables that therapist to gently redirect the patient to the group task (e.g., the therapist responds to an off-task remark by the patient by saying, "Can you hold that for now, George? I'd like you to watch Susan's role play right now and see which of the steps she does when practicing how to start up a conversation"). Second, disruptive patients who are difficult to redirect can be asked to leave the session for a brief period of time or the remainder of the session. This approach demonstrates to the patients clear standards of acceptable behavior in the group.

Attentional impairments are a limiting factor for most low functioning patients. Using briefer therapist modeling and role-play routines minimizes taxing patients' limited attentional capacity. It may be necessary to focus on smaller units of behavior to encourage small gains in skill. Furthermore, the liberal use of coaching (e.g., whispering a verbal content step of a skill) and nonverbal prompts (e.g., pointing the thumb up to increase voice volume) during role plays may elicit appropriate social responses that can be reinforced in subsequent rehearsals as the coaching or prompting is faded. Liberman, Massel, Mosk, and Wong (1985) developed a skills training procedure for extremely low-functioning patients who do not respond to standard skills-training procedures: attention-focusing social skills training. This approach is based on extensive verbal prompting and the use of primary reinforcers (e.g., soda and candy) to elicit the desired behaviors.

Young Chronic Patients

Schizophrenia tends to be a young persons' illness. The symptoms are most severe at an early age when there is the greatest denial of the illness and an associated noncompliance with the antipsychotic medication regimen. Substance abuse is more common in younger patients, who are also more vulnerable to suicide attempts. A final complicating factor is that many young schizophrenics live at home or are in close contact with relatives and may need better skills for managing conflicts at home. All of these factors may complicate the process of skills training and must be considered if one is to optimize outcome.

Noncompliance with the medication regimen is managed by a two-pronged approach. First, it is assumed that patients who are not compliant lack accurate information about the effects of the medication in both reducing acute symptoms and preventing symptom relapses, and hence rehospitalizations. In providing this information, it is *not* essential that the patients acknowledge that they have schizophrenia; rather, they should be informed that the medication helps them remain in the community instead of the hospital. Patients also need to be informed about the common side effects of the medication, to facilitate their recognition and management of these side effects. Second, patients often refuse to comply with a medication regimen because they lack the social skills to discuss and negotiate medication issues with their psychiatrist. Identifying and remediating social skill deficits in the ability to converse with the psychiatrist and to get specific concerns addressed is a viable strategy for most patients with compliance problems.

Substance abuse can interfere with learning social skills and it can increase patients' vulnerability to relapses. Ground rules need to be established early in treatment: patients will not be permitted to participate in training sessions if they arrive under the influence of drugs or alcohol. As in the case of medication noncompliance, substance-abusing patients are first informed about the negative effects of drug abuse on their illness. In addition, these patients usually benefit from learning social skills to decrease their propensity to abuse drugs. For example, patients benefit from training in assertiveness skills for refusing overtures to use drugs and in problem-solving skills to identify alternative behaviors for managing situations that place them at high risk for substance abuse.

Patients in high contact with relatives may be exposed to high levels of interpersonal stress, and skills training should be directed at teaching patients how to avoid or lower these sources of stress. Research has found that schizophrenic patients are impaired in their ability to perceive negative emotions in others and in their ability to manage conflict situations, regardless of the presence of strong negative affect in the other person (Bellack, Mueser, Wade, Sayers, & Morrison, 1992). Practicing the recognition of different negative emotions can aid patients in recognizing conflict situations. Specific skills useful in resolving conflicts include expressing negative feelings, making requests, active listening, assertiveness, compromise and negotiation, and problem solving. Some patients also benefit from learning how to excuse themselves from highly stressful interactions in order to continue the discussion at a later time, when the intense negative feelings have subsided. If immediate relatives of the patient have not been engaged in behavioral or educational family treatment, it is helpful to conduct some family sessions devoted to explaining the symptoms of schizophrenia, the early warning signs of a relapse, and the effects of stress and medication on the course of the illness.

Generalization and Maintenance Problems

Problems in the generalization and maintenance of social skills or a lack of impact of the skills on domains of social functioning is frequently encountered in the treatment of schizophrenia. Poor generalization of a targeted social skill from the hospital or clinic to the patients' natural environment is often not the result of faulty learning; rather, it is due to the lack of adequate social reinforcement available to the patients. A fundamental assumption of social skills training is that, if a patient learns a skill through behavioral rehearsal and feedback, this skill will be maintained through the naturally occurring social reinforcement in the patient's environment. Skills training is effective only to the extent that patients have opportunities to use their newly acquired social skills and that others respond positively to these skills. In many cases, in order to ensure that people in daily contact with patients (e.g., family members or board-and-care operators) will be supportive of the goals of skills training, they must be informed about the nature of the targeted skills and encouraged to prompt and reinforce these skills whenever possible. Most significant others respond positively to efforts to involve them in planning treatment and supporting improvements in social behavior.

The transfer of social skills from training to the natural environment can be maximized by considering in advance which skills are most relevant to patients' current needs or needs for the near future. For example, there is little point in training in job-interviewing skills if a patient does not plan to look for a job in the immediate future. Most schizophrenic patients do not actively seek out social skills training. It is therefore vital that patients who are engaged in treatment appreciate the relevance of the targeted skills to their personal goals in order to harness their motivation to use the skills outside the training sessions.

Patients with cognitive deficits, such as memory and attentional impairments, or chronic positive symptoms tend to show greater difficulty in transferring skills to their living environment. Several strategies are useful in enhancing the transfer of social skills. Homework assignments to practice the skill need to be explicit and within the patient's capability. It is better to make the assignment too easy than to make it too difficult. Requesting patients to paraphrase the homework assignment provides a check on their understanding of the assignment. When giving homework, the therapist also helps the patient anticipate when the assignment will be completed and what obstacles may be encountered. Rehearsing the homework assignment in the session and numerous rehearsals of the skill may also improve the chances of a successful behavior transfer.

Another strategy for enhancing the generalization of skills is to vary the site of the skills training and to conduct *in vivo* skills training on field trips into the community. *In vivo* social skills training, which follows active rehearsal of the skills in the session, combines the advantage of therapist prompting and observation with actual social reinforcement from people in the community. It also enables therapists to determine whether patients' environments are sufficiently socially reinforcing of the new skills.

A final problem common to many schizophrenic patients who receive social skills training is that the skills are maintained for only a limited time after training has ended. The maintenance of social skills can be improved by fading the frequency of skills training sessions (e.g., twice weekly sessions to weekly sessions) and by conducting "booster" sessions (e.g., monthly) after the end of treatment. Booster sessions enable therapists to identify when a patient's ability to use a skill has deteriorated, and to remediate the deficit before significant social consequences occur. Some schizophrenic patients may require long-term social skills training and may fail to maintain gains when treatment is stopped, regardless of the duration of the treatment. The optimal duration of skills training has not yet been established, but it is likely that the chronic nature of schizophrenia will require long-term social learning interventions, just as long-term pharmacological treatment is an accepted standard treatment for the illness.

SUMMARY

Schizophrenia is a chronic psychiatric illness that is characterized by difficulties in the perception of reality, cognitive deficits, and social impairments that impede the ability to enjoy relationships and work and to care for oneself. The etiology of the disorder is primarily biological, but environmental stress and substance abuse can worsen the episodic course, resulting in frequent symptom relapses and rehospitalizations. Patient coping skills, such as social skills and the ability to manage chronic symptoms, can mediate the negative effects of stress on symptoms, thereby lowering the risk of relapses. The principles of treatment are to lower the biological vulnerability by reducing substance abuse and fostering compliance with antipsychotic medication regimens, to minimize environmental stress, and to improve patients' coping abilities.

Behavioral interventions for schizophrenia focus on reducing stress in patients' ambient environment, modifying the inpatient environment in order to systematically reinforce prosocial behaviors (e.g., the token economy), teaching social skills to improve patients' social functioning and lower their propensity toward substance abuse (i.e., social skills training), and teaching strategies to cope with chronic symptoms such as hallucinations. The most widely used behavioral treatment for schizophrenia is social skills training. This approach involves the identification and remediation of specific deficits in social skills (e.g., initiating conversations and assertiveness) that are functionally related to areas of social functioning (e.g., the quality of relationships). The main techniques used to improve social skills are therapist modeling, behavioral rehearsal, social reinforcement, and programmed generalization with homework assignments. Skills training is usually conducted in a group, although it may also be provided individually, with multiple weekly training sessions held over a period of at least several months. Problems frequently encountered in skills training include difficulties in learning the targeted skills because of cognitive impairments or severe psychotic symptoms, poor motivation to participate in treatment, and limited generalization and maintenance of the skills in the natural environment. Controlled research supports the clinical efficacy of social skills training for schizophrenia. Long-term social learning treatment appears to be necessary for significant clinical gains to accrue and to be maintained. Significant advances have been made in the psychosocial treatment of schizophrenia since the early 1970s, indicating that behavioral interventions have an important role in helping patients to overcome the pervasive social impairments of the illness and to manage its chronic, distressful symptoms.

REFERENCES

Alterman, A. I., Erdlen, D. L., Laporte, D. J. & Erdlen, F. R. (1982). Effects of illicit drug use in an inpatient psychiatric population. *Addictive Behaviors*, 7, 231–242.

American Psychiatric Association. (1987). *Diagnostic and statistical manual of mental disorders* (3rd ed., rev.; DSM-III-R). Washington, DC: Author.

Andreasen, N. C. (1982). Negative symptoms in schizophrenia: Definition and reliability. *Archives of General Psychiatry*, 39, 784–788.

Andreasen, N. C., & Olsen, S. (1982). Negative vs. positive schizophrenia: Definition and validation. *Archives of General Psychiatry*, 39, 789–794.

Andreasen, N. C., Flaum, M., Swayze, V. W., Tyrrell, G., & Arndt, S. (1990). Positive and negative symptoms in schizophrenia. *Archives of General Psychiatry*, 47, 615–621.

Angermeyer, M. C., & Kuhn, L. (1988). Gender difference in age at onset of schizophrenia: An overview. *European Archives of Psychiatry and Neurological Sciences*, 237, 351–364.

Ayllon, T., & Azrin, N. (1968). *The token economy: A motivation system for therapy and rehabilitation*. New York: Appleton-Century-Crofts.

Bellack, A. S., & Mueser, K. T. (1986). A comprehensive treatment program for schizophrenia and chronic mental illness. *Community and Mental Health Journal*, 22, 175–189.

Bellack, A. S., Hersen, M., & Turner, S. M. (1976). Generalization effects of social skills training in chronic schizophrenics: An experimental analysis. *Behavior Research and Therapy*, 14, 391–398.

Bellack, A. S., Turner, S. M., Hersen, M., & Luber, R. F.(1984). An examination of the efficacy of social skills training for chronic schizophrenic patients. *Hospital and Community Psychiatry*, 35, 1023–1028.

Bellack, A. S., Morrison, R. L., & Mueser, K. T. (1989). Social problem solving in schizophrenia. *Schizophrenia Bulletin*, 15, 101–116.

Bellack, A. S., Morrison, R. L., Mueser, K. T., Wade, J. H., & Sayers, S. L. (1990a). Role play for assessing the social competence of psychiatric patients. *Journal of Consulting and Clinical Psychology*, 2, 248–255.

Bellack, A. S., Morrison, R. L., Wixted, J. T., & Mueser, K. T. (1990b). An analysis of social competence in schizophrenia. *British Journal of Psychiatry*, 156, 809–818.

Bellack, A. S., Mueser, K. T., Wade, J., & Sayers, S. (1992). The ability of schizophrenics to perceive and cope with negative affect. *British Journal of Psychiatry*, 160, 473–480.

Benton, M. K., & Schroeder, H. E. (1990). Social skills training with schizophrenics: A meta-analytic evaluation. *Journal of Consulting and Clinical Psychology*, 58, 741–747.

Blanchard, J. J., Mueser, K. T., & Bellack, A. S. (in press). Mood and the prediction of thought disorder in schizophrenia: A longitudinal investigation. *Journal of Psychopathology and Behavioral Assessment*.

Brown, G. W., Birley, J. L. T., & Wing, J. K. (1972). Influence of family life on the course of schizophrenic disorders: A replication. *British Journal of Psychiatry*, 121, 241–258.

Buchsbaum, M. S. (1990). The frontal lobes, basal ganglia, and temporal lobes as sites for schizophrenia. *Schizophrenia Bulletin*, 16, 379–389.

Caldwell, C. B., & Gottesman, I. I. (1990). Schizophrenics kill themselves too: A review of risk factors. *Schizophrenia Bulletin, 16*, 571–590.

Carr, V. (1988). Patients' techniques for coping with schizophrenia: An exploratory study. *British Journal of Medical Psychology, 61*, 339–352.

Ciompi, L. (1985). Aging and schizophrenic psychosis. *Acta Psychiatrica Scandinavica, 71*, 93–105.

Cohen, C. I., & Kochanowicz, N. (1989). Schizophrenia and social network patterns: A survey of black inner-city outpatients. *Community Mental Health Journal, 25*, 197–207.

Cohen, L. J., Test, M. A., & Brown, R. L. (1990). Suicide and schizophrenia: Data from a prospective community treatment study. *American Journal of Psychiatry, 147*, 602–607.

Corrigan, P. W., Liberman, R. P., & Engle, J. D. (1990). From noncompliance to collaboration in the treatment of schizophrenia. *Hospital and Community Psychiatry, 41*, 1203–1211.

Crow, T. J. (1980). Molecular pathology of schizophrenia: More than one disease process? *British Medical Journal, 280*, 66–68.

Crow, T. J. (1990). Meaning of structural changes in the brain in schizophrenia. In A. Kales, C. N. Stefanis, & J. Talbott (Eds.), *Recent advances in schizophrenia* (pp. 81–94). New York: Springer-Verlag.

Cutting, J., & Murphy, D. (1990). Impaired ability of schizophrenics, relative to manics or depressives, to appreciate social knowledge about their culture. *British Journal of Psychiatry, 157*, 355–358.

Derogatis, L. R. (1977). *SCL-90-R* (revised version). Baltimore: Johns Hopkins University School of Medicine.

Donahoe, C. P., & Driesenga, S. A. (1988). A review of social skills training with chronic mental patients. In M. Hersen, R. M. Eisler, & P. M. Miller (Eds.), *Progress in behavior modification*. Newbury Park, CA: Sage.

Douglas, M. S., & Mueser, K. T. (1990). Teaching conflict resolution skills to the chronically mentally ill. *Behavior Modification, 14*, 519–547.

Dow, M. G., Verdi, M. B., & Sacco, W. P. (1991). Training psychiatric patients to discuss medication issues. *Behavior Modification, 15*, 3–21.

Drake, R. E., Osher, F. C., Noordsy, D. L., Hurlbut, S.C., Teague, G. B. & Beaudett, M. S. (1990). Diagnosis of alcohol use disorders in schizophrenia. *Schizophrenia Bulletin, 16*, 57–67.

Endicott, J., & Spitzer, R. L. (1978). A diagnostic interview: The schedule for affective disorders and schizophrenia. *Archives of General Psychiatry, 35*, 837–844.

Escobar, J. I., & Randolph, E. T. (1981). *Social Network Inventory*. Veterans Administration Health Sciences Research and Development Project IIR 81–633. Los Angeles.

Falloon, I. R. H., & Talbot, R. E. (1981). Persistent auditory hallucinations: Coping mechanisms and implications for management. *Psychological Medicine, 11*, 329–339.

Foxx, R. M., & Faw, G. D. (1990). Problem-solving skills training for psychiatric inpatients: An analysis of generalization. *Behavioral Residential Treatment, 5*, 159–176.

Glynn, S. M. (1990). Token economy approaches for psychiatric patients: Progress and pitfalls over 25 years. *Behavior Modification, 14*, 383–407.

Glynn, S., & Mueser, K. (1986). Social learning for chronic mental inpatients. *Schizophrenia Bulletin, 12*, 648–668.

Grahame, P. S. (1984). Schizophrenia in old age. *British Journal of Psychiatry, 145*, 493–495.

Greden, J. F., & Tandon, R. (Eds.). (1991). *Negative schizophrenic symptoms: Pathophysiology and clinical implications*. Washington, DC: American Psychiatric Press.

Harding, C. M., Brooks, G. W., Ashikaga, T., Strauss, J. S., & Breier, A. (1987). The Vermont longitudinal study of persons with severe mental illness: 1. Methodology, study sample, and overall status 32 years later. *American Journal of Psychiatry, 144*, 718–726.

Heinrichs, D. W., Hanlon, T. E., & Carpenter, W. T. (1984). The Quality of Life Scale: An instrument for rating the schizophrenic deficit syndrome. *Schizophrenia Bulletin, 10*, 388–398.

Hogarty, G. E., Schooler, N. R., Ulrich, R., Mussare, F., Ferro, P., & Herron, E. (1979). Fluphenazine and social therapy in the aftercare of schizophrenic patients. *Archives of General Psychiatry, 36*, 1283–1294.

Hogarty, G. E., Anderson, C. M., Reiss, D. J., Kornblith, S. J., Greenwald, D. P., Javna, C. D., & Madonia, M. J. (1986). Family psycho-education, social skills training and maintenance chemotherapy: 1. One year effects of a controlled study on relapse and expressed emotion. *Archives of General Psychiatry, 45*, 797–805.

Hogarty, G. E., Anderson, C. M., & Reiss, D. J. (1987). Family psychoeducation, social skills training, and medication in schizophrenia: The long and short of it. *Psychopharmacology Bulletin, 23*, 12–13.

Holzman, P. S., & Matthysse, S. (1990). The genetics of schizophrenia: A review. *American Psychological Society, 1*, 279–286.

Johnson, A. B. (1990). *Out of Bedlam: Myths of deinstitutionalization*. New York: Basic Books.

Kane, J. M. (1985). Compliance issues in outpatient treatment. *Journal of Clinical Psychopharmacology, 5*, 22–27.

Kay, S. R., Fiszbein, A., & Opler, L. A. (1987). The positive and negative syndrome scale (PANSS) for schizophrenia. *Schizophrenia Bulletin, 13*, 261–276.

Lehman, A. F. (1988). A quality of life interview for the chronically mentally ill. *Evaluation and Program Planning, 11*, 51–62.

Levitt, A. J., Hogan, T. P., & Bucosky, C. M. (1990). Quality of life in chronically mentally ill patients in day treatment. *Psychological Medicine, 20*, 703–710.

Lewine, R. R. J. (1990). A discriminant validity study of negative symptoms with a special focus on depression and antipsychotic medication. *American Journal of Psychiatry, 147*, 1463–1466.

Liberman, R. P., & Corrigan, P. W. (in press). Designing new psychosocial treatments for schizophrenia. *Psychiatry: Interpersonal and Biological Processes.*

Liberman, R. P., & Mueser, K. T. (1989). In H. I. Kaplan & B. J. Sadock (Eds.), *Comprehensive textbook of psychiatry* (Vol. 5, pp. 792–806). Baltimore: Williams & Wilkins.

Liberman, R. P., Wallace, C. J., Teigen, J., & Davis, J. (1974). Interventions with psychotics. In K. S. Calhoun & H. E. Adams (Eds.), *Innovative treatment methods in psychopathology* (pp. 323–412). New York: Wiley.

Liberman, R. P., Massel, H. K., Mosk, M. D., & Wong, S. E. (1985). Social skills training for chronic mental patients. *Hospital and Community Psychiatry, 36*, 396–403.

Liberman, R. P., Mueser, K. T., & Wallace, C. J. (1986). Social skills training for schizophrenic individuals at risk for relapse. *American Journal of Psychiatry, 143*, 523–526.

Linn, M. W., Caffey, E. M., Klett, C. J., Hogarty, G. E., & Lamb, H. R. (1979). Day treatment and psychotropic drugs in the aftercare of schizophrenic patients. *Archives of General Psychiatry, 36*, 1055–1066.

Marneros, A., & Tsuang, M. T. (Eds.). (1986). *Schizoaffective psychoses*. Berlin: Springer-Verlag.

Meltzer, H. Y. (1985). Dopamine and negative symptoms in schizophrenia: Critique of the type I-II hypothesis. In M. Alpert (Ed.), *Controversies in schizophrenia* (pp. 110–136). New York: Guilford Press.

Meyer, N. G. (1976). Provisional patient movement and administrative data, state and county psychiatric inpatient services, 7/1/74–6/30/75. *Mental Health Statistical Note, 132*. Rockville, MD: National Institute of Mental Health.

Monti, P. M., Curran, J. P., Corriveau, D. P., & DeLancey, A. L. (1980). Effects of social skills training groups and sensitivity training groups with psychiatric patients. *Journal of Consulting and Clinical Psychology, 48*, 241–248.

Morrison, R. L., Bellack, A. S., & Mueser, K. T. (1988). Deficits in facial-affect recognition and schizophrenia. *Schizophrenia Bulletin, 14*, 67–83.

Mueser, K. T. (1989). Behavioral family therapy. In A. S. Bellack (Ed.), *A clinical guide for the treatment of schizophrenia*. New York: Plenum Press.

Mueser, K. T., Bellack, A. S., & Brady, E. U. (1990). Hallucinations in schizophrenia. *Acta Psychiatrica Scandinavica, 82*, 26–29.

Mueser, K. T., Bellack, A. S., Morrison, R. L., & Wade, J. H. (1990a). Gender, social competence, and symptomatology in schizophrenia: A longitudinal analysis. *Journal of Abnormal Psychology, 99*, 138–147.

Mueser, K. T., Bellack, A. S., Morrison, R. L., & Wixted, J. T. (1990b). Social competence in schizophrenia: Premorbid adjustment, social skill, and domains of functioning. *Journal of Psychiatric Research, 24*, 51–63.

Mueser, K. T., Yarnold, P. R., Levinson, D. F., Singh, H., Bellack, A. S., Kee, K., Morrison, R. L., & Yadalam, K. G. (1990c). Prevalence of substance abuse in schizophrenia: Demographic and clinical correlates. *Schizophrenia Bulletin, 16*, 31–56.

Mueser, K. T., Bellack, A. S., Douglas, M. S., & Morrison, R. L. (1991). Prevalence and stability of social skill deficits in schizophrenia. *Schizophrenia Research, 5*, 167–176.

Mueser, K. T., Bellack, A. S., Douglas, M. S., & Wade, J. H. (1991). Prediction of social skill acquisition in schizophrenic and major affective disorder patients from memory and symptomatology. *Psychiatry Research, 37*, 281–296.

Mueser, K. T., Douglas, M. S., Bellack, A. S., & Morrison, R. L. (1991). Assessment of enduring deficit and negative symptom subtypes in schizophrenia. *Schizophrenia Bulletin, 17*, 565–582.

Overall, J. E., & Gorham, D. R. (1962). The Brief Psychiatric Rating Scale. *Psychological Reports, 18*, 799–812.

Parker, G., & Hadzi-Pavlovic, D. (1990). Expressed emotion as a predictor of schizophrenic relapse: An analysis of aggregated data. *Psychological Medicine, 20*, 961–965.

Paul, G. L., & Lentz, R. J. (1977). *Psychosocial treatment of chronic mental patients: Milieu versus social-learning programs*. Cambridge: Harvard University Press.

Piatkowska, O. E., & Farnill, D. (in press). Self-control in schizophrenia. *Schizophrenia Bulletin.*

Rosen, A. J., Sussman, S., Mueser, K. T., Lyons, J. S., & Davis, J. M. (1981). Behavioral assessment of psychiatric inpatients and normal controls across different environmental contexts. *Journal of Behavioral Assessment, 3*, 25–36.

Roy, A. (1986). Suicide in schizophrenia. In A. Roy (Ed.), *Suicide* (pp. 97–112). Baltimore: Williams & Wilkins.

Schooler, N., Hogarty, G., & Weissman, M. (1979). Social Adjustment Scale II (SAS-II). In W. A. Hargreaves,

C. C. Atkisson, & J. E. Sorenson (Eds.), *Resource materials for community mental health program evaluations* (pp. 290–303). Publication No. (ADM) 79328, DHEW. Rockville, MD: Department of Health, Education, and Welfare.

Schulz, S. C., Conley, R. R., Kahn, E. M., & Alexander, J. (1989). In S. C. Schulz & C. A. Tamminga (Eds.), *Schizophrenia: Scientific progress*. New York: Oxford University Press.

Selzer, J. A., Lavelle. J., Frechen, K. A., Goldstein, G. A., & Lauve, S. (1990). *Psychoactive substance use in schizophrenics*. Paper presented at the annual meeting of the American Psychiatric Association, New York, May.

Sharfstein, S. S. (1984). Sociopolitical issues affecting patients with chronic schizophrenia. In A. S. Bellack (Ed.), *Schizophrenia: Treatment, management, and rehabilitation*. Orlando, FL: Grune & Stratton.

Spitzer, R. L., & Williams, J. B. W. (1985). *Instruction manual for the Structured Clinical Interview for DSM-III*. Biometrics Research Department, New York State Psychiatric Institute.

Stephens, P. (1990). A review of clozapine: An antipsychotic for treatment-resistant schizophrenia. *Comprehensive Psychiatry*, *31*, 315–326.

Strauss, J. S., & Carpenter, W. T. (1977). Prediction of outcome in schizophrenia. *Archives of General Psychiatry*, *34*, 159–163.

Sumner, J. H., Mueser, S. T., Hsu, L., & Morales, R. G. (1974). Overcorrection treatment for radical reduction of aggressive-disruptive behavior in institutionalized mental patients. *Psychological Reports*, *35*, 655–662.

Tarrier, N. (in press). Management and modification of residual psychotic symptoms. In M. Birchwood & N. Tames (Eds.), *Innovations in the psychological management of schizophrenia: Assessment, treatment, and services*. Chichester: Wiley.

Taylor, A., & Dowell, D. A. (1986). Social skills training in board and care homes. *Psychosocial Rehabilitation Bulletin*, *10*, 55–69.

Test, M. A., Knoedler, W. H., & Allness, D. J. (1985). In L. I. Stein & M. A. Test (Eds.), *The Training in Community Living Model: A decade of experience* (pp. 17–27). San Francisco: Jossey-Bass.

Turner, S. M., Hersen, M., & Bellack, A. S. (1977). Effects of social disruption, stimulus interference, and aversive conditioning on auditory hallucinations. *Behavior Modification*, *1*, 249–258.

Turner, W. M., & Tsuang, M. T. (1990). Impact of substance abuse on the course and outcome of schizophrenia. *Schizophrenia Bulletin*, *16*, 87–95.

Urey, J. R., Laughlin, C., & Kelly, J. A. (1979). Teaching heterosocial conversational skills to male psychiatric inpatients. *Journal of Behavior Therapy and Experimental Psychiatry*, *10*, 323–328.

Vaillant, G. E. (1978). A 10-year followup of remitting schizophrenics. *Schizophrenia Bulletin*, *4*, 78–85.

Ventura, J., Nuechterlein, K. H., Lukoff, D., & Hardesty, J. P. (1989). A prospective study of stressful life events and schizophrenic relapse. *Journal of Abnormal Psychology*, *98*, 407–411.

Volavka, J., & Krakowski, M. (1989). Schizophrenia and violence. *Psychological Medicine*, *19*, 559–562.

Walker, E., & Lewine, R. J. (1990). Prediction of adult-onset schizophrenia from childhood home movies of the patients. *American Journal of Psychiatry*, *147*, 1052–1056.

Wing, J. K., Cooper, J. E., & Sartorius, N. (1974). *The measurement and classification of psychiatric symptoms*. London: Cambridge University Press.

Wong, S. E., Massel, H. K., Mosk, M. D., & Liberman, R. P. (1986). Behavioral approaches to the treatment of schizophrenia. In G. D. Burrows, T. R. Norman, & G. Rubinstein (Eds.), *Handbook of studies on schizophrenia, Part 2* (pp. 79–99). Amsterdam: Elsevier Science Publishers BV.

Wykes, T., & Sturt, E. (1986). The measurement of social behaviour in psychiatric patients: An assessment of the reliability and validity of the SBS schedule. *British Journal of Psychiatry*, *148*, 1–11.

Zigler, E., & Glick, M. (1986). *A developmental approach to adult psychopathology*. New York: Wiley.

Zubin, J., & Spring, B. (1977). Vulnerability: A new view of schizophrenia. *Journal of Abnormal Psychology*, *86*, 103–123.

15

Alcohol Abuse and Dependence

STEPHEN A. MAISTO, TIMOTHY J. O'FARRELL,

MARK WORTHEN, and KIMBERLY WALITZER

INTRODUCTION

A variety of terms—globally including *alcohol problems*, *alcohol abuse*, *problem drinking*, *alcohol dependence*, and *alcoholism*—have been used to refer to a disorder that has cost individuals and the societies they live in dearly. For example, one study provided the conservative estimate that, in 1980, problems attributable to alcohol use cost U.S. citizens almost $90 billion (Harwood, Napolitano, Kristiansen, & Collins, 1984). Of course, such financial cost in no way addresses the major pain and suffering that individuals experience directly or indirectly because of alcohol abuse. In keeping with these staggering human and financial costs, considerable investment has been made in finding ways to effectively modify, or treat, harmful alcohol use.

In this chapter, we review the behavioral assessment and treatment of alcohol dependence in the hospital setting, which remains a major context of alcohol treatment. It is important to note here that we are not including detoxification in this chapter, although it is commonly a part of an individual's alcohol treatment in the hospital. Detoxification in the hospital consists essentially of medical management of the alcohol withdrawal syndrome and of referral to alcohol rehabilitation programs. Behavioral assessment and treatment procedures typically play little role in medically based alcohol detoxification programs. Therefore, we are concerned here with alcohol rehabilitation procedures, which are usually applied immediately following detoxification.

The chapter begins by describing the disorder alcohol dependence, with a brief overview of attempts at its definition. Two major sections follow, one on assessment and the other on treatment. Both sections have two subparts. The first of these covers prototypical, meaning ideal, behavioral procedures. The second covers actual, or typical, practice (of assessment or treatment) in the hospital setting. In the "actual" parts of these sections segments of case material are used for illustration. The chapter concludes with suggestions for the directions of future work on the behavioral assessment and treatment of alcohol dependence.

STEPHEN A. MAISTO • VA Medical Center, Brockton, Massachusetts 02401, and Brown University Medical School.   **TIMOTHY J. O'FARRELL** • VA Medical Center, Brockton, Massachusetts 02401, and Harvard Medical School.   **MARK WORTHEN and KIMBERLY WALITZER** • VA Medical Center, Brockton, Massachusetts 02401.

Handbook of Behavior Therapy in the Psychiatric Setting, edited by Alan S. Bellack and Michel Hersen. Plenum Press, New York, 1993.

Difficulties in Defining Alcohol Problems

In alcohol treatment, specifying what is the target of the treatment has been controversial for many years. This controversy is reflected in the first paragraphs of this chapter, where we used several terms (e.g., *alcoholism* and *problem drinking*) as labels for the disorder. As we show below, in current thinking, at least in the United States, the term *alcohol dependence* is used to refer to the symptoms and behavioral changes associated with the regular use of alcohol. Such changes are viewed as undesirable in virtually all cultures (American Psychiatric Association, 1987).

Traditionally, efforts to define what we will call *alcohol dependence* have been hampered by two problems. The first has been, and continues to be, the dominance of a disease conception of alcohol dependence (the classic reference is Jellinek, 1960). The disease model is, essentially, one that emphasizes physiological factors in the development and maintenance of alcohol dependence. The difficulty is the emphasis on one set of factors to the exclusion of others that have been shown to be important in etiology and maintenance. Unfortunately, such single-factor models or theories have characterized the alcohol field for years (e.g., Skinner, 1981a) and have restricted the viewpoints of researchers and clinicians alike.

Another difficulty that has been an obstacle to arriving at a generally accepted definition is the strong influence of culture on the manifestation of alcohol dependence. As a result, any definitions of alcohol dependence that have emphasized the consequences of use that societies judge to be harmful or undesirable are necessarily limited to the specific society under consideration. For example, common terms like *alcohol abuse* or *alcohol misuse* emphasize the negative consequences of regular alcohol use over some period of time, but typically, they have been bound to the culture that is doing the defining. Illustrative is Blum's definition (1984) of abuse (of drugs, including alcohol) as "the use of a drug that is not legally or socially sanctioned, without proper regard for its pharmacologic actions. Such an abuse would undoubtedly result in effects that are harmful to the individual and to the society" (p. 17).

Criticizing attempts to define alcohol dependence has been relatively easy, but arriving at a generally accepted definition that has heuristic value is another matter. First, researchers' and clinicians' realization in the 1960s and 1970s that alcohol dependence is a multifactorial disorder, rather than a single-factor disorder, led to more sophisticated and productive models of etiology, maintenance, and treatment (Pattison, Sobell, & Sobell, 1977). This advance was probably best formalized in the diagnostic criteria published by the National Council on Alcoholism (NCA; 1972). In these extensive criteria, individuals are identified as having alcohol dependence according to their standing on two tracks. Examples of Track I, physiological and clinical criteria, are evidence of alcohol withdrawal symptoms, alcoholic blackouts, or alcohol-related medical illnesses, such as alcoholic hepatitis or chronic gastritis. The behavioral, psychological, and attitudinal (i.e., Track II) criteria include drinking despite strong medical contraindications and the individual's complaint of loss of control over alcohol consumption. Each criterion is assigned a weight (1, 2, or 3) according to its diagnostic "level."

The NCA criteria have not been used widely in practice, largely because application of the criteria in making real diagnoses is difficult. Furthermore, in application, the criteria result in a large percentage of false-positive diagnoses (Skinner, 1981a). However, the NCA criteria were important in providing a formal integration of biological, psychological, and social factors in the diagnosis of alcohol dependence.

The next major advance in defining alcohol dependence in the United States was the publication of the third edition of the *Diagnostic and Statistical Manual of Mental Disorders of the American Psychiatric Association* (DSM-III; American Psychiatric Association, 1980). In that diagnostic system, alcohol dependence is considered one type of substance use disorder. Three distinctions are made regarding the consumption of alcohol: substance use, substance abuse, and substance dependence. Abuse is defined according to pattern of pathological use, social or occupational dysfunction caused by pathological use, and duration. Alcohol dependence is considered a more extreme form of alcohol abuse. It is defined by two criteria: a pattern of pathological use or impairment in social or occupational functioning, as defined for abuse, and evidence of either tolerance or physical dependence on alcohol.

The DSM-III definition has some difficulties, primarily in the ambiguity of some criteria or subparts of criteria, and the social-cultural boundedness of important terms like *pathological use* and *social-occupational impairment*. However, the DSM-III strengths are its reflection of the multifactorial complexity of alcohol dependence and the use of relatively well-specified descriptive criteria. This system has been highly influential in the practice of alcohol treatment in the United States.

The Alcohol Dependence Construct

About the same time that the DSM-III was being developed, the idea of the alcohol-dependence syndrome construct was published (Edwards & Gross, 1976). The essential advance in this work is separation of an alcohol dependence syndrome from the disabilities that may result from regular use of alcohol. In this construct, the syndrome consists of several elements, including alterations in the behavioral, subjective, and psychological levels, the leading symptom being diminished control over the use of alcohol. Not all of these elements must be present or present in some degree, but with greater intensity there is a higher likelihood of co-occurrence of symptoms. Another point is that the occurrence of this syndrome is in degree rather than in an all-or-none manner. Furthermore, how the symptoms are manifested is presumed to be shaped by personality and culture.

The dependence syndrome is considered one axis of identification; the other axis is disabilities that may result from use of alcohol over time. Such a disability is defined by an impairment in physical, mental, or social functioning that can be reasonably attributed to alcohol use.

The alcohol-dependence-syndrome construct is important because it addresses difficulties in the definition of both the multifactorial complexity and the culture-boundedness of describing alcohol use patterns and their consequences. The construct has also been shown to have empirical support (Edwards, 1986). Finally, the idea of the drug (including alcohol) dependence syndrome was highly influential in the revision of the third edition of the *Diagnostic and Statistical Manual of Mental Disorders* (DSM-III-R; American Psychiatric Association, 1987).

DSM-III-R Definition

The DSM-III-R, like its DSM-III predecessor, is the most influential diagnostic system in treating alcohol dependence in the United States. It fully incorporates the idea of the drug dependence syndrome. In the DSM-III-R, alcohol dependence is one type of "psychoactive substance use disorder." For an individual to receive a diagnosis of alcohol dependence, he or she must be judged to meet at least three of nine descriptive criteria. The criteria center on behavioral and psychological patterns surrounding alcohol use, "loss of control" of alcohol use being the leading symptom. Importantly, although tolerance to and physical dependence on alcohol underlie a few of the criteria, the patient does not have to meet these criteria to receive the alcohol dependence diagnosis. Thus, the DSM-III-R is set apart from DSM-III and from traditional uses of the term *alcohol dependence* or *alcoholism*. Another point is that, in the DSM-III-R, alcohol abuse is a residual rather than a major diagnostic classification, again a major step away from the DSM-III and other ideas on diagnosis. A final point is that, in keeping with the alcohol-dependence-syndrome construct, in the DSM-III-R dependence is viewed as having different degrees of severity, and the system includes guidelines for mild, moderate, and severe dependence, and for dependence in partial or full remission.

Summary

The description and definition of patterns of alcohol use that are maladaptive have proved to be extremely difficult. In this chapter, we use the DSM-III-R terminology and criteria because they are based on the most current thinking on the diagnosis of substance use disorders and have some empirical support. The DSM-III-R system is also the one used in hospital-based alcohol treatment in the United States.

PROTOTYPICAL BEHAVIORAL ASSESSMENT

Behavioral Assessment of Individuals with Alcohol Use Disorders

The prototypical behavioral approach to assessment in the alcohol area follows a multivariate model. For example, Donovan (1988) noted the increasing recognition that alcohol use develops and is maintained by multiple internal and external factors. This multifactorial approach substantially expands earlier behavioral approaches to alcohol and drug use, which tended to focus on the response of substance use and the mechanisms of its acquisition and modification (e.g., Maisto, 1985).

Within the multivariate model of the assessment of alcohol use, there are several important features of the behavioral approach. First, assessment is viewed as a process that occurs continuously during the entire course (before, during, and following) of treatment (Sobell, Sobell, & Nirenberg, 1988). Assessment, therefore, gives a good description of the individual and his or her problems and is the basis of treatment planning and the course of treatment. Assessment also sets the criteria for evaluating how effective such treatment is. Importantly, evaluation of a treatment's efficacy is a continuous process and provides the information required to make decisions about modification of the treatment plan.

A second hallmark of behavioral assessment is that it is objective (Lawson & Boudin, 1985). Thus, the assessment measures that are used hold up to traditional psychometric criteria of reliability and validity. The third point, related to the second, is that assessment covers multiple areas of functioning and includes multiple methods of measurement. The idea of assessing multiple areas of functioning follows directly from the biopsychosocial (multivariate) model of alcohol use. Multiple methods are important because they allow greater confidence in the accuracy (or validity) of the information gathered. The assessment of many variables relevant to treatment planning in the alcohol and drug areas has no "gold standard" of measurement. Rather, multiple methods (physiological, subjective, and behavioral) of measuring a variable give converging evidence about the accuracy of the information collected (Maisto, McKay, & Connors, 1990; O'Farrell & Maisto, 1987; Sobell & Sobell, 1990).

Table 1 lists the multiple areas of functioning that are important to assess in individuals presenting for the treatment of alcohol use disorders. The information listed in Table 1 is adapted from Sobell *et al.* (1988) and shows the wide range of the variables that constitute a complete assessment of individuals in alcohol treatment. Although it is impossible to review in this chapter, there is considerable empirical evidence supporting the importance of assessing each of these areas of functioning (Donovan & Marlatt, 1988; Sobell *et al.*, 1988). Furthermore, many of the variables listed in Table 1 can be assessed by more than one method. For example, quantity and frequency of drinking can be assessed by an individual's self-report and various physiological measures (Maisto & Connors, 1990). Other variables can be assessed by the same method but from a different, independent source. An illustration is an assessment of an individual's legal status by his or her self-report and by the report of a collateral source (e.g., spouse or probation officer).

A final important feature of behavioral assessment is that its sole purpose is the planning and evaluation of treatment specifically geared to the individual (Donovan, 1988). Therefore, the selection and administration of measures always should rest on the rationale that they will advance an individual's treatment.

Summary. The current behavioral approach to assessment of alcohol use disorders follows a multivariate model. It involves the objective, multimethod measurement of an individual's functioning in a wide range of areas. The goal of assessment specifically is treatment planning and evaluation. With this model there are important considerations of clinical application.

Additional Considerations in Assessment of Alcohol Use Disorders

Although a multivariate (systems) approach (Schwartz, 1982) to alcohol use disorders is consistent with the empirical evidence, it does pose a problem in assessment. As Barrios (1988) noted in regard to behavioral assessment in general, assessment on the systems level can create a data base that is difficult to integrate and refine for treatment planning. Thus, the question is raised whether taking a mutivariate view meets the criterion of effective assessment. That is, does it result in an efficient and effective treatment plan and intervention?

Skinner (1981a) outlined important questions that clinicians should ask themselves that will help them to make assessment efficient and yet multidimensional. He proposed a sequential or stage approach to assessment, and at each stage, it is determined if the necessary treatment decisions can be made or if additional assessment is needed. The three stages go from general to specific and from least to most costly.

Stage 1 is best thought of as screening and is used to identify general problem areas. Stage 2 may be viewed as basic assessment (Donovan, 1988) and has the goals of defining the nature and extent of the pattern of alcohol use in a way that is descriptive, that shows its full functional properties, as in a functional analysis (Maisto, 1985), and that leads to diagnostic conclusions. Stage 2 assessment occurs in individuals who have been identified in Stage 1 assessment as having a problem with alcohol and is the first stage of assessment of most individuals who are admitted to hospital-based alcohol treatment programs. Another goal of Stage 2 assessment is to develop hypotheses about what factors maintain the abusive drinking. The most specific and precise level of assessment is Stage 3. In this stage, typically, hypotheses about alcohol use

Table 1. Areas to Assess in Individuals Presenting
for Treatment of Alcohol Dependence[a]

- Specific quantities of alcohol and other drugs used and the frequency of use
- Predominant mood states and situations antecedent to and consequent on substance use
- Usual and unusual substance (alcohol or drug) use circumstances and patterns
- History of alcohol and other drug withdrawal symptoms
- Medical problems associated with or exacerbated by substance use
- Identification of possible difficulties that the client may encounter in initially refraining from substance use
- Extent and severity of previous substance abuse or dependence
- Multiple drug use
- Reports of frequent thoughts or urges to drink or take drugs
- History of previous responses to alcohol or drug treatment and self-initiated periods of abstinence
- Review of the positive consequences of substance use
- Other life problems
- Indicants of tolerance
- Past or present indicants of liver dysfunction
- (For alcohol use) risks associated with considering a nonabstinent treatment goal

[a]Based on information presented in Sobell, Sobell, and Nirenberg (1988, pp. 23–26).

generated in Stage 2 assessments are evaluated across physical, psychological, and social-environmental dimensions (Donovan, 1988). This specialized assessment is the basis of specific treatment interventions.

Reviewing Skinner's stages of assessment (1981a) not only gives an outline of a guide to the practical use of broad-based multimodal assessment but also emphasizes another important aspect of behavioral assessment. In this regard, the clinician is viewed as actively deciding what assessment information to collect and then using it for subsequent treatment and assessment decisions. The model is one of empirically based treatment decisions made through ongoing planning, administration, and evaluation.

ACTUAL BEHAVIORAL ASSESSMENT

Any consideration of the behavioral assessment of alcohol use disorders in the psychiatric hospital requires a description of four major factors. These are, not necessarily in order of influence, the Joint Commission on Accreditation of Health Care Organizations (JCAHO) Standards for Alcohol Treatment; the hospital organization; the theoretical base of the treatment program; and the program setting, structure, and intensity. We discuss each of these factors in turn, and then their consequences for behavioral assessment in hospital alcohol programs.

JCAHO Standards

The JCAHO, which is the major hospital accreditation agency in the United States, distinguishes alcohol (and other drug) use disorders by maintaining separate sets of standards of assessment and treatment delivery. The commission's standards of assessment of individuals who present for treatment of alcohol use disorders are extensive. From the *Accreditation Manual for Hospitals* (JCAHO, 1991), section on alcoholism and other drug dependence services, the following two standards are most relevant to this chapter:

- AL.2. A comprehensive assessment of the biopsychosocial needs and spiritual orientation of the patient is conducted.
- AL.2.1. The assessment includes a history of alcohol and other drug use, including age of onset, duration, patterns, and consequences of use; use of alcohol and other drugs by family members; and types of responses to previous treatment. (pp. 20–22)

The JCAHO standards then continue to specify what additional information should be included in the physical, psychiatric-psychological, and social parts of the assessment.

Several features of the JCAHO assessment standards are important to note. The most apparent is that the assessment must be comprehensive, covering literally all major areas of an individual's functioning. A second feature is that assessments are done in a multidisciplinary fashion. That is, representatives from the major disciplines (e.g., psychiatry, nursing, psychology, and social work) conduct the part of the assessment that is most relevant to their specialized training. An implication of this multivariate-multidisciplinary approach is that it is essential to integrate the diverse information for effective treatment planning. It is also clear that the JCAHO views assessment as the underpinning of planning patients' treatment.

Hospital Organization

The important parts of the hospital organization in assessment concern program leadership responsibilities, staff constitution, and formal relationships among staff members. In the hospital setting, alcohol treatment programs are typically led by a physician, although there are exceptions. The program director, or chief, commonly oversees the activities of a multidisciplinary treatment team. This team approach, which follows from the JCAHO criteria, has become standard practice in hospital-based alcohol treatment programs in the United States. In the hospital setting, the range of discipline representatives in a program varies according to program size and other factors and may include a psychiatrist (or other physician, such as an internist, or both), a physician's assistant, a psychologist, a social worker, and nursing staff. Nursing staff are extremely important and include RNs, LPNs, and nursing assistants. Commonly, at least in inpatient programs, nursing staff deliver the bulk of the day-to-day counseling and other assessment and treatment activities. Nursing personnel may or may not have formal credentials relevant to alcohol treatment, such as certified counselor status. Programs may also have other staff members, such as education coordinators or occupational therapists, but these positions are less consistently represented.

The program chief or coordinator is responsible for overall supervision of the program and staff, but the supervision is typically done through each respective discipline. For example, if a psychiatrist program director wishes to give a program assignment to a nursing staff person, she or he typically does so, not directly, but through the program's head nurse. This working "down and across" disciplines, known as *matrix management*, is common hospital structure.

The multidisciplinary team "treats" individual cases. In practice, each case is assigned to a team member who serves as case manager. The case manager coordinates the patient's treatment and is responsible for communicating information (assessment and otherwise) about the patient to the team. The team, in turn, directs information that may be relevant to a patient's treatment to his or her case manager. Case managers also typically are responsible for any individual therapy or counseling a patient may receive as part of his or her alcohol treatment.

Theoretical Base of the Program

Alcohol treatment in the United States is dominated by what is known as the *disease model* of alcoholism (Brower, Blow, & Beresford, 1989; McCrady, 1986). Essentially, this model posits that alcoholism is a biologically based disease that can be arrested but not cured. Important for assessment purposes is that the model also suggests that abstinence from alcohol is the primary alcohol-treatment-outcome goal. The result is less emphasis on or interest in specifying patterns of alcohol or other drug use. Rather, the emphasis is on whether substances are used at all. Another important point for assessment is that problems in other areas of functioning, such as vocational functioning or psychological functioning, are viewed as secondary to and, by some, as independent of drinking. Therefore, treatment personnel frequently see a person's drinking patterns as a product of his or her "alcoholism" and not of an identifiable set of personal or social determinants. However, the independence is not viewed bilaterally. For example, good vocational or psychological functioning is deemed to be impossible without abstinence from alcohol or other drugs. Finally, the disease model suggests that all alcoholics are essentially alike when it comes to their disease of alcoholism.

Although there are hospital-based behavioral alcohol treatment programs, they make up a small minority (Dickerson, 1989). Behavioral programs differ from disease model programs in assessment practices in a few important ways. First, there is a major interest in specifying patterns of alcohol and drug use, their determinants, and their consequences. This functional analytic approach is the basis of decisions about treatment goals in a variety of areas. Another important point follows from the first: The relationship between alcohol or drug use is not assumed to relate to other areas of functioning in any one way. Rather, the patterns of relationships must be defined individually. One implication of this approach is that assessment data become essential to individual treatment planning.

Program Setting, Intensity, and Structure

Alcohol rehabilitation programs commonly take place in inpatient, partial hospital, or outpatient settings. Because of alcohol and drug treatment insurers' demands for cost containment, inpatient and partial hospital programs are tending toward shorter lengths of stay, and there is a program setting trend in general toward outpatient care.

The setting that a treatment program occurs in tends to be confounded with time in treatment, treatment intensity, and the structuredness of treatment. Inpatient and partial hospital rehabilitation programs tend to last 10–28 treatment days but are very intense, offering a range of therapeutic activities on daily, multiactivity schedules. Furthermore, programs in these settings tend to be highly structured in that all program participants receive the same treatment care, which occupies the majority of their time in treatment. Outpatient treatment, on the other hand, typically takes place on a far less intense, less structured schedule. Typically, an individual comes for treatment one time a week, and interventions focus on his or her unique needs. Furthermore, time in outpatient treatment often ranges from several sessions over one or two months to many sessions over a few years.

As we show below, these program settings and structure features have direct consequences for behavioral assessment.

Consequences of Four Factors for Behavioral Assessment

Table 2 presents a summary of the four factors and their effects on the use of behavioral assessment in hospital alcohol treatment programs. Most alcohol treatment programs use the three phases of assessment that Skinner (1981a) defined (Maisto & Nirenberg, 1986). It is practical for structured programs to use behavioral principles of assessment in all three phases if the disciplines that constitute the treatment team are united on a behavioral orientation (see, for example, Maisto & Connors, 1990, for a thorough description of the assessment methods that can be used). Programs that are heavily based on a disease model, on the other hand, probably provide most opportunity for the use of behavioral assessment in Phase 2 (specification of problem areas) and Phase 3 (hypothesis testing). Such an assessment would occur through a behavioral case manager's individual sessions with his or her patient. The information gathered is

Table 2. Influence of Four Factors on Behavioral Assessment
in Hospital Alcohol Treatment Programs[a]

Factor	Implications for behavioral assessment
JCAHO standards	Multivariate model of alcohol dependence consistent with behavioral approach, as is view of assessment as basis of treatment planning.
	Assessments proceed rapidly in first days of treatment and cover multiple areas of functioning.
Hospital organization	Multiple disciplines constitute treatment team. Each discipline contributes to the patient's assessment.
	Integration of assessment required. In practice, left primarily to case manager.
	Influence of any treatment team member on assessment practices formally achieved laterally and vertically through other disciplines.
Program's theoretical base	Compared to behavioral programs, disease model programs place less emphasis and value on patterns of alcohol and drug use, on a functional analysis of alcohol and drug use, and on individual specification of relationships among alcohol and drug use and other areas of functioning.
Program intensity, setting, and structure	More structured programs tend to treat individuals largely alike, giving assessment less overall influence on treatment.
	Outpatient programs offer the most latitude in assessment practices and application of data.

[a]JCAHO = Joint Commission on Accreditation of Health Care Organizations.

then communicated to the rest of the treatment team in a way that is compatible with their belief systems and language about alcohol dependence.

Summary. In principle, as Table 2 shows, accreditation standards are highly consistent with the practice of behavioral assessment. However, other system factors in the hospital setting may work in varying degrees to restrict or advance behavioral assessment practice in alcohol treatment programs. It seems that the extent of the use of behavioral assessment procedures depends on the clinician's awareness of the workings of system factors and his or her communication with staff in a way that is clear and nonthreatening.

Case Illustration

The following is a description of the assessment portions of treating an individual in an inpatient, structured alcohol-treatment program. The program and its staff strongly follow a disease model of alcohol dependence, and program assessment and treatment practices are accordingly influenced. The exception is the program psychologist (Stephen A. Maisto) and interns whom he supervises. The case described below was treated by Mark Worthen while he was completing an internship in clinical psychology.

History. M was a 36-year-old white, divorced, unemployed male referred to the alcohol treatment unit from an area hospital following a suicide attempt. According to M and the hospital records, he swallowed about 35 Xanax and 5–10 Halcion tablets and drank at least a quart of vodka in this suicide attempt. Before the suicide attempt, M was living with his parents, both in their 70s, helping to care for his infirm mother and "looking for a job." M reported that he was drinking one quart of vodka a day and taking between one and four .025-mg Xanax tablets a day. The Xanax had been prescribed three years previously for the treatment of a panic disorder without agoraphobia. M had sought outpatient psychotherapy at that time for what he came to learn were panic attacks. Unfortunately, the only treatment M received for the panic attacks was a referral to his family physician for medication (the Xanax), and the treating professionals did not inquire into his drinking habits.

As a patient on the alcohol treatment unit, M underwent the standard series of interview assessments given by psychiatry, nursing, and social work services. The physician's assistant on the unit also conducted a physical examination. This series of assessments provided abundant background information on M. However, none of the nonmedical evaluations could be called behavioral, nor did they yield precise information about M's alcohol and drug use patterns or about other areas of his functioning. Individual sessions with M did give the opportunity to apply behavioral principles by interview and other self-report methods.

A functional analysis of M's substance use revealed that he had begun drinking in the Navy (age 18 or 19). During his late teens and early 20s, he experimented with LSD (12–13 times total), and he began to smoke marijuana daily for a total of about four years, with only occasional use thereafter. M used cocaine for the first time in 1980. He said that he used coke a total of about 50 times in the early to mid-1980s, primarily intranasally, although he said he had "free-based" on one occasion. M denied intravenous use of cocaine or other drugs. M's alcohol use had been continuous and progressive since his late teens. He had experienced several symptoms of physical dependence on alcohol, including tolerance and withdrawal symptomatology.

This information on alcohol and other drug use, obtained in interview, was elaborated on by the use of Annis' 1986 Inventory of Drinking Situations (IDS) to help specify the antecedents of M's alcohol use. The IDS revealed that the situations in which M drank most frequently were Social Pressure to Drink (4.00 on a scale of 1 to 4); Social Drinking (4.00); Negative Emotional States (3.75); and Positive Emotional States (3.75). It should be noted that all of the IDS categories, with the exception of Work Problems (2.33), were 3.00 or above, indicating that M "frequently" or "almost always" drank heavily in virtually every situation. This finding was most likely a reflection of the severity of M's alcohol dependence; before admission, he had been drinking from the time he got up until he went to bed at night.

The interview was also used to specify M's problem of panic disorder. In the first session, M reported that he was experiencing symptoms of panic attacks (heart palpitations, sweating, shakiness, fear of other people's noticing his anxiety, rapid breathing, derealization and depersonalization, and fear of impending doom). M was asked by his individual therapist to keep a "panic attack diary" (Stanford Panic Attack Diary, in Taylor & Arnow, 1988). Use of the diary showed that, during the first week of treatment, M experienced one panic attack or limited-symptom attack a day. The diary was used throughout the course of M's inpatient stay to monitor panic symptoms and to evaluate different interventions to control them.

PROTOTYPICAL BEHAVIORAL TREATMENT

The application of behavioral principles to the treatment of alcohol problems began over 50 years ago. The earliest methods involved the use of chemical or electrical aversion in a classical conditioning paradigm to decrease the desirability of alcohol. Such procedures, therefore, focused on the drinking response and were not derived from a behavioral model of the etiology and maintenance of abusive drinking. Later, Conger's tension-reduction hypothesis (1956) provided a behavioral theory of the etiology of alcohol problems. However, the implications of this drive-reduction theory for treatment were still relatively narrow.

As we mentioned above in discussing prototypical assessment, current behavioral models of alcohol use disorders are far more complex than previous models in their inclusion of multiple factors in the development, maintenance, and modification of harmful drinking patterns. The current behavioral approach includes the assumption that drinking is a voluntary response and that definable antecedents and consequences contribute to its maintenance. Thus, the antecedents and consequences of alcohol use are multidimensional, and both may include physiological, psychological, and social and environmental variables. Since the mid-1970s, some behavioral researchers and clinicians have also incorporated cognitive factors as mediators of alcohol use (Maisto, 1985; Pattison, Sobell, & Sobell, 1977). The current behavioral model of alcohol use disorders may be applied in each of three main parts of the treatment process that occur in the hospital setting: treatment planning, the application of treatment techniques or methods, and relapse prevention and intervention.

Treatment Planning

The prototypical behavioral treatment plan, which usually is developed in the first few days or sessions of treatment, has several features. First, the treatment plan is individualized or written specifically for the unique circumstances, needs, and goals of a given person. Second, this degree of specificity is possible because the plan follows directly from a comprehensive behavioral assessment of the individual (see above).

A third point about the treatment plan is that it consists of clearly defined and operationalized goals regarding alcohol use and other areas of life functioning that are to be addressed in treatment. Such clear definition is a feature of behavioral goal setting in general (Bellack & Hersen, 1988). Furthermore, it is important to include both short-term and long-term goals in treatment planning. The inclusion of both ranges of goals helps to sustain the patient's motivation in following the treatment plan, which is of particular importance in work with alcohol patients (Sobell et al., 1988).

Finally, treatment plans are regularly reviewed and modified according to the progress toward goal attainment and new information obtained from ongoing formal and informal assessment of the individual. Life events such as the death of a loved one or a job change may also require adjustment in the treatment plan.

Application of Treatment Techniques

Specific behavioral interventions are often vehicles of achieving behavioral treatment goals. Like behavior therapies in general since the early 1970s (Bellack & Hersen, 1985), alcohol treatment techniques have grown in number and diversity. This growth is a result of what we earlier noted was the expansion of behavioral models to include multidimensional antecedents and consequences of alcohol use (also see Lawson & Boudin, 1985).

Several review articles or chapters (Lawson & Boudin, 1985; Nirenberg, Ersner-Hershfield, Sobell, & Sobell, 1981; Riley, Sobell, Leo, Sobell, & Klajner, 1987) provide overviews of the major behavioral alcohol-treatment techniques. For a description of these techniques, the reader is referred to these articles; space limitations preclude our describing them in any detail. Behavioral alcohol techniques include aversive conditioning; relaxation training and related procedures of stress management; skills training (including drinking skills, social skills, vocational skills, cognitive skills, and marital-family training); contingency management, including community reinforcement; extinction techniques; and self-management. Very frequently, several of these procedures are used as parts of one treatment plan to form a "multimodal" treatment.

Scanning these treatment techniques shows that their base is primarily in classical conditioning (e.g., aversive conditioning) and operant conditioning (e.g., contingency management) principles, or in their combination (e.g., extinction procedure of cue exposure and response prevention). This listing also shows how varied the techniques are. But in discussing prototypical behavioral treatment, it is essential to evaluate which, if any, of the treatment techniques has empirical support. Miller and Hester's excellent review (1986) and integration of the alcohol treatment outcome data helps to address this question. In their thorough review of the many and diverse medical and psychosocial interventions that are used in alcohol rehabilitation programs, Miller and Hester concluded that the best empirical support is available for chemical aversion methods, behavioral self-control training, community reinforcement, marital and family therapy, stress management, and social skills training. Therefore, as individual techniques, behavioral methods are relatively effective means of achieving the desired treatment outcomes in alcohol programs.

However, Miller and Hester (1986) further refined their conclusions about treatment effectiveness to suggest that a multimodal approach may yield the best sustained treatment outcomes. In this regard, they argued that aversive conditioning and self-control training are best in modifying drinking patterns to moderation in or abstinence from alcohol. Another set of interventions that focus on environmental contingencies for alcohol use and sobriety as well as other life problems is most useful in maintaining treatment gains. These procedures include, for example, skills training, stress management, and marital-family therapy. Miller and Hester suggested that a selection of procedures from each category is the best tactic for reaching and maintaining treatment goals. It is notable that the community reinforcement approach (Azrin, 1976; Hunt & Azrin, 1973) is the multicomponent treatment package that best fits this strategy.

A final point about the prototypical application of treatment techniques is implied by the idea of individualized assessment and treatment. That is, treatments are matched to individuals. Although this idea seems simple and logical enough, matching has not been a common practice of alcohol treatment, especially in inpatient programs. Currently, major empirical studies of alcohol-treatment-patient matching are under way, as the question reached a prominent position in the field during the 1980s (e.g., Finney & Moos, 1986; Skinner, 1981b).

Relapse Prevention and Intervention

The last primary feature of prototypical behavioral alcohol treatment concerns relapse prevention, as well as intervention if a relapse should occur. In the context of alcohol use disorders, relapse may be broadly defined as a discrete violation of a rule or a set of rules regulating the rate or pattern of alcohol use (Marlatt & Gordon, 1980). Addressing relapse as part of a good behavioral treatment of alcohol use disorders recognizes the consistent finding that a high percentage of individuals relapse within the first three months after inpatient alcohol treatment (Marlatt & Gordon, 1985) and that the natural course of alcohol problems shows individuals cycling in and out of harmful drinking patterns over time (Polich, Armor, & Braiker, 1981; Valliant, 1983).

Behavioral researchers and clinicians (e.g., Annis & Davis, 1986; Marlatt & Gordon, 1985) have led the alcohol treatment field in providing a theoretical base for the empirical study of relapse and for making relapse a common part of hospital-based treatment programs. In this respect, procedures for preventing relapse or for dealing with it if it occurs are part of inpatient, structured treatment programs or of outpatient treatment. In addition, an important feature of inpatient treatment, called *aftercare planning* (often a course of outpatient treatment), follows from a general awareness in the field that the problem of relapse must be addressed.

Behavioral approaches to relapse show little difference in principle or practice from our discussion above of the behavioral assessment and treatment of alcohol problems in general. Currently, behavioral methods follow from Marlatt's cognitive behavioral model of relapse (Marlatt & Gordon, 1985), which suggests the importance of identifying "high-risk" (for harmful alcohol use) situations and having nonalcohol (or other drug) ways of dealing with them (also see Annis, 1986; Annis & Davis, 1986). This typically involves the application of, for example, the various skills training or stress management techniques that we referred to above. Another feature of this model is beliefs and expectancies about the effects of alcohol, particularly how it can help a person cope with a given situation, as well as cognitive processes (such as cognitive dissonance) that may occur following a first drink. These presumed cognitive mediators imply the importance of educating a person about the actual effects of alcohol and of the person's self-efficacy (Bandura, 1977). Furthermore, it is important to reframe relapse for the individual, from a "major personal failure" to a common event among individuals with alcohol problems that can be used as a learning experience (Sobell *et al.*, 1988).

Summary.   Current behavioral models of alcohol use disorders have clear implications for treatment planning and practices. The actual application of the model, however, depends on several factors.

ACTUAL BEHAVIORAL TREATMENT

The four factors we identified above as affecting the practice of behavioral assessment in hospital alcohol-treatment programs also influence the practice of behavior therapy. In this section, we cite the central aspects of alcohol treatment and behavior therapy and discuss what happens in practice in hospital alcohol programs. In the course of the discussion, we describe the effects on practice of the four factors.

The Use of Empirically Supported Treatment Methods and the Content of Treatment

Earlier, we discussed Miller and Hester's summary (1986) of what alcohol treatment techniques have the best empirical support. Their review also summarizes what treatment techniques or methods are used as "standard practice" in alcohol treatment, including Alcoholics Anonymous (AA); alcoholism education; confrontation; disulfiram (Antabuse); group therapy; and individual counseling.

The gap is considerable between what is standard practice in alcohol treatment and what methods, primarily behavioral, are empirically supported (see Miller & Hester, 1986). Although several possible reasons for the discrepancy have been proposed, a program's theoretical base seems to be most important. In this regard, the disease model of alcohol dependence underlies the vast majority of alcohol treatment programs in the United States and drives the content of the programs, especially in their 12-step AA model emphasis.

The treatment setting is another important factor. Programs that are less structured and that occur in the outpatient setting typically allow more latitude for the use of a given treatment method by a clinician, regardless of the stated theoretical basis of a program. In an outpatient setting, a behavioral approach may constitute the majority of the treatment, with some exceptions, that the patient receives in a disease model program. Therefore, the application of behavioral treatment methods in alcoholism treatment is most difficult in structured disease-model programs. The behavioral clinician working in such programs may use behavioral methods in treating his or her patient, mostly through the vehicle of individual treatment (or counseling) sessions. However, such treatment will constitute only a minor portion of a patient's total treatment content and time.

The case of M, whom we described above in the section on actual assessment, provides a good illustration. We noted in our initial description of M that he was participating in a strong disease-model, 12-step, structured, inpatient alcohol-treatment program. In fact, the programs' treatment activities closely followed the standard program that Miller and Hester (1986) characterized, with a particularly heavy emphasis on alcohol education and AA's 12-step program. However, the individual therapist also was able to use behavioral methods to constitute part of M's treatment activities, as we illustrate below.

In the first week of his treatment, M's panic attack diary showed that he had experienced one panic attack or limited-symptom attack a day. His treatment for this problem included stress management and cognitive techniques, as well as some education. M complied with suggestions to eliminate his intake of caffeinated beverages, to practice relaxation and breathing exercises that he had previously found helpful, and to practice some cognitive techniques (e.g., letting the panic attack "peak and pass," taking an "observer" position and watching the symptoms come and go, and challenging negative cognitions such as "Everyone can tell I'm losing it"). M was told that the panic attacks were most likely exacerbated by benzodiazepine withdrawal, as he had been taking a benzodiazepine for most of the last two to three years, and it therefore might take some time for the attacks to subside. By the end of M's four-week stay, his panic attacks had decreased in intensity (to only limited-symptom attacks) and frequency (two or three times in a week).

Another part of M's individual therapy while he was in inpatient treatment was use of the initial functional analysis and Inventory of Drinking Situations (IDS) data as bases of developing skills to cope with problem situations without using alcohol or drugs. Some therapy sessions focused on ways to prevent relapse, such as recognizing internal and external situations (e.g., from the IDS) that had seemed to lead to drinking in the past and developing new techniques to cope with these situations (e.g., challenging negative cognitions, remembering what had happened the last time M drank and the despair he felt as the result of his drinking, practicing assertion skills when others tried to pressure him, calling his AA sponsor or therapist when he felt "shaky," challenging the thought that drinking would help him when he experienced panic attacks, and practicing other coping techniques with the anxiety symptoms).

Although disease model programs are the most prevalent in hospital-based alcohol treatment, there are also programs based on a behavioral model. One example is a structured program begun at Butler Hospital (Providence, Rhode Island) by Barbara McCrady and colleagues (Dean, Dubreuil, McCrady, Paul, & Swanson, 1979). The program continues at Butler, primarily in a partial hospital setting. The major differences between the current version of the program and the original are the greater importance of AA and the self-help model in general; an individually determined length of stay compared to the earlier, more standard one of 17–20 treatment days; and education about drugs of abuse other than alcohol. (The last has been a change in many programs, regardless of theoretical orientation, because of the increased frequency of poly-substance abuse among patients presenting for alcohol treatment since the early 1980s.)

However, the current Butler Hospital alcohol and drug treatment program retains many of its behavioral qualities. These are represented, first, in a series of "functional analysis" treatment groups, in which the antecedents and consequences of alcohol and drug use are reviewed individually in a group setting. Alternatives to substance use are also covered in these groups. Information covered in these functional analysis groups is applied in another group on relapse that is based on the Marlatt and Gordon (1985) model. Another group pertains to helping individuals set and define realistic short-term and long-term behavioral treatment goals. There also are two social-skills training-group sessions a week, as well as a stress-management training group each week. Individual therapy sessions occur at least once a week and are used to amplify group therapy activities as needed by each patient.

Considerations for a Behaviorist Working in a 12-Step Alcohol Treatment Program

The behavioral clinician needs to be aware of three major points in practicing alcohol treatment in a 12-step program. We realize that we have referred to such programs repeatedly in this chapter. However, this repetition reflects the import of such programs in the field and the need for the behavioral clinician to be sensitive in several critical areas of treatment.

Influence of Research on Relapse. Many 12-step structured programs now contain information about relapse prevention and treatment. We noted earlier that this inclusion is a result largely of the empirical work of behavioral clinicians and researchers. Although the treatment planning and content related to relapse may not be presented in strictly behavioral terms in 12-step programs, the problem of relapse gives the behavioral clinician an important opportunity in two ways. First, as a treatment team member, he or she can help to inform, plan, and guide others in strategies of treatment that may only loosely follow from a behavioral model of relapse. Second, relapse is a topic for which a behavioral clinician can more easily use a behavioral model in planning and implementing a standard program treatment group, without clashing significantly with the overall program treatment philosophy and goals.

Drinking Outcome Goals. For years, the possibility of a moderate or "controlled" drinking treatment goal has created a major controversy in the alcohol field (Cook, 1989; Heather & Robertson, 1983). The controversy is due to a major premise of the disease model, that individuals who are physically dependent on alcohol can never safely drink alcohol. A behavioral model, on the other hand, makes no assumption about what drinking outcomes are possible for an individual who presents for alcohol treatment. However, the empirical evidence is that individuals with more severe alcohol dependence are less likely to achieve controlled drinking.

In previous years, primarily the 1970s, behavioral clinicians and researchers in the alcohol field took a firm stance on the question of drinking outcomes. However, the disease model has had a major influence on defining treatment program standards and practices in the United States. As a result, it has been virtually impossible politically and practically to use a drinking outcome goal other than abstinence for a given patient, regardless of program philosophy, setting, or structure (McCrady, 1986). Currently, therefore, behavioral clinicians working in alcohol treatment programs based in hospitals (or elsewhere) must use an abstinence as the goal for their patients. Fortunately, behavioral methods of alcohol treatment are highly compatible with achieving abstinence.

Language Used in Communicating with the Treatment Team. A major difficulty that a behavioral clinician may face when working in a 12-step treatment program is communicating ideas about behavioral treatment methods in a way that meshes with the 12-step model or that emphasizes the similarities between the behavioral and disease models. A major goal is to be able to work with the language of AA, which greatly colors the process and content of treatment given by most alcoholism counselors. O'Farrell (1987) gave three examples in a paper he presented on the use of a behavioral group in a 12-step treatment program.

- "Don't blame people, places, and things for your drinking" was an AA slogan used by some patients and staff to object to our individualized situational analysis and skills building group therapy program. It helped when we made the distinction that yes, we agree with AA that no matter what the situation, it is the alcoholic's responsibility not to drink; and that some situations are more risky for drinking than other situations.
- "H.A.L.T." (**H**ungry-**A**ngry-**L**onely-**T**ired) as the answer to high risk situations and no need to search for any others. We labeled these as negative physical and emotional states, agreed they are important relapse precipitants especially among chronic alcoholics, and went on to describe other important possible types of high risk situations (e.g., social pressure to drink) that the clients could relate to.
- "Call someone" was the major AA suggested alternative coping response to recognition of an urge to drink. Again by accepting this and building on it, we decreased resistance successfully. (p. 2)

Individualized Nature of Treatment Goals

Accreditation requirements have played a major role in including behavioral objectives and short- and long-term treatment goals for each identified problem area as part of the medical record in hospital alcohol-treatment programs. This practice is highly consistent with behavioral methods of treatment. How individualized these goals are, another behavioral ideal, depends on the degree of program structure: more structure means less variance in treatment goals. This rule pertains especially to what is considered the "alcohol rehabilitation" portion of a person's treatment. In a typical structured alcohol-treatment program there is little room for variance in the stated treatment goals (e.g., abstinence; attending AA meetings, say, five times a week; and taking Antabuse, if medically cleared) because the primary alcohol-based part of treatment is the same for everyone. What individualization occurs results primarily from the efforts of a patient's individual therapist, who is in the best position to notice the unique, directly alcohol-related problems and goals of a patient and to communicate them to the rest of the treatment team.

We should note that, even in structured treatment programs, problem areas other than those that staff typically see as directly alcohol-related (such as other psychiatric symptoms, physical problems, and vocational problems) are given much more room for the individualization of treatment goals. Hospital alcohol programs are usually in an excellent position to have these problems treated by consultation once they are identified in a patient.

Individualized Nature of Treatment Intervention

We have covered information relevant to the behavioral ideal of individualized treatment in different parts of this chapter. In essence, more individualized treatment is possible in less structured programs. Within structured programs individualized treatment tends to occur more often in behavioral programs. For example, we described earlier the behaviorally based Butler Hospital program. In that program, even standard treatment groups focus on individuals and the unique determinants of their alcohol and other drug use, and its consequences. Such individualization in a treatment group is far less likely to occur in disease model programs. We have argued in this chapter that, regardless of theoretical base, in structured alcohol programs much of the individualized treatment that does occur depends on the patient's assigned individual therapist or counselor.

Consistent with what we said about treatment goals, individualized treatment for problems other than what is viewed as centering on alcohol occurs far more readily. As noted above, the multiple-discipline consultation service network that characterizes many hospital settings is well suited to treatment of an array of personal needs. Integrating such interventions with the alcohol-centered part of a person's treatment is an important job of the alcohol treatment team.

SUMMARY

In this chapter we have reviewed the prototypical behavioral assessment and treatment of alcohol use disorders and the way they actually occur in hospital programs. Our review shows that what happens in hospital alcohol-treatment programs is often not consistent with behavioral models. We have argued that this inconsistency is due to the theoretical base of programs, accreditation requirements, hospital organizations, and program structure and setting. However, we have also shown that it is possible to integrate behavioral methods into alcohol treatment, even when working in a structured program with treatment staff who strongly adhere to the disease model of alcohol dependence.

Probably the best way to increase the influence of behavioral methods on alcohol treatment is exemplified by the problem of relapse, that is, to continue to emphasize the behavioral tradition of deriving treatment methods that are based in experimental research and then empirically evaluating them to demonstrate their effectiveness.

ACKNOWLEDGMENTS. Preparation of this chapter was supported by the Department of Veterans Affairs. Mark Worthen now is at the Department of Substance Abuse Services, Alexandria, Virginia, and Kimberly Walitzer is at the Research Institute on Alcoholism, Buffalo, New York. Correspondence about this chapter should be sent to Stephen A. Maisto, VA Medical Center (116B), 940 Belmont Street, Brockton, Massachusetts 02401.

REFERENCES

American Psychiatric Association. (1980). *Diagnostic and statistical manual of mental disorders* (3rd ed.; DSM-III). Washington, DC: Author.

American Psychiatric Association. (1987). *Diagnostic and statistical manual of mental disorders* (3rd ed., rev.; DSM-III-R). Washington, DC: Author.

Annis, H. M. (1986). A relapse prevention model for treatment of alcoholics. In W. R. Miller & N. Heather (Eds.), *Treating addictive behaviors* (pp. 407–473). New York: Plenum Press.

Annis, H. M., & Davis, C. S. (1986). Assessment of expectancies. In D. M. Donovan & G. A. Marlatt (Eds.), *Assessment of addictive behaviors* (pp. 84–111). New York: Guilford Press.

Azrin, N. H. (1976). Improvements in the community-reinforcement approach to alcoholism. *Behavior Research and Therapy, 14*, 339–348.

Bandura, A. (1977). *Social learning theory*. Englewood Cliffs, NJ: Prentice-Hall.

Barrios, B. A. (1988). On the changing nature of behavioral assessment. In A. S. Bellack & M. Hersen (Eds.), *Behavioral assessment* (3rd ed., pp. 3–41). New York: Pergamon Press.

Bellack, A. S., & Hersen, M. (Eds.). (1985). *Dictionary of behavior therapy techniques*. New York: Pergamon Press.

Bellack, A. S., & Hersen, M. (Eds.). (1988). *Behavioral assessment* (3rd ed.). New York: Pergamon Press.

Blum, K. (1984). *Handbook of abusable drugs*. New York: Gardner Press.

Brower, K. J., Blow, F. C., & Beresford, T. P. (1989). Treatment implications of chemical dependency models: An integrative approach. *Journal of Substance Abuse Treatment, 6*, 147–157.

Conger, J. J. (1956). Alcoholism: Theory, problem, and challenge: 2. Reinforcement theory and dynamics of alcoholism. *Quarterly Journal of Studies on Alcohol, 17*, 147–157.

Cook, D. R. (1989). A reply to Maltzman. *Journal of Studies on Alcohol, 50*, 484–486.

Dean, L., Dubreuil, E., McCrady, B. S., Paul, C., & Swanson, S. (1979). *The Problem Drinker's Program manual.* Unpublished manuscript, Butler Hospital.

Dickerson, F. (1989). Behavior therapy in private hospitals: A national survey. *The Behavior Therapist, 12*, 158.

Donovan, D. M. (1988). Assessment of addictive behaviors: Implications of an emerging biopsychosocial model. In D. M. Donovan & G. A. Marlatt (Eds.), *Assessment of addictive behaviors* (pp. 3–50). New York: Guilford Press.

Donovan, D. M., & Marlatt, G. A. (Eds.). (1988). *Assessment of addictive behaviors.* New York: Guilford Press.

Edwards, G. (1986). The alcohol dependence syndrome: A concept as stimulus to enquiry. *British Journal of Addiction, 81*, 171–183.

Edwards, G., & Gross, M. M. (1976). Alcohol dependence: Provisional description of a clinical syndrome. *British Medical Journal, 1*, 1058–1061.

Finney, J. E., & Moos, R. H. (1986). Matching patients with treatment: Conceptual and methodological issues. *Journal of Studies on Alcohol, 47*, 122–134.

Harwood, H. J., Napolitano, D. M., Kristianśen, P. L., & Collins, J. J. (1984). *Economic costs to society of alcohol and drug abuse and mental illness: 1980.* Report submitted to the Alcohol, Drug Abuse, and Mental Health Administration (Contract No. ADM 283-83-0002), Rockville, MD.

Heather, N., & Robertson, I. (1983). *Controlled drinking* (rev. ed.). London: Methuen.

Hunt, G. M., & Azrin, N. H. (1973). A community-reinforcement approach to alcoholism. *Behavior Research and Therapy, 1*, 91–104.

Jellinek, E. M. (1960). *The disease concept of alcoholism.* New Brunswick, NJ: Hillhouse.

Joint Commission on Accreditation of Health Care Organization (1991). *Accreditation manual for hospitals.* Chicago: Author.

Lawson, D. M., & Boudin, H. M. (1985). Alcohol and drug abuse. In M. Hersen & A. S. Bellack (Eds.), *Handbook of clinical behavior therapy with adults* (pp. 293–316). New York: Plenum Press.

Maisto, S. A. (1985). Behavioral formulation of cases involving alcohol abuse. In I. D. Turkat (Ed.), *Behavioral case formulation* (pp. 43–86). New York: Plenum Press.

Maisto, S. A., & Connors, G. J. (1990). Clinical diagnostic techniques and assessment tools in alcohol research. *Alcohol Health and Research World, 14*, 232–238.

Maisto, S. A., & Nirenberg, T. D. (1986). *The relationship between assessment and alcohol treatment.* Paper presented at the 94th Annual Meeting of the American Psychological Association, as part of the symposium, "The matching hypothesis in alcohol treatment: Current status, future directions," Washington, DC, August.

Maisto, S. A., McKay, J. R., & Connors, G. J. (1990). Self-report issues in substance abuse: State of the art and future directions. *Behavioral Assessment, 12*, 117–134.

Marlatt, G. A., & Gordon, J. R. (1980). Determinants of relapse: Implications for the maintenance of behavior change. In P. O. Davidson & S. M. Davidson (Eds.), *Behavioral medicine: Changing health lifestyles* (pp. 410–452). New York: Brunnel/Mazel.

Marlatt, G. A., & Gordon, J. R. (Eds.). (1985). *Relapse prevention.* New York: Guilford Press.

McCrady, B. S. (1986). Implications for behavior therapy of the changing alcoholism health care delivery system. *The Behavior Therapist, 9*, 171–174.

Miller, W. R., & Hester, R. K. (1986). The effectiveness of alcoholism treatment: What research reveals. In W. R. Miller & N. Heather (Eds.), *Treating addictive behaviors* (pp. 121–174). New York: Plenum Press.

National Council on Alcoholism. (1972). Criteria for the diagnosis of alcoholism. *American Journal of Psychiatry, 129*, 127–135.

Nirenberg, T. D., Ersner-Hershfield, S., Sobell, L. C., & Sobell, M. B. (1981). Behavioral treatment of alcohol problems. In C. K. Prokop & L. A. Bradley (Eds.), *Medical psychology: Contributions to behavioral medicine* (pp. 267–290). New York: Academic Press.

O'Farrell, T. J. (1987). *Behavioral and disease model perspectives on alcoholism.* Presented at the 21st annual meeting of the Association for the Advancement of Behavior Therapy, Boston.

O'Farrell, T. J., & Maisto, S. A. (1987). The utility of self-report and biological measures of alcohol consumption in alcoholism treatment outcome studies. *Advances in Behavior Research and Therapy, 9*, 91–125.

Pattison, E. M., Sobell, M. B., & Sobell, L. C. (Authors/Eds.). (1977). *Emerging concepts of alcohol dependence.* New York: Springer.

Polich, J. M., Armor, D. J., & Braiker, H. B. (1981). *The course of alcoholism: Four years after treatment.* New York: Wiley.

Riley, D. M. Sobell, L. C., Leo, G. I., Sobell, M. B., & Klajner, F. (1987). Behavioral treatment of alcoholic problems: A review and a comparison of behavioral and nonbehavioral studies. In W. M. Cox (Ed.), *Treatment and prevention of alcohol problems: A resource manual* (pp. 73–115). New York: Academic Press.

Schwartz, G. E. (1982). Testing the biopsychosocial model: The ultimate challenge facing behavioral medicine. *Journal of Consulting and Clinical Psychology, 50,* 1040–1053.

Skinner, H. A. (1981a). Assessment of alcohol problems. In Y. Israel, F. B. Glaser, H. Kalant, R. E. Popham, W. Schmidt, & R. G. Smart (Eds.), *Research advances in alcohol and drug problems* (Vol. 6, pp. 319–369). New York: Plenum Press.

Sobell, L. C., & Sobell, M. B. (1990). Self-report issues in alcohol abuse: State of the art and future directions. *Behavioral Assessment, 12,* 77–90.

Sobell, L. C., Sobell, M. B., & Nirenberg, T. D. (1988). Behavioral assessment and treatment planning with alcohol and drug abusers: A review with emphasis on clinical approach. *Clinical Psychology Review, 8,* 19–54.

Taylor, C. B. & Arnow, B. (1988). *The nature and treatment of anxiety disorders*. New York: Free Press.

Valliant, G. E. (1983). *The natural history of alcoholism*. Cambridge: Harvard University Press.

16

Bulimia Nervosa

J. SCOTT MIZES

INTRODUCTION

Behaviorally, the essential features of bulimia nervosa are frequent binge eating and some form of purging or marked calorie restriction. Though it has only recently been identified as a distinct disorder, there is evidence that the condition has existed for some time. For example, the Greek physician Galen reported the disorder in the second century A.D., and in the mid-1800s French writers noted that bulimia occurred in diabetics (Stein & Laakso, 1988). Partly because of an article by Boskind-Lodahl & White (1978), in which they described a disorder they termed "bulimarexia," interest in bulimia surged in the late 1970s. Most encouragingly, significant research progress has occurred so that much more is known about the essential psychopathology of the disorder as well as about the components of successful treatment.

Diagnostic Issues

The specific diagnostic criteria have been the topic of some debate, which has led to gradual refinements over time. The diagnostic entity was formally established in the third edition of the *Diagnostic and Statistical Manual* (DSM-III; American Psychiatric Association, 1980) under the term *bulimia*. The DSM-III criteria led to immediate concerns because they resulted in alarmingly high prevalence rates of nearly 10% of females (Fairburn, Phil, & Beglin, 1990). The criteria were viewed as overinclusive: purging was not necessary for the diagnosis, and there were no minimal criteria for the frequency or duration of binging. The result was a tightening of the diagnostic criteria in the revised third edition of the DSM (DSM-III-R; American Psychiatric Association, 1987). This version, which adopted the label *bulimia nervosa*, resulted in prevalence rates among adolescent and young adult women of approximately 1% (Fairburn *et al.*, 1990), mainly because of the specification of minimum binge frequency and duration.

Problems with the diagnosis still remain. One problem is the definition of a binge. An eating binge is not defined in the criteria by the amount of food consumed, the period of time that elapses during the binge, the rapidity of food consumption, or the types of food ingested. The criterion of a sense of loss of control is often not helpful in defining a binge. Bulimics often deny

J. SCOTT MIZES • Department of Psychiatry, MetroHealth Medical Center, Case Western Reserve University School of Medicine, Cleveland, Ohio 44109.

Handbook of Behavior Therapy in the Psychiatric Setting, edited by Alan S. Bellack and Michel Hersen. Plenum Press, New York, 1993.

311

feeling a loss of control. Patients often plan a binge or, alternatively, do nothing to prevent a binge that is about to occur in a specific situation. Also, some patient's binges are not characterized by rapid consumption. Many patients equate loss of control with rapid consumption.

Another problem is that the criteria vary along a continuum and are highly prevalent in nonclinical populations. Fasting, frequent dieting, and overemphasis on weight clearly occur in nonclinical females (Klesges, Mizes, & Klesges, 1987). Women in the North American culture have also been described as suffering from a "normative discontent" about their weight and bodies (Rodin, Silberstein, & Striegel-Moore, 1984). Thus, overconcern about body shape and weight is particularly difficult to assess in terms of what level of severity satisfies the criteria for a clinical case of bulimia nervosa.

The diagnostic criteria have also been criticized for what they do not include. Unlike those for anorexia, the criteria do not directly specify body image distortion and fear of weight gain as part of the disorder (Williamson, 1990). Indeed, bulimics have been shown to suffer from both fear of weight gain (Cutts & Barrios, 1986) and body image distortion (Mizes, 1988b; Wiliamson, Kelley, Davis, Ruggiero, & Blouin, 1985). These omissions are of theoretical importance as some have argued that both disorders are best viewed as two syndromes with a common underlying dysfunction, that is, body image disturbance and an intense fear of weight gain (Fairburn & Garner, 1986).

The distinction between anorexia and bulimia nervosa is often unclear. Body weight that is 15% or more under what is normative, the absence of binging, and amenorrhea for three consecutive months are the distinguishing criteria in the DSM-III-R. Though the distinction is not directly reflected in the criteria, anorectics have long been divided clinically into "restrictors" and "binge purgers" (Garner, Garfinkel, & O'Shaughnessy, 1985). In the DSM-III-R, restricting anorectics would be diagnosed with anorexia nervosa, normal-weight binge-purgers with bulimia nervosa, and binge-purge anorectics with both disorders.

The lack of diagnostic clarity is due, in part, to deficiencies in the criteria and to many patients' shifting from one disorder to the other. Often, these patients are diagnosed as having an eating disorder not otherwise specified (NOS). This category is defined only by the requirement that the patient does not fit into one of the specific eating-disorder diagnoses. A study (Mitchell, Pyle, Hatsukami, & Eckert, 1986) in which 10% of the sample was diagnosed as NOS found that most patients fell into one of two groups. One group did not meet the criteria for bulimia nervosa. They were of normal weight and they purged, but they ate only small amounts of foods before purging. The second group failed to meet the criteria for anorexia in that their weight was not low enough and/or they did not have amenorrhea.

At present, the NOS group also includes a group often referred to as *compulsive overeaters* (Williamson, 1990). These patients are typically obese and have frequent periods of binge eating but do not use extreme purgative methods. It is estimated that 20%–40% of obese persons suffer from frequent binge eating (Marcus & Wing, 1987). It is important to distinguish this group from those who are simply obese because obese binge eaters relapse more (Gormally, Rardin, & Black, 1980) and drop out of treatment more frequently (Marcus, Wing, & Hopkins, 1988). There is also preliminary evidence that compulsive overeaters can be distinguished from bulimia nervosa patients on key psychological dimensions (Davis, Williamson, Goreczny, & Bennett, 1989).

Description of Core Psychopathology

The key features in bulimia nervosa are the binge and purge behaviors. Research on the topography of these responses was summarized by Mizes (1985). Binging and purging 1 or 2 times a day is common. The consumption of 1,300 kilocalories of grains, cereals, snack foods, and deserts is typical (Davis, Freeman, & Garner, 1988). Episodes most often occur at home, while the patient is alone, in the late afternoon or early evening. By late afternoon bulimics are calorie-deprived because they tend either to skip or to have a small breakfast and lunch. Also, separate from their binges, they tend to eat only 70% of what normal females consume in a day (Arbitell & Mizes, 1988). Binging is most often preceded by negative affect, and ingestion of "forbidden" binge foods elicits much subjective distress (Mizes & Arbitell, 1991; Schlundt, Johnson, & Jarrell, 1986; Williamson, Goreczny, Davis, Ruggiero, & McKenzie, 1988). Although purging lessens this distress, bulimics' emotional state after purging is still poor (Johnson & Larson, 1982). By far, the most common form of purging is self-induced vomiting, the use of laxatives being second. The use of diuretics is also common, and occasionally, a patient reports rumination or spitting of food. Thought not purging *per se*, intense exercise after eating and the use of diet pills are also common.

Several authors have described what is hypothesized to be the "core psychopathology" of bulimia nervosa. Garner and Bemis (1982) suggested that bulimics' cognitions are characterized by rigid beliefs about weight regulation, seeking approval via low weight, and basing self-esteem on self-control of weight. Fairburn (1985) noted that, in bulimia nervosa, weight has become the most important, if not the exclusive, determinant of self-esteem. Mizes (1985) suggested that bulimics have the global difficulty of basing self-esteem on external approval and performance accomplishments, resulting in efforts to achieve low weight in order to gain the approval of others for physical attractiveness and the accomplishment of self-control of weight.

Closely associated with these cognitive perspectives is the concept of dietary restraint (Polivy & Herman, 1987). In fact, one hypothesis is that the preceding cognitive schema are the genesis of dietary restraint. Dietary restraint involves setting a low, biologically unrealistic boundary for food consumption. Keeping one's eating under this boundary requires significant self-regulatory effort. Breaking of the boundary occurs either in the face of small violations of the boundary, such as the consumption of a "forbidden food," or in the presence of negative affect. Both result in a weakening of self-regulatory effort, and a binge ensues in what is described as *counterregulatory eating*. The rigidity of the boundary sets up the conditions for the abstinence violation effect, a black-and-white sense of being "in control" or having "blown it" by consuming small amounts of forbidden foods. Although bulimics suffer from dietary restraint (Johnson, Corrigan, Crusco, & Schlundt, 1986), they may respond somewhat differently from obese bingers to violations of the dietary boundary (Duchmann, Williamson, & Stricker, 1989).

The construct of body image disturbance has been conceptually unclear and the subject of much debate (Cash & Brown, 1987). Nonetheless, several studies suggest significant body image disturbance in bulimics (Mizes, 1988b; Whitehouse, Freeman, & Annandale, 1986; Willmuth, Leitenberg, Rosen, Fondacaro, & Gross, 1985). Bulimics have shown a strong preference for thinness and a tendency to overestimate their body size relative to nondisturbed persons (Williamson, Davis, Goreczny, & Blouin, 1989a). Mizes (1992a) found that, on average, bulimics wished to weigh 5.9 kg less than their current weight and 8.2 kg less than acceptable normative weights.

The general personality features of bulimics are characterized by self-regulatory problems, social discomfort and sensitivity to rejection, and high achievement expectations (Yates, 1989). Mizes' theoretical model (1985) suggests that central difficulties in bulimia are excessive concerns about approval, excessively high external criteria as the basis of self-worth, and basic self-control deficits. Studies have found excess approval concerns (Mizes, 1988b; Ruderman, 1986), high expectations (Katzman & Wolchik, 1984; Mizes, 1988b), and self-control deficits (Heilbrun & Bloomfield, 1986; Mizes, 1988b). Though there is some evidence of generalized difficulties with social discomfort (Larson & Johnson, 1985), other research has not been consistent in this contention (Mizes, 1988b).

Associated Psychopathology

Bulimia nervosa is often accompanied by other psychological dysfunction, including depression, anxiety, personality disorder, interpersonal difficulties, poor heterosexual relationships, sexual difficulties, and difficulties in the family of origin. Other research has pointed to problems with substance and sexual abuse. There has been debate on the relationship between core and associated psychopathology. Some authors have suggested that, although significant concomitant psychopathology may be present, mild cases may be relatively free of global difficulties (Williamson, Prather, Upton, Davis, Ruggiero, & Van Buren, 1987). Other authors have suggested that global difficulties may be a consequence of bulimia rather than a reflection of the basic pathology of the disorder (Garner, Olmsted, Davis, Rockert, Goldbloom, & Eagle, 1990). Finally, it is possible that the presence of bulimia and other diagnoses represents a co-occurrence of disorders rather than a reflection of a common pathology.

Research on associated pathology has to be judged cautiously because it is highly dependent on the clinical referral base of a particular clinical research center. Also, the focus on cases presenting for treatment may blind us to the relative lack of associated pathology in less severe cases. Nonetheless, it is useful to describe the pathology that may be associated with bulimia so as to prepare the clinician for a variety of clinical presentations.

Bulimia is frequently accompanied by dysphoria and major depression. Although it has been suggested that bulimia is a variant of affective disorder, most of the evidence suggests that depression is secondary to the eating disruption (Hinz & Williamson, 1987). Bulimics also experience significant anxiety (Mizes, 1988b) that may be due partly to their fear of weight gain and partly to general anxiousness in response to life events (Shatford & Evans, 1986). This anxiety sometimes reflects an anxiety disorder, and some evidence points to a high prevalence of obsessive-compulsive characteristics (Hudson, Pope, Yurgelun-Todd, Jones, & Frankenburg, 1987).

Personality disorders are also frequently associated with bulimia nervosa; different studies point to different diagnoses (Head, Williamson, Duchmann, & Bennett, 1988; Yates, Bowers, Carney, & Fulton, 1990). Because bulimics with borderline personality disorder (BPD) may have a poorer prognosis (Garner et al., 1990), increasing attention has been paid to this diagnosis. Although it appears that BPD does often occur in bulimics (Johnson, Tobin, & Enright, 1989), this frequency may be due more to comorbidity with affective disorder and substance abuse (Pope & Hudson, 1989).

Bulimics often have significant disruptions in interpersonal relationships. Early theorists often emphasized assertion deficits, although there was little supportive research (Mizes, 1985). Mizes (1989) found that bulimics did not suffer from behavioral assertion-skills deficits but did have assertion-inhibiting cognitions. Bulimics are often observed to have difficulties in their primary heterosexual relationships. For example, bulimics experience significant marital distress (Van Buren & Williamson, 1988). Bulimics often have poor sexual adjustment and experience less enjoyment of sexual relationships, more difficulty in expressing sexual desires, more fear of not satisfying their partner, and a greater belief that their sexual enjoyment would improve if they were slimmer (Allerdissen, Florin, & Rost, 1981).

The family of origin of bulimic women often reflects unhealthy functioning, being characterized by hostility, conflict, isolation, and disorganization, and lacking in nurturance, support, and understanding (Strober & Humphrey, 1987). In addition, it appears that bulimics and bulimic anorexics have more pathological families than restricting anorexics (Strober & Humphrey, 1987). Consistent with the cognitive perspectives that suggest that bulimics' self-schema is built on a shaky, externally based foundation, it has been suggested that the family environment of bulimics hampers the development of a stable identity, self-efficacy, and autonomy (Strober & Humphrey, 1987).

Some have suggested that there is an association between bulimia and substance and sexual abuse. As cautioned earlier, this research must be interpreted carefully given the potential sample biases. For example, one study (Hudson *et al.*, 1987) found a lifetime prevalence of substance abuse (alcohol and other drugs) of 49%, and another (Bulik, 1987) found alcohol abuse in 49%, dependence in 23%, drug abuse in 26%, and dependence in 34%. On the other hand, other research has found that bulimics consume less alcohol than same-aged controls (Arbitell & Mizes, 1988). Regarding sexual abuse, case studies have highlighted the potential for histories of sexual abuse (Sloan & Leichner, 1986). One study reported a prevalence of sexual abuse of 24%–26%, depending on the definition of abuse used (Oppenheimer, Howells, Palmer, & Chaloner, 1985). It is not clear how these prevalence rates compare with those in other disorders, or with those in nondisordered populations.

Medical Complications

Bulimia has the potential for medical complications due either to low weight or to purging. The most severe problem is low potassium, resulting in hypokalemia. Most commonly, hypokalemia results in muscle weakness and lethargy. However, it can also lead to cardiac arrhythmias and arrest. There are several case reports of unusual and severe physical complications; however, these are rare events. The other problems that are of concern to the clinician include esophageal burning, parotid gland enlargement, dental caries and enamel erosion, constipation, orthostatic hypotension, coldness, menstrual irregularities, dry skin, and hair breakage (Mizes, 1985). Although there are few studies of the prevalence of medical problems in bulimics, one study found that most patients were in good health (Jacobs & Schneider, 1985). In this study, only 2% were found to have severely depressed potassium levels, and 8% had mildly decreased levels that were of much less concern. Decreased potassium levels were associated with low weight. Palpitations were found in 8%, dental problems in 13%, menstrual irregularity in 18%, and parotid gland enlargement in 8%.

The occurrence of bulimia in persons with insulin-dependent diabetes presents significant potential for medical problems (Hillard & Hillard, 1984). Binge eating of high-calorie food clearly runs counter to the need for strict dietary control. Also, some patients attempt to control their weight by reducing their insulin intake, an action that has serious health risks. One study of diabetic women found that 58% reported eating binges, and 39% reported "insulin purging" (Stancin, Link, & Reuter, 1989). Nearly 14% reported "traditional" purging, such as vomiting, and 12% appeared to be bulimic according to the DSM-III criteria. Alarmingly, bulimic diabetics were much more likely to have been hospitalized for diabetic problems and to have had episodes of ketoacidosis.

PROTOTYPICAL ASSESSMENT

The ideal assessment of an uncomplicated case of bulimia nervosa includes a clinical interview, self-monitoring of eating and purging behavior, questionnaire measures of eating-disorder and global psychopathology, an evaluation of body image, and an assessment of the actual avoidance of eating forbidden foods. Most writers recommend a medical evaluation that involves a routine checkup as well as laboratory tests of potassium levels (Jacobs & Schneider, 1985). However, because most bulimics are in good health, the degree and urgency of a medical evaluation may be influenced by the presence of physical symptoms, low weight, frequent purging, other significant health problems, a distant last physical exam and positive results, and the lack of an ongoing relationship with a physician. Referral to a dentist may also be considered for an assessment of enamel erosion and caries.

Clinical Interview

Two good sources describe a bulimia clinical interview and the reader is referred to them: Johnson (1985) and Williamson (1990). A cognitive behavioral orientation results in particular emphases during the interview, including a functional analysis of the binge-purge episodes. This will include an assessment of typical thoughts and emotions before and after binging and purging, typical precipitating events, typical times and places, and a clear delineation of the foods and amounts consumed during binges. There should also be a clear assessment of forbidden foods. Patients often have difficulty identifying their forbidden foods. One problem is that some foods have been off limits for so long that they fail to mention them. One way to address this is to ask patients which foods, if eaten, they would have difficulty keeping down. Another difficulty is that patients often have complex rules about appropriate eating, so that a specific food is not always in the forbidden category. These rules may include the amount of food eaten during the day, eating to the point of feeling full in the stomach, or the time of day of eating.

Questionnaire Assessment of Global and Specific Psychopathology

An assessment of global psychopathology most often includes the Minnesota Multiphasic Personality Inventory (MMPI). Bulimics most often show elevations on the hypochondriasis, depression, hysteria, psychopathic deviate, and psychasthenia scales (Mizes, 1988a; Williamson *et al.*, 1985). The MMPI is helpful in screening for depression, anxiety, personality disorder, and, to a lesser extent, the risk of substance abuse. Several questionnaires are available for the assessment of eating-disorder-specific psychopathology: the Bulimia Test (Smith & Thelen, 1984), whose assessment is based on the DSM-III criteria for bulimia; the Eating Disorders Inventory (EDI; Garner & Olmsted, 1984), which the assesses behavioral and cognitive characteristics of bulimia and anorexia as well as associated psychopathology; and the Eating Attitudes Test (Garner, Olmsted, Bohr, & Garfinkel, 1982), which assesses attitudes and behaviors in anorexia and bulimia. Although all these scales have been found to be valid and reliable, none are uniquely useful for differential diagnosis of the eating disorders (Williamson, 1990). Also, it is not clear if any of these scales add to the incremental validity of a diagnosis established via clinical interview, or if they add assessment refinements that assist in clinical treatment decisions. If used, they are probably best viewed as supporting the diagnosis made from the clinical interview, and they may have a role in documenting clinical change for external reviewers.

Recently, a few questionnaires that measure cognitions in bulimia have been introduced: the Bulimia Cognitive Distortions Scale (Schulman, Kinder, Powers, Prange, & Gleghorn, 1986), the Bulimic Thoughts Questionnaire (Phelan, 1987), and the Mizes Anorectic Cognitions Questionnaire (MAC; Mizes & Klesges, 1989). Although all of these scales are clearly in an initial developmental phase, the MAC has had the most investigation of its reliability and validity. The MAC has shown concurrent validity, criterion-related validity, high internal consistency, cross-validation of the factor structure, good test-retest reliability, construct validity, and sensitivity to clinical change due to treatment (Kettlewell, Mizes, & Wasylyshyn, 1992; Mizes, 1988b, 1990, 1991a, 1992b; Mizes & Klesges, 1989). However, much further work is needed on the MAC before it can be recommended for widespread clinical use.

Another useful questionnaire is the Forbidden Foods Survey (FFS; Ruggiero, Williamson, Davis, Schlundt, & Carey, 1988). The FFS assesses five food groups (milk, meat, fruit and vegetables, grains, and beverages) at high, low, and medium calorie levels. The FFS is useful in developing a hierarchy of forbidden foods to be gradually integrated into the patient's diet, or for exposure and response prevention.

The assessment of body image is controversial because of problems with the validity, reliability, and practicality of various measures (Cash & Brown, 1987). It appears that measures of the attitudinal rather than the perceptual distortion of body image are more useful because they more consistently discriminate eating-disordered from non-eating-disordered groups (Cash & Brown, 1987; Mizes, 1991b, 1992a). Increasingly, there is an emphasis on body dissatisfaction, which is often defined as the discrepancy between the self-perception of one's body and an ideal vision (Williamson, 1990). The Body Dissatisfaction subscale of the EDI has often been used to assess body dissatisfaction. The Body Image Assessment (BIA) procedure appears to be a valid measure (Williamson *et al.*, 1985). Although not a questionnaire, it is a useful self-report assessment procedure. This method uses nine cards that depict body silhouettes of various weights. The subjects pick one card to represent their perception of their own current size and another to represent the ideal. The discrepancy between the two represents the degree of body dissatisfaction. Height- and weight-referenced norms have been developed to provide an index of how realistic the patient's perception of current and ideal size are (Williamson, Davis, Goreczny, Bennett, & Gleaves, 1989). Major advantages of the approach are that it does not require extensive equipment and takes less than a minute to administer.

Behavioral Assessment

Although the clinical interview may provide initial information in the functional analysis of binge-purge episodes, self-monitoring is usually necessary for adequate specification of the relevant variables. Self-monitoring may occur on specially designed forms; good examples are provided by Fairburn (1985) and Williamson (1990). Self-monitoring is often accomplished just as adequately by means of a spiral notebook diary. Compliance with self-monitoring is often poor. Some bulimics are disorganized and overwhelmed, some fear they will be discovered via their records, and others are upset by seeing their behavior recorded in "black and white." Discussing these potential difficulties from the outset often lessens these problems.

Williamson (1990) advocated the use of test meals as another method of identifying the bulimic's forbidden foods. Research shows that, when purging is prevented, bulimics avoid consuming forbidden foods (Rosen, Leitenberg, Fondacaro, Gross, & Willmuth, 1985). This behavioral avoidance can be assessed by presenting patients with standard meals consisting of a normal portion of a food from each of the major food groups, with a strict prohibition on purging after the meal. Avoidance is measured in terms of the amount of the food consumed, and subjective measures of anxiety and the urge to purge are taken. The test meal procedure may be particularly helpful in the assessment of a patient who denies difficulties with eating behavior.

Assessment Complications

The prototypical assessment assumes that the patient is without other serious psychopathology, is compliant with the assessment, and is motivated for treatment, and that unlimited professional resources are available. When other psychopathology is found, it must be assessed in the manner appropriate for the type(s) of pathology discovered. A difficult clinical decision is whether to attend more to the eating disorder or the other psychopathology and is highly dependent on the type of psychopathology and the conceptualization of the relationship between it and the bulimia. For example, if the patient has a dependent personality disorder, it may be noted secondarily as a factor that will affect the therapeutic relationship. If BPD is present, it often becomes the primary target of the assessment.

Practical time constraints and third-party reimbursement issues result in choices' being made from the list of ideal assessment procedures. Often, all that it is realistic to accomplish is a clinical interview, self-monitoring, and a few supplementary questionnaires.

One of the more difficult challenges is the patient who denies that there is a problem and/or is very ambivalent about treatment. Often, this patient is brought to treatment by parents or a spouse, sometimes with latent or clearly stated threats. Under these circumstances, control issues, anger directed at the therapist, and viewing the therapist as "the enemy" are all potential problems. Ambivalent patients may directly or indirectly express that they are not ready to give up their eating disorder. This is not surprising because regulation of weight has become central to their self-esteem. A commonly expressed fear is that treatment means that they will have to gain weight. Most often, they can be reassured that treatment will result in no or only a few pounds weight gain. However, this gain may still be perceived as threatening. Patients with severe personality disorders (particularly borderlines) and current or past anorexic tendencies are the ones most likely to present these challenges.

Under these circumstances, it is important to defer the systematic assessment of eating pathology and shift the focus to the patient's ambivalence, active resistance, and fears. Thus, the therapist may quickly defer more threatening assessment procedures such as self-monitoring or test meals. Often, the focus is best shifted to gaining the patient's trust and establishing the therapeutic relationship, as well as managing interpersonal issues of the patient and the therapist. It is not at all uncommon for patients to "hit and run," that is, attend a session or two, drop out for a while, and reapproach. Being too quick to impose structure will often frighten these patients away. The task becomes one of assessing and treating not bulimia, but the patient's ambivalence and resistance. This task involves careful and difficult clinical decisions on the balance of patience, warmth, and building of trust versus confrontation on the seriousness of the disorder and lack of progress.

The initial assessment is often complicated by parents and spouses. Fueled by unrealistic fears via the media about the potentially serious medical consequences, some families are understandably frantic to have something done and may be quite demanding. This desperation may result in extreme efforts by the family to monitor and regulate the patient's eating and purging behavior. For example, one patient's family placed a padlock on the refrigerator door. Although these behaviors may reflect dysfunctional family processes, in some families these behaviors represent understandable responses to unrealistic fears. Often, all that is required is reassurance that their child is not going to die, as well as a clear statement that extreme monitoring of eating is not helpful and may be counterproductive. Of course, family members with their own psychopathology have more difficulty in responding to these directives, and family therapy is required.

Inpatient Assessment

Although most bulimic patients are treated as outpatients, some are best seen as inpatients. The inpatient setting offers advantages and disadvantages. The clear disadvantage is that it is impossible to accurately gauge the frequency of binge-purge episodes because of the restrictions on these behaviors in the hospital. Also, it is not possible to assess the typical situational and emotional precipitants and consequences of binging and purging in the home setting. On the plus side, it is possible to get a better assessment of daily caloric intake, food- and weight-related rituals, food avoidance, emotional responses to the ingestion of forbidden foods, and poor eating habits. The opportunity to observe these features may be particularly helpful in the assessment of the patient who denies eating difficulties.

PROTOTYPICAL TREATMENT

The overwhelming majority of cognitive behavioral treatment (CBT) outcome studies of bulimia nervosa are of outpatient services and may be divided into two groups: (1) multicomponent individual and group treatment and (2) exposure and response prevention (ERP).

Garner, Fairburn, and Davis (1987) reviewed both individual and group CBT of bulimia. Overall, on average, the treatment resulted in approximately an 80% reduction in the frequency of binging and purging. At the end of treatment, approximately 30% of the subjects were abstinent from binging and purging, and at follow-up, 45% were abstinent. Equally encouraging, there was clear evidence of improvement in other psychopathology, such as depression. However, it should be noted that improvement did not always result in scores that were in the normal range.

The typical duration of individual treatment was 15–20 weeks, usually with weekly sessions, although some programs included more frequent treatment at the beginning of therapy. In group treatment, the sessions occurred one or two times a week, and often lasted 6–7 weeks. Unfortunately, approximately 25% of the patients dropped out of treatment. Factors purportedly associated with dropout include a higher frequency of binging and purging, depression, severe personality disorder, and ambivalence about treatment. It should be noted, however, that these factors are based on clinical observations, as none of the studies had a large enough sample for empirical analysis.

Because all of these studies were multicomponent and included varying interventions, it is not clear what are the essential components of successful treatment. Three procedures stood out as the most frequently used in the studies reviewed by Garner *et al.* (1987). All studies included at least some form of cognitive restructuring of distorted attitudes regarding food, weight, and body shape. Moreover, all studies included self-monitoring of binge-purge episodes. Approximately 90% of the studies used extensive self-monitoring, that is, assessing thoughts, emotions, situational cues, and foods associated with binging and purging. Specific meal planning, which usually focused on eating three meals a day, as found in 85% of the studies. This meal planning often included directives to eat balanced meals, which for most bulimics resulted in a gradual expansion of the range of foods consumed and not avoided.

Several notable interventions were included in about half the studies. Somewhat surprisingly, *extensive* cognitive restructuring of food- and weight-related attitudes occurred in only 47% of the studies. However, it is important to note that a cognitive intervention is not the only way, and perhaps not always the best way, to effect cognitive change. Thus, behavioral prescriptions to normalize eating may also effect marked cognitive change as patients accrue behavioral evidence that their food-related fears are not realistic.

Half of the studies included assertiveness and social-skills training, or relaxation training. Although relaxation training has been shown to result independently in modest improvements (Mizes & Fleece, 1986; Mizes & Lohr, 1983), Garner *et al.* (1987) regarded both of these interventions as peripheral compared to treatments that focus more directly on eating behavior and distorted attitudes toward weight and food. They argued that, although interpersonal problems and negative emotions may precipitate binge-purge episodes, the more fundamental problem is the chronic dieting due to cognitive distortions. Reducing negative moods may take the "pressure" off bulimics' dietary restraint so that they break down less and binge less. However, the continued presence of chronic dieting and distorted beliefs puts bulimics at continual risk of a relapse when negative emotions inevitably occur.

Given the extensive research on formalized ERP, it is interesting that nearly 40% of the studies included some prescription that gradually included forbidden foods in the patients' diets. One could hypothesize that this prescription functioned as unsupervised "mini"-ERP, as opposed to the supervised, extensive procedures characteristic of the formal procedure.

There are insufficient data concerning whether group or individual treatment is more effective (Garner *et al.*, 1987). Conclusions are difficult to draw because there are few direct comparisons of individual and group treatment, most group studies include concomitant individual treatment, and group studies are often of less severe cases. There is also some suggestion that the dropout rate is higher for group treatment (Freeman, Sinclair, Turnbull, & Annandale, 1985). Clinically, many have the opinion that individual treatment is preferred over group treatment, especially for more severe bulimics (Garner *et al.*, 1987).

Exposure and Response Prevention

ERP is a procedure derived from the behavioral treatment of anxiety disorders. ERP is based on the hypothesized fear of weight gain and the anxiety model of bulimia (Rosen & Leitenberg, 1985). The anxiety model posits that the consumption of forbidden foods elicits much anxiety, and that vomiting serves as an escape response that provides anxiety relief. This anxiety relief tends both to increase the anxiety associated with forbidden food ingestion and to strengthen the vomiting response. Also, it is hypothesized that vomiting, and not binging, "drives" the binge-purge chain. That is, vomiting removes the inhibitions that moderate excessive eating.

The basics of ERP are that the patient, under the therapist's direction, is instructed to eat a variety of forbidden foods with a specific prohibition on vomiting or other purging afterward. Target foods or meals are usually presented one per session, and over sessions, increasingly threatening foods are selected from a hierarchy foods. The presentation of the foods may focus not only on the specific foods, but also on consuming increasing amounts of food. This food ingestion elicits strong emotion and associated cognitions; thus, cognitive restructuring of these distorted weight- and food-related attitudes occurs. An important component is the tracking of anxiety over time during the session. The purpose is to show patients that their anxiety gradually decreases within and between sessions, even in the absence of vomiting. Before ERP treatment, most bulimics view vomiting as the only way to reduce their discomfort after the ingestion of forbidden food. In the classic protocol, ERP occurs in two to three sessions a week that may last as long as 2½ hours. As the patients' anxiety lessens, the length and frequency of treatment are decreased. The common number of ERP sessions is approximately 20.

Rosen's review of ERP (1987) clearly suggests that it is an effective treatment. On average, patients experience a 70%–80% reduction in vomiting frequency, and nearly half of the patients are abstinent. These improvements generalize to other dimensions of the disorder and seem to be maintained over time. However, as in other CBT approaches, treatment refusal or dropout is a problem in approximately 15%–25% of patients. It is important to note that ERP is not intended to be a stand-alone treatment and is offered as a potentially useful adjunct to standard treatment.

There has been heated debate on the necessity of adding ERP to standard CBT (Agras, Schneider, Arnow, Raeburn, & Telch, 1989; Leitenberg & Rosen, 1989). At this time, the verdict is not yet in. Comparisons between ERP and standard CBT are complicated by treatment overlap. CBT often includes directives to gradually incorporate more forbidden foods into the diet, which may be conceptualized as "miniexposure" practices. Also, there is much overlap in the cognitive restructuring aspects of ERP and standard CBT. In summary, although the ERP treatment package is clearly effective, the essential effective components remain unknown. Also, it is possible that ERP may be more effective with some patients, such as high-frequency purgers.

ACTUAL TREATMENT

The outcome research on CBT must be understood within the constraints of clinical outcome research lest practicing clinicians become discouraged when they experience lower success rates. Often, the inclusion requirements of outcome studies result in relatively "clean" patients, that is, the effective screening out of some of the difficult patients whom the practicing clinician inevitably treats. For example, in one of the most successful studies (Fairburn, Kirk, O'Connor, & Cooper, 1986), patients were excluded from participation if they were of low weight, had a coexisting psychiatric disorder other than anxiety or depression, suffered from chemical abuse or dependency, were suicide risks, or otherwise needed psychiatric hospitalization. Treatment suggestions for some of these difficult patients, and other management issues, follows.

Treatment with Antidepressants

Antidepressants may be used with bulimics in at least two ways: to reduce binging and purging and/or to treat concurrent depression. Regarding the former, it should be noted that the vast majority of CBT studies have not included drug treatment. Increasingly, caution is being suggested regarding the use of antidepressants as a first-line intervention in bulimia (Mitchell, 1988). Though antidepressants appear to result in short-term reductions in binge-purge frequency, little is known about long-term effects, and relapse after stopping drugs is common. High dropout rates and difficulties with medication compliance are common, and there are concerns about using monoamine oxidase (MAO) inhibitors, which require strict compliance with a tyramine-free diet because of the risk of hypertensive crisis. For bulimics managed over a long period, frequent medication changes are often needed. Interestingly, improvement in binge-purge frequencies does not appear to be due to improvement in depression.

Antidepressants can be profitably used when there is a coexisting depression (Fairburn, 1985), though this recommendation is based only on clinical observation. Along with the enthusiasm for the antidepressant fluoxetine, there has been much speculation on its potential usefulness in bulimia, mainly because, unlike the tricyclics, fluoxetine does not tend to increase appetite and spur weight gain (Fava, Herzog, Hamburg, Riess, Anfang, & Rosenbaum, 1990). There is some preliminary evidence that it does reduce binge-purge frequencies (Fava et al., 1990), and its antidepressant effect is well established. Interestingly, there is some evidence that bulimics on tricyclics do not experience weight gain or increases in appetite (Mitchell, 1988). Thus, it remains to be seen if this characteristic of fluoxetine really does provide any advantages.

Management of Diabetes and Bulimia

The treatment of coexisting bulimia and diabetes requires much greater input from the patient's physician and often the guidance of a nutritionist with expertise in diabetes. To coordinate the amount and timing of meals with insulin administration, the typical prescription for bulimics to eat three meals a day becomes even more important. Whereas the typical bulimic is often encouraged to loosen the controls on food intake by eventually stopping dieting, counting calories, and avoiding certain foods, these recommendations are often not appropriate for the diabetic bulimic. Essentially, these patients should be encouraged to replace one set of rigid, inaccurate food rules with a set that is appropriate to their diabetic condition. Often, a diabetic food-exchange program is recommended. Medical limitations on the foods consumed may result in modification in the foods selected for formal or informal ERP. CBT often teaches that no food is a forbidden food, whereas brittle diabetics must clearly avoid certain foods. This stricture may result in difficult treatment decisions when a subjectively defined forbidden food is a frequent binge food, and it is also one that should be avoided because of diabetic limitations. In cases where dietary chaos is leading to substantial diabetic complications, it may be necessary to hospitalize the patient to achieve dietary and diabetic control. Also, severe diabetics often have clinically dysfunctional families, who may add to the problems of bulimic diabetics. Because of dietary limitations, subclinical binging is of much greater medical concern in diabetics and may merit treatment.

Management of Medical Complications

For the normal-weight bulimic, the medical complications of the disorder do not usually provide significant management problems. Potassium replacement therapy is straightforward, and in fact, some patients make an effort to eat high-potassium foods on their own. Dental problems and parotid enlargement are often effectively managed by having patients rinse the mouth and/or brush their teeth after purging. Constipation after stopping laxatives is common, and is best managed by increasing water intake, prescribing stool softeners, and advocating patience. Patients should be forewarned of the fluid retention that may follow reducing or stopping purging, so that their panic about weight gain will be reduced.

Bulimics and Borderline Personality Disorder

Bulimic borderlines represent a significant treatment challenge, although there are no published studies at present to guide treatment. Indeed, borderline personality disorder has only lately received the attention of cognitive behavioral researchers. Linehan (1987) described a cognitive behavioral conceptualization of BPD. She described three behavioral syndromes associated with BPD. The first, vulnerability versus invalidation, refers to the inability to regulate emotional responses, as well as the tendency for significant others to invalidate the borderline's emotions. Emotional dysregulation may precipitate numerous bulimic episodes. Because of the structured nature of CBT, there is a great risk that cognitive restructuring for food and weight attitudes, for example, may be perceived by the patient as invalidating and may result in extreme emotional reactions. Thus, the therapist must carefully balance supportive-accepting and confrontation-action interventions.

A second dimension is the active passivity syndrome, represented, on one hand, by extreme interpersonal dependency in the face of emotional distress. Thus, a frequent theme may be providing bulimic borderlines reassurance that the therapist "is there for them" and at the same time carefully encouraging the self-regulation skills characteristic of CBT. The other side of the coin is that borderlines may appear more competent than they are, and the therapist may be led to set up expectations that are unrealistic for the patient. The patient may perceive these expectations as overwhelming and often reacts with extreme anger and guilt.

Borderlines are also described as experiencing unrelenting crises versus emotional inhibition. The former refers to the tendency to be overwhelmed by minor stresses and not being able to "bounce back." To cope, borderlines may shut down their emotional responding. The most challenging aspect of this syndrome is suicidal behavior. Thus, the therapist must be vigilant for signs of distress in what otherwise might be perceived as mild stressors for a nonborderline bulimic. Also, when in crisis, the borderline bulimic is unable to implement focused behavioral interventions related to the eating disorder *per se*. At these times, the bulimic requires significant support and encouragement to attempt problem-solving strategies for the crisis at hand.

Linehan (1987) suggested that functioning as a consultant to the borderline, rather than as an intervener, often manages the "staff-splitting" behavior characteristic of these patients. Thus, the therapist teaches borderlines how to interact with others on the treatment team, rather than allowing the borderlines to expect the therapist to intervene with others on their behalf. This approach is highly relevant in that staff splitting may be a significant problem in both inpatient and outpatient treatment.

Turner (1989) described a treatment approach for BPD that is intensive and extensive. The treatment frequency is initially three times a week, eventually shifts to twice weekly, and lasts approximately one year. The treatment includes drug therapy (alprazolam) and a variety of strategies for improving emotional dysregulation and interpersonal relating. Because it is often advisable to focus more on the borderline facets of the bulimic borderline, Turner's work suggests that frequent, extended psychotherapy as well as pharmacotherapy be pursued for bulimic borderlines.

Inpatient Treatment

Inpatient treatment is sometimes required for patients with severe depression, suicidal behavior, BPD, medical complications, poor treatment compliance, or frequent binging and purging that has failed to respond to outpatient treatment. It is estimated that only 20%–30% of patients require inpatient treatment (Giles, Young, & Young, 1985; Williamson *et al.*, 1989b). For failed outpatients, Giles *et al.* (1985) offered more intensive therapy, including medication and, eventually, if needed, hospitalization. Approximately 67% of these difficult patients eventually improved. Wiliamson *et al.* (1989b) reported an uncontrolled comparison of inpatient versus outpatient treatment of bulimia. Patients improved substantially in both treatments. Inpatients tended to experience more rapid improvement but tended to relapse after discharge. Outpatients tended to show gradual improvements that were maintained. Because of the lack of random assignment, several explanations of this pattern of results may be plausible. However, the authors did conclude that outpatient therapy should be the treatment of choice in less difficult cases. However, inpatient treatment clearly has value for severe bulimics.

In addition to the intensity of therapies offered in the inpatient therapeutic milieu, this treatment modality does provide excellent control of eating behavior. Thus, it may be easier to achieve consumption of three regular meals a day with a focus on expanding the range of foods consumed. Purging behavior is also better controlled. For example, a behavioral program may include observation of the patient for one or two hours after meals to prevent purging, as well as limitations on unsupervised access to the bathroom or the patient's room. Limits on exercise is common. The limits on purging substantially slow binging; however, binging may still occur if the patient can devise a way to purge undetected. Also, food avoidance may occur, such as surreptitiously throwing food away and eating only the least fattening portions of meals. Like that of anorexics, bulimics' compliance with the treatment program is often facilitated by a contingency management program, typical reinforcers being unsupervised access to their room, therapeutic pass privileges, and other unit privileges. Care has to be taken to design a contingency program that is not punitive or coercive and in which compliance can be accurately monitored.

SUMMARY

Though bulimia nervosa has been recognized only recently as a distinct disorder, substantial progress has occurred since the early 1980s. Greater clarification of the diagnostic criteria has occurred, and there has been progress in the specification of the topography of binging and purging. Much is now known about the specific and global pathology and the medical complications of the disorder. Several new and promising assessment strategies have been developed, including questionnaires about specific eating-disorder pathology, as well as behavioral assessment such as test meals. The research since the early 1980s has led to the development of effective treatments, including multicomponent individual and group therapy and ERP. However, certain subsets of patients, particularly bulimic borderlines, await the development of effective interventions in the years to come.

REFERENCES

Agras, W. S., Schneider, J. A., Arnow, B., Raeburn, S. D., & Telch, C. F. (1989). Cognitive-behavioral treatment with and without exposure plus response prevention in the treatment of bulimia nervosa: A reply to Leitenberg and Rosen. *Journal of Consulting and Clinical Psychology, 57,* 778–779.

Allerdissen, R., Florin, I., & Rost, W. (1981). Psychological characteristics of women with bulimia nervosa (bulimarexia). *Behavioral Analysis and Modification*, *4*, 314–317.

American Psychiatric Association. (1980). *Diagnostic and statistical manual of mental disorders* (3rd ed.; DSM-III). Washington, DC: Author.

American Psychiatric Association. (1987). *Diagnostic and statistical manual of mental disorders* (3rd ed., rev.; DSM-III-R). Washington, DC: Author.

Arbitell, M. R., & Mizes, J. S. (1988). *Typographical and descriptive variables in bulimia nervosa: A controlled comparison*. Paper presented at the Southeastern Psychological Association Convention, New Orleans.

Boskind-Lodahl, M., & White, W. C. (1978). The definition and treatment of bulimarexia in college women: A pilot study. *Journal of the American College Health Association*, *27*, 84–97.

Bulik, C. M. (1987). Drug and alcohol abuse by bulimic women and their families. *American Journal of Psychiatry*, *144*, 1604–1606.

Cash, T. F., & Brown, T. A. (1987). Body image in anorexia nervosa and bulimia nervosa. *Behavior Modification*, *11*, 487–521.

Cutts, T. F., & Barrios, B. A. (1986). Fear of weight gain among bulimic and nondisturbed females. *Behavior Therapy*, *17*, 626–636.

Davis, C. J., Williamson, D. A., Goreczny, A. J., & Bennett, S. M. (1989). Body-image disturbances and bulimia nervosa: An empirical analysis of recent revisions of the DSM-III. *Journal of Psychopathology and Behavioral Assessment*, *11*, 61–69.

Davis, R., Freeman, R. J., & Garner, D. M. (1988). A naturalistic investigation of eating behavior in bulimia nervosa. *Journal of Consulting and Clinical Psychology*, *56*, 273–279.

Duchmann, E. G., Williamson, D. A., & Stricker, P. M. (1989). Bulimia, dietary restraint, and concern for dieting. *Journal of Psychopathology and Behavioral Assessment*, *11*, 1–13.

Fairburn, C. G. (1985). A cognitive-behavioral treatment of bulimia. In D. M. Garner & P. E. Garfinkel (Eds.), *Handbook of psychotherapy for anorexia nervosa and bulimia* (pp. 160–192). New York: Guilford Press.

Fairburn, C. G., & Garner, D. M. (1986). The diagnosis of bulimia nervosa. *International Journal of Eating Disorders*, *5*, 403–419.

Fairburn, C. G., Kirk, J., O'Connor, M., & Cooper, P. J. (1986). A comparison of two psychological treatments for bulimia nervosa. *Behaviour Research and Therapy*, *24*, 629–643.

Fairburn, C. G., Phil, M., & Beglin, S. J. (1990). Studies of the epidemiology of bulimia nervosa. *American Journal of Psychiatry*, *147*, 401–408.

Fava, M., Herzog, D. B., Hamburg, P., Riess, H., Anfang, S., & Rosenbaum, J. F. (1990). Long-term use of fluoxetine in bulimia nervosa: A retrospective study. *Annals of Clinical Psychiatry*, *2*, 53–56.

Freeman, C., Sinclair, F., Turnbull, J., & Annandale, A. (1985). Psychotherapy for bulimia: A controlled study. *Journal of Psychiatric Research*, *19*, 473–478.

Garner, D. M., & Bemis, K. M. (1982). A cognitive-behavioral approach to anorexia nervosa. *Cognitive Therapy and Research*, *6*, 123–150.

Garner, D. M., & Olmsted, M. P. (1984). *Eating Disorder Inventory manual*. Odessa, FL: Psychological Assessment Resources.

Garner, D. M., Olmsted, M. P., Bohr, Y., & Garfinkel, P. E. (1982). The Eating Attitudes Test: Psychometric features and clinical correlates. *Psychological Medicine*, *12*, 871–878.

Garner, D. M., Garfinkel, P. E., & O'Shaughnessy, M. (1985). The validity of the distinction between bulimia with and without anorexia nervosa. *American Journal of Psychiatry*, *142*, 581–587.

Garner, D. M., Fairburn, C. G., & Davis, R. (1987). Cognitive-behavioral treatment of bulimia nervosa: A critical appraisal. *Behavior Modification*, *11*, 398–431.

Garner, D. M., Olmsted, M. P., Davis, R., Rockert, W., Goldbloom, D., & Eagle, M. (1990). The association between bulimic symptoms and reported psychopathology. *International Journal of Eating Disorders*, *9*, 1–15.

Giles, T. R., Young, R. R., & Young, D. E. (1985). Behavioral treatment of severe bulimia. *Behavior Therapy*, *16*, 393–405.

Gormally, J., Rardin, D., & Black, S. (1980). Correlates of successful response to a behavioral weight control clinic. *Journal of Counseling Psychology*, *14*, 701–704.

Head, S. B., Williamson, D. A., Duchmann, E. G., & Bennett, R. T. (1988, November). *Bulimia nervosa: Association with Axis I and Axis II disorders*. Paper presented at the Association for the Advancement of Behavior Therapy Convention, New York.

Heilbrun, A. B., & Bloomfield, D. L. (1986). Cognitive differences between bulimic and anorexic females: Self-control deficits in bulimia. *International Journal of Eating Disorders*, *5*, 209–222.

Hillard, J. R., & Hillard, P. J. A. (1984). Bulimia, anorexia nervosa, and diabetes: Deadly combinations. *Psychiatric Clinics of North America*, *7*, 367–379.

Hinz, L. D., & Williamson, D. A. (1987). Bulimia and depression: A review of the affective variant hypothesis. *Psychological Bulletin, 102*, 150–158.

Hudson, J. I., Pope Jr., H. G., Yurgelun-Todd, D., Jones, J. M., & Frankenburg, F. R. (1987). A controlled study of lifetime prevalence of affective and other psychiatric disorders in bulimic outpatients. *American Journal of Psychiatry, 144*, 1283–1287.

Jacobs, M. B., & Schneider, J. A. (1985). Medical complications of bulimia: A prospective evaluation. *Quarterly Journal of Medicine, 54*, 177–182.

Johnson, C. (1985). Initial consultation for patients with bulimia and anorexia nervosa. In D. M. Garner & P. E. Garfinkel (Eds.), *Handbook of psychotherapy for anorexia nervosa and bulimia* (pp. 19–54). New York: Guilford Press.

Johnson, C., & Larson, R. (1982). Bulimia: An analysis of moods and behavior. *Psychosomatic Medicine, 44*, 341–351.

Johnson, C., Tobin, D., & Enright, A. (1989). Prevalence and clinical characteristics of borderline patients in an eating disordered population. *Journal of Clinical Psychiatry, 50*, 9–15.

Johnson, W. G., Corrigan, S. A., Crusco, A. H., & Schlundt, D. G. (1986). Restraint among bulimic women. *Addictive Behaviors, 11*, 351–354.

Katzman, M. A., & Wolchik, S. A. (1984). Bulimia and binge eating in college women: A comparison of eating patterns and personality characteristics. *Journal of Consulting and Clinical Psychology, 52*, 423–428.

Kettlewell, P. W., Mizes, J. S., & Wasylyshyn, N. (1992). A cognitive behavioral group treatment of bulimia. *Behavior Therapy, 23*.

Klesges, R. C., Mizes, J. S., & Klesges, L. M. (1987). Self-help dieting strategies in college males and females. *International Journal of Eating Disorders, 6*, 409–417.

Larson, R., & Johnson, C. (1985). Bulimia: Disturbed patterns of solitude. *Addictive Behaviors, 10*, 281–290.

Leitenberg, H., & Rosen, J. (1989). Cognitive-behavioral therapy with and without exposure plus response prevention in treatment of bulimia nervosa: Comment on Agras, Schneider, Arnow, Raeburn, and Telch. *Journal of Consulting and Clinical Psychology, 57*, 776–777.

Linehan, M. M. (1987). Dialectical behavior therapy for borderline personality disorder. *Bulletin of the Menninger Clinic, 51*, 261–276.

Marcus, M. D., & Wing, R. R. (1987). Binge eating among the obese. *Annals of Behavioral Medicine, 9*, 23–27.

Marcus, M. D., Wing, R. R., & Hopkins, J. (1988). Obese binge eaters: Affects, cognitions and responses to behavioral weight control. *Journal of Consulting and Clinical Psychology, 56*, 433–439.

Mitchell, J. E., Pyle, R. L., Hatsukami, D., & Eckert, E. D. (1986). What are atypical eating disorders? *Psychosomatics, 27*, 21–28.

Mitchell, P. B. (1988). The pharmacological management of bulimia nervosa: A critical review. *International Journal of Eating Disorders, 7*, 29–41.

Mizes, J. S. (1985). Bulimia: A review of its symptomatology and treatment. *Advances in Behavior Research and Therapy, 7*, 91–142.

Mizes, J. S. (1988a). Controlled comparisons of bulimics and noneating disordered controls on the MMPI-168. *International Journal of Eating Disorders, 7*, 425–428.

Mizes, J. S. (1988b). Personality characteristics of bulimic and non-eating-disordered female controls: A cognitive behavioral perspective. *International Journal of Eating Disorders, 7*, 541–550.

Mizes, J. S. (1989). Assertion deficits in bulimia nervosa: Assessment via behavioral, self-report and cognitive measures. *Behavior Therapy, 20*, 603–608.

Mizes, J. S. (1990). Criterion-related validity of the Anorectic Cognitions questionnaire. *Addictive Behaviors, 15*, 153–163.

Mizes, J. S. (1991a). Construct validity and factor stability in the Anorectic Cognitions questionnaire. *Addictive Behaviors, 16*, 89–93.

Mizes, J. S. (1991b). Validity of the Body Image Detection Device. *Addictive Behaviors, 16*, 411–417.

Mizes, J. S. (1992a). The Body Image Detection Device versus subjective measures of weight dissatisfaction: A validity comparison. *Addictive Behavior, 17*, 125–136.

Mizes, J. S. (1992b). Validity of the Mizes Anorectic Cognitions scale: A comparison between anorectics, bulimics, and psychiatric controls. *Addictive Behavior, 17*, 283–289.

Mizes, J. S., & Arbitell, M. R. (1991). Bulimics' perceptions of emotional responding during binge-purge episodes. *Psychological Reports, 69*, 527–532.

Mizes, J. S., & Fleece, E. L. (1986). On the use of progressive relaxation in the treatment of bulimia: A single-subject design study. *International Journal of Eating Disorders, 5*, 169–176.

Mizes, J. S., & Klesges, R. C. (1989). Validity, reliability, and factor structure of the Anorectic Cognitions questionnaire. *Addictive Behaviors, 14*, 589–594.

Mizes, J. S., & Lohr, J. M. (1983). The treatment of bulimia (binge-eating and self-induced vomiting): A quasi-experimental investigation of the effects of stimulus narrowing, self-reinforcement and self-control relaxation. *International Journal of Eating Disorders*m 2, 59–65.

Oppenheimer, R., Howells, K., Palmer, R. L., & Chaloner, D. A. (1985). Adverse sexual experience in childhood and clinical eating disorders: A preliminary description. *Journal of Psychiatric Research, 19*, 357–361.

Phelan, P. W. (1987). Cognitive correlates of bulimia: The Bulimic Thoughts Questionnaire. *International Journal of Eating Disorders, 6*, 593–607.

Polivy, J., & Herman, C. P. (1987). Diagnosis and treatment of normal eating. *Journal of Consulting and Clinical Psychology, 55*, 625–635.

Pope, H. G., & Hudson, J. I. (1989). Are the eating disorders associated with borderline personality disorder? A critical review. *International Journal of Eating Disorders, 8*, 1–10.

Rodin, J., Silberstein, L., & Striegel-Moore, R. (1984). Women and weight: A normative discontent. In T. B. Sonderegger (Ed.), *Psychology and gender: Nebraska Symposium on Motivation* (pp. 267–307). Lincoln: University of Nebraska Press.

Rosen, J. C. (1987). A review of behavioral treatments for bulimia nervosa. *Behavior Modification, 11*, 464–486.

Rosen, J. C., & Leitenberg, H. (1985). Exposure plus response prevention treatment of bulimia. In D. M. Garner & P. E. Garfinkel (Eds.), *Handbook of psychotherapy for anorexia nervosa and bulimia* (pp. 193–209). New York: Guilford Press.

Rosen, J. C., Leitenberg, H., Fondacaro, K. M., Gross, J., & Willmuth, M. (1985). Standardized test meals in assessment of eating behavior in bulimia nervosa: Consumption of feared foods when vomiting is prevented. *International Journal of Eating Disorders, 4*, 59–70.

Ruderman, A. J. (1986). Bulimia and irrational beliefs. *Behavior Research and Therapy, 24*, 193–197.

Ruggiero, L., Williamson, D., Davis, C. J., Schlundt, D. G., & Carey, M. P. (1988). Forbidden food survey: Measure of bulimic's anticipated emotional reactions to specific foods. *Addictive Behaviors, 13*, 267–274.

Schlundt, D. G., Johnson, W. G., & Jarrell, M. P. (1986). A sequential analysis of environmental, behavioral, and affective variables predictive of vomiting in bulimia nervosa. *Behavioral Assessment, 8*, 253–269.

Schulman, R. G., Kinder, B. N., Powers, P. S., Prange, M., & Gleghorn, A. (1986). The development of a scale to measure cognitive distortions in bulimia. *Journal of Personality Assessment, 50*, 630–639.

Shatford, L. A., & Evans, D. R. (1986). Bulimia as a manifestation of the stress process: A LISREL causal modeling analysis. *International Journal of Eating Disorders, 5*, 451–473.

Sloan, G., & Leichner, P. (1986). Is there a relationship between sexual abuse or incest and eating disorders? *Canadian Journal of Psychiatry, 31*, 656–660.

Smith, M. C., & Thelen, M. H. (1984). Development and validation of a test for bulimia. *Journal of Consulting and Clinical Psychology, 52*, 863–872.

Stancin, T., Link, D. L., & Reuter, J. M. (1989). Binge eating and purging in young women with IDDM. *Diabetes Care, 12*, 601–603.

Stein, D. M., & Laakso, W. (1988). Bulimia: A historical perspective. *International Journal of Eating Disorders, 7*, 201–210.

Strober, M., & Humphrey, L. L. (1987). Familial contributions to the etiology and course of anorexia nervosa and bulimia. *Journal of Consulting and Clinical Psychology, 55*, 654–659.

Turner, R. M. (1989). Case study evaluations of a bio-cognitive-behavioral approach for the treatment of borderline personality disorder. *Behavior Therapy, 20*, 477–489.

Van Buren, D. J., & Williamson, D. A. (1988). Marital relationships and conflict resolution skills of bulimics. *International Journal of Eating Disorders, 7*, 735–741.

Whitehouse, A. M., Freeman, C. L., & Annandale, A. (1986). Body size estimation in bulimia. *British Journal of Psychiatry, 149*, 98–103.

Williamson, D. A. (1990). *Assessment of eating disorders: Obesity, anorexia, and bulimia nervosa*. New York: Pergamon Press.

Williamson, D. A., Kelley, M. L., Davis, C. J., Ruggiero, K., & Blouin, D. C. (1985). Psychopathology of eating disorders: A controlled comparison of bulimic, obese, and normal subjects. *Journal of Consulting and Clinical Psychology, 53*, 161–166.

Williamson, D. A., Prather, R. C., Upton, L., Davis, C. J., Ruggiero, L., & Van Buren, D. (1987). Severity of bulimia: Relationship with depression and other psychopathology. *International Journal of Eating Disorders, 6*, 39–47.

Williamson, D. A., Goreczny, A. J., Davis, C. J., Ruggiero, L., & McKenzie, S. J. (1988). Psychophysiological analysis of the anxiety model of bulimia nervosa. *Behavior Therapy, 19*, 1–9.

Williamson, D. A., Davis, C. J., Goreczny, A. J., & Blouin, D. C. (1989a). Body-image disturbances in bulimia nervosa: Influences of actual body size. *Journal of Abnormal Psychology, 98*, 97–99.

Williamson, D. A., Prather, R. C., Bennett, S. M., Davis, C. J., Watkins, P. C., & Greenier, C. E. (1989b). An uncontrolled evaluation of inpatient and outpatient cognitive-behavior therapy for bulimia nervosa. *Behavior Modification*, *13*, 340–360.

Wiliamson, D. A., Davis, C. J., Goreczny, A. J., Bennett, S. M., & Gleaves, D. H. (1992). Development of a simple procedure for assessing body image disturbances. *Behavioral Assessment*, *11*, 433–446.

Willmuth, M. E., Leitenberg, H., Rosen, J. C., Fondacaro, K. M., & Gross, J. (1985). Body size distortion in bulimia nervosa. *International Journal of Eating Disorders*, *4*, 71–78.

Yates, A. (1989). Current perspectives on the eating disorders: 1. History, psychological and biological aspects. *Journal of the American Academy of Child and Adolescent Psychiatry*, *28*, 813–828.

Yates, W. R., Bowers, W. A., Carney, C. P., & Fulton, A. I. (1990). Is bulimia nervosa related to alcohol abuse? A personality analysis. *Annals of Clinical Psychiatry*, *2*, 23–27.

17

Personality Disorders

ELIZABETH J. WASSON and MARSHA M. LINEHAN

INTRODUCTION

It is only since 1980 that behaviorists have begun to venture publicly into the treatment of personality disorders (Beck & Hersen, 1990; Padesky, 1986; Pretzer, 1983, 1990; Turner, 1981, 1983, 1984, 1989; Young, 1983, 1988). This phenomenon may be attributed both to changes in diagnostic practices and to developments in personality research (Linehan & Wasson, 1990). The third edition of the *Diagnostic and Statistical Manual* (DSM-III; American Psychiatric Association, 1980) operationalized criteria for psychiatric diagnoses, thus shifting closer to the behavioral paradigm in which an empirical validation of results is essential. Out of the DSM-III, for example, have come several semistructured interviews for the personality disorders that have obtained respectable levels of reliability (Loranger, Oldham, Russakoff, & Susman, 1984; Pfohl, Stangl, & Zimmerman, 1983; Spitzer & Williams, 1985; Widiger, 1985).

The efficacy of behavioral treatments for personality disorders is, to all intents and purposes, untested but promising. The few controlled studies conducted to date, mostly with avoidant and borderline personalities, report favorable outcomes (eight summarized in Shea, 1990b). Behavioral treatments for individual symptoms, such as anger management, anxiety, and impulse control, have been available for some time (O'Leary & Wilson, 1987), and there is some evidence of their efficacy in the treatment of personality-disordered samples (reviewed in Kellner, 1986). Given the prevalence of personality disorders—up to 10% of adults in the general population and over 50% of clinical cases (Merikangas & Weissman, 1986; Spitzer, Forman, & Nee, 1979)—and the positive findings cited, the treatment of personality disorders would seem a fertile area for behavioral exploration.

In this chapter, we present an assessment and treatment package developed for borderline personality disorder, Dialectical Behavior Therapy (Linehan, 1984, in press). Because this treatment has been found effective in this population (Linehan, 1987b; Linehan *et al.*, 1991) and attrition has been low even in so difficult a population (16.7% compared to 58.3% in a "treatment-as-usual" community control group), we feel there may be value in exploring its generalizability to other personality disorders.

ELIZABETH J. WASSON and MARSHA M. LINEHAN • Department of Psychology, University of Washington, Seattle, Washington 98195.

Handbook of Behavior Therapy in the Psychiatric Setting, edited by Alan S. Bellack and Michel Hersen. Plenum Press, New York, 1993.

ELIZABETH J.
WASSON and
MARSHA M.
LINEHAN

According to the DSM-III (American Psychiatric Association, 1980) and the third edition, revised, of the DSM (DSM-III-R; American Psychiatric Association, 1987), the diagnosis of a personality disorder requires the presence of "inflexible" and "maladaptive" traits or behaviors that cause either significant impairment in occupational or social functioning, or self-reported distress. The criterion behaviors or traits must have been in evidence since early adulthood, must be characteristic of the person's recent and long-term functioning, and must not be symptomatic of a discrete episode of an Axis I disorder. *Recent* is defined as occurring within the past year.

The phrase "behaviors or traits" used in the DSM-III and DSM-III-R indicates the host of knotty conceptual problems that beleaguer these diagnoses at every turn. Are traits and behaviors to be understood as equivalent? *Trait* can be understood as a term summarizing observed behavior or as referring to some underlying structure that is seen as responsible for apparent consistency (Paulhus & Martin, 1987). The authors of the DSM-III and DSM-III-R asserted an atheoretical stance, but clearly, the decisions of what to observe and what words best describe these observations cannot be completely separated from the theories that inspired them (Meehl, 1978; Widiger & Trull, 1987).

Defining *personality* requires a level of inference much greater than the labels of the Axis I disorders. In the absence of a direct correspondence to some physical entity, decisions concerning the definition of this term are theoretically based. Thus, it is not surprising that the ongoing tension between psychoanalytic inference and the behaviorally based operationalism out of which the recent DSM editions have evolved is in striking evidence in the personality disorders sections. Further, in the absence of a consistent, organizing theoretical perspective, it is probably no coincidence that controversy surrounds all aspects of these diagnoses, empirically and theoretically, from the type and validity of classification system used to what and how criteria are selected (Livesley, 1987; Millon, 1987a; Morey, 1988a).

The choice of personality disorder categories may have consensual validity inasmuch as the opinions of the members of the DSM-III personality disorders task force represented those of clinicians at large. However, using a card-sorting task, Blashfield and Haymaker (1988) found that 30% of the DSM-III-R personality disorder criteria failed to be sorted into their appropriate category by the majority of clinician participants. Although the sample size was small ($n = 20$), numerous other studies have found great overlap between personality diagnoses (Livesley & Jackson, 1986; Mellsop, Varghese, Joshua, & Hicks, 1982; Morey, 1988c; Pfohl, Coryell, Zimmerman, & Stangl, 1986) and low discriminability of criteria (Livesley & Jackson, 1986). In fact, the amount of overlap has dramatically increased with the DSM-III-R, according to a study by Morey (1988c). His finding of a decrease in the use of the "Other Personality Disorder" category, however, suggests that the coverage in the DSM-III-R has increased as well.

Problems with overlap raise questions concerning the goodness of fit of the personality disorder categories with the existing data. For example, is schizotypal personality better conceptualized as a subdromal phase of schizophrenia (Millon, 1990)? Similarly, is borderline personality disorder more accurately viewed as a part of a spectrum of affective disorders (Akiskal, 1981) or as a final common pathway of multiple disorders (Reich, 1987)? Perhaps compulsive, avoidant, and antisocial personality disorders also share spectrum relationships with other Axis I disorders (Marin, Widiger, Frances, Goldsmith, & Kocsis, 1989).

Among the criteria, a range of inconsistencies is apparent. The theoretical mix is evident in the listing, side by side, of concrete behavioral observations, such as self-mutilating activity, and unoperationalized trait labels and psychoanalytically rooted terms, such as *overidealization* or *egocentricity*. Some criteria exhibit internal redundancy (Millon, 1987a); others, a range of globality (Livesley, 1987). Terms such as *aloof* and *exploitative*, for example, cover aggregations of behavior but are left unspecified. Little wonder that the reliabilities of DSM-III Axis II diagnoses have been low (Mellsop *et al.*, 1982; Spitzer *et al.*, 1979). Nevertheless, many commentators warn against increasing reliability by developing better operationalized terms because of the danger of prematurely restricting diagnostic definitions at a time when the conceptualization of these disorders is still so uncertain (Michels, 1987; Millon, 1987a; Widiger & Frances, 1985; Widiger & Trull, 1987).

An additional problem is the weighting of criteria. All of the Axis II diagnoses in the DSM-III-R are prototypical (compared to the DSM-III's 8 out of 11). In contrast to a "classical" classification system, members of a prototypical system differ in what features they share because each is an approximation of the best example (prototype) of that category. The DSM-III-R personality diagnoses are assigned as if all criteria were equally weighted (i.e., "any 5 out of 8" or "4 out of 7"). However, it is likely that the criteria represent a range of diagnostic efficiencies (e.g., Widiger, Frances, Warner, & Bluhm, 1986, on the borderline diagnosis). What these different efficiencies are for individual criteria or combinations of criteria is unknown, both because of an absence of data and because the diagnostic efficiency of the criteria change depending on the comparisons being made (Frances & Widiger, 1986; Millon, 1987a; Morey, 1988c).

Like the choice of diagnostic categories, the current criteria for the personality disorders were selected informally through a limited and unsystematic sampling of expert opinion (Livesley, 1987; Livesley, Jackson, & Schroeder, 1989). One improvement in the DSM-III-R over the DSM-III is that a criterion used in more than one diagnosis now appears with the same wording across diagnoses.

PROTOTYPICAL ASSESSMENT

Behavioral assessment plays a crucial role in all instances of behavior therapy. How this assessment is applied to personality disorders is based on the particular theory of personality that one holds. Although there are a number of different behavioral perspectives, the assessment and treatment paradigm presented here is based on that of Linehan (in press), who, in turn, drew from both Wallace (1966) and Staats (1975).

Personality is regarded as a set of behavioral capabilities (Wallace) or repertoires (Staats). Wallace distinguished between response predisposition, inherent in notions of the "drives" and "traits" that guide (predispose one to) certain ways of responding, and response capability. Such a conceptualization has the advantage over traditional trait approaches in distinguishing between the ability to perform a response and the actual performance of the response (Paulhus & Martin, 1987; Wallace, 1966). An additional distinction between response ability and response capability is useful. Paulhus and Martin (1987) theorized that *ability* refers to knowing what and how to perform a skill (i.e., having the response in one's repertoire), whereas *capability* refers to ease of performance.

This distinction allows access to another set of variables influencing performance. Capability is affected by conditioned emotional responses such as anxiety, by perceptions of ability, and by performance expectations. Thus, even when the situational incentives are high to act assertively, the individual with high assertion ability but low capability may behave passively. An individual's tendency to display a behavior is a function of the ability to perform the behavior, the capability of performing it, and the existence of situational reinforcers. Failure to perform may be due to lack of ability, response inhibition (performance is associated with high aversive emotionality, such as anxiety or guilt), or absence of incentive (performance is not reinforced).

The distinctions between performance, abilities, and capabilities have clear implications for treatment. In addition, the information generated is relatively unique in that it is not contained in the diagnosis itself. The diagnostic criteria for the personality disorders are based on trait conceptions and thus do not specify whether the behavior patterns listed are considered instances of deficient or excessive abilities, behavioral inhibitions or disinhibitions, or faulty situational control of behavior (Linehan, in press).

In examining abilities, capabilities, and possible deficits in these areas, it is useful to use a tripartite view of human functioning. Behavioral responses are divided into three general subsystems: (1) the overt-motor system; (2) the physiological-emotional system; and (3) the cognitive-verbal system (Staats, 1975).

During a behavioral assessment, the clinician scrutinizes each of the response systems in the tripartite organization in order to elicit as exact and detailed an account of the problem behavior, with its precipitants and consequences, as possible. Current and potential controlling variables as they are manifested in each of the three systems are assessed for duration, pervasiveness, frequency, and severity. A chain of events is gradually constructed accounting for as many of the thoughts, feelings, physical sensations, action urges, and behaviors as the patient can remember. The analysis includes the reciprocal interaction of the environment and the patient's responses. Historical settings for the behavior, as well as current situational determinants and their interaction with behavioral responses, are examined.

As the chain analysis unfolds, the information coming to light is also considered from a functional perspective. Possible reinforcing contingencies for the problem behavior are noted and used in generating hypotheses concerning the variables influencing or maintaining the behavior. Implicit in the hypotheses suggested by this functional analysis are alternative response patterns.

Generating solutions, an important step in problem-solving treatment strategies, involves a careful consideration of personal and environmental variables that may enhance or interfere with problem solutions. Given that problem behavior is thought of in terms of the presence or absence of abilities, the primary assessment question at this stage is whether or not patients can emit the needed behavior. If they can, are they inhibited from emitting it? The patients' assets and deficiencies in relevant areas—physical, aptitude, interests, and so forth—are considered, as are the environmental assets and deficits. Is there a history of conditioned negative reinforcement connected to the needed response, or are incentives lacking, or does the patient have faulty rules? The answer to each question points to an intervention. If the patient is unable to perform the response, then skills training is indicated.

The more episodes of a particular problem behavior subjected to this kind of analysis, the greater the confidence patient and clinician will have in their hypotheses and the greater the opportunity for fine-tuning alternative solutions. Frequently, other problem behaviors, including beliefs, thoughts, and/or overt action patterns, are functionally related to the problem behavior. In these instances, it is quite possible that the assessment process must be repeated for the other problem behaviors. However, such an analysis should be done less intensively until it becomes clear that these associated behaviors are critical in the maintenance of the targeted problem behavior (Linehan, 1984).

Diagnostic Assessment

Driven by behavioral assessment, treatment is idiographic. However, individual case conceptualizations and the blend of treatment strategies are based on categorical notions suggesting a "common thread" or common characteristics that distinguish the various personality-disordered patients from each other and from non-personality-disordered patients. Although the DSM-III-R Axis II diagnoses can be challenged on many grounds, this category-based system does provide a concise organization of data that facilitates communication between professionals. In addition, despite its conceptual and empirical problems, the system retains some validity. Fairly good convergence and internal consistency have been found for the 11 DSM-III-R definitions (Livesley & Jackson, 1986; Morey, 1988a,c), and prototypes have been identified for 6 of the DSM-III personality disorders (Blashfield, Sprock, Pinkston, & Hodgin, 1985).

The relationship between behavioral assessment and diagnostic assessment is complementary and reciprocal. Whereas behavioral assessment provides a description of the house a particular patient lives in, diagnosis describes the neighborhood. Obtaining the diagnosis of avoidant personality may suggest the use of exposure or skill-training techniques (Alden, 1989; Renneberg, Goldstein, Phillips, & Chambless, 1990), but assessment will determine to which stimuli the patient needs exposure or the specific skills in need of remediation. Diagnosis provides hypotheses, and behavioral assessment tests the match. In turn, through its idiographic approach, behavioral assessment clarifies the diagnostic confusion resulting from the fuzzy boundaries and heterogeneous membership of the current Axis II categories.

By allowing access to the clinical and research literature, diagnosis plays a vital role in treatment planning and management. Treating alcoholism in a schizotypal personality, for example, is different from the treatment for a nonschizotypal alcoholic (Kroll & Ryan, 1983). Given the accumulating number of studies suggesting that characterological difficulties are a major moderating variable in treatment, this point should not underemphasized. The presence of personality disorder has affected treatment response and has required a modification of the strategies used in the treatment of obsessive-compulsive disorder (Jenike, Baer, & Carey, 1986; Minichiello, Baer, & Jenike, 1987); alcoholism (Kroll & Ryan, 1983; Poldrugo & Forti, 1988); depression (Black, Bell, Hulbert, & Nasrallah, 1988; Pfohl, Stangl, & Zimmerman, 1984; Pilkonis & Frank, 1988; Shea, Pilkonis, Beckham, & Collins, 1990; Thompson, Gallagher, & Czirr, 1988); social anxiety (Turner, 1987); panic disorder (Mavissakalian & Hamann, 1987; Reich, 1988); bulimia (Brotman, Herzog, & Hamburg, 1988); and mental retardation (Reid & Ballinger, 1987); as well as in pharmacotherapy (antidepressants—antipanic medications) (Green & Curtis, 1988; Shawcross & Tyrer, 1985).

The use of several assessment devices allows for intrarater reliability checks, which are particularly important because self-report inventories have shown a tendency to record far more pathology than is diagnosed in clinical interviews (Pfohl, Coryell, Zimmerman, & Stangl, 1987; Piersma, 1987; Repko & Cooper, 1985; Wetzler & Dubro, 1990). This gap raises many intriguing possibilities, including those of patient exaggeration on self-report inventories and underdiagnosis of personality disorders by clinicians. Despite the great overlap among Axis II disorders, researchers have noted that, in everyday practice, chart reviews rarely reveal a diagnosis of more than one personality disorder for an individual patient (Pfohl *et al.*, 1986). The categorical nature of the classification system may prejudice clinicians against multiple diagnoses. Then again, there may be a halo effect, so that the first diagnosis that appears to fit colors other symptoms, and those incongruent with the first diagnosis are less likely to be perceived as significant (Widiger & Frances, 1987). Still another explanation comes from recent findings that clinicians do not follow the DSM-III criteria closely; rather, they invoke their own decision rules when diagnosing personality disorders, weighting some criteria more than others and applying idiosyncratic exclusion rules (Morey & Ochoa, 1989).

Accurate diagnostic assessment may be facilitated by diagnostic instruments. For clinical purposes, multiscale interviews and inventories are recommended, given the possibility of finding features of more than one disorder. However, two caveats are in order. The agreement among structured interviews has been only fair, a finding suggesting that interviews are not interchangeable (Hyler, Skodol, Kellman, Oldham, & Rosnick, 1990; O'Boyle & Self, 1990), and in addition, diagnoses may vary depending on whether the interview is based on the DSM-III or the DSM-III-R. Many patients who formerly met the criteria for schizotypal personality disorder in the DSM-III, for example, now meet the DSM-III-R diagnoses for schizoid personality (Morey, 1988c). In general, Morey (1988b) found the criteria in the DSM-III-R less restrictive than those in the DSM-III.

Listed here are the four semistructured interviews that correspond most closely to the DSM-

III and the DSM-III-R and that have been in use longest and therefore have some track record in terms of reliability and validity. Because all have been updated or are in the process of being updated for use with the DSM-III-R, the most recent versions are referenced here: the Structured Clinical Interview for DSM-III Personality Disorders (SCID-II; Spitzer & Williams, 1987); the Personality Disorder Examination (PDE; Loranger, 1988); the Structured Interview for the DSM-III Personality Disorders (SIDP; Pfohl *et al.*, 1983); and the Personality Interview Questions II (PIQ-II; Widiger, 1987). The SCID-II has the advantage of being the only structured interview with an Axis I instrument *and* a self-report inventory (the PDQR; see below) designed to complement it.

The best known self-report inventories are the Minnesota Multiphasic Personality Inventory (MMPI; Hathaway & McKinley, 1943), the Millon Clinical Multiaxial Inventory (MCMI; Millon, 1983), and the Personality Diagnostic Questionnaire Revised (PDQR; Hyler & Rieder, 1984). Even without recent revisions, the long research traditions of both the MMPI and the MCMI make them valuable assessment tools. Recently, both have been modified to better accommodate DSM-III-R diagnoses. The MMPI now has personality disorder scales (Morey, Waugh, & Blashfield, 1985), and the MCMI-II (Millon, 1987b), in addition to some modifications in older scales (antisocial and compulsive), includes two new scales equivalent to the proposed DSM-III-R "self-defeating" and "sadistic" personality disorders.

For comprehensive reviews of instruments pertaining to Axis II, the reader is referred to Reich (1987, 1989) and Widiger and Frances (1987).

Actual Assessment

The evaluation of a new patient, including an assessment of suicidal or homicidal risk, involves some additional considerations.

As always, practical concerns, such as the evaluation of the patient's living situation and financial arrangements, are paramount in assessing the feasibility of treatment. For example, long commutes for already emotionally overtaxed patients may decrease the chances of regular attendance and may prove a dangerous obstacle in emergencies. A highly suicidal patient living in an isolated area without a phone may present an unacceptable risk that must be changed before treatment can begin. A discussion of such aspects of the patient's current living situation enables the patient and the therapist to create as treatment-enhancing a context for beginning therapy as is reasonable and possible for that patient. Other potential hazards in the continuation of therapy may become goals of treatment (see "Hierarchy of Targets" under "Prototypical Treatment" below), for example, helping the patient to gain employment or federal assistance to mitigate financial strains.

Especially helpful in evaluating a new patient for treatment is information concerning previous therapy experiences. Details concerning what patients have found helpful and unhelpful, their reactions to previous therapists, and their perceptions of therapist's reactions to them are data important in developing a treatment approach that will survive a difficult patient.

Background information, such as recent losses or disruptions, pattern of past parasuicides and suicide attempts, the amount of social support versus isolation, and the presence or absence of current substance abuse, figures significantly in assessing near-term and long-term parasuicide and suicide risk (Linehan, 1981; Motto, 1988).

Other factors cited as indicators of near-term (within 60 days) suicide risk are prominent suicidal ideation and impulses (Gutierrez, Russakoff, & Oldham, 1988; Linehan, 1981; Motto, 1988); lethality and number of prior attempts (Gutierrez *et al.*, 1988; Linehan, 1981; Modestin, 1989; Motto, 1988); the presence of affective disorders (Gutierrez *et al.*, 1988; Linehan, 1981; Modestin, 1989; Petronis, Samuels, Moscicki, & Anthony, 1990); poor or variable results of prior attempts to get help (Motto, 1988); indifference to treatment (Linehan, 1981); hopelessness (Gutierrez *et al.*, 1988; Linehan, 1981); severe guilt, shame, or remorse (Motto, 1988); and links with significant others who have parasuicided (Kreitman, Smith, & Tan, 1970). With respect to psychotic symptoms, ideas of reference and/or persecution have been flagged as significant risk factors for both near- and long-term (within two years) risk (Motto, 1988; inpatient sample).

An assessment of imminent suicide risk should include an evaluation of past and current patterns of self-injury with respect to the lethality and availability of method(s), which may include knowledge of prescribed as well as over-the-counter medications and medication compliance; the degree of premeditation or impulsivity usually involved; the characteristic degree of concealment or deception in terms of timing and place; and characteristic environmental conditions associated with suicidal responding. Clearly, a note written or in progress, patient arrangements for his or her own death such as giving away possessions, and indirect references to his or her own death are all serious signs of imminent self-destructive behavior.

An assessment of the potential for aggressive acting out similarly involves a knowledge of past patterns and methods, including the availability of weapons, customary or intended victims, and disinhibiting drugs or alcohol. Other situational variables to be considered are the characteristics of the patient's family, peer group, and job (Goldstein & Keller, 1987).

With new patients, performing the behavioral assessments required to elicit the kind of detailed information recommended here necessitates keeping the client on track with tact, persistence, and sensitivity to the particular response biases intrinsic in different personality syndromes (Shea, 1990). For example, exaggeration may be displayed by individuals with histrionic patterns of behavior; denial, by those with narcissistic diagnoses; withholding, by those with paranoid tendencies; and acquiescence, by those with dependent patterns. A matter-of-fact style of interviewing and asking for examples of other people's responses to and opinions of the patient may be useful in sorting through these and other forms of distortion. Being alert for the influence of mood as well as response biases will help in obtaining a clearer picture both situationally and diagnostically.

Prototypical Treatment

Like most behavior therapies, dialectical behavior therapy (DBT) is directive and intervention-oriented. Standard behavioral techniques such as exposure, skills training, shaping, and cognitive modification are used. Differing from traditional behavior therapy, however, DBT focuses on dialectical process, acceptance, and validation of behavior as it is in the moment; on treating behaviors that interfere with therapy; and on the therapeutic relationship as essential to the treatment.

Dialectical behavior therapy consists of sets of strategies applied to a hierarchy of targets. The heart of the treatment lies in the ongoing tension between problem-solving and validation strategies, which represent the central dialectic between change and acceptance.

The dialectical underpinning of DBT stresses the inherent wholeness and interrelatedness of reality. Encompassing systems theories, a dialectical view emphasizes the dynamic, ongoing interaction of parts and whole that constantly creates and re-creates new relationships among parts and of parts to the whole (Linehan & Wasson, 1990). Person and environment exert reciprocal influences.

Dialectical thinking recognizes that all statements contain within themselves their own opposition. Reality is constantly evolving and exists in an ongoing state of tension, each element or propositional truth being balanced by its complement. Thus, rather than involving a relativistic position that would see oppositional truths as existing side by side, equally but separately true, dialectical thinking involves a synthesis that engenders a new set of tensions. Unlike traditional cognitive therapy, a dialectical view does not seek to verify one side of an argument. Truth is not an absolute. Clinging to either extreme of a dialectic increases polarization and inhibits growth and change. An impasse is reached. Looking for what is being left out or is missing helps reclaim the dialectic and allows continued movement (Linehan, in press).

Dialectical thinking permeates all levels of the treatment. It is a mode of conceptualizing that guides the therapist's thinking; for example, problem behaviors are targets for change and are also appreciated as attempts to solve problems in their own right. On another level, the dialectic guides the process of a session as the therapist balances change and acceptance strategies in order to maintain a collaborative relationship. More substantively, dialectics inform specific interventions such as paradox, metaphor, and storytelling, which appeal to experiential knowledge, and finally, dialectics enter the content of sessions directly as the patient is taught to think dialectically through cognitive restructuring, questioning, and modeling.

The overarching dialectic of change and acceptance is represented by the problem-solving and validation strategy sets. Problem solving always begins with behavioral analysis. Because identifying the factors precipitating a problem is not always easy, the patient learns to use dysfunctional behaviors as signals of a problem to be solved. Behavior analysis is then used to identify the controlling factors, to formulate hypotheses, and to generate alternative solutions.

Questions concerning abilities, capabilities, and deficits take center stage. If the patient lacks the ability to make a more adaptive response, the skills necessary to remedy this situation are taught. If the patient has the ability but the reinforcement contingencies are not set up to increase the probability of adaptive responses, then contingency management strategies are used. Are adaptive responses punished, or is maladaptive behavior reinforced? If so, again, contingency management strategies are appropriate.

If the adaptive response is, within the patient's repertoire, the next issue is capability. Is adaptive responding inhibited by anxiety or guilt? Is the patient emotion-phobic? If so, an exposure-based treatment is appropriate. Finally, if appropriate responses are available, faulty expectations, beliefs, or assumptions that may impede performance are probed. If they are in evidence, cognitive modification may be undertaken. For example, the therapist may need to help the patient learn what she can reasonably expect from both the therapist and her immediate environment.

Contingency management involves arranging or highlighting the therapist's responses in a way that reinforces adaptive behaviors and extinguishes maladaptive behaviors. Concurrently, the therapist helps the patient begin to arrange contingencies in her life productively. Thus, in our clinic, therapists do not allow phone conversation (other than to ensure appropriate medical care) for 12 hours following a parasuicide because the patient has already "coped" with the problem. In contrast, in phone calls received *before* any urges have been acted on, therapists are fully engaged, sympathetic, and working hard to help patients apply their skills and generate more adaptive coping responses.

DBT teaches a range of general behavioral skills, some of which are typically taught in many instances of behavior therapy. The skills include mindfulness, distress tolerance, emotion regulation, and interpersonal effectiveness. Mindfulness skills are the building blocks for all of the other skill sets and are a behavioral adaptation of Eastern meditation practices. The specific skills are observing, describing, and participating nonjudgmentally, attentively, and effectively. Mindfulness practice seeks to increase awareness and control of attentional processes. The learning of the skills is presented to the patient as learning to control one's own mind. An assumption is that participation without awareness is characteristic of impulsive and mood-dependent behaviors (Linehan, in press). Mindfulness requires attending no matter what distressing events may be occurring. Thus, mindfulness practice is also the basis of exposure techniques and can be used to facilitate the extinction of automatic avoidance and fear responses.

Mindfulness skills teach, in addition, that observing is separate from what is being observed. In particular, practice in observing teaches that events and one's responses to those events are not identical. Feeling as if the world is out of control does not necessarily mean that it is. Distinguishing between events and one's thoughts, feelings, and actions concerning them is essential to communication as well as to self-control. Describing—that is, the ability to apply verbal labels to internal, behavioral, and environmental events—helps underline this difference. Participating allows total, unselfconscious involvement in whatever is needed to be effective or aware with one's entire self in the moment. Mindfulness is *participating* with attention to the task at hand.

Distress tolerance skills assume that some pain is unavoidable in life and that the refusal to accept this pain exacerbates distress. In addition, the ability to tolerate distress is necessary for change in order that impulsive responses not interfere with efforts to establish new patterns of responding. However, an essential point is that an acceptance of reality as it is does not imply approval of that reality and, conversely, that wishing reality were different does not make it so. For change to occur, one has to know what needs changing; this knowledge implies acceptance of one's current state.

Emotion regulation skills teach nonjudgmental observation and description of one's current emotional responses as well as a range of methods for coping with or reducing unwanted emotions. Behavioral analysis of the events precipitating a strong emotion helps identify the feelings and generate alternative coping responses. Interpersonal effectiveness skills involve many standard assertiveness-training techniques as well as interpersonal problem solving. Learning to ask for what one needs, saying no, accepting no, and coping with interpersonal conflict are all included here.

Countering the push for change represented by the problem-solving strategies and skills training is constant validation, the acceptance pole of the dialectic. Like client-centered therapies, validation is the attempt by the therapist to observe nonjudgmentally, to reflect accurately, and to find and communicate the inherent value or wisdom of the patient's cognitive, emotional, or overt behavior. The therapist communicates a belief in the patient's desire to grow and change as well as in his inherent ability to do so. The therapist conveys understanding and empathetic acknowledgment of the patient's sense of desperation. It is important in DBT to remember to validate the emotional response to the emotion (Linehan, 1984). There may be panic at the first signs of anxiety, shame over anger, humiliation over feeling dependent. Emotional pain is normalized: Many or most people would feel that way under those circumstances; given the patient's learning history, it makes perfect sense that she would respond that way.

Use of the validation strategies counteracts therapists' all-too-frequent tendencies to focus prematurely on change when patients present with intolerable pain or suffering. Often, therapists' invalidation of the patient's feelings arises from their overanxious attempts to make the patient feel better right now. Telling patients they need not feel a certain way, praising the behaviors or opinions they feel badly about, or too quickly focusing on changing emotions is not helpful. Such quick reassurance conflicts with the teaching of distress tolerance skills; that is, teaching that aversive feelings are both understandable and tolerable. In contrast, helping patients to observe can bring them closer to accepting and eventually being able to validate their own feelings, opinions, and behavioral decisions.

Case management strategies hinge on the consultant and environmental intervention strategies. In DBT, the therapist is seen as a consultant to the patient, not to other professionals. The therapist works with the patient to help the patient interact more effectively with outside agencies or professionals. Problems with and inappropriate behavior on the part of other mental health professionals are viewed as opportunities for learning. As a consequence, not only is an active problem-solving stance reinforced, but validation, the therapist's belief in the patient, is behaviorally communicated.

Part of the patient's task is to learn to adjust to an inconsistent and variable world. As a problem solver, the therapist does not work to rescue patients from what may be the natural consequences of their behavior. For this reason, rather than advising other professionals on how to deal with one's patients, the DBT therapist suggests that other professionals follow their normal procedures.

An important exception to the consultant strategy occurs when outside agencies or people are unwilling to modify their treatment, substantial harm may come to the patient as a result, and the patient clearly does not have the ability to influence the outcome. Involuntary commitment and public assistance are two systems where intervention by a high-power person is often needed. This kind of intervention is an example of environmental intervention.

A last set of strategies describes two styles of communication found useful in working with borderlines: irreverent communication and reciprocal vulnerability. Irreverent communication involves a matter-of-fact, irreverent attitude toward dysfunctional problem solving, including parasuicide. These problems are accepted as normal consequences of individual learning histories and current operating factors in the individual's life. The therapist's reactions are sometimes experienced as "off the wall" and involve the therapist's framing the issue under consideration in a context different from the patient's. The patient is pushed off balance so a new balancing can occur (Linehan, in press).

For example, while eliciting an initial commitment to treatment, a therapist says in passing, "You do realize that if you don't drop out for a year, that really does, if you think about it logically, rule out suicide for a year?" Again, still working on commitment, the therapist says firmly, after discussing numerous instances in which the patient's behavior appears mood-dependent, "So I see as our number one priority getting you to agree—sincerely, of course—to follow through on staying alive and not harming yourself and not attempting suicide no matter what kind of mood you're in."

In contrast, reciprocal vulnerability is warm, empathetic, and directly responsive to the patient's vulnerability. It includes therapeutic self-disclosure as a vehicle for modeling both mastery of and coping with problems. Because many borderline patients have difficulty directly expressing feelings or discussing interpersonal conflict, this mode of therapist communication becomes a form of reinforcement, models normative responses to everyday situations, and is inherently validating. For example, in response to a patient who has been able to recognize and acknowledge feeling hurt (with subsequent mild self-destructive urges) because of something the therapist said, the therapist acknowledges, "People have told me I'm very direct, sometimes too direct. I think you're right about that, but you know, if you can deal with someone like me, it's probable you can deal with almost anyone."

Hierarchy of Targets

DBT orders treatment goals or targets—that is, behaviors to be increased and behaviors to be decreased—hierarchically according to importance. In order of importance the targets are suicidal behaviors, behaviors that interfere with therapy, behaviors that interfere with quality of life, behavioral skills, posttraumatic stress responses, respect of oneself, and, finally, any other goals the patient may have.

From session to session, the priority target varies depending on what behaviors the patient has been engaging in. Whenever high-risk suicidal behaviors, including threats, parasuicidal acts, or serious suicidal ideation, are occurring, they take precedence over all other problems. If suicidal behaviors are not a current problem, the priority target becomes any current behaviors that interfere with the giving and receiving of effective therapy. In the absence of any of these behaviors, the session focuses on quality-of-life issues, such as substance abuse or financial problems.

The rationale for the hierarchy is both pragmatic and theoretically compatible with Staats's conception of cumulative hierarchical learning (Staats, 1986). Common sense suggests that therapy with dead or terminated patients will be ineffective. Similarly, it may be difficult to acquire essential skills for improved interpersonal relationships and self-management if the patient usually attends sessions in an intoxicated state or if crises such as no housing or food or imminent threat of jail require attention. Staats (1986) pointed out that many responses depend on the successful acquisition of other smaller response units for their mastery. If a patient is unable to cope with aversive feelings about everyday life without self-mutilation or drinking excessively, uncovering trauma from the past is unlikely to lead to a better quality of life, or perhaps any life at all, until sufficient emotion-regulation skills have been acquired to deal with the aversive feelings in more adaptive ways.

Unlike the behavioral case formulation method of Turkat (Turkat & Maisto, 1985), it should be noted that the highest priority targets are not so much those "primary" problems that may be seen as giving rise to all other symptoms, but those problems that embody the gravest immediate threat to continued life, continued therapy, and a minimal quality of life, in that order. From the DBT point of view, any problem will soon lead to the "core" problem through the interrelationships of behavioral systems and across problems that emerge through repeated behavioral analyses.

Some comments on less obvious aspects of the targets and on less traditional targets follow. Suicidal behavior, in addition to intentional self-injury and suicide crisis behavior, includes suicidal ideation, suicide-related expectancies and beliefs, and suicide-related affect, all of which may lead to self-destructive behavior (Linehan, in press). Suicide-related affect is a positive emotional response, such as relief or calmness, that may reinforce suicidal or parasuicidal thoughts, images, fantasies, and acts. Examples of short-term expectancies of suicide or parasuicide are getting help, making others sorry, escaping an intolerable life situation, restarting or terminating relationships, or getting others to take one's problems seriously. Because many of these expectancies are accurate, DBT focuses on long-term rather than short-term expectancies.

Therapy-interfering behavior is behavior by either patient or therapist that jeopardizes effective therapy. It is crucial in DBT that the therapist take seriously both the patient's behaviors that interfere with comfort or therapeutic outcome and the therapist's own behaviors that interfere with the patient's satisfaction or progress. On the patient's side, these behaviors range from behaviors that prevent the patient from receiving treatment, including behaviors that lead to therapist burnout, to behaviors that interfere with other patients' receiving treatment. Examples include not attending sessions, dropping out, excessive hospital admissions that result in missed sessions, dissociating, lying, withdrawing, digressing constantly from priority targets, physical violence, not keeping agreements made with the therapist, and refusing to agree to essential treatment goals.

In group and inpatient settings, patients have a significant impact on each other and on the therapy. Behaviors that interfere with other patients' receiving treatment include hostile, critical, or judgmental remarks to other patients, as well as behavior that threatens the physical safety or the emotional sense of safety of the environment, such as angry acting out involving throwing or breaking property or attempts or threats to injure others. On the other hand, a goal of DBT is to help patients become more comfortable with conflict. Inability to tolerate negative feedback appropriately given by another patient would therefore be considered therapy-interfering, as would negative feedback given at an ill-timed moment or insistent attempts to problem-solve an interpersonal situation with another patient.

Therapists, however, can also interfere with therapy, such as by doing ineffective or harmful therapy. For convenience, these therapist behaviors are divided into two categories: those that interfere with the balance between acceptance and change in therapy and those that are disrespectful of the patient. Examples are excessive anger, hostility, and/or frustration directed at the patient; "blaming-the-victim" attitudes; unrealistic beliefs about what is possible in the moment and correspondingly unrealistic expectations of the patient; taking care of patients rather than teaching patients to care for themselves (often because it is easier for the therapist); rigidity and refusal to change treatment methods or too frequent changes in approach; too much self-disclosure; and forgetting appointments, coming late, acting tired in the session, not returning phone calls, and forgetting important information.

A common and very debilitating therapist-interfering behavior is the inability to tolerate a patient's distress in the present, which can lead to ameliorating efforts that reinforce dysfunctional behavior in the long run. This kind of behavior indicates therapist burnout, either in general or with that particular patient. In DBT, therapists must be willing to admit errors and must be open to repairing and changing response patterns when necessary.

The third target is behaviors that interfere with quality of life. These behaviors include behaviors that, if not changed, preclude the likelihood of a reasonable quality of life. Although many behaviors, such as severe substance dependence, having no housing or income, or engaging in criminal activity likely to lead to jail, can be taken as interfering in themselves, a recognition of the problems they cause may be the first step toward change. The determination of other quality-interfering behaviors is, at times, somewhat idiosyncratic and therefore must be discussed by patient and therapist, for example, whether to stay on public assistance. Often, case conferences and supervision will help the therapist sort through his or her values and gain clarity on how differences in values between the patient and the therapist may be affecting treatment.

The fourth target is skills training, which targets the skill sets described above and may also include any additional skills necessary for progress in treatment. In structured therapy settings, such as inpatient groups, there may be little opportunity to tailor the skills being taught to the individual needs of patients; in other settings, individual behavioral assessments may dictate which skills need the most time and attention. In either case, independent of the specific skill, behavioral skills training in DBT communicates to patients that problems can be solved, even if the solution is simply greater acceptance, a solution that has itself been arrived at by assuming an active problem-solving stance.

Fifth on the hierarchy are post-traumatic stress behaviors. These are relevant whenever there is a history of abuse (sexual, emotional, or physical) or significant loss or traumatic threat of loss. These behaviors fall in the hierarchy because the trauma associated with even therapeutic exposure to abuse-related cues is high. A solid alliance, a stable life situation, and working behavioral skills must be well in place if the patient is to cope with the stress and to avoid counterproductive decompensation.

The sixth target is respect for oneself and involves the ability to care for, value, believe in, validate, and trust one's own self (Linehan, in press). This target involves learning to evaluate one's own responses and to hold on to self-evaluations independent of what important others may think. The ability to feel close to and appropriately depend on others without invalidating one-self is an important target of DBT.

ACTUAL TREATMENT

In considering the possible application of DBT to other personality disorders, we focus on those aspects that may be potent in fostering work with difficult patients. Because there are few published behavioral treatments for personality disorders, let alone empirically confirmed approaches, and we have not attempted DBT with other than borderline patients, the sections that follow should be taken in the spirit of a thought experiment. Where some evidence exists for the efficacy of a particular intervention, it is noted.

Treatment Parameters

DBT uses several modes of therapy, including individual, group, and phone calls for the patients and consultation groups for the therapist. All modes of therapy revolve around the individual therapy, which is held once a week. Skills-training groups use a psychoeducational format and run 2 to 2½ hours once a week. Consultation meetings are held once a week and include all therapists in a particular setting who are interested in applying DBT principles.

In complicated cases, it is difficult to attend to the many pressing problems that arise in sessions and teach skills at the same time. Therefore, it is useful to provide skills training either in a group or as a tutorial with another clinician. The individual therapist is responsible for seeing that the skills are integrated with daily functioning. On an inpatient unit with skills-training groups, where there may be no individual therapist *per se*, this role could be assumed either by a designated person or by which ever person is assigned to the patient at a particular time. In one setting, developed by C. Swenson at New York Hospital, this role is assumed by a unit skills consultant who has regular office hours that patients can use for help in applying their skills.

Therapist and patient contract (and recontract) for the length of time they will work together. At the Suicidal Behaviors Research Clinic at the University of Washington, borderline patients and their therapists typically make an initial six-month to one-year commitment. From the initial outcome studies (Linehan, 1987b), it appears that parasuicidal behavior can begin to come under control within the first four months of therapy, but that stable gains in reducing both parasuicide and therapy-interfering behaviors may take up to a year. Bringing suicidal behavior and therapy-interfering behavior under control maximizes the patient's chances of being accepted into treatment elsewhere at the end of the year and of benefiting from that treatment, and it increases the chances that both the DBT therapist and the patient will wish to continue beyond their first year.

A firm operational definition of "dropping out" is an important part of the contract. Although the notion of a limit was originally defined for research purposes, it proved so clinically useful that it has been retained as a part of DBT. At the Suicidal Behaviors Clinic, four consecutive sessions missed for any reason (with more than one session a week counting as only one session) are taken to indicate termination. In order to work with mood-dependent behaviors, it has been important to ensure that patients will not be terminated by the therapist simply because they have said that they have quit. Having such an operationalized definition allows latitude for working with the patient's avoidance at these difficult junctures. The therapist may choose to actively pursue the patient, especially in the early stages of treatment when the patient does not yet have many alternative modes of dealing with aversive situations.

The frequency of the sessions may vary, depending on the therapist's assessment of the patient's needs. With borderline patients, twice-a-week sessions at the beginning of therapy and during crisis periods have been helpful. The frequency and length of phone calls are determined by the ongoing process of therapists' observing their limits. Session length may also vary depending on the tasks to be accomplished and the difficulty of the patient in opening up and then closing up emotionally. Desensitization techniques using imaginal situational hierarchies may require 1½-hour sessions for some patients, and for others, shorter, more frequent sessions may be most useful.

DBT is based on a voluntary treatment contract. Depending on the circumstances and the legal restrictions, failure to agree may lead to referral to other resources or to other programs or treatment modalities within the same setting. Essential to the initial therapy contract is the patient's agreement to work on the behaviors that most obstruct his or her future well-being or quality of life (i.e., those behaviors that are of top priority in the hierarchy). Determination of these behaviors is based on information obtained during the initial assessment. In settings where patients cannot be rejected from treatment, a special program-within-a-program may be needed so that patients can be rejected (Linehan, in press). Agreements to work on other target goals are developed as therapy progresses. Patients' agreements to the terms of DBT are always brought up when they later try to violate the rules or to get the rules changed. During the first year with very dysfunctional patients, recommitment to the initial agreement must be sought repeatedly.

Hierarchy of Targets

Most poorly functioning patients with personality disorders can be expected to enter treatment with quality-of-life-interfering behavior (Target 3), therapy-interfering behavior (Target 2), or even suicidal behavior (Target 1).

Clearly, patients with life-threatening habits, such as parasuicidal behavior, must agree to work on these habits. Intentional self-injury appears to cut across disorders, but some recent evidence suggests that the combination of personality disorder and depression is a significant risk factor in parasuicide and suicide (Black *et al.*, 1988; Modestin, 1989; Pfohl *et al.*, 1984). Findings are mixed, however, regarding whether particular clusters of personality disorders are more likely than others to include suicidal behaviors. In addition to suicidal behavior, other circumstances that may assume life-threatening proportions are promiscuity without proper precautions, certain criminal activities, remaining in a severely abusive relationship, or not undergoing proper medical care.

Patients who repeatedly burn out therapists or fail to comply with treatment regimes, as is characteristic of lower functioning borderline patients, must agree to work on those therapy-interfering aspects of their interpersonal style. Patterns that interfere with the ability to accept feedback from the therapist are included here. The extreme fear of social evaluation in a paranoid patient (Turkat & Maisto, 1985) may be of therapy-threatening proportions and may need to be targeted, including an agreement to make in-session occurrences of the problem a therapy focus. The sensitivity to criticism displayed by avoidant, narcissistic, and compulsive patients may be similarly therapy-interfering. Other examples and the personality styles with which they may be associated are not asking for help or withdrawing (schizoid, schizotypal, or avoidant); constant verbal abuse of the therapist (antisocial or narcissistic); tantrumming (histrionic or narcissistic); threats to sue (paranoid, narcissist, or borderline antisocial); setting up for therapy failure through constant unreasonable therapy demands (obsessive-compulsive, narcissistic, or paranoid); bringing weapons to sessions (antisocial or paranoid); and not complying with treatment recommendations or following through on agreements with the therapist (passive-aggressive, antisocial, or narcissistic).

Behaviors that fall under the category of therapy-interfering must be distinguished from interpersonal behaviors in general. Whereas problem interpersonal behaviors are probably always positive indicators of a need for skills training, therapy-threatening behavior is a type or frequency of behavior that truly either seriously interferes with therapy being received (e.g., avoidance of exposure in exposure-based treatment) or threatens either the therapist or the patient with burnout (e.g., constantly criticizing or judging the other).

Quality-of-life-interfering behaviors include the difficulty with delay of gratification shown by antisocial, narcissistic, and histrionic individuals. Poor impulse control with respect to social or legal conventions, substance use, gambling, food, driving, financial expenditure, and so forth may impair quality of life. Similarly, the limited range of daily activities, social contact, and—for higher functioning patients—emotional experience that characterizes patients with schizoid and schizotypal patterns (Liebowitz, Stone, & Turkat, 1986; Stone, 1985) fall under this target, as would the overly eccentric social presentation of a schizotypal or severely histrionic person. The procrastination or indecisiveness that is often a part of a passive-aggressive, compulsive, or dependent picture may reach quality-of-life-threatening proportions when interfering with job performance, financial affairs, or relationships.

With increased functioning, skills training may be the expected entry target for most personality-disordered patients. Thus, the assertiveness training encompassed by DBT's interpersonal effectiveness skills would be appropriate for people with dependent (Livesley, Schroeder, & Jackson, 1990) and avoidant diagnoses (Alden, 1989; Renneberg *et al.*, 1990). Turkat and Maisto (1985) described the successful use of assertiveness training to help a paranoid patient give feedback without others' feeling attacked and therefore provoked to counterattack. Social-skills training has also been conceptualized as helpful with histrionic patients (Brantley & Callon, 1985). Working on time management issues (passive-aggressive patterns), prioritizing demands and balancing "wants" with "shoulds" (obsessive-compulsive styles), and working on realistic goals (narcissistic patterns) are other skills targeted in interpersonal effectiveness training. Distress tolerance skills are a target for dependent or histrionic individuals to ameliorate difficulties in being alone or without reassurance, to help an antisocial person tolerate boredom, to help an obsessive-compulsive individual with inefficiency and fallibility, and to help a narcissistic person with feeling weak or insignificant. Emotion regulation skills are a target for all disorders because of the training they offer in coping with anger, feelings of emptiness, anxiety, dysphoria, panic, and so forth.

In addition to targeting the more standard skills described above, DBT considers strengths and weaknesses in patients' mindfulness skills. These basic skills of observing, describing, and participating allow patients to identify their feelings and thoughts; to distinguish between feelings and facts; to slow down escalating chains of distress-eliciting thoughts, feelings, and action urges; and, through increasing observation, to learn that feelings don't come "out of the blue." Clearly, these lessons have application across disorders.

For example, increasing mindful observation may be an important target for patients with histrionic and dependent patterns in order to help them begin monitoring their need for reassurance. As they become more aware of their internal state, including prompting events and cognitions, they may more easily develop strategies to use when they are alone to soothe or reinforce themselves. Similarly, paranoia and boredom can be observed. Fluctuations in intensity will be noticed that can provide toeholds for the regulation of feelings that previously were experienced as monolithic and overwhelming. Individuals with a diagnosis of schizoid personality disorder might be asked to come up with a description of their usual state and then observe this state for variations, which over time and through continued observation may become amplified into a greater range of emotional experience. Observing and describing external stimuli with schizotypal patients may help them to anchor their thoughts and feelings to facts rather than idiosyncratic "special" meanings. Individuals with obsessive-compulsive, avoidant, and paranoid diagnoses may benefit from observing judgmentalness.

The targets may be modified to fit a number of treatment settings. For example, on inpatient units, the treatment targets may be a blend of general targets for all patients and individualized targets for each patient. Each patient may have his or her own set of targeted quality-of-life-interfering behaviors. In our experience, an important life-interfering behavior that can be usefully targeted on acute inpatient units is passivity with respect to finding affordable housing or coping with other crisis survival situations.

An inpatient unit is often an ideal environment for beginning the work of treating post-sexual-abuse stress, especially when the treatment involves exposure to abuse-related cues, because of the risk of suicidal behavior when the patient is beginning this work. An important guideline in DBT, however, has to do with who treats serious suicidal behavior when and if it emerges. DBT suggests that these behaviors be treated directly by one designated member of the treatment team. Other members of the team do the minimal amount to keep the patient safe and may use parasuicidal crises as opportunities to implement new skills, but the chief responsibility for dealing extensively with parasuicide resides with one person or role (Linehan, in press). Thus, when such behaviors occur or are threatened, patients are referred to the designated team member for an in-depth application of behavioral analyses and other problem-solving strategies.

It should be noted that the DBT target hierarchy subsumes comorbidity problems as long as the personality disorder is the primary diagnosis and the problems associated with comorbidity are sufficiently severe. Agoraphobia in a dependent or avoidant patient may well constitute a quality-of-life-threatening behavior, as would major depression in a schizotypal or an untreated or maltreated serious medical condition, such as may be found in borderlines or possibly histrionic patients. Severe substance abuse, such as may be associated with various disorders, from antisocial and schizotypal (Bornstein, Klein, Mallon, & Slater, 1988) to dependent (Greenberg & Bornstein, 1988), qualifies as quality-of-life-threatening. When less serious, it may fall much later in the hierarchy under "other targets."

It is easy to feel overwhelmed by the life chaos of very dysfunctional patients. The hierarchy helps the therapist maintain focus and continuity in the treatment. It may be difficult to achieve the control of the session necessary to follow the hierarchy. One aid, emphasized in DBT and many behavioral treatments, is the use of diary cards on which patients monitor relevant behaviors. Diary cards give both therapist and patient a quick summary of the week's activities and current targets. Also, glancing at a card is a quick way to monitor very-low-frequency behaviors without having to ask about them constantly.

DBT attaches great importance to following the hierarchy. All too often, therapists and patients find "heart-to-hearts" reinforcing because of the positive feelings they generate. However, these feelings may have little to do with solving the patient's problems and may be more on the order of unhelpful "gratification" in the older psychoanalytic sense of the term. Borderline patients often want to "process" the relationship, for example. However, such processing sometimes represents a collusion of the therapist with the avoidance strategies of the patient. Examining in minute detail the chain of events leading to a drinking binge is much less pleasant.

The Relationship

From a dialectical perspective, attending to the therapist end of the relationship is as important as attending to the patient end. The therapist–patient interpersonal relationship is considered a "real" relationship, in which the patient responds to the therapist rather than to projections from the past (Linehan, 1987a). Thus, the therapist and the patient are each constantly challenged to recognize their own therapy-interfering behaviors and to address these straightforwardly as problems arise. It is assumed that patients are doing the best they can, even when their behavior is exasperating and unmanageable. Patients cannot fail, but the therapy and/ or the therapist may.

The therapist works to create a caring, supportive environment that enhances patient self-esteem by acknowledging the competent, enjoyable aspects of the patient (Swenson, 1989). At the same time, the therapist is not neutral or unconditionally accepting but functions more as a gentle and benign goad. During crises, the therapist constantly nudges patients to use their skills while sticking close to them with encouragement and helpful suggestions. Even though patients may not have caused all of their problems, they are still responsible for solving them. If patients' behaviors are pushing termination, the therapist warns of the danger, allowing enough time for patients to make the necessary changes, and assists them in making those changes. The therapist is caring but pragmatic: He or she is unable to save the patients; therefore, the patients must accept help to learn to save themselves.

Therapy can last only as long as therapist and patient continue to meet. Teaching patients behaviors that will keep their therapists wanting to work with them is therefore considered a legitimate goal in DBT. With diligence and perseverance, patients *can* get their therapists to reject them. Increasing behaviors that consolidate the working alliance (such as asking for help rather than parasuiciding) and trying out strategies suggested by the therapist are therefore important. Equally important but rarely discussed in the clinical literature is therapists' clarity regarding their own personal limits.

Observing limits is one of the most important contingency management strategies available to the therapist in DBT. In contrast to the arbitrary limits suggested by such diagnostic labels as *borderline* or by the theoretical discipline of the therapist, DBT stresses the observation of natural limits. Every therapist has personal limits that restrict both what she or he is willing to do for the patient and what she or he can tolerate from the patient. These limits vary, depending on the phase of treatment and on individual factors in the therapist's life. Unfortunately, identifying one's own limits is difficult for therapists because of a tendency to attribute these behaviors either to the pathology of the patient or to the inadequacies of the therapist. Both explanations shift the focus away from the patients' behaviors.

Therapy with borderline and suicidal patients is particularly noted for bringing up issues of therapists' limits in conducting treatment. Behaviors that often push therapists' limits include patients' not accepting treatment plans that the therapist views as essential to progress in therapy; phoning too much; going to the therapist's house; demanding solutions to problems that the therapist cannot solve; initiating interactions with the therapist's family members; and/or threatening harm to the therapist or the therapist's family members. Again, there are no *a priori* limits that must be observed. The targeted behaviors vary, depending on the capabilities of the patient as well as on the therapist's limits.

To maintain the stance of patient validation and constant therapist self-examination with difficult patients is extremely stressful, and for this reason, treatment of the therapist through consultation groups is essential. Although in many ways similar to the usual case conference or therapy team meetings, where information is exchanged and treatment plans are made, DBT consultation meetings differ in at least one important respect. The goal of the meetings is to assist therapists in applying the guidelines of DBT. Thus, the general assumption is that all members of the consultation group have previously agreed to a DBT framework as the treatment guide. In non-DBT or nonbehavioral settings, therefore, one may want to set up a second, optional team meeting for all those who wish to apply DBT (or any other consistent treatment philosophy).

Strategies

Dialectical Strategies. Given the cognitive and behavioral rigidity characteristic of the personality disorders by definition, as well as the extreme emotions involved, it is likely that DBT's dialectical approach will generalize. Dialectics help balance the therapist's perceptions by eliciting the whole range of stimuli impinging on behavior that Akhtar (1987, 1990) categorized as "overt" and "covert." The dialectic can bridge the gap between the patient's perceptions and those of others in the world by continually reminding the therapist and ultimately the patient of "the other side." Thus, Akhtar (1987) pointed out that, whereas the schizoid individual appears to others as aloof and withdrawn, the patient's own experience may be one of intense sensitivity to and curiosity about others. Similarly, where the paranoid person may appear outwardly demanding and stubborn, her or his inside view may be of feelings of inferiority and self-doubt (Akhtar, 1990). Whereas both borderline and narcissistic patients may appear competent and "in charge," thinking dialectically will facilitate the therapist's recognition of these patients' extreme sensitivity to criticism, helplessness, or fear of showing a weak side, which may color their internal states.

Use of the dialectic helps soften the impact of patients' aversive behaviors by reminding the therapist of their functional aspects. The therapist can avoid power struggles by accepting the patient's modus operandi and at the same time allowing for the possibility that the picture is incomplete. Rather than expecting obsessive-compulsive patients to change their rational approach to life, the dialectic adds a complementary dimension of spontaneity. While validating a histrionic individual's range of emotional expression and sensitivity to social cues, a therapist can also nudge these patients toward a more thoughtful, linear analysis of the problem (Joines, 1986; Liebowitz *et al.*, 1986).

Among the dialectics useful in guiding therapists' performance in DBT are irreverent communication versus reciprocal vulnerability, stability of treatment approach versus flexibility, and, most important, the balance between acceptance and change. The positioning of the therapist fulcrum along these continua will vary across personality disorders, individual patients, and phases of treatment.

Irreverent Communication versus Reciprocal Vulnerability Strategies. Irreverent communication around the passive-aggressive patient's ability to best authority, for example, can be helpful in coaxing observation and acknowledgment of dysfunctional patterns

(Cole, 1984; Joines, 1986). On the other hand, irreverent communication should probably be avoided in moderate or severe paranoid cases during the early stages of treatment, because of the high probability of being misunderstood. The rigidity of paranoid as well as compulsive individuals makes the kind of mental agility necessary to appreciate humor difficult and thus heightens the chances of misunderstandings (Akhtar, 1990). In dialectical thinking, however, the rigid cognitive set would be validated as a natural response to stress and appreciated for permitting such highly focused attention, as well as being targeted for change.

Patients sensitive to indirect communication, such as covert evaluation or rejection (found in avoidant, paranoid, dependent, schizoid, and obsessive-compulsive disorders), "game playing" (antisocial), or magical signs (schizotypal) may respond more to reciprocal vulnerability strategies. With paranoid personalities, for example, this strategy may validate a perception: "I think you're concerned about my feeling critical toward you because my tone of voice changed. That change meant I was becoming more businesslike in trying to solve the problem we have been discussing." With disorders such as passive-aggressive personality, straightforward therapist disclosure may be used to model "backing down" or being "mistaken"(Cole, 1984). With obsessive-compulsive, paranoid, and narcissistic patients, reciprocal vulnerability may model coping with error or imperfection or, for schizoid individuals, the verbal expression of a range of emotions. However, for both schizoid and schizotypal individuals, reciprocal vulnerability would probably be most effective when applied with a light, matter-of-fact touch, respecting these patients' real discomfort and the ease with which they may be intimidated by interpersonal closeness (Liebowitz *et al.*, 1986; Stone, 1985).

Flexibility versus Stability. In considering the dimension of flexibility and stability, it is likely that with those whose disorders make them prone to crisis behaviors and looking to others for solutions, such as borderline, dependent, histrionic, and narcissistic, the therapist must be the "Buddha in the road." Having assessed the patient's capabilities, the therapist maintains a firm but sympathetic stance in doing her best to pull self-care from the client. With borderlines, a fair amount of time must be spent on any one strategy before progress will occur. The same is probably true of those with dependent, histrionic, and antisocial disorders. Under stress, DBT says, "Now is the time to learn new ways of coping—not later, when the patient feels better."

With other diagnoses, however, flexibility may be the key to reinforcing essential reaching out or asking for help. Encouraging such behavior is extremely important in avoidant, schizoid, compulsive, passive-aggressive, and, sometimes, paranoid personality disorders. With paranoid disorders, however, flexibility may introduce more objects of misperception. However, an unbending stance, in addition to overlooking potentially positive behaviors, also runs the risk of not recognizing the true limitations and need for more support and nurturing of some patients or real problems with a particular therapeutic approach that requires reassessment. The essential point is that strategies are switched for theoretical reasons and not because of the mood of either the patient or the therapist (Linehan, in press).

Problem Solving versus Validation. Considered dimensionally, the personality disorders offer ample opportunity for standard behavioral interventions. Any of these interventions fall well within the realm of DBT, which unabashedly seeks to use whatever technologies have proved effective. Skill training, contingency management, exposure, and cognitive modification, the four main problem-solving approaches in DBT, are all useful in dealing with the problems of emotional control, cognitions, and interpersonal behaviors that characterize the various personality disorders. Behavioral analyses clarify what combination of skills training and exposure will be most reasonable to start with as well as what skill areas need to be addressed.

Those individuals with disorders involving social anxiety—for example, avoidant, dependent, paranoid, obsessive-compulsive, schizotypal, and schizoid disorders—may well benefit from desensitization techniques. Using single-subject designs, Turkat and Maisto (1985) reported success in improving independent decision making in a dependent patient by using anxiety hierarchies with progressive relaxation and other anxiety-management skills. They also reported success in reducing a paranoid patient's extreme fear of social evaluation by using systematic covert exposure to imaginal scenes. Similarly, several group studies of avoidant patients have reported successful outcomes and have cited *in vivo* exposure with relaxation techniques, skills training, and psychoeducational discussions as the significant factors in inducing change (Alden, 1989; Renneberg *et al.*, 1990; Stravynski, Lesage, Marcouiller, & Elie, 1989). Similar exposure techniques may well be helpful in dealing with the social anxiety and sensitivity to criticism of schizotypal patients (Liebowitz *et al.*, 1986). By extrapolation, anxiety management techniques may also prove helpful in dealing with the obsessive-compulsive individuals' anxiety about imperfection and social criticism.

Impulse control problems like those characteristic of antisocial, narcissistic, and histrionic (and, of course, borderline) patterns may also benefit from desensitization techniques. Urge hierarchies, both imaginal and *in vivo*, as well as stress inoculation, have been found helpful in treating narcissistic patients (Turkat & Maisto, 1985) and antisocial patients (Kellner, 1986). It should be noted that behavioral analyses involve a fair amount of imaginal exposure and thus, in and of themselves, may help patients come to grips with the anxiety and fear that play a role in so many of the personality disorders.

Cognitive therapy techniques are useful when faulty beliefs are helping to maintain behavior. Beck and his associates have described the application of these techniques across personality disorders (Beck, 1990; Young, 1983, 1988). Rumination, such as occurs in obsessive-compulsive and some borderline individuals, may be reduced with thought stopping and techniques used in response prevention, as suggested by Liebowitz *et al.* (1986).

In addition to the skills and interventions described above, DBT offers an approach to implementation. The view of problem behaviors as maladaptive solutions removes the judgmental tone of the term *problems* and therefore allows the therapist to more easily validate the patient's efforts. The emphasis on validation in DBT naturally leads to a more ready integration and recognition of the patient's strengths, which are helpful in generating possible reinforcers and alternate coping strategies. Therapist and patient work collaboratively to develop solutions. There are no failures on either side, only an ever-expanding data base that provides new information concerning response contingencies, which, in turn, generates new potential solutions.

The nonjudgmental stance and view of the patient–therapist relationship as a real relationship with its own sets of contingencies increase the probability of the therapist's becoming a reinforcer, a function essential in working with the high-risk addictive behaviors frequently encountered in borderline and antisocial patients (Linehan, in press; Sutker & King, 1985).

Problem emotions, behaviors, and thoughts can all be used as signals of a problem that needs tracking. The choice of signal depends on what is most immediately accessible to (and workable for) the patient. For some patients, thoughts or action urges are more easily observed than feelings in the early stages of treatment. Thus, going blank, mind reading (of the therapist and others), and needing to interrupt an ongoing activity in an avoidant individual (Padesky & Beck, 1988) may become focal experiences around which behavioral analyses are done. In the process, a more accurate understanding of an emotion regulation problem, an impulse control problem, a social isolation problem, and so on may emerge as well as a decrease in the maladaptive signal for coping.

Possible triggers for behavioral analyses in other disorders are feelings of failure, flashes of anger, or breaking social rules (e.g., cutting into a line) in narcissistic patients; boredom and "soap opera" behavior in histrionic patients; indecision or depression in dependent individuals; impulsive behavior and anger in antisocial patients; self-doubt, "needing to finish," or indecisiveness in obsessive-compulsive individuals; suicidal ideation or becoming vague in schizoid patients; odd cognitions in schizotypal patients; procrastination in passive-aggressive patients; and judgmental thoughts, panic attacks, or anger in paranoid patients.

The active problem-solving stance stresses the step-by-small-step approach to change. Patients are given diary cards on which they can monitor their use and mastery of skills. Each step taken toward applying skills is reinforced. Thus, at first, simply thinking about the new skill(s) is recognized, then thinking about them and wanting to try them out, but not doing so. Next, patients may think about, want to try, and do so but fail because of lack of mastery. Eventually, patients more frequently find themselves trying skills with mastery and bringing about a positive outcome.

At the same time, it is important to recognize that tolerance of change and the extent of change vary dramatically. Acceptance of the solitary and anhedonic life experience of people who exhibit severe schizoid or schizotypal patterns may be crucial in preventing nonproductive decompensation and in maintaining enough of an alliance so that some experimentation with an increased range and variety of activities is possible, including—especially for schizoid patients—some social activities (Karakashian, 1988; Liebowitz et al., 1986; Stone, 1985).

Disorders also vary in their tolerance of feedback. Borderlines, for example, may have difficulty with negative feedback; hence, a more effective focus is on shaping and providing positive contingencies for successive approximations of the goal behaviors (Linehan, 1988). The same is true of other personality styles that share exquisite sensitivity to social evaluation and/or approval, such as the avoidant, schizoid, compulsive, paranoid, narcissistic, passive-aggressive, and histrionic styles. Validation, praise, and encouragement reinforce the shaping of assertiveness behavior in avoidant (Alden, 1989; Renneberg et al., 1990) and obsessive-compulsive patients (Kaplan, 1987), self-directed behavior in passive-aggressive patients (Cole, 1984; Joines, 1986), the forays into social activities of schizoid patients (Liebowitz et al., 1986), and the increased range of activities of schizotypal patients (Stone, 1985), and are generally more effective than threats in improving the performance of antisocial personalities (Sutker & King, 1985). Experience with dependent and histrionic borderline patients suggests that validation may also become an important mode of teaching self-soothing through the modeling provided by the therapist of "talking oneself down" in times of distress and thus may apply to more "pure" dependent and histrionic patterns.

Case Management Strategies: Consultation versus Environmental Intervention.   Congruent with an active problem-solving approach is the consultant strategy, which is extremely important in validating the ability of dependent, histrionic, and passive-aggressive patients to be self-directed and to care for themselves. The hardest part for the therapist is letting the patient fail at times when life-or-death is not at issue (Cole, 1984; Linehan, 1984, in press). Learning occurs through trial and error, and a certain amount of struggle may be inevitable while the patient tries to figure out how to grab hold. Antisocial individuals may also need a firm but caring and alert therapist to permit them to discover that they can get what they need by straightforward means (Joines, 1986; Sutker & King, 1985). At the other end of the continuum, environmental strategies, such as intervention for financial assistance or housing may well be needed by and clinically appropriate for low-functioning schizotypal patients.

Ancillary Treatments.   Patients in DBT may participate in other ancillary treatments, such as pharmacotherapy, vocational counseling, Alcoholics Anonymous (AA), day treatment, or acute hospitalization. Pharmacotherapy is often a useful adjunct when moderate to severe depression, anxiety, or insomnia is a symptom, as well as when explosive rage or psychotic symptoms are present. With some exceptions, DBT does not favor hospitalization because it removes patients from the environment in which they need to learn new skills. Day treatments may be very helpful in modifying the social isolation of schizotypal and schizoid patients and may provide the necessary structure for borderline patients. Groups may be helpful in providing safe social exposure for avoidant patients, a broader base of support for dependent and histrionic patients, and normalizing for some schizoid patients. Family or couples sessions may be helpful in cases where the larger system is clearly maintaining a dysfunctional pattern. Where substance abuse is an issue, AA, Narcotics Anonymous, or any other community support organization will be useful.

In DBT, patients are held responsible for the ancillary professional's staying on track regarding the referral question. Members of the DBT treatment team, such as the group and individual therapists, are in constant contact. From the point of view of DBT, staff splitting is a problem of treatment professionals rather than of the patient. The weekly consultation meetings are a forum in which problems with patients and/or other treating professionals can be aired and understood. Dialectical strategies are emphasized in these meetings, and problems are approached with the same blend of active problem-solving with plenty of validation and acceptance of the inevitability of the difficulties, stress, and frustration integral to therapy sessions.

SUMMARY

Personality disorders offer a tremendous challenge, from their diagnostic classification and assessment to their treatment. Conceptualizing personality in terms of behavioral abilities and capabilities opens the door to tried-and-true behavioral methods such as skills training, exposure techniques, contingency management, and cognitive restructuring. Behavioral analysis becomes the pivotal intervention, providing both a powerful assessment procedure and a treatment intervention.

Standard techniques, however, must be embedded in a relationship of sufficient strength and resiliency to endure the tremendous stresses inherent in work with problems that are long-standing and intransigent. Dialectical behavior therapy was developed for use with patients with just such problems. To the treatment of other personality disorders, it is hoped that DBT can contribute several features that may facilitate a healthy working alliance and effective treatment. These features are a dialectical perspective that appreciates the importance of acceptance as well as change, and that remains sensitive to what is not said or shown as well as to the outward manifestations of thoughts, feelings, or behaviors; a recognition of therapy-interfering behavior as a legitimate target of therapy; a recognition that therapists as "real" people contribute to problems that may arise in treatment and thus themselves need treatment and support; a recognition of possible patient deficits in the skills essential for engaging in psychotherapy, such as observing, describing, and participating; and the importance of constant problem assessment in order to develop effective interventions.

REFERENCES

Akhtar, S. (1987). Schizoid personality disorder: A synthesis of developmental, dynamic, and descriptive features. *American Journal of Psychotherapy, 41*, 499–518.

Akhtar, S. (1990). Paranoid personality disorder: A synthesis of developmental, dynamic, and descriptive features. *American Journal of Psychotherapy, 44*, 5–25.

Akiskal, H. S. (1981). Subaffective disorders: Dysthymic, cyclothymic and bipolar II disorders in the "borderline" realm. *Psychiatric Clinics of North America, 4*, 25–46.

Alden, L. (1989). Short-term structured treatment for avoidant personality disorder. *Journal of Consulting and Clinical Psychology, 57*, 756–764.

American Psychiatric Association. (1987). *Diagnostic and statistical manual of mental disorders* (3rd ed., rev.; DSM-III- R). Washington: Author.

Beck, A. T. (1990). *Cognitive therapy of personality disorders*. New York: Guilford Press.

Black, D. W., Bell, S., Hulbert, J., & Nasrallah, A. (1988). The importance of Axis II in patients with major depression: A controlled study. *Journal of Affective Disorders, 14*, 115–122.

Blashfield, R. K., & Haymaker, D. (1988). A prototype analysis of the diagnostic criteria for DSM-III-R personality disorders. *Journal of Personality Disorders, 2*, 272–280.

Blashfield, R., Sprock, J., Pinkston, K., & Hodgin, J. (1985). Exemplar prototypes of personality disorder diagnoses. *Comprehensive Psychiatry, 26*, 11–21.

Bornstein, R. F., Klein, D. N., Mallon, J. C., & Slater, J. F. (1988). Schizotypal personality disorder in an outpatient population: Incidence and clinical characteristics. *Journal of Clinical Psychology*, *44*, 322–325.

Brantley, P. J., & Callon, E. B. (1985). Histrionic personality: A behavioral formulation. In I. D. Turkat (Ed.), *Behavioral Case Formulation* (pp. 199–251). New York: Plenum Press.

Brotman, A. W., Herzog, D. B., & Hamburg, P. (1988). Long-term course in 14 bulimic patients treated with psychotherapy. *Journal of Clinical Psychiatry*, *49*, 157–160.

Cole, M. (1984). How to make a person passive-aggressive or the power struggle game. *Transactional Analysis Journal*, *14*, 191–194.

Frances, A., & Widiger, T. A. (1986). Methodological issues in personality disorder diagnosis. In T. Millon & G. L. Klerman (Eds.), *Contemporary directions in psychopathology* (pp. 381–400). New York: Guilford Press.

Goldstein, A. P., & Keller, H. R. (1987). *Aggressive behavior: Assessment and intervention*. New York: Pergamon Press.

Green, M. A., & Curtis, G. C. (1988). Personality disorders in panic patients: Response to termination of antipanic medication. *Journal of Personality Disorders*, *2*, 303–314.

Greenberg, R. P., & Bornstein, R. F. (1988). The dependent personality: 1. Risk for physical disorders. *Journal of Personality Disorders*, *2*, 126–135.

Gutierrez, H. O., Russakoff, L. M., & Oldham, J. M. (1988). The prediction of suicide: Dilemmas for training. In D. Lester (Ed.), *Proceedings of the 21st Annual Meeting of the American Association of Suicidology*, Washington, April 1988.

Hathaway, S. R., & McKinley, J. C. (1943). *The Minnesota Multiphasic Personality Inventory*. Minneapolis: University of Minnesota Press.

Hyler, S. E., & Rieder, R. C. (1984). *Personality Diagnostic Questionnaire Revised* (PDQR). New York: New York State Psychiatric Institute.

Hyler, S. E., Skodol, A. E., Kellman, D., Oldham, J. M., & Rosnick, L. (1990). Validity of the Personality Diagnostic Questionnaire—Revised: Comparison with two structured interviews. *American Journal of Psychiatry*, *147*, 1043–1048.

Jenike, M. A., Baer, L., & Carey, R. J. (1986). Concomitant obsessive-compulsive disorder and schizotypal personality disorder. *American Journal of Psychiatry*, *143*, 530–532.

Joines, V. (1986). Using redecision therapy with different personality adaptations. *Transactional Analysis Journal*, *16*, 152–160.

Kaplan, A. H. (1987). Obsessive compulsive phenomena in adult obsessionality, compulsive personality disorder and obsessive compulsive disorder (neurosis). *Psychiatric Journal of the University of Ottawa*, *12*, 214–221.

Karakashian, S. J. (1988). Differential diagnosis of the borderline personality: The first step in treatment. *Transactional Analysis Journal*, *18*, 178–184.

Kellner, R. (1986). Personality disorders. *Psychotherapy and Psychosomatics*, *46*, 58–66.

Kreitman, N., Smith, P., & Tan, E. (1970). Attempted suicide as language: An empirical study. *British Journal of Psychiatry*, *116*, 465–473.

Kroll, P., & Ryan, C. (1983). The schizotypal personality on an alcohol treatment unit. *Comprehensive Psychiatry*, *24*, 262–270.

Liebowitz, M. R., Stone, M. H., & Turkat, I. D. (1986). Treatment of personality disorders. In R. E. Hales & A. J. Frances (Eds.), *The American Psychiatric Association annual review* (Vol. 5, pp. 356–393). Washington, DC: American Psychiatric Press.

Linehan, M. M. (1981). A social-behavioral analysis of suicide and parasuicide: Implications for clinical assessment and treatment. In H. G. Glazer & J. F. Clarkin (Eds.), *Depression: Behavioral and directive intervention strategies* (pp. 229–294). New York: Garland Press.

Linehan, M. M. (1984). *Dialectical behavior therapy for treatment of parasuicidal women: Treatment manual*. Unpublished manuscript, University of Washington, Seattle.

Linehan, M. M. (1987a). Dialectical behavior therapy: A cognitive behavioral approach to parasuicide. *Journal of Personality Disorders*, *1*, 328–333.

Linehan, M. M. (1987b). Dialectical behavior therapy for borderline personality disorder: Theory and method. *Bulletin of the Menninger Clinic*, *51*, 261–276.

Linehan, M. M. (1988). Perspectives on the interpersonal relationship in behavior therapy. *Journal of Integrative and Eclectic Psychotherapy*, *7*, 278–290.

Linehan, M. M. (in press). *Comprehensive treatment for borderline personality disorder*. New York: Guilford Press.

Linehan, M. M., & Wasson, E. J. (1990). Behavior therapy for borderline personality disorder. In M. Hersen & A. S. Bellack (Eds.), *Handbook of comparative treatments for adults disorders* (pp. 420–435). New York: Wiley.

Linehan, M. M., Armstrong, H. E., Suarez, A., & Allmon, D. J. (1991). Cognitive behavioral treatment of chronically parasuicidal borderline patients. *Archives of General Psychiatry, 48*, 1060–1064.

Livesley, W. J. (1987). Theoretical and empirical issues in the selection of criteria to diagnose personality disorders. *Journal of Personality Disorders, 1*, 88–94.

Livesley, W. J., & Jackson, D. N. (1986). The internal consistency and factorial structure of behaviors judged to be associated with DSM-III categories of personality disorders. *American Journal of Psychiatry, 143*, 1473–1474.

Livesley, W. J., Schroeder, M. L., & Jackson, D. N. (1990). Dependent personality disorder and attachment problems. *Journal of Personality Disorders, 4*, 131–140.

Livesley, W. J., Jackson, D. N., & Schroeder, M. L. (1989). A study of the factorial structure of personality pathology. *Journal of Personality Disorders, 3*, 292–306.

Loranger, A. W., Russakoff, I. M., Oldham, J. M., & Susman, V. L. (1984). *Personality Disorders Examination: A structured interview for DSM-III-R Axis II diagnosis.* White Plains: The New York Hospital-Cornell Medical Center, Westchester Division.

Loranger, A. W. (1988). *Personality Disorder Examination (PDE) Manual.* Yonkers, NY: DV Communications.

Marin, D. B., Widiger, T. A., Frances, A. J., Goldsmith, S., & Kocsis, J. (1989). Personality disorders: Issues in assessment. *Psychopharmacology Bulletin, 25*, 508–514.

Mavissakalian, M., & Hamann, M. S. (1987). DSM-III personality disorder in agoraphobia: 2. Changes with treatment. *Comprehensive Psychiatry, 28*, 356–361.

Meehl, P. E. (1978). Theoretical risks and tabular asterisks: Sir Karl, Sir Ronald, and the slow progress of soft psychology. *Journal of Consulting and Clinical Psychology, 46*, 806–834.

Mellsop, G., Varghese, F., Joshua, S., & Hicks, A. (1982). The reliability of Axis II of DSM-III. *American Journal of Psychiatry, 139*, 1360–1361.

Merikangas, K. R., & Weissman, M. M. (1986). Epidemiology of DSM-III Axis II personality disorders. In R. H. Hales & A. J. Frances (Eds.), *The American Psychiatric Association annual review* (Vol. 5, pp. 258–278). Washington, DC: American Psychiatric Press.

Michels, R. (1987). How should the criteria for personality disorders be formulated? *Journal of Personality Disorders, 1*, 95–99.

Millon, T. (1983). *Millon Clinical Multiaxial Inventory* (3rd ed.). Minneapolis: National Computer Services.

Millon, T. (1987a). Personality disorder criteria: Empirical or theoretical—introduction. *Journal of Personality Disorders, 1*, 71–72.

Millon, T. (1987b). *Millon Clinical Multiaxial Inventory—II* (MCMI-II). Minneapolis: National Computer Services.

Millon, T. (Ed.). (1990). Schizotypy: Theory and commentary (Special Issue). *Journal of Personality Disorders, 4*(1).

Minichiello, W. E., Baer, L., & Jenike, M. A. (1987). Schizotypal personality disorder: A poor prognostic indicator for behavior therapy in the treatment of obsessive-compulsive disorder. *Journal of Anxiety Disorders, 1*, 273–276.

Modestin, J. (1989). Completed suicide in personality disordered inpatients. *Journal of Personality Disorders, 3*, 113–121.

Morey, L. C. (1988a). The categorical representation of personality disorder: A cluster analysis of the DSM-III-R features. *Journal of Abnormal Psychology, 97*, 314–321.

Morey, L. C. (1988b). Personality disorders under DSM-III and DSM-III-R: Convergence, coverage, and internal consistency. *American Journal of Psychiatry, 145*, 573–577.

Morey, L. C. (1988c). A psychometric analysis of the DSM-III-R personality disorder criteria. *Journal of Personality Disorders, 2*, 109–124.

Morey, L. C., & Ochoa, E. S. (1989). An investigation of adherence to diagnostic criteria: Clinical diagnosis of the DSM-III personality disorders. *Journal of Personality Disorders, 3*, 180–192.

Motto, J. A. (1988). Empirical indicators of near term suicide risk. In D. Lester (Ed.), *Proceedings of the 21st Annual Meeting of the American Association of Suicidology*, Washington, April 1988.

O'Boyle, M., & Self, D. (1990). A comparison of two interviews for DSM-III-R personality disorders. *Psychiatry Research, 32*, 85–92.

O'Leary, K. D., & Wilson, G. T. (1987). *Behavior therapy: Application and outcome.* Englewood Cliffs, NJ: Prentice-Hall.

Padesky, C. A. (1986, September). *Personality disorders: Cognitive therapy into the 90's.* Paper presented at the 2nd International Conference on Cognitive Psychotherapy, Umea, Sweden.

Padesky, C. A., & Beck, J. S. (1988). Cognitive therapy treatment for avoidant personality disorders. In C. Perris & M. Eisemann (Eds.), *Cognitive psychotherapy: An update* (pp. 121–125). Umea, Sweden: DOPUU Press.

Paulhus, D. L., & Martin, C. L. (1987). The structure of personality capabilities. *Journal of Personality and Social Psychology, 52,* 354–365.

Petronis, K. R., Samuels, J. F., Moscicki, E. K., & Anthony, J. C. (1990). An epidemiologic investigation of potential risk factors for suicide attempts. *Social Psychiatry and Psychiatric Epidemiology, 25,* 193–199.

Pfohl, B., Stangl, D. A., & Zimmerman, M. (1983). *Structured interview for DSM-III personality disorders* (SIDP, 2nd ed.). Iowa City: University of Iowa, College of Medicine.

Pfohl, B., Stangl, D., & Zimmerman, M. (1984). The implications of DSM-III personality disorders for patients with major depression. *Journal of Affective Disorders, 7,* 309–318.

Pfohl, B., Coryell, W., Zimmerman, M., & Stangl, D. (1986). DSM-III personality disorders: Diagnostic overlap and internal consistency of individual DSM-III criteria. *Comprehensive Psychiatry, 27,* 21–34.

Pfohl, B., Coryell, W., Zimmerman, M., & Stangl, D. (1987). Prognostic validity of self-report and interview measures of personality disorder in depressed inpatients. *Journal of Clinical Psychiatry, 48,* 468–472.

Piersma, H. L. (1987). The MCMI as a measure of DSM-III axis II diagnoses: An empirical comparison. *Journal of Clinical Psychology, 43,* 478–483.

Pilkonis, P. A., & Frank, E. (1988). Personality pathology in recurrent depression: Nature, prevalence, and relationship to treatment response. *American Journal of Psychiatry, 145,* 435–441.

Poldrugo, F., & Forti, B. (1988). Personality disorders and alcoholism treatment outcome. *Drug and Alcohol Dependence, 21,* 171–176.

Pretzer, J. L. (1983, August). *Borderline personality disorder: Too complex for cognitive therapy?* Paper presented at the American Psychological Association Annual Convention, Anaheim, CA.

Pretzer, J. L. (1990). Borderline personality disorder. In A. Freeman (Ed.), *Clinical applications of cognitive therapy*. New York: Plenum Press.

Reich, J. H. (1987). Instruments measuring DSM-III and DSM-III-R personality disorders. *Journal of Personality Disorders, 1,* 220–240.

Reich, J. H. (1988). DSM-III personality disorders and the outcome of treated panic disorder. *American Journal of Psychiatry, 145,* 1149–1152.

Reich, J. H. (1989). Update on instruments to measure DSM-III and DSM-III-R personality disorders. *Journal of Nervous and Mental Disease, 177,* 366–370.

Reid, A. H., & Ballinger, B. R. (1987). Personality disorder in mental handicap. *Psychological Medicine, 17,* 983–987.

Renneberg, B., Goldstein, A. J., Phillips, D., & Chambless, D. L. (1990). Intensive behavioral group treatment of avoidant personality disorder. *Behavior Therapy, 21,* 363–377.

Repko, G. R., & Cooper, R. (1985). The diagnosis of personality disorder: A comparison of MMPI profile, Millon inventory and clinical judgment in a workers' compensation population. *Journal of Clinical Psychology, 41,* 867–881.

Shawcross, C. R., & Tyrer, P. (1985). Influence of personality on response to monoamine oxidase inhibitors and tricyclic antidepressants. *Journal of Psychiatric Research, 19,* 557–562.

Shea, M. T. (1990, November). *Psychosocial treatment of personality disorders*. Paper presented at National Institutes of Mental Health conference on personality disorders, Williamsburg, VA.

Shea, M. T., Pilkonis, P. A., Beckham, E., Collins, J. F., Elkein, I., Sotsky, S. M., & Docherty, G. P. (1990). Personality disorders and treatment outcome in the NIMH treatment of depression collaborative research program. *American Journal of Psychiatry, 147,* 711–718.

Spitzer, R. L., Williams, J. B., et al. (1985, March 1). *Structured Clinical Interview for DSM-III personality disorders* (SCID-II). New York: Biometrics Research Department, New York State Psychiatric Institute.

Spitzer, R. L., & Williams, J. B. W. (1987). *Structured Clinical Interview for DSM-III-R personality disorders* (SCID-III). New York: Biometrics Research Department, New York State Psychiatric Institute.

Spitzer, R. L., Forman, J. B. W., & Nee, J. (1979). DSM-III field trials: 1. Initial interrater diagnostic reliability. *American Journal of Psychiatry, 136,* 815–187.

Staats, A. W. (1975). *Social behaviorism*. Homewood, IL: Dorsey Press.

Staats, A. W. (1986). Behaviorism with a personality: The paradigmatic behavioral assessment approach. In R. O. Nelson & S. C. Hayes (Eds.), *Conceptual foundations of behavioral assessment* (pp. 242–296). New York: Guilford Press.

Stone, M. (1985). Schizotypal personality: Psychotherapeutic aspects. *Schizophrenia Bulletin, 11,* 576–589.

Stravynski, A., Lesage, A., Marcouiller, M., & Elie, R. (1989). A test of the therapeutic mechanism in social skills training with avoidant personality disorder. *Journal of Nervous and Mental Disease, 177,* 739–744.

Sutker, P. B., & King, A. R. (1985). Antisocial personality disorder. In I. D. Turkat (Ed.), *Behavioral case formulation* (pp. 111–153). New York: Plenum Press.

Swenson, C. (1989). Kernberg and Linehan: Two approaches to the borderline patient. *Journal of Personality Disorders, 3*, 26–35.

Thompson, L. W., Gallagher, D., & Czirr, R. (1988). Personality disorder and outcome in the treatment of late-life depression. *Journal of Geriatric Psychiatry, 21*, 133–146.

Turkat, I. D., & Maisto, S. A. (1985). Personality disorders: Application of the experimental method to the formulation and modification of personality disorders. In D. H. Barlow (Ed.), *Clinical handbook of psychological disorders* (pp. 502–570). New York: Guilford Press.

Turner, R. M. (1983). Behavioral therapy with borderline patients (Carrier Foundation letter, #88). Belle Mead, NJ: Carrier Foundation.

Turner, R. M. (1984, November). *Assessment and treatment of borderline personality disorder*. Paper presented at the 18th Meeting of the Association for the Advancement of Behavior Therapy, Philadelphia.

Turner, R. M. (1987). The effects of personality disorder diagnosis on the outcome of social anxiety symptom reduction. *Journal of Personality Disorders, 1*, 136–143.

Turner, R. M. (1989). Case study evaluations of a bio-cognitive-behavioral approach for the treatment of borderline personality disorder. *Behavior Therapy, 20*, 477–489.

Turner, R. M., & Hersen, M. (1987). Disorders of social behavior: A behavioral approach to personality disorders. In S. M. Turner, K. S. Calhoun, & H. E. Adams (Eds.), *Handbook of clinical behavior therapy* (pp. 103–124). New York: Wiley.

Wallace, J. (1966). An abilities conception of personality: Some implications for personality measurement. *American Psychologist, 21*, 132–138.

Wetzler, S., & Dubro, A. (1990). Diagnosis of personality disorders by the Millon clinical multiaxial inventory. *Journal of Nervous and Mental Disease, 178*, 261–263.

Widiger, T. A. (1985). *Personality Interview Questions* (PIQ). Unpublished manuscript, University of Kentucky, Lexington.

Widiger, T. A. (1987). *Personality Interview Questions II* (PIQ-II). Lexington: University of Kentucky.

Widiger, T., & Frances, A. (1985). The DSM-III personality disorders: Perspectives from psychology. *Archives of General Psychiatry, 42*, 615–623.

Widiger, T. A., & Frances, A. (1987). Interviews and inventories for the measurement of personality disorders. *Clinical Psychology Review, 7*, 49–75.

Widiger, T. A., & Trull, T. J. (1987). Behavioral indicators, hypothetical constructs, and personality disorders. *Journal of Personality Disorders, 1*, 82–87.

Widiger, T. A., Frances, A., Warner, L., & Bluhm, C. (1986). Diagnostic criteria for the borderline and schizotypal personality disorders. *Journal of Abnormal Psychology, 95*, 43–51.

Young, J. (1983, August). *Borderline personality: Cognitive therapy and treatment*. Paper presented at the American Psychological Association Annual Convention, Philadelphia.

Young, J. (1988, April). *Schema-focused cognitive therapy for personality disorders*. Paper presented at the Society for the Exploration of Psychotherapy Integration, Cambridge, MA.

18

Geriatric Patients

JANE E. FISHER, LAURA L. CARSTENSEN,
SUSAN E. TURK, and JAMES P. NOLL

INTRODUCTION

The elderly population in Western countries is growing at an unprecedented rate, and a proportionate increase in the geropsychiatric inpatient population is expected during the next 30 years. The basic principles of treatment for the problems that this group faces are essentially the same as those for young adults. However, there are several important considerations unique to the elderly. Medical problems, for example, frequently complicate the diagnostic picture, and complex medication regimens may obscure or exacerbate symptom profiles. Cognitive impairment may hinder assessment (e.g., limit knowledge of the patient's personal history), and treatment may be impeded by the reduced behavioral repertoires associated with physical impairment or limited working memory.

In spite of these very real complications, the treatment of geriatric patients is as effective as treatment efforts directed toward the young (Carstensen, 1988). Indeed, in some ways, age has a beneficial effect on the positive symptomatology associated with psychotic illness. In a study of patients hospitalized for 28 years or longer, for example, Lawton (1972) described patients as "less agitated, less disorganized and more conforming" (p. 141) than indicated in earlier records. This pattern was also observed in nonhospitalized schizophrenics (Ciompi, 1985). One potentially negative consequence of this diminution of symptoms, however, is that patients are more likely to fall between the cracks of the mental health system, particularly when mental professionals believe that effective treatment is futile. In this chapter, we provide descriptive information about the geropsychiatric population, review general treatment considerations, note factors that restrict access to treatment, and provide an overview of several common disorders.

JANE E. FISHER and JAMES P. NOLL • Department of Psychology, Northern Illinois University, DeKalb, Illinois 60115-2892.   **LAURA L. CARSTENSEN and SUSAN E. TURK** • Department of Psychology, Stanford University, Stanford, California 94305.

Handbook of Behavior Therapy in the Psychiatric Setting, edited by Alan S. Bellack and Michel Hersen. Plenum Press, New York, 1993.

Until the early 1980s, researchers and laypeople alike believed that mental health problems increased linearly with age (e.g., Butler & Lewis, 1982; Pfeiffer & Busse, 1973). However, more recent epidemiological studies (Myers, Weissman, Tischler, Holzer, Leaf, Orvachel, Anthony, Boyd, Burke, Kramer, & Stoltzman, 1984) and longitudinal studies (Aldwin, Spiro, Levenson, & Bosse, 1989) suggest that the mental health of the general elderly population is as good as or better than that of younger generations. This is particularly true of initial-onset psychiatric disturbance. In the absence of a psychiatric history, the likelihood of a major psychiatric disturbance in late life is quite low (LaRue, Dessonville, & Jarvik, 1985).

The singular, but notable, exception to the positive mental-health age trends is organic brain syndrome, that is, Alzheimer's disease and related disorders (ADRD). ADRD is indubitably more prevalent with increasing age. In the over-65 age group, the incidence of ADRD is 5%. In the over-85 age group, the incidence is generally estimated to be 20%. One recent study of a community sample in East Boston suggested that rates may be as high as 47% (Evans, Funkenstein, Albert, Scherr, Cook, Chown, Hebert, Hennekens, & Taylor, 1989).

About one third of geriatric state-hospital admissions are based on organic mental disorders (Moak & Fisher, 1990). Some of these patients are long-term psychiatric patients who have developed dementia in late life. Others are new admissions precipitated by dementia-related problems. Mei-Tal and Meyers (1986) analyzed the records of 112 consecutive admissions to a geriatric psychiatric inpatient unit and found that 53% of patients had been admitted for depression; dementia had been diagnosed in 32%; 8% had been admitted for mania associated with bipolar disorder; and 33% had a schizophrenic or paranoid disorder. Of the patients with dementia, 30% had associated depression. The majority (82%) of the patients were found to have at least one coexisting medical and/or neurological condition requiring intervention. Eighteen percent of the patients had presented with acute organic brain syndromes. The causes of these acute organic brain syndromes included metabolic and endocrine disturbances, cardiovascular disorders, nutritional deficiencies, infectious states, substance-induced toxic states, and localized brain dysfunctions. A high prevalence of cognitive impairment among geriatric psychiatric inpatients was also reported by LaRue, Spar, and Hill (1986), who found that over 20% of elderly depressed patients scored in the cognitively impaired range on a mental status examination. Delusions and high anxiety and agitation levels were more prevalent in the cognitively impaired group, and the prognosis for these patients was found to be significantly worse than that for nonimpaired patients.

A selection bias operates so that ADRD patients placed in psychiatric facilities are relatively obstreperous. Consequently, the geriatric inpatient population comprises both withdrawn, passive patients and agitated patients who are behaviorally disruptive.

Overall, the older inpatient population essentially comprises four distinct groups: chronically mentally ill patients grown old, previously normal people who have become demented, chronically mentally ill patients with a secondary diagnosis of dementia, and patients suffering from late-onset psychosis. The vast majority of older inpatients fall into the first category: chronically mentally ill patients. These people generally suffer from a cognitive and functional deterioration associated with the primary disorder, which is frequently compounded by the iatrogenic effects of psychotropic medication and long-term institutionalization.

CHANGES IN THE MENTAL HEALTH SYSTEM

The quality and type of care provided to the elderly suffering from major mental illness has varied tremendously over the past 50 years and because most of the current cohort of chronically mentally ill elderly lived through these changes, they merit mention. At different historical times, the elderly have been more and less likely than younger people to receive inpatient treatment. Today, older patients receive disproportionately more inpatient services than out-patient services.

Before the 1960s older people were frequently committed to state hospitals if their ability to live independently became severely impaired and family alternatives were exhausted. However, the deinstitutionalization movement of the 1960s changed things considerably. Although, in spirit, the movement was intended to shift the burden of care from institutions to communities, community-based services never appeared at a satisfactory level. The failure of the movement was particularly pronounced for older patients. Many faced extreme isolation and a subsequent exacerbation of symptoms. From 1950 to 1975, the rates of psychiatric admissions of individuals over the age of 65 in the United States fell by 71%, even though the admissions of younger patients increased over the same period (Kahn, 1975). Instead, nursing homes proliferated and came to be the locus of care for the chronically mentally ill elderly. Although some contend that there may be advantages in nursing-home placement over psychiatric placement—such as reduced social stigma and geographical proximity to the community—the disadvantages prevail. Most notably, nursing homes had (and have) virtually no mental health professionals, and consequently, care is almost entirely custodial. Thus, nursing-home residents with psychiatric histories who have been admitted to nursing homes over the past 40 years have received minimal or no psychiatric treatment.

In 1987, Congress passed federal legislation under the Omnibus Budget Reconciliation Act (OBRA) to reduce the number of inappropriate placements of psychiatric patients and mentally retarded people in nursing homes. OBRA mandates the preadmission review of all nursing-home applicants and the annual review of nursing-home residents suffering from "serious mental illness" in an effort to determine if nursing-home placement is appropriate. However, even though some 60% of nursing-home residents have psychiatric histories, the legal criteria used to define "mental illness" in OBRA is such that only 2.5%–5.7% of nursing-home residents are affected (Lair, Smyer, Goldman, & Arons, 1989). Patients suffering from Alzheimer's disease or related disorders are exempted from this review.

Not only are elderly people more likely to be treated with inpatient than with outpatient mental health services, a pattern that very likely reflects better Medicare and Medicaid reimbursement for inpatient than outpatient services (Gatz & Smyer, 1990), but also the average length of stay for geropsychiatric inpatients is double that of younger patients, that is, approximately 27 versus 12 days (Knight & Carter, 1990). Currently, admission rates to private psychiatric hospitals and psychiatric units of general hospitals are comparable for older and younger people (Gatz & Smyer, 1990), whereas admission rates to state mental hospitals and Veterans Administration Medical Centers are disproportionately low for younger patients. Older patients account for only 21% of the state-hospital patient population nationwide (NIMH, 1987). There is also a current trend, motivated by hospitals' ability to recover insurance remuneration for services, toward the hospitalization of geropsychiatric patients on nonpsychiatric wards of general hospitals (Kiesler & Sibulkin, 1987). Thus, usage trends, coupled with demographic age trends, augur substantial increases in the numbers of geropsychiatric inpatients treated in traditional psychiatric settings, nursing homes, and general hospitals.

TREATMENT CONSIDERATIONS

The most important consideration in designing interventions for older adults is health. Although individuals over the age of 65 represent 12% of the total population in the United States, they use one third of the hospital beds and consume 40% of all prescription drugs (Rowe, 1977). Physical illness frequently produces psychological symptoms, most commonly confusion, disorientation, depression, and psychosis. In many cases, psychological symptoms are entirely accounted for by physical infirmity. In addition, physical problems may exacerbate preexisting psychological symptoms. Thus, the anticipation of potential limitations due to health or cognitive impairment must be considered carefully in the assessment and treatment of the elderly, particularly for new admissions, in whom the psychological disorder itself may be secondary to physical illness. Chronically mentally ill patients are at particular risk of malnutrition and the subsequent exacerbation of preexisting symptoms (Basu & Schorah, 1982). Low body weight and long-term nutritional deficiencies often characterize newly admitted patients (Hancock, Hullin, Alward, King, & Morgan, 1985; Morgan & Hullin, 1982). Delirium caused by a deficiency in nicotinic acid may mimic dementia. Thiamine deficiency may exacerbate symptoms of Wernicke's syndrome (Sier, Hartnell, Morley, Guiliano, Kaiser, & Frankl, 1988). Severe psychological disorders resulting from nutritional deficits, such as scurvy, although rare, have also been detected in elderly populations (Milner, 1963).

Sier *et al.* (1988) argued that "almost all metabolic disorders can cause psychiatric disturbances in the elderly" (p. 164). They further stated that three psychiatric disturbances—delirium, dementia, and depression—are commonly caused by underlying physical illness (see Table 1 for a list of medical ailments that can lead to psychological symptoms). One example of an illness that can lead to a plethora of psychological symptoms is primary hyperparathyroidism, diagnosed at 188.5 per 100,000 in women and 92.2 cases per 100,000 in men in the United States (Heath, Hodgson, & Kennedy, 1980). This medical disorder is accompanied by personality changes, nervousness, affective disorders, delirium, memory problems, and cognitive deficits at rates of 1% to 25% (Aarcon & Franceschini, 1984). Because, with surgery, these psychological symptoms generally improve, screening is essential (Heath *et al.*, 1980).

A number of other potentially treatable physical and psychiatric illnesses may resemble dementia in the older population (Fox, Topel, & Huckman, 1975; Smith & Kiloh, 1981). Renvoize, Gaskell, and Klar (1985) administered a battery of psychological and biological tests to elderly psychiatric inpatients diagnosed with dementia and discovered that 4.7% had reversible dementia.

The existence of a physical illness in and of itself is associated with mood and anxiety disorders among elderly inpatients. The prevalence of depression among hospital inpatients is estimated at 15%–45% (Okimoto, Barnes, Veith, Raskind, Inui, & Carter, 1982; Waxman & Carner, 1984). High anxiety levels have been found to be associated with several medical

Table 1. Metabolic Causes of Psychiatric Disturbances in the Elderly[a]

Delirium	Dementia	Depression
Hypoxemia	Hypoxemia	Hypokalema
Electrolyte disturbances	Electrolyte disturbances	Apathetic thyrotoxicosis
Acid–base abnormalities	Hyperlipidemia	Hypothyroidism
Uremia	Hypothyroidism	?Diabetes mellitus
Hepatic failure	Hypoglycemia	Hyperparathyroidism
Thyroid disorders	Diabetes mellitus	Cushing's disease
Hypoglycemia	Hypoparathyroidism	Addison's disease
Hypoparathyroidism	Hyperparathyroidism	?Malnutrition
Hyperparathyroidism	Hypoadrenalism	Pernicious anemia
Hypoadrenalism	Malnutrition	
Hypopituitarism	Pernicious anemia	
Exogenous corticosteroids	Folate deficiency	
Thiamine deficiency	Dehydration	
Pellagra		
Porphyria		

[a]From H. C. Sier, J. Hartnell, J. Morley, A. Giuliano, F. Kaiser, and D. Frankl. (1988). Primary hyperparathyroidism and delirium in the elderly. *Journal of the American Geriatrics Society, 36*, 157–170. © by Williams & Wilkins, 1988.

conditions, including hypertension, kidney or bladder disease, stomach ulcers, hardening of the arteries, stroke, and diabetes (Himmelfarb & Murrell, 1984). Urinary incontinence, a common health problem in elderly populations (Diokno, Brock, Brown, & Herzog, 1986), has also been associated with depression and anxiety (Norton, 1982; Wells, 1984).

Side effects of medication must be considered as well, especially because physicians regularly prescribe neuroleptics for relatively mild behavioral problems in elderly populations (Buck, 1988). Typically, medication regimes are not overseen by psychiatrists or geriatricians, yet the side effects of drugs include symptoms that resemble ADRD, depression, and psychosis. Tardive dyskinesia, a disorder directly related to long-term use of major psychotropic medications, afflicts as many as 50% of chronically treated patients. In spite of dangerous side effects, major psychotropic medication is commonly used to manage behavioral aggressiveness, wandering, and sleepless in nursing homes. In fact, Gurian, Baker, Jacobson, Lagerbom, and Watt (1990) surveyed inpatient communities and found that 68% of elderly patients on a psychiatric unit and 44% of nursing-home residents took neuroleptics; 67% of the nursing-home residents did not exhibit thought disorder but were given neuroleptics to control aggressive and undesired behavior. The effectiveness and legality of using neuroleptics solely to control the behavior of the elderly are being reassessed in accordance with laws on patients' right to consent. For a further discussion of the ethics of neuroleptics, see Gurian *et al.* (1990).

Normal age-related changes also demand modification of interventions. For examples, interventions involving memory may need to be modified to incorporate written materials or standard stimuli enlarged to accommodate poor vision. Similarly, interventions that involve physical efforts must be adjusted so that goals are realistic.

Finally, beliefs and stereotypes about aging held by mental health professionals may seriously hinder treatment efforts. Although attitude-behavior relationships between client and therapist remain unclear (Gatz & Pearson, 1988), we do know that older psychiatric patients are less likely than younger people to be referred for treatment (Kucharski, White, & Schratz, 1979; Rapp, Parisi, Walsh, & Wallace, 1988) and that, when treating older adults, professionals prefer pharmacotherapy to behavior therapy in spite of evidence that behavior therapy is as effective with the old as with the young (Burgio & Sinnott, 1990).

TREATMENT OF HIGH-PREVALENCE DISORDERS

In discussing the treatment of common disorders and problems experienced by the elderly, we focus on age-associated differences that affect the treatment process and outcome.

Depression

The majority of epidemiological studies indicate that the prevalence rates of mood disorders are lower in older adults than in younger groups (Myers *et al.*, 1984; Robins *et al.*, 1984). Although most older adults do not experience significant psychological distress, of the problems that are experienced, depression is the most common. A recent review of the records of 168 elderly patients (mean age 69.7 years) admitted to the psychiatric unit of a general hospital found that the large majority of patients (76%) had mood disorders. Dementia was the second most prevalent diagnosis, occurring in 41% of the patients (Conwell, Nelson, Kim, & Mazure, 1989).

As mentioned earlier, depression is often found in elderly medical patients. A recent survey of admissions to an acute geriatric assessment unit found that 23.4% of the patients screened had depression of a clinically significant degree, and that another 10.8% were experiencing depression with a coexisting organic brain disorder (O'Riordan, Hayes, Shelley, O'Neill, Walsh, & Coakley, 1989). These findings point to the complex nature of problem assessment in this population. It is often necessary to conduct daily mental status assessments in order to identify fluctuating cognitive deficits associated with toxic or metabolic conditions (Mei-Tal & Meyers, 1986).

Although rates of depression among the aged are low, suicide rates are disproportionately high when compared with those in the general population. Suicide rates increase with age and peak past age 65 (Osgood & Brant, 1991). Currently, individuals over the age of 65 make up 12% of the population and account for 17% of suicides (McIntosh, 1985). When the suicide rates of the elderly as a group are examined, we find that those between the ages of 75 and 84 are at the greatest risk (Osgood & Brant, 1991). These statistics point to the importance of a careful assessment of suicide risk when treating elderly individuals suffering depression. Caucasian men commit the vast majority of suicides in this age group. The following factors have also been found to be associated with suicide among the aged: depression, being divorced or widowed, chronic illness, isolation and loneliness, relocation, and alcohol abuse (Osgood & Brant, 1991).

The rate of depression among the institutionalized elderly has been found to be much higher than the rate among the community-residing elderly (Zimmer, Watson, & Treat, 1984). Only one study has systematically examined suicide rates in long-term-care facilities. Although Osgood and Brant (1991) found lower rates of suicide among the elderly residing in long-term-care facilities than among those living in the community, she argued that suicide among the institutionalized elderly is grossly underreported. Deaths certified as "natural" often result from intentional self-starvation and failure to follow prescribed medical treatment (Osgood & Brant, 1991). For the institutionalized frail elderly, more efficient means of suicide may be inaccessible or physically impossible.

The characteristics of institutions that were associated with increased suicide risk included the size of the facility (i.e., the number of residents) and staff turnover. Facilities with over a 100 residents or with a staff turnover rate greater than 50% were significantly more likely to experience some form of suicidal behavior than smaller institutions or institutions with lower staff-turnover rates (Osgood & Brant, 1991).

Many of the risk factors for suicide in the elderly are associated with a loss of control. It has been suggested, for example, that, when compared to other demographic groups, elderly white men experience the greatest losses of power, status, and role relationships, primarily through retirement (McIntosh & Santos, 1981). When these losses are coupled with declines in physical health, the development of depression is not surprising. When such depression results in hospitalization, the risk of suicide may initially be even higher as the hospitalization may be perceived as further evidence of a loss of control.

Behavior Therapy for Depression. In the 1980s several studies appeared supporting the efficacy of behavior therapy in the treatment of depression in elderly outpatients (Gallagher & Thompson, 1982, 1983; Steuer *et al.*, 1984). There have been few treatment studies of depression in elderly inpatients; operant interventions, involving social reinforcement of activity (Hussian & Lawrence, 1981) and a combination of operant and cognitive therapy (Hussian, 1983), have been found to be effective in reducing depression in elderly inpatients.

Behavior therapy offers several attractive features for the treatment of depression in older adults. First, antidepressant medications may be contraindicated because of other medications being taken or because of physical disorders. Tricyclics, for example, are associated with anticholinergic and cardiovascular effects that significantly limit their utility in the aged. Further, although monoamine oxidase inhibitors (MAOIs) have been found to be more effective for the elderly than for younger groups, the risks associated with the ingestion of tyramine and the concomitant use of other medications may be very serious (Crook, 1982). The use of MAOIs by elderly individuals with memory or attention deficits may, in fact, be very dangerous.

The therapist's active role in behavior therapy, the brief nature of behavior therapy, and the focus on current functioning are particularly appealing in the treatment of the problems of the elderly. Behavioral theories and therapies for depression emphasize the roles of reinforcement and control in depression (e.g., Beck, 1972; Lewinsohn, 1974). Efforts to replace lost sources of reinforcement and the empowerment of individuals through skills training are particularly powerful aspects of behavior therapy for depressed older adults.

When designing interventions for elderly individuals, it is important to remember that there are more similarities between older clients as a group and younger clients than there are differences. One area where there may be differences is cognitive functioning. Characterization of cognitive deficits is important in treatment planning. For instance, individuals with memory impairment may not be appropriate candidates for more complex cognitively oriented therapies. It has also been suggested that therapy may progress more slowly because of age-associated intellectual decline and health problems (Steuer & Hammen, 1983).

Certain dysfunctional cognitive themes have been found to be common among the depressed elderly (Emery, 1981; Gallagher & Thompson, 1983). Elderly individuals often say that they are too old to change and may believe that old age brings inherent limitations. In reviewing their lives, older people may focus on a negative aspect of their lives and draw generalizations about their personal worth. In examining the role of cognitions in depression in the elderly, it has been found that depression is often associated with negative cognitions involving fears of rejection and avoidance by others. Further, when compared with the nondepressed elderly, the depressed elderly held lower expectations of the probability of positive events occurring and higher expectations regarding the recurrence of negative events (Fry & Grover, 1982).

Anxiety

Elderly individuals are rarely seen as inpatients for the treatment of anxiety alone. Anxiety is, however, often associated with medical illness in the elderly (Himmelfarb & Murrell, 1984). Given the strong empirical support for the efficacy of behavior therapy for anxiety, its application with the chronically ill elderly is particularly attractive because reduction of anxiety has been found to be associated with decreases in the length of hospital stay and with the facilitation of recovery (Mumford, Schlesinger, & Glass, 1982).

Behavioral Treatment of Anxiety in the Elderly. Few studies have evaluated the efficacy of behavior therapy or other nonpharmacological treatments for anxiety in the elderly, and none has dealt with an elderly inpatient psychiatric population. The data that are available provide little support for the necessity of making significant modifications in standard behavioral therapies for anxiety when they are applied to the elderly. Some speculate, however, that exposure therapy for phobias may be contraindicated for the elderly because of the potential impact of anxiety on cognitive performance in this age group (McCarthy, Katz, & Foa, 1991).

Evidence supporting other approaches has emerged from work with nursing-home elderly. Hussian (1981) described the treatment of four elderly nursing-home residents who were phobic of elevators. The treatment included instruction in relaxation, positive self-talk and imagery, and *in vivo* exposure. At a two-month follow-up, all subjects were able to ride the elevator with only minimal anxiety.

A case study of a 67-year-old individual with a 45-year history of obsessive-compulsive disorder found an almost complete elimination of ritualistic behavior following an eight-session treatment program (Rowan, Holburn, Walker, & Siddique, 1984). The intervention included both *in vivo* exposure and response prevention. The treatment gains had been maintained at an 18-month follow-up.

Paranoid and Schizophrenic Disorders

Paranoia is the second most commonly occurring disorder and the most commonly occurring psychotic disorder observed in the elderly (Fisher, Zeiss, & Carstensen, 1992; Pfeiffer, 1977). It has been estimated that at least 10% of elderly psychiatric inpatients are admitted because of paranoid behavior (Jorgensen & Monk-Jorgensen, 1985; Kay & Roth, 1961; Roth &

Kay, 1962). However, accurate estimates of the prevalence of paranoid disorders and schizophrenia in the elderly are difficult to obtain because the development of paranoid behaviors and their relationship to other disorders in the elderly have not been adequately investigated (Fisher *et al.*, 1992).

Behavioral and nonbehavioral researchers have agreed, in general, that paranoid behaviors are characterized by "unshakable" false beliefs (delusions) and/or hallucinations (e.g., Post, 1987). Delusional behaviors appear in numerous diagnostic categories in the revised third edition of the *Diagnostic and Statistical Manual* (DSM-III-R; American Psychiatric Association, 1987). Diagnosis is a function, in part, of the content of the delusional verbal behavior and the age of onset (Post, 1987; Raskind, 1982). When paranoid delusions remain nonbizarre and do not have serious consequences, an elderly individual is rarely seen by a mental health professional. Typically, only when the delusional behavior has serious consequences or is very bizarre are mental health professionals consulted (Post, 1987).

Concomitants and/or causes of delusional behavior in the elderly include seclusion, sensory impairment, memory impairment, and physical disorders. In addition, several drugs can produce paranoid or psychotic behaviors, including anti-Parkinson medication, antihypertensive medication, antiarrhythmic medication, gastrointestinal steroids, antidepressants (e.g., tricyclics and MAOIs), minor tranquilizers (benzodiazepines), and lithium carbonate. Moreover, the withdrawal of some medications may induce psychotic behavior. The assessment of psychotic behavior in the elderly should always include an examination of the patient's medication regime. A functional analysis of paranoid and psychotic disorders should also include an assessment of organic disorders, especially if the elderly inpatient has a history of physical illness or if there is an abrupt change in the frequency or intensity of paranoid or psychotic behaviors (Hussian, 1981).

Behavior Therapy for Paranoid and Schizophrenic Behaviors. To date, there have been few treatment studies of paranoid behaviors in elderly inpatients, regardless of the type of therapy implemented. Most treatment studies have been limited to the evaluation of pharmacological agents. Not surprisingly, insight-oriented therapy has not been particularly successful in the treatment of paranoid behaviors in the elderly (Post, 1987). However, studies examining the effects of behavioral treatments on delusional behavior have shown promise relative to other treatment approaches.

Early studies examining the effects of behavioral treatments on delusional behavior have been conducted mostly with patients diagnosed with schizophrenia. In fact, delusional behavior is among the most widely investigated psychotic targets in behavior modification research (Stahl & Leitenberg, 1976). Therefore, the treatment of the delusional behavior of patients diagnosed with schizophrenia may be extrapolated to the treatment of the delusional behavior of nonschizophrenic patients at the level of the specific target behavior, which is, of course, delusional verbal behavior.

One of the earliest studies of delusional verbal behavior in an elderly patient was that of Rickard and colleagues (Rickard, Dignam, & Horner, 1960; Rickard & Dinoff, 1962). The subject was a 60-year-old male inpatient. The treatment was implemented during thirty-five 45-minute sessions. The treatment involved positive reinforcement consisting of interest in or approval of nondelusional verbal behavior and extinction of delusional verbal behavior. Rickard *et al.* (1960) reported a 100% increase in nondelusional verbalizations. However, because the authors did not report the rate of delusional verbal behavior, it is not possible to determine whether the rate of delusional verbal behavior increased as well, so that the subject was simply talking more frequently.

Using a similar approach, Carstensen and Fremouw (1981) examined the effects of a behavioral treatment on the delusional verbal behavior of a 68-year-old female nursing-home resident. The researchers instructed nursing-home staff to ignore the subject's delusional speech by having the staff state that someone was coming to talk to the subject about her concerns and then changing the topic. The staff were also instructed to initiate conversation with the subject when she was not emitting delusional verbal behavior. The subject was seen in 14 weekly individual sessions, which allowed the therapist to establish a trusting relationship with the subject while applying the same procedures of extinction and reinforcement as the nursing-home staff. The subject's delusional verbal behavior was essentially nonexistent by the end of the second week of treatment. At the end of treatment, the subject rarely emitted delusional verbal behavior or anxiety and/or fear responses associated with the delusional behavior.

In a recent study, Foxx, McMorrow, Davis, and Bittle (1988) examined the effects of a stimulus control approach on the delusional verbal behavior and the social behavior of a 69-year-old man diagnosed with schizophrenia. The researchers used the "cues, pause, point" procedure (see Foxx, McMorrow, Faw, Kyle, & Bittle, 1987), in which appropriate verbal stimuli were presented to the subject on a card. Responses from the client were classified as delusional, correct, or incorrect. Access to reinforcement was made contingent on the emission of a correct response in the presence of social-interaction environmental cues (i.e., the cards containing written words). The researchers found that the subject's delusional speech was replaced with appropriate verbal responses learned by the use of the social interaction stimuli. The results also showed generalization across experimenters, settings, and time, and at the 15-month follow-up, correct responding averaged 75% and delusional verbal behavior was almost nonexistent (i.e., only one delusional verbal response was emitted).

Generalization from case studies or from studies in which the subjects have been diagnosed with disorders other than delusional disorder (e.g., schizophrenia) must be done cautiously. However, extrapolations can be useful in demonstrating the utility that behavioral treatments have to offer in altering the frequency of delusional behaviors observed in elderly inpatients.

Elderly patients seen in psychiatric settings may not fit the criteria for delusional disorder but may exhibit more chronic disorders, such as schizophrenia. Treatment planning based on specific diagnostic distinctions between delusional disorder and schizophrenia is probably not justified based on the success of behavioral interventions in the alteration of target behaviors common to both diagnoses.

Mental health professionals working in geropsychiatric settings must be sensitive to the role of sensory impairment and drug reactions in the exhibition of paranoid and schizophrenic behavior observed in elderly inpatients. These factors may mediate the frequency, duration, and/or magnitude of the response under investigation. For example, interventions involving stimulus control procedures should compensate for decreases in visual acuity or auditory function; that is, discriminative stimuli may need to be increased in intensity or saliency (Hussian, 1981). In addition, research with elderly populations has shown that these individuals may present slower rates of acquisition and greater response rates during extinction than younger populations, although these differences may be small (Hussian, 1981). For example, delusional response rates may be resistent to changes in reinforcement contingencies, so that the reduction in delusional verbal behavior may progress more slowly in elderly individuals.

Agitation

Agitation is often a precipitant of institutionalization for older adults. A study (Moak, 1990) involving 124 demented and nondemented patients admitted to a psychogeriatric unit of a state mental hospital found that assaultive behavior was the most common reason for admission. Among dementia patients, who comprised 29% of the cases, assaultiveness, wandering, and disruptive behavior were the top three reasons for admission. Among nondemented patients, assaultiveness, inability to care for themselves, and disruptive behavior were the most common reasons for admission. The sample of dementia patients included a disproportionately high number of men (67%), indicating that men with dementing disorders who are aggressive may be particularly threatening to caregivers (Moak, 1990).

Coping with aggressiveness is extremely stressful for caregivers and, in fact, is often described by institutional staff and family members as the most difficult behavior problem to manage (Fisher, Fink, & Loomis, in press; Haley, Brown, & Levine, 1987). Nursing-home staff are often not adequately prepared to deal with agitated behavior in patients and tend to transfer an assaultive patient to a psychiatric hospital. In the sample described by Moak (1990), 47.2% of the demented patients and 25% of the nondemented patients admitted to the state psychiatric unit were admitted from nursing homes. The demented patients were more likely to remain in long-term care in the state hospital than nondemented patients. Fifty percent of the dementia patients were released to long-term care psychogeriatric units of state hospitals. Thirty percent were released to nursing homes. These findings suggest that inpatient psychiatric units can provide brief active treatment to geriatric patients.

In recent years, evidence has accumulated in support of the role of environmental influences on the occurrence of agitation and wandering in dementia patients. Previously, these behaviors were believed to be solely the result of organic impairment and hence untreatable except through pharmacological intervention or physical restraint. Statistics from a variety of sources indicate that chemical and physical restraint are the most common interventions for agitation (Evans & Stumpf, 1989; Garrard *et al.*, 1991). A review of the literature on physical restraint use found prevalence rates ranging from 25% to 85% (Evans & Strumpf, 1989). A recent longitudinal study (Tinetti, Liu, Marottoli, & Ginter, 1991) of 12 skilled-nursing facilities found that 67% of the residents were restrained at some point during the year, unsteadiness (72%), disruptive behavior (41%), and wandering (20%) being the most frequently cited reasons for the initiation of restraints. Unfortunately, physical restraints have been found to be associated with a number of physical problems, including muscle atrophy, osteoporosis, limb ischemia, and strangulation (Dube & Mitchell, 1986; Lofgren, MacPhersons, Grenieri, Myllenbeck, & Sprafka, 1989; McLardy-Smith, Burge, & Watson, 1986).

A recent observational study of agitation among nursing-home residents found that, in comparison to the number of agitated behaviors observed when restraints were not applied, the residents exhibited either the same amount or more agitation than when not restrained (Werner, Cohen-Mansfield, Braun, & Marx, 1989). Furthermore, restraint use did not reduce the number of falls experienced by the subjects. The results of this study suggest that restraint use leads to increased rather than decreased agitation. This finding is consistent with Hussian's report (1981) of a positive correlation between dementia patients' time in restraint and time spent wandering. These findings suggest that wandering and agitation may be, in part, schedule-induced. Falk (1969) described schedule-induced responses or "adjunctive behaviors" (e.g., aggression) as showing significant increases when a patient is subjected to a scheduled presentation of reinforcement of noxious stimuli (e.g., physical restraint). He noted that adjunctive behaviors have certain properties in common: (1) they occur in the presence of a deprivation state in the organism; (2) they are excessive and persistent; (3) they consistently occur as postreinforcement phenomena; and (4) they occur as unprogrammed responses independent of other response contingencies. This paradigm has not been explored by behavioral researchers studying aggression and wandering. It may prove useful in clarifying the environmental control of these behaviors.

Chemical restraint also has serious side effects that limit its usefulness. Drugs that are commonly used to reduce agitation and wandering include neuroleptics, beta blockers, antidepressants, lithium, and anticonvulsants (Salzman, 1988). All of these drugs have been found to be only moderately effective in managing wandering and agitation, and all may have considerable side effects. Further, age-related physiological changes alter the response of the older patient to psychotropic drugs. These age-related changes result in a reduction of clinical effectiveness, increases in toxicity, and a prolongation of both clinical and toxic effects (Salzman, 1982). These side effects and an overreliance on chemical restraints have resulted in new Health Care Finance Administration guidelines for nursing homes. Effective October 1,

1990, the new rules restrict neuroleptic use on an as-needed basis and require systematic efforts to reduce the dose and to replace neuroleptics with behavioral programming and environmental modification.

A few studies suggest that behavioral interventions, focusing on the modification of discriminative stimuli, can provide less restrictive alternatives to physical and chemical restraint. Although wandering, for example, is often conceptualized as random and purposeless, behavioral research has demonstrated that this behavior is often controlled by environmental stimuli. Hussian (1981) observed that patients ($n = 13$) exhibited less wandering and more stationary time in places that provided much stimulation and potential reinforcement. Patients tended to stop near other persons, in rooms where others were located, and at windows, water fountains, and untended food trays. In mapping the routes of the subjects, it was clear that each had developed consistent patterns. Finally, Hussian observed a direct relationship between the duration patients were held in restraints and the subsequent time spent wandering. When patients were provided with periods of free ambulation, the subsequent duration of and distance covered decreased significantly.

Another behavioral approach to controlling wandering involves the use of exaggerated discriminative stimuli. Hussian (1987) proposed that simple architectural cues (e.g., wall color and floor coverings) are used by dementia patients when they navigate through the environment. He demonstrated that this information can be used to reduce wandering. Wanderers ($n = 3$) were trained to attend to very simple stimuli (colored arrows) and learned to return to their rooms by following the arrows; they were reinforced by either food, access to television, or cigarettes. The subjects also participated in training sessions during which stimuli of other colors were paired with aversive events (e.g., a loud noise). These stimuli were then placed strategically at points of potential danger (e.g., stairwells) or exit locations around the facility. Following intervention, Hussian reported no change in rates of ambulation but a reduction of ambulation into hazardous areas. Booster training sessions were needed within two months of treatment termination.

Capitalizing on the observation that many dementia patients perceive two-dimensional patterns as barriers, Hussian and Brown (1987) proposed a restraint-free intervention that involved placing masking tape in varying grid patterns in front of the exits on a geriatric ward of a state psychiatric hospital. The authors found that placing eight horizontal strips ending 57.2 cm from the door was effective in preventing most exits. For seven of the eight patients studied, crossings were eliminated for over 60% of opportunities.

When stimulus control techniques are applied in the treatment of wandering, the patient is not restrained, and care providers are not burdened with continuous monitoring of the wanderer. Further, once established, stimulus-response relationships are difficult to dissolve. This phenomenon may prove useful in maintaining behavior among dementia patients.

To date, few controlled studies have examined behavioral interventions for managing agitation in the elderly. Not surprisingly, the largest proportion of treatment research on agitation has focused on the effectiveness of pharmacological agents. A reduced stimulation unit for patients with Alzheimer's disease and related disorders was found to be effective in reducing agitation levels from 1.7 to .8 points on a 4-point scale (Cleary, Clamon, Price, & Shullaw, 1988). Haley (1983) reported the successful application of a behavioral self-management program in the treatment of agitation in an elderly woman. The intervention included role playing, assertion training, cognitive restructuring, and progressive muscle relaxation. In addition, Mishara and Kastenbaum (1973) demonstrated the effectiveness of a token economy program in the treatment of self-injurious behavior among elderly long-term psychiatric-hospital patients.

Given the prevalence and costs of agitation among both community-residing and institutionalized elderly, the paucity of well-controlled treatment outcome studies is remarkable. Studies comparing the effects of behavioral interventions and pharmacotherapy in managing agitation are critically needed. The emphasis of behavior therapy on direct observation and functional analysis produces a particularly powerful methodology for improving our understanding of one of the most serious problems confronting geriatric inpatients and their care providers. Behavior therapy holds great promise for replacing physician and chemical restraint with less restrictive interventions that promote elderly patients' basic rights.

SUMMARY

A review of the findings from research on behavior therapy with elderly psychiatric patients is encouraging. Most studies to date indicate that there are few differences in the efficacy of behavior therapies for older adults and for younger adults. When differences are identified, they usually involve the rate of behavior change and the necessity of examining the roles of sensory deficits and chronic illness in the etiology and treatment of problems. Although these factors complicate assessment and treatment, they do not preclude the effective application of behavioral interventions with the elderly.

REFERENCES

Aarcon, R., & Franceschini, J. (1984). Hyperparathyroidism and paranoid psychoses. Case report and review of the literature. *British Journal of Psychiatry*, *145*, 477–486.

Aldwin C. M., Spiro, A., III, Levenson, M. R., & Bosse, R. (1989). Longitudinal findings from the normative aging study: 1. Does mental health change with age? *Psychology and Aging*, *4*, 295–306.

American Psychiatric Association. (1987). *Diagnostic and statistical manual of mental disorders* (3rd ed., rev.; DSM-III-R). Washington, DC: Author.

Basu, T. K., & Schorah, C. J. (1982). *Vitamin C in health and disease*. London: Croom Helm.

Beck, A. T. (1972). *Depression: Causes and treatment*. Philadelphia: University of Pennsylvania Press.

Buck, J. A. (1988) Psychotropic drug practice in nursing homes. *Journal of the American Geriatric Society*, *36*, 409–418.

Burgio, L., & Sinnott, J. (1990). Behavioral treatments and pharmacotherapy: Acceptability ratings by elderly individuals in residential settings. *The Gerontologist*, *30*, 811–816.

Butler, R. N., & Lewis, M. I. (1982). *Aging and mental health* (3rd ed.). St. Louis, MO: Mosby.

Carstensen, L. L. (1988). The emerging field of behavioral gerontology. *Behavior Therapy*, *19*, 259–281.

Carstensen, L. L., & Fremouw, W. J. (1981). The demonstration of a behavioral intervention for late life paranoia. *The Gerontologist*, *21*, 329–333.

Ciompi, L. (1985). Aging and schizophrenic psychosis. *Acta Psychiatrica Scandinavia*, *71*, 93–105.

Cleary, T. A., Clamon, C., Price, M., & Shullaw, G. (1988). A reduced stimulation unit: Effects on patient with Alzheimer's disease and related disorders. *The Gerontologist*, *28*, 511–514.

Conwell, Y., Nelson, J. C., Kim, K., & Mazure, C. M. (1989). Elderly patients admitted to the psychiatric unit of a general hospital. *Journal of the American Geriatrics Society*, *37*, 35–41.

Crook, T. (1982). Diagnosis and treatment of mixed anxiety depression in the elderly. *Journal of Clinical Psychiatry*, *43*, 35–43.

Diokno, A. C., Brock, B. M., Brown, M. B., & Herzog, A. R. (1986). Prevalence of urinary incontinence and other urological symptoms in the non-institutional elderly. *The Journal of Urology*, *136*, 1022–1025.

Dube, A. H., & Mitchell, E. K. (1986). Accidental strangulation from vest restraints. *Journal of the American Medical Association*, *256*, 2725–2726.

Emery, G. (1981). Cognitive therapy with the elderly. In G. Emery, S. D. Hollon, & R. C. Bedrosian (Eds.), *New directions in cognitive therapy: A casebook* (pp. 84–98). New York: Guilford Press.

Evans, D. A., Funkenstein, H., Albert, M. S., Scherr, P. A., Cook, N. R., Chown, M. J., Hebert, L. E., Hennekens, C. H., & Taylor, J. O. (1989). Prevalence of Alzheimer's disease in a community population of older persons. *Journal of the American Medical Association*, *262*, 2551–2556.

Evans, L. K., & Strumpf, N. E. (1989). Tying down the elderly: A review of the literature on physical restraint. *Journal of the American Geriatrics Society*, *37*, 65–74.

Falk, J. L. (1969). Conditions producing psychogenic polydipsia in animals. *Annals of the New York Academy of Sciences*, *157*, 569–593.

Fisher, J. E., Fink, C. M., & Loomis, C. C. (in press). *Prevalence and severity of behavior problems among dementia patients in long term care*. Clinical Gerontologist.

Fisher, J. E., Zeiss, A. M., & Carstensen, L. L. (1992). Psychopathology in the aged. In P. B. Sutker & H. E. Adams (Eds.), *Comprehensive handbook of psychopathology* (2nd ed.). New York: Plenum Press.

Fox, J. H., Topel, J. L., & Huckman, M. S. (1975). Dementia in the elderly: A search for treatable illnesses. *Journal of Gerontology, 30*, 557–564.

Foxx, R. M., McMorrow, M. J., Faw, G. D., Kyle, M. S., & Bittle, R. G. (1987). Cues-pause-point language training: Structuring trainer statements to provide students with correct answers to questions. *Behavioral Research and Treatment, 2*, 103–115.

Foxx, R. M., McMorrow, M. J., Davis, L. A., & Bittle, R. G. (1988). Replacing a chronic schizophrenic man's delusional speech with stimulus appropriate responses. *Journal of Behavior Therapy and Experimental Psychiatry, 19*, 43–50.

Fry, P. S., & Grover, S. (1982). Cognitive appraisals of life stress and depression in the elderly: A cross-cultural comparison of Asians and Caucasians. *International Journal of Psychology, 17*, 437–454.

Gallagher, D., & Thompson, L. W. (1982). Treatment of major depressive disorder in older adult outpatients with brief psychotherapies. *Psychotherapy: Theory, Research, and Practice, 19*, 482–490.

Gallagher, D., & Thompson, L. W. (1983). Effectiveness of psychotherapy for both endogenous and nonendogenous depression in older adult outpatients. *Journal of Gerontology, 38*, 707–712.

Garrard, J., Makris, L., Dunham, T., Heston, L. L., Cooper, S., Ratner, E. R., Zelterman, D., & Kane, R. L. (1991). Evaluation of neuroleptic drug use by nursing home elderly under proposed Medicare and Medicaid regulations. *Journal of the American Medical Association, 265*, 463–467.

Gatz, M., & Pearson, C. G. (1988). Ageism-revised and the provision of psychological services. *American Psychologist, 43*, 184–188.

Gatz, M., & Smyer, M. S. (1990, August). *The mental health system and older adults in the 1990's.* Invited address to Division 20 at the meetings of the American Psychological Association, New Orleans.

Gurian, B. S., Baker, E. H., Jacobson, S., Lagerbom, B., & Watt, P. (1990). Informed consent for neuroleptics with elderly patients in two settings. *Journal of the American Geriatrics Society, 38*, 37–44.

Haley, W. E. (1983). Behavioral self-management: Application to a case of agitation in an elderly chronic psychiatric patient. *Clinical Gerontologist, 6*, 25–34.

Haley, W. E., Brown, S. L., & Levine, E. G. (1987). Family caregiver appraisals of patient behavioral disturbance in senile dementia. *Clinical Gerontologist, 6*, 25–34.

Hancock, M. R., Hullin, R. P., Alward, P. R., King, J. R., & Morgan, D. B. (1985). Nutritional state of elderly women on admission to mental hospital. *British Journal of Psychiatry, 147*, 404–407.

Heath, H., Hodgson, S., & Kennedy, M. (1980). Primary hyperparathyroidism: Incidence, morbidity, and potential economic impact in a community. *New England Journal of Medicine, 302*, 189–193.

Himmelfarb, S., & Murrell, S. A. (1984). Prevalence and correlates of anxiety symptoms in older adults. *Journal of Psychology, 116*, 159–167.

Hussian, R. A. (1981). *Geriatric psychology: A behavioral perspective.* New York: Van Nostrand Reinhold.

Hussian, R. A. (1983). A combination of operant and cognitive therapy for geriatric patients. *International Journal of Behavioral Geriatrics, 1*, 57–61.

Hussian, R. A. (1987). Wandering and disorientation. In L. L. Carstensen & B. A. Edelstein (Eds.), *Handbook of clinical gerontology* (pp. 177–189). New York: Pergamon Press.

Hussian, R. A., & Brown, D. C. (1987). Use of two dimensional grid patterns to limit hazardous ambulation in demented patients. *Journal of Gerontology, 42*, 558–560.

Hussian, R. A., & Lawrence, P. S. (1981). Social reinforcement of activity and problem-solving training in the treatment of depressed institutionalized elderly patients. *Cognitive Therapy and Research, 5*, 57–69.

Jorgensen, P., & Monk-Jorgensen, P. (1985). Paranoid psychosis in the elderly: A follow-up study. *Acta Psychiatrica Scandinavica, 72*, 358–363.

Kahn, R. L. (1975). The mental health system and the future aged. *The Gerontologist, 15* (Suppl.), 24–31.

Katz, L., Weber, F., & Dodge, P. (1981). Patient restraint and safety vests: Minimizing the hazards. *Dimensions of Health Services, 58*, 10–11.

Kay, D. W. K., & Roth, M. (1961). Environmental and hereditary factors in the schizophrenias of old age ("late paraphrenia") and their bearing on the general problem of causation in schizophrenia. *Journal of Mental Science, 107*, 649–686.

Kiesler, C. A., & Sibulkin, A. E. (1987). *Medical hospitalization: Myths and facts about a national crisis.* Newbury Park, CA: Sage.

Knight, B. G., & Carter, P. M. (1990). Reduction of psychiatric inpatient stay for older adults by intensive case management. *The Gerontologist, 30*, 510–515.

Kucharski, L. T., White, R. M., & Schratz, M. (1979). Age bias, referral for psychological assistance, and the private physician. *Journal of Gerontology, 34*, 423–428.

Lair, T. J., Smyer, M. A., Goldman, H. H., & Arons, B. (1989, November). *Mental illness and the impact of nursing home reform: Estimates from the National Medical Expenditures Survey.* Paper presented at the annual meetings of the Gerontological Society of American, Minneapolis.

LaRue, A., Dessonville, C., & Jarvik, L. (1985). Aging and mental disorders. In J. E. Birren & K. W. Schaie (Eds.), *Handbook of the psychology of aging* (pp. 664–702). New York: Van Nostrand Reinhold.

LaRue, A., Spar, J., & Hill, C. D. (1986). Cognitive impairment in late-life depression: Clinical correlates and treatment implications. *Journal of Affective Disorders, 11,* 179–184.

Lawton, P. (1972). Schizophrenia forty-five years later. *Journal of Genetic Psychology, 121,* 133–143.

Lewinsohn, P. M. (1974). A behavioral approach to depression. In R. M. Friedman & M. M. Katz (Eds.), *The psychology of depression: Contemporary theory and research.* New York: Wiley.

Lofgren, R. P., MacPhersons, Grenieri, R., Myllenbeck, S., & Sprafka, J. M. (1989). Mechanical restraints on the medical wards: Are protective devices safe? *American Journal of Public Health, 79,* 735–738.

McCarthy, P. R., Katz, I. R., & Foa, E. B. (1991). Cognitive-behavioral treatment of anxiety in the elderly: A proposed model. In C. Salzman & B. D. Lebowitz (Eds.), *Anxiety in the elderly* (pp. 197–204). New York: Springer.

McIntosh, J. L. (1985). Suicide among the elderly: Levels and trends. *American Journal of Orthopsychiatry, 55,* 188–193.

McIntosh, J. L., & Santos, J. F. (1981). Suicide among the elderly: A review of issues with case studies. *Journal of Gerontological Social Work, 4,* 63–74.

McLardy-Smith, P., Burge, P. D., & Watson, N. A. (1986). Ischemic contracture of the instinsic muscles of the hands: A hazard of physical restraint. *Journal of Hand Surgery, 11,* 65–67.

Mei-Tal, V., & Meyers, B. (1986). Empirical study on an inpatient psychogeriatric unit: Diagnostic complexities. *International Journal of Psychiatry in Medicine, 15,* 91–109.

Milner, G. (1963). Ascorbic acid in chronic psychiatric patients: A controlled trial. *British Journal of Psychiatry, 109,* 294–299.

Mishara, B., & Kastenbaum, R. (1973). Self-injurious behavior and environmental change in the institutionalized elderly. *International Journal of Aging and Human Development, 4,* 133–145.

Moak, G. S. (1990). Characteristics of demented and nondemented geriatric admissions to a state hospital. *Hospital and Community Psychiatry, 41,* 799–801.

Moak, G. S., & Fisher, W. H. (1990). Alzheimer's disease and related disorders in state mental hospitals: Data from a nationwide survey. *The Gerontologist, 30,* 798–802.

Morgan, D. B., & Hullin, R. P. (1982). The body composition of the chronically mentally ill. *Human Nutrition Clinical Nutrition, 360,* 439–448.

Mumford, E., Schlesinger, H. J., & Glass, G. V. (1982). The effects of psychological intervention recovery from surgery and heart attacks: An analysis of the literature. *American Journal of Public Health, 72,* 141–151.

Myers, J. K., Weissman, M. M., Tischler, G. L., Holzer, C. E., Leaf, P. H., Orvachel, H., Anthony, J. C., Boyd, J. H., Burke, J. D., Kramer, M., & Stolzman, R. (1984). Six-month prevalence of psychiatric disorders in three communities. *Archives of General Psychiatry, 41,* 959–967.

National Institute of Mental Health. (1987). *Additions and resident patients at end of year, state and county mental hospitals, by and diagnosis, by state, United States, 1984.* Rockville, MD: National Institute of Mental Health, Division of Biometry and Applied Sciences, Survey and Reports Branch.

Norton, C. (1982). The effects of urinary incontinence in women. *International Rehabilitation Medicine, 4,* 9–14.

Okimoto, J. T., Barnes, R. F., Veith, R. C., Raskind, M. A., Inui, T. S., & Carter, W. B. (1982). Screening for depression in geriatric medical patients. *American Journal of Psychiatry, 139,* 799–802.

Omnibus Budget Reconciliation Act of 1987, Section 4201, Subtitle C U.S.C.

O'Riordan, T. G., Hayes, J. P., Shelley, R., O'Neill, D., Walsh, J. B., & Coakley, D. (1989). The prevalence of depression in an acute geriatric medical assessment unit. *International Journal of Geriatric Psychiatry, 4,* 17–21.

Osgood, N. J., & Brant, B. A. (1991). Suicide among the elderly in institutional and community settings. In M. S. Harper (Ed.), *Management and care of the elderly: Psychosocial perspectives* (pp. 37–71). Newbury Park, CA: Sage Publications.

Pfeiffer, E. (1977). Psychopathology and social pathology. In J. E. Birren & K. W. Schaie (Eds.), *Handbook of the psychology of aging* (pp. 650–671). New York: Van Nostrand Reinhold.

Pfeiffer, E., & Busse, E. W. (1973). Affective disorders. In R. W. Busse & E. Pfeiffer (Eds.), *Mental illness in later life* (pp. 107–144). Washington, DC: American Psychiatric Association.

Post, F. (1987). Paranoid and schizophrenic disorders among the aging. In L. L. Carstensen & B. A. Edelstein (Eds.), *Handbook of clinical gerontology* (pp. 43–56). New York: Pergamon Press.

Rapp, S., Parisi, S. A., Walsh, D. A., & Wallace, C. E. (1988). Detecting depression in elderly medical inpatients. *Journal of Consulting and Clinical Psychology, 56*, 509–513.

Raskind, M. (1982). Paranoid syndromes in the elderly. In C. Eisdorfer & W. E. Fann (Eds.), *Treatment of psychopathology in the aging* (pp. 184–191). New York: Springer.

Renvoize, E. B., Gaskell, R. K., & Klar, H. M. (1985). Results of investigations in 150 demented patients consecutively admitted to a psychiatric hospital. *British Journal of Psychiatry, 147*, 204–205.

Rickard, H. C., & Dinoff, M. (1962). A follow-up note on "Verbal manipulation in a psychotherapeutic relationship." *Psychological Reports, 11*, 506.

Rickard, H. C., Dignam, P. J., & Horner, R. F. (1960). Verbal manipulation in a psychotherapeutic relationship. *Journal of Clinical Psychology, 16*, 364–367.

Robins, L. N., Helzer, J. E., Weissman, M. M., Orvaschel, H., Greenberg, E., Burke, J. D., & Regier, D. A. (1984). Lifetime prevalence of specific disorders in three sites. *Archives of General Psychiatry, 41*, 949–958.

Roth, M., & Kay, D. W. K. (1962). Social, medical, and personality factors associated with vulnerability to psychiatric breakdown in old age. *Gerontological Clinics, 4*, 147–160.

Rowan V. C., Holburn, S. W., Walker, J. R., & Siddique, A. (1984). A rapid multi-component treatment for an obsessive-compulsive disorder. *Journal of Behavior Therapy and Experimental Psychiatry, 15*, 347–352.

Rowe, J. (1977). Clinical research on aging: Strategies and directions. *New England Journal of Medicine, 297*, 1332–1336.

Salzman, C. (1982). Key concepts in geriatric psychopharmacology: Altered pharmokinetics and polypharmacy. *Psychiatric Clinics of North America, 5*, 181–190.

Salzman, C. (1988). Treatment of the agitated demented elderly patient. *Hospital and Community Psychiatry, 39*(11), 1143–1144.

Sier, H. C., Hartnell, J., Morley, J., Giuliano, A., Kaiser, F., & Frankl, D. (1988). Primary hyperparathyroidism and delirium in the elderly. *Journal of the American Geriatrics Society, 36*, 157–170.

Smith, J. S., & Kiloh, L. G. (1981). The investigation of dementia: Results in 200 consecutive admissions. *Lancet, 1*, 824–827.

Stahl, J. R., & Leitenberg, H. (1976). Behavioral treatment of the chronic mental hospital patient. In H. Leitenberg (Ed.), *Handbook of behavior modification and behavior therapy* (pp. 211–241). Englewood Cliffs, NJ: Prentice-Hall.

Steuer, J. L., & Hammen, C. L. (1983). Cognitive-behavioral group therapy for the depressed elderly: Issues and adaptations. *Cognitive Therapy and Research, 7*, 285–296.

Steuer, J. L., Mintz, J., Hammen, C. L., Hill, M. A., Jarvik, L. F., McCarley, T., Motoike, P., & Rosen, R. (1984). Cognitive-behavioral and psychodynamic group psychotherapy in treatment of geriatric depression. *Journal of Consulting and Clinical Psychology, 2*, 180–189.

Tinetti, M. E., Liu, W. L., Marotioli, R. A., & Ginter, S. F. (1991). Mechanical restraint use among residents of skilled nursing facilities: Prevalence, patterns, and predictors. *Journal of the American Medical Association, 265*, 468–471.

Waxman, H. M., & Carner, E. A. (1984). Physicians' recognition, diagnosis, and treatment of mental disorders in elderly medical patients. *The Gerontologist, 24*, 593–597.

Wells, T. J. (1984). Social and psychological implications of incontinence. In J. C. Brocklehurst (Ed.), *Urology in old age* (pp. 107–126). New York: Churchill Livingstone.

Warner, P., Cohen-Mansfield, J., Braun, J., & Marx, M. S. (1989). Physical restraints and agitation in nursing home residents. *Journal of the American Geriatrics Society, 37*, 1122–1126.

Zimmer, J. G., Watson, N., & Treat, A. (1984). Behavioral problems among patients in skilled nursing facilities. *American Journal of Public Health, 74*, 1118–1121.

III
TREATMENT OF CHILDHOOD AND ADOLESCENT DISORDERS

19

Medical Issues in the Care of Child and Adolescent Inpatients

JOHN V. CAMPO

INTRODUCTION

"In the last analysis, we see only what we are ready to see, what we have been taught to see. We eliminate and ignore anything that is not a part of our prejudices."

Charcot (Prugh, 1983, p. 115)

It surprises very few mental health workers that emotional and behavioral disorders in children and adolescents are often underdiagnosed and undertreated or inappropriately treated in traditional medical and pediatric settings, where the focus of patient, family, and physician is generally on physical symptoms or complaints (Costello, Edelbrock, Costello, Dulcan, Burns, & Brent, 1988). Conversely, in the mental health setting, where the focus is generally on "psychological" suffering, the presence of a predisposing, precipitating, or coexisting medical illness may be overlooked or undervalued, or it may be treated with a great deal of uneasiness. The mind-body problem that has plagued Western medicine and philosophy does not appear likely to go away any time soon. Although some have derided the "false boundary between mind and brain" (Detre, 1987, p. 621), our real limitations in examining, identifying, and studying the somatic underpinnings of psychological states are all too evident from a practical perspective. In our day-to-day dealings with patients, we are confronted with a "practical dualism" (McHugh & Slavney, 1983; Schiffer, Klein, & Sider, 1988). In order to ensure adequate care, we must view our patients as both subjective agents (who experience and do things) and objective organisms (who are diagnosed, studied, and "have" things, like diseases) (Schiffer *et al.*, 1988). Nevertheless, an integrated understanding of our patients is desirable, and in many instances, the relationship between the "psychological" and the "organic," the subjective and the objective, can be sorted out, at least in part. In some instances, there appears to be evidence that a biological lesion or vulnerability may require a subsequent stressor in order to become manifest (Kruesi, 1990). In addition, although our impressions about the direction of causality (i.e.,

JOHN V. CAMPO • Department of Psychiatry, Allegheny General Hospital and Medical College of Pennsylvania, Pittsburgh, Pennsylvania 15212.

Handbook of Behavior Therapy in the Psychiatric Setting, edited by Alan S. Bellack and Michel Hersen. Plenum Press, New York, 1993.

373

whether psychological distress precedes physical illness or vice versa) are often of clinical relevance, and words like *psychosomatic* or *somatopsychic* slip easily off the tongue, it is difficult to imagine a truly "nonpsychosomatic" disorder (Lask & Fosson, 1989).

The importance of comprehensive medical evaluation and physical assessment in the child or adolescent psychiatric inpatient cannot be minimized. Furthermore, in a setting where the focus is often first and foremost on the emotional and behavioral, it is essential that mental health workers appreciate and pay attention to the complex relationship between psyche and soma, a relationship that has been of interest to clinicians since the beginnings of Western medicine (Schiffer *et al.*, 1988). Despite the limitations of categorical thinking, it seems useful from a pragmatic standpoint to consider how physical illness and emotional or behavioral disorders can relate in the clinical setting. While we realize that the categorizations are not absolute, that the boundaries between categories are often blurred, and that the state of our current knowledge is inadequate, physical illness or suffering becomes an issue in the inpatient setting in a number of ways:

1. Previously undiagnosed medical illness may present with psychological symptoms or complaints.
2. Patients with known medical illnesses or a history of such difficulties may suffer from psychological difficulties that may coexist with the medical illness or develop in relation to it.
3. Child and adolescent psychiatric patients may develop or manifest physical illnesses during their treatment.
4. Psychiatric disorders may present with or manifest prominent physical symptoms or complaints.

DIFFERENTIAL DIAGNOSIS IN PSYCHIATRY: PSYCHIATRIC PRESENTATIONS OF MEDICAL ILLNESS

The multiaxial classification used in the revised third edition of the *Diagnostic and Statistical Manual of Mental Disorders* (DSM-III-R; American Psychiatric Association, 1987) recognizes the interrelationship of clinical psychiatric presentations, developmental issues, psychosocial issues, and physical disorders.

The DSM-III-R devotes an entire section to organic mental syndromes and disorders, their essential feature being a psychological or behavioral abnormality associated with transient or permanent dysfunction of the brain. *Organic mental syndrome* refers to a constellation of psychological or behavioral symptoms without reference to etiology (i.e., delirium, dementia, amnestic syndrome, organic delusional syndrome, organic hallucinosis, organic mood syndrome, organic anxiety syndrome, organic personality syndrome, intoxication, and withdrawal). *Organic mental disorder* refers to a particular organic mental syndrome of which the etiology is known or presumed (i.e., an explanatory Axis III physical diagnosis is present) (American Psychiatric Association, 1987; Gudex & Werry, 1990). There is good evidence from the adult literature that many patients who present with psychiatric disorders have previously unrecognized physical illness that may account for their symptoms, and that is detectable on routine medical history, physical examination, and laboratory evaluation (Hall, 1980; Koranyi, 1979; Lazare, 1989). The psychological symptoms presented by physical illness are often not distinguishable phenomenologically from those of so-called functional psychiatric disorders, or those psychiatric disorders in which an organic etiology of the difficulties observed is not identifiable (Schiffer *et al.*, 1988).

While *delirium* or *cognitive impairment* may be important clues to the presence of an unstable medical condition or an organic etiology, it is a misconception to believe that the absence of cognitive impairment rules out a medical or organic etiology for a particular psychiatric symptom or symptom complex. Other related misconceptions include the belief that the nature of the psychological symptom presented allows a reliable distinction between "purely" medical or psychological disorders, that the presence of psychosocial stressors in temporal conjunction with the development of psychological symptoms "proves" that the symptoms are psychogenically determined, and that specific physical diseases cause only a handful of psychiatric syndromes (Schiffer *et al.*, 1988; Sternberg, 1986). Indeed, a given medical illness may be responsible for a variety of different psychiatric presentations in different patients, or even in the same patient.

The misconceptions mentioned may help fuel staff rationalizations that careful medical and physical evaluation may be passed over lightly or neglected. There are probably a number of reasons for such dangerous rationalizations, including the likelihood that many mental health care workers may be quite uneasy or frightened by medical issues and thus may avoid the procedures necessary in a high-quality physical assessment (Schiffer *et al.*, 1988). *There is no substitute for a comprehensive physical evaluation and assessment of each child and adolescent admitted to an inpatient setting.* These must be an integral part of the initial assessment from both a conceptual and a practical perspective. Adequate space and equipment must be provided for such an assessment, and direct-care workers should be comfortable with the fundamentals of physical evaluation.

The initial physical evaluation and examination may be an efficient use of the psychiatrist's time, and concern that such an assessment may be psychologically harmful is largely unjustified, the benefits appearing to far outweigh any potential risks (Schiffer *et al.*, 1988; Summers, Munoz, & Read, 1981). At the very least, a physician skilled in physical assessment and sensitive to psychological issues must be involved in the assessment of each patient, as early as possible. Communication with referring physicians or clinicians should be emphasized, as they are often a source of important psychosocial as well as medical information. Aside from its importance in providing information necessary to the diagnosis and treatment of medical illness, the physical assessment itself may be helpful in eliciting information important to a psychological assessment of the patient. In many cases, such information may be elicited naturally in the context of the physical examination. For example, physical findings such as scars may provide important clues in questioning about physical abuse or past traumas such as accidents or surgeries, and a history of accident-proneness may provide evidence that supports the diagnosis of an impulsive behavioral disorder such as attention-deficit hyperactivity disorder (ADHD).

The hypothesis that the psychiatric presentation may be caused or worsened by a concurrent medical illness should be considered in every patient. It is useful and realistic to consider the current state of psychiatric diagnosis syndromic, with the major categories, such as delirium, psychosis, and depression, signifying a symptom complex that may have a number of different and specific etiologies. The discipline involved in such an approach is frequently rewarded, and when physical illness is detected, it may have extremely important implications for prognosis, treatment planning, and outcome (Hall, 1980; Koranyi, 1979). Szymanski (1988) reported that, with the use of the DSM-III-R suggested approach to diagnosing organic mental disorders, such disorders were noted to be present in 5% of nonretarded and 4% of retarded patients, emphasizing that such disorders are of relevance before adulthood. The fact that the patient is cared for by a pediatrician or a family physician does not ensure that a satisfactory medical work-up has taken place, nor does a patient's being granted "medical clearance" guarantee that a contributing medical illness is not present. In patients with a known medical condition, it is extremely important to recognize that their psychiatric presentation may be related to that illness, to its treatment, or to complications (Hall, 1980; Koranyi, 1979; Lazare, 1989). Although it is true that a given medical illness may present in a variety of ways, and it also appears to be true that comorbidity in psychiatric presentations is more the rule than the exception, the following categories of symptoms may provide a useful starting point in generating a differential diagnosis in selected patients.

Delirium

Delirium is generally the most important clue to the presence of an underlying physical disorder (Stoddard & Wilens, 1990). Although the absence of delirium hardly confirms that a given presentation is not caused by medical illness, the presence of delirium should alert the clinician to the likelihood of an unstable or serious medical condition (Schiffer *et al.*, 1988). The essential finding in delirium is an impairment in arousal or consciousness; the DSM-III-R highlights a "reduced ability to maintain attention to external stimuli and to appropriately shift attention to new external stimuli" (p. 100). Such a *reduced ability to maintain or shift attention* is often demonstrated by the patient's inability to focus on the interview, by the need for repetitive questioning, or by perseverations by the patient in answering previously asked questions. Associated findings include *disorganized thinking*, which may appear fragmented, disjointed, or lacking in goal-directedness. Speech may be rambling, irrelevant, or incoherent, and *fluctuations in the patient's level of consciousness* may be evidenced by drowsiness, as well as marked *changes in activity level*, such as lethargy and/or agitation.

Disorientation is common, disorientation to time being the earliest to appear and the most sensitive indicator. *Memory impairment* may be evidenced by deficits in short-term memory on the mental status examination, by the inability to learn new material, and by the inability to remember past events. *Perceptual disturbances* are common, and patients often misinterpret or distort sensory input or frankly hallucinate, visual hallucinations being the most common. *Sleep-wake cycle disturbance* may manifest itself by insomnia or daytime sleepiness. *Emotional disturbance* is commonly present, with a variety of symptoms including extreme fearfulness or anxiety, irritability, anger, depression, or apathy. *Abnormal movements*, such as *tremor* or *asterixis*, may be present, depending on the underlying cause of the delirium (American Psychiatric Association, 1987; Stoddard & Wilens, 1990).

Patients at the extremes of the life cycle appear to be at special risk for delirium, and patients with known structural brain disease are at especially high risk. Although little formal research has been done on delirium in children and adolescents, it is common in sick children and may be an early sign of a rapidly deteriorating medical condition (Prugh, Wagonfeld, Metcalf, & Jordan, 1980). Such patients are often fearful, "on guard," and afraid of losing control. Commonly, delirium develops acutely, and the course fluctuates, the symptoms often being worse at night. Such patients may be dangerous to themselves or to others. Prugh *et al.* (1980) concluded that the diagnostic criteria for delirium in adults were applicable to children, but that mild delirium is often missed in younger patients. These patients present special difficulties in assessment as a result of developmental issues, including problems with formal cognitive testing. Delirium in children may be mistaken for "naughty" behavior (Gudex & Werry, 1990).

Delirium may be produced by virtually any serious medical illness that is significantly advanced, and its presence should be assumed to be organic in nature, necessitating a full medical evaluation and work-up. Though some "functional" psychiatric disorders such as mania or schizophrenia may, rarely, be severe enough to produce the symptom complex of delirium, this possibility should be considered only after a careful medical work-up. The EEG may assist in diagnosis, as it often reveals generalized slowing, though in some patients such slowing may not be evident if a premorbid EEG is not available, as a patient whose baseline tracing is at the high end of the normal range may show a tracing that appears to be within the normal range, even though it is actually somewhat slowed with reference to the baseline for that patient (Fenichel, 1988; Lipowski, 1988a; Stoddard & Wilens, 1990).

A detailed listing of the possible medical causes of delirium is beyond the scope of this chapter, though factors in delirium of childhood and adolescence may include *metabolic derangements* (e.g., hypoxia, hypoglycemia, diabetic ketoacidosis, hypoperfusion/dehydration, electrolyte imbalance, uremia, inborn errors of metabolism, and hepatic failure); *infections* (e.g., sepsis, and meningoencephalitis); *toxins* (e.g., alcohol, heavy metals, hydrocarbons, and drugs such as anticholinergics, anticonvulsants, hallucinogens, sedatives, and psychotropics); *withdrawal states*; *endocrine disorders* (e.g., hypo- or hyperthyroidism); *CNS disorders* (e.g., epilepsy, trauma, increased intracranial pressure of any etiology, intracranial mass lesion, and cerebrovascular disease); *nutritional deficiency* (e.g., B-12, folate, and thiamine); serious *systemic disease*; and environmental causes such as *sensory deprivation* or prolonged *sleep deprivation* (Volow, 1983).

In addition to appropriate medical work-up and intervention, such patients should be carefully observed and supervised to prevent self-injury, and increased contact with staff and family is generally helpful, with attention being paid to frequently orienting the patient to time and place. Preventing the patient from being overwhelmed by extraneous sensory input is often helpful, such as the elimination of unnecessary noise or stimulation, as overstimulation may encourage distortions or misperceptions. Dim lighting is often advocated during the evening, though this choice is often an individual matter. Low doses of neuroleptic medication such as haloperidol may also be helpful (Stoddard & Wilens, 1990). Depending on the underlying condition, such patients may require a transfer to an acute-care medical setting.

Psychosis

Psychosis is characterized by a serious or gross impairment in reality testing; the psychotic patient makes incorrect inferences about reality as a result of distortions of perception, thought, or consciousness (Maltbie, 1983). Psychosis is generally accompanied by bizarre behavior of some sort. Delirious patients may be considered psychotic, but psychotic patients need not meet the criteria for a diagnosis of delirium, though delirium is an important clue to the presence of an organic etiology. Indeed, the majority of psychotic patients seen in psychiatric settings are not delirious, but it remains important to evaluate these patients for medical causes of their thought disorder, even when a careful examination for signs or symptoms of delirium is negative.

The presence of *hallucinations* or *delusions* provides direct evidence of a psychotic process, though the term may be used when a patient shows evidence of a *formal thought disorder* characterized by logical errors or incoherence in thinking (Manschrek & Keller, 1989a; Schiffer *et al.*, 1988). Often, a patient's behavior may appear so disorganized or bizarre that a disturbance in reality testing can be inferred (American Psychiatric Association, 1987). *Hallucinations* may be defined as sensory misperceptions not related to external stimuli (Maltbie, 1983). Other perceptual disturbances may be present, including *distortions*, in which, although a real object is present as the stimulus for a particular perception, that perception is altered. *Illusions* are misinterpretations of stimuli that arise from an external object (Manschrek & Keller, 1989b). A detailed discussion of the evaluation of hallucinations in children and adolescents is beyond the scope of this chapter but is available elsewhere (Burke, DelBeccaro, McCauley, & Clark, 1985; Pilowsky & Chambers, 1986). Hallucinations may occur in any of the sensory modalities and may be a symptom of a variety of medical conditions and psychiatric disorders.

Organic hallucinosis refers to a syndrome of recurrent or persistent hallucinations, occurring with a full preservation of consciousness, that is referable to organic factors (Lishman, 1987). *Isolated visual hallucinations should strongly suggest the presence of an organic etiology.* Though visual hallucinations may occur in purely psychiatric disorders, they are generally accompanied by other types of hallucinations, such as auditory hallucinations (Manschrek & Keller, 1989b). With visual hallucinations, the more complex or formed the hallucination, the more likely is it to be referable to a dysfunction of the temporal or occipital association cortex (Schiffer *et al.*, 1988). Auditory hallucinations are most often seen in "functional" psychiatric disorders, though chronic auditory hallucinations may be related to alcohol or may occur with other substance-induced psychoses, such as those caused by amphetamines and cocaine (Lishman, 1987). Temporal lobe disorders may also produce such hallucinations. *Olfactory, gustatory, tactile, or somatic hallucinations should arouse suspicion of organic illness.* Tactile hallucinations in the form of formication, the sensation that bugs are crawling on the skin, may be seen in cocaine or amphetamine intoxication (Manschrek & Keller, 1989b).

Delusions are false personal beliefs based on incorrect inferences about external reality and firmly sustained in spite of what almost everyone else in the culture believes, and in spite of what constitutes incontrovertible and obvious evidence to the contrary (American Psychiatric Association, 1987). *Organic delusional disorder* is a psychotic syndrome, in which delusional thinking occurs in the absence of impairment of consciousness, and which is judged to be the result of a specific organic factor (Lishman, 1987).

See Table 1 for a listing of the drugs that may be associated with psychosis. Also, see Table 2 for a listing of some medical conditions associated with psychosis.

The evaluation of each patient who presents with psychosis should be individualized, though persistent psychotic symptoms in a child or adolescent often justify a structural brain study, such as a CT scan or an MRI scan of the head, as well as a sleep-deprived EEG. Diagnostic and laboratory evaluation should be directed by the careful evaluation of a skilled physician.

Table 1. Drugs Associated with Psychosis

Alcohol	Asparaginase	Hallucinogens
Amantadine	Atropine, anticolenergics	Mescaline
Aminocaproic acid	Baclofen	LSD
Amiodarone	Benzodiazepines	PCP
Amphetamines	Beta-adrenergic blockers	Psilocybin
Anabolic steroids	Bromocriptine	THC
Anticonvulsants	Caffeine	H2-blockers
Barbiturates	Captopril	Cimetidine
Carbamazepine	Chlorambucil	Ranitidine
Ethosuximide	Clomiphene	Interferon
Primidone	Clonidine	Isosorbide Dinitrate
Valproic acid	Cocaine	Levodopa
Antidepressants	Corticosteroid	Lidocaine
Bupropion	Cyclobenzaprine (Flexeril)	Methyldopa
Monoamine oxidase inhibitors	Cycloserine	Methylphenidate
Trazodone	Cyclosporine	Methysergide
Tricyclic antidepressants	Dapsone	Metoclopramide (Reglan)
Antihistamines	Decongestants	Metrizamide (Contrast)
Antimicrobial/antiviral agents	Oxymetazoline (Afrin)	Narcotics
Acyclovir	Phenylephrine	Nonsteroidal anti-inflammatory drugs
Cephalosporins	Phenylpropanolamine	Podophyllin
Ethionamide	Pseudoephedrine	Prazosin
Gentamicin	Deet (bug spray)	Promethazine (Phenergan)
Isoniazid	Digitalis	Quinidine
Ketoconazole	Disopyramide	Salicylates
Metronidazole	Disulfiram	Thyroid hormone
Nalidixic acid	Dronabinol	Verapamil
Procaine penicillin and other procaine derivatives	Ephedrine	Vincristine
Quinine derivatives		
Tobramycin		
Trimethoprim-sulfamethoxazole		
Zidovudine		

Depression

Depression is one of the most common reasons for psychiatric referral in adults (Koranyi, 1979) and has come to be recognized as a significant problem in children and adolescents (Kovacs, 1989; Puig-Antich, 1986). Aside from delirium proper, depression may be the second most common psychiatric symptom whose etiology is ultimately determined to be organic in nature (Barreira, 1989; Hall, 1980). An *organic mood disorder* is said to be present when a specific organic factor is judged to be etiologically related to the mood disturbance (American Psychiatric Association, 1987). Determining the presence of an organic factor is often much more difficult than it sounds. As with other psychiatric symptoms, a long list of agents and disorders has been associated with depression, most often on the basis of case reports, with their obvious limitations. In addition, medical or neurological illness may produce symptoms of lassitude, fatigue, and discomfort that may be difficult to sort out diagnostically from depressive symptoms *per se* (Schiffer *et al.*, 1988). In addition, drug-induced psychomotor slowing, sedation, or decreased exercise tolerance, such as that observed with propranolol, may be mistaken for depression.

These caveats aside, *medications* appear to be the factor most likely to be associated with depression and mood disorders in general, though most patients with drug-associated mood disorders appear to have a vulnerability to mood disorder such as that suggested by a previous history of mood disorder or a positive family history of such disorders (Spar, 1989). It was reported (Brent, Crumrine, Varma, Allan, & Allman, 1987) that epileptic patients treated with phenobarbital had a much higher prevalence of major depressive disorder and suicidal ideation than did those patients treated with carbamazepine. In addition, the study also suggested that phenobarbital disturbed mood only in those patients judged vulnerable to mood disorder on the basis of a family history of major affective disorder among first-degree relatives. The use of

Table 2. Medical Conditions Associated with Psychosis

Drugs/withdrawal	Neurological/CNS
(See Table 1)	Epilepsy (partial complex epilepsy)
Toxins	Cerebrovascular disease (stroke, hemorrhage,
Heavy metals	hematoma)
Organic fluorides	Intracranial mass lesion (tumor, arteriovenous
Organic phosphates	malformation [AVM])
Carbon disulfide	Trauma
Metabolic	Neurodegenerative disorders (e.g., Huntington's
Electrolyte imbalance	chorea, spinocerebellar degeneration)
Hypercalcemia, hypocalcemia	Multiple sclerosis
Hypoglycemia	Nutritional
Hepatic failure/hyperamnonemia	Zinc deficiency
Inborn errors of metabolism (e.g., acute intermittent	Thiamine deficiency
porphyria, Wilson's disease, homocystinuria)	B-12, folate deficiency
Endocrine	Nicotinic acid deficiency (pellagra)
Hypo- or hyperthyroidism	Pyridoxine deficiency
Hyper- or hypoparathyroidism	Systemic illness
Hyperadrenalism	Systemic lupus erythematosus, collagen-
Hypoadrenalism	vascular disease
Infectious	Sleep or sensory deprivation
CNS infection (e.g., viral meningoencephalitis,	Postoperative states
parasitosis)	Systemic malignancy
Neurosyphilis	
HIV infection	
Systemic infection	

anticonvulsant medication may result in folate deficiency, which may contribute to the development of depression (Edeh & Toone, 1985).

Depressive symptoms may appear early after the introduction of medication, but may not appear for several months in some instances (Schiffer *et al.*, 1988). In many cases, a trial period off medication may be the only way to determine its contribution to the patient's depression. In some instances, unfortunately, such a trial period may be difficult or impossible to arrange, particularly in the treatment of life-threatening or chronic conditions when alternative agents may not be available. A number of different agents have been associated with depression, including antihypertensives, anticonvulsants, psychotropic agents such as benzodiazepines or neuroleptics, corticosteroids, and oral contraceptive pills (Medical Letter, 1989). Because many adolescents fail to mention that they are on oral contraceptives when a routine medication history is taken it is especially important to ask—specifically adolescent girls—about such medications. Prenatal exposure to diethylstilbestrol (DES) has also been associated with depressive and anxiety symptoms (Vessey, Fairweather, Norman-Smith, & Buckley, 1983).

Structural brain lesions appear to be more likely than medications to produce affective symptoms in patients without a clear-cut predisposition to mood disorder; *endocrine disorders* occupy an intermediate position between medications and structural brain disorders in terms of being associated with mood disorder in patients not previously thought to be vulnerable (Spar, 1989; Whitlock, 1982). *Thyroid dysfunction* appears to be the most common endocrine disturbance associated with depression (Schiffer *et al.*, 1988). Endocrine disorder may also exacerbate psychiatric conditions, such as appears to be the case with thyroid abnormalities and rapidly cycling bipolar disorder; rapid cycling appears to be associated more frequently with thyroid abnormalities when these patients are compared with bipolar patients who are not rapid cyclers (Bauer, Whybrow, & Winokur, 1990). *Hypoadrenalism*, though rare, deserves mention, particularly that resulting from Addison's disease. Such patients may present with profound fatigue, weakness, hypoglycemia, hypotension, and hyperpigmentation (Schiffer *et al.*, 1988).

Viral infection may also be a factor in psychiatric illness; most commonly, the depressive symptoms are described following infection with a variety of agents, including influenza and the Epstein-Barr virus (Meijer, Zakay-Rones, & Morag, 1988). This is currently an area of much controversy, and public interest in "chronic fatigue syndrome" as a manifestation of a previously undiagnosed viral illness is on the rise (Wessely, 1990). Despite this interest, hard evidence supporting a viral etiology for the "chronic fatigue syndrome" is lacking when the methodological issues in the available studies are considered, and many have noted similarities between the recent interest in chronic fatigue and the history of neurasthenia, a disorder that rapidly diminished in popularity when it came to be viewed as psychologically, rather than medically, based (Greenberg, 1990; Wessely, 1990). See Tables 3 and 4 for a list of drugs and medical disorders associated with depression, though a myriad of medical conditions or medications should be considered capable of such an association in the individual patient. Tests of thyroid function and thyroid-stimulating hormone (TSH) should be done on virtually all patients who present with serious depression. Patients should be questioned carefully about alcohol or substance abuse, given its association with mood disorders, as well as the clinically recognized improvement in mood noted in many patients who stop drinking or using drugs.

Mania

Mania may occur as a result of physical illness or specific organic factors. Such "secondary mania" (Krauthammer & Klerman, 1978) may occur concurrently with the onset of a medical disorder or insult, but it may also be delayed; manic symptoms sometimes follow stroke or trauma by several years (Massion & Benjamin, 1989). Approximately 50% of adult patients who appear to develop mania secondary to organic factors have had a history of previous depression, and 25% have a family history of affective illness (Massion & Benjamin, 1989). This finding

Table 3. Drugs Associated with Depression

Acyclovir	Disulfiram	Metronidazole
Amphetamines	Ethambutol	Nalidixic acid
Anabolic steroids	Ethionamide	Narcotics
Asparaginase	Etretinate	Neuroleptics
Baclofen	Halothane	Nifedipine (Procardia)
Barbiturates	H2-blockers	Nonsteroidal anti-inflammatory agents
Benzodiazepines	Cimetidine	Norfloxacin
Beta-adrenergic blockers	Ranitidine	Oral contraceptives, estrogens
Bromocriptine	Interferon	Pergolide
Clonidine	Isoniazid	Phenylephrine
Cocaine	Isosorbide Dinitrate	Prazosin
Corticosteroid	Isotretinoin (Accutane)	Procaine derivatives
Cycloserine	Levodopa	Reserpine
Dapsone	Methyldopa	Thiazide diuretics
Digitalis	Metoclopramide (Reglan)	Thyroid hormone
Diltiazem	Metrizamide (Contrast)	Trimethoprim-sulfamethoxazole
Disopyramide		

Table 4. Medical Conditions Associated with Depression

Drugs/withdrawal
  (See Table 3)
  Prenatal exposure to diethylstilbestrol (DES)
Toxins
  Heavy metals
Metabolic
  Electrolyte imbalance
  Uremia
  Anemia
  Hepatic failure
  Hypocalcemia, hypercalcemia
  Hypomagnesemia
  Wilson's disease
Endocrine
  Hypo- or hyperthyroidism
  Hypopituitarism
  Adrenal insufficiency (Addison's disease)
  Hyperadrenalism (Cushing's syndrome)
Hyperparathyroidism
  Hyperaldosteronism
  Hyperinsulinism
Infectious
  HIV infection
  Encephalitis
  Neurosyphilis
  Hepatitis
  Influenza
  Infectious mononucleosis
  Malaria

Infectious (*Cont.*)
  Brucellosis
  Tuberculosis
Neurological/CNS
  Intracranial mass lesion (tumor, arteriovenous
    malformation)
  Cerebrovascular disease (stroke, hemorrhage,
    hematoma)
  Trauma
  Neurodegenerative disorders
  Epilepsy (especially partial complex epilepsy)
  Migraine
Nutritional
  B-12, folate deficiency
  Thiamine deficiency
  Nicotinic acid deficiency (pellagra)
  Iron deficiency
  Malnutrition, protein deficiency
  Vitamin C deficiency
  Zinc deficiency
Systemic Disease
  Systemic malignancy (e.g., lymphoma)
  Carcinoid syndrome
  Sarcoidosis
  Systemic lupus erythematosus, rheumatoid arthritis,
    collagen-vascular disease
  Inflammatory bowel disease
  Sleep deprivation, obstructive sleep apnea

suggests a possible interaction between organic factors and an underlying vulnerability to mood disorder. The list of drugs and disorders that can produce mania is considerable and is summarized in Tables 5 and 6; *drugs* are the most common precipitant (Schiffer *et al.*, 1988). Drugs that upregulate CNS catecholamines, such as antidepressants, bronchodilators, decongestants, and psychostimulants, are especially important to consider, as are corticosteroids (Medical Letter, 1989; Schiffer *et al.*, 1988). The withdrawal of antidepressant medications has also been associated with mania (Dilsaver & Greden, 1984).

Immunological disorders such as systemic lupus erythematosus and multiple sclerosis have also resulted in the development of the manic syndrome (Schiffer *et al.*, 1988). *Infections* are also of concern; neurosyphilis and human immune deficiency virus (HIV) infections are especially relevant (Massion & Benjamin, 1989). A case report of HIV infection presenting with mania as the initial CNS feature highlights the importance of considering HIV infections in patients with psychiatric presentations (Gabel, Barnard, Norko, & O'Connell, 1986). *Hyperadrenalism* or *Cushing's syndrome* is rare in childhood, but these patients may suffer from mania or other mood disorders; the physical findings include obesity, decreased growth velocity, hirsutism, and hypertension (Frank & Doerr, 1989). *Structural brain lesions* are also of importance in secondary mania, especially lesions in the right hemisphere and the right temporal lobe (Starkstein, Mayberg, Berthier, Fedoroff, Price, Dannals, Wagner, Leiguarda, & Robinson, 1990).

Disruptive Behavior Disorders

Disruptive behavior disorders are those characterized by socially disruptive behavior and "externalizing" symptoms. The DSM-III-R includes Attention-Deficit Hyperactivity Disorder (ADHD), Oppositional Defiant Disorder, and Conduct Disorder within this category (American Psychiatric Association, 1987). For purposes of differential diagnosis in a broad sense, patients with intermittent episodes of explosiveness or aggression will be considered in this category, as well. This category almost certainly includes a heterogeneous population of patients, and although it has been easier to demonstrate an association of such disorders, particularly hyperactivity, with environmental factors such as social disadvantage, large family size, and overcrowding than it has been to demonstrate a link with organic factors when these patients are considered together as a group, organic or physical factors appear to be of importance in

Table 5. Drugs Associated with Mania

Amantadine	Baclofen	Isoniazid
Amphetamines	Beta-adrenergic blockers	Levodopa
Anabolic steroids	Bromocriptine	Metoclopramide (Reglan)
Anticholenergics, atropine	Corticosteroid	Metrizamide (Contrast)
Anticonvulsants	Cyclobenzaprine (Flexeril)	Niridazole
Antidepressants	Cyclosporine	Nonsteroidal anti-inflammatory agents
Bupropion	Dapsone	Procarbazine
Fluoxetine	Decongestants	Quinine derivatives
Monoamine oxidase inhibitors	Deet (bug spray)	Theophylline
Trazodone	Hallucinogens	Thyroid hormones
Tricyclic antidepressants	LSD	Yohimbine
Antihypertensives	PCP	Zidovudine
Captopril	H2-blockers	
Clonidine	Cimetidine	
Hydralazine	Ranitidine	
Clonidine		

individual patients or in subgroups of patients (Greenhill, 1990; Rubinstein & Shaffer, 1985; Rutter, Tizard, & Whitmore, 1970).

Organic personality syndrome refers to a change in temperament or a change in characteristic patterns of reacting to events or to other people that is judged to be secondary to a specific organic factor, and that takes place in the absence of an obvious disruption in intellect or cognition (Lishman, 1987). When patients with *neurological difficulties* such as *epilepsy* are considered as a group, they do appear to be at higher risk for psychiatric disturbance, but there is little evidence of specific psychiatric sequelae, and these patients suffer from the full spectrum of psychiatric disorders seen in the general population (Breslau, 1990a; Rutter *et al.*, 1970). Physical or organic factors can be viewed as predisposing factors in some patients with disruptive behavioral disorders, essentially inducing vulnerabilities or directly causing the disorders. Though this is generally far from clear, there is some suggestion of a direct effect of brain dysfunction (Breslau, 1990b).

Psychiatric disturbance has been observed as a consequence of serious *head trauma*, the development of behavioral difficulties being related to the severity of the injury (Brown, Chadwick, Shaffer, Rutter, & Traub, 1981). Social disinhibition, impulsivity, inappropriate behavior, inattention, poor concentration, and overfamiliarity have traditionally been associated with *frontal lobe* lesions, though a variety of brain lesions may result in personality change (Yudofsky, Silver, & Yudofsky, 1989). Such patients may be irritable or explosive, may exhibit difficulties in controlling emotions or impulses, and may evidence significant deficits in social judgment or motivation (Yudofsky *et al.*, 1989).

Malnutrition and *very low birth weight* appear to be risk factors for disruptive behavioral difficulties, though confounding variables such as socioeconomic status and other environmental factors have been difficult to control for in studies of this etiology (Kruesi, 1990). Studies of psychiatric sequelae of *central nervous system infections*, such as meningitis or meningoencephalitis, have suggested an association with later behavioral difficulties, though similar methodological problems are present here as well (Kruesi, 1990).

Some have suggested an association between minor physical anomalies, attributes, or characteristics and disruptive behavioral disorders such as hyperactivity and conduct disorder (Rapoport, 1980). Rosenberg and Kagan (1987) showed a statistical association between the

Table 6. Medical Conditions Associated with Mania

Drugs/withdrawal	Infectious (*Cont.*)
(See Table 4)	Epstein-Barr virus infection
Toxins	Influenza
Manganese	HIV infection
Copper	Neurologic/CNS
Vanadium	Multiple sclerosis
Bromides	Intracranial mass lesion (especially right-side lesions)
Metabolic	Cerebrovascular disease (stroke, hemorrhage, hematoma)
Hypocalcemia	Trauma
Hemodialysis encephalopathy	Epilepsy
Hepatic failure	Neurodegenerative disease
Wilson's disease	Myasthenia gravis
Endocrine	Nutritional
Hyperthyroidism	B-12 deficiency
Hyperadrenalism (Cushing's disease)	Nicotinic acid deficiency (pellagra)
Infectious	Systemic illness
Neurosyphilis	Systemic lupus erythematosus
Meningoencephalitis	Multiple lentigines syndrome (leopard syndome)
Cryptococcal meningitis	

degree of iris pigmentation in white children and the degree of behavioral inhibition; the inhibited behavior was associated with blue eyes, and relatively disinhibited behavior was associated with brown eyes. A variety of *chromosomal abnormalities* have been associated with behavioral and developmental difficulties (Kruesi, 1990), the more common disorders including Turner's syndrome (45 XO; McCauley, Ito, & Kay, 1986), Klinefelter's syndrome (47 XXY; Bancroft, Axworthy, & Ratcliffe, 1982), XXY syndrome (Pitcher, 1981), and the fragile-X syndrome (Bregman, Dykens, Watson, Ort, & Leckman, 1987). The Prader-Willi syndrome, often associated with abnormalities of chromosome 15, is characterized by marked obesity, hypogonadism, small hands and feet, and learning difficulties. Many of these patients have severe problems with disruptive behavior, including abnormal eating behaviors and bizarre foragings for food (Fenichel, 1988).

A variety of foods and dietary factors are popularly believed to be associated with behavioral difficulties in childhood and adolescence (Rosén & Beyers, 1990). *Food sensitivity* may be broadly defined as a clinically abnormal reaction to a food or a food additive, whereas *food allergy* refers to the development of an immunological response to a specific food (Raiten, 1990). Artificial colors and flavors, salicylates, and other food additives have been suggested as being responsible for hyperactivity and learning difficulties in many children (Feingold, 1975). Although research seems to indicate that food sensitivity is not the cause of hyperactivity in most cases, there does appear to be a small subgroup of children who are affected by food additives (Raiten, 1990; Rosén & Beyers, 1990). It appears that Feingold's claims (1975) are greatly exaggerated, and his elimination diet should not be considered a form of treatment for hyperactive children in general (Rosén & Beyers, 1990). Other dietary factors that have generated interest have included sugar and aspartame. More research appears to be necessary, as several studies have found behavioral changes with sugar ingestion that are contradictory: some show adverse effects, and others show beneficial effects, but most show no significant behavioral reactions (Rosén & Beyers, 1990). Although the role of aspartame as a significant agent probably requires further investigation, it appears reasonable on nutritional grounds alone to question the exclusive use of this substance in childhood because it is certainly not an essential nutrient (Raiten, 1990). In any case, the role of dietary factors appears to be much less significant than is generally believed by the public (Rosén & Beyers, 1990).

Metabolic abnormalities have been associated with disruptive behavior disorders. Some have associated low activity of the enzyme dopamine beta-hydroxylase with conduct disturbance (Rogeness, Hernandez, Macedo, Amrung, & Hoppe, 1986). Another example is phenylketonuria (PKU), which has been associated with symptoms of attention-deficit hyperactivity disorder (Realmuto, Garfinkel, Tuchman, Tsai, Chang, Fisch, & Shapiro, 1986). *Wilson's disease* or *hepatolenticular degeneration* is a rare inherited disorder linked to abnormalities in copper metabolism, which affects both the central nervous system and the liver, and which has been associated with emotional and behavioral disturbance. The onset is usually in childhood or adolescence, and the initial presentation may be psychiatric. Approximately 20% of patients in one study had seen a psychiatrist before the diagnosis of Wilson's disease was made (Dening & Berrios, 1989). Approximately 50% of patients will have some psychopathological findings at the time of diagnosis, with disorders of behavior, irritability, aggression, and personality change being most frequent, though other symptoms, including depression and anxiety, are sometimes reported. Psychosis may occur, though it is less likely in Wilson's disease than was previous believed, and only a small proportion of patients present with psychotic symptoms (Dening & Berrios, 1989). Such patients are sometimes viewed as suffering from somatoform illness. A number of psychiatric symptoms in Wilson's disease appear to be associated with neurological symptoms, particularly dysarthria, dysphasia, drooling, and rigidity (Dening & Berrios, 1989). Patients may be referred because of deterioration in school performance, outbursts of abnormal behavior, or strange disorders in movement (Lishman, 1987). Cognitive impairment is relatively common in such patients as well. This disorder is important to identify, as it is treatable with the copper-chelating agent D-penicillamine (Lishman, 1987). On physical examination, brown, green, or yellow pigmentation as a ring at the periphery of the cornea may be present in up to 90% of patients with Wilson's disease; these rings are known as *Kayser-Fleischer rings* (Schiffer *et al.*, 1988). These are best identified by slit-lamp examination by an ophthalmologist. A low serum ceruloplasmin level is of great diagnostic importance, and this is probably the best screen for Wilson's disease. Though false negatives may occur in a small percentage of patients (Crumley, 1990), a ceruloplasmin level higher than 30 mg/dl is usually convincingly negative. Serum copper may be decreased, urinary copper may be elevated, and liver enzymes may show elevations, as well, but these elevations are nonspecific. If liver enzymes are elevated and a suspicion of Wilson's disease remains, measurement of urinary copper is indicated, even if ceruloplasmin is low normal (i.e., between 20 mg/dl and 30 mg/dl) (Crumley, 1990). Structural studies of the brain, such as CT scans or MRI scans, may also show abnormalities (Lishman, 1987; Schiffer *et al.*, 1988).

Environmental toxins such as *lead* should also be considered, particularly in urban children. The work of Needleman, Gunnoe, Leviton, Reed, Peresie, Maher, and Barrett (1979) has suggested that low-level lead exposure may result in distractibility, frequent off-task behavior, and poor academic performance. Lead levels above 30 micrograms per deciliter have been associated with a variety of behavioral and neurological symptoms, including symptoms of attention deficit and hyperactivity, irritability, fatigue, and behavioral change (Lishman, 1987). Surveys have shown that 3.9% of all American children under age 5 had lead levels of 30 micrograms per deciliter or more, and children of urban African-American families with very low incomes in the core of large cities showed an 18.6% incidence of lead levels of 30 micrograms per deciliter or more (Hanesian, Paez, & Williams, 1988; U.S. Department of Health and Human Services, 1985). Lower income white children also show a similar trend toward a greater likelihood of lead exposure (U.S. Department of Health and Human Services, 1985). Patients with *iron deficiency anemia* may also show evidence of inattention, poor school performance, irritability, and behavioral difficulties (Oski, 1979). Prenatal exposure to alcohol, drugs, or toxins may be of great significance, and the *fetal alcohol syndrome* has been associated with attentional problems, hyperactivity, and behavioral difficulties (Spohr & Steinhausen, 1987).

The history of the behavioral difficulties is often of relevance, as patients with Attention-deficit Hyperactivity Disorder are reported to have difficulties from at least their early school years, and most often from their preschool years. A more acute onset of symptoms that appears to be consistent with the hyperactivity syndrome should especially alert the clinician to the possibility of organic factors. Such factors include *medications*, particularly barbiturates and other anticonvulsants; bronchodilators such as theophylline; and anabolic steroids (Medical Letter, 1989; Rachelefsky, Wo, Adelson, Mickey, Spector, Katz, Siegel, & Rohr, 1986). *Hyperthyroidism* may occasionally present with symptoms of hyperactivity; these patients often appear tall or at least show an increasing growth velocity in addition to other signs and symptoms of the disorder. Because disruptive behavior may be associated with *epilepsy*, particularly with partial complex seizures, neurological evaluation and EEG studies may be of benefit in patients suspected of seizure disorder on clinical grounds. *Sleep disorder* or *sleep deprivation* should also be considered, as patients with *obstructive sleep apnea* have been noted clinically to manifest problems with hyperactivity, behavioral difficulties, irritability, and personality change (Dahl, 1992). Parents may report that such patients snore loudly and are restless sleepers. Obese children may be at special risk (Mallory, Fiser, & Jackson, 1989).

Anxiety

Anxiety is an especially common symptom among psychiatric patients, and most mental health workers are well aware of the frequency with which anxiety symptoms may be misperceived by the patient as indicating physical illness. This is especially true of panic anxiety. In this common scenario, it is often easy to forget that anxiety may be the result of physical illness or organic factors. A listing of the physical factors associated with anxiety is extensive, and the major categories are included in Tables 7 and 8.

Dietary factors and *medications* are among the most common causes of organically associated anxiety symptoms (Schiffer *et al.*, 1988). A carefully dietary history is often helpful, as it may reveal excessive *caffeine ingestion*, which has been associated with reversible anxiety disorders in some patients (Greden, Fontaine, Lubetsky, & Chamberlin, 1978). *Monosodium glutamate* (MSG) has also been associated with anxiety symptoms (Lawlor & Lazare, 1989). *Drugs of abuse*, such as cocaine, amphetamines, and hallucinogens (e.g., phencyclidine), have also been associated with anxiety and other psychiatric symptoms, as has *withdrawal* from alcohol, sedatives, or beta-blockers (Schiffer *et al.*, 1988).

Of the endocrine disorders associated with anxiety, *hyperthyroidism* appears to be the most common. Such patients may present with a variety of physical symptoms, including tachycardia, fine tremor, diaphoresis, exophthalmos, and hyperreflexia, among others. Such patients may complain of heat intolerance, fatigue, palpitations, increased appetite, and weight loss. Essentially, they are hypermetabolic and tend to have an elevated pulse. The presence of an enlarged thyroid gland is also suggestive, and thyroid function tests should confirm the diagnosis (Schiffer *et al.*, 1988).

Pheochromocytoma is a rare catecholamine-secreting tumor that may present with anxiety symptoms, particularly episodic panic attacks (Schiffer *et al.*, 1988; Starkman, Zelnik, Nesse, & Cameron, 1985). Such patients experience their anxiety most often in association with headache, excessive sweating, palpitations, and hypertension (Starkman *et al.*, 1985). Though rare, this disorder is important to detect, as the antidepressant medications used to treat panic anxiety may often exacerbate the hypertension and enhance the effect of the excessive catecholamines secreted by the tumor (Schiffer *et al.*, 1988). Diagnosis is confirmed by a demonstration of elevated urinary levels of vanillylmandelic acid (VMA) (Bravo, Tarazi, Gifford, & Stewart, 1979).

Hypoglycemia is often mentioned as a cause of anxiety and a myriad of other psychiatric symptoms, though the public's concern regarding functional or reactive hypoglycemia appears to be greatly exaggerated, as true hypoglycemia is quite rare in the absence of a known medical disorder such as adrenal insufficiency or diabetes, where insulin use may result in hypoglycemia (Lawlor & Lazare, 1989). Though rare, patients with intracranial mass lesions may present with anxiety symptoms and/or school refusal (Blackman & Wheler, 1987). Though the nature of the relationship is far from clear, an association between *mitral valve prolapse* and anxiety, including panic anxiety, has been suggested (Casat, Ross, Scardina, Sarno, & Smith, 1987; Schiffer *et al.*, 1988).

Another rare metabolic disorder that has been associated with anxiety symptoms and other unexplained physical and psychiatric symptoms is *acute intermittent porphyria* (AIP) (Boon &

Table 7. Drugs Associated with Anxiety

Amphetamines	Cycloserine	Nifedipine
Anticholinergics, atropine	Decongestants	Nonsteroidal anti-inflammatory agents
Antihistamines	Dronabinol	Norfloxacin
Baclofen	Inrerferon	Pergolide
Bromocriptine	Metrizamide (Contrast)	Procaine derivatives
Caffeine	Monoamine oxidase inhibitors	Promethazine (Phenergan)
Captopril	Nabilone	Quinine derivatives
Cocaine	Narcotics	Theophylline, bronchodilators

Ellis, 1989). AIP is an autosomal dominant inherited enzymatic disorder of porphyrin metabolism in which acute "attacks" of symptoms, often including abdominal pain, occur episodically (Lishman, 1987). The course is chronic, but intermittent, and psychiatric and neurological symptoms often follow the abdominal pain, although they sometimes occur as the initial presentation (Schiffer *et al.*, 1988). In addition to anxiety, the psychiatric symptoms include depression, agitation, psychosis, and frank delirium (Boon & Ellis, 1989). Attacks may be precipitated by starvation, infection, endogenous steroids related to the menstrual cycle, alcohol, and, most important, drugs (Lishman, 1987; Schiffer *et al.*, 1988). Drugs that are especially dangerous in patients with acute intermittent porphyria include barbiturates and most anticonvulsants, sulfonamides, synthetic estrogens and progestogens, amphetamines, metoclopramide, theophylline, and griseofulvin (Boon & Ellis, 1989). Patients with this disorder may be considered "hysterical" because of the intermittent nature of the symptoms, and the diagnosis may be missed (Barkowsky & Schady, 1982). Diagnosis is important, as some patients have died during fulminant attacks (Lishman, 1987). Blood studies from such patients should show a reduction in porphobilinogen deaminase of at least 50% as compared to normal controls, and 24-hour urine collection for porphyrins may be abnormal during attacks (Schiffer *et al.*, 1988).

Migraine headache is a highly prevalent condition, which may be associated with a variety of gastrointestinal and neurological symptoms, as well as symptoms of psychiatric disorder. Merikangas, Angst, and Isler (1990) demonstrated a strong association between migraine and anxiety disorders, as well as migraine and depression. Migraine was more strongly associated with anxiety syndromes than with depression. The onset of anxiety often occurred during childhood and generally preceded the onset of the migraine headaches. The onset of depression tended to occur after the development of headaches, generally several years later. It is of interest that antidepressant medications and lithium carbonate have been reported to be effective in the treatment of migraine or cluster headaches as well (Merikangas *et al.*, 1990).

Table 8. **Medical Conditions Associated with Anxiety**

Drugs/withdrawal	Infectious (*Cont.*)
(See Table 7)	Infectious mononucleosis
Prenatal exposure to diethylstilbestrol (DES)	Tuberculosis
Toxins	Malaria
Heavy metals	Brucellosis
Metabolic	CNS/neurological
Inborn errors of metabolism (acute	Multiple sclerosis
intermittent porphyria)	Intracranial mass lesion
Electrolyte imbalance	Cerebrovascular disease
Hypoxia	Trauma
Hypoperfusion/anemia	Epilepsy
Hypoglycemia	Neurodegenerative disorders
Wilson's disease	Myasthenia gravis
Endocrine	Nutritional
Hyperthyroidism	B-12 deficiency
Hyperadrenalism (Cushing's syndrome)	Nicotinic acid deficiency (pellagra)
Hypoparathyroidism	Zinc deficiency
Hypoadrenalism (adrenal insufficiency)	Systemic illness
Pheochromocytoma	Systemic lupus erythematosus, collagen-vascular disease
Infectious	Supraventricular tachycardia
Neurosyphilis	Mitral valve prolapse
Encephalitis	Malignancy
Hepatitis	

Dementia

Dementia is an acquired global impairment of intellect, memory, and personality that occurs without impairment of consciousness. The DSM-III-R emphasizes an impairment in short- and long-term memory in the context of a general loss of intellectual functioning that is sufficient to cause disability (American Psychiatric Association, 1987). An underlying organic etiology is assumed for dementia, and dementia is distinguished from delirium by a relative preservation of arousal and generally a more chronic course. In general, such patients require a careful medical work-up in consultation with a neurologist. Dementia is uncommon, but not unheard of, in younger patients, and a variety of *neurodegenerative disorders* such as Huntington's chorea and inherited enzymatic defects may occasionally present with psychiatric symptoms in children and adolescents. Disorders of lysosomal enzymes, such as the mucopolysaccharidoses, Gaucher's disease, Niemann-Pick disease, and metachromatic leukodystrophy, may present with psychiatric symptoms in the context of psychomotor regression (Fenichel, 1988). We recently diagnosed Niemann-Pick disease, Type C, in a teenager who presented with psychotic symptoms, but who was found to be demented on cognitive examination, with significant impairments in short- and long-term memory. Other rare inherited disorders include adrenoleukodystrophy, ceroid lipofuscinosis, mitochondrial encephalomyopathies, and Wilson's disease (Fenichel, 1988).

Human immune deficiency virus (HIV) infections are being diagnosed more frequently in children and adolescents, and the development of the AIDS-dementia complex is not unheard of, the patients manifesting progressive cognitive impairment, spasticity, and weakness (Krener & Miller, 1989). Behavioral signs or symptoms may predominate in the early phase of the illness, with symptoms suggestive of depression, apathy, withdrawal, or psychosis (Krener & Miller, 1989).

Toxic exposures, such as to lead, should also be considered in dementia (Gudex & Werry, 1990).

Enuresis

Enuresis is a common problem in child and adolescent inpatient work and is occasionally the result of a medically treatable condition, though only in a small percentage of patients. Enuretic patients are sometimes distinguished from one another on the basis of whether their enuresis is considered "primary," meaning that dryness has never been achieved for six months or longer, or "secondary," meaning that the patient has been dry for six months or longer and has then relapsed.

Patients with congenital abnormalities that result in enuresis are most likely to present as "primary" enuretics, though it would be incorrect to assume that most primary enuretics suffer from a medically caused disorder. Patients with both daytime and nighttime incontinence may also be somewhat more likely to manifest an organic etiology than those with nocturnal enuresis alone. *Urinary tract infection* and early *diabetes mellitus* are the most common medical causes, though some patients have *structural disorders of the genitourinary tract*, such as urethral valves that cause poor urinary stream and dribbling. *CNS abnormalities*, such as disorders of the spinal cord (e.g., myelomeningocele and spinal dysraphism), hydrocephalus, degenerative neurological disorders, or seizures, may also result in enuresis (Landman, 1990). *Diabetes insipidus* that is central, or that is nephrogenic, such as that caused by *lithium carbonate*, may also result in enuresis. Patients with *sickle cell anemia* may be prone to renal concentration disorders (Tunnessen, 1988). In addition to lithium, other *medications*, such as caffeine, theophylline, and antipsychotic drugs, may cause or contribute to enuresis. Clinically, some feel that *chronic constipation* may be associated with enuresis, and some patients show an improvement after the constipation is corrected (Tunnessen, 1988). Urinalysis and urine culture constitute a reasonable initial work-up in patients with enuresis, unless further investigation is suggested by history or physical examination.

Encopresis

Encopresis is most often associated with *chronic constipation*, but it may be caused in some patients by specific medical disorders, such as *Hirschsprung's disease, hypothyroidism, spinal cord lesions*, or *lead poisoning*, and may be mimicked by *diarrheal disorders* or *inflammatory bowel disease* (Landman, 1990). A history and physical examination, including a rectal examination, are most helpful in directing medical evaluation and treatment. Patients with Hirschsprung's disease generally have symptoms dating to infancy, tend to have problems with growth and development, are rarely incontinent, and most often have thin, ribbonlike stools (Landman, 1990). A rectal biopsy to rule out Hirschsprung's disease should be performed only on carefully selected patients, and in consultation with a pediatric gastroenterologist. Depending on the clinical evaluation, an abdominal flat-plate X ray may be helpful in evaluating the degree of stool retention and in monitoring treatment response. Indeed, encopresis is a particularly striking example of the impossibility of separating the physical and the psychological in the understanding of a condition or in its treatment.

In summary, a careful and complete medical history and physical assessment should be performed on each patient on admission, with additional assessments being performed in directed fashion as issues arise. The *past medical history* should be reviewed, including a *past history of illnesses, accidents*, and *surgeries*, and an *immunization history* is often useful in providing an index of early caretaking, as well as having obvious utility in confirming whether the patient has been properly immunized. Questions about whether a patient has had the common illnesses of childhood, such as chicken pox, or has been recently exposed to such illnesses are often of great practical importance, as the admission of a newly exposed patient may result in the infection of inpatients who have not been exposed and may essentially shut down an inpatient service to new admissions. *Current and past medications* need to be determined, as many commonly used drugs can cause serious psychiatric symptoms, either directly, on withdrawal, or in interaction with other drugs (Medical Letter, 1989). *A history of allergies or sensitivities* to medications or other substances should be taken. This is another area where medical questioning may provide additional information relevant to the psychological evaluation of the patient. Patients who report or whose families report food allergy show a high incidence of psychiatric disorders, even when the presence of such an allergy cannot be objectively confirmed (Rix, Pearson, & Bentley, 1984; Rubinstein & Shaffer, 1985). A medical *review of systems* may be rewarding, as well.

A careful *family history* of medical disorders is also of particular importance, especially in the assessment of children and adolescents, because inherited metabolic or neurological disorders, such as acute intermittent porphyria or Huntington's chorea, may elicit psychiatric symptoms or complaints, even though the family members may not make this connection. *Alcohol and substance abuse* may result in psychiatric symptoms or may have significant medical complications and should be considered in the assessment of each patient. Withdrawal from such substances may result in medical and psychiatric complications, as well as a confounding clinical picture, that are best anticipated. *Drug screens* should be performed on appropriate patients where the history or presentation suggests the possibility of substance abuse.

A physical examination should be performed, and *height, weight*, and *head circumference* should be obtained on each patient, with the age-specific percentile rank on each of these measures. Short stature is a common finding, and psychosocial dwarfism, though unusual, may be underdiagnosed. Determining the *stage of pubertal development* is important, and an appropriate Tanner stage should be assigned. Abbreviated screenings of vision and hearing on initial evaluation should help direct the need for further investigations. The results of the initial medical history and physical examination should be carefully recorded in the patient's chart and should be readily accessible. It is wise to call prominent attention to any special allergies, medications, or illnesses by specially labeling the chart.

Although laboratory and diagnostic evaluations are best generated by clinical judgment following an appropriate history and physical examination, and opinions may differ about what the "routine" laboratory evaluation of psychiatric inpatients should be, it seems reasonable that the initial laboratory evaluation should include drawing blood for electrolytes, urea nitrogen, creatinine, glucose, calcium, liver function tests, a complete blood count with differential and platelet count, an erythrocyte sedimentation rate (ESR), and tests for thyroid function and TSH. Testing for lead level also seems reasonable, especially in urban children. A urinalysis should be obtained on admission, and urine cultures should be ordered for enuretic children who have not been previously evaluated or in whom the presence of urinary tract infection seems likely. If syphilis is suspected, a specific antibody test, such as the fluorescent treponemal antibody absorption test (FTA-ABS), should be ordered, as such tests are both sensitive and specific and have fewer false positives than serological tests such as the rapid plasma reagin (RPR) and the Venereal Disease Research Laboratories (VDRL) tests. Studies to consider for selected patients include antinuclear antibodies (ANA) in patients with suspected systemic lupus erythematosus, ceruloplasmin and urine copper in patients with suspected Wilson's disease, and HIV titers in patients with suspected HIV infections. *Chromosomal studies*, including fragile-X determinations, should be obtained based on physical assessment and clinical suspicion. *Drug screening* should be considered for many patients, especially adolescents. Specific studies such as the *EEG*, *structural studies* (CT and MRI scans), and *sleep studies* should be obtained on the basis of clinical evaluation and judgment. *Neuropsychological testing* may also be of help when organic factors are known or suspected (Selz & Reitan, 1979).

CHRONIC MEDICAL ILLNESS AND PSYCHIATRIC DISORDER

It is estimated that 10%–12% of children and adolescents in the United States suffer from a chronic physical condition; that physical condition causes significant functional impairment in approximately 1%–3% of that total population (Garrison & McQuiston, 1989). A recent study suggested that 9% of U.S. children aged 4–17 had at least 1 of 19 different chronic physical conditions, and that approximately 25% of these children appeared to be functionally limited (Gortmaker, Walker, Weitzman, & Sobol, 1990). The estimated prevalence of selected chronic conditions in this population is shown in Table 9.

A number of studies have suggested that chronic medical conditions in children and adolescents are risk factors for psychiatric disorder and psychosocial morbidity (Breslau, 1990a; Gortmaker *et al.*, 1990; Rutter *et al.*, 1970). These chronic physical conditions appear to be a significant risk factor independent of sociodemographic factors, and these patients also appear to be at increased risk for school problems and for placement in special education (Gortmaker *et al.*, 1990). Functional impairment as a result of chronic illness is felt to convey additional risk. Further, the severity of the illness has also been thought to be a significant factor. However, both of these factors appear to be less powerful predictors than might be expected (Breslau, 1990a; Garrison & McQuiston, 1989). A predisposition to psychiatric disorder may well be an important factor in determining which children with chronic illness are ultimately psychosocially impaired. The presence of a documented brain disorder such as epilepsy appears to be an especially important risk factor in the development of a mental disorder. In the Isle of Wight study (Rutter *et al.*, 1970), mental disorder was found in 34% of 9- to 11-year-old children with a documented brain disorder such as epilepsy, as compared to 12% of children with non-brain-related physical disorders, and to 7% of children without a physical disorder. This finding was supported by subsequent studies (Gortmaker *et al.*, 1990). Indeed, as reviewed by Breslau

(1990a), the relative risk of psychiatric disorder conveyed by conditions that do not involve the brain appears to be of marginal significance when compared to the risk in children with documented brain abnormalities. Thus, the type of chronic illness suffered is of significance from the psychiatric perspective. Most studies of chronically ill children have documented low referral rates to mental health personnel, and mental health services for such patients are often fragmented (Gortmaker *et al.*, 1990; Sabbeth & Stein, 1990).

Patients with chronic medical illness present special challenges to mental health workers, particularly in the inpatient psychiatric setting. Such patients may generate considerable anxiety in staff. These factors and the special needs of this population have encouraged the development of specialty programs, like our own, focusing specifically on the psychiatric inpatient treatment of children and adolescents with physical and psychiatric disorders. Chronically ill children and adolescents exhibit the gamut of psychiatric disorders experienced in children and adolescents who are not medically ill. Though less well studied, psychiatric disorder in the patient or in the family appears to be capable of becoming a significant issue in that patient's medical care. Essentially, just as chronic illness may be a risk factor for psychiatric disorder, psychiatric disorder in the patient or family may result in the exacerbation and possibly even the precipitation of medical illness. Emotional distress, family distress, and/or a diagnosable psychiatric disorder in the patient or a family member may have medical consequences, generally by affecting the disease process psychophysiologically or by affecting treatment adherence or compliance (Dunbar & Waszak, 1990; White, Kolman, Wexler, Polin, & Winter, 1984). Emotional distress or psychiatric disorder in patients or in the families of patients with diabetes mellitus has been implicated as a factor in poor medical compliance, poor metabolic control, and even the precipitation of recurrent diabetic ketoacidosis (Helz & Templeton, 1990).

Table 9. Estimated Prevalence of Selected Chronic Conditions
among Children and Adolescents Aged 4–17 Years[a]

	Estimated prevalence per 1,000
Arthritis	3.4
Asthma	9.3
Blindness	3.3
Cancer (any kind)	0.6
Cardiac: Rheumatic fever, rheumatic or congenital heart disease	0.7
Cerebral palsy	0.9
Cystic fibrosis	0.3
Deafness	5.4
Deformed body part: back, foot, leg, fingers, hand, arm, other deformities	19.4
Diabetes	1.0
Ear, nose, throat: Cleft palate, harelip	0.4
Epilepsy: Convulsions (repeated), seizures (repeated)	3.0
Gastrointestinal: Colitis, ulcer (excluding skin)	1.6
Hearing: Trouble hearing/one ear, trouble hearing/both ears	6.1
Missing body part: Finger, hand, arm, toe, foot, leg	2.1
Orthopedic: Curvature of spine, clubfoot	9.6
Paralysis	0.3
Sickle cell anemia	0.9
Vision: Cataracts, trouble seeing/one eye, trouble seeing/both eyes, other trouble seeing	8.4
Any of 19 chronic condition groups	89.0

[a]From "Chronic Conditions, Socioeconomic Risks, and Behavioral Problems in Children and Adolescents" by S. L. Gortmaker, D. K. Walker, M. Weitzman, and A. M. Sobol, 1990, *Pediatrics*, 85, p. 269. Copyright 1990 by the American Academy of Pediatrics. Adapted by permission.

Exacerbation of asthma, and even death from asthma, have been associated with psychological factors (Mrazek & Miller, 1987; Strunk, Mrazek, Wolfson, & LaBrecque, 1985). Family factors have also been associated with treatment adherence (Steidl, Finkelstein, Wexler, Feigenbaum, Kitsen, Kliger, & Quinlan, 1980).

In addition to the problems inherent in the medical care of such patients during their stay in the psychiatric setting, difficulties in assessment may be faced as well. For example, the diagnosis of depression may be difficult in such patients, the clinical impression being that depression is often underdiagnosed in this population. The symptoms of the medical disorder, particularly somatic symptoms such as pain and fatigue, may be difficult to separate from the somatic symptoms of depression, and vice versa, conceivably resulting in errors in the direction of underdiagnosis and possibly overdiagnosis of depression in the medically ill (Katon, 1982; Rodin & Voshart, 1990). Pain in medical illness is frequently accompanied by depressive symptoms, just as depression may be manifested in painful somatic complaints. It is important to remember that depression may present in the patient with chronic medical illness through the expression of pain, through somatization, through medical noncompliance, or through outright refusal of medical treatment (Rodin & Voshart, 1990). Staff and medical caretakers may dismiss depressive symptoms as a likely consequence of the disorder. Depression may be left undiagnosed and untreated because of the belief that patients with such illnesses "ought to be depressed." Such attitudes may be modified by equating serious depressive symptoms with physical suffering. The fact that many conditions result in physical pain which is "explainable" and "expected" should not prevent the use of analgesics. The same approach holds true with serious psychic pain: It deserves active treatment. Chronic medical illness may also precipitate and foster intense separation fears, and families may adopt rigid coping styles that interfere with age-appropriate development (Drotar & Bush, 1985).

A review of the treatment of psychiatric disorders in the chronically ill child or adolescent is clearly beyond the scope of this chapter, though several principles of treatment and approach to the patient should be highlighted (Drotar & Bush, 1985).

Associated psychiatric disorders should be treated aggressively, and mental health workers should pay special attention to the possible physical complications of treatment (whether that treatment is psychological or medical in the form of medication). Close involvement with the referring medical caretakers should be maintained, as such caretakers often become part of the family system and, on that basis alone, cannot be ignored. In addition, such communication allows for disease-related education and management, which is in keeping with the care of the patient and the family following discharge. The patient and the family should be encouraged to take an active role in their relationships with caregivers in both the medical and the mental health setting, as opposed to their behaving as passive recipients of treatment.

Treatment should be framed as a joint process, as this approach communicates mutual respect and conjoint responsibilities. Shared decision making and responsibility also provide the indirect suggestion that patient and family have the power to manage the situation. Moreover, they enhance the development of appropriate autonomy and competence for both the patient and the family. This enhanced sense of control may be exceedingly important to patients when their medical condition has resulted in a significant loss of control over many areas of their lives. A focus on the strengths of the patient and the family communicates a sense of hope and optimism, when appropriate, and fosters the development of enhanced competence and responsibility. Rather than focusing on the various deficits associated with the chronic illness, a rehabilitative stance is essential, centering on how the patient and the family can manage a chronic disease. This approach includes finding ways in which they can obtain some sense of mastery over the illness (e.g., putting illness "in its place" in relation to the patient's whole life). The patient's and the family's coping strategies must be evaluated within the context of the patient's entire life, rather than with an exclusive focus on the illness. This proviso applies to adherence to medical regimens as well. Adherence is an area where conflict may arise with referring caretakers, who may feel that it is unacceptable for the patient to be working toward anything less than full compliance with the medical regimen. Here, again, focus on the patient's life rather than on the disease is generally beneficial.

Advocacy is important in the care of such patients and their families (Drotar & Bush, 1985; Garrison & McQuiston, 1989). Working closely with schools when the patient is discharged from the hospital is of great importance, and clear, concise recommendations about the patient's physical abilities, the special procedures necessary in the school setting, medication administration, and behavioral management are often very much appreciated by and very helpful to the school personnel. The education of teachers and school nurses by appropriate medical and mental health personnel can play an essential role in helping the patient to be integrated into a more functional lifestyle. Although homebound instruction or tutoring is often popular in the care of chronically ill patients, it should generally be avoided unless absolutely necessary as a result of the physical condition, as it may well have negative long-term effects on the patient's socialization, self-esteem, and development of autonomy (Drotar & Bush, 1985). Homebound instruction may serve as a way of maintaining the profound separation fears that often plague such patients.

Advocacy for the patient for outpatient mental health treatment is also essential, and staff at community mental health centers often benefit from information about the patient's medical and psychiatric illnesses and the ways in which the disorders may interact (Drotar & Bush, 1985). Specialized outpatient programs for children and adolescents are often extremely helpful in this regard, and we have had the good fortune to be part of a comprehensive system of mental health care for children and adolescents with physical disorders (Sabbeth & Stein, 1990). Enhancing socialization with peers is an important part of any treatment regimen and is best accomplished in the hospital through a high-quality, structured group-therapy program. Many such patients have not had the opportunity to speak with other children or adolescents with chronic medical illnesses, and the results are often extremely gratifying. Such patients can benefit from the opportunity to be of support and help to other youngsters who suffer from a chronic physical disorder, and such opportunities enhance the patient's sense of control, autonomy, and self-esteem.

Though the use of traditional individual psychotherapy and play therapy is common, it is poorly studied, and there is limited empirical literature at this time (Garrison & McQuiston, 1989). A variety of behavioral treatment methods have demonstrated efficacy in the treatment of difficulties confronted by patients with chronic medical illness, particularly in the areas of treatment adherence and disease management (Garrison & McQuiston, 1989; LaGreca, 1988; Melamed & Johnson, 1981; Werry & Wollersheim, 1989). For example, stress reduction techniques such as biofeedback, hypnosis, and relaxation training have resulted in enhanced metabolic control in some diabetic patients, though not in all studies (Boehnert & Popkin, 1986; Helz & Templeton, 1990; Nathan, 1985). Individual psychotherapy has been reported to be effective in improving metabolic control in patients with diabetes mellitus, as well as in patients with recurrent diabetic ketoacidosis (Helz & Templeton, 1990). Techniques such as biofeedback, relaxation training, and operant conditioning are of proven relevance and effectiveness in dealing with the psychiatric and physical complications of chronic illness (Garrison & McQuiston, 1989). As mentioned above, group psychotherapy has a number of advantages. Indeed, it has been shown to improve compliance and metabolic control in diabetic patients (Helz & Templeton, 1990). The importance of family therapy and a systems perspective has also been stressed by a number of authors and confirmed by our own clinical experience (Kazak, 1989; Minuchin, Baker, Rosman, Liebman, Milman, & Todd, 1975).

PHYSICAL ILLNESS DEVELOPING IN THE PSYCHIATRIC SETTING

Child and adolescent inpatients, like youngsters everywhere, are subject to a variety of physical illnesses, most of them self-limited. Staff in the psychiatric setting should be alert to the development of physical disorders in their patients. Viral illnesses are especially common. Injuries to the extremities are also common, either as a result of falls, athletic injuries, and so on, or as a result of self-inflicted injuries, such as the boxer's fracture sustained by the patient who punches a seclusion room wall. Staff must also be prepared to deal with the complications of psychiatric treatment, such as allergic drug reactions and medication-related side effects. A routine should be established for the following of vital signs, and there should be increased monitoring of patients in special circumstances, such as those being managed on tricyclic antidepressants. Access to a physician who is well trained and comfortable with common physical disorders in children and adolescents is indispensable in such a setting. Weight should be monitored at least weekly, as many patients demonstrate a significant weight change while in the hospital. Access to appropriate dietary and nutritional evaluation and advice is extremely beneficial, particularly in dealing with patients who have known medical illnesses or who are obese.

PHYSICAL SYMPTOMS AS A PRESENTATION OF PSYCHIATRIC DISORDER

Physical or somatic symptoms are especially common in the general population (Kellner, 1985, 1986), as well as in psychiatrically hospitalized children (Livingston, Taylor, & Crawford, 1988). The evaluation and handling of such physical complaints in the psychiatric setting may be especially difficult because of the power of such symptoms and the social messages and obligations that they may imply. Much has been written about the social aspects of the "sick role," and it is clear that being "sick" can change a person's position in the world. For example, illness "releases" an individual from societal obligations, such as school, work, or interpersonal duties, and the sick person often becomes the object of special duties and attention from those around them (Parsons, 1964; Slavney, 1990). The sick role can be extremely powerful socially, as it can confer benefits and lift burdens, but only after the patient's "sick" role is legitimized by a physician, who in our society is regarded as the final arbiter of who "deserves" that label.

Pilowsky (1969, 1978) developed the concept of "abnormal illness behavior" to describe situations in which "the physician does not believe that the patient's objective pathology entitles him to be placed in the type of sick role he expects, for the reasons which he claims it" (p. 347), but the patient continues in this expectation despite being told by the physician that it is inappropriate. Attempting to understand the patient's motivations in pursuing the sick role under such circumstances becomes important clinically, as conflicts related to autonomy, responsibility, and motivation may be exhibited in the patient's pursuit of the sick role or unwillingness to give it up. The "sick" can expect that they will not be held responsible for their condition, and that others will not see the illness as surmountable simply by an act of will (Parsons, 1964; Slavney, 1990). Goldberg and Bridges (1988) considered "blame-avoidance" a key function of somatization because it allows patients to avoid the stigma of mental illness and possibly allows them to avoid the experience of more intense emotional distress or depression (Pilowsky, 1990).

Motivations for the sick role under conditions of "abnormal illness behavior" have been conceptualized in a variety of ways. Physical symptoms have also been understood as a means of indirect or symbolic communication. Sometimes they allow communication with important persons in the environment, without the "sick" individual's having to face the possible or feared unpleasant consequences of direct communication (Slavney, 1990). Henderson (1974) championed the concept of "care-eliciting behavior," which is described as "a pattern of activity on the part of one individual which evokes from another responses which give comfort" (p. 172). Thus, physical symptoms, like depressive symptoms and anxiety symptoms may elicit nurturant or protective responses from others in the environment and maintain the physical proximity of the patient and important attachment figures.

Traditionally, unexplained physical symptoms believed to be psychogenically derived have been understood through the concepts of *primary gain* and *secondary gain*. Primary gain may be understood as the advantage conveyed by keeping an internal conflict, need, impulse, or memory (as in traumatic memory) out of awareness. It is essentially the relief of emotional distress by symptom production (Lask & Fosson, 1989). Freud (1953) noted that "falling ill involves a saving of psychical effort" (p. 43). *Somatization* itself has been defined as the experience and expression of emotional or psychological distress in physical terms (Lipowski, 1988c). Secondary gain is the benefit conveyed by a symptom in allowing the patient to avoid a "noxious" activity or responsibility, and/or to get support that might not otherwise be forthcoming (Slavney, 1990).

Though the focus here is on somatoform illness, a number of disorders may present with unexplained physical symptoms.

Undiagnosed Medical Illness

Undiagnosed medical illness must be a consideration, as a substantial number of patients with so-called functional complaints may ultimately be diagnosed as having a physical illness that is proved by physical examination, laboratory evaluation, or other diagnostic tests at a later date (Kellner, 1985). The presence of a psychosocial stressor that is temporally associated with the development of a symptom should not automatically result in that symptom's being labeled functional.

Somatoform Disorder

Somatoform disorder is a broad category in the DSM-III-R encompassing patients who suffer from physical symptoms with no demonstrable organic findings or known pathophysiological mechanisms, when there is a strong presumption that the symptoms are linked to psychological factors (American Psychiatric Association, 1987). According to the DSM-III-R criteria, somatoform disorders are not intentionally produced. The most common complaint in children younger than 7 years is abdominal pain; headaches and limb pain tend to become more predominant during adolescence (Apley, 1975; Goodyer & Mitchell, 1989). Symptoms suggesting abnormalities in neurological function, such as those of gait, faints, and pseudoseizures, appear to become more likely with increasing age (Goodyer & Mitchell, 1989). Though these disorders have not been especially well studied in children and adolescents, a variety of subcategories of somatoform disorder within the DSM-III-R are worth reviewing from both a practical and conceptual standpoint.

Somatoform Pain Disorder. This disorder appears to be the most common of the somatoform disorders. It is regarded as a somatoform disorder where the preoccupation is with pain in the absence of physical findings that account for the presence or intensity of pain (American Psychiatric Association, 1987). *Recurrent abdominal pain* in children is an extremely common example: up to 15% of school-aged children report recurrent abdominal discomfort that is associated with academic or social dysfunction, and only 10% of these children have a demonstrable organic etiology (Apley, 1975; Garber, Zeman, & Walker, 1990). These patients have been shown in a number of studies to have higher rates of anxiety and depressive disorders than normal controls, separation fears and school refusal being particularly common (Garber *et al.*, 1990; Hodges, Kline, Barbero, & Flanery, 1985; Wasserman, Whitington, & Rivara, 1988). Mothers of such patients have also been reported to be significantly more anxious and depressed than mothers of healthy controls, and a preponderance of somatization disorder has also been noted in the families of such patients (Garber *et al.*, 1990; Hodges *et al.*, 1985; Routh & Ernst, 1984; Walker & Greene, 1989). One study (Routh & Ernst, 1984) also suggested increased rates of alcoholism, antisocial personality, conduct disorder, and attention deficit disorder in the families of patients with functional abdominal pain.

Conversion Disorder. This disorder is an alteration in or loss of physical functioning that suggests a physical disorder, but that appears to express a psychological conflict or need (American Psychiatric Association, 1987). The presenting physical complaints include pseudo-seizures, other movement difficulties such as gait disturbance or paralysis, and sensory problems, though all manner of motor and sensory symptoms have been noted (Klykylo, McConville, & Maloney, 1990; Volkmar, Poll, & Lewis, 1984). Conversion symptoms, particularly pseudo-seizures, have been associated in the literature with sexually traumatic events, and examiners should be alert to the possibility of previous psychological trauma in such patients (Goodwin, Simms, & Bergman, 1979; Gross, 1979; Volkmar et al., 1984). Conversion symptoms have also been associated with depression in children and adolescents (Lesse, 1981; Weller & Weller, 1983).

Hypochondriasis. This disorder is the fear of having or the belief that one has a serious disease. This belief persists despite medical reassurance to the contrary (American Psychiatric Association, 1987). Transient hypochondriasis is common in response to stressful life events (Kellner, 1985), and it may be based on interpreting physical signs or sensations as evidence of physical illness. Such patients often amplify normal sensory input and incorrectly assess and misinterpret normal bodily sensations or signs of emotional arousal (Barsky, Goodson, Lane, & Cleary, 1988). Like other somatoform disorders, hypochondriasis is often associated with anxiety and depressive symptoms (Kellner, 1986).

Somatization Disorder. This disorder is a syndrome at the extreme end of somatoform illness, the diagnosis being based on recurrent and multiple somatic complaints of several years' duration, for which medical care has been sought, but which are not apparently due to a diagnosable physical disorder (American Psychiatric Association, 1987). Somatization disorder has also been referred to as *Briquet's syndrome* and *hysteria*. The majority of diagnosed cases are female in the adult literature. Though the disorder is felt to begin relatively early in life, and Briquet's original paper described 20% of cases beginning before puberty (Mai & Merskey, 1980), diagnosis of the full-blown disorder is relatively uncommon in children. Because of the number of symptoms necessary to make this rather specific diagnosis, it is more common during adolescence (Klykylo et al., 1990). Somatization disorder has been diagnosed in prepubertal children, though rarely, and there is much interest in identifying which child and adolescent patients with somatoform illness will go on to develop full-blown somatization disorders (Ernst, Routh, & Harper, 1984; Goodyer & Mitchell, 1989; Livingston & Martin-Cannici, 1985).

Undifferentiated Somatoform Disorder. This diagnosis is made in the DSM-III-R when somewhat chronic multiple somatic complaints are present that do not meet the criteria for a diagnosis of somatization disorder proper. Children and adolescents with multiple functional somatic complaints are most likely to be placed within this category, when the diagnosis is properly applied.

Body Dysmorphic Disorder. This disorder is a preoccupation with some imagined defect in a normal-appearing person or excessive concern over a slight physical abnormality or anomaly (American Psychiatric Association, 1987). These patients often present in their teenage years or early 20s and may suffer from an additional serous psychiatric illness, such as schizophrenia, severe personality disorder, or obsessive-compulsive disorder (Thomas, 1985). Occasionally, patients with a serious eating disorder may present with concerns about a particular body area. These patients may actively pursue cosmetic surgery.

Factitious Disorder with Physical Symptoms

Factitious disorder with physical symptoms is a disorder in which the physical symptoms are feigned or intentionally produced, the goal being the attainment of the sick role (American Psychiatric Association, 1987). The patient may present factitious illness in three ways: by giving a factitious history, by simulating the signs of a disease, and by actively creating a physical illness (Eisendrath, 1989). Factitious disorder has been known by a variety of different names, including *Munchausen syndrome*, and cases have been described of *Munchausen syndrome by proxy*, in which children present with unexplained physical symptoms that have been intentionally produced or feigned by a caretaker (Meadow, 1982). These patients often have a history of emotional and physical deprivation, abuse, neglect, or hospitalization early in childhood (Eisendrath, 1989; Palmer & Yoshimura, 1984).

Malingering

Malingering is the intentional production or feigning of physical symptoms for an external purpose, such as obtaining financial compensation, obtaining drugs, or avoiding school, work, prosecution, or other obligations (American Psychiatric Association, 1987). These patients tend to have serious conduct disorders or antisocial personality traits.

Psychophysiological Disorders

Psychophysiological disorders (psychological factors affecting a medical condition) are disorders in which psychologically meaningful environmental stimuli are temporally related to the initiation or exacerbation of a specific physical condition or disorder (American Psychiatric Association, 1987). Examples are tension headaches, some migraine headaches, some patients with recurrent diabetic ketoacidosis, and some cases of asthma, as well as a myriad of other disorders. In the past, many of these disorder were referred to as *psychosomatic disorders*. There may well be a significant overlap between patients classified as having psychophysiological disorders, those patients with chronic illness who are suffering from treatment failure, and patients with somatoform illness (significant depressive and anxiety symptoms are common to all three groups). In a study by Garber *et al.* (1990), young patients with an organic explanation of their abdominal discomfort (generally peptic ulcer disease or inflammatory bowel disease) had rates of anxiety and depressive disorders similar to those of patients with somatoform pain. All of these patients had significantly more anxiety and depression than healthy controls. These findings suggest that somatoform illness and psychophysiological illness are linked in some way, though other explanations certainly are possible. It is of interest that the lifetime prevalence of depressive illness was significantly greater in patients with inflammatory bowel disease when these patients were compared with a control group of chronically ill children with cystic fibrosis (Burke, Meyer, Kocoshis, Orenstein, Chandra, Nord, Sauer, & Cohen, 1989).

Primary Psychiatric Disorders

Primary psychiatric disorders, particularly anxiety and depressive disorders, are frequently associated with physical symptoms. Livingston *et al.* (1988) explored unexplained somatic complaints in 95 psychiatrically hospitalized children aged 6–12. Headaches, food intolerance, abdominal pain, buzzing in the ears, nausea, and dizziness were each reported by at least 25% of the patients. Most were not associated with a particular psychiatric diagnosis, though abdominal pain appeared to be specifically associated with depression, separation anxiety, and psychosis, which in this study was most often the likely result of psychotic depression. Palpitations were common symptoms in separation anxiety disorder and psychosis. Other uncommon symptoms of neurological disorder, such as pseudoseizures and paralysis were most often reported by children with psychosis and possible somatization disorder, as determined by a structured psychiatric interview. Psychiatric diagnoses of somatization disorder, psychosis, and separation anxiety disorder were associated with significantly greater mean numbers of somatic symptoms, though physical symptoms were common in a variety of different psychiatric disorders. Girls tended to report more physical symptoms than boys, and the absolute number of somatic symptoms also appeared to be associated with a history of sexual abuse (Livingston, 1987; Livingston et al., 1988).

Others have reported increased somatic and behavioral difficulties in patients with a history of sexual abuse months to years after the abuse was reported and had supposedly ended (Rimza, Berg, & Locke, 1988). Recent evidence that vulnerability to anxiety and depressive disorders may be linked genetically or developmentally is of great interest (Merikangas, Prusoff, & Weissman, 1988), and the possibility that somatoform disorders and psychophysiological disorders are related to the anxiety and depressive disorders should also be kept in mind, given the frequent clinical association of anxiety, depression, and somatic complaints.

The remaining discussion focuses primarily on the somatoform disorders. Vulnerability to somatoform disorder may be conceptualized in terms of predisposing, precipitating, or perpetuating factors (Kellner, 1985, 1986). The *predisposing factors* appear to include genetic and familial variables. In many patients, the functional somatic symptom may resemble the symptoms of other family members. A child's attentiveness to a given symptom may be related to the amount of interest shown in that symptom by the caretakers (Kriechman, 1987; Lehmkuhl, Blanz, Lehmkuhl, & Braun-Scharm, 1989; Robinson, Alverez, & Dodge, 1990; Steinhausen, Aster, Pfeiffer, & Gobel, 1989; Volkmar et al., 1984). Parental bereavement in childhood has been associated with somatic complaints later in life, and patients from lower socioeconomic groups and with less education tend to be at greater risk. Some studies have shown that certain cultural groups, such as American Hispanics, are especially prone to somatization (Escobar, Rubio-Stipec, Canino, & Karno, 1989). In addition, the presence of an actual physical disease may predispose the patient to functional somatic complaints, organic brain disease, as in epilepsy, being an especially notable risk factor (Kellner, 1986). A significant proportion of patients with pseudoseizures also suffer from actual epilepsy (Shapiro & Rosenfeld, 1987; Williams & Hirsch, 1988).

Precipitating factors have also been noted in somatoform illness. The attention in the literature has been on stressful life events such as recent bereavement, physical disease, and other significant psychological trauma (e.g., sexual abuse) (Kellner, 1986; Rimsza et al., 1988; Volkmar et al., 1984). In bereavement, the physical symptoms may resemble the symptoms of the lost individual.

Perpetuating or maintaining factors may largely be encompassed by the concept of secondary gain. The symptoms may be perpetuated by performing unnecessary tests, giving an inappropriate diagnosis, or by the patient's being granted special status or some degree of financial compensation or disability benefit (Kellner, 1986).

The *treatment* of patients with somatoform illness should follow a careful medical and physical evaluation. Information about treatment methods and outcome in somatoform illness in children and adolescents is limited (Shapiro & Rosenfeld, 1987; Werry & Wollersheim, 1989). Unnecessary laboratory tests or diagnostic procedures should be avoided (Leslie, 1988; Shapiro & Rosenfeld, 1987). The possibility that psychological factors may be involved in the symptom should be presented early to the patient and should generally be included in the differential diagnosis. Once a clear clinical impression is derived, it should be discussed frankly and clearly with the patient and the family. Ambiguous diagnostic statements should be avoided, and it should be emphasized that the diagnosis of a somatoform disorder is not simply one of exclusion. The reality of the symptom should not be challenged, and the patient's suffering should be acknowledged (Klykylo et al., 1990). Most workers in the field advocate symptom removal, followed by some treatment of the underlying psychopathology, the idea being that the symptom must be viewed as less threatening if treatment is to proceed (Kellner, 1986; Klykylo et al., 1990). It is important to avoid the promise of a "cure." Instead, the focus should be on patient and staff's working together to keep the troubling physical symptom or symptoms from seriously interfering with the patient's life. This rehabilitative approach is extremely useful, as it is essential that secondary gain be minimized (Blackwell, Merskey, & Kellner, 1989).

Behavioral methods are often extremely helpful in this regard. Some patients are able to return to their usual responsibilities and functioning only gradually (Werry & Wollersheim, 1989). The expectation that the patient will return to the usual responsibilities should be communicated matter-of-factly, and with a reassuring tone. Such an approach acknowledges the patient's suffering but avoids sanctioning secondary gain, and in the end, it is probably the most compassionate approach in most instances. With children and adolescents, this approach is helpful in convincing the patient (and often the family) that he or she is "strong enough" to overcome the problem. Associated psychiatric disorders should be diagnosed and treated appropriately in such patients, and antidepressant or antianxiety agents may be especially helpful (Kellner, 1985).

Psychotherapy may take a variety of forms, and many patients respond to a supportive approach characterized by reassurance and education that clarifies misconceptions of the patient related to bodily perceptions or to previously made physical diagnoses. Physical exercise may be usefully prescribed when available and appropriate, and other techniques that enable the patient to take control of the situation are especially helpful, such as relaxation training, biofeedback, and hypnosis (Olness, 1986; Werry & Wollersheim, 1989; Williamson, McKenzie, Goreczny, & Faulstich, 1987). Cognitive behavioral strategies (Salkovskis, 1989) have been used, as well as psychodynamically oriented psychotherapy, group therapy (Kellner, 1986), and family therapy (Minuchin et al., 1978). Specialized inpatient treatment programs for refractory patients have been developed in adult psychiatry (Lipowski, 1988b), and programs for children and adolescents like our own are becoming more common. Although patients with somatoform disorders have often been painted as having a bad prognosis, the available evidence suggests that, in a large number of patients, the outcome is very good (Apley & Hale, 1973; Kellner, 1985). Good prognostic factors are felt to include an acute onset of the symptoms, a shorter duration of the illness, diagnosable anxiety or depression, the absence of personality disorder, higher socioeconomic status, younger age, the absence of organic disease, and few previous referrals to medical physicians (Kellner, 1985, 1986).

SUMMARY

Medical issues become important in the psychiatric setting in a variety of ways, though it should be understood that the physical and the psychological cannot truly be separated, other than conceptually. Physical illness may present with symptoms of psychiatric disorder, and patients with medical illness may suffer all varieties of psychiatric disturbance and may be especially vulnerable to it. Physical complaints and injuries arise commonly in hospitalized children and adolescents. Unexplained physical complaints are common in child and adolescent psychiatric patients and may reflect symptoms of a variety of psychiatric disorders. The importance of careful medical and physical assessment cannot be overemphasized, and access to appropriate medical treatment and maintenance is essential, particularly for the chronically ill. Collaboration with a physician trained in the medical problems of children and adolescents is mandatory, but staff should also have a working familiarity and sense of comfort with medical assessment and treatment.

ACKNOWLEDGMENTS.   The clerical assistance of Ms. June Husar and the editorial comments of Dr. Judith Marsh and Dr. Deborah Moss are gratefully acknowledged.

REFERENCES

American Psychiatric Association. (1987). *Diagnostic and statistical manual of mental disorders* (3rd ed., rev.; DSM-III-R). Washington, DC: Author.
Apley, J. (1975). *The child with abdominal pain*. Oxford: Blackwell.

Apley, J., & Hale, B. (1973). Children with recurrent abdominal pain: How do they grow up? *British Medical Journal, 3*, 7–9.

Bancroft, J., Axworthy, D., & Ratcliffe, S. (1982). The personality and psychosexual development of boys with the 47XXY chromosome constitution. *Journal of Child Psychology and Psychiatry, 23*, 167–180.

Barkowsky, H., & Schady, W. (1982). Neurologic manifestations of acute porphyria. *Seminars in Liver Disease, 2*, 108–124.

Barreira, P. J. (1989). Depression. In A. Lazare (Ed.), *Outpatient psychiatry: Diagnosis and treatment* (2nd ed., pp. 252–255). Baltimore: Williams & wilkins.

Barsky, A. J., Goodson, J. D., Lane, R. S., & Cleary, P. D. (1988). The amplification of somatic symptoms. *Psychosomatic Medicine, 50*, 510–519.

Bauer, M. S., Whybrow, P. C., & Winokur, A. (1990). Rapid cycling bipolar affective disorder: 1. Association with grade I hypothyroidism. *Archives of General Psychiatry, 47*, 427–432.

Blackman, M., & Wheler, G. H. T. (1987). A case of mistaken identity: A fourth ventricular tumor presenting as school phobia in a 12 year old boy. *Canadian Journal of Psychiatry, 32*, 584–587.

Blackwell, B., Merskey, H., & Kellner, R. (1989). Somatoform pain disorders. In American Psychiatric Association Task Force on Treatments of Psychiatric Disorders, *Treatments of psychiatric disorders* (pp. 2120–2138). Washington, DC: American Psychiatric Association.

Boehnert, C. E., & Popkin, M. K. (1986). Psychological issues in treatment of severely noncompliant diabetics. *Psychosomatics, 27*, 11–20.

Boon, F. F. L., & Ellis, C. (1989). Acute intermittent porphyria in a children's psychiatric hospital. *Journal of American Academy of Child and Adolescent Psychiatry, 28*(4), 606–609.

Bravo, E. L., Tarazi, R. C., Gifford, R. W., & Stewart, B. H. (1979). Circulatory and urinary catecholamines pheochromocytoma: Diagnosis and pathophysiologic implications. *New England Journal of Medicine, 301*, 682–686.

Bregman, J. D., Dykens, E., Watson, M., Ort, S. I., & Leckman, J. F. (1987). Fragile-X syndrome: variability of phenotypic expression. *Journal of the American Academy of Child and Adolescent Psychiatry, 26*, 463–471.

Brent, D. A., Crumrine, P. K., Varma, R. R., Allan, M., & Allman, C. (1987). Phenobarbital treatment and major depressive disorder in children with epilepsy. *Pediatrics, 80*, 909–917.

Breslau, N. (1990a). Chronic physical illness. In B. J. Tonge, G. D. Burrows, & J. S. Werry (Eds.), *Handbook of studies on child psychiatry*, (pp. 371–384). New York: Elsevier.

Breslau, N. (1990b). Does brain dysfunction increase children's vulnerability to environmental stress? *Archives of General Psychiatry, 47*, 15–20.

Brown, G., Chadwick, D., Shaffer, D., Rutter, M., & Traub, M. (1981). A prospective study of children with head injuries: 3. Psychiatric sequelae. *Psychological Medicine. 2*, 63–78.

Burke, P., DelBeccaro, M., McCauley, E., & Clark, C. (1985). Hallucinations in children. *Journal of American Academy of Child Psychiatry, 24*(1), 71–75.

Burke, P., Meyer, V., Kocoshis, S., Orenstein, D. M., Chandra, R., Nord, D. H., Sauer, J., & Cohen, E. (1989). Depression and anxiety in pediatric inflammatory bowel disease and cystic fibrosis. *Journal of American Academy Child and Adolescent Psychiatry, 28*(6), 948–951.

Casat, C. D., Ross, B. A., Scardina, R. Sarno, C., & Smith, K. E. (1987). Separation anxiety and mitral valve prolapse in a 12 year old girl. *Journal of American Academy of Child and Adolescent Psychiatry, 26*(3), 444–446.

Costello, E. J., Edlebrock, C., Costello, A. J., Dulcan, M. K., Burns, B. J., & Brent, D. (1988). Psychopathology in pediatric primary care: the new hidden morbidity. *Pediatrics, 82*(3), 415–424.

Crumley, F. E. (1990). Pitfalls of diagnosis in the early stages of Wilson's disease. *Journal of American Academy of Child and Adolescent Psychiatry, 29*(3), 470–471.

Dahl, R. E. (1992). Child and adolescent sleep disorders. In D. M. Kaufman (Ed.), *Neurology for child psychiatrists*. Baltimore: Williams & Wilkins.

Dening, T. R., & Berrios, G. E. (1989). Wilson's disease. *Archives of General Psychiatry, 46*, 1126–1134.

Detre, T. (1987). The future of psychiatry. *American Journal of Psychiatry, 144*, 621–625.

Dilsaver, S. C., & Greden, J. F. (1984). Antidepressant withdrawal-induced activation (hypomania and mania): Mechanism and theoretical significance. *Brain Research, 319*, 29–48.

Drotar, D., & Bush, M. (1985). Mental health issues and services. In N. Hobbs & J. M. Perrin (Eds.), *Issues in the care of children with chronic illness* (pp. 514–550). San Francisco: Jossey-Bass.

Dunbar, J., & Waszak, L. (1990). Patient compliance: Pediatric and adolescent populations. In A. M. Gross & R. S. Drabman (Eds.), *Handbook of clinical behavioral pediatrics* (pp. 365–382). New York: Plenum Press.

Edeh, J., & Toone, B. K. (1985). Anti-epileptic therapy, folate deficiency, and psychiatric morbidity: A general practice survey. *Epilepsia, 26*(5), 434–440.

Eisendrath, S. J. (1989). Factitious disorder with physical symptoms. In American Psychiatric Association Task Force on Treatments of Psychiatric Disorders, *Treatments of psychiatric disorders* (pp. 2159–2164). Washington, DC: American Psychiatric Association.

Ernst, A. R., Routh, D. K., & Harper, D. C. (1984). Abdominal pain in children and symptoms of somatization disorder. *Journal of Pediatric Psychology*, 9, 77–86.

Escobar, J. I., Rubio-Stipec, M., Canino, G., & Karno, M. (1989). Somatic symptom index (SSI): A new abridged somatization construct. *Journal of Nervous and Mental Diseases*, 177, 140–146.

Feingold, B. F. (1975). Hyperkinesis and learning disabilities linked to artificial food flavors and colors. *American Journal of Nursing*, 75, 797–803.

Fenichel, G. M. (1988). *Clinical pediatric neurology*. Philadelphia: W. B. Saunders.

Frank, R., & Doerr, H. G. (1989). Mania in a girl with cushing's disease. *Journal of American Academy for Child and Adolescent Psychiatry*, 28(4), 610–611.

Freud, S. (1953). Fragment of an analysis of a case of hysteria. In J. Strachey (Ed.), *The standard edition of the complete psychological works of Sigmund Freud* (Vol. 7, pp. 1–122). London: Hogarth Press.

Gabel, R. H., Barnard, N., Norko, M., & O'Connell, R. A. (1986). AIDS presenting as mania. *Comprehensive Psychiatry*, 27, 251–254.

Garber, J., Zeman, J., & Walker, L. S. (1990). Recurrent abdominal pain in children: Psychiatric diagnoses and parental psychopathology. *Journal of the American Academy of Child and Adolescent Psychiatry*, 29, 648–656.

Garrison, W. T., & McQuiston, S. (1989). *Chronic illness during childhood and adolescence: Psychological aspects*. Newbury Park, CA: Sage.

Goldberg, D. P., & Bridges, K. (1988). Somatic presentations of psychiatric illness in the primary care setting. *Psychosomatic Research*, 32, 136–144.

Goodwin, J., Simms M., & Bergman, R. (1979). Hysterical seizures in 4 adolescent girls. *American Journal of Orthopsychiatry*, 49, 698–703.

Goodyer, I. M., & Mitchell, C. (1989). Somatic emotional disorders in childhood and adolescence. *Journal of Psychosomatic Research*, 33, 681–688.

Gortmaker, S. L., Walker, D. K., Weitzman, M., & Sobol, A. M. (1990). Chronic conditions, socioeconomic risks, and behavioral problems in children and adolescents. *Pediatrics*, 85, 267–276.

Greden, J. F., Fontaine, P., Lubetsky, M., & Chamberlin, K. (1978). Anxiety and depression associated with caffeinism among psychiatric inpatients. *American Journal of Psychiatry*, 135, 963–966.

Greenberg, D. B. (1990). Neurasthenia in the 1980's: Chronic mononucleosis, chronic fatigue syndrome, and anxiety and depressive disorders. *Psychosomatics*, 31, 129–137.

Greenhill, L. L. (1990). Attention deficit hyperactivity disorder in children. In B. D. Garfinkel, G. A. Carlson, & E. P. Weller (Eds.), *Psychiatric disorders in children and adolescents* (pp. 149–170). Philadelphia: W. B. Saunders.

Gross, M. (1979). Incestuous rape: A cause for hysterical seizures in 4 adolescent girls. *American Journal of Orthopsychiatry*, 49, 704–708.

Gudex, M., & Werry, J. S. (1990). Organic and substance use disorders. In B. J. Tonge, G. D. Burrows, & J. S. Werry (Eds.), *Handbook of studies on child psychiatry* (pp. 107–122). New York: Elsevier.

Hall, R. C. W. (1980). Medically induced psychiatric disease—An overview. In R. C. W. Hall (Ed.), *Psychiatric presentations of medical illness: Somatopsychic disorders* (pp. 3–11). New York: Spectrum.

Hanesian, H., Paez, P., & Williams, D. T. (1988). The neurologically impaired child and adolescent. In C. J. Kestenbaum & D. T. Williams (Eds.), *Handbook of clinical assessment of children and adolescents* (pp. 415–445). New York: New York University Press.

Helz, J. W., & Templeton, B. (1990). Evidence of the role of psychosocial factors in diabetes mellitus: A review. *American Journal of Psychiatry*, 147, 1275–1282.

Henderson, S. (1974). Care eliciting behavior in man. *Journal of Mental and Nervous Disease*, 159, 172–181.

Hodges, K. Kline, J. J., Barbero, G., & Flanery, R. (1985). Depressive symptoms in children with recurrent abdominal pain and in their families. *Journal of Pediatrics*, 107, 622–626.

Katon, W. (1984). Depression: Relationship to somatization and chronic medical illness. *Journal of Clinical Psychiatry*, 45, 4–11.

Kazak, A. E. (1989). Families of chronically ill children: A systems and social-ecological model of adaptation and challenge. *Journal of Consulting and Clinical Psychology*, 57, 25–30.

Kellner, R. (1985). Functional somatic symptoms and hypochondriasis. *Archives of General Psychiatry*, 42, 821–833.

Kellner, R. (1986). *Somatization and hypochondriasis*. New York: Praeger.

Klykylo, W. M., McConville, B. J., & Maloney, M. J. (1990). Somatoform and eating disorders. In B. J. Tonge,

G. D. Burrows, & J. S. Werry (Eds.), *Handbook of studies on child psychiatry*, (pp. 243–263). New York: Elsevier.

Koranyi, E. K. (1979). Morbidity and rate of undiagnosed physical illness in a psychiatric clinic population. *Archives of General Psychiatry*, *36*, 414–419.

Kovacs, M. (1989). Affective disorders in children and adolescents. *American Psychologist*, *44*, 209–215.

Krauthammer, C. & Klerman, G. L. (1978). Secondary mania: Manic syndromes associated with antecedent physical illness or drugs. *Archives of General Psychiatry*, *35*, 1333–1339.

Krener, P., & Miller, F. B. (1989). Psychiatric response to HIV spectrum disease in children and adolescents. *Journal of American Academy of Child and Adolescent Psychiatry*, *36*, 414–419.

Kriechman, A. M. (1987). Siblings with somatoform disorders in childhood and adolescence. *Journal of the American Academy of Child and Adolescent Psychiatry*, *26*, 226–231.

Kruesi, M. J. P. (1990). Biological risk factors in the etiology of childhood psychiatric disorders. In B. J. Tonge, G. D. Burrows, & J. S. Werry (Eds.), *Handbook of studies on child psychiatry* (pp. 13–28). New York: Elsevier.

LaGreca, A. N. (1988). Adherence to prescribed medical regimens. In D. K. Routh (Ed.), *Handbook of pediatric psychology* (pp. 299–320). New York: Guilford Press.

Landman, G. B. (1990). Disorders of elimination: Encopresis and enuresis. In F. A. Oski (Ed. in chief), C. D., DeAngelis, R. D. Feigin, & J. B. Warshaw (Eds.), *Principles and practice of pediatrics* (pp. 690–697). Philadelphia: J. B. Lippincott.

Lask, B., & Fosson, A. (1989). *Childhood illness: The psychosomatic approach*. New York: Wiley.

Lawlor, T., & Lazare, A. (1989). Anxiety. In A. Lazare (Ed.), *Outpatient psychiatry: Diagnosis and treatment* (2nd ed., pp. 246–251). Baltimore: Williams & Wilkins.

Lazare, A. (1989). Medical disorders in psychiatric populations. In A. Lazare (Ed.), *Outpatient psychiatry: Diagnosis and treatment* (2nd ed., pp. 240–245). Baltimore: Williams & Wilkins.

Lehmkuhl, G., Blanz, B., Lehmkuhl, U., & Braun-Scharm, H. (1989). Conversion disorder: Symptomatology and course in childhood and adolescence. *European Archives of Psychiatry and Neurological Sciences*, *238*, 155–160.

Leslie, S. A. (1988). Diagnosis and treatment of hysterical conversion reactions. *Archives of Diseases of Children*, *63*(5), 506–511.

Lesse, S. (1981). Hypochondriacal and psychosomatic disorders masking depression in adolescents. *American Journal of Psychotherapy*, *35*, 356–367.

Lipowski, Z. J. (1988a). Delirium (acute confusional states). *Journal of American Medical Association*, *258*, 1789–1792.

Lipowski, Z. J. (1988b). An inpatient program for persistent somatizers. *Canadian Journal of Psychiatry*, *32*, 275–278.

Lipowski, Z. J. (1988c). Somatization: The concept and its clinical application. *American Journal of Psychiatry*, *145*, 1358–1368.

Lishman, W. A. (1987). *Organic psychiatry: The psychological consequences of cerebral disorder* (2nd ed.). Oxford: Blackwell Scientific.

Livingston, R. (1987). Sexually and physically abused children. *Journal of the American Academy of Child and Adolescent Psychiatry*, *26*, 413–415.

Livingston, R., & Martin-Cannici, C. (1985). Multiple somatic complaints and possible somatization disorder in prepubertal children. *Journal of the American Academy of Child Psychiatry*, *24*, 603–607.

Livingston, R., Taylor, J. L., & Crawford, S. L. (1988). A study of somatic complaints and psychiatric diagnosis in children. *Journal of the American Academy of Child and Adolescent Psychiatry*, *27*, 185–187.

Mai, F., & Mersky, H. (1980). Briquet's treatise on hysteria: A synopsis and commentary. *Archives of General Psychiatry*, *37*, 1401–1405.

Mallory, G. B., Fiser, D. H., & Jackson, R. (1989). Sleep associated breathing disorders in morbidly obese children and adolescents. *Journal of Pediatrics*, *115*, 892–897.

Maltbie, A. A. (1983). Psychosis. In J. O. Cavenar & H. K. H. Brodie (Eds.), *Signs and symptoms in psychiatry* (pp. 413–432). Philadelphia: J. B. Lippincott.

Manschreck, T. C., & Keller, M. B. (1989a). Disturbances of thinking. In A. Lazare (Ed.), *Outpatient psychiatry: Diagnosis and treatment* (2nd ed., pp. 267–273). Baltimore: Williams & Wilkins.

Manschreck, T. C., & Keller, M. B. (1989b). Perceptual disturbances. In A. Lazare (Ed.), *Outpatient psychiatry: Diagnosis and treatment* (2nd ed., pp. 274–279). Baltimore: Williams & Wilkins.

Massion, A. O., & Benjamin, S. (1989). Manic behavior. In A. Lazare (Ed.), *Outpatient psychiatry: Diagnosis and treatment* (2nd ed., pp. 256–266). Baltimore: Williams & Wilkins.

McCauley, E., Ito, J., & Kay, T. (1986). Psychosocial functioning in girls with Turner's syndrome and short stature:

Social skills, behavior problems and self concept. *Journal of the American Academy of Child Psychiatry, 25,* 105–112.

McHugh, P. R., & Slavney, P. R. (1983). *The perspectives of psychiatry.* Baltimore: Johns Hopkins University Press.

Meadow, R. (1982). Munchausen syndrome by proxy. *Archives of Diseases of Children, 60,* 92–98.

Medical Letter. (1989). Drugs that cause psychiatric symptoms. *Medical Letter on Drugs and Therapeutics, 31,* 113–118.

Meijer, A., Zakay-Rones, Z., & Morag, A. (1988). Post influenzal psychiatric disorder in adolescents. *Acta-Psychiatra Scandinavian, 78,* 176–181.

Melamed, B. G., & Johnson, S. B. (1981). Chronic illness: Asthma and juvenile diabetes. In E. J. Mash & L. G. Tertal (Eds.), *Behavioral assessment of childhood disorders* (pp. 529–572). New York: Guilford Press.

Merikangas, K. R., Prusoff, B. A., & Weissman, M. M. (1988). Parental concordance for affective disorders: Psychopathology in offspring. *Journal of Affective Disorders, 15,* 279–290

Merikangas, K. R., Angst, J., & Isler, H. (1990). Migraine and psychopathology. *Archives of General Psychiatry, 47,* 849–853.

Minuchin, S., Baker, L., Rosman, B. L., Liebman, R., Milman, L., & Todd, T. C. (1975). A conceptual model of psychosomatic illness in children. *Archives of General Psychiatry, 32,* 1031–138.

Mrazek, D. A., & Miller, B. D. (1987). The pediatric patient with severe asthma and psychiatric illness: Diagnostic and therapeutic considerations. *Seminars in Respiratory Medicine, 8,* 347–352.

Nathan, S. W. (1985). Psychological aspects of recurrent diabetic ketoacidosis in preadolescent boys. *American Journal of Psychotherapy, 39,* 193–205.

Needleman, H. L., Gunnoe, C., Leviton, A., Reed, R., Peresie, H., Maher, C., & Barrett, P. (1979). Deficits in psychologic and classroom performance of children with elevated dentine lead levels. *New England Journal of Medicine, 300,* 689–695.

Olness, K. N. (1986). Hypnotherapy in children: New approach to solving common pediatric problems. *Postgraduate Medicine, 79,* 95–105.

Oski, F. A. (1979). The nonhematologic manifestations of iron deficiency. *American Journal of Diseases of Children, 133,* 315.

Palmer, A., & Yoshimura, G. J. (1984). Munchausen syndrome by proxy. *Journal of the American Academy of Child Psychiatry, 23,* 503–508.

Parsons, T. (1964). *Social structure and personality.* New York: Free Press.

Pilowsky, D., & Chambers, W. (Eds.). (1986). *Hallucinations in children.* Washington, DC: American Psychiatric Press.

Pilowsky, I. (1969). Abnormal illness behavior. *British Journal of Medical Psychology, 42,* 347–351.

Pilowsky, I. (1978). A general classification of abnormal illness behaviors. *British Journal of Medical Psychology, 51,* 131–137.

Pilowsky, I. (1990). Neurosis manifesting in physical symptoms. *Current Opinion in Psychiatry, 3,* 204–210.

Pitcher, D. (1981). Sex chromosome disorders. *CRC Critical Reviews in Clinical Laboratory Sciences, 13,* 241–282.

Prugh, D. G. (1983). *The psychosocial aspects of pediatrics.* Philadelphia: Lea & Febiger.

Prugh, D., Wagonfeld, S., Metcalf, D., & Jordan, K. (1980). A clinical study of delirium in children and adolescents. *Psychosomatic Medicine, 42,* 177–195.

Puig-Antich, J. (1986). Psychobiological markers: Effects of age and puberty. In M. Rutter, C. E. Izard, & P. B. Read (Eds.), *Depression in young people: Developmental and clinical perspectives* (pp. 341–381). New York: Guilford Press.

Rachelefsky, G. S., Wo, J., Adelson, J., Mickey, M. R., Spector, S. L., Katz, R. M., Siegel, S. C., & Rohr, A. S. (1986). Behavior abnormalities and poor school performance due to oral theophylline use. *Pediatrics, 78,* 1133–1138.

Raiten, D. J. (1990). The medical basis for nutrition and behavior. In B. D. Garfinkel, G. A. Carlson, & E. D. Weller (Eds.), *Psychiatric disorders in children and adolescents* (pp. 410–427). Philadelphia: W. B. Saunders.

Rapoport, J. L. (1980). Congenital anomalies, appearance and body build. In M. Rutter (Ed.), *Scientific foundations of developmental psychiatry* (pp. 40–47). London: Heinemann Medical Books.

Realmuto G. M., Garfinkel, D. D., Tuchman, M., Tsai, M. Y., Chang, P., Fisch, R. O., & Shapiro, S. (1986). Psychiatric diagnosis and behavioral characteristics of phenylketonuric children. *Journal of Nervous and Mental Disease, 174,* 536–540.

Rimsza, M. E., Berg, R. A., & Locke, C. (1988). Sexual abuse: Somatic and emotional reactions. *Child Abuse and Neglect, 12,* 201–208.

Rix, K. H. B., Pearson, D., & Bentley, S. (1984). A psychiatric study of patients with supposed food allergy. *British Journal of Psychiatry, 145,* 121–126.

Robinson, J. O., Alverez, J. H., & Dodge, J. A. (1990). Life events and family history in children with recurrent abdominal pain. *Journal of Psychosomatic Research, 34,* 171–181.

Rodin, G., & Voshart, K. (1990). Depression in the medically ill: An overview. *American Journal of Psychiatry, 143,* 696–705.

Rogeness, G. A., Hernandez, J. M., Macedo, C. A., Amrung, S. A., & Hoppe, S. K. (1986). Near zero plasma dopamine beta hydroxylase and conduct disorder in emotionally disturbed boys. *Journal of the American Academy of Child Psychiatry, 25,* 521–527.

Rosèn, L. A., & Beyers, J. A. (1990). Allergies: Behavioral effects and treatment implications. In A. M. Gross & R. S. Drabman (Eds.), *Handbook of clinical behavioral pediatrics* (pp. 267–278). New York: Plenum Press.

Rosenberg, A., & Kagan, J. (1987). Iris pigmentation and behavioral inhibition. *Developmental Psychobiology, 20,* 377–392.

Routh, D. K., & Ernst, A. R. (1984). Somatization disorder in relatives of children and adolescents with functional abdominal pain. *Journal of Pediatric Psychology, 9,* 427–437.

Rubinstein, B., & Shaffer, D. (1985). Organicity in child psychiatry: Signs, symptoms, and syndromes. *Psychiatric Clinics of North America, 8*(4), 755–777.

Rutter, M., Tizard, J., & Whitmore, K. (1970). *Education, health and behavior.* London: Longman Group.

Sabbeth, B., & Stein, R. E. K. (1990). Mental health referral: A weak link in comprehensive care of children with chronic physical illness. *Journal of Developmental and Behavioral Pediatrics, 11,* 73–78.

Salkovskis, P. M. (1989). Somatic problems. In K. Hawton, P. M. Salkovskis, J. Kirk, & D. M. Clark (Eds.), *Cognitive behaviour therapy for psychiatric problems: A practical guide* (pp. 235–276). New York: Oxford University Press.

Schiffer, R. B., Klein, R. F., & Sider, R. C. (1988). *The medical evaluation of psychiatric patients.* New York: Plenum Press.

Selz, M., & Reitan, R. M. (1979). Neuropsychological test performance of normal, learning disabled, and brain damaged older children. *Journal of Nervous and Mental Diseases, 167,* 298–302.

Shapiro, E. G., & Rosenfeld, A. A. (1987). *The somatizing child.* New York: Springer-Verlag.

Slavney, P. R. (1990). *Perspectives of "hysteria."* Baltimore: Johns Hopkins University Press.

Spar, J. E. (1989). Organic mood syndrome: In American Psychiatric Association Task Force on Treatments of Psychiatric Disorders, *Treatments of psychiatric disorders* (pp. 853–856). Washington, DC: American Psychiatric Association.

Spohr, H. L., & Steinhausen, H. C. (1987). Follow-up studies of children with fetal alcohol syndrome. *Neuropediatrics, 18,* 13–17.

Starkman, M. N., Zelnik, T. C., Nesse, R. M., & Cameron, O. G. (1985). Anxiety in patients with pheochromocytomas. *Archives of Internal Medicine, 145,* 248–252.

Starkstein, S. E., Mayberg, H. S., Berthier, M. L., Fedoroff, P., Price, T. R., Dannals, R. F., Wagner, H. N., Leiguarda, R., & Robinson, R. G. (1990). Mania after brain injury: Neuroradiological and metabolic findings. *Annals of Neurology, 27,* 652–659.

Steidl, J. H., Finkelstein, F. O., Wexler, J. P., Feigenbaum, H., Kitsen, J., Kliger, A. S., & Quinlan, D. M. (1980). Medical condition, adherence to treatment regimens, and family functioning. *Archives of General Psychiatry, 37,* 1025–1027.

Steinhausen, H. C., Aster, M. V., Pfeiffer, E., & Gobel, D. (1989). Comparative studies of conversion disorders in childhood and adolescence. *Journal of Child Psychology and Psychiatry, 30,* 615–621.

Sternberg, D. E. (1986). Testing for physical illness in psychiatric patients. *Journal of Clinical Psychiatry, 47,* 3–9.

Stoddard, F. J., & Wilens, T. E. (1990). Delirium. In M. S. Jellinek & D. B. Herzog (Eds.), *Psychiatric aspects of general hospital pediatrics* (pp. 254–259). Chicago: Year Book.

Strunk, R. C., Mrazek, D A., Wolfson, G. S., & LaBrecque, J. F. (1985). Physiological and psychological characteristics associated with deaths from asthma in childhood: A case controlled study. *Journal of the American Medical Association, 254,* 1193–1198.

Summers, W. K., Munoz, R. A., & Read, M. R. (1981). The psychiatric physical examination: 1. Methodology. *Journal of Clinical Psychiatry, 42,* 95–98.

Szymanski, L. S. (1988). The retarded child and adolescent. In C. J. Kestenbaum & D. T. Williams (Eds.), *Handbook of clinical assessment of children and adolescents* (pp. 446–468). New York: New York University Press.

Thomas, C. S. (1985). Dysmorphophobia or monosymptomatic hypochondriasis. *British Journal of Psychiatry, 146,* 672–673.

Tunnessen, W. W. (1988). *Signs and symptoms in pediatrics* (2nd ed.). Philadelphia: J. B. Lippincott.

U. S. Department of Health and Human Services. (1988). *Preventing lead poisoning in young children.* Second revision of the statement by the Centers for Disease Control.

Vessey, M. P., Fairweather, D. V., Norman-Smith, B., & Buckley, J. (1985). A randomized double blind controlled trial of stilbestrol therapy in pregnancy: Long term follow-up of mothers and their offspring. *British Journal of Obstetrics and Gynecology, 90*, 1007–1017.

Volkmar, F. R., Poll, J., & Lewis, M. (1984). Conversion reactions in children and adolescents. *Journal of the American Academy of Child Psychiatry, 23*, 424–430.

Volow, M. R. (1983). Delirium, dementia, and other organic mental syndromes. In J. O. Cavenar & H. K. H. Brodie (Eds.), *Signs and symptoms in psychiatry* (pp. 511–551). Philadelphia: J. B. Lippincott.

Walker, L. S., & Greene, J. W. (1989). Children with recurrent abdominal pain and their parents; More somatic complaints, anxiety and depression than other patient families? *Journal of Pediatric Psychology, 14*, 231–243.

Wasserman, A. L., Whitington, P. F., & Rivara, F. P. (1988). Psychogenic basis for abdominal pain in children and adolescents. *Journal of the American Academy of Child and Adolescent Psychiatry, 27*, 179–184.

Weller, E., & Weller, R. (1983). Case report of conversion symptoms associated with major depressive disorder in a child. *American Journal of Psychiatry, 140*, 1079–1080.

Werry, J. S., & Wollersheim, J. P. (1989). Behavior therapy in children and adolescents: A 20 year overview. *Journal of the American Academy of Child and Adolescent Psychiatry, 28*, 1–18.

Wessely, S. (1990). Old wine in new bottles: Neurasthenia and "M.E." *Psychological Medicine, 220*, 35–53.

White, K., Kolman, M. L., Wexler, P., Polin, G., & Winter, R. J. (1984). Unstable diabetes and unstable families: A psychosocial evaluation of diabetic children with recurrent ketoacidosis. *Pediatrics, 73*, 749–755.

Whitlock, F. A. (1982). *Symptomatic affective disorder.* New York: Academic Press.

Williams, D. T., & Hirsch, G. (1988). The somatizing disorders: somatoform disorders, factitious disorders, and malingering. In Kestenbaum, C. & Williams, D. T. (Eds.), *Handbook of clinical assessment of children and adolescents* (pp. 743–768). New York: New York University Press.

Williamson, D. A., McKenzie, S. J., Goreczny, A. J., & Faulstich, M. (1987). Psychophysiological disorders. In Hersen, M. & Van Hasselt, V. B. (Eds.), *Behavior therapy with children and adolescents* (pp. 279–300). New York: Wiley.

Yudofsky, S. C., Silver, J., & Yudofsky, B. (1989). Organic personality disorder, explosive type. In American Psychiatric Association Task Force on treatments of psychiatric disorders, *Treatments of psychiatric disorders* (pp. 839–852). Washington, DC: American Psychiatric Association.

20

Separation Anxiety Disorder

ANNETTE M. FARRIS and ERNEST N. JOURILES

INTRODUCTION

This chapter highlights issues faced by mental health professionals who operate in psychiatric settings and deliver services to children exhibiting problems consistent with the diagnosis of separation anxiety disorder (SAD; American Psychiatric Association, 1980, 1987). In the first section of the chapter, diagnostic issues are briefly covered. In subsequent sections, prototypical behavioral assessment and treatment approaches are described, and the application of these practices within psychiatric settings is discussed.

DIAGNOSTIC ISSUES AND CONTROVERSIES

SAD is a relatively new diagnostic category, first created for the third edition of the *Diagnostic and Statistical Manual* (DSM-III; American Psychiatric Association, 1980), and replicated in the revision of the third edition (DSM-III-R; American Psychiatric Association, 1987). The primary feature of SAD is excessive anxiety, for at least two weeks, on the part of a child when he or she anticipates or experiences separation from significant attachment figures. Specific problems include unrealistic worries about being permanently abandoned because of unforeseen catastrophes (e.g., parents being hurt or the child being kidnapped), refusal to attend school, persistent avoidance of being alone (e.g., clinging to the parents even at home), nightmares involving separation themes, the use of somatic complaints to avoid separation, excessive temper tantrums or complaints during departure scenes, and an excessive need to return to or contact the parents during separation (e.g., through phone calls). The behavior therapist should immediately appreciate that, contrary to "medical" diagnoses, psychiatric diagnoses such as SAD are explicitly *not* based on underlying pathogenic mechanisms that are linked to specific treatments (Garfield, 1984). However, in recent years, attempts have been made to confirm the clinical usefulness of psychiatric diagnoses by gathering data to establish their reliability and their differential validity in client description, prognosis, and treatment.

ANNETTE M. FARRIS and ERNEST N. JOURILES • Department of Psychology, University of Houston, Houston, Texas 77204-5341.

Handbook of Behavior Therapy in the Psychiatric Setting, edited by Alan S. Bellack and Michel Hersen. Plenum Press, New York, 1993.

ANNETTE M. FARRIS
and ERNEST N.
JOURILES

Reliability

Recent research indicates that SAD can be diagnosed with adequate interrater reliability by the use of semistructured diagnostic interviews, such as the Interview Schedule for Children (ISC; Last, Strauss, & Francis, 1987d; Last, Francis, Hersen, Kazdin, & Strauss, 1987a), the Schedule of Affective Disorders and Schizophrenia for School-Age Children (KIDDIE-SADS; Chambers, Puig-Antich, Hirsch, Paez, Ambrosini, Tabrizi, & Davies, 1985; Last & Strauss, 1990), and the Diagnostic Interview Schedule for Children (DISC; Anderson, Williams, McGee, & Silva, 1987; Edelbrock, Costello, Dulcan, Kalas, & Conover, 1985). In addition, SAD is one of the few diagnoses for which acceptable reliability can be reached based on the typical assessment procedures used in psychiatric hospitals (i.e., case presentations at ward rounds) provided that a sufficient number of cases are available to test for reliability (Werry, Methven, Fitzpatrick, & Dixon, 1983).

In terms of prevalence, Table 1 displays the results from research on general-population outpatient, or hospitalized samples in which SAD was specifically diagnosed. As would be expected, lower prevalence estimates were generally reported in studies using more stringent criteria to identify a child with SAD (e.g., examining both child and parent reports, and requiring clinically significant impairment in functioning). Also, the prevalence of SAD appears to vary as a function of the reporter, with children appearing somewhat more likely to report SAD symptoms than parents. In sum, the prevalence of SAD in the general population ranges from 1.3% to 13%. In outpatient settings, the range of children meeting threshold SAD criteria varies from 20% to 55%. In inpatient populations, SAD consistently occurs at about 14%. Finally, in studies reporting these data, strikingly high levels of comorbidity exist between SAD and at least one other psychiatric diagnosis (52%–91%), including a wide range of anxiety, affective, and externalizing disorders. Thus, SAD occurs predominantly with other diagnoses, although a clear pattern of specific concurrent problems is not readily discernible.

Differential Validity Evidence

A major diagnostic controversy pertains to whether a psychiatric label provides useful differential information about children exhibiting the disorder. That is, are children with SAD different from those with other diagnoses, and do these differences relate to treatment planning or outcome?

In terms of simple descriptive data, substantial evidence indicates that SAD children are likely to be younger than children with other types of anxiety disorders, particularly overanxious disorder (OAD) and non-separation-related school phobia (Bowen, Offord, & Boyle, 1990; Kashani & Orvaschel, 1990; Last, Hersen, Kazdin, Finkelstein, & Strauss, 1987b; Last & Strauss, 1990). Also, children with SAD are more likely to exhibit concurrent somatic complaints than children with other types of psychiatric illnesses, with the exception of somatization disorder or psychosis (Livingston, Taylor, & Crawford, 1987). Although girls do not appear to be more likely than boys to be diagnosed with SAD in samples referred to an anxiety clinic (Francis, Last, & Strauss, 1987; Last et al., 1987d), an epidemiological study on the general population in New Zealand found girls four times more likely than boys to exhibit SAD (Anderson et al., 1987).

Almost all of the available controlled research fails to substantiate that children with SAD differ from children with other psychiatric diagnoses on dimensions of functioning (e.g., anxiety- and fear-rating scales, depression scales, and rates of externalizing problems) not directly reflected in the diagnosis of SAD itself. Clinical accounts frequently underscore a prior traumatic separation incident(s) as a causal precursor of SAD, and Gittelman-Klein and Klein (1980) reported that 80% of children with separation anxiety had recently suffered a major disruption in their lives (e.g., the death of a loved one). It is equally apparent, however, that such stressful events rarely lead to long-term or severe separation problems in most children (Campbell, 1986; Gittelman, 1986). In sum, as is characteristic of childhood diagnoses in general (for reviews, see Reeves, Werry, Elkind, & Zametizin, 1987; Werry, Elkind, & Reeves, 1987a), there is a dearth of information about the factors that differentiate children with SAD from those with other diagnoses. The exception to this rule is research on patterns of parental psychopathology. Last, Hersen, Kazdin, Francis, and Grubb (1987c) found a higher lifetime incidence of any adult anxiety disorder in mothers of children presenting to a clinic with SAD (68%), OAD (86%), or both SAD and OAD (94%) compared to mothers of children with externalizing psychiatric disorders (40%; e.g., oppositional defiant disorder [ODD], conduct disorder [CD], and/or attention deficit disorder [ADD]).

Interestingly, some evidence suggests that it is the presence of concurrent diagnoses, and not SAD alone, that predicts increased severity of anxiety and/or depressive symptoms, or of family problems. For example, children identified with a "pure anxiety disorder," such as SAD, have been found to exhibit fewer anxiety and depressive symptoms than children with a concurrent depressive disorder (Bernstein & Garfinkel, 1986; Strauss, Last, Hersen, & Kazdin, 1988). Similarly, children with a pure depressive disorder exhibit fewer anxiety and depressive symptoms than children with a coexisting anxiety disorder such as SAD (Bernstein & Garfinkel, 1986). In addition, children with only SAD appear to be less likely than those with both SAD and OAD to have mothers with a history of anxiety disorders (64% vs. 86%; Last et al., 1987c). Likewise, Kashani, Vaidya, Soltys, Dandoy, Katz, and Reid (1990) concluded that, as the severity and comorbidity of specific childhood anxiety disorders increases (SAD was not differentiated), so do parental rates of a wide range of psychiatric symptoms.

SAD and School Phobia

Though not a formal diagnosis, school phobia has received considerable attention in the behavioral literature and is characterized by intense fear and/or avoidance of the school environment. Theoretical views on the relationship between separation anxiety and school phobia have a fairly complex history. Early psychodynamic thinkers emphasized underlying separation fears, whereas behavioral proponents tended to focus on the school avoidance *per se* (see Ollendick & King, 1990, for summary). Contrary to early estimates that 75%–80% of school-phobic children suffer underlying SAD (Waldron, Shrier, Stone, & Tobin, 1975), recent empirical work suggests that SAD accompanies school phobia 33%–50% of the time (Bernstein & Garfinkel, 1986; Bernstein, Svinger, & Garfinkel, 1990; Last & Strauss, 1990), and a variety of other DSM-III-R diagnoses are represented in school-phobic samples as well (Bernstein et al., 1990; Last & Strauss, 1990). In addition, although school avoidance is a common aspect of SAD, children with SAD avoid a wide range of situations, other than school, in which their attachment figure is unavailable. The partial overlap of SAD and "school phobia" indicates that, at times, the two problems reflect identical etiological processes (e.g., operant reinforcement), but, that, on other occasions, school avoidance may be unrelated to generalized separation anxiety (e.g., a conditioned fear of specific stimuli on the way to or at school).

In an attempt to clarify the relationship between school phobia and SAD, Last et al. (1987a) compared school-avoidant children with SAD to those with a non-separation-related school phobia. They found SAD children more likely to be prepubertal, female, and from families with lower socioeconomic backgrounds, as well as more likely to meet the criteria for an additional DSM-III diagnosis (92% vs. 63%). In addition, mothers of children with SAD were four times more likely to have an affective disorder than mothers of school-phobic children, but both groups shared the same prevalence of maternal anxiety disorders. Last and Strauss (1990) also reported that school refusers with generalized SAD are more likely than children with school-focused fears to have mothers with a history of school refusal problems themselves. These researchers suggested tentatively that school refusal associated with separation anxiety may be functionally

ANNETTE M. FARRIS
and ERNEST N.
JOURILES

Table 1. Prevalence and Comorbidity Data on SAD

Study	Sample characteristics	Diagnostic tools and source(s)	Rates of SAD	Comorbidity with other disorders
Epidemiological studies				
Anderson *et al.* (1987)	792 11-year-olds representative of general population in New Zealand	Clinician ratings based on DISC with children and Rutter's Child Scale with parents and teachers; three levels of severity of diagnosis given: (1) strong, pervasive; (2) situational; and (3) weak, pervasive.	3.5% of sample met SAD criteria using all levels of severity. 1.3% had strong, pervasive SAD; 1.6% had situational SAD; and .6% had weak, pervasive SAD.	Of 59 anxiety cases, 39% had concurrent disorders 19% had 1 additional disorder including attention deficit disorder (ADD) or conduct disorder/opposition and defiant disorder (CD/ODD); 3% had 2 additional disorders; 17% had 3 or more additional disorders.
Bird *et al.* (1988)	843 4- to 16-year-old children representative of Puerto Rico	Clinician rating based on DISC with children and parents. Also used a cutoff of 61 on Global Assessment Scale, an adaptive functioning scale, to designate cases as clinically severe.	6.8% of sample met SAD criteria; 4.7% were defined as clinically severe.	Of 81 anxiety diagnoses, 67% had concurrent disorders: 42% had 1 additional; 20% had 2 additional; 5% had 3 or more additional disorders. 39% had concurrent CD/ODD; 21% concurrent ADD; 17% concurrent affective.
Bowen *et al.* (1990)	1,299 12- to 16-year-old adolescents representative of Ontario	SAD diagnosis based on 7 items from a modified behavior-problem checklist completed by youths and parents. The match between the two sets of symptoms was limited because some symptoms on checklist were more liberal than DSM-III-R.	2.4% of sample had SAD according to youths using most stringent critera. 2.7% of sample had SAD according to parents using moderately stringent thresholds.	In 23 cases of SAD without OAD, 22% also had externalizing problems, 9% had depression, and 4% had externalizing and depression. In 8 cases of SAD with OAD, 50% had depression, and 13% had depression and externalizing disorder.
Kashani and Orvaschel (1990)	Stratified random sampling of 210 children aged 8, 12, and 17 in equal numbers from a U.S. sample	Clinician rating based on child asessment schedule (CAS) with child and mother.	13% of sample met SAD criteria.	Only comorbidity of anxiety disorders reported. Of 27 SAD cases, 52% had concurrent anxiety disorders: 44% had 1 additional disorder; 7.5% had 2 additional disorders.
Outpatient data				
Costello *et al.* (1985)	40 7- to 11-year old children referred to a psychiatric clinic, also matched with pediatric population in U.S.	Clinician rating based on DISC with parent and child. Authors divided DISC diagnoses into two categories of "mild to moderate" severity, just above diagnostic threshold, and "severe" level.	With parent reports, 20% of psychiatric sample had minimal SAD and 5% had severe SAD; 5% pediatric sample had minimal SAD and 0% had severe SAD. With child self-reports, 55% of psychiatric sample had minimal SAD and 32.5% had severe SAD; 32.5% of pediatric sample met minimal SAD criteria and 12.5% had severe SAD.	Data not reported.

Last et al. (1987a)	91 5- to 18-year-old children referred to oupatient anxiety disorder clinic for children and adolescents in U.S.	Clinical rating based on ISC interviews with child and parent.	47% of sample met criteria for SAD; 24% had SAD without overanxious disorder (OAD), and 23% had SAD with OAD.	91% of children with SAD without OAD had additional disorders, including avoidant disorder (5%); major depression (MD) (32%); ADD (23%); ODD (27%). 95% of children with SAD and OAD had a wide range of other diagnoses.
Last et al. (1987b)	73 5- to 18-year-olds referred to an outpatient anxiety disorder clinic for children and adolescents in U.S.	Clinician rating based on ISC interviews with child and parent.	33% of sample exhibited SAD as a *primary* diagnosis (SAD was most common primary disorder); 4% had SAD as a *secondary* diagnosis	Of primary SAD cases, 25% had 1 additional diagnosis, 33% had 2 additional diagnoses, and 21% had 3 or more concurrent diagnoses. The most common comorbid diagnoses were OAD (33%); ODD (17%); ADD (17%); MD (12.5%); dysthymia (12.5%); simple phobia (12.5%).
Inpatient data				
Livingston et al. (1988)[a]	95 6- to 12-year-old psychiatrically hospitalized children in U.S.	Clinician rating based on diagnostic interview for children and adolescents (DICA) with child.	14% of sample met criteria for SAD.	Children with SAD had a significant number of somatic symptoms, with an average of 8.5. The most comon were abdominal pain and palpitations.
Kashani et al. (1990)	100 7- to 12-year-old psychiatrically hospitalized children in U.S.	Clinician ratings based on DICA with child and parent. Agreement between sources required for diagnosis to be given.	15% of sample met stringent criteria for SAD.	Only comorbidity of anxiety disorders reported. 67% of SAD involved and 33% had phobia & OAD; 20% had phobia only; 13% had OAD only.
Werry et al. (1983)	195 5- to 14-year-old psychiatrically hospitalized children and adolescents in U.S.	Clinical diagnosis based on typical hospital weekly case presentation.	14% of sample were given SAD diagnosis.	Data not reported.
Weinstein et al. (1988)	163 12- to 15-year-old psychiatrically hospitalized adolescents in U.S.	Compared typical hospital diagnoses to DISC-based rating with child.	13% had SAD based on DISC. 0% had SAD with typical clinical diagnostic process.	No data.

[a]Focus of study was on comorbid somatic complaints in a hospitalized psychiatric sample.

tied to the mother-child relationship because of instructional learning and operant reinforcement (i.e., the mother communicating separation concerns and reinforcing the child for anxiety behavior). In contrast, the etiology of phobic-related school refusal may be related to specific circumstances or events in the school environment (e.g., academic and/or social fears).

Distinguishing SAD from Normal Separation Anxiety

Typically, childhood fears are considered abnormal when they (1) are out of proportion to the demands of the situation; (2) cannot be explained or reasoned away; (3) are beyond voluntary control; (4) lead to avoidance of the feared situation; (5) persist over an extended period of time; (6) are unadaptive; and (7) are not age- or stage-specific (Marks, 1969; Miller, Barrett, & Hampe, 1974). Empirical work has documented the normal escalation and decrease of many childhood fears that helps prevent inappropriate diagnostic labeling (see reviews by King, Hamilton, & Ollendick, 1988; Morris & Kratochwill, 1983). Interestingly, however, very little behavioral literature has examined how the emergence and resolution of normal "separation anxiety" at 8–24 months may relate, if at all, to later manifestations of abnormal separation problems. During this developmental stage, virtually all children exhibit distress (e.g., crying and clinging) at separation and show apprehension when anticipating separation from their mothers, although the duration and intensity of the reactions vary with age, the quality of the mother-infant attachment, the situation, and prior experiences with separation (see the review by Campbell, 1986). Developmental psychopathologists have expanded on Bowlby's neoanalytic-ethological theory of attachment (1969) and have hypothesized that parent responses during the normal stage of separation anxiety may predispose a child to later problems (Belsky & Nezworski, 1990). Empirical work supports a link between early parent-child attachment patterns and later child functioning (see the review by Paterson & Moran, 1988), but considerable controversy surrounds the interpretation of these data (Lamb, Thompson, Gardner, Charnov, & Estes, 1984). The largest problem from a diagnostic perspective is that the "vulnerability" associated with poor attachment patterns has been used to explain the later emergence of the entire gambit of childhood clinical problems, thereby leaving considerable questions about the specific link between normal separation anxiety and SAD.

Prototypical Assessment

The foregoing abbreviated review highlights the scarcity of useful clinical or differential validity information on SAD as well as the high degree of comorbidity between SAD and other childhood problems. Thus, although the diagnostic criteria for SAD provide a summary description of the problems a child may have, in practice clinicians must (1) use a theory-based functional assessment to identify the various possible mechanisms (e.g., classical and operant conditioning, modeling, and cognitive processes) contributing to SAD and (2) extrapolate from theory to guide their interventions. A theme in the rest of this chapter is how the consideration of multiple theoretical processes can guide a behavior therapist from the global psychiatric diagnosis of SAD toward treatment-focused assessment and intervention. Efforts are made to avoid perpetuating a "uniformity myth" (Kielser, 1966), in which a single causal mechanism is presumed to be responsible for SAD. In addition, because the symptoms of different psychiatric disorders may be maintained by identical antecedents or consequences, the identification of theoretical processes can help clinicians understand the comorbidity often associated with SAD.

Generally, conventional behavioral assessment has emphasized the systematic analysis and operationalization of a presenting clinical problem and its situational determinants (e.g., its antecedents and consequences). An additional goal is the generation of hypotheses about an appropriate match between the problem behaviors and interventions (King *et al.*, 1988; Mash &

Terdal, 1981). Ollendick and Hersen (1984) also emphasized that empirically validated, multiline assessment methods should be used to gain the best "picture of a child," including sensitivity to developmental processes and a solicitation of information from the child as well as relevant adults. Currently, unstructured and semistructured clinical interviews and informal *in vivo* behavioral observation constitute the primary methods available for gathering information about SAD, as empirically validated rating scales for this particular disorder do not exist (Ollendick & King, 1990). Detailed descriptions of the available methods can be found in general texts on childhood behavioral assessment (King *et al.*, 1988; Mash & Terdal, 1981), and in reviews of SAD by Thyer and Sowers-Hoag (1988) and Ollendick and King (1990).

The major distinction between behavioral and more traditional forms of psychological assessment lies not in the technique *per se* (i.e., both may use interviews or observation), but in the theoretical assumptions driving the assessment. Generally, the behavioral approach tends to emphasize current interactions between a child and her or his environment, whereas traditional assessment approaches tend to focus on identifying the general traits of the child. From a behavioral perspective, classical, operant, and vicarious conditioning represent the theoretical processes traditionally invoked to explain and treat childhood anxiety problems (King *et al.*, 1988; Morris & Kratochwill, 1983; Ollendick & King, 1990; Ollendick & Mayer, 1984). More recently, in accordance with Bandura's social learning model (1977), some have argued that the "final common pathway" that accounts for child anxiety problems involves cognitive processes that mediate the influence of environmental events, particularly learned self-efficacy expectations (Ollendick & King, 1990; Wilson & O'Leary, 1980). To explore the processes that apply to a given case, four content areas need to be assessed, including (1) targeted clinical phenomena, which are often conveniently divided into the three response systems of overt avoidance or distress behavior, physiological arousal, and maladaptive cognitive processes; (2) the antecedents that elicit targeted response components; (3) the consequences of the targeted problem behavior; and (4) the assets available to children or families to implement alternative coping strategies when they are faced with a triggering antecedent. These four areas are covered below to illustrate how a behavior therapist might assess the processes involved in maintaining SAD.

The first assessment task is to identify, differentiate, and quantify the targeted excesses and deficits of concern within and across the three response systems. For example, when separated or anticipating separation from a parent, a child with SAD may exhibit excessive avoidance or distress behaviors, cognitive preoccupation or worries, somatic complaints (e.g., stomachaches and headaches), or some combination of all three reactions. Several goals can be accomplished by identifying specific targets of change within each response system, including the establishment of a baseline by which to judge interventions, as well as possible treatment matching of techniques with problems (e.g., relaxation for excessive physiological arousal and cognitive restructuring for worries). Moreover, given the incongruity that seems to exist across changes in various response components (Barlow, 1988; Hodgson & Rachman, 1974), a therapist cannot take it for granted that getting a child with SAD to stay in school by using an operant intervention will relieve his or her subjective cognitive distress when separated from an attachment figure.

The next step is to clarify the specific antecedents that elicit maladaptive responses. External cues, such as a mother walking toward an exit, have been emphasized in the behavioral literature, but internal processes (e.g., anxiety-provoking thoughts and images) may also be activated by idiosyncratic cues and may begin a self-perpetuating, internal cycle of anticipatory physiological arousal and cognitive worries. In addition, more temporally distant but relevant antecedents, so-called setting events, may also help set the stage for maladaptive reactions. For example, a child may be particularly prone to separation distress when fatigued, or when dealing with concurrent stresses (e.g., fights with siblings or a strange environment).

A third major target of assessment in a behavioral framework is how a child's behavior is reinforced. Parents may inadvertently instigate or maintain SAD symptomatology with consequences (e.g., attention, concern, comfort, letting a chid stay with the parent and play, or continued avoidance of separation) that act as positive and/or negative reinforcers. In other words, these parental responses may provide pleasant events for the child in addition to terminating the fear-provoking situation itself. Unfortunately, a vicious circle of interactive reinforcement may operate within a dyad to maintain both the parent's reinforcing responses and the child's separation anxiety. For example, the child's dependent behavior may make a parent feel especially needed (i.e., give positive reinforcement) and may also negatively reinforce the parent by relieving his or her fears about leaving the child with alternative caretakers. This bidirectional process may be more likely if the child has genuine medical problems or has been accidentally or intentionally harmed by others in the absence of the parent. Finally, although exceptionally difficult to pinpoint, important "indirect contingencies" within a family may operate to maintain SAD (Kennedy, 1983; King *et al.*, 1988). For example, a child's clinging to a mother may draw attention away from other family problems, such as marital conflict.

Finally, the resources available to a child and his or her family should be assessed to guide the choice or the therapeutic technique. For example, a child must have the requisite cognitive abilities to use systematic desensitization (e.g., imaginal skills and concentration). Likewise, an intervention based on systematic reinforcement by caretakers requires behaviorally oriented parenting skills and considerable motivation on the part of the parents. In conclusion, it is important to emphasize that the various theoretical processes discussed above may operate simultaneously and synergistically in a given case.

ACTUAL ASSESSMENT

This section features previously overlooked objectives that a behavioral therapist may have when assessing SAD in a psychiatric setting. The first, and perhaps most critical, decision that a behavior therapist faces when conducting an assessment in psychiatric settings is whether a child requires inpatient hospitalization. Hospitalization has several potential deleterious consequences that must be seriously considered when deciding whether to take this treatment route: (1) a child's negative reaction to hospitalization, which may aggravate SAD; (2) the disruption of the child's family and community relationships; (3) substantial expense; (4) the reinforcement of parental uninvolvement, denial, or guilt; (5) confused and distorted perceptions by the patient's siblings; (6) removal of the child from a regular education system; (7) the predictable stigmatism of labeling; and (8) the potential for unresolved dependency on the institution (Stone, 1979). Also, psychiatric hospitalization has been associated with the placement of a large proportion of children (54%) in more restrictive educational settings after release, although objective differences in intellectual and academic achievement did not exist between hospitalized and disturbed nonhospitalized children (Barack, 1986). Finally, complex issues are involved in ensuring that the ethical and legal rights of parents, and especially minors are fully respected in the course of hospitalization (Appelbaum, 1989; Brewer & Faitak, 1989). Most notably, a thorough and appropriate informed consent should be provided both to the parents and to minor clients about the implications of hospitalization and about the nature of all assessment and treatment procedures used in that environment.

Given the significant possible negative ramifications of psychiatric hospitalization, a heavy burden is placed on the assessor to determine clearly whether this action is necessary. Various commentators seem to concur about the circumstances that warrant hospitalization (Connell, 1985; Hersov & Bentovim, 1985; Dalton, Muller, & Forman, 1989). Connell's (1985) comprehensive criteria are (1) the need for diagnostic work that cannot be obtained on an outpatient basis; (2) severe problems that preclude parental management within the home (e.g., suicide attempts or severe aggression); (3) impaired physical status of the child that requires skilled nursing care (e.g., anorexia nervosa); (4) adverse environmental circumstances that preclude the child's improvement within the home; (5) gross overprotection by the parents or encouragement of infantilism after an injury; and (6) school refusal that cannot be managed on an outpatient basis (Dalton *et al.*, 1989; Dalton & Forman, 1987). The overarching issue appears to be unequivocally establishing that hospitalization represents the most efficient and least invasive available therapeutic approach to remedying the clinical problems. Interestingly, limited data suggest that the decision to hospitalize minors is frequently tied to a critical precipitating event that convinces the family, social agencies, or medical providers of the urgency of hospitalization, rather than a thorough weighing of all options (Barack, 1986). In addition, critics have noted that the decision to hospitalize minors may often be a product of convenience, third-party reimbursement, or pressure to maintain the financial well-being of a hospital or clinician instead of the most rational choice of treatment (Dalton & Foreman, 1987).

Substantiating that hospitalization represents the most sensible treatment option when SAD is the primary problem may be particularly difficult. Case studies indicate that quite severe cases of separation anxiety can be successfully remedied on an outpatient basis (see Garvey & Hegrenes, 1966; Montenegro, 1968; Neisworth, Madle, & Goeke, 1975; Stokes, Boggs, & Osnes, 1989). Additional indirect evidence of the utility of outpatient treatment comes from a quasi-experimental one-year follow-up outcome study of adolescent school refusers who had received either a comprehensive behavioral treatment approach (BTA), traditional psychiatric hospitalization (HU), or in-home tuition and counseling (HT) (Blagg & Yule, 1984). BTA demonstrated clear superiority over hospitalization in terms of both continued school attendance one year after treatment (93.3% versus 37.5%) and cost-effectiveness; the BTA treatment took an average of 2.5 weeks, and hospitalization lasted an average of 4.5 weeks. Although this study has some design flaws (e.g., lack of random assignment and unknown raters' bias in the outcome measures) and may not be generalizable to cases involving pervasive separation anxiety, the results suggest the efficacy and efficiency of outpatient behavioral approaches over hospitalization for school avoidance. School avoidance is a prevalent symptom of SAD that often seems to necessitate drastic intervention attempts. We strongly advocate aggressively pursuing outpatient behavioral interventions and clearly establishing that such methods are ineffective before resorting to hospitalization for SAD.

Because hospitalization seems unwarranted in uncomplicated cases of SAD, a child hospitalized with SAD can be expected to be experiencing serious medical or psychiatric disorders that call for hospitalization (e.g., suicidality or anorexia). Thus, the second major assessment objective that a psychologist in a psychiatric hospital setting has when assessing children with SAD is to identify concurrent psychological and/or medical problems and to assign priorities to the various targets of intervention. To accomplish this goal, a behavioral therapist will need to evaluate parent-child interaction patterns and other relevant family problems.

Based on the data reviewed earlier, there is no clear pattern in the kinds of child problems that coexist with SAD. Comorbid child psychosocial deficits may include other anxiety problems, depressive symptomatology, oppositional or conduct problems, academic skills deficiencies, and underdeveloped peer relationships. Any or all of these may interact synergistically with SAD symptomatology and/or may be maintained by similar processes. By conducting a comprehensive evaluation of possible concurrent child behavior problems, the clinician should be in a better position to make an informed decision regarding the priorities of treatment.

A child with SAD may also have concurrent medical problems. Difficult assessment decisions involve whether physiological arousal (e.g., an asthma attack) and avoidance of separation from the caregiver function to maintain unnecessary dependency, or if the child requires assistance from a caretaker. Indeed, many medical problems make separation difficult for the child and the parent alike, and mixed messages may be given by various medical specialists who simultaneously encourage and discourage a parent from being highly accessible to the child. Thus, a psychologist should carefully assess the amount of education a parent has had about the child's medical versus psychological problems. Then, the psychologist should work with the family's physicians to provide clear guidelines regarding when physiological symptomatology is indicative of underlying medical problems and when a child is reinforced by exaggerating medical symptoms to procure parental companionship. Parents may be willing to stop reinforcing SAD symptomatology if given consistent prescriptions by medical specialists and psychologists (e.g., Hersen, 1968). On the other hand, parents may remain extremely ambivalent about enforcing contingencies that would facilitate independent functioning on the part of a medically impaired child. Thus, parent's willingness to change the way they handle their children's medical problems requires careful assessment. In a related vein, behavioral therapists should be aware of the medication(s) a child may be receiving and investigate whether these substances may increase physiological arousal, thereby increasing the likelihood of panic reactions when a parent departs.

Other family factors make up a third area of potentially complicating concurrent problems, especially because a child with SAD does often not require hospitalization unless the parents are unusually overprotective, disorganized, or somehow invested in maintaining the problem. Most obviously, some mothers and fathers may lack an understanding of the parenting skills necessary to alter their unwitting operant reinforcement of excessive dependency. In addition, parents may fail to implement such skills even after they are taught. Many factors may account for resistance to altering parent-child interaction patterns, and the beliefs and contingencies underlying the parents' behavior patterns require thorough investigation. For example, some parents may derive pleasure from being needed by the child (i.e., a positive reinforcement) or may use the child's dependency as an excuse to avoid work or being alone with their spouse (i.e., a negative reinforcement). Alternatively, some parents may suffer considerable generalized anxiety themselves when away from the child because they worry about what could happen to the child. It may be recalled that parents of children with SAD are likely to have anxiety problems themselves. In severe cases, then, an assessment of parental functioning may be warranted. For example, unless a parent finds other ways to gain positive reinforcement and/or to cope with the issues that the child's SAD allows him or her to avoid (e.g., other worries, loneliness, marital discord or fear of working), he or she may subvert intervention attempts.

In terms of the methodology used to gather information in a psychiatric setting, one will probably begin by conducting thorough clinical interviews with the parents and the child (and other relevant parties if they are available), making sure to cover concurrent problems and the history of SAD. In addition, direct observation of the three classic facets of anxiety are likely to be fruitful in establishing baseline functioning, in conducting ongoing monitoring, and in doing a follow-up of the treatment. For SAD, direct observation includes (1) overt behavior and arousal during departure scenes; (2) the use of somatic complaints to attract companionship or to avoid separation; and (3) self-reports of worries or nightmares about harm to the self or to others. Also, direct behavioral observation of departure scenes may provide valuable information about the kinds of maladaptive modeling or subtle positive reinforcement that a parent provides a child during departure. Of course, immediate observation will probably not reveal "indirect" contingencies in the family structure that maintain a child's SAD symptomatology. In addition, one can arrange naturalistic situations to observe parents' basic skills, especially their delivery and enforcement of commands and their use of praise to encourage independent child activities. This information will hopefully aid in targeting antecedent conditions that perpetuate a cycle of separation anxiety.

Finally, one should consider using a general behavioral checklist, such as the Child Behavior Checklist (Achenbach & Edelbrock, 1983) or the Behavior Problem Checklist (Quay & Peterson, 1979) as a very systematic and efficient way of identifying problem areas to inquire into during interviews, and as a reliable method of measuring treatment efficacy. In addition, normative data are available on these instruments to help the clinician gauge the severity of impaired functioning across various ages. Similarly, standardized measures of anxiety or fears, such as the Revised Manifest Anxiety Scale (Reynolds & Richmond, 1978) or the Fear Survey

Schedule for Children—Revised (Ollendick, 1983), represent useful and empirically validated methods of identifying and differentiating the severity of coexisting anxiety problems and fears across ages, and of assessing posttreatment changes.

Before closing this section, we should note that SAD may sometimes emerge *during* hospitalization for other problems. In this case, careful functional assessment of the ongoing hospital environment and child-staff interactions may uncover antecedents and consequences that maintain overly dependent behavior (e.g., inappropriate attending by the staff to SAD symptomatology). SAD symptomatology may also occasionally emerge following discharge because the child or adolescent craves the attention and care she or he received from hospital staff. Careful monitoring may alert a psychologist to the likelihood of this outcome so that preventive steps can be taken. For example, the transition from hospital to home and school may be eased by ensuring that someone will be available to provide the child with consistent attention in his or her normal environment.

PROTOTYPICAL TREATMENT

This section reviews the recommended behavioral treatment strategies for SAD that are supported by case reports of generalized separation fears, as well as an extrapolation of theory and research on specific phobias, especially school phobia (Ollendick & King, 1990; Thyer & Sowers-Hoag, 1988). The interventions are based on classical, vicarious, and operant conditioning principles, and may be categorized, respectively, as follows: (1) counterconditioning or extinction of anxiety responses; (2) modeling and instruction of appropriate behaviors during departure scenes and parental absence; and (3) reorganization of reinforcers in the child's environment to encourage the child to approach and be exposed to situations without his or her attachment figure. Cognitive techniques aimed solely at alleviating internal aspects of SAD symptomatology, such as obsessive worries, have not been reported in published case studies but may also be useful, especially with older children and adolescents (Ollendick & Frances, 1990). Ultimately, all of the above techniques aim at successful *exposure* to the feared circumstances (i.e., being without a particular attachment figure) because this appears to be critical in overcoming anxiety problems. Of course, aspects of these interventions have appeared in the literature of other theoretical orientations, but different underlying mechanisms are hypothesized to account for results (see the review in Blagg, 1987). Typically, these behavioral treatment components are discussed separately to facilitate training, but they are probably best applied within a flexible and integrative treatment program matched to the child's needs (Blagg, 1987; Ollendick & King, 1990). Further, although case studies tend to emphasize the predominant use of one technique, a combination of classical and operant principles often appears to be needed, especially in cases where extinction is used to diminish the anxiety response and operant reinforcement is simultaneously used to reward nonfearful behavior.

Ten published behavioral studies were located that clearly involved generalized separation anxiety—not only school avoidance—as the child's central presenting problem. Table 2 summarizes the major features of these articles. All of the studies consist of narrative reports, and only three used formal single-subject research designs. This heavy reliance on case studies mirrors the scarcity of controlled treatment-outcome research on childhood anxiety disorders in general (see King *et al.*, 1988; Morris & Kratochwill, 1983). In particular, only two between-group outcome studies are available on the efficacy of behavioral approaches for school phobia (Blagg & Yule, 1984; Kennedy, 1965; see the thorough review in Blagg, 1987). Below, selected case studies are summarized to illustrate the behavioral techniques available to alleviate generalized separation anxiety.

Counterconditioning procedures consist of presenting a specific feared stimulus to a child (in the presence of alternative stimuli) that elicits responses incompatible with anxiety reactions. Thus, anxiety responses are thought to be counterconditioned when the child engages in the antagonistic response. The most familiar counterconditioning technique is systematic desensitization, as developed by Wolpe (1958). Here, the client is first taught how to self-induce a deep muscular relaxation response. Then, a highly detailed and graduated hierarchy of anxiety cues is carefully explicated, and the anxiety provoking situations are incrementally paired with the relaxation response. Systematic desensitization may be conducted *in vivo* or imaginally with children. Although systematic desensitization classically involves relaxation as the competing response (Lazarus, 1960; Miller, 1972), counterconditioning has also been accomplished with children by using food (Montenegro, 1968) or a therapist's presence (Garvey & Hegrenes, 1966) to elicit antagonistic responses. Another potential form of counterconditioning for children involves the use of "emotional imagery" to negate anxiety responses (King *et al.*, 1988; Ollendick & King, 1990). Here, the therapist uses imagery scenes believed to arouse feelings of self-assertion, pride, affection, happiness, and so on to counter anxiety responses. Care needs

Table 2.   Published Studies on Separation Anxiety

Article	# of cases	Age in yrs.	Gender	No. of sessions	Treatment time	Research design	Treatment	(Pre)-school attendance	Follow-up and school attendance
Lazarus (1960)	1	9½	F	5	10 days	Case report	Imaginal CC[a]	Yes	15 mos.; yes
Patterson (1965)	1	7	M	23	6 wks.	Case report	Gradual exposure and operant[b]	Yes	3 mos.; yes
Garvey and Hegrenes (1966)	1	10	M	20	6 wks.	Case report	Gradual *in vivo* CC and operant	yes	2 yrs.; yes
Montenegro (1968)	2	6	M	10	16 days	Case report	Gradual *in vivo* CC	Yes	1 mo.; yes
Miller (1972)	1	10	M	Not clear	Approx. 16 wks.	A-B	Imaginal and *in vivo* CC	Yes	18 mos.; yes
Neisworth *et al.* (1975)	1	4	M	18	18 days	A-B	Gradual exposure and operant	Yes	6 mos.; yes
Martin and Korte (1978)	1	7	F	7	7 days	Case report	Operant	Yes	—
Bornstein and Knapp (1981)	1	12	M	Not clear	56 days	MBL[c] across problems	Self-guided imaginal SD	Not targeted	12 mos.; yes
Phillips and Wolpe (1981)	1	12	M	88	2 yrs.	Case report	Imaginal and *in vivo*; operant	Yes	—
Stokes *et al.* (1989)	1	10	M	12	Not clear	Case report	Operant	Yes	2 mos. and 2 yrs.; yes

[a]CC = counterconditioning, which involved with food or muscular relaxation as the counterconditioning agent.
[b]Operant = negative and positive reinforcement for appropriate behaviors in attachment figures' absence.
[c]MBL = multiple baseline.

to be taken to match the image with the child's age, verbal abilities, and individual fantasies. This technique has been reported in two cases of school phobia (Lazarus & Abramovitz, 1962; Van der Plog, 1975), but there are no reports of its use with generalized separation anxiety.

As an illustrative case study, Lazarus (1960) used imaginal systematic desensitization for a 9-year-old girl, Carol, who developed numerous severe SAD symptoms following three traumatic incidents involving sudden death (she witnessed a fatal car accident, a school friend drowned, and a playmate died suddenly of meningitis). A seven-step hierarchy was developed of increasing lengths of separation time. Five desensitization sessions were conducted over the course of 10 days with successful dissipation of all symptoms, after which Carol agreed to go to school. At a 15-month follow-up, she remained satisfactorily adjusted. By comparison, Garvey and Hegrenese (1966) reported a successful use of *in vivo* counterconditioning in the treatment of a 10-year-old boy, Jimmy, who developed school refusal, somatic symptoms, and intense fears and fantasies of losing his mother, which appeared vicariously reinforced by the mother (e.g., "Some day I'll be dead, and you'll wish you had me!"). After six months of conventional psychotherapy had failed to resolve his separation anxiety or to foster school attendance, the authors developed a 13-step desensitization hierarchy beginning with a therapist and Jimmy's sitting in the car outside school and culminating with Jimmy's sitting in a full classroom. Although the therapist used praise to reinforce Jimmy's progress while he accompanied Jimmy through the course of the hierarchy, the authors primarily viewed the therapist as a counterconditioning agent who invoked positive affective responses from Jimmy that offset anxiety responses. After 20 consecutive days of 20–40 minutes of treatment, Jimmy remained in school alone, and at two-year follow-up, he exhibited no manifestations of the original fears.

Extinction procedures constitute another set of treatment strategies based on the principle of classical conditioning, which, in theory, may be applied to SAD. Rather than introduce a competing coping response (e.g., relaxation) to reciprocally inhibit children's anxiety responses, the conditioned fear stimuli may simply be presented repeatedly in the absence of negative consequences for the child. Presumably, a child's anxiety response will dissipate after repeated trials as he or she comes to learn that there is really nothing to be afraid of in the absence of the attachment figure. Rapid *in vivo* extinction is often referred to as flooding. With SAD, this technique would consist of forcing the child to be separated despite protests, so that the child learns the feared sequelae, such as harm to the self or others, will not occur. Implosion, a variant of flooding, is carried out in the individual's imagination and frequently involves extremely intense or exaggerated scenes regarding the feared object or event. Although hospitalization may be conceived of as a form of flooding for separation anxiety, to date, behavioral clinicians have not reported or recommended the use of this type of extinction technique to resolve pervasive separation fears.

Vicarious conditioning principles have also been used in the treatment of child phobias and may be applied to SAD. Corresponding interventions include the use of video modeling, live modeling, and/or participant modeling of appropriate responses in the face of anxiety-provoking stimuli (for reviews, see Graziano, DeGiovanni, & Garcia, 1979; King *et al.*, 1988). With SAD, a child's learning history may include an absence of productive observational learning or the presence of poor role models who have vicariously taught dysfunctional ways of dealing with separation anxiety. In particular, if poor modeling on the part of parents occurs during departure scenes, parents can be taught how to control their own anxiety reactions and give their children clear instructions about appropriate behavior during separation.

Procedures based on operant conditioning principles involve the use of positive and negative reinforcement to shape a child's approach feared situations. Most often, gradual, step-by-step *in vivo* shaping procedures are used. This method is distinguished from counterconditioning because new behavior is maintained by contingent reinforcement, not just by concurrent anxiety-inhibiting responses (e.g., relaxation). Efforts are made to teach caregivers to stop inadvertently reinforcing separation problems with positive attention and removal of the child from the feared situation. Instead, caretakers are taught to provide positive attention for the desired behavior. Several case studies portray the contingency management of separation anxiety (Martin & Korte, 1978; Neisworth et al., 1975; Patterson, 1965; Stokes et al., 1989). Stokes et al. (1989) described an especially well-articulated treatment plan focused exclusively on altering a couple's management of their 10-year-old son, Barry, who insisted that his mother accompany him to school, experienced severe physiological reactions when she was not present (e.g., was initially taken to an emergency room for uncontrolled shaking), and spent less than 30 minutes per day out of her sight. Before treatment, Barry readily elicited physical affection and parental attention with SAD symptomatology and mild oppositional behavior. Over the course of 12 weeks, several types of operant interventions were used. First, Barry self-monitored the length of his separation from his mother both at school and at home. The therapist contingently rewarded Barry for improvements with attention, games, and treats in session. Second, his parents carefully monitored the distribution of their attention, such as conversation or hugs, on a daily basis. They became highly skilled at attending to appropriate behavior and ignoring mild misbehavior, an area in which they had previously had major deficits. Third, Barry systematically received tangible, inexpensive rewards from his parents as the time he spent away from his mother increased. This system contrasted with the parents' prior use of disproportionate and inconsistent prizes for good behavior (e.g., a colt for allowing the mother to leave school one day). After his mother stopped going to school, Barry's three daily phone calls home were also gradually eliminated with praise and concrete awards. Two months after termination, the parents showed evidence of generalizing their skills by shaping Barry's willingness to remain at home alone for reasonable periods of time. Two years after his initial presentation, Barry displayed normal adjustment when separated from his parents at home, at school, and in public settings.

A final treatment strategy for SAD involves altering irrational beliefs about separation. The assumption underlying "cognitive restructuring" is that cognitive patterns and self-statements themselves sustain maladaptive physiological arousal and behavioral responses (Barlow, 1988). Several overlapping sets of cognitive techniques have been developed for adults to modify untenable beliefs and expectations, including Ellis's rational-emotive therapy (RET; 1970), Beck's cognitive therapy (1976), and Meichenbaum's self-instructional training (1977). Application of these intervention to children or adolescents who specifically have anxiety disorders is currently based only on "cumulative wisdom" gleaned from clinical experience, rather than on controlled studies (King et al., 1988). Nonetheless, in some cases of SAD, youngsters may be helped by being taught to provide themselves with systematic reassurance (e.g., positive self-statements), and to pay attention to their abilities to handle various activities instead of relying on attachment figures for guidance. As a brief illustrative example, RET with an adolescent with SAD might involve having the client identify the irrational beliefs that underlie statements such as "I can't do it unless she is with me." Irrational beliefs may include fear of rejection if failure occurs, fear of disappointing a parent unless a situation (e.g., school or camp) is handled exactly according to his or her specifications, or subtle threats of disapproval if the adolescent does indeed establish independent competency and "proves" he or she no longer needs the parent's overprotective support. Homework assignments may involve generating alternative explanations for "automatic thoughts" or testing the credibility of assumptions with real-life experiments.

ACTUAL TREATMENT

As with assessment, the conventional literature on behavioral therapy has tended to neglect some of the complications of delivering treatment for SAD in psychiatric settings. This section depicts the application of behavioral treatment in complex cases of SAD when one is working within psychiatric hospitals. However, it is first helpful to understand some typical aspects of inpatient hospitalization for children.

According to a review by Dalton *et al*. (1989), corroborated by Hersov and Bentovim (1985), the following four components represent classic structural features of inpatient hospital settings for minors:

1. Individual and concrete treatment planning by a treatment team, with the goal of reuniting the child or adolescent with his or her family and normal routine as efficaciously and quickly as possible and with appropriate outpatient after care used to continue improvement.
2. A "milieu" atmosphere, that is, a structured, consistent activity routine (e.g., set mealtime, wake-up time, bedtime, and school and therapy schedule) and a clear specification of the rules and consequences of misconduct; also, a tangible privilege or token reward system is often in place to facilitate compliance with prescribed activities and to facilitate improvement.
3. Therapeutic activities, including several peer groups per week focused on promoting social support and insight into maladaptive patterns of behavior, recreational therapy, art therapy, and play therapy; In addition, an individual staff member may be assigned to each patient to provide individual psychotherapy.
4. A school environment where academic needs and deficits are addressed.

In addition to these four elements, the direct involvement of the parents throughout the course of the hospitalization of minors appears to be gaining some support in the psychiatric community (Dalton *et al*., 1989; Hersov & Bentovim, 1985). Although routine family services (e.g., a weekly or biweekly parent's group) may be insufficient to help families alter maladaptive interaction patterns that are unresponsive to prior outpatient intervention, psychologists may be able to take advantage of changing hospital policies to encourage parents' in-depth involvement in their child's treatment.

Besides the structural aspects of inpatient hospitalization, it is crucial to recognize the process of service delivery in psychiatric settings. A behavioral therapist may play a heavy role in planning treatment for clients, but he or she will often have fairly limited contact with the child relative to other staff. Paraprofessionals, interns, and nurses are responsible for the vast majority of daily contacts with a child. Thus, major challenges involve soliciting the support of such personnel and carefully training and supervising them in carrying out treatment recommendations.

Treatment of Two Hypothetical SAD Cases

As should be obvious from earlier sections, a variety of mechanisms may maintain a particular child's SAD symptomatology. Here, two hypothetical situations are discussed to illustrate the complications of delivering treatment to children with SAD in psychiatric settings.

One common scenario involves an older child or early adolescent who is hospitalized for severe depression, including suicide attempts, with concurrent separation fears. A detailed analysis of the case might identify all of the following as target problems: (1) intense conditioned fear of being left alone; (2) high base levels of physiological arousal and tension; (3) somatic problems consistent with both depression and SAD; (4) a lack of confidence in being able to solve problems without the help of a safety figure; (5) actual deficits in problem-solving and reasoning skills; (6) poor interpersonal skills that interfere with obtaining social support from peers; and (7) a conviction that the family would be better off without his or her burdensome presence. Naturally the treatment plan would involve hypothesizing the manner in which classical, vicarious, and operant principles might individually or interactively account for the development and maintenance of these problems. In addition, cognitively based principles might be helpful in conceptualizing the case. For example, distortions in cognitive processing, failure to engage in appropriate cognitive mediating activity, and maladaptive expectations may all contribute to a spiral of anxiety (for a full discussion of the application of cognitive therapy to anxious children, see Kendall, Howard, & Epps, 1988).

Psychosocial treatment in a case like the one described above would require a careful prioritization and clear operationalization of the seven target areas so that the relevant overt behavior or subjective feelings and thoughts could be reliably observed and intervened upon in a systematic fashion. For example, the area of interpersonal skills might be divided into the specific treatment targets of improving eye contact, using a prosocial body posture, and increasing other-focused questioning. To help the youth gain mastery over separation experiences and to learn to be self-sufficient without an attachment figure present in a hospital setting, a number of techniques might be applied, depending on the conceptualization of what underlying mechanisms appeared to maintain particular deficits. These strategies include imaginal counterconditioning, shaping and reinforcement of adaptive functioning with tangible and meaningful rewards, the use of vicarious role modeling, and the delivery of concrete interpersonal skills training. Of course, *in vivo* practice of separating from the attachment figure would ultimately need to be conducted. Here, the interventions would also require altering the negative and positive reinforcement that the parent provided the child for displaying depressive symptomatology or separation distress, as well as training the parent in how to request adaptive behavior and not criticize or berate the child for mistakes. As discussed in the section on assessment, complicating circumstances may interfere with parents' commitment to altering parent-child interaction patterns. For example, parental fears of a child's becoming self-sufficient may need to be alleviated with desensitization or cognitive restructuring. Alternatively, parents may need help in resolving issues that their child's problems allow them to avoid (e.g., marital difficulties, career decisions, and loneliness). Thus, family therapy aimed at parental resistance may be indicated.

A treatment plan for the above case would also need to address the source and role of somatic symptoms, especially given the propensity of psychiatric settings to prescribe tricyclic antidepressants, like imipramine, for severe child depression (see the review by Simeon & Ferguson, 1985). Based on two studies, some researchers have also recommended the short-term use of imipramine for separation anxiety and school phobia, but these investigators have also emphasized that medication alone is insufficient to overcome such anxiety problems and have recommended concurrent behavioral treatment (Gittelman-Klein & Klein, 1971; Rapoport & Mikkelsen, 1978). In addition, the precise dosage and general effectiveness of antidepressants for children is far from well established (Simeon & Ferguson, 1985). Furthermore, although benzodiazepines are frequently used for sedation, there are no controlled studies of their effects on children with anxiety diagnoses, and few data are available on how this class of drugs alters mood and subjective feelings, learning, and cognitive and brain functioning in children and adolescents (Simeon & Ferguson, 1985). Also, it should be kept in mind that sudden withdrawal of these commonly used drugs can cause intense rebound anxiety, which may trigger or exacerbate SAD.

Another complex situation encountered in psychiatric settings is that of a younger child admitted because separation anxiety seriously interacts with a medical condition (e.g., asthma or arthritis), so that it is difficult for the parent to determine if and when the child is malingering to gain attention. For example, it may be difficult for a parent to resist a child's plea to be brought home from school after he or she has worked himself or herself into a full asthmatic and concurrent panic attack. In such cases, both the parent's and the child's physicians may be uncertain about the legitimacy of the child's call for help without careful monitoring of the child's behavior in the parent's absence. Just as it is hypothesized that panic attacks in some adults may escalate because of an oversensitivity to internal somatic cues (Barlow, 1988), some children may be hypervigilant to physiological symptoms that rapidly escalate into a full-blown panic, which has historically been alleviated by the parent's administration of medication and/or comfort.

A behavioral analysis of cases complicated by medical problems might involve careful observation of the child's physiological arousal levels. Assuming that some kind of escalation process is occurring in response to somatic cues, a child could be trained to become aware of the internal physiological signals that he or she is experiencing immediately before anxiety reactions intensify. Then, the treatment might involve counterconditioning the child to internal cues that trigger panic and push the child to seek attachment figures. Also, the child could be taught and positively reinforced for self-monitoring his or her medical status and using appropriate coping strategies. For example, a child who has asthmatic attacks may learn to offset initial problems by using relaxation and deep breathing and may also be subsequently reinforced for his or her attempt to short-circuit the hyperventilation process. In addition, the child could be provided with vicarious and participant modeling that show how to deal with medical symptoms and could be positively reinforced for handling such stressors with new skills. Finally, careful assessment and monitoring of medication, including dosage size and side effects, may also help to teach the child to anticipate typical reactions to medication (e.g., increased irritability) and to avoid misinterpreting somatic cues. It is also critical for parents to learn to differentiate the child's malingering from "true" medical symptoms.

SUMMARY

As is obvious, a monolithic or integrated theory of the assessment and treatment of children with SAD is currently unavailable. Instead, multiple mechanisms and environmental circumstances may account for the etiology and maintenance of this psychiatric diagnosis. Furthermore, whereas Barlow (1988) provided an excellent cognitive-behavioral framework for comparing and contrasting the basic mechanisms that may underlie adult anxiety diagnoses, similar work on the children await development. Rather than lament the current status of the empirical research and the scarcity of clinical accounts of complex cases involving SAD, the behavioral therapist is hopefully in the position to critically analyze and adequately test various hypotheses. This process of case conceptualization and ongoing empirical verification is the very heritage of behavioral therapy.

REFERENCES

Achenbach, T. M., & Edelbrock, C. S. (1983). *Manual for the child behavior checklist*. Available from T. M. Achenbach, University of Vermont, Burlington.

American Psychiatric Association. (1980). *Diagnostic and statistical manual of mental disorders* (3rd ed.; DSM-III). Washington, DC: Author.

American Psychiatric Association. (1987). *Diagnostic and statistical manual of mental disorders* (3rd ed. rev.; DSM-III-R). Washington, DC: Author.

Anderson, J. C., Williams, S., McGee, R., & Silva, P. A. (1987). DSM-III disorders in preadolescent children. *Archives of General Psychiatry*, 44, 69–80.

Appelbaum, P. (1989). Admitting children to psychiatric hospitals: A controversy revived. *Hospital and Community Psychiatry*, 40, 334–335.

Bandura, A. (1977). *Social learning theory*. Englewood Cliffs, NJ: Prentice-Hall.

Barack, R. S. (1986). Hospitalization of emotionally disturbed children: Who gets hospitalized and why. *American Journal of Orthopsychiatry*, 56, 317–319.

Barlow, D. (1988). *Anxiety and its disorders*. New York: Guilford Press.

Beck, A. T. (1976). *Cognitive therapy and the emotional disorders*. New York: International Universities Press.

Belsky, J., & Nezworski, T. (1990). *Clinical implications of attachment*. Hillsdale, NJ: Erlbaum.

Bernstein, G. A., & Garfinkel, B. D. (1986). School phobia: The overlap of affective and anxiety disorders. *Journal of the American of Child Psychiatry*, 26, 527–531.

Bernstein, G. A., Svinger, P. H., & Garfinkel, B. D. (1990). School phobia: Patterns of family functioning. *Journal of American Academy of Child and Adolescent Psychiatry, 29*, 24–30.

Bird, H. R., Canino, G., Rubio-Stipec, M., Gould, M. S., Ribera, J., Sesman, M., Woodbury, M., Huertas-Goldman, S., Pagan, A., Sanchez-Lacay, A., & Moscoso, M. (1988). Estimates of the prevalence of childhood maladjustment in a community survey in Puerto Rico. *Archives of General Psychiatry, 45*, 1120–1126.

Blagg, N. R. (1987). *School phobia and its treatment.* London: Croom Helm.

Blagg, N. R., & Yule, W. (1984). The behavioral treatment of school refusal: A comparative study. *Behavior Research and Therapy, 22*, 119–127.

Bornstein, P. H., & Knapp, M. (1981). Self-control desensitization with a multi-phobic boy: A multiple-baseline design. *Journal of Experimental Psychiatry and Behavior Therapy, 12*, 281–285.

Bowen, R. C., Offord, D. R., & Boyle, M. H. (1990). The prevalence of overanxious disorder and separation anxiety disorder: Results from the Ontario Child Health Study. *Journal of American Academy Child and Adolescent Psychiatry, 29*, 753–758.

Bowlby, J. (1969). *Attachment and loss: Vol. 1. Attachment.* New York: Basic Books.

Brewer, T., & Faitak, M. T. (1989). Ethical guidelines for the inpatient psychiatric care of children. *Professional Psychology: Research and Practice, 20*, 142–147.

Campbell, S. B. (1986). Developmental issues in childhood anxiety. In R. Gittelman (Ed.), *Anxiety disorders of childhood* (pp. 24–57). New York: Guilford Press.

Chambers, W. J., Puig-Antich, U., Hirsch, M., Paez, P., Ambrosini, J. J., Tabrizi, M. A., & Davies, M. (1985). The assessment of affective disorders in children and adolescents by semistructured interview. *Archives of General Psychiatry, 42*, 696–702.

Connell, H. M. (1985). *Essentials of child psychiatry.* Melbourne: Blackwell Scientific Publications.

Costello, E. J., Edelbrock, C., & Costello, A. J. (1985). Validity of the NIMH Diagnostic Interview Schedule for children: A comparison between psychiatric and pediatric referrals. *Journal of Abnormal Child Psychology, 13*, 579–595.

Dalton, R., & Forman, M. A. (1987). Conflict of interest associated with the psychiatric hospitalization of children. *American Journal of Orthopsychiatry, 57*, 12–14.

Dalton, R., Muller, B., & Forman, M. A. (1989). The psychiatric hospitalization of children: An overview. *Child Psychiatry and Human Development, 19*, 231–244.

Edelbrock, C., Costello, A. J., Dulcan, M. K., Kalas, R., & Conover, N. C. (1985). Age differences in the reliability of the psychiatric interview of the child. *Child Development, 56*, 265–275.

Ellis, A. (1970). *The essence of rational psychotherapy: A comprehensive approach to treatment.* New York: Institute for Rational Living.

Francis, G., Last, C. G., & Strauss, C. C. (1987). Expression of SAD: The roles of age and gender. *Child Psychiatry and Human Development, 18*, 82–89.

Garfield, S. L. (1984). Methodological problems in clinical diagnosis. In H. E. Adams & P. B. Sutker (Eds.), *Comprehensive handbook of psychopathology* (pp. 27–46). New York: Plenum Press.

Garvey, W., & Hegrenes, J. (1966). Desensitization techniques in the treatment of school phobia. *American Journal of Orthopsychiatry, 36*, 147–152.

Gittelman, R. (1986). Childhood anxiety disorders: Correlates and outcome. In R. Gittelman (Ed.). *Anxiety disorders of childhood* (pp. 101–125). New York: Guilford Press.

Gittelman-Klein, R., & Klein, D. F. (1971). Controlled imipramine treatment of school phobia. *Archives of General Psychiatry, 25*, 204–207.

Gittelman-Klein, R., & Klein, D. F. (1980). Separation anxiety in school refusal and its treatment with drugs. In L. Hersov & I. Berg (Eds.), *Out of school* (pp. 321–341). London: Wiley.

Graziano, A. M., DeGiovanni, I. S., & Garcia, K. A. (1979). Behavioral treatment of children's fears: A review. *Psychological Bulletin, 86*, 804–830.

Hersen, M. (1968). A treatment of a compulsive and phobic disorder through a total behavioural therapy program: A case study. *Psychotherapy, 5*, 220–225.

Hersov, L., & Bentovim, A. (1985). In-patient and day-hospital units. In M. Rutter & L. Hersov (Eds.), *Child and adolescent psychiatry* (pp. 766–779). London: Blackwell.

Hodgson, R., & Rachman, S. (1974). Desynchrony in measures of fear. *Behavior Research and Therapy, 12*, 319–326.

Kashani, J. H,. & Orvaschel, H. (1990). A community study of anxiety in children and adolescents. *American Journal of Psychiatry, 147*, 313–318.

Kashani, J. H., Vaidya, A. F., Soltys, S. M., Dandoy, A. C., Katz, L. M., & Reid, J. C. (1990). Correlates of anxiety in psychiatrically hospitalized children and their parents. *American Journal of Psychiatry, 147*, 319–323.

Kendall, P. C., Howard, B. L., & Epps, J. (1988). The anxious child: Cognitive-behavioral treatment strategies. *Behavior Modification, 12*, 281–310.

Kennedy, W. A. (1965). School phobia: Rapid treatment of 50 cases. *Journal of Abnormal Psychology, 70*, 285–289.

Kennedy, W. A. (1983). Obsessive-compulsive and phobic reactions. In T. O. Ollendick & M. Hersen (Eds.), *Handbook of Child Psychopathology* (pp. 277–291). New York: Plenum Press.

Kielser, D. (1966). Some myths of psychotherapy research and the search for a paradigm. *Psychological Bulletin, 65*, 110–136.

King, N. J., Hamilton, D. I., & Ollendick, T. H. (1988). *Children's phobias: A behavioral perspective*. London: Wiley.

Lamb, M. E., Thompson, R. A., Gardner, W. P., Charnov, E. L., & Estes, D. (1984). Security of infantile attachment as assessment in the "strange situation": Its study and biological interpretation. *The Behavioral and Brain Sciences, 7*, 127–147.

Last, C. G., & Strauss, C. C. (1990). School refusal in anxiety-disordered children and adolescents. *Journal of the American Academy of Child and Adolescent Psychiatry, 29*, 31–35.

Last, C. G., Francis, G., Hersen, M., Kazdin, A. L., & Strauss, C. C. (1987a). Separation anxiety and school phobia: A comparison using DSM-III criteria. *American Journal of Psychiatry, 144*, 653–657.

Last, C. G., Hersen, M., Kazdin, A. L., Finkelstein, R., & Strauss, C. C. (1987b). Comparison of DSM-III separation anxiety and overanxious disorders: Demographic characteristics and patterns of comorbidity. *Journal of the American Academy of Child Psychiatry, 26*, 527–531.

Last, C. G., Hersen, M., Kazdin, A. L., Francis, G. F., & Grubb, H. J. (1987c). Psychiatric illness in the mothers of anxious children. *American Journal of Psychiatry, 144*, 1580–1583.

Last, C. G., Strauss, C. C., & Francis, G. F. (1987d). Comorbidity among childhood anxiety disorders. *Journal of Nervous and Mental Disease, 175*, 726–730.

Lazarus, A. A. (1960). The elimination of children's phobias by deconditioning. In H. J. Eysenck (Ed.), *Behavior therapy and the neuroses* (pp. 114–122). New York: Pergamon Press.

Lazarus, A. A., & Abramovitz, A. (1962). The use of emotive imagery in the treatment of children's phobias. *Journal of Mental Science, 108*, 191–195.

Livingston, R., Taylor, L. J., & Crawford, L. S. (1988). Study of somatic complaints and psychiatric diagnoses in children. *Journal of the American Academy of Child and Adolescent Psychiatry, 27*, 185–187.

Marks, I. (1969). *Fears and phobias*. New York: American Press.

Martin, C. A., & Korte, A. O. (1978). An application of social learning principles to a case of school phobia. *School Social Work Journal, 2*, 77–82.

Mash, E. J., & Terdal, L. G. (Eds.). (1981). *Behavioral assessment of childhood disorders*. New York: Guilford Press.

Meichenbaum, D. H. (1977). *Cognitive-behavior modification*. New York: Plenum Press.

Miller, L. C., Barrett, C. L., & Hampe, E. (1974). Phobias of childhood in a prescientific era. In A. Davids (Ed.), *Child personality and psychopathology: Current topics* (Vol. 1, pp. 89–134). New York: Wiley.

Miller, P. M. (1972). The use of visual imagery and muscle relaxation in the counterconditioning of a phobic child: A case study. *Journal of Nervous and Mental Disease, 154*, 457–460.

Montenegro, H. (1968). Severe separation anxiety in two preschool children: Successfully treated by reciprocal inhibition. *Journal of Child Psychology and Psychiatry, 9*, 93–103.

Morris, R. J., & Kratochwill, T. R. (1983). *Treating children's fears and phobias*. New York: Pergamon Press.

Neisworth, J. T., Madle, R. A., & Goeke, K. E. (1975). "Errorless" elimination of separation anxiety: A case study. *Journal of Behavior Therapy and Experimental Psychiatry, 6*, 79–82.

Ollendick, T. H. (1983). Reliability and validity of the revised Fear Survey Schedule for Children (FSS CR-R). *Behavior Research and Therapy, 21*, 685–692.

Ollendick, T. H., & Francis, G. (November, 1990). *Behavioral assessment and treatment of childhood phobia and childhood anxiety disorders*. Workshop at the 24th Annual Convention of Association for Advancement of Behavior Therapy, San Francisco.

Ollendick, T. H., & Hersen, M. (1984). An overview of child behavioral assessment. In T. H. Ollendick & M. Hersen (Eds.), *Child behavioral assessment: Principles and procedures* (pp. 3–19). New York: Pergamon Press.

Ollendick, T. H., & King, N. J. (1990). School phobia and separation anxiety. In H. Leitenberg (Ed.), *Handbook of social anxiety* (pp. 179–214). New York: Plenum Press.

Ollendick, T. H., & Mayer, J. A. (1984). School phobia. In S. M. Turner (Ed.), *Behavioral theories and treatment of anxiety* (pp. 367–412). New York: Plenum Press.

Paterson, R. J., & Moran, G. (1988). Attachment theory, personality development, and psychotherapy. *Clinical Psychology Review, 8*, 611–636.

Patterson, G. R. (1965). A learning theory approach to the treatment of school phobic child. In L. P. Ullman & L. Krasner (Eds.), *Case studies in behavior modification* (pp. 279–285). New York: Holt, Rinehart & Winston.

Phillips, D., & Wolpe, S. (1981). Multiple behavioural techniques in severe separation anxiety of a twelve-year-old. *Journal of Behavior Therapy and Experimental Psychiatry, 12*, 329–332.

Quay, H. C., & Peterson, D. R. (1979). *Manual for the Behavior Problem Checklist.* Published by authors at 59 Fifth St., Highland Park, NJ 08904.

Rapoport, J. L., & Mikkelsen, E. J. (1978). Antidepressants. In J. S. Werry (Ed.), *Psychopharmacology* (pp. 208–233). New York: Brunner/Mazel.

Reeves, J. C., Werry, J. S. Elkind, G. S., & Zametizin, A. (1987). Attention deficit, conduct, oppositional and anxiety disorders in children: 2. Clinical characteristics. *Journal of the American Academy of Child Psychiatry, 26*, 144–155.

Reynolds, C. R., & Richmond, B. O. (1978). What I think and feel: A revised measure of children's manifest anxiety. *Journal of Abnormal Child Psychology, 6*, 271–280.

Simeon, J. G., & Ferguson, H. B. (1985). Recent developments in the use of antidepressant and anxiolytic medications. *Psychiatric Clinics of North American, 8*, 893–907.

Stokes, T. F., Boggs, S. R., & Osnes, P. G. (1989). Separation anxiety disorder and school phobia. In M. C. Robert & C. E. Walker (Eds.), *Casebook of child and pediatric psychology* (pp. 71–93). New York: Guilford Press.

Stone, L. (1979). Residential treatment. In S. I. Harrison (Ed.), *Basic handbook of child psychiatry* (pp. 231–262). New York: Basic Books.

Strauss, C. C., Last, C. G., Hersen, M., & Kazdin, A. L. (1988). Association between anxiety and depression in children and adolescents with anxiety disorders. *Journal of Abnormal Child Psychology, 16*, 57–68.

Thyer, B. A., & Sowers-Hoag, K. M. (1988). Behavior therapy for separation anxiety disorder. *Behavior Modification, 12*, 205–233.

Van der Plog, H. M. (1975). Treatment of frequency of urination by stories competing with anxiety. *Journal of Behavior Therapy and Experimental Psychiatry, 6*, 165–166.

Waldron, S., Shrier, D. K., Stone, B., & Tobin, S. (1975). School phobia and other childhood neuroses: A systematic study of children and their families. *American Journal of Psychiatry, 132*, 802–308.

Weinstein, S. R., Stone, K., Noam, G. G., Grimes, K., & Schwab-Stone, M. (1989). Comparison of DISC with clinicians' DSM-III diagnoses in psychiatric inpatients. *Journal of the American Academy of Child Adolescent Psychiatry, 28*, 53–60.

Werry, J. S., Methven, R. J., Fitzpatrick, J., & Dixon, H. (1983). The interrater reliability of DSM-III in children. *Journal of Abnormal Child Psychology, 11*, 341–354.

Werry, J. S., Elkind, G. S., & Reeves, J. C. (1987a). Attention deficit, conduct, oppositional, and anxiety disorders in children: 1. A review of the research on differentiating characteristics. *Journal of the American Academy of Child Psychiatry, 26*, 133–143.

Werry, J. S., Elkind, G. S., & Reeves, J. C. (1987b). Attention deficit, conduct, oppositional, and anxiety disorders in children: 3. Laboratory differences. *Journal of Abnormal Child Psychology, 15*, 409–428.

Wilson, G. T., & O'Leary, K. D. (1980). *Principles of behavior therapy.* Englewood Cliffs, NJ: Prentice-Hall.

Wolpe, J. (1958). *Psychotherapy by reciprocal inhibition.* Stanford, CA: Stanford University Press.

21

Depression

KEVIN D. STARK, JOHN A. CHRISTOPHER, and MARGARET DEMPSEY

INTRODUCTION

A significant number of children and adolescents who are hospitalized for psychiatric reasons are suffering from depressive disorders. Although the figures vary widely from study to study, between 6.2% (Olsen, 1961) and 17.8% (Strober, Green, & Carlson, 1981) of inpatient adolescents, and between 37% (Alessi, 1986) and approximately 59% (Carlson & Cantwell, 1980; Kashani, Husain, Shekim, Hodges, Cytryn, & McKnew, 1981b; Petti, 1978) of inpatient children have been diagnosed as having a depressive disorder.

Youths who are hospitalized because of a psychological disturbance commonly are experiencing multiple disorders. This may be especially true of youngsters who are experiencing a depressive disorder. Depressive disorders during childhood and adolescence commonly co-occur with other disorders (Anderson, Williams, McGee, & Silva, 1987), which may greatly complicate the clinical picture. Among inpatient samples, a relatively large proportion of depressed children present with concurrent externalizing disorders (Asarnow, 1988). Especially common are conduct disorders among adolescents (Carlson & Cantwell, 1979; Jensen, Burke, & Garfinkel, 1988; Marriage, Fine, Moretti, & Haley, 1986; Rutter, Tizard, & Whitmore, 1970) and attention-deficit hyperactivity disorder (ADHD) among children (Biederman & Steingar, 1989). However, among children with ADHD, the depressive disorder is often secondary to the ADHD. Consequently, the clinician is faced with a variety of questions that must be addressed before or during treatment. Is the depressive disorder the primary concern, or is it secondary to another disorder? Is the depressive disorder a reaction to the loss of self-esteem associated with having another disorder such, as ADHD, or does it stem from the limitations in functioning that result from having an anxiety disorder or a phobia? If one treats the depression, will the other pathology disappear? If one treats the other presenting pathology, will the depression dissipate? Is the prototypical treatment of one disorder antithetical to the treatment of the other co-occurring disorder, as is the case in a child or adolescent with a combination of a depressive disorder and a conduct disorder? Will multiple pharmacological interventions be required,

KEVIN D. STARK, JOHN A. CHRISTOPHER, and MARGARET DEMPSEY • Department of Educational Psychology, University of Texas at Austin, Austin, Texas 78712.

Handbook of Behavior Therapy in the Psychiatric Setting, edited by Alan S. Bellack and Michel Hersen. Plenum Press, New York, 1993.

or may just one disorder be the primary focus of intervention? The clinical picture is further complicated if the youngster is abusing drugs and alcohol. Is the youngster self-medicating, or is the depression secondary to the physiological damage that results from the substance abuse? Furthermore, the hospital milieu may or may not be conducive to the unique treatment needs of depressed youths, as hospital procedures are commonly designed to manage youths with acting-out disorders. This is not surprising, as the majority of children hospitalized for psychiatric reasons are suffering from externalizing disorders.

The focus of this chapter is the behavioral assessment and treatment of depression in the hospital setting when it is the primary disturbance. Although anxiety disorders may be the most common disorders co-occurring with depression, perhaps the most difficult combination for which to devise treatment plans is a depressive disorder in combination with ADHD in a child, or a depressive disorder in combination with a conduct disorder in an adolescent. Youngsters presenting with either of these mixed clinical pictures require modifications in the prototypical treatment plan for depressed youth. In addition to describing the prototypical treatment for depressed youths and the modifications needed to deal with the mixed clinical picture, we offer suggestions for enhancing the hospital milieu for depressed youths. However, we begin with a brief description of the expression of depression during childhood and then discuss the prototypical assessment of depression during childhood.

Nature of Depression during Childhood

Depression during childhood is manifested in a similar fashion to depression during the adult years (Kaslow & Rehm, 1983). However, it is expressed in a developmentally appropriate fashion. Depression is a syndrome (Carlson & Cantwell, 1980) that comprises a number of symptoms that co-occur in reliable fashion. Although the definitive symptoms are affective, the syndrome also involves symptoms that can be grouped into the cognitive, motivational, and physical domains (Kovacs & Beck, 1977). Because of space limitations, the description of the symptoms here is quite brief. The interested reader is referred to Stark (1990) for a more detailed description of the clinical picture of depression during childhood.

Of course, the quintessential symptom of depression is dysphoric mood. However, a large number of children and adolescents report anger as the primary mood disturbance. Perhaps more children than adults report anger as their primary mood disturbance (Brumback, Dietz-Schmidt, & Weinberg, 1977). Other affective symptoms include anhedonia, loss of the mirth response, diminished self-esteem, excessive weepiness, a sense of worthlessness, feeling unloved, self-pity, and negative evaluations.

Included among the cognitive symptoms are negative self-evaluations, hopelessness, morbid ideation, poor concentration, and indecisiveness. Most of these symptoms are expressed overtly in a variety of ways in the classroom and other settings. Negative self-evaluations are commonly expressed in the child's verbalizations, such as "I'm no good at that." Hopelessness may also be expressed verbally in such statements as "Why bother to try? I can't do it anyway." Morbid ideation is often evident in the youngster's essays, diary entries, and choice of reading materials. Poor concentration is often evident in the child's short attention span and "spaciness." Indecisiveness is evident when the youngster is given a choice about what to do, and he or she takes an extraordinarily long time to make a decision or makes a decision and then regrets it. Excessive guilt, which is presumed to reflect an internalizing attributional style, is the final cognitive symptom.

The motivational symptoms of depression include social withdrawal, decreased academic performance, and suicidal ideation and behavior. Depressed youngsters withdraw from both family members and friends. They often withdraw to their bedrooms, preferring to listen to music rather than to go out to play. The impact of depression on academic performance is unclear: some studies find a negative impact (e.g., Hollon, 1970), and others (e.g., Stark,

Livingston, Laurent, & Cardenas, 1991d) have found a minimal impact. Children do attempt and commit suicide (Carlson & Cantwell, 1982) although it occurs very infrequently; however, the rate is much higher among adolescents.

Among the physical symptoms are fatigue, changes in appetite and/or weight, sleep disturbance, psychomotor retardation and agitation, and psychosomatic complaints. Sleep disturbance, especially initial insomnia, is relatively common among depressed youngsters (Kashani, Barbero, & Bolander, 1981a). Fatigue and aches and pains, especially headaches and stomachaches, are also relatively common (Brumback *et al.*, 1977). Psychomotor disturbances and extreme weight gains appear more frequently among the severely depressed.

PROTOTYPICAL ASSESSMENT

The prototypical assessment of youths with a suspected depressive disorder involves more than simply assessing for the presence and severity of depressive symptoms. It also involves an assessment of therapeutically relevant constructs, such as hopelessness, the child's automatic thoughts, and the child's way of constructing his or her perceptions. In addition to assessing the child, it is important to evaluate the child's parents for psychopathology as well as their parenting style and skills. Furthermore, the family's beliefs, rules, and interaction patterns are assessed. Finally, following the behavioral tradition, it is important to assess the severity of the client's depressive symptoms over the course of treatment to determine whether the treatment is effective.

Assessment of the Child's Depression

Because depression is a highly subjective disorder, self-report measures are an integral part of the assessment process. A variety of paper-and-pencil self-report measures of depression have been developed. However, they have not demonstrated the ability to discriminate between depressive disorders and other disorders or general maladjustment (Kendall, Cantwell, & Kazdin, 1989). Thus, they should not be used as anything more than screening tools (Reynolds & Stark, 1987). It is critical to use a clinical interview to assess for the presence and severity of depressive symptoms and to obtain a diagnosis (Kazdin, 1988).

A variety of semistructured clinical interview schedules are available, including the Child Assessment Schedule (Hodges, McKnew, Cytryn, Stern, & Kline, 1982), the Diagnostic Interview for Children and Adolescents (Herjanic & Reich, 1982), the Diagnostic Interview Schedule for Children (Costello, Edelbrock, & Costello, 1985), the Interview Schedule for Children (Kovacs, 1978), and the Schedule for Affective Disorders and Schizophrenia for School-Age Children (Puig-Antich & Ryan, 1986). These measures have been described elsewhere, so the current discussion is limited to the interview that we have chosen to use (cf. Kazdin, 1988; Kendall *et al.*, 1989). At this time, our preference is the Schedule for Affective Disorders and Schizophrenia for School-Age Children (Kiddie-SADS or K-SADS), because it has demonstrated solid psychometric properties (e.g., Ambrosini, Metz, Prabucki, & Lee, 1989; Apter, Orvaschel, Laseg, Moses, & Tyano, 1989) and diagnostic reliability (Ambrosini *et al.*, 1989; Last & Strauss, 1990; Mitchell, McCauley, Burke, Calderon, & Schloredt, 1989). In addition, it assesses a breadth of depressive symptoms as well as the symptoms that comprise most of the other major disorders in the American Psychiatric Association's *Diagnostic and Statistical Manual of Mental Disorders*.

The K-SADS interview consists of an unstructured portion, followed by a structured portion. During the unstructured portion, or the interview, rapport is established, and identifying information and relevant historical data are gathered. In addition, the interviewer and the child collaboratively define emotional labels and identify the child's problem affects. Also, the time of onset of the symptoms as well as the time when the symptoms were most severe over the previous year is identified. Such preliminary information sets the stage for the rest of the interview. Based on the clinical picture that emerges during the unstructured portion of the interview, the interviewer goes on to the relevant portion of the structured interview and assesses the child for the presence and severity of symptoms.

During the structured portion of the interview, the symptoms of depression are assessed at two potentially different points in time, including the past week and when the disturbance was at its most severe over the previous year. Because depressive disorders are episodic, this procedure can give the interviewer a broader perspective of the course of the child's depressive disorder. However, for many children below the age of 11, the distinction between last week and the most severe time becomes blurred. A strength of the K-SADS is that the anchors that make up the rating scale for each symptom are well defined and provide the interviewer with useful information about the frequency, duration, and intensity of each manifestation of each symptom. The interviewer then combines all of this information with his or her clinical judgment to construct an overall severity rating for each symptom. This same interview format is followed in assessing the presence and severity other co-occurring disorders.

Another advantage of this interview is that, with a minimum of changes in the wording of the items, the interview can be administered to the youngster's parents as a means of assessing the severity of the child's symptoms. The standard procedure is to interview the parent(s) first and then the child.

Related Constructs

A number of variables that are related to depression should be assessed, as they have implications for the treatment of the youngster. Especially important are hopelessness and self-evaluations.

Hopelessness.   Hopelessness is the expectation that one's life is not going to get any better or that it is only going to get worse. Because hopelessness is highly related to suicidal behavior (Kazdin, French, Unis, Esveldt-Dawson, & Sherick, 1983) and to the individual's belief that treatment can help, it is useful to assess the child's level of hopelessness. If the child is hopeless, is agitated, has adequate energy, and has suicidal ideation, his or her safety must be ensured, which often means hospitalization. A very brief 17-item measure has been developed by Kazdin and colleagues (1983) that assesses the severity of hopelessness. This measure has demonstrated acceptable psychometric properties (Kazdin, Colbus, & Rogers, 1986), and it can be completed in 5–10 minutes by most children who have at least a second-grade reading level.

Self-Evaluations.   A youngster's self-evaluations are highly related to depression (Kendall, Stark, & Adam, 1990) and suicidal ideation (Robbins & Alessi, 1985), and they are a target of treatment because they often are unrealistically negative (Kendall, Stark, *et al.*, 1990). We (Stark, Adam, & Best, 1990a) have developed a 30-item measure that assesses (1) the child's self-evaluations; (2) his or her ideal standards; and (3) the child's perceptions of parental standards for the child. The evaluations are completed in 10 areas of importance to 8- to 13-year-old children (e.g., school performance, popularity, and athletic prowess). On the first 10 items, the child rates how well he or she would have to do in order to feel absolutely satisfied with himself or herself. The items are then repeated, and the child is instructed to rate how well his or her parents expect him or her to do. The items are repeated a third time, and the child is instructed to rate how well he or she is now doing in these same areas. The ratings are made on an 11-point Likert scale. The instrument yields five scores: (1) an indication of the magnitude of the standards the child sets; (2) a measure of the perceived parental standards; (3) the child's self-evaluation; (4) a discrepancy score between self-imposed standards and self-evaluations; and (5) the perceived parentally imposed standards and the child's self-evaluations. Finally, the child rank-orders the 10 areas from most to least personally important.

The treatment program described later is based on a cognitive-behavioral model of depression (Stark, Rouse, & Livingston, 1990c). Therefore, in addition to maladaptive behaviors and symptoms of depression, the youngster's automatic thoughts, processing errors, and schemata are prime targets for intervention. To assess the youngster's cognitions, we have used both paper-and-pencil self-report measures and projective techniques, as well as the client's statements during treatment sessions.

Automatic Thoughts. The frequency of depressive thoughts has been found to be related to depression in children (Kendall, Rowe, & Ronan, in press; Stark, Humphrey, Livingston, Christopher, & Laurent, 1991c). Kendall *et al.* (in press) and Stark, Best, and McCabe (1991a) have modified Hollon and Kendall's Automatic Thoughts Questionnaire (1980) for use with children. The Kendall *et al.* (in press) measure consists of 42 items and the Stark *et al.* (1991a) measure consists of 30 items. On both measures, the child reads each item and indicates how frequently he or she has the thought on a 5-point Likert scale. Both teams of researchers have reported acceptable internal consistency reliability. Kendall *et al.* (in press) reported that their measure separates identified cases of depressed children from nondepressed children, and Stark *et al.* (1991a) reported that their measure separates depressed from anxious and normal control children. A measure of automatic thoughts is used primarily for its clinical utility. The clinician can review the client's responses to determine which ones occur most frequently and to determine any themes that may exist within the depressive thoughts that the child endorses. For example, the child may endorse negative thoughts about herself or himself or about social situations. Such a measure may also be used to assess treatment effectiveness if it is administered repeatedly over the course of treatment.

Social Skills. Our own research (Linn & Stark, 1991) indicates that depressed children experience a deficit in social skills that is due in part to a disturbance in their thoughts in social situations as well as aversive emotional arousal. It is unclear whether the youngster's disturbance in social behavior is a reflection of a skills deficit or of distortions in thinking and aversive emotional arousal. Nonetheless, it is useful to identify deficient or maladaptive social skills for intervention, as noted later in this chapter. A number of social skills measures exist, but we have used the Matson Evaluation of Social Skills for Youths (MESSY; Matson, Rotatori, & Helsel, 1983). The MESSY is a paper-and-pencil measure that can be completed either by the child and/or by his or her teacher. The items were derived from a number of the most widely accepted measures for assessing social behavior, including the Child Behavior Checklist (Achenbach, 1978), the School Behavior Checklist (Miller, 1972), the Social Performance Survey Schedule for Adults (Lowe & Cautela, 1978), and the Peer Nomination Inventory (Wiggens & Winder, 1961). The self-report scale consists of 62 items that cover five factors: appropriate social skills, inappropriate assertiveness, impulsive/recalcitrant, overconfident, and jealousy/withdrawal. The teacher report version consists of two scales, appropriate social skills and inappropriate assertiveness. The MESSY has demonstrated acceptable psychometric properties (Kazdin, Matson, & Esveldt-Dawson, 1984; Matson *et al.*, 1983) and the appropriate-social-skills, inappropriate-assertiveness, and impulsive/recalcitrant scales have been shown to be related to depression in children (Helsel & Matson, 1984; Kennedy, Spence, & Hensley, 1989; Stark *et al.*, 1991d).

RATINGS COMPLETED BY SIGNIFICANT OTHERS

Although the child is usually the best source of information about his or her subjective experience of depressive symptoms, the youngster's parents may be more accurate reporters of time-related information, such as when the current episode began, how long it has lasted, how often symptoms are present over an average week, and for how long they last over the course of the day. The parents can also report time-related information about previous episodes. In some instances, when the child believes that it is in his or her best interest to report inaccurate information, such as when the youngster is trying to avoid hospitalization, the child's parents may be the only reliable source of information. Thus, it is important to interview the child's parents with the K-SADS.

ASSESSMENT FOR PARENTAL PSYCHOPATHOLOGY

Depressed youths are at greater risk of having a parent with a psychological disorder, especially a depressive disorder. Research indicates that depressed parents are likely to be more irritated by their child's behavior and more punitive, and that they do not have the energy and the proper emotional state to provide their child with adequate nurturance. A parent who is not feeling good about himself or herself, the world, and the future is likely to communicate such messages to his or her child. Consequently, it is important to assess the youngster's parents to determine whether either one is currently suffering from, or has suffered from, a psychological disorder. If the parent is currently experiencing a psychological disorder, then the parent will also need therapy and the family system is likely to be more severely disturbed. In addition to gathering the usual demographic information from the parents, we commonly ask them to complete the Beck Depression Inventory (Beck, Ward, Mendelson, Mock, & Erbaugh, 1961) and the 1990 version of the Minnesota Multiphasic Personality Inventory (MMPI-2).

ASSESSMENT OF FAMILY PATHOLOGY

Although a variety of measures have been developed for assessing the family milieu, we have relied on the combination of a paper-and-pencil measure and observations to gain an initial understanding of the family's functioning. The paper-and-pencil measure is completed by each family member who is old enough to do so and is used to gain an understanding of that member's perceptions of the family. Observations of the family during therapy sessions are the primary assessment tool and are compared with each member's perceptions.

To assess each family member's perception of the family, we have used the Self-Report Measure of Family Functioning (SRMFF; Bloom, 1985). It consists of 75 items that were selected from the Family Environment Scale (Moos & Moos, 1981), the Family-Concept Q Sort (Van der Veen, 1965), the Family Adaptability and Cohesion Evaluation Scales (Olson, Bell, & Portner, 1978), and the Family Assessment Measure (Skinner, Steinhauer, & Santa-Barbara, 1983) as the result of a series of investigations of the psychometric properties of these measures. The resultant measure consists of three dimensions and 15 scales. Each scale contains five items. The Relationship dimension consists of 6 scales (cohesion, expressiveness, conflict, family sociability, family idealization, and disengagement) that describe various characteristics of the relationships among family members. The Value dimension consists of 3 scales (intellectual/cultural orientation, active-recreational orientation, and religious emphasis). The third dimension, System Maintenance, consists of 6 scales (organization, external locus of control, democratic family style, laissez-faire family style, authoritarian family style, and enmeshment) that describe the management style of the parents and the family's perceptions of who controls their lives. The wording of the original SRMFF was modified for children by simplifying the language in the directions and items, removing double negatives, and simplifying the descriptive anchors (Stark, Humphrey, Lewis, Crook, & Dempsey, 1991b). Stark and colleagues reported that 12 of the original 15 scales demonstrated acceptable levels of internal consistency reliability, whereas the external-locus-of-control, disengagement, and laissez-faire-family-style scales did not and therefore have been excluded.

Because family interactions are so complex, the primary form of assessment involves joining the family, observing, and interpreting the interactions. Of primary interest are the messages that the child receives from his or her family that lead to and maintain the child's sense of herself or himself, the world, and the future. These messages may be communicated verbally or more subtly through patterns of behaviors. The therapist is also concerned about determining what thoughts and beliefs underlie various maladaptive behaviors of the family members. In addition to observing other family members, the clinician observes the child-patient to identify the behaviors that he or she is enacting that contribute to the maladaptive sequence of interactions.

When observing and interacting with the family, it is important to try to identify maladaptive rules that may be governing the family's interactions and communications. These rules have to be deduced from observing and interacting with the family.

Research with families of depressed children (e.g., Stark, Humphrey, Crook, & Lewis, 1990b) indicates that a number of additional variables need to be assessed. It is important to be vigilant for conflict within the family. It may not be clear whether the conflict is between the depressed child and another family member, between the marital partners, or between other family members. Another very important consideration is the activity level of the family. Does the family restrict its recreational activities, social interactions, religious activity, and involvement in intellectual or cultural activities? Does the family do anything for fun? It is also important to determine how the parents manage the family. Families of depressed children are described within the literature as being managed in a significantly less democratic fashion. In addition, do the parents rely on punitive and guilt-inducing methods of managing their children's behavior, or do they appear to be uncaring?

A number of structural characteristics of the family must also be evaluated (Stark & Brookman, 1992). The structural characteristics of interest include the subsystems, boundaries, alignment, and power within the family. We have hypothesized that the families of depressed children are characterized by a weak marital subsystem, diffuse parent-child boundaries, low levels of supportive alliance behaviors, and stable and detouring coalitions, and that these interaction patterns are inflexible.

Ongoing Assessment

An assessment of the impact of treatment during the course of the intervention is important because it allows the therapist to know whether the treatment program is effective and whether any changes should be made. In addition, it alerts the therapist to any setbacks that the child is experiencing and any changes in the clinical picture. In the adult literature, a number of investigators have reported administering the Beck Depression Inventory at the beginning of each session. We have tried to duplicate this procedure when treating depressed children. However, children have reacted very negatively to both weekly and biweekly administrations of the Children's Depression Inventory (CDI). Consequently, we have created a 20-item symptom checklist (see Table 1). The child indicates which symptoms he or she has experienced between sessions by placing a check mark in front of the symptom.

Informal assessment is completed throughout treatment, as the therapist is continually vigilant for examples of depressogenic thoughts, processing errors, maladaptive expectancies and attributions, and themes in the child's thinking and behavior that reflect schemata. Especially important is an assessment of the child's self-schema, as it is assumed that this is the core schema, and that changing it will produce additional changes in schematic functioning and consequently alleviate the symptoms of depression. In addition to attending to the youngster, the therapist attends to his or her own reactions to the child and uses a negative reaction as a cue to pay particular attention to the child's interpersonal behavior in an attempt to identify excesses and deficits that have led to the therapist's reaction. It is assumed that the child's behaviors and the therapist's reactions to them are a microcosm of the behaviors exhibited by the child and of the typical reactions of others to the child in other social situations.

ACTUAL ASSESSMENT

Our experience with psychiatric hospitals suggests that a fair amount of the prototypical assessment is completed. The youngster and his or her parent(s) are interviewed. However, there is typically no structure beyond the interviewer's knowledge of psychopathology guiding the interview. Usually, it is only in university or medical school hospitals, where research is being conducted, that a semistructured interview such as that noted above is used. During the interview, the clinician obtains a psychosocial history, completes a mental status examination, and forms his or her impressions of both the youngster and his or her parent(s) and family. Following the interview, the hospital often contracts with a clinician to perform a psychological assessment. The parents are often asked to complete a rating scale, such as the Child Behavior Checklist. Parents rarely complete a formal assessment as a matter of procedure. They may be evaluated after the therapist or hospital staff member working with the child and/or his or her family recognizes some disturbance. Once again, only in a research institution have the related constructs and treatment-relevant constructs been assessed. Ongoing assessment is usually based on the clinician's and/or the clinical team's judgment of the client as he or she works through the hospital program. Weekly assessments of symptom severity are rare.

PROTOTYPICAL TREATMENT

The prototypical treatment program we describe here has evolved over the years as a result of continued empirical evaluation, related research, and expanded clinical application. The program was originally designed (Stark, Reynolds, & Kaslow, 1987) as a school-based intervention that was modeled after self-control treatment programs for depressed adults (Rehm, Kaslow, & Rabin, 1985) and impulsive children (Kendall & Braswell, 1985). While maintaining an emphasis on helping the youngsters to obtain skills for coping with depressive symptoms, the treatment program has been greatly expanded (Stark, 1990). As a result of clinical experience and research (e.g., Kendall *et al.*, 1990; Stark *et al.*, 1990b), techniques from Beck's cognitive therapy for depression (Beck, Rush, Shaw, & Emery, 1979) have been integrated into the

Table 1. Symptom Checklist

Please read each statement carefully. If the statement is true about how you felt over the last week, circle the number of that statement. If the statement is not true about you over the last week, then just read it and go on to the next statement.

1. I felt sad, or down, or unhappy, or like crying.	11. I couldn't sit still.
2. I was angry.	12. I felt as if I was moving in slow motion.
3. I felt guilty.	13. I wanted to be by myself.
4. I felt as if no one loved me.	14. Nothing seemed fun.
5. I didn't like myself.	15. I had trouble sleeping.
6. I felt as if life was harder on me than on other people.	16. I slept longer than usual.
7. I had aches and pains.	17. I didn't feel like eating.
8. I worried about my health.	18. I ate more than usual.
9. I was tired.	19. I tried to hurt myself.
10. I had trouble concentrating.	20. I thought about hurting myself.

program, as have parent training (Barkely, 1987; Phillips & Bernstein, 1989) and cognitive-behavioral family-therapy procedures (e.g., Epstein, Schlesinger, & Dryden, 1988). As the program began to be applied within the hospital setting, the importance of the therapeutic milieu and a more active staff with a different and more positive philosophy became apparent.

The effectiveness of the treatment approach outlined briefly above, and in more detail below, is in part based on the opportunities provided for implementing the procedures within the child-patient's environment. The therapeutic milieu created within the hospital setting has a number of advantages and poses a few limitations in the treatment of depressed youths. The primary advantage is that a coordinated treatment program can be devised that combines individual (both psychological and psychiatric) and group therapy that is delivered within an environment that encourages, and reinforces, the use of new ways of thinking and behaving. Furthermore, the focus of the treatment program can be expanded to include the child-patient's parents and family, and these changes can be further fostered and supported through multifamily meetings.

The discussion of the treatment program is divided into the primary modes of delivering therapy: individual, group, family, and parent training. In addition, as the hospital milieu is so critical to the overall effectiveness of the treatment, this component receives a good deal of attention.

Pharmacotherapy

Individual therapy with a depressed child or adolescent involves both pharmacological and psychological interventions. Although it is common practice in psychiatric hospitals to medicate depressed children and adolescents, we know very little about the effectiveness and potential long-term side effects of this practice. There is a paucity of double-blind studies of the effectiveness of antidepressants with depressed children and adolescents. Most of our knowledge of their effectiveness is based on case studies. There are two basic approaches to pharmacotherapy; one involves polymedicating, and the other, more conservative approach is using a single medication. The assumption underlying the use of multiple medications is that one medication may potentiate the effectiveness of the other. To date, there is no research to support or obviate either practice.

The most commonly prescribed antidepressant for depressed youths is imipramine, a tricyclic. It is assumed to work through its impact on norepinephrine uptake receptors. However, there are a number of competing theories, none of which has predominated. Although Prozac is gaining widespread use with depressed adults, it is rarely used with children, although it is being prescribed with increasing frequency for adolescents. Although all antidepressants have similar side effects, they vary in their relative emphasis of each one. The most common side effects are cardiac change, increased blood pressure and pulse rate, dysrhythmia, drowsiness, loss of appetite, dry mouth, and orthostatic hypertension. Drowsiness, loss of appetite, and dry mouth subside with time, and orthostatic hypertension can be compensated for by getting up from a sitting or lying position more slowly and carefully.

Before putting a child on an antidepressant, it is imperative to complete an EKG to identify any cardiac problems that would rule out the use of such a drug (see Elliott, Popper, & Frazier, 1990). Once the child begins to take the medication, his or her vital signs are checked daily, and blood plasma levels are checked at least biweekly, or more frequently if the dosage and rate of titration are high. However, this conservative procedure may be necessary only when (1) the patient is not responding to reasonable levels of medication, and (2) it becomes important to rule out or exclude the possibility of drug-related toxicity. Typically, it takes four to six weeks to identify the most effective dosage and for the medication to work at its maximum.

The pharmakinetics (how the medication is circulated and metabolized by the body) is different in adults and children. Children differ from adults in the rate of absorption, distribution within the body, metabolization, and excretion. Children have very active livers and thus may need proportionately higher doses. The half-life of the drugs is shorter in children, so they need to take the medication more frequently, commonly three times a day, whereas adolescents may need to take the medication only twice a day.

As noted earlier, depression commonly co-occurs with other disorders. This fact creates problems in the medication of depressed youngsters. Antidepressants are less effective in children who are suffering from concurrent disorders. If the combination is a depressive disorder plus ADHD, then the treatment of choice remains Tofranil, as it improves impulse control and concentration. However, if the co-occurring problem is a conduct disorder, there is no additional or alternative course of medication that will alleviate both disturbances. In other cases, polypharmacy may be indicated to determine a combination that works for the youngster.

Psychotherapy

The psychological intervention begins with the establishment of a solid therapeutic relationship and affective education. The therapeutic relationship is of critical importance because of its own therapeutic value, and because it helps the child to have the courage to try out the new skills that he or she is being taught and to challenge his or her comfortable way of thinking and behaving. Furthermore, in a program where therapeutic homework is so crucial, the therapeutic relationship serves as the leverage that enables the child to complete it. Moreover, many of the cognitive procedures cannot be used with maximum efficiency without an empathic understanding of the youngster.

Cognitive behavioral therapists are paying greater attention to the role of, and the modification of, maladaptive affect in psychological disorders. The primary mode of intervention has been affective education, which is the first therapeutic procedure used in the treatment of depressed youths. It is used as a means of helping youngsters gain an understanding of the relationship among their thoughts, feelings, and behaviors, and it helps them to learn the cognitive-behavioral conceptualization of depression and how to treat depression. In addition, affective education serves as a fairly nonthreatening avenue for building a relationship with the child, establishing trust, and teaching the child that he or she is expected to play an active role in the treatment process.

A series of games can be used as the medium for teaching a depressed youngster about his or her emotions. Participation in the games enables the child to learn the names of a variety of emotions and to learn that emotions are experienced along a continuum of intensity. The child learns how to recognize when he or she is experiencing these emotions as well as the cues of what others look like when they are experiencing them. A series of five games, which we refer to as Emotional Vocabulary, Emotional Vocabulary II, Emotion Charades, Emotion Statues, and Emotion Expression, can be used. Through these games, the child is taught that his or her emotions are associated with what he or she is thinking and how he or she is behaving.

Because depressed youths often find most activities boring, it is important to be creative and to devise methods other than the clinical interview to engage the child-patient in treatment. With one particularly secretive child who became angry when the attention was focused solely on her during sessions, I had to carry on the treatment one step removed from the child. We created a set of cartoon characters (dragons and unicorns) and a fantasy world that they lived in (Dragonville). The child's problems, including her extreme defensiveness, were projected onto the main character (Princess Erika) in the story, and the child and I led the characters through learning to trust others, and me (King Johnah) in particular. In addition, Princess Erika learned skills and strategies for coping with depression and altering how she thought about herself.

As the child is learning to understand his or her emotions and rapport is being established, we commonly introduce self-monitoring of pleasant events. This is done to produce some symptom relief, to teach the child a coping skill, and as a means of restructuring the thought that

"Nothing good happens in my life." In addition, it is a nice way to introduce the child to therapeutic homework. The child can be told that he or she is going to be asked to complete a homework assignment, and after the usual sighs, the therapist can tell the child that his or her assignment is to try to do something fun and then remember to tell the therapist about it.

The first step in the self-monitoring procedure involves the therapist and the child collaboratively developing a list of activities that the child enjoys or enjoyed before the current depressive episode. The youngster's parents may be asked to add to the list any activities that they remember the child enjoying. The list is then typed, along with a number of blanks to create a personalized pleasant-events schedule. An example can be found in Figure 1. An 11-point Likert scale representing the continuum of the child's mood is typed at the bottom of the page, and multiple copies of the schedule are made and placed in a binder. The child is instructed to self-monitor his or her engagement in pleasant activities each day between sessions by checking off each pleasant activity that he or she participated in during that day. When the child engages in a pleasant activity that is not on the list, he or she writes down a description of the activity in one of the blanks. At the end of the day, before going to bed, the child rates how he or she felt in general over the course of the day. One form is completed each day. During subsequent sessions, the therapist and the child use problem solving to devise ways to increase the number and variety of pleasant activities in which the child engages. In addition, contracting can be used as a means of ensuring that the child will increase his or her activity level. Most children can increase their activity level without the need for external contingencies. However, it is somewhat more difficult to get the children to complete the self-monitoring forms. This often requires an external contingency that can be established through a contract. Within the hospital, the youngster can earn points or steps up a level system for completing the self-monitoring.

Engaging in pleasant activities is a problem for children who are in a psychiatric hospital because their activities and access to pleasant events are greatly restricted, often for the child's own safety. In addition, the child's access to various activities may be made contingent on ward behavior as part of a token economy system. Moreover, the child's ability to travel to places outside the hospital is restricted for obvious reasons. Thus, it is necessary to be creative in the use of hospital resources that have potential reinforcing value. For example, the hospital gymnasium may be used for more than the equivalent of a physical education class. Some children enjoy such sporting activities enough so that they would like access to these activities at other times. Because it is especially useful for the child to engage in activities that require rigorous physical exercise, access to the hospital gymnasium and pool is important. In addition, more indoor activities have to be identified. These may take the form of access to art therapy materials and board games as well as video games. Finally, the child may enjoy group outings, which are often very difficult to arrange but are very powerful reinforcers.

In addition to having the child self-monitor his or her engagement in pleasant activities, the youngster is commonly asked to monitor a number of additional variables that are relevant to changing his or her schemata. For example, a child who believes that his parents always "gripe" at him would be asked to keep track of how many times this occurs over the next week. Before being instructed to do this, he would be asked to define "griping," and the definition would be written down to use as a comparison to determine whether the parent's behavior qualifies as "griping." Commonly, in such a case the parent would be asked to self-monitor his or her own relevant behavior.

Depressed youngsters may also be instructed to monitor the occurrence of positive self-statements. Commonly occurring positive self-statements, or positive self-statements that have been identified during treatment as being true, can be added to the list of pleasant activities, and the child is instructed to check them off as they are noticed. Or the youngster may be asked to write them down as they occur.

Later in treatment, as the child has gained some distance from his or her thinking and has mastered a number of coping skills, self-monitoring is used as an assessment tool to identify

---

Activity Diary

Date _____

As often as possible, check-off the *things that happen, that you do and think* each day. Try your best to remember to carry these diary sheets to school and back home again. If you do something fun, or if you think about or have something good happen that is not on your list, check-off "Other" and write it down. At the end of the day, compare the right side of your list with your mom and dad's list, and then rate how you felt in general over the entire day.

_____ Help out at school	_____ **I'm me and that's all I have to be to be loved.**
_____ Play cards	_____ Mom and Dad said nice things to me.
_____ Play with friends	_____ Mom and Dad hugged and kissed me.
_____ Go to a concert	_____ Mom and Dad gave me a choice.
_____ Go to a play	_____ Mom and Dad played with me.
_____ Ride bikes	_____ Mom and Dad listened to me.
_____ Play with Jasmine	_____ Mom and Dad said "I love you."
_____ Play with friends	_____ Mom and Dad said something nice to me.
_____ Play board games	_____ Thought about good things
_____ Help Mom cook	_____ Asked for attention
_____ Latch-hook	_____ Asked for love
_____ Draw	_____ Asked for a "Good job"
_____ Roller skating	_____ Taught my family to have fun
_____ Go to a party	_____ Told myself that I'm good
_____ Practice basketball	_____ Expressed affection
_____ Go to the mall	_____ Noticed I was being nice
_____ Go grocery shopping	_____ Did the special things that make me me
_____ Go to the bookstore	
_____ Go to the library	
_____ Do something with dad	
_____ Go to the pet store	
_____ Play catch with Brandy	
_____ Make bracelets	
_____ Build forts	
_____ Hobby kit	
_____ Jump rope	
_____ Run track	
_____ Other	

Worst ever					OK				On top of the world	
0	1	2	3	4	5	6	7	8	9	10

Figure 1. Sample Self-Monitoring Diary.

depressogenic thoughts and to serve as a cue for using cognitive restructuring. The youngster is commonly instructed to use a change in mood to focus on his or her thinking and then to write down what he or she is thinking. Particularly difficult situations that are associated with dysphoria may also be used by the child as cues to tune into his or her thoughts and to write them down.

Because of the depressed youngster's proclivity for distorting information in a negative way, it is important for the therapist to remain actively involved in the self-monitoring process as he or she helps the child process the results. For example, the child may very accurately record the occurrence of a variety of pleasant events over the course of a day. When asked for an evaluation of how the day went, the child replies, "Awful! Nothing went right," and proceeds to describe a disappointing event. A closer look at the child's pleasant-events diary reveals that a variety of positive things also happened. However, because of the processing error of selective abstraction, the youngster has focused on the one negative thing that happened and has excluded the positives. The therapist can correct this error and help the youngster recognize other times when the error occurs through the cognitive restructuring procedures described below. With the pervious example of the "awful" day, the therapist might first ask the child to define an awful day. Then, based on the definition, the therapist and the child would check the child's diary for the evidence to determine whether it was an "awful" or OK day. Countless opportunities for using cognitive procedures present themselves during these discussions.

After the youngster has learned self-monitoring and he or she has been independently applying it to increase engagement in pleasant activities and to identify positive events occurring in his or her life, he or she is taught self-reinforcement. Self-reinforcement is used (1) as a means of enhancing mood; (2) to reinforce the child's use of coping skills; (3) as a motivational bridge between acquiring and using skills and the natural reinforcement of symptom improvement; and (4) as a procedure that remediates the deficit in self-reinforcement that typically exists among depressed youths. The youngsters are taught to reinforce themselves after completing the steps of a therapeutic homework assignment, after enacting an adaptive behavior, and to enhance mood.

The first step in the procedure is to identify rewards for the child, including favored activities, snacks, beverages, people, objects, and positive thoughts. The important feature of the rewards to be identified is that they should be readily available to the child for self-administration.

Availability may be a problem for a depressed child in a psychiatric hospital for many of the same reasons noted previously in connection with identifying pleasant activities. In addition to the previously noted limitations surrounding access to enjoyable activities, there are often strict limitations on who can visit the child and when he or she can visit, and there are restrictions on the youngster's access to snacks, beverages, and other treats. Once the rewards are identified, permission for access to them has been secured, and the staff have been notified, a reward menu is constructed with the child. Next, the child is taught a number of basic principles: (1) rewards should be administered immediately following the occurrence of the desired behavior; (2) rewards are to be administered contingent on enactment of a desired behavior; and (3) rewards can be administered on occasion just for the fun of it.

Subsequently, the child and the therapist review the reward menu and arrange them according to their reward value. Highly desirable rewards are administered for difficult tasks and less desirable rewards are self-administered for easier tasks. Most nondepressed children can learn to use self-reinforcement in a few sessions. Depressed children seem to take substantially longer, in part because of an intense belief that they do not deserve a reward. Thus, self-reinforcement has to be used in coordination with cognitive restructuring procedures. It takes quite a while for a depressed child to be able to effectively use self-reinforcement, and the child's efforts have to be closely monitored and processed with him or her.

As noted above in the descriptions of the use of self-monitoring and self-reinforcement, cognitive restructuring procedures are used throughout treatment and may be used in every session, beginning with the first one. Cognitive restructuring is initially used tentatively, because youngsters are rarely willing or able initially to benefit from the procedures. Instead, they tend to be unable to believe schema-inconsistent information. In addition, they tend to talk right over what the therapist tries to say, or they simply seem unable to hear what the therapist says.

A few rules guide the use of cognitive restructuring: First, the therapist initially takes the responsibility for identifying and helping the child modify depressogenic thoughts. Second, as therapy progresses, the child is taught to identify and restructure his or her own maladaptive thoughts. Third, the therapist and the child progress from applying the techniques to individual thoughts to applying them to themes in the youngster's thinking. Finally, the most powerful way of changing the child's thinking is through behavioral assignments that directly test the premises that underlie his or her maladaptive beliefs.

A number of cognitive restructuring procedures are used including: What's the evidence? What's another way of thinking about it? And what if? (Beck *et al.*, 1979; Stark, 1990). The essence of the procedures is that they are designed to help the youngster acquire a more adaptive and realistic way of thinking about himself or herself, the world, and the future. Over time, within the sessions, most children seem to respond with some symptom relief to the therapist's attempts at cognitive restructuring. However, the improvement is short-lived, as youngsters return to their comfortable and maladaptive ways of thinking shortly after leaving the therapist's office. The goal is to help children to complete cognitive restructuring outside the office. It seems as though children require some extra structure to be able to do this on their own. This structure can be provided by giving them a form that facilitates the identification and restructuring process (see Figure 2). In addition to using this form, we have used Beck's two-column technique quite effectively with adolescents (see Figure 3).

A good deal of time must be spent working with the child to help him or her identify the situations that typically elicit depressogenic thoughts and to identify the thoughts that occur most frequently and that are associated with depressive symptoms. These situations serve as cues for the child to tune into his or her thinking and for then using cognitive restructuring. It is useful for the child and the therapist to review the situations that have come up in therapy to date as particularly causing problems and to keep a running list of them. We commonly go as far as writing down the situations on the forms before giving them to the child, and then the child is given the specific homework assignment to pay attention to his or her thinking in those situations. Typically, the child monitors his or her thinking in only one type of situation at a time.

Because many of the problem situations involve other family members or classmates, the hospitalized child is not as likely to find himself or herself in those situations. Thus, times that the youngster is out on a pass or in a family therapy session should be very closely monitored and planned for.

In addition to the spontaneous use of cognitive restructuring that goes on throughout treatment, a number of sessions are devoted to teaching the chid how to tune into his or her thoughts and to use cognitive restructuring. The child can learn to self-monitor by tuning into his or her thoughts during the sessions. The child is instructed to pay attention to changes in mood during the sessions and to use changes in mood as a cue to pay attention to his or her thoughts. The therapist can help the child recognize mood changes by pointing out that he or she looks as if, or is acting as if, he or she has experienced a change in mood. Then the child is asked to think out loud as a means of becoming used to attending to his or her thinking. Once the child is able to tune into his or her thinking, the therapist educates the child about how to use cognitive restructuring.

To facilitate the independent use of cognitive restructuring outside the office, the child and the therapist rehearse restructuring the thoughts that the child typically has in a particular situation. For some children, it is useful to write down these examples so that they can refer to them as needed. Commonly, children are unable to restructure all of their thoughts, so they bring

Thought Record

Remember to complete this form each time that you feel sad or angry and to bring your booklet to group.

I was feeling _____

What was happening.

What I was doing.

My thoughts were.

The evidence.

Alernative ways of thinking
1.
2.
3.
4.
5.

What might happen.

The thought I choose to believe.

Figure 2. Example of a thought record.

the monitoring sheets back incomplete. Subsequently, the child and the therapist work together to restructure the difficult thoughts. Many children report that, over time, they begin to hear the therapist asking the questions that lead to restructuring.

A couple of procedures can further facilitate the independent use of cognitive restructuring. One procedure is to use the analogy of being a detective who looks for the evidence for certain thoughts and for other interpretations of the thoughts. As noted below, the therapeutic milieu may facilitate cognitive restructuring as the staff help the child tune into his or her thoughts and to restructure them. Finally, parents can be trained to help the child identify and restructure his or her thinking.

Another cognitive procedure that is introduced shortly after the youngster has acquired the self-monitoring and self-reinforcement skills is problem solving. Problem solving is used both as a means of helping the child learn to overcome everyday problems and as a means of trying to solve the problem of experiencing depressive symptoms. Problem solving seems to help the child gain a sense of self-efficacy and hope. In addition, it serves as a means of loosening up the

Automatic thought	More realistic thought
1	1
2	2
3	3
4	4
5	4
6	6
7	7
8	8

Figure 3. Two-column technique form.

child's thinking. The problem-solving training procedure has been described elsewhere (e.g., Stark, 1990), so it will not be described here.

After the child has acquired the aforementioned skills, self-evaluation training is introduced. It is introduced later in treatment because of the heavy overlay of distorted thinking surrounding the child's self-evaluations. There are two primary objectives in the self-evaluation training: (1) the identification and modification of standards and self-evaluations and (2) working toward self-improvement. By this point in treatment, the youngster has acquired a number of valuable coping skills that can be used to produce additional improvements in the youngster's life. The therapist and the child work together to identify areas where the child would like to change and where it is realistic to expect some change. Subsequently, the therapist works with the child to identify the areas where the child would like to improve. This desire is translated into objective goals and then broken down into subgoals. The child and the therapist then create a plan for achieving the subgoals and bring all of the relevant skills that the child has acquired to bear on achieving the goals. Then, they work together to monitor the child's progress and modify the plans as needed. This process may be quite lengthy.

Group Therapy

Group therapy is an integral part of the treatment of depressed youths in the hospital. However it is important to recognize some of the limitations of group therapy with depressed youngsters. They seem to be less effective in groups because of their symptoms (especially pessimism and egocentricism). It often appears to be difficult for them to decenter enough to be able to support and empathize with other group members. These limitations may be further exacerbated when depressed children are included in groups with children who have other disorders. The other youngsters often find it difficult to understand the depressed child's problems and fragile self-concept. Other group members' confrontations may be misunderstood by the depressed youngster as personal attacks that confirm a negative self-image, and direct cutting comments may be devastating to a depressed child. Some of these difficulties can be moderated by structuring the groups and setting specific rules that prohibit personal attacks.

In addition to conventional group therapy, we have a hospital group that meets specifically with the goal of helping its members identify and restructure their maladaptive automatic thoughts and schemata. This group seems both to be facilitated by and to facilitate individual therapy. There seem to be some advantages in combining group cognitive therapy with individual cognitive therapy. Initially, it seems easier for the youngsters to identify distortions in others' thinking than in their own. The group also seems to help children obtain some distance from their own thinking so that they can identify and restructure their own thoughts. Furthermore, once a youngster has been successful in helping other children identify and restructure their thoughts, this success can be used as evidence that she or he can, in fact, do it.

Consistent with individual therapy, group sessions are structured and oriented toward problem solving. The primary objective is to identify the thoughts and schemata that underlie each group member's problem behaviors and symptoms. The therapist's behavior is also similar to that in individual sessions. The therapist is very active, focusing the group on the members' problems and asking questions that help the youngsters identify their thoughts and schemata. As sessions progress, the therapist becomes less active, and the youngsters take greater responsibility for these tasks. Because the children do not stay in the hospital for more than a few weeks, and new group members are continually joining the group, there is usually at least one group member who can model the process for others. The therapist and the other group members observe each other for changes in affect and then use this observation as an opportunity to have the child verbalize his or her thoughts.

Homework is an integral part of group treatment as well. The group can work along with the therapist to develop the homework assignments. Because homework is often highly structured, such as writing down automatic thoughts, and because compliance with homework assignments is maintained through a review and discussion at the beginning of each session, it is useful to have a cotherapist who can review the homework while the other therapist prompts the group to develop an agenda for the day. Then the therapists can lead the group through a review of the homework and note any important trends or events.

Groups also seem to be the ideal medium for teaching the youngsters social and assertiveness skills. Because groups represent an interpersonal situation, they provide a natural medium for assessing and teaching social skills. Not only can the actual social behaviors be taught, but the distorted cognitions that occur before, during, and after interpersonal situations and the accompanying aversive physiological arousal can be addressed while they are occurring.

Social skills training in the group can be coordinated with individual therapy to maximize the impact of both. Interpersonal skills deficits can be identified during group sessions, and a personalized program can be developed during individual sessions and subsequently enacted during future group sessions. Feedback can be provided to the child during both forms of therapy, and the skills can be refined during individual sessions. Frequently, the most powerful feedback about new social behavior is that provided by other group members rather than the therapist.

The content of the group sessions may be based on a predetermined curriculum or more loosely based on what transpires during the group sessions. Commonly, we combine the two approaches and have a set curriculum that teaches both macroscopic social skills, such as making and keeping friends, joining a conversation, ending a conversation, and solving conflicts, and more microscopic skills, such as appropriate eye contact and voice tone and recognizing personal space.

Therapeutic Milieu

The importance of the therapeutic milieu in the treatment of depressed youths became keenly apparent as we began working with such youngsters in psychiatric hospitals. Commonly, the behavior management programs are not designed to deal with the depressed youths' self-denigrating style of processing information, nor are the staff used to the more active role they need to assume in the depressed patients' programs. Rather, they have been used to dealing with the acting-out patient, such as youths with a conduct disorder.

From our perspective, the overriding goal is to establish a hospital environment that is positive and nurturant, that is oriented toward problem solving, and that offers enough communication between hospital staff and other mental health professionals to individualize the program. When we talk about a positive environment, we are referring to one in which the staff are both vigilant for the children's strengths and reinforce them for appropriate and therapeutically targeted behavior. This approach contrasts with the more traditional management system, which is passive and reacts to a child's misbehavior with punishment and to appropriate behavior with delayed positive consequences such as greater privileges. On certain days of the week, the youngsters can petition the staff to move up a level and receive additional privileges. Within the positive approach, the staff are trying to modify the youngster's behavior through the systematic use of social rewards (praise) to shape more adaptive behavior. The objective is to "catch the child being good" and to overtly recognize this. Thus, an environment that is very rich in social reinforcement is created.

In addition to the social reinforcement, a point system is in effect in which the youngsters earn points for specific positive behaviors and target behaviors that are of therapeutic relevance. Desired hospital and interpersonal behaviors are operationally defined for both the staff and the children, and an observational form that lists the behaviors and the time intervals is created. The staff actively monitor the children using a partial interval recording system, and they record whether or not the desired behaviors occurred during each half-hour interval. If the behaviors occurred at any time during the half hour, the child earns a point (only 1 point per interval for each behavior), and the staff member praises the child in specific terms immediately following the occurrence of the behavior (e.g., "I like the way you complimented Susan"). Each staff member monitors the behavior of four youngsters.

At the end of the half hour, each child's point sheet is reviewed with the youngster as a means of helping him or her become aware of his or her behavior and how to evaluate it. The staff member asks the child whether he or she remembered whether the behavior occurred during the half hour. If the child's self-observation agrees with the staff member's recorded observation, the child earns an additional agreement point for each behavior on which there is agreement.

This system also helps the staff and the youngsters pay specific attention to the occurrence of therapeutically relevant target behaviors. A target behavior identified during either individual or group therapy is added to each youngster's monitoring sheet, and this targeted behavior is placed on a continuous schedule of reinforcement. Its occurrence is recorded by means of a frequency recording procedure. Thus, the child earns a point for each occurrence of that behavior, and each time it occurs, it is recorded with a tally mark. For example, a child may have a goal of using problem solving to handle conflicts better in social situations. The child would earn a point for each time he or she approached an assigned staff member and completed the problem-solving steps.

At the beginning of each shift (eight hours of staff time) during which the children are awake, the children meet as a community, and each youngster states how many points he or she is going to try to earn during that shift. The staff have to work with the children to help them set realistic and achievable goals, as personal success is desired. In addition, each youngster reviews his or her target behavior with the staff. At the end of the shift, the community meets again to review each youngster's accomplishments. The community as a whole praises each youngster's efforts. Effort rather than accomplishment is emphasized.

The points the children earn acquire their reward value because they determine which set of activities the children may engage in during activity periods. In order to participate in the more desirable activities, the youngsters have to earn more points between activity periods. For example, access to Nintendo games requires more points than access to board games.

A nurturant environment is one in which staff members are sensitive to each child's individual needs and developmental status and try to provide the children with support, affection, appropriate physical affection (e.g., a handshake or a pat on the shoulder), and an empathic relationship, along with unconditional positive regard. Regardless of how difficult the youngster may be, the staff work to find the positive qualities in the child and to support the growth of these qualities.

To help depressed youths overcome their sense of helplessness and loss of control, the environment is designed to be problem-solving-oriented. The goal is to help the youngsters acquire a problem-solving philosophy toward life. In other words, the children learn to approach everyday problems, disappointments, and depressive symptoms with the attitude that they just represent problems that can at least be coped with and in some instances actually solved. This attitude is accomplished through direct education, modeling, coaching, shaping, and self-monitoring. The children are taught a five-step problem-solving sequence during individual and group sessions, and the steps also are strategically posted throughout the ward (see Table 2). The staff model this five-step problem-solving sequence when required. In addition, during group sessions, when interpersonal problems arise, the therapist asks group members to problem-solve so that the process can be modeled for all group members. The therapist and the staff members are vigilant for occasions when the youngsters can use problem solving. When such situations arise, they help the youngsters recognize that a problem exists and then coach them through the problem-solving process. As the children become more proficient in problem solving, they monitor their own use of it and offer examples during the end-of-the-shift community meetings.

Our experience is that there are some limitations in regimenting the problem-solving process. The youngsters may begin simply to parrot the problem-solving steps rather than actually thinking them through. Furthermore, they may state the socially appropriate and adaptive solution to a problem but may fail to enact it in the same situations in the future. To counter this problem, when the staff see a pattern of not following through on the previously established most adaptive solution, this pattern is brought to everyone's attention during community meetings. Subsequently, the child will earn problem-solving points only if he or she enacts that solution the next time it occurs.

In order to help youngsters carry out their individual and group homework assignments, it is important for the staff who have daily contact with them to be aware of the assignments. Then they can prompt the youngsters to remember to complete the task and can reward the youngsters when the task has been carried out. For example, a child may be asked to record her thoughts whenever she begins to display the overt signs of anger. A staff member can remind the youngster to make a record when he first sees the early signs of anger. With progression of treatment, this same child may be helped by the staff to use coping statements, relaxation, problem solving, and/or alternative interpretations to control her anger.

Another important characteristic of the hospital milieu that we try to establish for depressed youngsters is that the day is highly scheduled with activities, including academic, art, music, athletic, and recreational activities, in addition to therapy. It is important for the youngsters to learn that they can distract themselves as a means of decreasing their depressive symptoms. We try to emphasize strenuous physical exercise on a daily basis as part of a philosophy of developing good health behavior. We believe that this is important because research on depressed adults indicates that exercise in and of itself is an effective treatment for depression.

Table 2.   Problem-Solving Sequence

1. Problem definition
2. Generation of alternative solutions
3. Consequential thinking
4. Monitoring and evaluating the chosen action
5. Self-reinforcement or coping statements

Family

We consider family therapy an extremely important part of the treatment of depressed youths. Our own research (e.g., Stark *et al.*, 1990b) and experience have pointed to its importance. We have described this portion of the intervention in much more depth elsewhere (Fine & Carlson, 1992). The overarching goal of family intervention is to identify and help the family alter the interaction patterns, communications, and family rules that support the child's maladaptive behavior and thinking. Treatment begins by working with family members to help them understand how they fit into a cognitive behavioral model of depression. The therapist observes the family, waits for examples of maladaptive interactions, and provides feedback. In addition, the therapist explores the thoughts and beliefs of the family member who is involved in the maladaptive interactions in an attempt to help that individual change his or her contribution to the maladaptive behavior pattern. The family, like the depressed youngster, is given specific homework assignments to carry out between meetings.

Based on the therapist's knowledge of the depressed child's maladaptive cognitive structures and core beliefs, the therapist looks for behaviors and verbalizations of other family members, especially the parents, that may have led to the development and that currently support the child's maladaptive beliefs. Once these behaviors and verbalizations are identified, the therapist may use a variety of procedures, including therapeutic directives, education, coaching, modeling, feedback, behavioral rehearsal, and contracting, to help the family change. Conflict resolution skills appear to be especially important (Stark *et al.*, 1990b). In some very inactive families, activity scheduling may be used to increase their involvement in pleasant endeavors.

Parent Training

Part of the hospital treatment program involves an evening of parent training each week. During this time, the parents are taught basic parenting skills that we have borrowed from Barkley (1987) and Phillips and Bernstein (1989). In addition, they are provided the opportunity to ask questions about specific situations that they are facing with their children. They are taught to use a more positive approach to managing their depressed children's behavior. An attempt is made to teach the parents to create an environment at home that is similar to the therapeutic environment in the hospital. They are taught to praise and reward their children for desirable behavior, and they are also taught to help their youngsters use problem solving to overcome difficulties and disagreements that come up at home. In addition, the parents are instructed how to use problem solving themselves to deal with problems that arise within the family.

ACTUAL TREATMENT

Although the actual treatment program that we use with depressed youths is similar to the one described above, and although it varies to fit the client's individual needs, such a behavioral approach is not typically followed by many other mental health workers in a psychiatric hospital. Commonly, the treatment of depressed youngsters in the hospital involves individual, group, and family therapy. Individual therapy is dominated by psychiatric treatment. The approach to psychotherapy often varies across youngsters depending on the training of the therapist, but it is frequently psychodynamic because this approach is more consistent with the training of the psychiatrists and the psychiatric nursing staff. A traditional approach to group therapy that relies on the group process is used. The nature of the family therapy also seems to vary widely, depending on the individual therapist's training. As noted earlier, the therapeutic milieu is based on a level system in which the youngsters earn privileges for appropriate behavior and effort in therapy.

Bob was a 13-year-old boy who was originally referred to the first author for aggressive acting-out behavior at home and in school, and for suspected substance abuse. Bob lived with his single mother; his father was a drug addict who had physically abused his mother. His parents had been divorced when Bob was 5 years old; however, he had vivid memories of the abuse. Bob and his mother moved frequently, and he had had a number of additional male father figures in his life, who typically stayed with the family for a short time. Bob was originally diagnosed as ADHD when he was 7 and as having dysthymic disorder at age 9. He was hospitalized with major depression when he was 11 years old. The hospitalization ended after three months, when his mother withdrew him against medical advice.

Bob was a reluctant participant in the initial assessment, as his mother had to "trick" him into coming along with her to the office. Bob appeared to be depressed; he maintained minimal eye contact, showed no emotionality other than some anger, and had a generally unkempt appearance. On the K-SADS, he acknowledged no depressive symptoms, but he reported the symptoms associated with a conduct disorder. In contrast to the interview with Bob, during the K-SADS interview with his mother she reported that Bob was experiencing a severely depressed mood and anger that did not appear to be associated with any specific environmental events. There appeared to be a diurnal variation in the mood disturbance, as it was worse in the morning. In addition to the mood disturbance, Bob's mother reported that he was experiencing the following symptoms: negative self-image, feeling unloved, hopelessness, self-pity, somatic complaints, anhedonia, fatigue, difficulty in concentrating, psychomotor retardation including decreased speech, and difficulty in falling asleep.

Bob was on probation following a two-week stay in a juvenile detention center for shoplifting, truancy from school, and threatening his mother's life. He rarely attended school, and when he did, he would arrive after 11:00 in the morning. With one other youngster, he was in a special program for adolescents who were out of control and unmanageable. They were assigned to a self-contained classroom with an isolation room attached to it. The day before the initial assessment, Bob had thrown a chair through the window, had tried to break the window bars, and had threatened the principle's life with a piece of the broken glass. His mother reported that he frequently drank and that he stole anything that she had that was of value. She stated that she had lost all control over his behavior and suspected that he was abusing drugs.

Bob was hospitalized within a couple days of his initial assessment. While outside of the hospital, his primary presenting problem was his antisocial behavior, especially his stealing, vandalism, and oppositional behavior. Following hospitalization, oppositional and destructive behavior was kept in check to the extent possible, and the episode of major depression became the primary focus of treatment. In addition, it became apparent that he had a rather extensive history of substance abuse, especially inhalants, alcohol, and marijuana. Thus, his chemical dependency became a focus of treatment.

A couple of days after admission, Bob was evaluated by a neuropsychologist who contracts with the hospital. It was determined that Bob had above-average intelligence and was not suffering from any learning disabilities, and that there were no apparent lasting neurological effects from his substance abuse. The diagnoses of major depression and conduct disorder were given for the client. A treatment team was formed that included a psychiatrist, a psychologist to conduct individual therapy, and another psychologist to conduct individual therapy with Bob's mother and also family therapy with Bob and his mother. The hospital program staff, including his teacher, the head nurse on the adolescent unit, and the group leader for the substance abuse program, formed the rest of the treatment team.

Pharmacological treatment (20 mg Prozac) was initiated on Bob's entry to the hospital. After three weeks, the dosage was increased to 40 mg. During the initial individual psychological treatment sessions, most of the therapist's efforts were directed toward establishing a relationship with Bob and assessing his maladaptive schemata. The following were identified: "I will become whomever I am around or talk to; therefore, I don't interact with anyone," "Everything I do is wrong or bad;" "People should know me without my having to communicate with them;" "I can't have people screaming at me;" "I can't tolerate being bugged;" "I would be better off living alone;" "My mother is the source of all of my problems;" "I don't have to do anything that I don't want to do;" "Drugs are a great escape from my problems;" "You mess with me and I'll get even;" "School is stupid;" "People should just let me be who I am;" "I am the best that I can be now;" "I can't control my anger;" and "You know someone loves you if they cry about you." He also demonstrated a variety of processing errors that supported these maladaptive schemata, including a propensity for black-and-white thinking, selective abstraction, and magnification.

Bob evinced three coping skills for dealing with stress, all of which represented a form of escape. Sleep was one of his primary coping mechanisms. It seemed to have its genesis in the beatings his mother withstood while he was a young child. They were terrifying and he was powerless to stop them, so he would withdraw to his room and try to sleep. Another form of escape was drug abuse. He noted that he felt good only when he was high; otherwise, he constantly felt bad. The third coping mechanism was self-abuse. He found that he could distract himself from his psychic pain through focusing on physical pain. The more intense the psychic pain, the more severe the self-induced physical pain. He would punch his head, bang it against the wall, or cut himself on the arms.

Bob's social skills were extremely poor. He had two primary styles of interacting with others: sarcasm and arguing. In addition, he had little ability to take someone else's perspective.

Continuing to build a healthy relationship between Bob and the therapist remained a major goal throughout treatment, as he clearly had not established a healthy relationship with other authority figures. In addition, the therapeutic relationship was considered a microcosm of the relationships he had with other people. Thus, it offered the therapist an opportunity to model appropriate interpersonal behavior and to coach Bob to behave more appropriately. In addition, the therapist systematically praised Bob for approximations of more appropriate behaviors. The therapeutic relationship also provided Bob with the necessary base of trust and support to be able to attempt to carry out a new way of thinking and behaving.

In addition to working on the therapist–patient relationship, treatment focused on Bob's poor self-concept. This focus was accomplished through the use of "What's the evidence," alternative interpretations, and the assignment to self-monitor with special attention paid to things that he did well and liked about himself. A list of positive qualities was constructed, reviewed, and added in each therapy session. For the first four to six sessions, the therapist had to devise the items on the list. Subsequently, Bob was more effective in thinking about his positive attributes.

In order to ensure that Bob would receive positive feedback from the hospital environment, the staff were instructed to try to reinforce Bob when he was behaving appropriately. Indeed, Bob responded very positively to this approach. Concurrently, his belief that the hospital staff were all mean "jerks" who were out to get him was consistently challenged. In addition, to help ensure more positive interactions, Bob and the therapist took turns role playing (as Bob and the unit staff) as a means to help him assume the perspective of the staff. This was a very enlightening experience for Bob, and he quickly altered his approach to interacting with the staff. He adopted more appropriate behaviors that had been role-played during the individual sessions.

Bob's anger, which easily turned to rage, became the next target of intervention. He was initially taught to use deep-muscle relaxation as a means of coping with his anger. A Walkman and relaxation tape were left at the nursing station for Bob to use at least twice a day, and especially when he began to experience anger. In addition, he was taught to use relaxation as a substitute for getting high. As a means of controlling his anger, he was also taught to alter his internal dialogue when he was getting upset.

Bob was not interacting with the other adolescents on the unit, especially during group therapy, because he thought that they were "nerds" and that if he talked to them he would become a "nerd." This belief was repeatedly challenged, and he was given homework assignments to try talking with others on the unit.

Individual treatment continued in a similar fashion, changing maladaptive schemata and identifying and altering additional unhealthy schemata. In addition, prosocial skills that were in direct contrast to arguing and being sarcastic were taught. Moreover he was taught to be overtly supportive of his peers. This process took a great deal of time, as he was painfully deficient in even the most basic skills.

Family therapy and individual therapy were coordinated. Bob's belief that the only way that someone could demonstrate love for him was to cry was attacked. Bob's mother was also taught positive ways of expressing affection. As a consequence, Bob's behavior changed, as he began to elicit responses from her by positive means. In addition, Bob and his mother were taught how to spend leisure time together. Finally, they were taught how to develop mutual contracts to promote appropriate behaviors at home.

The therapeutic milieu, which consisted of a level system, was altered for Bob. A system that responded more quickly to Bob's behavior was devised. At the beginning of each shift, he contracted with the staff to behave in the desired fashion and to display specific target behaviors. The target behaviors were clearly defined and coordinated with individual and group therapy. He earned additional pleasant activity time after each two hours of appropriate, compliant behavior. In addition, his prosocial behavior was praised by the staff. The staff's interactions became more positive as they learned to reframe Bob's sarcasm and argumentative interactions as a reflection of the only way he knew how to interact, rather than as belligerence.

Bob's group therapy was not conducted by any of the authors, so the specifics are a bit sketchy. Nevertheless, Bob participated in a group for substance abusers in which they worked through a 12-step program, and in a cognitive distortions group that was modeled on rational emotive therapy. Reports from the group leaders indicated that his initial distance and sarcastic interpersonal style inhibited participation in the group. However, over time, as he evinced improved social skills, he contributed to the groups in a meaningful way.

At this time, Bob's treatment continues, and he has moved into a day treatment program. Thus, the final outcome is unknown. A recent administration of the K-SADS to Bob and his mother indicated that Bob's depression is under control, and the focus of intervention has switched to dealing with his antisocial behaviors and concurrently further improving his interpersonal skills. Family therapy is focusing on teaching his mother how to control his behavior.

SUMMARY

In this chapter, we have described a behavioral approach to the assessment and treatment of depression in children and young adolescents. It has been our experience that it is both possible and desirable to conduct such comprehensive assessment and treatment programs in hospital settings. However, they appear to be uncommon, perhaps because of the continued dominance of alternative theoretical and applied clinical orientations. Consequently, our description of the actual assessment and treatment of depressed youths has reflected these alternative orientations, rather than the behavioral approach, because they represent common practice.

The assessment of depression in youths involves more than an evaluation of the child's depressive symptoms. It also involves an assessment of the constructs that are relevant to treatment and an evaluation of the child's parents and family. The primary tool for assessing the presence and severity of depressive symptoms is the clinical interview. It is important to interview both the child and his or her primary caretaker in a semistructured clinical interview. In addition to assessing the child for depression, the child's hopelessness and self-evaluations are evaluated because they have implications for treatment and the degree of suicidal risk. Depressive cognitions are assessed, and the results serve as a guide to cognitive restructuring efforts. Although the children are considered the primary source of information about their experience of depressive symptoms, their parents are a valuable source of information about the duration and onset of the current episode of depression. In addition, when the child is defensive or resistant, the parents may be the only reliable source of information. The parents' own level of depression and other psychological disorders is assessed both because there is a great likelihood that they are disturbed and because, if such a disorder exists, it must be addressed in the overall treatment plan. The family's beliefs, rules, and interaction patterns are assessed with an eye to identifying the variables that produce and maintain depressive symptoms and maladaptive cognitive structures. Finally, we advocate ongoing assessment to determine progress in treatment.

The prototypical behavioral treatment of depression in youths includes individual, group, and family therapy, and it emphasizes creating a therapeutic environment that is positive and nurturant, that is oriented toward problem solving, and that meets the children's individual needs. Individual therapy involves both pharmacological and psychological interventions. The psychological intervention includes training in self-control, social skills, problem solving, and cognitive restructuring. Group therapy is coordinated with individual therapy and emphasizes cognitive restructuring and the attainment of adaptive social skills. Hospital staff are taught to use positive reinforcement as the primary tool for shaping appropriate behavior. A point system is used to reinforce prosocial and therapeutically relevant behaviors. The number of points the children earn determines which activities they will have access to during recreational periods. Finally, we emphasized the importance of creating a busy schedule in which the youngsters have little idle time.

References

Achenbach, T. M. (1978). The Child Behavior Profile-1. Boys Aged 6–11. *Journal of Consulting and Clinical Psychology, 46*, 478–488.

Alessi, N. E. (1986). *DSM III diagnosis associated with childhood depressive disorders.* Paper presented at the American Academy of Child Psychiatry, Los Angeles.

Ambrosini, P. J., Metz, C., Prabucki, K., & Lee, J. (1989). Videotape reliability of the third revised edition of the K-SADS. *Journal of the American Academy of Child and Adolescent Psychiatry, 28*, 723–728.

Anderson, J. D., Williams, S., McGee, R., & Silva, P. A. (1987). DSM-III disorders in preadolescent children: Prevalence in a large sample from the general population. *Archives of General Psychiatry, 44*, 69–76.

Apter, A., Orvaschel, H., Laseg, M., Moses, T., & Tyano, S. (1989). Psychometric properties of K-SADS-P in an Israeli adolescent inpatient population. *Journal of the American Academy of Child and Adolescent Psychiatry, 28*, 61–65.

Asarnow, M. H. (1988). Peer status and social competence in child psychiatric inpatients: A comparison of children with depressive, externalizing, and concurrent depressive and externalizing disorders. *Journal of Abnormal Child Psychology, 18*, 151–162.

Barkley, R. A. (1987). *Defiant children: A clinician's manual for parent training.* New York: Guilford Press.

Beck, A. T., Ward, C. H., Mendelson, M., Mock, J., & Erbaugh, J. (1961). An inventory for measuring depression. *Archives of General Psychiatry, 4*, 561–571.

Beck, A T., Rush, A. J., Shaw, B. F., & Emery, G. (1979). *Cognitive therapy of depression.* New York: Guilford Press.

Biederman, J., & Steingar, R. (1989). Attention-deficit hyperactivity disorder in adolescents. *Psychiatric Annals, 19*, 587–596.

Bloom, B. (1985). A factor analysis of self-report measures of family functioning. *Family Process, 24*, 225–239.

Brumback, R. A., Dietz-Schmidt, S. G., & Weinberg, W. A. (1977). Depression in children referred to an educational diagnostic center: Diagnosis and treatment and analysis of criteria and literature review. *Diseases of the Nervous System, 38*, 529–535.

Carlson, G. A., & Cantwell, D. P. (1979). A survey of depressive symptoms in a child and adolescent psychiatric population: Interview data. *Journal of the American Academy of Child Psychiatry, 18*, 587–599.

Carlson, G. A., & Cantwell, D. P. (1980). Unmasking masked depression in children and adolescents. *American Journal of Psychiatry, 137*, 445–449.

Carlson, G. A., & Cantwell, D. P. (1982). Suicidal behavior and depression in children and adolescents. *Journal of the American Academy of Child Psychiatry*, *21*, 361–368.

Costello, E. J., Edelbrock, C. S., & Costello, A. J. (1985). Validity of the NIMH Diagnostic Interview Schedule for Children: A comparison between psychiatric and pediatric referrals. *Journal of Abnormal Child Psychology*, *13*, 579–595.

Elliott, G. R., Popper, C. W., & Frazier, S. H. (1990). Tricyclic antidepressants: A risk for 6–9 year olds? *Journal of Child and Adolescent Psychopharmacology*, *1*, 105–106.

Epstein, N., Schlesinger, S., & Dryden, W. (1988). *Cognitive-behavior therapy with families*. New York: Brunner/ Mazel.

Helsel, W. J., & Matson, J. L. (1984). The assessment of depression in children: The internal structure of the Child Depression Inventory (CDI). *Behavior Research and Therapy*, *22*, 289–298.

Herjanic, B., & Reich, W. (1982). Development of a structure psychiatric interview for children: Agreement between child and parent on individual symptoms. *Journal of Abnormal Child Psychology*, *10*, 307–324.

Hodges, K., McKnew, D., Cytryn, L., Stern, L., & Kline, J. (1982). The Child Assessment Schedule (CAS) Diagnostic Interview: A report on reliability and validity. *Journal of the American Academy of Child Psychiatry*, *21*, 468–473.

Hollon, S. D., & Kendall, P. C. (1980). Cognitive self-statements in depression: Development of an automatic thoughts questionnaire. *Cognitive Therapy and Research*, *4*, 383–395.

Hollon, T. H. (1970). Poor school performance as a symptom of masked depression in children and adolescents. *American Journal of Psychotherapy*, *24*, 258–263.

Jensen, J. B., Burke, N., & Garfinkel, B. D. (1988). Depression and symptoms of attention deficit disorder with hyperactivity. *Journal of American Academy of Child and Adolescent Psychiatry*, *27*, 742–747.

Kashani, J. H., Barbero, G. J., & Bolander, F. D. (1981a). Depression in hospitalized pediatric patients. *Journal of the American Academy of Child Psychiatry*, *20*, 123–134.

Kashani, J. H., Husain, A., Shekim, W. O., Hodges, K. K., Cytryn, L., & McKnew, D. H. (1981b). Current perspectives on childhood depression: An overview. *American Journal of Psychiatry*, *138*, 143–153.

Kazdin, A. E. (1987). Children's Depression Scale: Validation with psychiatric inpatients. *Journal of Child Psychology and Psychiatry*, *28*, 29–41.

Kazdin, A. E. (1988). Childhood depression. In J. C. Witt, S. N. Elliott, & F. M. Gresham (Eds.), *Handbook of behavior therapy in education* (pp. 739–772). New York: Plenum Press.

Kazdin, A. E., French, N. J., Unis, A. S., Esveldt-Dawson, K., & Sherick, R. B. (1983). Hopelessness, depression, and suicidal intent among psychiatrically disturbed children. *Journal of Consulting and Clinical Psychology*, *51*, 504–510.

Kazdin, A. E., Matson, J. L., & Esveldt-Dawson, K. (1984). The relationship of role-play assessment of children's social skills to multiple measures of social competence. *Behavioral Research and Therapy*, *22*, 413–437.

Kazdin, A. E., Colbus, D., & Rodgers, A. (1986). Assessment of depression and diagnosis of depressive disorders among psychiatrically disturbed children. *Journal of Abnormal Child Psychology*, *14*, 499–515.

Kendall, P. C., & Braswell, L. (1985). *Cognitive-behavioral therapy for impulsive children*. New York: Guilford Press.

Kendall, P. C., Cantwell, D. A., & Kazdin, A. E. (1989). Depression in children and adolescents: Assessment issues and recommendations. *Cognitive Therapy and Research*, *13*, 109–146.

Kendall, P. C., Stark, K. D., & Adam, T. (1990). Cognitive deficit or cognitive distortion in childhood depression. *Journal of Abnormal Child Psychology*, *18*, 255–270.

Kendall, P. C., Rowe, M., & Ronan, K. (in press). Development and cross-validation of a Children's Automatic Thoughts Questionnaire. *Cognitive Therapy and Research*.

Kennedy, E., Spence, S. H., & Hensley, R. (1989). An examination of the relationship between childhood depression and social competency amongst primary-school children. *Journal of Child Psychology and Psychiatry and Allied Disciplines*, *30*, 561–573.

Kovacs, M. (1978). *Interview Schedule for Children* (ISC) (10th rev.). Pittsburgh: University of Pittsburgh School of Medicine.

Kovacs, M., & Beck, A. T. (1977). An empirical-clinical approach toward a definition of childhood depression. In J. G. Schluterbrandt & A. Raskin (Eds.), *Depression in childhood: Diagnosis, treatment and conceptual models* (pp. 1–25). New York: Raven Press.

Last, C. G., & Strauss, C. C. (1990). School refusal in anxiety disordered children and adolescents. *Journal of the American Academy of Child and Adolescent Psychiatry*, *29*, 31–35.

Linn, J. L., & Stark, K. D. (1991). *Childhood depression and social skill deficits*. Manuscript in preparation.

Lowe, M. R., & Cautela, J. R. (1978). A self-report measure of social skills. *Behavior Therapy*, *9*, 535–544.

Marriage, K., Fine, S., Moretti, M., & Haley, G. (1986). Relationship between depression and conduct disorder in children and adolescents. *Journal of the American Academy of Child Psychiatry*, *25*, 687–691.

Matson, J. L., Rotatori, A. F., & Helsel, W. J. (1983). Development of a rating to measure social skills in children: The Matson Evaluation of Social Skills with Youngsters (MESSY). *Behavioral Research and Therapy, 41,* 335–340.

Miller, L. C. (1972). A school behavior checklist: An inventory of deviant behavior for elementary school children. *Journal of Consulting and Clinical Psychology, 38,* 134–144.

Mitchell, J., McCauley, E., Burke, P., Calderon, R., & Schloredt, K. (1989). Psychopathology in parents of depressed children and adolescents. *Journal of the American Academy of Child and Adolescent Psychiatry, 28,* 352–357.

Moos, R. H., & Moos, B. S. (1981). *Family Environment Scale Manual.* Palo Alto, CA: Consulting Psychologist Press.

Olsen, T. (1961). Follow-up study of manic-depressive patients whose first attack occurred before the age of 19. *ACTA Psychiatry Scandinavia, 162,* 45–51.

Olson, D. H., Bell, R., & Portner, J. (1978). *FACES Item Booklet.* St. Paul: Family Social Science, University of Minnesota.

Petti, T. A. (1978). Depression in hospitalized child psychiatry patients: Approaches to measuring depression. *Journal of Child Psychiatry, 17,* 49–59.

Phillips, D., & Bernstein, F. (1989). *How to give your child a great self-image.* New York: Random House.

Puig-Antich, J., & Ryan, N. (1986). *Schedule for Affective Disorders and Schizophrenia for School-Age Children.* Pittsburgh: Western Psychiatric Institute and Clinic.

Rehm, L. P., Kaslow, N. J., & Rabin, A. S. (1985). Cognitive and behavioral targets in a self-control therapy program for depression. *Journal of Consulting and Clinical Psychology, 55,* 60–67.

Reynolds, W. M., & Stark, K. D. (1987). School-based intervention strategies for the treatment of depression in children adolescents. *Special Services in the Schools, 1,* 69–85.

Robbins, D. R., & Alessi, N. E. (1985). Depressive symptoms and suicidal behavior in adolescents. *American Journal of Psychiatry, 142,* 588–592.

Rutter, M., Tizard, J., & Whitmore, K. (1970). *Education, health and behavior.* New York: Wiley.

Skinner, H. A., Steinhauer, P. D., & Santa-Barbara, J. (1983). The Family Assessment Measure. *Canadian Journal of Community Mental Health, 2,* 91–105.

Stark, K. D. (1990). *Childhood depression: School based intervention.* New York: Guilford Press.

Stark, K. D., Reynolds, W. M., & Kaslow, N. J. (1987). A comparison of the relative efficacy of self-control therapy and a behavioral problem-solving therapy for depression in children. *Journal of Abnormal Child Psychology, 15,* 91–113.

Stark, K. D., Adam, T., & Best, L. (1990a). *My Standards Questionnaire—Revised.* Unpublished manuscript, University of Texas, Austin.

Stark, K. D., Humphrey, L. L., Crook, K., & Lewis, K. (1990b). Perceived family environments of depressed and anxious children: Child's and maternal figure's perspectives. *Journal of Abnormal Child Psychology, 18,* 527–547.

Stark, K. D., Rouse, L., & Livingston, R. (1990c). Treatment of depression during childhood and adolescents: Cognitive-behavioral procedures for the individual and family. In P. C. Kendall (Ed.), *Child and adolescent therapy: Cognitive-behavioral procedures* (pp. 165–208). New York: Guilford Press.

Stark, K. D., Best, L., & McCabe, N. (1991a). *Development of a depressive cognitions questionnaire for children.* Manuscript submitted for publication.

Stark, K. D., Humphrey, L. L., Crook, K., Lewis, K., & Dempsey, M. (1991b). *The Self-Report Measure of Family Functioning for Children: Preliminary investigation of its psychometric properties.* Manuscript submitted for publication.

Stark, K. D., Humphrey, L. L., Livingston, R., Christopher, J., & Laurent, J. (1991c). *Cognitive, behavioral, and family variables in childhood depression.* Manuscript submitted for publication.

Stark, K. D., Livingston, R. Laurent, J. L., & Cardenas, B. (1991d). *Achievement, performance in school, and depressive and anxiety disorders during childhood.* Manuscript submitted for publication.

Stark, K. D., & Brookman, C. (1992). Childhood depression: Theory and family-school intervention. In M. Fine & C. Carlson (Eds.), *Handbook of family-school intervention: A systems perspective.* Orlando, FL: Grune & Stratton.

Strober, M., Green, J., & Carlson, G. (1981). Phenomenology and subtypes of major depressive disorder in adolescence. *Journal of Affective Disorders, 3,* 281–290.

Van Der Veen, F. (1965). The parent's concept of the family unit and child adjustment. *Journal of Counseling Psychology, 12,* 196–200.

Wiggins, J. S., & Winder, C. L. (1961). The Peer Nomination Inventory: An empirically derived sociometric measure of adjustment in pre-adolescent boys. *Psychological Reports, 9,* 643–677.

22

Alcohol and Drug Abuse

OSCAR G. BUKSTEIN and VINCENT B. VAN HASSELT

INTRODUCTION

The 1980s witnessed a dramatic upsurge of clinical and investigative interest in the assessment, prevention, and treatment of substance abuse in children and youth (see reviews by Horan & Straus, 1987; Kaminer & Bukstein, 1992). The impetus toward increased activity in this area is, in part, based on epidemiological findings documenting the scope and magnitude of the problem. Indeed, despite recent evidence of diminished usage rates of some substances (tobacco, cocaine) in younger populations, levels of use and abuse in the United States are still the highest of any nation in the world (Holden, Moncher, & Schinke, 1990). Another reason for the acceleration of efforts directed toward this problem is the burgeoning body of research attesting to the deleterious consequences of substance abuse in children and adolescents (Newcomb & Bentler, 1988). Specifically, data have accumulated that document the relationship between high rates of substance use and a wide range of social, emotional, academic, and behavior problems in youth (Kandel, Davies, Karus, & Yamaguchi, 1986).

Behavioral clinicians and researchers have been focusing greater attention on the problem of adolescent substance abuse (e.g., Bry & Krinsley, 1990; Schinke, Botvin, & Orlandi, 1991). In particular, applications of behavioral strategies for the prevention of substance use in both children and youth have proliferated (cf. Botvin, 1986; Botvin, Baker, Renick, Filazzda, & Botvin, 1984; Pentz, Cormack, Flay, Hansen, & Johnson, 1986; Schinke & Gilchrist, 1984). However, since the mid-1980s, there has been an acceleration of efforts directed toward the treatment of substance abuse in young persons as well. The purpose of this chapter is to provide an overview of behavioral approaches for adolescent substance abusers that have demonstrated utility in the psychiatric setting. Because the current work in this field is at the nascent stage, we must include discussions of case reports and program descriptions as well as relevant clinical research on the topic. In addition, we will provide illustrations of the use of behavioral interventions with substance-abusing adolescents from our own efforts in the Adolescent Drug Abuse and Psychiatric Treatment (ADAPT) inpatient program at the University of Pittsburgh School of Medicine.

OSCAR G. BUKSTEIN • Department of Psychiatry, University of Pittsburgh School of Medicine, Pittsburgh, Pennsylvania 15213.   VINCENT B. VAN HASSELT • School of Psychology, Nova University, Fort Lauderdale, Florida 33314.

Handbook of Behavior Therapy in the Psychiatric Setting, edited by Alan S. Bellack and Michel Hersen. Plenum Press, New York, 1993.

In describing the disorder of substance abuse in adolescents, the continuum of substance use behaviors (from the use of specific and multiple substances to abuse and eventually dependence) must be examined.

Defining behaviors and symptoms that constitute substance abuse or dependence is difficult. Past and current efforts to establish diagnostic criteria are based on research with adults. Despite the almost universal application of these same criteria to adolescents, many differences exist between adolescents and adults in a variety of substance use characteristics, including their use patterns and the consequences (Blane, 1979; Weschler, 1979). The tendency to view adult and adolescent substance abuse as fundamentally the same disorder is questionable in light of the evidence of a discontinuity in problem drinker status between adolescence and young adulthood (Jessor, 1984). Specifically, frequent heavy drinking in adolescents and the problems resulting from their drinking appear to be self-limiting and are not highly predictive of alcoholism in adults (Blane, 1979). Similarly, patterns of involvement with marijuana and other illicit drugs peak in late adolescence (Kandel & Logan, 1984).

In the revised third edition of the *Diagnostic and Statistical Manual* (DSM-III-R; American Psychiatric Association, 1987), psychoactive substance use disorders (see Table 1) represent a broadening of the concept of dependence to include clinically significant behaviors, cognitions, and symptoms that indicate a substantial degree of involvement with a psychoactive substance (Rounsaville, Snitzer, & Williams, 1986). Many adolescents formerly meeting the criteria in the third edition of the DSM (American Psychiatric Association, 1980) for a diagnosis of substance abuse now meet the DSM-III-R criteria for psychoactive substance dependence. Elimination of the DSM-III reliance on the physical parameters of tolerance and/or withdrawal as necessary for a diagnosis of dependence allows the clinician to exercise appropriate clinical judgment in the diagnosis of psychoactive substance abuse and dependence in adolescents.

The criteria for DSM-III-R diagnoses of psychoactive substance dependence and abuse are listed in Tables 1 and 2, respectively. The criteria for psychoactive substance abuse are consistent across all substances and are met by a maladaptive pattern of use. Such a maladaptive pattern is indicated by continued use despite recurrent or persistent social, psychological, or physical problems or recurrent use in physically hazardous situations. Psychoactive substance dependence contains criteria involving a cluster of cognitive behavioral and physiological symptoms that reflect impaired control of substance use and continued use despite adverse consequences. Because the physiological symptoms of addiction and withdrawal from addictive substances are rare in adolescents (Vingilis & Smart, 1981), the increased emphasis on a variety of substance-seeking and substance-taking behaviors is more relevant to adolescents. Research has not established either the validity or the clinical utility of the DSM-III-R psychoactive substance use disorders in adolescents. The presence of social, occupational, or psychological dysfunction as the basis for a substance abuse diagnosis is especially problematic.

Table 1.   Psychoactive Substance Dependence DSM-III-R[a]

At least 3
  • Taken in larger amounts or over longer period than planned.
  • Persistent desire to cut down and/or previous unsuccessful efforts to control use.
  • Lots of time spent in getting, taking or recovering from substance.
  • Intoxication or withdrawal when expected to fulfill major role obligations.
  • Give up important social, occupational or recreational activities due to use.
  • Continued use despite having social, psychological, or physical problem(s).
  • Marked tolerance.
  • Characteristic withdrawal symptoms.
  • Use to relieve or avoid withdrawal symptoms.
Symptoms have persisted for at least one month.

[a]From American Psychiatric Association (1987).

These areas of dysfunction may be the result of coexisting psychopathology, or, social and environmental circumstances that are highly correlated with adolescent substance abuse, but not necessarily the direct result of abuse. For example, the work of Donovan and Jessor (1978) points to problem drinking as only a part of a larger syndrome of deviant behavior in adolescents. Substance use in these individuals is almost always illicit. Certain negative consequences follow from this illegality rather than from the properties of the substance being used or from the substance use behavior.

Additional work is needed to establish a useful diagnostic system for adolescent substance abuse. For the clinician, an understanding of the progression of adolescent substance use behaviors is essential. For most adolescents, experimental use without significant consequences is common. A significant proportion progress to a level of abuse or "problem use," that is, use producing significant negative consequences in one or more areas of psychosocial functioning. At this level, the use of the term *abuse* is reasonable, as an identifiable clinical threshold has been reached. Eventually, a small portion of youth become dependent on substances with more compulsive use and devote increasing time and attention to obtaining and using substances and recovering from their effects.

Epidemiology of Substance Use

The most accurate estimates of current adolescent substance use patterns are derived from two national surveys. Since 1974, the National Senior Survey (NSS) has provided annual data on the drug and alcohol use of high school seniors (Johnston, O'Malley, & Bachman, 1987). The National Household Survey, funded by the National Institute on Drug Abuse, is administered every two to three years. Both are self-report surveys with consistent, reliable results (Oetting & Beauvais, 1990). Unfortunately, the NSS does not include the approximately 15%–20% of a class cohort that leaves school early. This group of dropouts contains high-risk youth and corresponding elevated rates of substance use and abuse.

Lifetime annual and monthly prevalence data from the NSS reveal interesting trends over the 1980s (Johnston, 1991). Although the use of most drugs by high school seniors (as defined by lifetime prevalence) increased from the mid-1970s to the early 1980s, there has been a subsequent decline in the proportion of high school seniors using marijuana, cocaine, crack, stimulants, and sedatives. In 1990, one third (33%) of all high school seniors claimed they had taken at least one illicit drug during the past year. This represents a substantial decrease from the peak of 54% in 1979. Daily usage rates for cocaine, stimulants, and marijuana were down an estimated 75% from peak levels.

Although seniors reported modest declines in the use of alcohol, its use among youth remains widespread. From a peak of 72% of seniors reporting alcohol use in the prior month in 1980, the rate had fallen to 57% in 1990. Of the 1990 seniors, 32% reported at least one occasion of drinking in the prior two weeks; this rate was down from a peak of 41% in 1983. Daily use of alcohol declined from a peak of 6.9% in 1979 to 3.7% in 1990.

Even though the purchase and use of alcohol are illegal for all adolescents in this country, alcohol experimentation is normative. Substantial portions of adolescents use alcohol with

Table 2. Psychoactive Substance Abuse DSM-III-R[a]

1. Maladaptive pattern of use:
   - Continued use despite social, occupational, psychological, or physical problem(s).
   - Recurrent use in physically hazardous situations.
2. Symptoms have persisted for at least one month or have occurred repeatedly over a longer period.
3. Does not meet criteria for psychoactive substance dependence.

[a]From American Psychiatric Association (1987).

few or no problems or impairment. A large portion of youth also experiment with a variety of other agents, again without significant clinical consequences. Unfortunately, we have no current data pertaining to the prevalence of adolescent's substance abuse in the general population.

Risk Factors and Stages of Use

Identifying the presence of risk or antecedent factors correlated with increased adolescent use and abuse is important not only so that we can describe the range of pathological substances, but so that we can conduct a comprehensive assessment of the adolescent. Environmental antecedents are among the most robust predictors of adolescent substance use, and parental attitudes and behavior are the most significant among these factors (Kandel, 1982). In addition to parental role modeling, the quality and consistency of family communication and parental behavior management are strong predictors of adolescent use (Donovan & Jessor, 1978; Kandel, Kessler, & Margulies, 1978).

Among the peer-related factors predicting adolescent use are peer drug-use behaviors and attitudes (Kandel, Kessler, & Margulies, 1978) and the perceived use of substances by peers (Jessor & Jessor, 1977). Reported peer drinking has the strongest relationship with adolescent drinking. Indeed, individual adolescent drinking behavior resembles that of peers. The more that peers use, the greater the likelihood that an adolescent will initiate use and progress to heavier levels (Donovan & Jessor, 1978; White, Johnson, & Horwitz, 1986).

Individual factors, including beliefs, attitudes, substance use expectancies, and preexisting psychopathology, also are implicated as antecedents of adolescent substance use and abuse. Prior and current beliefs about alcohol are associated with current drinking patterns (Christiansen, Goldman, & Inn, 1982). Favorable attitudes concerning drug use preceding initiation appear to facilitate initiation into drug use (Kandel et al., 1978). Substance-use-related expectancies (i.e., effects attributed to a substance that the individual anticipates when using that substance) are related to future substance use (Brown, 1985) as well as to current use patterns (Christiansen, Goldman, & Brown, 1985).

Preexisting as well as coexisting psychopathology in the adolescent often predicts use. For example, antisocial behavior often predicts adolescent substance use (Johnston et al., 1987; Kandel et al., 1978), the delinquency occurring before substance use. Other studies suggest that depression (Christie, Burke, Regier, Rae, Boyd, & Locke, 1988; Deykin, Lory, & Wells, 1987) and attention deficit disorder (Gittleman, Mannuzza, Shenker, & Bonagura, 1985) precede substance use or abuse.

A number of researchers have used these risk factors to construct theories explaining adolescent substance use and progression to abuse. Kandel (1982) proposed four developmental stages of use: (1) beer and wine; (2) cigarettes and/or hard liquor; (3) marijuana; and (4) other elicit drugs. Participation in each stage is a necessary but insufficient condition for progression to a later stage. There are stage-specific predictors of initiation into various legal and illegal drugs. For involvement in alcohol, both peer and especially parental influences (e.g., modeling) are critical. Peer influences are more important in predicting marijuana use. The use of illicit drugs other than marijuana is influenced by parental use, poor family relationships, and psychological distress.

PROTOTYPICAL ASSESSMENT

A clinically relevant and valid assessment forms the basis for effective treatment interventions. Ideally, a standardized instrument would obtain relevant data that allow appropriate comparisons with both clinical and normal populations. Despite several research-based measures, there are no standardized devices linking the assessment of substance abuse in adolescents to treatment (Tarter, 1990). A number of investigators have developed questionnaires for use in epidemiology (Singh, Kandel, & Johnson, 1975) and measuring the quantity, frequency, and context of drug use (Jessor, 1976). The Adolescent Alcohol Involvement Scale (AAIS; Mayer & Filstead, 1979) represents an attempt to develop an adolescent-specific screening instrument for alcohol. The Rutgers Alcohol Problem Index (RAPI; White & Labouvie, 1989) is a self-report instrument designed to evaluate adolescent problem drinking. However, its utility for clinical or substance-abusing populations has not been demonstrated.

Unfortunately, there is dissatisfaction with one or more elements of the currently available screening and interview instruments (Tarter, 1990; Winters, 1990). Several structured and semistructured diagnostic interviews, such as the children's version of the Schedule for Affective Disorders and Schizophrenia (K-SADS; Chambers, Puig-Antich, Hirsh, Paez, Ambrosini, Tabrizi, & Davies, 1985) and the Diagnostic Interview for Children and Adolescents (DICA; Herjanic & Reich, 1982), cover substance abuse, although the relevant sections do not have established psychometric properties.

More recently, several more comprehensive instruments have been developed with prospective clinical application. The Personal Experience Inventory (PEI; Henly & Winters, 1988) measures the quantity, frequency, and history of use and evaluates the environmental circumstances and personality characteristics of the adolescent. Tarter (1990) proposed the Drug Use Screening Inventory (DUSI) for systematically screening and identifying areas of disturbance that are frequently concomitant with drug use in adolescence. The DUSI consists of 10 domains in key areas of health, psychiatric, and psychosocial disturbances. The purpose of the DUSI is to screen and identify areas for further, more detailed evaluation. The domains suggested by Tarter (1990) for evaluation (see Table 3) provide an excellent outline for any broad-spectrum approach to the assessment of substance abuse in adolescents. A survey of quantity and frequency data on the substances used is not sufficient to determine pathological use or to identify associated areas of dysfunction or risk. The prototypical assessment must evaluate areas that place the adolescent at risk of starting and continuing substance abuse and areas of disturbance amenable to treatment intervention.

Substance Use

Each of the instruments previously mentioned has quantity-frequency data questions. Many treatment centers have developed their own assessment devices to gather such objective data. The Chemical Dependency Assessment Scale (CDAS) is a self-administered, computer-scored measure that comprehensively describes and quantifies adolescent substance use behavior (Oetting, Beauvais, Edwards, & Waters, 1984). The Substance Use Disorders Diagnostic Schedule (SUDDS) was constructed by the Chemical Abuse/Addiction Treatment Outcome Registry, which offers a proprietary service for evaluation and a follow-up of treatment outcome (Harrison & Hoffman, 1985). This instrument provides quantity, frequency, and age-of-onset data as well as brief sections on stress and depression. Whether relying on a simple instrument

**Table 3. Domains for Assessment[a]
of Adolescent Use and Abuse**

I. Substance Use Behavior	VI. Family System
II. Behavior Patterns	VII. School
III. Health Status	VIII. Work
IV. Psychiatric Disorder	IX. Peer Relationship
V. Social Skill	X. Leisure and Recreation

[a]From Tarter (1990), by courtesy of Marcel Dekker Inc.

measuring quantity, frequency, and age-of-onset data or a comprehensive interview or device tapping several domains, the prototypical substance use assessment should examine (1) the direct consequences of use, withdrawal, or physical symptoms due to use and (2) cognitive and behavioral evidence of dependence.

Behavior Patterns and Adaptive Functioning

The Child Behavior Checklist (CBCL) is a widely-used self-report instrument assessing a wide range of behavior problems (Achenbach & Edelbrock, 1983). The self-report form and the parent and teacher informant versions include behavior-rating scales focusing on an evaluation of psychopathology. Each version also includes items relevant to the assessment of adaptive functioning or social competence. A number of other measures assessing adaptive function are available in a variety of methods of administration (see Orvaschel & Walsh, 1984).

Health Status

Every adolescent inpatient should have a complete medical history and physical examination as part of a comprehensive assessment. Indeed, preexisting medical conditions may influence the course of substance use or abuse and may heighten the potential consequences of use. A number of medical conditions (e.g., hepatitis, AIDS, lung disease, and liver disease) result from substance abuse. Laboratory testing is useful in identifying relevant medical problems. Suggested tests include a complete blood count with differential, liver function tests, a urine drug screen, and a pregnancy test. Depending on the patient's sexual history, tests for human immunodeficiency virus (HIV-1), syphilis, gonorrhea, and chlamydia may be indicated.

The use of drug-screening tests (urine and serum) may be very useful or may be abused. The clinician should be aware of the indications for the use of drug screens (Gold & Dachis, 1986) as well as of the factors affecting the validity and reliability of screens, such as sample collection, handling and protection against contaminants, and mislabeling.

Psychiatric Disorder

Psychopathology coexisting with substance abuse in adolescents is often encountered in a variety of clinical settings (Bukstein, Brent, & Kaminer, 1989). Psychiatric disorders, such as mood disorders, conduct disorder, attention-deficit hyperactivity disorder (ADHD), and anxiety disorder, appear to have an important role in the etiology of or vulnerability to substance use problems in adolescents.

Structured and semistructured psychiatric interviews, such as the Childhood Schedule for Affective Disorders and Schizophrenia (K-SADS), mentioned earlier, can be administered to children and a parent informant to yield Axis I diagnoses. The clinician should use parent informants and attempt to elicit the age of onset of each comorbid disorder. Information regarding past psychiatric treatment and response should be gathered as well.

A number of instruments for specific disorders, such as ADHD, depression, eating disorders, and obsessive-compulsive disorder, are available for an evaluation of the severity of symptoms in adolescents (Rapoport & Connors, 1985). Scales measuring behaviors and symptoms in specific areas can provide a baseline as well as a measurement of change after treatment.

Family

Family variables account for many of the most robust psychosocial determinants of risk of substance abuse in adolescents. The literature points to a genetic contribution to alcoholism and related problems (Goodwin, 1979). Children of alcoholic parents show increased rates of psychopathology and alcoholism (Earles, Reich, Jung, & Cloninger, 1988; West & Printz, 1987). In view of the genetic risks and the frequent familial nature of alcoholism, drug abuse, and other forms of psychopathology (e.g., depression), the clinician should obtain a detailed family history of both psychiatric disorders and substance use and abuse.

For evaluating social and environmental factors, a number of instruments are available to (1) provide a baseline assessment; (2) identify areas in need of intervention; and (3) ascertain treatment outcome. The Family Environment Scale (FES; Moos & Moos, 1981), the Parent-Adolescent Relationship Inventory (PARI; Robin & Foster, 1988), and the Family Assessment Measure (FAM; Skinner, Steinhauer, & Santa-Barbara, 1983) are questionnaires for evaluating family adjustment. The FES examines the family in three primary domains: relationship, personal growth, and system maintenance. The FAM provides an assessment of several important family characteristics: risk accomplishment, values and norms, role performance, communication, affective expression, affective involvement, and control. For a more specific assessment of parent-child conflict, the Conflict Behavior Questionnaire (CBQ; Foster, Prinz, & O'Leary, 1983) provides data concerning conflict and negative communication among family members. Although each of the representative family assessment instruments reflects different conceptual models, they all pertain to several adolescent substance abuse risk factors.

School and Occupational Performance

School is the occupation of most adolescents. Their performance, in both grades and behavior, is a critical measure of psychosocial functioning. School records, grades, teacher observations, and disciplinary records provide important objective data. Several instruments, such as the Child Behavior Checklist (Achenbach & Edelbrock, 1983a) and the Conners Scale (Conners, 1969), have versions for teachers.

Peer Relationships and Social Skills

Increased attention has been directed to the assessment of interpersonal skills and social adjustment in adolescents in general (see the review by Christoff & Myatt, 1987) and substance-abusing youth in particular (Van Hasselt, Null, & Bukstein, 1992). The impetus for the efforts in this area is a considerable body of research attesting to the association between social dysfunction in the early years and a host of difficulties (depression, substance abuse, antisocial behavior, and relationship problems) later in life (Cowen, Pederson, Babigan, Izzo, & Trost, 1973; King & Young, 1981; Roff, 1961; Roff, Sells, & Golden, 1972). Consequently, a number of social-skills-assessment strategies have been developed for this population. Representative self-report measures are the Social Experience Inventory (Brodsky, 1976), the Adolescent Problems Inventory (Freedman, Rosenthal, Donahoe, Schlundt, & McFall, 1978), the Assertiveness Schedule (Rathus, 1973), the Children's Assertive Behavior Scale (Michelson & DiLorenzo, 1981), and the Social Behavior Inventory (Galejs & Stockdale, 1982). These measures generally require adolescents to indicate how they would respond in various interpersonal situations. Some ask the respondents to describe how they feel about themselves and what their responses would be in a range of social encounters.

Ratings of adolescents' social behavior by adults and teachers have also been used. Some of these instruments are the Social Behavior Rating Scale (Csapo, 1983), the Positive Social Behavior Scale (Greenwood, Walker, Todd, & Hops, 1979), Kohn's Social Competence Scale (Kohn & Rosman, 1972), and the Walker Problem Behavior Checklist (Walker, 1976). These instruments are useful in providing a convergence of data (from multiple sources) regarding the adolescent's level of social adjustment.

Finally, role-play tests (i.e., laboratory or clinic-based simulations of real-world social situations) have been used to assess social competence in children and youth. These devices have measured a wide variety of social skills (e.g., assertion, conversational skills, and dating skills) that are difficult to evaluate through more naturalistic methods (Van Hasselt, Hersen, & Milliones, 1978). Although previous investigations have questioned the correspondence between role-play performance and *in vivo* behavior (Kazdin, Matson, & Esveldt-Dawson, 1984; Van Hasselt, Hersen, & Bellack, 1981), the clinical utility of such strategies with adolescents has been supported (Christoff & Myatt, 1987). For example, we are currently developing a role-play test to assess four areas of social functioning in substance-abusing adolescents: (1) conversational skill; (2) positive assertion (giving and receiving compliments and expressing praise and appreciation); (3) negative assertion—general (standing up for one's rights and denying unreasonable requests); and (4) negative assertion—drug refusal (refusing substances and leaving high-risk situations). We have found this role-play strategy to be useful in selecting specific treatment targets and in evaluating the impact of social skills training.

ACTUAL ASSESSMENT

Although multiple self-reports, observational scales, and structured interviews may provide a comprehensive assessment of an adolescent who abuses substances, the clinician may not have the time or resources to manage such an endeavor. A less structured assessment should evaluate each relevant domain of an adolescent's psychosocial functioning. Also, an understanding of the importance of engaging the adolescent should assist in obtaining valid and reliable information.

In approaching an adolescent substance abuser (or suspected abuser), the clinician must realize that such adolescents rarely present voluntarily for evaluation or intervention. Because they are usually "on guard," a less confrontational approach often serves to engage the adolescent and provides important and valid data as well. A suggested strategy is to inquire about the adolescent's current life circumstances (e.g., where he or she lives and goes to school, current academic progress, home composition, friends, and preferred activities). Adolescents will probably not view such questions as intrusive, as they are expecting a more confrontational, judgmental approach regarding their specific problem behaviors. Very often, such seemingly innocuous questions provide a natural opening for the exploration of deviant behavior (including substance abuse), family problems and functioning, or other difficulties. For example, when asked about peers and leisure activities, an adolescent may reveal that several of his or her friends have problems related to substance abuse. Adolescents frequently provide information concerning deviant behavior and substance abuse in anonymous friends although they are unwilling to reveal similar information pertaining to themselves. Inquiry into an adolescent's life circumstances should survey them for risk factors or correlates of adolescent substance use. By identifying the presence of such correlates, the clinician not only raises the suspicion of substance abuse but also identifies areas for possible treatment.

Eventually, an evaluation must assess the domain of substance abuse. Included should be questions regarding past and current substance use, frequency, and quantity. The age of onset for each substance ever used, as well as the age of regular use, is also important to ascertain. The clinician should understand that variability (in terms of quantity and frequency) of adolescent substance use is the *rule* rather than the exception. Additional assessment data should include both the direct and the perceived consequences of use, the context of use, expectancies, and the adolescent's reasons for use.

Rather than relying on the adolescent's acknowledgment of difficulties, the clinician should also ask about specific behaviors that endorse or imply direct consequences. Identification of negative consequences attributable to substance use forms the basis of the identification and diagnosis of substance abuse. The context of use constitutes the time and place of use, with whom the use occurs, peer use levels, and who acquires the substance. This is a functional analysis of substance use and includes the antecedents of the behavior, the context of the behavior, the specific behavior itself, and the result or consequences of the behavior. Questions or lines of questioning should be substance-specific and should include tobacco. The clinician must determine the use of each substance (e.g., alcohol, marijuana, cocaine, and sedatives) with subsequent, more detailed questions pertaining to each substance.

The remaining questions in the substance use domain follow the DSM-III-R criteria: Does the adolescent view use as a problem? Has the adolescent attempted to stop use? Has the adolescent given up role responsibilities to use? Does he or she spend more time than planned in obtaining and using substances? Does the adolescent feel compelled to use or does he or she lose control once an episode of use is started? Despite the lower prevalence of physical sequelae of use in adolescents, questions pertaining to the presence of tolerance or withdrawal symptoms are essential. These questions determine the presence of a psychological and/or a physical dependence. Urine drug screens can be used to validate the adolescent's report of recent use; however, they do little to confirm or deny actual abuse.

An assessment of psychiatric status is part of every comprehensive evaluation. The clinician must ask screening questions concerning depression, anxiety disorders or symptoms, attention-deficit hyperactivity disorder, eating disorders, and psychotic symptoms (with and without substance use). The presence of other psychiatric symptoms or behaviors preceding regular use or during periods of abstinence should provide evidence of a potentially treatable condition that is not necessarily "caused" by the adolescent's substance use. Although the clinician may have obtained information concerning family composition and interpersonal functioning during the initial portion of the interview, the family history of substance use and abuse (current use patterns and their attitudes about use) and psychiatric disorders should also be assessed. Questions about suicidal behavior, including current suicidal ideation, plan(s), or intent, as well as recent and past attempts, are essential. Substance-abusing adolescents, particularly those with depression, appear to be at higher risk for suicidal behavior (Crumley, 1990).

The clinician may need parents or other family members as informants. The use of parents, as well as teachers, friends, and other family members, is critical to confirm or contradict the adolescent's report. Other informants are especially valuable for reports on the range and severity of specific deviant behaviors, external evidence of psychiatric disorders, and a more reliable report of the adolescent's past treatment history and school functioning. Although parents may not be accurate or well-informed with regard to their child's substance use patterns, they may have evidence of substance use (e.g., finding bottles, cans, or drug-related paraphernalia around the house). They may also have observed the pharmacological effects of substances as demonstrated in strange behavior, personality change, different friends, and secretiveness. Asking both the adolescent and the parent informant about previous treatment efforts is helpful in ascertaining failed approaches to intervention and adolescent and parent engagement in treatment.

A multidomain assessment is critical in determining (1) the baseline functioning of the adolescent in his or her environment and (2) long-term change within each of the domains. Achieving abstinence from substance use may be of marginal overall benefit to the adolescent who remains depressed, socially isolated, academically inadequate, or active with a deviant peer group.

Prototypical Treatment

In the behavioral approach to alcoholism and drug addiction, substance abuse has been viewed as a multiply determined, learned behavioral disorder, which is "best understood through the empirically derived principles of social learning, cognitive psychology, and behavior therapies" (Marlatt & Donovan, 1982). The focus of behavioral strategies is on the observable aspects of substance use: the frequency and duration of substance abuse episodes, the amount consumed, and the difficulties associated with excessive use. Assessment consists of an examination of the situational and environmental antecedents, a past learning history, and previous experience with substances, as well as cognitive processes and expectations concerning drug and alcohol effects (Donovan & Marlatt, 1980). These variables serve as antecedent cues that may precipitate substance use. Also important are the consequences of substance use, as these maintain the maladaptive behavior.

In light of the multiple and interactive factors associated with the onset of substance abuse, behavior therapists have designed and implemented numerous treatment procedures to deal with the problem. Three of the most commonly used methods with adolescent substance abusers to date are aversion therapy, social skills training, and behavioral family therapy. Unfortunately, however, only a modicum of information is available regarding the application of behavioral interventions to adolescents using drugs or alcohol. Suggested applications of these treatment procedures, with illustrations drawn from extant although limited clinical research, are presented in the sections below.

Aversion Therapy

The purpose of aversion therapy is to reduce or eliminate the craving or desire for an illicit substance. Typically, unpleasant stimuli or events, such as nausea, electrical shock, and apnea, have been paired with urges to drink or use drugs (e.g., Rachman & Teasdale, 1969; Rimmele, Miller, & Dougher, 1989), as in the classical conditioning paradigm. The most common approaches have involved the induction of nausea through chemical aversion. Here, a drug (usually emetine hydrochloride or apomorphine) is administered during the tasting or swallowing of alcohol. Ingestion of the chemical at the time of drug use leads to violent emesis and nausea, which, with repeated pairings, diminish the positive valence of the targeted substance. Similarly, electrical aversion pairs a painful shock with the consumption of alcohol or drugs; this procedure eventually leads to decreased interest in the illicit substance.

Although the use of the above-mentioned painful stimuli has shown some clinical utility, problems inherent in their application include (1) the stressful nature of these aversive interventions; (2) the need for medical supervision, particularly with the use of chemical aversion; and (3) the high patient dropout rates (see Rimmele *et al.*, 1989). Aversion techniques using noxious stimuli are rarely used in adolescent treatment. An alternative to these methods is covert sensitization, which uses aversive imagery with imagery of drinking or drug use (e.g., Cautela, 1970; Maletzky, 1974) to produce nausea and/or imagined aversive consequences.

Duehn (1978) described one of the first applications of covert sensitization to adolescents (seven males 16–18 years of age) with long-term histories of amphetamine, LSD, and marijuana use. The treatment was applied in 11 group sessions over a six-week period. The following is an example of a covert sensitization scenario constructed to diminish LSD usage in participants:

> Picture yourself standing (with a friend) on the parking lot at (a shopping center). The sun has just gone down, the air feels cool and crisp. You feel a little nervous as you approach 3 longhairs from whom you are about to buy a hit of acid. The guys see you approaching and begin to talk to each other. As you near them, one turns and asks you what you want. You tell him you want a hit of acid. He reaches into the pocket of his blue jeans and pulls out a match box. He opens the box and picks out a "hit of acid" and hands it to you. As you pick it out of his hand, hot liquid squirts up into your throat and mouth. The hot liquid tastes sour. You try real hard to swallow it back down, but as you do this, small chunks of food you had for supper gush up into your mouth. As you raise your hand to your mouth with part of the tab in it, vomit fills your mouth. You try again to swallow it. Your hand shakes and you have difficulty placing the tab into your mouth. As the bland, chalky tasting tab touches your lips, the tab is suddenly swept out of your hand to the pavement below you by the vomit gushing from your mouth. The sour, bitter, slimy, sticky vomit covers your hands, shirt, arms, legs, and the pavement around you. You see the speck of a tab floating and melting

away in vomit below you. Your friend and the 3 longhairs stare at you in disgust as you stand there in your vomit. (pp. 487–488)

Duehn (1978) stated that patients were then instructed to imagine that they were escaping the situation by running away. As they ran, they were asked to image that "the vomit disappeared and that they felt better." The results of posttreatment evaluation indicated that all group members reported no LSD usage or desire to take LSD. Further, 6- and 18-month follow-up meetings showed that six of the patients had remained drug-free.

The benefits of using covert sensitization with substance-abusing adolescents await further empirical verification. However, this approach appears promising and appears to have several advantages (e.g., it requires no apparatus or drugs, it is less time-consuming, and it has the potential for self-administration) over other more painful and stressful aversive methods that have been used with adult populations.

Social Skills Training

Social skills training has been used with substance-abusing individuals (primarily adults) in both inpatient and outpatient settings. The rationale for skills interventions with this population is that social skill deficits have a role in substance abuse, in that the person drinks or uses drugs in order to (1) diminish social anxiety; (2) increase assertiveness; and (3) enhance perceptions of self-efficacy in interpersonal contexts (Van Hasselt *et al.*, 1978). Some reasons that have been offered for skill deficiencies in substance abusers include inadequate parental and peer role models of effective social responding, inadequate feedback regarding interpersonal behavior, and environmental deprivation (O'Leary, O'Leary, & Donovan, 1976). Consequently, numerous skill treatment strategies have been developed for substance abusers since the late 1970s (see reviews by Chaney, 1989; Van Hasselt *et al.*, 1978). The goals of these investigations have ranged from improving assertion skills (Ferrell & Galassi, 1981; Freedberg & Johnston, 1981) to social problem solving (i.e., decision making and the generation of alternatives in problem situations) (Chaney, O'Leary, & Marlatt, 1978; Intagliata, 1978) and coping skills (Sanchez-Craig & Walker, 1982).

Skills training has only recently been conducted with adolescent substance abusers. In one of the first such efforts, Hawkins, Catalano, and Wells (1986) applied "Project Skills," a combination of behavioral skills training, involvement in prosocial activities, and social network development, to substance-abusing adolescents and adults in therapeutic communities. The skills targeted for modification were social introductions and assertion (including drug and alcohol refusal), giving and receiving praise and criticism, structured problem solving, stress management, and social network development. The sessions incorporated the role playing of problem social encounters and multiple behavioral techniques (instructions, modeling, feedback, and group discussion) to affect behavior change. The results indicated improved performance in situations involving avoiding drug use, coping with relapse, social interaction, interpersonal problem solving, and coping with stressful events in treated subjects relative to an untreated control group.

Haggerty, Wells, Jenson, Catalano, and Hawkins (1989) described Project ADAPT, a treatment and aftercare program for institutionalized delinquents with significant drug or alcohol problems. This approach combines behavioral skill training, supportive network development, and involvement in prosocial activities to facilitate the community reintegration of adolescents following their placement in a residential facility. The skill-training component of Project ADAPT attempts to increase a range of social and behavioral skills requisite to successful community placement. Seven skill areas are included in this intervention: (1) consequential thinking—awareness of the antecedents and consequences of antisocial behavior and drug use; (2) self-control—resisting impulses and peer pressure (e.g., refusing drugs or alcohol);

(3) avoiding trouble—recognizing and avoiding high-risk situations; (4) social networking—determining prosocial activities and making new friends; (5) coping with authority—using negotiation and compliance to get along with authority figures (e.g., parents, teachers, and employers); (6) problem solving—generating effective and prosocial solutions in difficult situations; and (7) relapse coping—strategies for coping with substance use or delinquent behavior (e.g., positive self-statements). Haggerty *et al.* (1989) stated that Project ADAPT is a multiyear demonstration project; the results will be disseminated in the near future.

DeJong and Henrich (1980) used a multielement behavioral approach that included assertion, communication, and decision-making skills training with 89 drug addicts (31 female and 58 male) aged 16–27 years. The subjects were included in this study if they had attended a rehabilitation center for at least a week. Unfortunately, details regarding the skills training portion of the program were not provided. However, DeJong and Henrich reported that approximately one third of the total sample was drug-free up to two years following termination of the treatment. Moreover, among those completing the programs and receiving normal discharges, the success rate was 80%.

In our experience, a disproportionately high number of substance-abusing adolescents exhibit some form of social maladjustment. Of particular importance are recent data that we have accumulated attesting to the relationship between social skills deficits and depression in this population (Van Hasselt, Null, & Bukstein, 1991). This finding led to the development of a social skills intervention for patients in our own program (see "Actual Treatment" below). Although research and treatment efforts in this area are at the preliminary stage, social dysfunction in substance-abusing adolescents is a problem warranting increased clinical and investigative attention in future endeavors.

Behavioral Family Therapy

The role of the family in the etiology and maintenance of adolescent substance abuse has been well established (Bry, 1988; Hops, Tildesley, Lichtenstein, Ary, & Sherman, 1990). Indeed, parental substance abuse, poor monitoring and supervision of children, and coercive parental management practices have been associated with a high risk of substance use or abuse in offspring (Dishion, Patterson, & Reid, 1988). Therefore, family treatment must be viewed as a critical aspect of comprehensive behavioral intervention. Yet, few investigations of the implementation of behavioral family therapy with adolescent substance abusers are available. One of these is a case report by Frederiksen, Jenkins, and Carr (1976) that used contingency contracting to modify the interpersonal interactions between a polydrug-abusing 17-year-old male and his parents. The goals of the treatment were (1) improvement in family relationships; (2) decreased drug use; and (3) attending a vocational program. The contingency contract covered the aforementioned problem areas, and behaviors and consequences were specified for all family members. Assessment via family self-reports of happiness and urine drug screens of the patient revealed improved family adjustment and dramatically reduced drug use. Gains were maintained at a one-year follow-up.

Rueger and Liberman (1984) successfully used a contingency contract with a 15-year-old female marijuana user and her family. The contract detailed target behaviors (completing her chores and informing her parents of out-of-home activities), for which consistent positive consequences were provided. These investigators found reduced substance use and improved family relations as a result of the intervention. In one of the first applications of problem-solving-skills training (PSST) with adolescent substance abusers and their families, Bry, Conboy, and Bisgay (1986) adapted Robin and Foster's problem-solving approach (1988; identifying the desired changes, assessing the maintaining variables, generating solutions, and reinforcing positive changes) with three substance-abusing adolescents and their families. The treatment was conducted in weekly and biweekly sessions held over the course of a three- to four-month period. The PSST led to decreased drug use and school failure in the project participants, although lengthy delays before improvements and periodic recurrences of problem behaviors during follow-up reflected an "incomplete understanding of the variables" (p. 43).

Inpatient intervention with substance-abusing adolescents that fails to proactively involve the family in treatment is unlikely to yield significant short- or long-term improvements. Indeed, it is imperative that families learn and develop behavior management skills that will facilitate the maintenance and generalization of the gains made by adolescent patients during the inpatient admission.

ACTUAL TREATMENT

To provide an illustration of actual treatment of substance-abusing adolescents, we describe here the Adolescent Drug Abuse and Psychiatric Treatment (ADAPT) program at the University of Pittsburgh School of Medicine. ADAPT is a 14-bed inpatient treatment facility that offers specialized treatment for adolescents with a substance abuse problem as well as some form of psychiatric disorder (e.g., conduct disorder, major depressive disorder, or attention-deficit hyperactivity disorder). This program provides broad-spectrum behavioral intervention combined with chemical dependency treatment for these dually diagnosed adolescents. The program uses a multidisciplinary team approach to intervention and includes psychiatrists, psychologists, psychiatric nurses, social workers, a chemical dependency counselor, and developmental specialists. Further, although a wide variety of treatment components are available, the treatment is individualized, and the treatment plans are designed to meet the unique needs of each patient.

On admission to ADAPT, all patients undergo an initial comprehensive evaluation in a number of areas. First, all patients receive an extensive medical evaluation to determine their health status. This consists of a complete medical history and a physical examination (see the health status section above). Second, patterns of substance use, abuse, and dependency are assessed through a psychiatric interview about past and current substance use with the patient and the parents, as well as administration of the Diagnostic Inventory of Substance Use (DISU; Bukstein & Blasher, 1991). The DISU examines eight relevant domains of substance abuse: Control of Use, Effort to Quit, Involvement, Negative Consequence, Role Deterioration, Physical/Mental Problem Scale, Tolerance, and Withdrawal/Avoidance. The clinical value of this instrument lies in its ability to obtain DSM-III-R diagnoses of psychoactive substance use disorders in adolescents and in its identification of areas of dysfunction related to the use of drugs or alcohol.

Third, the social and emotional adjustment of the patient is assessed via a clinical assessment battery designed to tap important areas of functioning by using devices with demonstrated psychometric properties. The specific instruments that are administered to each adolescent during the first week of admission are listed in Table 4. In addition, the level of family adjustment is examined by means of multiple family-assessment measures (see Table 5). Further, family functioning is evaluated by the unit social workers, who obtain a detailed family history during the initial phase of the admission. An emphasis is placed on the identification of potential controlling variables (antecedents and consequences) of adolescent substance abuse within the family system. Records are obtained from any psychiatric centers and institutions where the adolescent was treated previously in order to gain as clear a picture as possible regarding family adjustment and involvement in current maladaptive behavior patterns.

Psychiatric diagnoses and problems are ascertained through structured interviews with the patients and their families. For this purpose, the K-SADS (mentioned earlier) is used to determine the presence of lifetime and current psychiatric disorders; it is also used to record the past treatment, age of onset, and number of episodes of any psychiatric disorder. Intellectual functioning and academic achievement are evaluated via standardized psychological and achievement tests. These are conducted by a school psychologist, who works closely with the unit developmental specialists in obtaining and examining prior school records and performance profiles to determine the adequacy of current school placements and the need for additional or alternative school services.

Once the assessment data are collected, the results are reviewed in the context of a unit diagnostic conference, in which the salient deficits and problems are identified and a treatment plan is formulated. As mentioned above, interventions are individually tailored so as to be relevant and appropriate to the adolescent patient. Moreover, in an effort to match the patients' need(s) with the most heuristic intervention, the evaluation data are used to assign the patients to treatment components. Each of the ADAPT program elements is described briefly in the sections below.

Social-Problem-Solving-Skills Training

As noted earlier, many substance-abusing adolescents appear to have deficits in interpersonal skills (Van Hasselt, Null, & Bukstein, 1992). The purpose of training in social problem-solving skills (SPSS) is to provide instruction in a variety of performance areas that have been implicated as being requisite for adequate social functioning: conversational skills, friendship-making skills, heterosocial (dating) skills, and positive assertion (expressing praise and appreciation and giving and receiving compliments), and negative assertion (denying unreasonable requests and standing up for one's rights). An important aspect of the latter category involves acquiring the skills necessary to refuse drugs or alcohol and to extricate oneself from high-risk situations. These skills are trained via a combination of direct instructions, performance feedback, behavioral rehearsal, and modeling. In addition, role-play procedures are incorporated as a vehicle for both skills assessment and skills treatment. Specifically, scenarios relevant to the adolescent patient are described and role-played to provide an opportunity for practice and instruction. For example, a role-play item involving negative assertion regarding alcohol use is as follows: "You are at a party with several of your friends and there's not too much happening yet. One of your friends from school comes over to you and says, 'Hey, I have a six-pack in my car. Why don't we go out, finish it off and come back to the party?'" The patient is initially asked to respond as he or she would if the situation were actually occurring. Then, skills training proceeds to shape an effective response.

Another target of SPSS training is problem solving. This involves teaching a four-step problem-solving sequence that can be applied across difficult or high-risk situations: (1) stop and think of the problem; (2) identify the goal; (3) generate possible solutions and determine the consequences of each solution; and (4) choose the most effective solution and self-reinforce for

Table 4.   Adolescent Assessment Battery

Beck Depression Inventory (Beck *et al.*, 1961)
Cognitive Negative Errors Questionnaire (Leitenberg *et al.*, 1986)
Beck Hopelessness Scale (Beck *et al.*, 1974)
Adolescent Assertion Expression Scale (Connor *et al.*, 1982)
Conflict Behavior Questionnaire (Prinz *et al.*, 1979)
Loneliness Scale (Asher *et al.*, 1984)
Novaco Provocation Inventory (Novaco, 1975)
Self-Esteem Scale (Rosenberg, 1965)
Coddington Life Events Record (Coddington, 1972a,b)
Youth Self Report (Achenbach & Edelbrock, 1987)
Diagnostic Inventory of Substance Use (Bukstein, 1990)
Area of Change Questionnaire (Weiss & Margolin, 1977)
Social Phobia and Anxiety Inventory (Turner *et al.*, 1989)

appropriate behavior. In addition, patients receive instruction in social perception (i.e., the ability to identify and understand the feelings and emotional states of others).

Anger Control Training

Numerous adolescents admitted to inpatient psychiatric facilities can be characterized as having difficulties with anger and impulse control. Indeed, many are hospitalized because of recent episodes of angry outbursts or aggressive episodes. The program in anger control training (ACT) that we developed is an adaptation of the anger control strategy described by Ecton and Feindler (1990) for adolescents displaying a chronic pattern of angry outbursts and related impulse-control problems. This approach incorporates a number of cognitive behavioral methods: (1) the identification of anger triggers (antecedents and consequences); (2) relaxation techniques—deep breathing, backward counting, and visual imagery; (3) the "broken-record" technique—the calm, monotone repetition of a request (e.g., "Please give me my radio back"); (4) empathic assertion—sensitive listening to the other person's feeling state (e.g., "I know you're upset that I haven't done my homework yet, but I got out of school late and I haven't had time to do it"); (5) escalating assertion—begin with a minimal assertive response and escalate to the final contract option, in which a consequence for noncompliance is presented (e.g., "Please let me have my book back" escalating to "If you don't give me my book now, I will tell the staff, and they will come and get it for me"); and (6) fogging—confusing the provoker with an agreement (e.g., "You're right, I am stupid").

Like SPSS training, training in anger control strategies involves the role playing of problem situations, the teaching of specific control techniques, and positive reinforcement from the staff for appropriate responding.

Behavioral Family Therapy

The behavioral family therapy (BFT) used in ADAPT is a combination of two behavioral treatment strategies that have enjoyed widespread application with dysfunctional families of adolescents. The initial phase of treatment is derived from functional family therapy (Alexander & Parsons, 1982), in which the therapist joins with the family in a series of reframing exercises in order to obtain maximal engagement and commitment from each family member without alienating any other family member. After engagement and clarification of the problems and goals that the family wants to achieve through therapy, the treatment proceeds to the behavioral component as developed by Bry *et al.* (1986), Patterson (1975), and Patterson and Forgatch (1987).

A strong emphasis is placed on four major areas. First, families are trained in *contingency management* skills, including instruction in (1) accurately identifying the problem behaviors and

Table 5. Family Assessment Battery

Child Behavior Checklist (Achenbach & Edelbrock, 1983)
Conflict Behavior Questionnaire (Prinz *et al.*, 1979)
Marital Adjustment Scale (Locke & Wallace, 1959)
Beck Depression Inventory (Beck *et al.*, 1961)
Areas of Change Questionnaire (Weiss & Margolin, 1977)
Coddington Life Events Record (Coddington, 1972a,b)
Child Abuse Potential Inventory (Milner, 1986)
Teacher Report Form (Achenbach & Edelbrock, 1983)

the controlling variables and (2) changing the consequences by providing consistent rules that reduce negative demands and commands, and by systematically reinforcing the desired behaviors while withdrawing reinforcement for negative ones.

Second, *communication skills* training focuses on a reduction in negative and coercive family interchanges and on increasing positive and constructive interactions. Here, families are taught to (1) clearly state their desires and preferences; (2) indicate their understanding of others' wants and needs; and (3) provide feedback to others in a nonpunitive fashion.

Third, *problem-solving-skills* training consists of instruction and rehearsal in those behaviors needed to solve problems and resolve conflicts. This process entails (1) defining the problem; (2) "brainstorming" for the generation of alternative solutions; (3) evaluating the costs and benefits of the solutions; (4) negotiating for an optimal solution; and (5) determining the strategies for implementation and providing positive reinforcement for effective problem solving.

Fourth, families receive instruction in designing *behavioral contracts*. The behavioral contract is a written document specifying the behaviors to be modified and the reinforcing consequences that have been agreed on by all members of the family. Contracts have been found to be particularly effective with adolescent problems because they provide clear and consistent positive consequences (through compromise) for the emission of previously identified and agreed-on behaviors (Nichols, 1984).

Cognitive Therapy

Cognitive therapy (CT) is

> a variety of therapeutic approaches whose major mode of action is modifying the patient's thinking and the premises, assumptions, and attitudes, underlying his cognitions. The focus of therapy is on the ideational content involved in the symptom, namely the irrational inferences and premises. (Meichenbaum, 1977, pp. 183–184)

CT has been widely applied in the treatment of depression (Beck, Rush, Shaw, & Emery, 1979). Although implementation of this approach with adolescent populations is a recent development (Lewinson, Clarke, Hops, & Andrews, 1990), the high prevalence of affective disorders in substance-abusing adolescents suggests the utility of CT with this group.

CT initially examines patients' irrational belief systems, faulty thinking styles, and deficient coping skills. Then, patients are systematically taught such skills as self-observation (in order to become aware of the association between thoughts and emotions) with attention directed to negative and irrational self-statements that occur in particular situations and that are related to depressed and/or anxious mood (Beck, 1976). Next, the validity of these maladaptive thoughts and self-statements are challenged, and more functional cognitions are gradually substituted.

The clinical utility of CT for substance-abusing adolescents awaits empirical verification. However, our preliminary evidence indicates that a significant portion of these individuals report cognitive distortions and negative internalized self-statements (Van Hasselt, Null, & Bukstein, 1992), and that CT is a much needed component in behavioral intervention.

Chemical Dependency Counseling and Self-Help Groups

An important component of treatment in ADAPT is chemical dependency counseling, which involves a review and discussion of problems and issues associated with drug and alcohol abuse. In addition, a relapse prevention model is used to teach patients how to anticipate and cope with the problem of relapse. This approach is based on the model developed by Marlatt and his colleagues (e.g., Marlatt, 1985; Marlatt & Gordon, 1985) and emphasizes the importance of (1) identifying high-risk situations for relapse and preparing the patient to handle them effectively; (2) dealing positively and constructively with relapse when it occurs; and (3) learning to view relapse as a learning experience rather than a serious personal failure or disaster.

Also as part of chemical dependency intervention, all patients participate in self-help groups such as Alcoholics Anonymous (AA) and Narcotics Anonymous (NA) over the course of the admission. These are referred to as 12-step programs because there are 12 defined steps in the program for recovery. It is generally acknowledged that these support groups view alcoholism and drug addition as physical, mental, and spiritual "diseases" to which lifelong abstinence is the only viable alternative. Members provide each other with strong support for abstinence and offer ideas for coping with stresses without abusing substances.

Although historically the philosophical differences between the self-support groups and behavior therapy have been emphasized, more recent formulations have cogently underscored the common features of both perspectives. For example, Brady & Irvine (1989) pointed out that both approaches stress

> avoiding drinking environments, developing interests and activities incompatible with drinking, developing skills to use in situations where alcohol is present, and having clearly defined behaviors to draw upon when experiencing a desire to drink. . . . On the important level of practice, the two approaches have many common goals and some common methods, such as stimulus control, and formal or informal covert sensitization. (p. 163)

We are in agreement with the viewpoint that self-help groups are a vital aspect of the treatment of the substance-abusing adolescent, primarily because many come from dysfunctional family systems that are unable to provide the supervision, support, or reinforcement needed to ensure that the patient will remain drug-free. Indeed, many adolescents referred for inpatient treatment no longer reside with their biological parents and are in foster care or some other out-of-home placement. In these cases, support groups can serve a crucial function in providing the necessary social and community supports. Thus, we clearly encourage involvement in support groups and view these as complementary to other aspects of inpatient behavioral intervention.

Milieu Behavior Management

ADAPT uses a behavioral level system that provides systematic and consistent consequences in the form of points (older adolescents) or stars (younger or cognitively limited patients) for attention at and participation in treatment groups and compliance with unit rules. In this four-tier system, patients advance from one level to the next based on increased percentages of points earned from one week of the admission to the next. For example, the requirements to maintain Level 1 status are at least 60% of all possible points earned. Progression to Level 2 requires a minimum of 70% of the points earned over the prior week. Each escalating level includes a greater number of privileges and reinforcers to enhance interest and motivation in the program.

The reason for using a token economic program with adolescent substance abusers is threefold. First, many of these individuals display antisocial behaviors (e.g., aggression and acting out). Considerable behavioral research since the early 1970s has documented the need for a structured therapeutic environment to manage such patients effectively (see Kazdin, 1987). Second, many adolescent inpatients have received attention only for deviant or maladaptive behavior. Positive reinforcement from families or peers for prosocial responding has often been lacking. Thus, the token economy provides an opportunity for such individuals to learn and respond to new and positive contingencies. Third, many inpatient facilities have limited staff available to carry out interventions. An advantage of token economies is their simplicity and objectivity, which generally reduce stress and confusion in the inpatient setting (see Kazdin, 1977).

Another important aspect of unit management is the development of a behavioral contract with the patient. The purpose of the behavioral contract is to identify specific areas of deficit that require remediation over the course of the admission. These contracts are individually tailored, and input is solicited from the patient and members of the treatment team. Multiple goals are typically determined weekly. Further, positive reinforcers are identified by both the patient and a staff member and are provided on goal completion. We have found the behavioral contract to be instrumental in (1) improving patient motivation in the milieu and (2) serving as a prompt for the patient to focus better on the treatment goals.

Integration of Treatment Modalities

In view of the multiple risk factors for the development of substance abuse problems in adolescents, the frequent presence of psychopathology, and the multiple deficits in social skills and family functioning, the use of multiple modalities is often required in the treatment of adolescent substance abusers. In addition to the primarily behavioral treatments noted previously in this chapter, psychotropic medications such as antidepressants and lithium may be useful, especially in the presence of a mood disorder or predominant mood symptoms. The use of multiple treatment modalities often dictates an intensive treatment setting, such as inpatient or partial hospitalization. The heterogeneity of adolescent substance abusers and their problems suggests a treatment-matching approach in which types of patients are matched with types and/or levels of interventions (McLellan, Woody, Luborsky, O'Brien, & Druley, 1983; Miller & Hester, 1986).

SUMMARY

Despite successful efforts to reduce recreational substance use among adolescents, the identification and treatment of significant substance abuse problems among youth remain a critical problem. The diagnosis of substance use disorders among adolescents requires a developmental perspective and a comprehensive examination of the adolescent's functioning in multiple domains beyond substance use alone. Similarly, treatment should be targeted at each identified deficit rather than directed only at abstinence. Substance abuse in adolescence is a complex problem that requires a comprehensive approach to assessment and treatments.

ACKNOWLEDGMENT.   Preparation of this chapter was supported in part, by the Center for Education and Drug Abuse Research (CEDAR), funded by the National Institute on Drug Abuse (No. DA05605). The authors would like to express their appreciation to Tracey Eck for her technical assistance in preparation of this manuscript.

REFERENCES

Achenbach, T. M., & Edelbrock, C. S. (1983a). Manual for the Child Behavior Checklist and Revised Child Behavior Profile. Burlington: University of Vermont, Department of Psychiatry.

Achenbach, T. M., & Edelbrock, C. S. (1983b). *Manual for the youth self-report and profile*. Burlington: University of Vermont, Department of Psychiatry.

Alexander, J. F., & Parsons, B. V. (1973). Short-term behavioral intervention with delinquent families: Impact on family process and recidivism. *Journal of Abnormal Psychology, 81*, 219–225.

American Psychiatric Association. (1980). *Diagnostic and statistical manual of mental disorders* (3rd ed.; DSM-III). Washington, DC: Author.

American Psychiatric Association. (1987). *Diagnostic and statistical manual of mental disorders* (3rd ed. rev.; DSM-III-R). Washington, DC: Author.

Ammerman, R. T., Lubetsky, M. J., Hersen, M., & Van Hasselt, V. B. (1988). Maltreatment of multihandicapped children and adolescents. *Journal of the Multihandicapped Person, 1*, 129–140.

Barned, Z., Rahan, G., & Teichman, M. (1987). The reliability and consistency of self-reports on substance use in a longitudinal study. *British Journal of Addictions*, *82*, 891–898.

Beck, A. (1976). *Cognitive therapy and the emotional disorders*. New York: International Universities Press.

Beck, A. T., Ward, C. H., Mendelson, M., Mock, J., & Erbaugh, J. (1961). An inventory for measuring depression. *Archives of General Psychiatry*, *4*, 561–571.

Beck, A. T., Weissman, A., Lefter, D., & Trexler, L. (1974). The measurement of pessimism: The Hopelessness Scale. *Journal of Consulting and Clinical Psychology*, *42*, 86865.

Beck, A. T., Rush, A. J., Shaw, B. F., & Emery, G. (1979). *Cognitive therapy of depression*. New York: Guilford Press.

Blane, H. (1979). Middle-aged alcoholics and young drinkers. In H. Blane, M. Chafetz (Eds.), *Youth, Alcohol and Social Policy* (pp. 5–38). New York: Plenum Press.

Botvin, G. J. (1986). Substance abuse prevention research: Recent developments and future directions. *Journal of School Heath*, *56*, 369–386.

Botvin, G. J., Baker, E., Renick, N. C., Filazzda, A. D., & Botvin, E. M. (1984). A cognitive-behavioral approach to substance abuse prevention. *Addictive Behaviors*, *9*, 137–147.

Brady, B. S., & Irvine, S. (1989). Self-help groups. In R. K. Hester & W. R. Miller (Eds.), *Handbook of alcoholism treatment approaches*. New York: Pergamon Press.

Brodsky, H. S. (1976). The assessment of social competence in adolescents. *Dissertation Abstracts International*, *36*, 4144B–4145B

Brown, S. A. (1985). Reinforcement expectancies and alcoholism outcome after a one year follow-up. *Journal of Studies on Alcohol*, *46*, 305–308.

Bry, B. H. (1988). Family-based approaches to reducing adolescent substance use: Theories, techniques, and findings. In E. R. Rahdert & J. Grabowski (Eds.), *Adolescent drug abuse: Analyses of treatment research* (NIDA Research Monograph No. 77). Washington, DC: U.S. Government Printing Office.

Bry, B. H., & Krinsley, K. E. (1990). Adolescent substance abuse. In E. L. Feindler & G. R. Kalfus (Eds.), *Adolescent behavior therapy handbook*. New York: Springer.

Bry, B. H., Conboy, C., & Bisgay, K. (1986). Decreasing adolescent drug use and school failure: Long-term effects of targeted family problem-solving training. *Child and Family Behavior Therapy*, *8*, 43–59.

Bukstein, O., & Blasher, J. (1991). Diagnostic inventory of substance use (DISU). Unpublished.

Bukstein, O. G., Brent, D. A., & Kaminer, Y. (1989). Comorbidity of substance abuse and other psychiatric disorders in adolescents. *American Journal of Psychiatry*, *146*, 1131–1141.

Cautela, J. R. (1970). The treatment of alcoholism by covert sensitization. *Psychotherapy: Theory, Research and Practice*, *7*, 86–90.

Chambers, W., Puig-Antich, J., Hirsh, M., Paez, P., Ambrosini, P. J., Tabrizi, M. A., & Davies, M. (1985). The assessment of affective disorders in children and adolescents by semi-structured interview: Test-retest reliability of the K-SADS-P. *Archives of General Psychiatry*, *42*, 696–702.

Chaney, E. F. (1989). Social skills training. In R. K. Hester & W. R. Miller (Eds.), *Handbook of alcoholism treatment approaches*. New York: Pergamon Press.

Chaney, E. F., O'Leary, M. R., & Marlatt, G. A. (1978). Skill training with alcoholics. *Journal of Consulting and Clinical Psychology*, *46*, 1092–1104.

Christiansen, B. A., Goldman, M. S., & Inn, A. (1982). Development of alcohol-related expectancies in adolescents: Separating pharmacological from social learning influences. *Journal of Consulting and Clinical Psychology*, *50*, 336–344.

Christiansen, B. A., Goldman, M. S., & Brown, S. A. (1985). The differential development of adolescent alcohol expectancies may predict adult alcoholism. *Journal of Addictive Behaviors*, *10*, 299–306.

Christie, K. A., Burke, J. D., Regier, D. A., Rae, D. S., Boyd, J. H., & Locke, B. Z. (1988). Epidemiologic evidence for early onset of mental disorders and higher risk of drug abuse in young adults. *American Journal of Psychiatry*, *145*, 971–975.

Christoff, K. A., & Myatt, R. J. (1987). Social isolation. In M. Hersen & V. B. Van Hasselt (Eds.), *Behavior therapy with children and adolescents: A clinical approach*. New York: Wiley.

Coddington, R. D. (1972a). The significance of life events as etiologic factors in the diseases of children. 1. A survey of professional workers. *Journal of Psychosomatic Research*, *16*, 7–18.

Coddington, R. E. (1972b). The significance of life events as etiologic factors in the diseases of children. 2. A study of a normal population. *Journal of Psychosomatic Research*, *16*, 205–213.

Connor, J. M., Dann, L. N., & Twentyman, C. T. (1982). A self report measure of assertiveness in young adolescents. *Journal of Clinical Psychology*, *38*, 101–106.

Cowen, E. L., Pederson, A., Babigan, H., Izzo, L. D., & Trost, E. A. (1973). Long term follow up of early detected vulnerable children. *Journal of Consulting and Clinical Psychology*, *41*, 438–446.

Crumley, F. E. (1990). Substance abuse and adolescent suicidal behavior. *Journal American Medical Association*, *263*, 3051–3056.

Csapo, M. (1983). Effects of social learning training with socially rejected children. *Behavioral Disorders*, *8*, 199–208.

DeJong, R., & Henrich, G. (1980). Follow-up results of a behavior modification program for juvenile drug addicts. *Addictive Behaviors*, *5*, 49–57.

Deykin, E. Y., Levy, J. C., & Wells, V. (1987). Adolescent depression, alcohol and drug abuse. *American Journal of Public Health*, *77*, 178–182.

Dishion, T. J., Patterson, G. R., & Reid, J. R. (1988). Parent and peer factors associated with drug sampling in early adolescence: Implications for treatment. In E. R. Rahdert & J. Grabowski (Eds.), *Adolescent drug abuse: Analyses of treatment research* (NIDA Research Monograph No. 77). Washington, DC: U.S. Government Printing Office.

Donovan, D. M., & Marlatt, G. A. (1980). A behavioral assessment of social and problematic drinking: A cognitive social learning formulation. *Journal of Studies on Alcohol*, *41*, 1153–1185.

Donovan, J. E., & Jessor, R. (1978). Adolescent problem drinking: Psychosocial correlates in a national sample study. *Journal Studies Alcohol*, *39*, 1506–1524.

Duehn, W. D. (1978). Covert sensitization in group treatment of adolescent drug abusers. *The International Journal of the Addictions*, *13*, 485–491.

Earles, F., Reich, W., Jung, K. O., & Cloninger, C. R. (1988). Psychopathology in children of alcoholic and antisocial parents. *Alcoholism: Clinical and Experimental Research*, *12*, 481–487.

Ecton, R. B., & Feindler, E. L. (1990). Anger control training for temper control disorders. In E. L. Feindler & G. R. Kalfus (Eds.), *Adolescent behavior therapy handbook*. New York: Springer.

Ferrell, W. L., & Galassi, J. P. (1981). Assertion training and human relations training in the treatment of chronic alcoholics. *The International Journal of the Addictions*, *16*, 959–968.

Foster, S. L., Prinz, R. J., & O'Leary, K. D. (1983). Impact of problem-solving communication training and generalization procedures on family conflict. *Child and Family Behavior Therapy*, *5*, 1–23.

Frederiksen, L. W., Jenkins, J. O., & Carr, C. R. (1976). Indirect modification of adolescent drug abuse using contingency contracting. *Journal of Behavior Therapy & Experimental Psychiatry*, *7*, 377–378.

Freedberg, E. J., & Johnston, W. E. (1981). Effects of assertion training within context of a multi-modal alcoholism treatment program for employed alcoholics. *Psychological Reports*, *48*, 379–386.

Freedman, B. J., Rosenthal, L., Donahoe, C. P., Schlundt, D. G., & McFall, R. M. (1978). A social-behavioral analysis of skill deficits in delinquent and nondelinquent adolescent boys. *Journal of Consulting and Clinical Psychology*, *46*, 1448–1462.

Galejs, I., & Stockdale, D. F. (1982). Social competence, school behaviors, and cooperative-competitive preferences: Assessments by parents, teachers, and school-age children. *Journal of Genetic Psychology*, *141*, 243–252.

Gittleman, R., Mannuzza, S., Shenker, R., & Bonagura, N. (1985). Hyperactive boys almost grown up: I. Psychiatric status. *Archives of General Psychiatry*, *42*, 937–947.

Gold, M.S., & Dachis, G. A. (1986). Role of laboratory in the evaluation of suspected drug abuse. *Journal of Clinical Psychiatry*, *47* (Suppl.), 17–23.

Goodwin, D. W. (1979). Alcoholism and heredity: A review and hypothesis. *Archives of General Psychiatry*, *36*, 57–61.

Greenwood, C. R., Walker, H. M., Todd, N. M., & Hops, H. (1979). Selecting a cost-effective screening measure for the assessment of preschool social withdrawal. *Journal of Applied Behavior Analysis*, *12*, 639–652.

Haggerty, K. P., Wells, E. A., Jenson, J. M., Catalano, R. F., & Hawkins, J. D. (1989). Delinquents and drug use: A model program for community reintegration. *Adolescence*, *24*, 439–456.

Harrison, P. A., & Hoffmann, H. G. (1985). The substance use disorders diagnostic schedule, St. Paul, MN, Ramsey Clinic.

Hawkins, J. D., Catalano, R. F., & Wells, E. A. (1986). Measuring effects of a skills training intervention for drug abusers. *Journal of Consulting and Clinical Psychology*, *54*, 661–664.

Henly, C., & Winters, K. (1988). Development of problem severity scales for the assessment of adolescent alcohol and drug abuse. *International Journal of the Addictions*, *23*, 65–85.

Herjanic, B., & Reich, W. (1982). Development of a structured psychiatric interview for children: Agreement between children and parent on individual symptoms. *Journal of Abnormal and Child Psychology*, *10*, 307–321.

Holden, G. W., Moncher, M. S., & Schinke, S. P. (1990). Substance abuse. In A. S. Bellack, M. Hersen, & A. E. Kazdin (Eds.), *International handbook of behavior modification and therapy*. New York: Plenum Press.

Hops, H., Tildesley, E., Lichtenstein, E., Ary, D., & Sherman, L. (1990). Parent-adolescent problem-solving interactions and drug use. *American Journal of Drug and Alcohol Abuse*, *16*, 239–258.

Horan, J. J., & Strauss, L. K. (1987). Substance abuse. In V. B. Van Hasselt & M. Hersen (Eds.), *Behavior therapy with children and adolescents: A clinical approach*. New York: Wiley.

Intagliata, J. C. (1978). Increasing the interpersonal problem-solving skills of an alcoholic population. *Journal of Consulting and Clinical Psychology, 46*, 489–498.

Jessor, R. (1976). Predicting time and onset of marijuana use: A developmental study of high school youth. *Journal of Consulting and Clinical Psychology, 44*, 125–134.

Jessor, R. (1984). Adolescent problem drinking: Psychosocial aspects and developmental outcomes. In L. H. Towle (Ed.), *Proceedings: NIAAA-WHO Collaborating Center Designation Meeting and Alcohol Research Seminar*. Washington, D.C.: Public Health Service.

Jessor, R., & Jessor, S. L. (1977). *Problem behavior and psychosocial development: A longitudinal study of youth*. New York: Academic Press.

Johnston, L. D. (1991). Press release University of Michigan Institute for Social Research.

Johnston, L., O'Malley, P., & Bachman, J. (1987). National trends in drug use and related factors among high school students and young adults. 1975–1986 (DHHS Pub. No. ADM 87–1535). Washington, D.C.: US Government Printing Office.

Kaminer, Y., & Bukstein, O. G. (1992). Substance abuse. In V. B. Van Hasselt & D. J. Kolko (Eds.), *Child and adolescent inpatient behavior therapy*. New York: Plenum Press.

Kandel, D. B. (1982). Epidemiological and psychosocial perspectives on adolescent drug abuse. *Journal of the American Academy of Child Psychiatry, 21*, 328–347.

Kandel, D. B., & Logan, J. A. (1984). Patterns of drug use from adolescence to young adulthood: I. periods of risk for initiation, continued use and discontinuation. *American Journal of Public Health, 74*, 660–666.

Kandel, D. B., Kessler, R. C., & Margulies, R. Z. (1978). Antecedents of adolescent initiation into stages of drug use: A developmental analyses. In D. B. Kandel (Ed.), *Longitudinal research on drug use: Empirical findings and methodological issues*. Washington, DC: Hemisphere (Halstead-Wiley).

Kandel, D. B., Davies, M., Karus, D., & Yamaguchi, K. (1986). The consequences in young adulthood of adolescent drug involvement. *Archives of General Psychiatry, 43*, 746–754.

Kazdin, A. E. (1977). *The token economy*. New York: Plenum Press.

Kazdin, A. E. (1987). *Conduct disorders in childhood and adolescence*. Newbury Park, CA: Sage.

Kazdin, A. E., Matson, J. L., & Esveldt-Dawson, K. (1984). The relationship of role-play assessment of children's social skills to multiple measures of social competence. *Behavior Research and Therapy, 22*, 129–139.

King, C. A., & Young, R. D. (1981). Peer popularity and peer communication patterns: Hyperactive versus active but normal boys. *Journal of Abnormal Child Psychology, 9*, 465–482.

Kohn, M., & Rosman, B. L. (1972). A social competence scale and symptom checklist for the preschool child: Factor dimensions, their cross instrument generality and longitudinal persistence. *Developmental Psychology, 6*, 430–444.

Lewinson, P. M., Clarke, G. N., Hops, H., & Andrews, J. (1990). Cognitive-behavioral treatment for depressed adolescents. *Behavior Therapy, 21*, 385–401.

Locke, H. J., & Wallace, K. M. (1959). Short marital adjustment and prediction tests. *Marriage and Family Living, 21*, 251–255.

Maletzky, B. M. (1974). Assisted covert sensitization for drug abuse. *International Journal of Addiction, 9*, 411–429.

Marlatt, G. A. (1985). Cognitive assessment and intervention procedures for relapse prevention. In G. Marlatt, G. A., & Donovan, D. M. (1982). Behavioral approaches to alcoholism. In E. M. Pattison & E. Kaufman (Eds.), *Encyclopedic handbook of alcoholism*. New York: Gardner Press.

Marlatt, G. A., & Gordon, J. R. (1985). *Relapse prevention*. New York: Guilford Press.

Mayer, J. E., & Filstead, W. J. (1979). Empirical procedures for defining adolescent alcohol abuse. *Journal of Studies on Alcohol, 40*, 291–300.

McLellan, A. T., Woody, G. E., Luborsky, L., O'Brien, C. P., & Druley, K. A. (1983). Increased effectiveness of substance abuse treatment: A prospective study of patient-treatment "matching." *Journal of Nervous and Mental Disorders, 171*, 597–605.

Meichenbaum, D. (1977). *Cognitive-behavior modification: An integrative approach*. New York: Plenum Press.

Michelson, L., & DiLorenzo, T. M. (1981). Behavioral assessment of peer interaction and social functioning in institutional and structured settings. *Journal of Clinical Psychology, 37*, 499–504.

Miller, W. R., & Hester, R. K. (1986). Matching problem drinkers with optimal treatments. In W. R. Miller & N. Heather (Eds.), *Treating addictive behaviors: Process of change* (pp. 175–203). New York: Plenum Press.

Milner, J. S., & Wimberly, R. C. (1979). An inventory for the identification of child abusers. *Journal of Clinical Psychology, 35*, 95–100.

Moos, R., & Moos, P. S. (1981). *Family environment scale: Manual*. Palo Alto, CA: Consulting Psychologists Press.

Newcomb, M. D., & Bentler, P. M. (1988). *Consequences of adolescent drug use*. Newbury Park, CA: Sage.

Nichols, M. (1984). *Family therapy: Concepts and methods*. New York: Gardner Press.

Novaco, R. W. (1975). *Anger control: The development and evaluation of an experimental treatment*. Lexington, MA: Lexington Books (DC Heath Co.).

Oetting, E. R., & Beauvais, F. (1990). Adolescent drug use: Findings of national and local surveys. *Journal of Consulting and Clinical Psychology, 58*, 385–394.

Oetting, E., Beauvais, F., Edwards, R., & Waters, M. (1984). *The drug and alcohol assessment system*. Rocky Mountain Behavioral Sciences Institute, Inc., Fort Collins, Colorado.

O'Leary, D. E., O'Leary, M. R., & Donovan, D. M. (1976). Social skill acquisition and psychosocial development of alcoholics: A review. *Addictive Behaviors, 1*, 111–120.

Orvaschel, H., & Walsh, G. (1984). *The assessment of adaptive functioning children: A review of existing measures suitable for epidemiological and clinical services research*. Washington, DC: Supt. of Docs., U.S. Govt Printing Off., DHHS Public No. (ADH) 84–1343.

Patterson, G. R. (1975). *Families: Applications of social learning to family life*. Champaign, IL: Research Press.

Patterson, G., & Forgatch, M. (1987). *Parents and adolescents: Living together*. Eugene, OR: Castalin.

Pentz, M. A., Cormack, C., Flay, B., Hansen, W. B., & Johnson, C. A. (1986). Balancing program and research integrity in community drug abuse prevention: Project STAR approach. *Journal of School Health, 56*, 389–393.

Prinz, R. J., Foster, S. L., Kent, R. N., & O'Leary, K. D. (1979). Multivariate assessment of conflict in distressed and nondistressed mother-adolescent dyads. *Journal of Applied Behavior Analysis, 12*, 691–700.

Rachman, S., & Teasdale, J. (1969). *Aversion therapy and behavior disorders: An analysis*. Coral Gables, FL: University of Miami Press.

Rapoport, J., & Conners, C. K. (Eds.). (1985). Rating scales and assessment instruments for use in pediatric psychopharmacology. *Psychopharmacology Bulletin, 21*, 713–1124.

Rathus, S. A. (1973). A 30-item schedule for assessing assertive behavior. *Behavior Therapy, 4*, 398–406.

Rimmele, C. T., Miller, W. R., & Dougher, M. J. (1989). Aversion therapies. In R. K. Hester & W. R. Miller, *Handbook of alcoholism treatment approaches*. New York: Pergamon Press.

Robin, A. L., & Foster, S. L. (1988). *Negotiating parent adolescent conflict: A behavioral-family systems approach*. New York: Guilford Press.

Roff, M. (1961). Childhood social interaction and young adult bad conduct. *Journal of Abnormal and Social Psychology, 63*, 333–337.

Roff, M., Sells, S. B., & Golden, M. (1972). *Social adjustment and personality development in children*. Minneapolis: University of Minnesota Press.

Rosenberg, M. (1965). *Society and the adolescent self-image*. Princeton, NJ: Princeton University Press.

Rounsaville, B. J., Snitzer, R. L., & Williams, J. B. W. (1986). Proposed changes in DSM-III substance use disorders: Description and rationale. *American Journal of Psychiatry, 143*, 463–468.

Rueger, D. B., & Liberman, R. P. (1984). Behavioral family therapy for delinquent and substance-abusing adolescents. *Journal of Drug Issues*, 403–418.

Sanchez-Craig, M., & Walker, K. (1982). Teaching coping skills to chronic alcoholics in a coeducational halfway house: 1. Assessment of programme effects. *British Journal of Addiction, 77*, 35–50.

Schinke, S. P., & Blythe, B. J. (1981). Cognitive-behavioral prevention of children's smoking. *Child Behavior Therapy, 3*, 25–42.

Schinke, S. P., & Gilchrist, L. D. (1984). *Life skills counseling with adolescents*. Austin, TX: Pro-Ed Press.

Schinke, S. P., Botvin, G. J.,& Orlandi, M. A. (1991). *Substance abuse in children and adolescents: Evaluation and intervention*. Newbury Park, CA: Sage.

Singh, E., Kandel, D., & Johnson, B. (1975). The internal validity and reliability of drug use responses in a large scale survey. *Journal of Drug Issues, 5*, 426–433.

Skinner, H. A., Steinhauer, P. S. & Santa-Barbara, J. (1983). The family assessment measure. *Canadian Journal of Community Mental Health, 2*, 91–105.

Tarter, R. E. (1990). Evaluation and treatment of adolescent substance abuse: A decision tree method. *American Journal of Drug Alcohol Abuse, 16*, 1–46.

Turner, S. M., Beidel, D. C., Dancu, C. V., & Stanley, M. A. (1989). An empirically derived inventory to measure social fears and anxiety: The social phobia and anxiety inventory. *Journal of Consulting and Clinical Psychology, 1*, 35–40.

Van Hasselt, V. B., Hersen, M., & Milliones, J. (1978). Social skills training for alcoholics and drug addicts: A review. *Addictive Behaviors, 3*, 221–233.

Van Hasselt, V. B., Hersen, M., & Bellack, A. S. (1981). The validity of role play tests for assessing social skills in children. *Behavior Therapy, 12*, 202–216.

Van Hasselt, V. B., Null, J., & Bukstein, O. G. (1992). Maltreatment of dually-diagnosed adolescent substance abusers: Case examples. *Journal of Family Violence*.

Vingilis, E., & Smart, R. G. (1981). Physical dependence on alcohol in youth. In F. B. Gleser & H. Kalant (Eds.), *Research advances in alcohol and drug problems* (pp. 197–215). New York: Plenum Press.

Walker, H. M. (1976). *Problem behavior identification checklist*. Los Angeles: Western Psychological Services.

Weiss, R. L., & Perry, B. A. (1979). *Assessment and treatment of mental dysfunction*. Eugene, OR: Oregon Mental Studies Program.

Weschler, H. (1979). Patterns of alcohol consumption among the young: High school, college, and general population studies. In H,. Blane & M. Chafetz (Eds.), *Youth, alcohol, and social policy*. New York: Plenum Press.

West, M. O., & Printz, R. J. (1987). Parental alcoholism and childhood psychopathology. *Psychological Bulletin*, *1102*, 204–218.

White, H. R., Johnson, V., & Horwitz, A. (1986). An application of three deviance theories to adolescent substance use. *International Journal of Addictions*, *21*, 347–366.

Winters, K. (1990). The need for improved assessment of adolescent substance involvement. *The Journal of Drug Issues*, *20*, 487–502.

23

Eating Disorders

DAVID M. GARNER and ALEXANDER H. SACKEYFIO

INTRODUCTION

Eating disorders are associated with a significant morbidity and, in the case of anorexia nervosa, a high risk of mortality (18%) over the course of the illness (Theander, 1985). Although it is widely accepted that the majority of eating-disordered patients can be managed effectively as outpatients, most clinicians would agree that there is a subgroup of patients who either require or greatly benefit from inpatient treatment. The main objectives of hospitalization for eating-disordered patients are (1) weight restoration, or the interruption of steady weight loss in the case of anorexia nervosa; (2) the interruption of unremitting binging and vomiting; (3) the evaluation and treatment of medical complications; (4) the management of associated conditions, such as severe depression, suicidal behavior, and substance abuse; (5) addressing the psychological and interpersonal factors that have initiated or maintained the eating disorder; and (6) occasionally, the disengagement of patients from a social system that both contributes to the maintenance of the disorder and disrupts outpatient treatment. Although there is still a divergence of opinion regarding the etiology of eating disorders, considerable agreement exists on the parameters of inpatient management (Andersen, 1985; Andersen, Morse, & Santmyer, 1985; Garfinkel & Garner, 1982; Mitchell, 1990; Russell, 1970; Strober & Yager, 1985; Vandereycken & Meermann, 1984).

From the onset, it is important to note that, in most cases, hospitalization alone does not lead to the resolution of an eating disorder. It must be considered only one facet of a sometimes lengthy and complex treatment process aimed primarily at seriously ill patients. Nevertheless, there are instances, particularly with pediatric patients, where hospitalization can achieve rather dramatic results in reversing the course of the eating disorder. In other situations, in which there is a prolonged therapeutic impasse, inpatient treatment may be a humane alternative to the tremendous emotional and financial expense of continued unproductive outpatient therapy, which cannot proceed past a certain point in the presence of the severe limits imposed by starvation or by unremitting binging and vomiting.

The primary goals of this chapter are to review the fundamental aspects of the inpatient

DAVID M. GARNER • Department of Psychiatry, Michigan State University, East Lansing, Michigan 48824-1316.   ALEXANDER H. SACKEYFIO • Eating Disorder Program, Beaumont Hospital, Royal Oak, Michigan 48073.

Handbook of Behavior Therapy in the Psychiatric Setting, edited by Alan S. Bellack and Michel Hersen. Plenum Press, New York, 1993.

care of the eating-disordered patient, beginning with a complete assessment. The application of these assessment and treatment principles will be highlighted by a case illustration indicating certain deviations from the prototypical plan. Before proceeding with the primary objectives of the chapter, we briefly describe eating disorders and their variants.

DESCRIPTION OF THE DISORDERS

Anorexia Nervosa

The requirements for a diagnosis of anorexia nervosa are (1) refusal to maintain a normal body weight (e.g., weight loss leading to the maintenance of a body weight 15% below norms, or failure to achieve expected weight during a period of growth); (2) intense fear of gaining weight or becoming fat, even though underweight; (3) disturbance in how body weight, size, or shape is experienced; and (4) amenorrhea in females (DSM III-R; American Psychiatric Association, 1987). Although the distinction is not made in the DSM-III-R criteria, anorexia nervosa patients have been differentiated into the *restricting subtype* (i.e., those who lose weight by rigidly restricting food intake) and the *bulimic subtype* (i.e., those whose stringent attempts to limit intake are punctuated by episodes of binge eating). Bulimic subtype patients tend to present at a heavier weight and with a more frequent premorbid and family history of obesity than the restricting subtype patients (Garner, Garfinkel, & O'Shaughnessy, 1985a).

Bulimia Nervosa

The essential features of bulimia nervosa are (1) recurrent episodes of binge eating (the rapid consumption of a large amount of food in a discrete period of time) occurring at least twice a week for the past three months; (2) a feeling of lack of control over eating behavior during these binges; (3) self-induced vomiting, the use of laxatives or diuretics, strict dieting or fasting, or vigorous exercising in order to prevent weight gain; and (4) persistent overconcern about body weight and shape (American Psychiatric Association, 1987; 1991).

Binge-Eating Disorder

There is increasing evidence that a significant proportion of obese individuals who present for weight loss treatment engage in binge-eating episodes. Although a small minority of these individuals meet the criteria for bulimia nervosa, others engage in binge eating but do not meet the other criteria for eating disorders (Spitzer, Devlin, Walsh, Hasin, Wong, Marcus, Stunkard, Wadden, Yanovski, Agras, Mitchell, & Nona, 1992). The criteria have not been established at this time, but initial discussions have focused on defining the disorder in terms of recurrent episodes of binge eating similar to those found in bulimia nervosa plus behavioral indicators that the behavior is associated with "loss of control" over eating. Although there is merit in adopting the binge-eating disorder into the diagnostic nomenclature, it is critical to remain aware that binge eating and the associated psychological symptoms, particularly in the obese, may be attributed to standard weight-loss treatments (Garner & Wooley, 1991).

The Relationships between Different Diagnostic Subgroups

Even though distinctions between the eating disorder syndromes have been emphasized, there are serious limitations in these nominal subtype designations. Eating-disordered patients tend to be more alike than different. There is extraordinary variability within each of these subgroups on a wide range of demographic, clinical, and psychological dimensions (Welch, Hall, & Renner, 1990), and patients have been observed to move between the two subtypes at different times (Russell, 1979). Many individuals present with some but not all of the features required for an eating-disorder diagnosis as specified by the DSM-III-R (i.e., insufficient weight loss, binging on *small* amounts of food, and engaging in self-induced vomiting). Although some of these individuals may be thought of as "subthreshold" cases, they deserve careful evaluation, because it may be only owing to improved recognition of eating disorders that they have been identified at an early stage in the course of their eating disorder. Even the most obvious distinction between anorexia nervosa and bulimia nervosa (i.e., absolute body weight) is blurred when one looks at the amount of body weight that bulimia nervosa patients have lost during the course of their disorder. These and other diagnostic issues have been discussed in detail elsewhere (Garner & Garfinkel, 1988; Garner, Shafer, & Rosen, 1992; Garner, Garner, & Rosen, in press).

Differential Diagnosis

Patients who do not suffer from anorexia nervosa, bulimia nervosa, or some variant may superficially resemble patients with an eating-disorder diagnosis. Patients with a severe affective disorder may display marked weight loss (due to loss of appetite) or hyperphagia. Schizophrenics may present with an aversion to eating and occasionally binge eating or purging. Vomiting and weight loss may also be associated with what has been described as a conversion disorder (Garfinkel, Kaplan, Garner, & Darby, 1983). A range of physical illnesses producing weight loss (e.g., inflammatory bowel disease, chronic hepatitis, Addison's disease, Crohn's disease, undiagnosed cystic fibrosis, diabetes mellitus, hyperthyroidism, tuberculosis, malignancies, malabsorption diseases, and other wasting diseases) should be ruled out as the primary diagnosis (Comerci, 1990).

Prototypical Assessment

Format and Context of the Initial Assessments

It is important that the format and style of initial or early interviews be aimed at the development of a sense of openness and trust between the patient and the assessing clinician. These early meetings are particularly crucial with eating-disordered patients, who may assume that the goal of assessment and treatment is to convince them to abandon certain symptoms that they view as necessary or even desirable. Under most circumstances, when assessments are being performed with young patients who are living at home, all members of the family should participate in the evaluation. When it is impractical or deemed clinically unnecessary for the siblings to be part of an initial assessment, they may play an important role in subsequent meetings. With older patients, it may be preferable to see the individual alone for all or at least part of the initial assessment. This privacy denotes respect for the patient's autonomy from the family of origin (even though significant enmeshment may still exist) and allows the clinician to gather information regarding eating symptoms that the patient may be reluctant to share in the presence of the parents or the spouse. The decisions about whether or not to perform the assessment and subsequent treatment with the individual alone, to include the spouse, to include current family members, or to involve members of the family of origin must depend on the specific clinical issues pertinent to the given case (Vandereycken, Kog, & Vanderlinden, 1989).

Various approaches to information gathering have been developed for the eating disorders, including standard clinical interviews, semistructured interviews, behavioral observation, standardized self-report measures, symptom checklists, clinical rating scales, self-monitoring procedures, and standardized test meals.

Content Areas for Assessment

Several specific content areas should be covered in the initial assessments of patients with eating disorders. These areas are briefly reviewed below; however, further details, as well as

DAVID M. GARNER
and ALEXANDER H.
SACKEYFIO

specific probe questions, have been provided elsewhere (Fairburn, 1987; Foreyt & McGavin, 1988; Garner, 1991).

Physical Complications. A medical evaluation of patients with eating disorders is necessary to determine the patients' overall physical status and to identify or rule out physical complications associated with starvation or with certain extreme weight-losing behaviors. Occasionally, a medical evaluation is necessary to determine if weight loss has been precipitated by an underlying physical disorder (Comerci, 1990; see "Differential Diagnosis" above). Symptoms such as hypotension, hypothermia, bradycardia, and overall reduced metabolic rate are common to starvation and may be evident in anorexia nervosa. Self-induced vomiting and purgative abuse may cause various symptoms or abnormalities, such as weakness, muscle cramping, edema, constipation, cardiac arrhythmias, and paresthesia. Additionally, general fatigue, constipation, depression, various neurological abnormalities, kidney and cardiac disturbances, swollen salivary glands, electrolyte disturbances, dental deterioration, finger clubbing or swelling, edema, and dehydration have been reported (Comerci, 1990; Mitchell, 1990; Mitchell & Boutacoff, 1986; Mitchell, Pomery, & Huber, 1988).

Weight History. A thorough weight history provides important information about the nature and the temporal sequence of events as they relate to the patient's struggle with weight. It is also a relatively nonthreatening area for early discussion that facilitates the development of rapport.

Overconcern about Weight and Shape. It has been suggested that one of the fundamental features of eating disorders is the tendency to use weight, shape, or thinness as the sole or predominant referent for inferring personal value or self-worth (Fairburn & Garner, 1988; Garner & Bemis, 1982). Directly flowing from an assessment of the weight history is an evaluation of the nature and intensity of patients' overconcern with weight and shape. Specific questions regarding weight and shape not only provide valuable information on this topic but also reveal the more general belief structure and conceptual style of the patient. Through this type of questioning, the meaning of weight and shape and the intensity of the patient's convictions can be explored.

Binge-Eating, Dieting, and Weight-Losing Behaviors. The frequency and intensity of the patient's binge eating, dieting efforts, and types of weight-losing behaviors should be assessed in an initial interview. A dietary history should pinpoint when dieting and binge eating first began as well as the different methods that have been used to reduce or control weight. Questions should be asked about weight-controlling behavior such as laxative and diuretic abuse, the use of diet pills or other drugs to control appetite, the use of emetics, chewing and spitting food out before swallowing, prolonged fasting, and vigorous exercise for the explicit purpose of controlling body weight.

Predisposing Factors. Individual, familial, and sociocultural background factors have collectively and in combination been implicated in the development of anorexia nervosa and bulimia nervosa. These background factors have formed the basis for different theoretical approaches to eating disorders, which have resulted in treatment orientations that may be characterized as primarily behavioral, cognitive behavioral, educational, psychodynamic, and family-system. A full discussion of the range of determinants and the psychological orientations that they represent is far beyond the scope of this chapter, and they have been reviewed elsewhere (Garfinkel & Garner, 1982; Garner & Garfinkel, 1985; Johnson & Connors, 1987; Vandereycken *et al.*, 1989). Although certain core features may be common to many eating-disordered patients, individual differences in premorbid personality and levels of psychological functioning contribute to major differences in the manifestation of the key symptoms (Tobin, Johnson, Steinberg, Staats, & Dennis, 1991). Moreover, it may not be apparent from the initial assessment whether psychological distress, cognitive impairment, and behavioral symptoms reported by anorexic and bulimic patients signal fundamental emotional disturbance or are secondary elaborations resulting from weight loss and chaotic dietary patterns (Fairburn, Cooper, Kirk, & O'Connor, 1985; Garner, Olmsted, Davis, Rockert, Goldbloom, & Eagle, 1990). In this sense, a valuable assessment tool is simply the patient's response to brief, educationally oriented therapy, because many patients show rapid improvement, including more consistent eating patterns and weight restoration (Olmsted, Davis, Rockert, Irvine, Eagle, & Garner, 1991).

The complete psychiatric assessment of eating-disordered patients should include measures of personality functioning, psychological distress, depression, anxiety, family functioning, history of sexual abuse, self-esteem, social and vocational adaptation, and impulse-related features that may be relevant to the development and maintenance of these syndromes. Careful assessment of these related areas is important in confirming DSM-III-R Axis II diagnoses and in treatment planning. Reassessment during the course of treatment is desirable as it may provide a more meaningful picture of personality dimensions that endure once the acute symptoms of the eating disorder are resolved.

ACTUAL ASSESSMENT

Presenting Complaints and Reason for Admission

Ms. R was a 26-year-old woman with a 10-year history of anorexia nervosa, bulimic subtype. She weighed 89 pounds at 5 feet 4 inches tall and was referred for admission following a suicide attempt in which she ingested approximately 100 aspirin tablets and ten 5-mg tablets of diazepam. She had been treated in the emergency ward of a local hospital and had been discharged under the proviso that she seek inpatient care. She was referred by her outpatient therapist, with whom she had been in treatment for over a year. R complained of general weakness and appeared wan, confused, despondent, and unanimated in the initial meeting. She explained that this had been her first suicide attempt, although she had increasingly experienced the impulse to harm herself over the past several months. She reported that this impulse was connected with hopelessness related to her belief that she would never be able to recover from her eating disorder. She felt that her individual therapy had initially been helpful, but she did not feel that she was making progress now. R had become increasingly depressed following her breakup a month earlier with a man whom she had been dating for the past year. She decided that ending her life was the only solution at this point.

Clinical and Psychometric Assessment

Space limitations permit only a sketch of this patient's background and highlights of the assessment. Essentially, the above "prototypical assessment" was followed and background material related to complications, eating behavior, weight history, and predisposing factors was gathered.

> R had been in individual therapy several times during the past 10 years, and she felt that it had never really led to improvement in her eating disorder. Her eating disorder had begun when she was 16 years old, shortly after she had dropped from 130 pounds to 85 pounds. Two years later she began binging and vomiting. She had experienced fluctuations in weight since that time, but her weight had never exceeded 105 pounds. She reported binge-eating and self-induced vomiting at least three times daily over the past year. She did not remember any days in the past six months during which she had not binged and vomited at least once. She also reported abusing laxatives, taking between 5 and 10 Ex-Lax tablets daily. She had begun drinking several years ago and would periodically "binge" on alcohol because she felt depressed and because she felt that drinking to a state of "oblivion" could keep her from giving in to her impulse to eat. There was no reported history of drug abuse. At least once a week, R described binging and vomiting 15 or more times in a day. The types of foods consumed on a "binge" usually consisted of those typically prohibited from her diet, such as desserts and other sweet foods that were high in fat content; however, she would also often binge-eat on

other foods that were not proscribed from her daily diet. Binge-eating episodes usually involved consuming more than 1,000 calories of food before vomiting; however, she also described vomiting after eating small amounts because of feeling "guilty" or "bloated."

Initially, R did not want to be admitted for treatment of her eating disorder, and her mental status at the time of the assessment interview did not make admission necessary. She became more interested in inpatient treatment with further discussion of the possible benefits of simply seeing how her mental state would improve with some weight gain and with the interruption of her binging, vomiting, and laxative abuse. She described being terrified of the possibility of weight gain but understood that she had only two unpleasant options to choose from: continuing to feel either depressed by her current circumstances or upset about confronting the possibility of addressing some of her symptoms in the hospital. Treatment was presented as an opportunity to separate her real psychological problems from the sequelae of starvation and chaotic eating.

At this point, R agreed to a comprehensive assessment. She was given a complete physical exam, electrocardiogram, and laboratory tests, including blood count, electrolytes, and blood urea nitrogen, all of which were within normal limits (Andersen, 1985; Comerci, 1990). R also completed psychological tests, including the Eating Disorder Inventory-2 (EDI-2), the EDI symptom checklist, the EAT, the Beck Depression Inventory, the Millon Clinical Multiaxal Inventory (MCMI; Millon, 1982), and the SCL-90. Her Eating Disorder Inventory EDI-2 (Garner, 1991) findings are presented in Figure 1 and indicate the typical profile of a chronically eating-disordered patient. The subscales concerned with eating and the body (Drive for Thinness, Bulimia, and Body Dissatisfaction) indicate prominent problems in these areas. The elevated Ineffectiveness, Interoceptive Awareness, Impulse Regulation, and Social Insecurity subscales also confirmed the clinical impression of serious psychological and interpersonal disturbances. Evidence of a personality disorder was indicated by elevated Borderline, Dysthymia, Alcohol Abuse, and Avoidant scales on the MCMI. Psychometric testing corroborated the clinical picture of a patient who was experiencing marked psychological and interpersonal distress with possible characterological disturbance.

R's family history revealed a past in which relationships were troubled and unpredictable. She was the first of four children (all girls) and was reminded repeatedly by her mother that pregnancy with R was the reason for the mother's entering into an unsatisfactory marriage. R described her mother as unhappy and rejecting. Her mother was unable to express feelings of warmth or tenderness toward her daughters and was described as incessantly pushing her children toward success, defined exclusively in terms of academics and autonomous functioning. The mother did not work outside the home. She was described as having a serious problem with alcohol. R's father was a highly successful executive who was idealized by his daughters and described by R as the "perfect father." He had extremely high standards of performance for himself and prided himself in his efficient use of virtually every moment of every day. He would frequently read reports from work while on an exercise bicycle listening to classical music through portable headphones. R reported feeling like a failure throughout her schooling even though she had performed well in the early grades and in high school. She had attended university after high school but withdrew after the first term. She attributed her inability to cope to her eating disorder and to her fear of failure in light of her recognition that the demands of the university might be more than she could meet. Her failure at the university resulted in further rejection by her mother, which worsened with the academic accomplishments of R's three siblings. R worked in an insurance company as a claims adjuster and, despite her eating disorder, had done well within her firm. R did not report any history of sexual abuse.

R did not report satisfying or sustained relationships with men before the relationship that had recently ended. She had had what she described as superficial relationships with various women at work, and her closest friend also had an eating disorder.

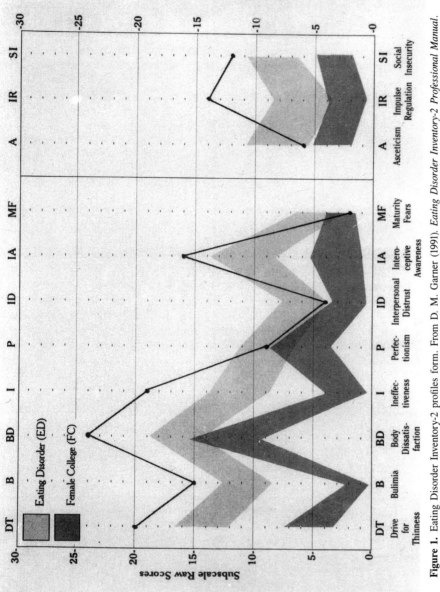

Figure 1. Eating Disorder Inventory-2 profiles form. From D. M. Garner (1991). *Eating Disorder Inventory-2 Professional Manual.* Psychological Assessment Resources, Odessa, Florida. Reproduced by permission.

DAVID M. GARNER
and ALEXANDER H.
SACKEYFIO

Preadmission Interview

Preadmission interviews provide a valuable opportunity for further assessment and for strategic interventions that may have a powerful effect on the course of hospitalization. The specific aims of the preadmission interview include (1) a further assessment of the patient and her family; (2) confirmation of the diagnosis of an eating disorder; (3) a description of the ward routine, with details of the program aimed at the normalization of eating and weight; (4) a confrontation of denial of the seriousness of the disorder; (5) explaining that the eating disorder serves a psychologically adaptive function and outlining common themes; (6) qualifying any formulations by emphasizing that current psychological and interpersonal experiences have very likely been clouded and distorted by starvation symptoms and metabolic disturbances caused by chaotic eating patterns; (7) addressing fears about hospitalization; and (8) building a therapeutic alliance that will enhance the patient's cooperation. The preadmission interview may be the first exposure to the staff with whom the patient will need to form trusting, empathic, and limit-setting relationships that will form the cornerstone of both symptom management and psychotherapy.

It must be emphasized that the aim of hospitalization is not just symptom management; it must deal with the psychological and family problems that have personal relevance to the patient. The interest in psychological issues may be underscored in the initial interviews through an overview of the adaptive functions or types of interactional themes, belief systems, or simplified "dynamics" that often operate in eating disorders (Garner & Bemis, 1985). Specific formulations regarding the patient's disorder are often premature at this time because the themes that appear to be fundamental at admission often change during the course of hospitalization. Many of the psychological and behavioral symptoms experienced by the patient may be reattributed to starvation (Garner, Rockert, Olmsted, Johnson, & Coscina, 1985b). This connection of some symptoms with starvation also provides the rationale for pursuing weight gain and symptom management as a precursor to attempting to completely understand or resolve the psychosocial issues underlying the eating disorder.

Treatment of the Eating Disorder versus Medical Management

The decision to implement hospitalization often involves the delicate philosophical balance between free will and determinism (Crisp, 1980; Goldner, 1989). On the one hand, the eating-disordered patient may be seen as free to choose the current way of life (i.e., anorexia nervosa, even if it involves suboptimal functioning). On the other, the patient may be seen as unable to exercise free choice because of supervalent psychological determinants that cloud the patient's judgment about the medical risks. Probably both points of view are correct, and there appears to be no consensus on the solution to the dilemma. However, Goldner (1989) provided a summary of recommendations designed to minimize treatment refusal, and they may be paraphrased as follows: seek a voluntary alliance, identify the reasons for treatment refusal, carefully explain the reasons for the treatment recommendations, remain flexible, show respect for the patient's belief in the importance of thinness, minimize intrusive interventions, weigh the risks and benefits of active treatment, avoid punitive interventions, involve the family where possible, and consider involuntary treatment only when nonintervention constitutes an immediate and serious danger.

Program Staff

Most eating-disorder inpatient programs are staffed by a multidisciplinary team, consisting of a psychiatrist, an internist, nurses, and a dietitian or nutritional staff as the core. Most programs also have ongoing consultants or full-time staff from occupational therapy, psychology, and social work. All programs should have trained clinicians who are familiar with the psychology of eating disorders and who enjoy working with eating-disordered patients.

The mortality risk and self-initiated nature of some of the symptoms in eating disorders may cause feelings of fear, anger, frustration, and helplessness among treatment staff (Brotman, Stern, & Herzog, 1984). The volitional nature of many of the symptoms displayed by eating-disordered patients may cause them to be perceived as having a less "legitimate" disorder than those occupying other medical wards in the hospital. Health professionals who work with eating-disordered patients may be affected by increased awareness of food, and of their own physical condition, appearance, and feelings about their own bodies (Shisslak, Gray, & Crago, 1989), which may have to be dealt with during supervision and in-service training. However, the staff may also respond with healthier attitudes toward eating and with job satisfaction (Sansone, Fine, & Chew, 1988).

In any event, inpatient treatment is complicated by the interpersonal exigencies inevitable when multiple staff members are involved in the care of a diverse group of patients. The differences among staff attitudes, the varied dynamics among patients, and the interplay between these factors have the potential for either heightening conflict or facilitating meaningful interpersonal goals of treatment. Staff require special training and supervision in order to fully appreciate the vulnerabilities of these patients as well as the potential for negative or inappropriate reactions to them (Hamburg & Herzog, 1990).

Sometimes, negative reactions to patients may be indirectly inferred from the language that is used to characterize the patients' behavior. For example, the term *splitting* is often used in inpatient settings to describe patients' interactions with staff surrounding the surreptitious disposal of food, dishonesty regarding vomiting or exercising, and other apparently manipulative attempts to avoid compliance with the program. Although intended as an explanatory concept, the term *splitting* often loses its original meaning and becomes an overused and pejorative euphemism for behavior that the staff sees as frustrating. A more parsimonious understanding of these apparent "deceptions" is that they simply reflect a dread of weight gain or "feeling fat." This dread is understandable, given the eating-disordered patient's frame of reference. In this sense, it is similar to the intense fear experienced by an elevator phobic who steps onto an elevator, except that the eating-disordered patient cannot escape the feared stimulus (i.e., her or his own body). In addition to this phobic avoidance stance, the eating-disordered patient's behavior is driven by the ego-syntonic belief that extreme dieting is virtuous (Garner, Garfinkel, & Bemis, 1982). Thus, as the staff develops a full understanding of the depth of eating-disordered patients' extraordinary fears of normal eating and weight gain, behaviors previously characterized as manipulative, uncooperative, and deceitful are viewed with more compassion. Once the staff becomes more knowledgeable, competent, and successful, negative responses are often replaced by pride, staff unity, and a sincere preference for treating eating-disordered patients.

General Principles

Several programs have offered a range of inpatient management strategies for the eating disorders. Some are shaped by a particular theoretical orientation toward the understanding of eating disorders. For example, Crisp (1980) emphasized the importance of bedrest and nutritional rehabilitation aimed at achieving a body weight associated with adult appearance and hormonal status. This approach is consistent with his conceptualization of the disorder as a means of avoiding a host of adolescent developmental challenges through the "psychobiological regression" resulting from weight loss. Other programs have relied less on strong theoretical guiding principles and have emphasized the value of interpersonal support and environmental structure within the hospital environment as safe and effective means of interrupting symptoms, facilitating renutrition, and helping the patient learn to regulate eating and weight (Anderson *et al.*, 1985).

Providing the conceptualization of treatment as following a "two-track" approach is helpful in making the patient and the family acutely aware of the interdependence of the physical and psychosocial aspects of functioning (Garner *et al.*, 1982). The first track distinguishes the therapy for eating disorders from the treatment of other disorders. It pertains to issues related to weight, binging, vomiting, extreme dieting, and other behaviors aimed at weight control. The second track is focused on the psychological and interpersonal context of the disorder. This track overlaps considerably with issues that are relevant to many patients who do not have eating disorders. The early phases of treatment tend to focus more on Track 1 themes, as it is very difficult to distinguish the patient's genuine psychological vulnerabilities from the sequelae of starvation and chaotic eating. As eating and weight become regulated, there is more emphasis on psychological and family interventions designed to address the individual, family, and social factors that may have played a role in the development and maintenance of the eating disorder.

The Therapeutic Relationship

The importance of the therapeutic relationship in promoting change has been emphasized in various approaches to the treatment of eating disorders (Andersen *et al.*, 1985; Bruch, 1973; Casper, 1987; Crisp, 1980; Garner *et al.*, 1982, 1985b; Guidano & Liotti, 1983; Stern, 1986; Vandereycken *et al.*, 1989), and the reader is encouraged to consult the original sources on the topic. Warmth, genuineness, empathy, honesty, and acceptance are qualities that should be part of the repertoire of all skilled therapists. These qualities are vital in the treatment of eating disorders, because the patients may begin the therapeutic process with the conviction that the goal of the therapeutic team is to deprive them of certain ego-syntonic symptoms (e.g., thinness, dieting, and weight control) that are viewed as vital to their well-being. Thus, the strength of the therapeutic relationship may be a major determinant of patients' willingness to engage in the terrifying prospects of eating and weight gain.

Explaining the Need to Impose External Controls and Limits

The initial phase of hospitalization tends to emphasize the use of external controls to help the patient begin eating and to inhibit symptomatic behavior. As soon as the patient has improved enough to be out of medical danger, has begun complying with the program of eating, has demonstrated a motivation to change, has developed a positive alliance with the staff, and has experienced some reduction in anxiety, depression, obsessionality, and resistance to weight gain, there is then a shift toward eating with less supervision. Before discharge, patients should be eating and maintaining their weight with only minimal external controls.

The controls imposed by hospitalization itself, as well as by certain rules regarding eating and weight management, may be seen at first blush as contradicting the goals of treatment, such as the development of autonomy, self-expression, and self-sufficiency. It is helpful to remind patients that, although autonomous functioning is the ultimate goal, their current state involves incredible confusion and loss of control over the vital functions of eating and weight management. Patients must temporarily turn control over to the staff, who will take responsibility for the refeeding and the symptom management process until the patients are able to regulate eating and weight on their own. Although there is some initial resistance to this notion, patients are usually quite relieved to no longer have to struggle every moment with decisions about whether or not to eat, exercise, or purge after eating. They may express concern that they will become accustomed to eating large amounts or the "wrong types" of foods and that they will "lose their will" to exercise. They need to be reminded that their current feelings and attitudes about the level of discipline required to hold eating in check and to control weight are occurring within the context of a marked disturbance in the biological mechanisms underlying normal weight regulation. Thus, truly "internal" regulation of eating and weight may take some time. In the meantime, on the road to internal control, they have to "mimic" normal eating and rely on others to help establish a proper weight.

The need for some of the controls and exposure to foods that have been avoided can be explained in behavioral or psychodynamic terms. Many of the avoidance behaviors have been maintained by negative reinforcement (i.e., the offset of aversive consequences), and the controls of a hospital can help patients to learn that some of the feared consequences may no longer be operational. The hospital may also be characterized as a "holding environment" that allows appropriate developmental experiences to occur (Goodsitt, 1985). Regardless of the rationale, when controls are imposed the patients need to be reassured that key objectives for the staff are to assist them with any psychosocial difficulties that they may be experiencing now or will experience in the future. Although reasonable attempts should be made to be firm and consistent in the treatment plan, the milieu should not be harsh, uncompromising, and unreal. It is not necessary to impose arbitrary rules because there is almost always a logical reason for prudent programmatic decisions. An approach in which there is a mixture of firmness in certain areas and flexibility in others is probably easiest for the staff and the patients to follow (Andersen, 1985; Stern, 1986; Touyz, Beumont, Glaun, Philips, & Cowie, 1984).

Normalizing Eating and Weight

It is now well recognized that addressing eating and weight is central to both inpatient and outpatient treatments of eating disorders. Because a detailed manual is available outlining various behavioral and cognitive behavioral methods aimed specifically at addressing Track 1 issues (Garner et al., 1985b), only the key topic areas are mentioned here.

Educational Material. Reviewing the studies illuminating starvation symptoms and the biological consequences of under- and overfeeding is useful in conveying the notion that body weight appears to be homeostatically regulated and that deviations from a certain level (i.e., "set point") result in the activation of powerful compensatory mechanisms designed to restore equilibrium (Garner et al., 1985b). These mechanisms occur not only in those at or below a statistically normal weight but also in those who are obese (Garner & Wooley, 1991).

Target Weight. There are no definitive standards for determining an appropriate goal weight; however, it should allow normal menstrual functioning and should be high enough so that it reduces some of the biological cravings for food. There is increasing agreement about the limited value of simply using weight norms as the gauge for any given individual, as they do not take into account the tremendous individual differences in genetic and constitutional factors (Garner et al., 1985b). Thus, a realistic goal-weight range should be no less than between three and five pounds above the patient's menstrual weight threshold and as close as can be tolerated to about 10% below her highest weight before the onset of the disorder. This guideline may have to be accomplished very gradually and modified periodically based on the patient's capacity for change.

Rate of Weight Gain. On an inpatient unit, the rate of weight gain should generally be between 1 and 2 kg (2.2–4.4 lb) per week. More weight may be gained during the first two weeks because of rehydration (particularly when there has been laxative abuse), and this should be explained to the patient in advance. The patient should be reassured that the staff will take weight gain that is too rapid as seriously as weight gain that is too slow.

Monitoring Weight. Weight should be monitored, but the schedule and format for weighing depend on the patient's individual needs. Patients should be weighed in the morning, before breakfast, by a nurse. Early in the hospitalization, it is advisable to weigh patients daily in order to assure them that the staff is not going to allow their weight to spiral out of control.

Daily weighing also allows staff to be alerted immediately to possible episodes of binge eating or surreptitious disposal of food. Finally, it allows the patient to examine the record later in the hospitalization in order to reinforce the idea that daily fluctuations in weight are common and that changes on any given day should not be overinterpreted. Some patients prefer to be informed immediately of their weight so that potential distress may be addressed in therapy, and others who become preoccupied with minute shifts in weight prefer to be "blind" to weighing and to be informed only if there is a consistent trend up or down over several days or even weeks. Later in hospitalization, weighing once or twice a week may be sufficient to monitor change and build trust in the fact that hypervigilance is not required to keep weight from changing unpredictably.

Behavioral Contingencies Related to Weight. Every effort should be made to make behavioral contingencies rational if they are imposed when weight falls outside the weight gain limits. First, there should be careful inquiry into the patient's understanding of the failure to gain weight. If the patient divulges a reasonable explanation for why progress has been slow (e.g., disposal of food or vomiting), the clinician should implement strategies for refraining from these behaviors rather than impose contingencies that may be seen as punitive (in light of the new information and the trust that it implies). Second, in the absence of a plausible explanation for failure to gain, calories should be systematically increased and activity levels restricted to bring the rate of weight gain in line with the projection of 1–2 kg per week. In rare cases, bed rest may have to be briefly reinstated if all else fails to produce a steady weight gain. Again, weight gain that exceeds the limits should result in a prompt reduction in calories. Striking a balance between firmness and leniency in the benevolent imposition of contingencies is a key to successful inpatient management. Touyz *et al.* (1984) found that both patients and staff react more favorably to a lenient or flexible behavioral approach than to a strict program. Rigidity in the management protocol leads to a harsh and repressive atmosphere, and too much indulgence leads to chaos as well as mistrust in light of perceived impotency on the part of the staff.

Planning Meals and Monitoring Eating. Dread and confusion surrounding food are characteristic of eating disorders. As indicated earlier, hospitalization provides the structure to assist patients in tolerating the guilt experienced when they deviate from their symptomatic eating behavior. Patients should be encouraged to eat previously avoided foods "mechanically" and to adhere precisely to predetermined guidelines for the quantity, quality, and spacing of the food consumed (Garner *et al.*, 1985b).

A set number of calories should be stipulated in order to achieve the trajectory of weight gain desired. For patients who have been subsisting on a highly restricted diet before hospitalization, it may not be realistic to consume more than 900 calories during the first several days. Again, they may gain weight quickly over the first several days because of rehydration. Increasing caloric intake gradually in 500-calorie increments to between 2,500 and 4,500 calories is usually necessary to sustain the desired rate of weight gain; however, intake has to be tailored to the individual needs of the patient. Patients with a history of obesity generally require fewer calories, and those from leaner genetic stock usually need more food. The individual differences in caloric needs among patients create distress for some patients. Patients who gain on fewer calories while still experiencing marked hunger have the most difficulty, although those who show metabolic resistance to weight gain despite consuming prodigious amounts of food also report distress.

There are several standard methods of selecting a diet. One that we prefer because of its simplicity and compatibility with a "nonanorexic" philosophy toward food involves permitting the patient to exclude no more than three specific foods (i.e., entire food groups like meats or sweets cannot be excluded) from the standard hospital meals provided. Food is "prescribed" like medicine. Patients often resist initially but are soon relieved by not having the onerous responsibility of choosing each meal. Considerable anxiety is experienced by some patients at the realization that they actually "enjoy" the less-than-sumptuous hospital cuisine. Their reactions to food, eating, and the changes in their bodies should be actively addressed by cognitive behavioral methods (Garner *et al.*, 1982, 1985b; Garner & Rosen, 1990).

Early in the hospitalization, the staff should scrupulously monitor meals. Although a careful monitoring of food and weight may be interpreted by the patient as a sign of distrust, it must be explained as "protection" against the relentless turmoil and ambivalence suffered at each meal if choices regarding diet are allowed too early in treatment. If patients *must* complete meals, they soon feel less guilt and apprehension around mealtime. Also, the completion of meals provides the staff and the patient with more reliable information about the number of calories that the patient actually requires to attain the expected rate of gain. If patients do not reliably consume a set number of calories, they never really learn that their weight can "regulate itself" at an appropriate level. This learning is an invaluable source of data for helping patients challenge self-defeating attitudes regarding their ability to maintain an appropriate weight without "dieting." Most patients need tremendous support during mealtime, as their commitment to the long-term goal of recovery from their eating disorder wanes at mealtime. Patients should be encouraged to refrain from "symptomatic eating," such as cutting food into small pieces or prolonged lingering over meals. Failure to complete meals or other attempts to avoid the steady weight gain should be interpreted with regard to the devastating long-term implications of continued symptomatic behavior (Garner, Garner & Rosen, 1990).

"Relearning" Hunger Cues. Some programs and popular books on eating disorders have emphasized the notion that eating in response to emotions is inherently abnormal and that patients should be encouraged to focus on recognizing and accurately responding to internal hunger cues. Helping patients to avoid eating vast amounts of food when they are emotionally distressed is very appropriate. However, spending inordinate amounts of time trying to teach patients to become attuned to subtle "internal cues" related to hunger is irrational and confusing, as these cues are unreliable for many months during the nutritional stabilization process. Semistarvation studies indicate that, for individuals exposed to just three months of moderate dietary restriction, well over a year may pass before the experience of hunger and satiety normalizes (cf. Garner *et al.*, 1985b). Chronically starved eating-disordered patients simply do not know when they are hungry; they are barraged by interoceptive miscues for hunger and satiety, which are then interpreted by distorted feelings about the "morality" of eating. Thus, such patients need to be gradually exposed to the evidence that dieting and weight suppression are responsible for the proclivity to "binge-eat" and for increased food cravings. Even if short-term nutritional needs appear to be adequate, these cravings may persist for many months.

There is another fallacy in the notion that heightened awareness of "internal cues" related to hunger should be a primary objective of treatment. Simple observation indicates that, although "internal cues" may be responsible for the long-term homeostatic regulation of body weight, there is little support for the notion that "normal eating" (both onset and termination of eating) is more than loosely connected to perceptible hunger cues. Moreover, there is little evidence that "turning to food" or "eating for emotional reasons" is always a sign of psychopathology. Most individuals eat because of social demands or because they are bored, depressed, happy, or sad, and to suggest that we should eat only when we feel "hunger pangs" is to impose obsessional control on a process that appears to be quite elastic in meeting dynamic physiological needs. Similarly, it would be absurd to view "drive reduction" as the only determinant of behaviors tied to other drives, such as sex, thirst, and sleep. Therefore, patients with eating disorders need to be gradually reassured that (1) their current cravings for food are aberrant and determined by chronic starvation and weight suppression; (2) they may need to depend on external controls (such as meal planning) for many months after they have assumed a healthy weight before their abnormal cravings and thoughts about food dissipate or disappear completely (this happens without special training in interoception); (3) they should not consider themselves "pathological" or "eating-disordered" if they occasionally or even often eat for nonnutritional reasons, as this behavior characterizes the eating of most non-eating-disordered individuals;

(4) once they are no longer starved, the amount they eat on these occasions will be relatively small; again, until that time, external and internal controls must be used to hold these increased cravings in check; and (5) they need to address their guilt about eating within the context of their extreme overconcern about weight and shape.

Bed Rest. Based on the conceptualization of anorexia nervosa as a "phobic" response to a normal body weight, Crisp (1980) recommended a hospital regimen in which patients are given a high-calorie diet while on complete bed rest for six to eight weeks, or until they reach their goal weight. This type of program may be impractical in many hospital settings, and this level of control is not necessary in order to achieve steady weight gain. Modified bed rest with a high-calorie diet has been recommended as an alternative for emaciated patients (Garfinkel & Garner, 1982; Lucas, Duncan, & Piens, 1976; Russell, 1970). One of the advantages of bed rest is that it is a rational starting point for evaluating and treating a patient who is sufficiently ill to warrant hospitalization. It may assist in breaking through denial by emphasizing that the staff consider the medical situation serious enough to require extreme caution. Patients should be told that they will be removed from bed rest as soon as the prescribed diet is being consumed and when they are out of medical danger. The inherent behavioral contingencies aimed at promoting completion of meals and weight gain are obvious, and we feel that they should be explained as reflecting a legitimate concern about the patient's medical welfare. It is not necessary for the duration of bed rest to be identical for all patients, as the medical and psychological considerations are quite varied across the heterogeneous patient population. Although some patients may protest about these inconsistencies in treatment, they are usually comforted by the fact that the treatment is tailored explicitly to their individual needs.

Tube Feeding. Although tube feeding and total parenteral nutrition (TPN) have been suggested in the past as an acceptable treatment for emaciated patients, most would agree with Russell's assertion (1973) that tube feeding "should be quickly dismissed as a crude method of forcing food into the patient and is no longer justified because of enlightened nursing methods" (p. 47). These treatments should be considered only in the rare instances in which the patient is in imminent physical danger and completely unresponsive to more conservative methods.

Control of Vomiting, Laxative Abuse, and Excessive Exercising. In the same way that vigilance and structure at mealtime protect patients from agonizing decisions about whether or not to eat the prescribed diet, structure in dealing with other behavioral symptoms of eating disorders is constructive, particularly in the early stages of hospitalization. Patients who vomit after meals should be routinely accompanied to the bathroom for up to 45 minutes after meals. They should be encouraged to discuss their emotional reactions to not being able to engage in inappropriate weight-controlling behaviors and should have access to staff familiar with appropriate cognitive therapy techniques (Garner et al., 1982, 1985b). Patients who engage in excessive exercise should be told that they will be closely monitored by designated staff who are interesting in the feelings and thoughts generated when symptomatic behavior is inhibited. These thoughts and feelings should also be discussed in the individual and group therapies throughout the hospitalization. The patients should be gradually given greater responsibility for controlling these symptoms as the hospitalization progresses. When changes in weight do not agree with the reports regarding behavior, greater external controls may have to be temporarily reinstated.

Integration of Different Therapies

Details of the various forms of individual, group, family, and drug treatments appropriate to inpatient treatment have been discussed in detail elsewhere and are beyond the scope of this chapter (Andersen et al., 1985; Garner et al., 1982; Mitchell, 1990; Russell, 1970; Stern, 1986; Strober & Yager, 1985; Vandereycken et al., 1989; Wooley & Wooley, 1985). These original sources, as well as others cited below, should be consulted in developing or modifying an inpatient program. We believe that one of the keys to treatment is the integration and sequencing of different forms of treatment based on the needs of the patient. Although Tobin and Johnson (1991) advocated integrating behavioral and psychodynamic approaches, indicating that they "have yet to see anyone specifically discuss this need for integration," there is actually a long history of attempts by behaviorally oriented writers (Garner *et al.*, 1982; Garner, Garfinkel, & Irvine, 1986; Geller, 1975; Giles, Young, & Young, 1985; Hersen & Detre, 1980), psychodynamically oriented writers (Andersen *et al.*, 1985; Crisp, 1980; Goodsitt, 1985; Kalucy, Gilchrist, McFarlane, & McFarlane, 1985; Stern, 1986; Strober & Yager, 1985; Wooley & Wooley, 1985), and family-oriented writers (Minuchin, Rosman, & Baker, 1978; Selvini-Palazzoli, 1974) to integrate symptom management with treatment principles designed to address the long-term needs of the patient.

Individual Therapy. It is our view that the same professional should coordinate symptom management plans and the psychotherapeutic aspects of the treatment program. This can be done within the context of cognitive therapy, psychodynamic psychotherapy, or some combination of both approaches. As indicated earlier, the range of individual treatment options is not reviewed here, as it has been summarized elsewhere (Garner *et al.*, 1982; Johnson, 1991).

Behavioral Therapy. Behavior modification is appealing in an inpatient setting because the technology is simple, easily taught, and readily mastered by staff. It has been over 25 years since initial reports indicated that both operant procedures (Bachrach, Erwin, & Mohr, 1965) and respondent procedures (Hallsten, 1965) can be used effectively in treating anorexia nervosa. These initial optimistic reports were tempered by concerns that behavioral methods may be mechanical, punitive, and coercive when they disregard other psychological needs of the patient (Bruch, 1974). However, it is very important to distinguish the simplistic application of rigid behavioral principles from the careful implementation of a behavioral program based on the systematic analysis of the contingencies that maintain the eating disorder (Bemis, 1987; Rosen, 1987). Moreover, the need to integrate behavioral principles with other individual and family treatments for eating disorders has long been recognized (Garner *et al.*, 1982; Geller, 1975; Hersen & Detre, 1980). Particularly when behavioral methods are integrated with other approaches for an adolescent population, positive results can be expected (Minuchin *et al.*, 1978).

Group Therapy. Group psychotherapy can play an important role as part of an inpatient or residential program (Andersen, 1985; Hall, 1985; Wooley & Wooley, 1985). Wooley and Wooley (1985) provided a detailed description of different treatment groups that have distinct aims and orientations. A task-oriented, relatively structured, "food and eating group" helps to encourage patients to deal with their aberrant eating behaviors and their attitudes about food. Interpersonal groups are also described as sharing many of the goals of traditional assertiveness or social-skills-training groups but add the richness of experiential techniques aimed at encouraging the development of honesty and intimacy in interpersonal relationships. Wooley and Wooley (1985) described body image groups that use a range of creative methods aimed at heightening an awareness of the nature and the derivation of body image disturbances. Once these disturbances are identified, specific techniques are proposed to further clarify feelings toward the body and to offer corrective experiences to redress hypothesized developmental deficits. The methods include guided imagery and movement, art, and dramatic exercises designed to create a more positive body image.

Family Therapy. Several modern pioneers in the area of family therapy have made enormous contributions to the understanding and treatment of eating disorders (Bruch, 1974; Minuchin *et al.*, 1978; Selvini-Palazzoli, 1974). These advancements have been amplified by more recent progress and refinements that have resulted in several comprehensive models in which family interactional patterns are linked to anorexia nervosa and bulimia nervosa (Humphrey, 1989; Minuchin *et al.*, 1978; Root, Fallon, & Friedrich, 1985; Schwartz, Barrett, & Saba,

1985; Strober & Humphrey, 1987; Vandereycken *et al.*, 1989). In the only controlled trial examining the efficacy of family therapy for anorexia nervosa, Russell, Szmukler, Dare, and Eisler (1987) found that family therapy was superior to individual therapy for younger patients. This study, as well as earlier reports of family therapy with younger patients, suggest that family therapy should be routinely used as one of the primary interventions for pediatric eating-disordered patients treated in an inpatient setting.

Medications. Many pharmacological agents have been tried, either as the primary mode of treatment or as adjuncts to other therapeutic methods (Garfinkel & Garner, 1987). Although we recognize the danger in condensing a complicated area of research, the following points summarize our current views on the role of pharmacological agents in the treatment of eating disorders:

1. Pharmacotherapy has a very limited value for emaciated anorexia nervosa patients and should never be the sole treatment (Garfinkel & Garner, 1982). Because depression and other emotional changes are often secondary to starvation, it is best to rely on food as the "medication of choice" in promoting weight gain. Occasionally, patients require medication to deal with overwhelming anxiety, severe depression, or intolerable gastric discomfort after meals, but these are the exceptions (Andersen, 1985; Garfinkel & Garner, 1982; Mitchell, 1988).

2. Although tricyclic antidepressants, such as imipramine, and the bicyclic fluoxetine may lead to reduced binging and vomiting in some outpatients, they appear to be less effective than psychotherapy and are associated with a high dropout rate (Mitchell, Pyle, Eckert, Hatsukami, Pomeroy, & Zimmerman, 1990). However, some inpatients whose depression is severe and unremitting may benefit from treatment with tricyclics or even monoamine oxidase inhibitors.

3. Research suggests that antidepressants are generally effective in holding binging and vomiting in check for as long as they are continued, but there is a high relapse rate once they are discontinued (Walsh, Hadigan, Devlin, Gladis, & Roose, 1991).

4. This reaction may be explained by recent research indicating that the mechanism of action of antidepressants in bulimia nervosa may be to temporarily lower appetite or suppress binge eating without changing the concerns about weight or shape that appear to be fundamental in maintaining most eating disorders (Craighead & Agras, 1991).

There are instances in which pharmacotherapy may be useful, particularly if psychotherapy is not effective; the reader is encouraged to consult primary sources for further details.

Need for Liaison with Outpatient Services

As indicated earlier, it is vital to recognize that hospitalization is just one component in the overall treatment strategy. For treatment to have the greatest likelihood of success, close cooperation must be maintained with outpatient clinicians. In most cases, it is optimal for the inpatient and outpatient facilities to be in close geographic proximity, and for management to be undertaken by cooperating clinicians. Except in large metropolitan centers, the ideal logistical circumstances are rarely achieved. Unless there is close contact between the inpatient and outpatient clinicians, treatment is routinely sabotaged in the transitions between outpatient care, the hospital, and the return to management in the community.

Relapse and Repeated Hospitalizations

Although hospitalization and subsequent outpatient care lead to complete recovery for many patients, there are some who relapse immediately or gradually once they are discharged. When hospitalization fails, the failure may not only generate feelings of hopelessness on the part of the patient but also cause the staff to become discouraged. Past treatment failures may even lead to reluctance to readmit a patient in clear need of inpatient care. It should be recognized that there is a subgroup of patients who show little sustained benefit from an initial hospitalization but who do very well following a second, third, or even many admissions. Some require a number of relapses for motivational change, and others require that the hospitalization be timed with particular changes or shifts in their interpersonal lives that make recovery possible. It is important to recognize the range of reasons for patients' initial refusal of treatment as well as of the principles that may assist patients in the choice of treatment when it is appropriate (Goldner, 1989). Finally, it is important to be aware of the subgroup of chronic patients who are often neglected because the prospects for recovery seem so dismal. These patients may do quite well in a "chronic patient group," where the goals are not recovery but close monitoring of their physical condition with brief admissions when their situation deteriorates. Occasionally, these groups break through the denial where other methods have failed, and the patients do well because they can no longer disavow in themselves the bleak future that they now see in others.

Residential and Day Care Programs

A review of residential and day care programs falls outside the scope of this chapter. However, it is important for the reader to be aware that day care and residential programs offer a very desirable and cost-effective alternative to hospitalization for many eating-disordered patients (Piran, Kaplan, Kerr, Shekter-Wolfson, Winocur, Gold, & Garfinkel, 1989).

ACTUAL TREATMENT

The primary aims of R's treatment were to (1) interrupt her binging and vomiting; (2) normalize her food intake; (3) promote steady weight gain; (4) further assess her suicide potential; (5) explore the psychological and social factors that led to the development and the maintenance of her eating disorder; (6) further assess the need for possible family therapy; and (7) determine the degree to which psychological features (depression and borderline features) were primary or secondary to her eating disorder.

R was given a standard 900-calorie diet, which was increased to 1,500 calories after the first week and 2,500 calories after the second week. An initial goal weight of 110 pounds was established, as it represented a weight that was above her likely menstrual threshold and was deemed the likely lowest "normal weight" that she could realistically hope to maintain. R indicated that she would agree to eat the prescribed meals but did not want to be placed on bed rest. Her request was agreed to with the proviso that she would spend the next day on bed rest if she was not able to complete any meal in the first week. On the first day that R was required to eat without vomiting, she reported overwhelming panic and requested to be discharged. After a two-hour meeting with the primary therapist, R agreed to try to complete her meal. She was successful in complying with this aspect of the program, and bed rest was never implemented. During the first week, R required extraordinary support and was tremendously distressed because she gained eight pounds. This gain was explained as a likely result of her discontinuation of laxatives, and she agreed to continue on the program for another week before the plan was altered. She gained one pound during the second week and was still upset by the continued weight gain but was reassured that the rate had diminished.

Discharge planning was initiated after the second week, with the understanding that hospitalization would last approximately six more weeks, assuming a weight gain of approximately three pounds a week, successful coping with *ad lib* eating for two weeks before discharge, and overall psychological improvement. R's outpatient therapist was contacted and agreed to follow up after discharge. The outpatient therapist attended weekly ward meetings and met with the inpatient therapist to discuss R's progress. There was no evidence of suicidal ideation after admission.

R participated in group therapy five days a week. In the mornings, she attended food groups aimed at education and eating management. The afternoon groups were less structured and addressed relevant developmental issues. They were also aimed at facilitating openness and self-expression in interpersonal relationships. A body image group met twice a week and focused on the nature and source of each member's body disparagement. Each member was encouraged to begin to challenge inappropriate cultural imperatives regarding weight. Individual therapy occurred three times a week and focused on both symptom management and psychological themes. After four weeks, it became clear that R's current feelings toward her parents were being fueled by ongoing interactions with the family, and it was decided that meetings with R and her parents might be helpful. In these meetings, the mother was able to identify and express feelings of sadness and anger about family responsibilities that had thwarted her own professional aspirations. R was seen as the symbol for her mother's failed ambitions. Both R and her mother were able to speak directly for the first time about feelings that had begun with the mother's pregnancy with R. R was also able to reevaluate her idealization of her father and see him as a man haunted by his fear of being less than outstanding in everything he attempted. R was able to see the connection between the strength of her loathing of her imperfect body and the pressure she felt to live up to the excessive performance standards in her family. The painful exploration of the feelings related to her mother's rejection and her father's neglect were repeated themes throughout the family meetings.

The characterization of R's psychological distress changed throughout her eight weeks of hospitalization. She was no longer confused and unanimated in meetings. Her sadness was replaced by a fear that she would be unable to cope with the weight gain. She was able to address issues with her parents that she had never put into words before. She was given complete control over her dietary intake during the last two weeks of hospitalization. She was still very concerned about gaining weight but was now equally distressed about the prospect of weight loss. She reported no wish to consume alcohol, but it was agreed this area should be closely followed after discharge. R was discharged at 110 pounds after eight weeks in the hospital. She began meeting with her outpatient therapist two weeks before discharge. Family therapy was continued after discharge.

SUMMARY

It is widely accepted that the majority of eating-disordered patients can be managed effectively as outpatients; however, this chapter has focused on the treatment of the small minority of difficult patients who either require or greatly benefit from inpatient treatment. The inpatient treatment of eating disorders is a complex task. A brief presentation of the treatment guidelines, with an illustrative case, is bound to miss the subtleties of treatment and the inevitable deviations from the protocol required with every patient.

This chapter has emphasized the importance of a thorough assessment before hospitalization. Specific content areas for assessment have been suggested in support of the main objectives of hospitalization: (1) weight restoration or the interruption of steady weight loss in the case of anorexia nervosa; (2) the interruption of unremitting binging and vomiting; (3) the evaluation and treatment of medical complications; (4) the management of associated conditions such as severe depression, suicidal behavior, and substance abuse; (5) addressing the psychological and interpersonal factors that have initiated or maintained the eating disorder; and (6) occasionally, the disengagement of patients from a social system that both contributes to the maintenance of the disorder and disrupts outpatient treatment.

ACKOWLEDGMENTS.   The authors wish to thank Dr. Lionel Rosen for thoughtful comments on a draft of this chapter and Ms. Mary Gowans for assistance in the preparation of the manuscript.

American Psychiatric Association (1987). *Diagnostic and statistical manual of mental disorders* (3rd ed.; DSM-III-R). Washington, DC: Author.

American Psychiatric Association (1991). *DSM-IV options book: Work in progress 9/1/91 task force of DSM-IV.* Washington, DC: Author.

Andersen, A. E. (1985). *Practical comprehensive treatment of anorexia nervosa and bulimia.* Baltimore: Johns Hopkins Press.

Andersen, A. E., Morse, C., & Santmyer, K. (1985). Inpatient treatment for anorexia nervosa. In D. M. Garner & P. E. Garfinkel (Eds.), *Handbook of psychotherapy for anorexia nervosa and bulimia.* New York: Guilford Press.

Bachrach, A. J., Erwin, W. J., & Mohr, J. P. (1965). The control of eating behavior in an anorexic by operant conditioning techniques. In L. P. Ullmann & L. Krasner (Eds.), *Case studies in behavior modification.* New York: Holt, Rinehart & Winston.

Bemis, K. M. (1987). The present status of operant conditioning for the treatment of anorexia nervosa. *Behavior Modification, 11*(4), 432–463.

Brotman, A. W., Stern, T. A., & Herzog, D. B. (1984). Emotional reactions of house officers to patients with anorexia nervosa, diabetes, and obesity. *International Journal of Eating Disorders, 3*, 71–77.

Bruch, H. (1973). *Eating disorders: Obesity, anorexia nervosa and the person within.* New York: Basic Books.

Bruch, H. (1974). Perils of behavior modification in treatment of anorexia nervosa. *Journal of American Medical Association, 230*, 1419–1422.

Casper, R. C. (1987). The psychopathology of anorexia nervosa: The pathological psychodynamic processes. In P. J. V. Beaumont, G. D. Burrows, & R. C. Casper (Eds.), *Handbook of eating disorders.* Amsterdam: Elsevier.

Comerci, G. D. (1990). Medical complications of anorexia nervosa and bulimia nervosa. *Medical Clinics of North America, 74*(5), 1293–1310.

Craighead, L. W., & Agras, W. S. (1991). Mechanisms of action in cognitive-behavioral and pharmacological interventions for obesity and bulimia nervosa. *Journal of Consulting and Clinical Psychology, 59*(1), 115–125.

Crisp, A. H. (1980). *Anorexia nervosa.* New York: Grune & Stratton.

Fairburn, C. G. (1987). The definition of bulimia nervosa: Guidelines for clinicians and research workers. *Annals of Behavioral Medicine, 9*, 3–7.

Fairburn, C. G., & Garner, D. M. (Eds.). (1988). *Diagnostic criteria for anorexia nervosa and bulimia nervosa: The importance of attitudes to shape and weight.* New York: Brunner/Mazel.

Fairburn, C. G., Cooper, P. J., Kirk, J., & O'Connor, M. (1985). The significance of the neurotic symptoms of bulimia nervosa. *Journal of Psychiatric Research, 19*, 135–140.

Foreyt, J. P., & McGavin, J. K. (1988). Anorexia nervosa and bulimia. In E. J. Marsh & L. G. Tudal (Ed.), *Behavioral assessment of childhood disorders* (pp. 776–805). New York: Guilford Press.

Garfinkel, P. E., & Garner, D. M. (1982). *Anorexia nervosa: A multidimensional perspective.* New York: Brunner/Mazel.

Garfinkel, P. E., & Garner, D. M. (1987). *Psychotropic drug therapies for eating disorders.* New York: Brunner/Mazel.

Garfinkel, P. E., Kaplan, A. S., Garner, D. M., & Darby, P. L. (1983). The differentiation of vomiting/weight loss as a conversion disorder from anorexia nervosa. *American Journal of Psychiatry, 140*, 1019–1022.

Garner, D. M. (1991). *Eating disorder inventory: 2. Professional manual.* Odessa, FL: Psychological Assessment Resources.

Garner, D. M., & Bemis, K. M. (1982). A cognitive-behavioral approach to anorexia nervosa. *Cognitive Therapy and Research, 6*, 123–150.

Garner, D. M., & Bemis, K. M. (1985). Cognitive therapy for anorexia nervosa. In D. M. Garner & P. E. Garfinkel (Eds.), *Handbook of psychotherapy for anorexia nervosa and bulimia* (pp. 107–146). New York: Guilford Press.

Garner, D. M., & Garfinkel, P. E. (1985). *Handbook of psychotherapy for anorexia nervosa and bulimia.* New York: Guilford Press.

Garner, D. M., & Garfinkel, P. E. (1988). *Diagnostic issues in anorexia nervosa and bulimia nervosa.* New York: Brunner/Mazel.

Garner, D. M., & Rosen, L. W. (1990). *Anorexia nervosa and bulimia nervosa* (pp. 805–817) In A. S. Bellack, M. Hersen, & A. E. Kazdin (Eds.), *International Handbook of Behavior Modification and Therapy* (2nd ed.). New York: Plenum Press.

Garner, D. M., & Wooley, S. C. (1991). Confronting the failure of behavioral and dietary treatments for obesity. *Clinical Psychology Review, 11*, 729–780.

Garner, D. M., Garfinkel, P. E., & Bemis, K. M. (1982). A multidimensional psychotherapy for anorexia nervosa. *International Journal of Eating Disorders, 1,* 3–46.

Garner, D. M., Garfinkel, P. E., & O'Shaughnessy, M. (1985a). The validity of the distinction between bulimia with and without anorexia nervosa. *American Journal of Psychiatry, 142,* 581–587.

Garner, D. M., Rockert, W., Olmsted, M. P., Johnson, C. L., & Coscina, D. V. (1985b). Psychoeducational principles in the treatment of bulimia and anorexia nervosa. In D. M. Garner & P. E. Garfinkel (Eds.), *Handbook of psychotherapy for anorexia nervosa and bulimia* (pp. 513–572). New York: Guilford Press.

Garner, D. M., Garfinkel, P. E. & Irvine, M. J. (1986). Integration and sequencing of treatment approaches for eating disorders. *Psychotherapy and Psychosomatics, 46,* 67–75.

Garner, D. M., Olmsted, M. P., Davis, R., Rockert, W., Goldbloom, D., & Eagle, M. (1990). The association between bulimic symptoms and reported psychopathology. *International Journal of Eating Disorders, 9,* 1–15.

Garner, D. M., Shafer, C. L., & Rosen, L. W. (1992). Critical appraisal of the DSM-III-R diagnostic criteria for eating disorders. In S. R. Hooper, G. W. Hynd, & R. E. Mattison (Eds.), *Child psychopathology, diagnostic criteria and clinical assessment* (pp. 261–303). Hillsdale, NJ: Erlbaum.

Garner, D. M. Garner, M. V., & Rosen, L. W. (in press). Anorexia nervosa "restrictors" who purge: Implications for subtyping anorexia nervosa. *International Journal of Eating Disorders.*

Geller, J. L. (1975). Treatment of anorexia nervosa by the integration of behavior therapy and psychotherapy. *Psychotherapy and Psychosomatics, 26,* 167–177.

Giles, T. R., Young, R. R., & Young, D. E. (1985). Case studies and clinical replication series: Behavioral treatment of severe bulimia. *Behavioral Therapy, 16,* 393–405.

Goldner, E. (1989). Treatment refusal in anorexia nervosa. *International Journal of Eating Disorders, 8,* 297–306.

Goodsitt, A. (1985). Self psychology and the treatment of anorexia nervosa. In D. M. Garner & P. E. Garfinkel (Eds.), *Handbook of psychotherapy for anorexia nervosa and bulimia* (pp. 55–84). New York: Guilford Press.

Guidano, V. F., & Liotti, G. (1983). *Cognitive processes and emotional disorders: A structural approach to psychotherapy.* New York: Guilford Press.

Hall, A. (1985). Group psychotherapy for anorexia nervosa. In D. M. Garner & P. E. Garfinkel (Eds.), *Handbook of psychotherapy for anorexia nervosa and bulimia* (pp. 213–239). New York: Guilford Press.

Hallsten, E. A., Jr. (1965). Adolescent anorexia nervosa treated by desensitization. *Behavior Research and Therapy, 3*(87), 87–91.

Hamburg, P., & Herzog, D. (1990). Supervising the therapy of patients with eating disorders. *American Journal of Psychotherapy, XLIV*(3), 369–380.

Hersen, M., & Detre, T. (1980). The behavioral psychotherapy of anorexia nervosa. In T. B. Karasu, & L. Bellak (Eds.), *Specialized techniques in individual psychotherapy* (pp. 295–304). New York: Brunner/Mazel.

Humphrey, L. L. (1989). Is there a causal link between disturbed family processes and eating disorders? In W. G. Johnson (Ed.), *Bulimia nervosa: Perspectives on clinical research and therapy.* New York: JAI Press.

Johnson, C. (1991). *Psychodynamic treatment of anorexia nervosa and bulimia.* New York: Guilford Press.

Johnson, C., & Connors, M. E. (1987). *The etiology and treatment of bulimia nervosa: A biopsychosocial perspective.* New York: Basic Books.

Kalucy, R. S., Gilchrist, P. N., McFarlane, C. M., & McFarlane, A. C. (1985). The evolution of a multitherapy orientation. In D. M. Garner & P. E. Garfinkel (Eds.), *Handbook of psychotherapy for anorexia nervosa.* New York: Guilford Press.

Lucas, A. R., Duncan, J. W., & Piens, V. (1976). The treatment of anorexia nervosa. *American Journal of Psychiatry, 133,* 1034–1038.

Millon, T. (1982). *Millon Clinical Multiaxial Inventory Manual* (3rd ed.). Minneapolis: National Computer Systems.

Minuchin, S., Rosman, B. L., & Baker, L. (1978). *Psychosomatic families: Anorexia nervosa in context.* Cambridge: Harvard University Press.

Mitchell, J. E. (1990). *Bulimia nervosa.* Minneapolis: University of Minnesota Press.

Mitchell, J. E., & Boutacoff, L. I. (1986). Laxative abuse complicating bulimia: Medical and treatment implications. *International Journal of Eating Disorders, 5,* 325–334.

Mitchell, J. E., Pomery, C., & Huber, M. (1988). A clinician's guide to the eating disorders medicine cabinet. *International Journal of Eating Disorders, 2,* 211–223.

Mitchell, J. E., Pyle, R. L., Eckert, E. D., Hatsukami, D., Pomeroy, C., & Zimmerman, R. (1990). A comparison study of antidepressants and structured intensive group psychotherapy in the treatment of bulimia nervosa. *Archives of General Psychiatry, 47,* 149–157.

Mitchell, P. B. (1988). The pharmacological management of bulimia nervosa: A critical review. *International Journal of Eating Disorders, 7*(1), 29–41.

Olmsted, M. P., Davis, R., Rockert, W., Irvine, M. J., Eagle, M., & Garner, D. M. (1991). Efficacy of a brief group psychoeducational intervention for bulimia nervosa. *Behavior Research and Therapy*, *29*, 71–83.

Piran, N., Kaplan, A., Kerr, A., Shekter-Wolfson, L., Winocur, J., Gold, E., & Garfinkel, P. E. (1989). A day hospital program for anorexia nervosa and bulimia. *International Journal of Eating Disorders*, *8*(5), 511–521.

Root, M. M. P., Fallon, P., & Friedrich, W. N. (1985). *Bulimia: A systems approach to treatment*. New York: W. W. Norton.

Rosen, J. C. (1987). A review of behavioral treatments for bulimia nervosa. *Behavior Modification*, *11*(4), 464–486.

Russell, G. (1979). Bulimia nervosa: An ominous variant of anorexia nervosa. *Psychological Medicine*, *9*, 429–448.

Russell, G. F. M. (1970). Anorexia nervosa: Its identity as an illness and its treatment. In J. H. Price (Ed.), *Modern trends in psychological medicine* (Vol. 2, pp. 131–164). London: Butterworth's.

Russell, G. J. M. (1973). The management of anorexia nervosa. In *Symposium on Anorexia Nervosa and Obesity* (pp. 44–62). Edinburgh: Royal College of Physicians.

Russell, G. F. M., Szmukler, G. I., Dare, C., & Eisler, I. (1987). An evaluation of family therapy in anorexia nervosa and bulimia nervosa. *Archives of General Psychiatry*, *44*, 1047–1056.

Sansone, R. A., Fine, M. A., & Chew, R. (1988). A longitudinal analysis of the experiences of nursing staff on an inpatient eating disorders unit. *International Journal of Eating Disorders*, *7*(1), 125–131.

Schwartz, R. C., Barrett, M. J., & Saba, G. (1985). Family therapy for bulimia. In D. M. Garner & P. E. Garfinkel (Eds.), *Handbook of psychotherapy for anorexia nervosa and bulimia*. New York: Guilford Press.

Selvini-Palazzoli, M. P. (1974). *Self-starvation*. London: Chaucer Publishing.

Shisslak, C. M., Gary, N., & Crago, M. (1989). Health care professionals' reactions to working with eating disorder patients. *International Journal of Eating Disorders*, *8*(6), 689–694.

Spitzer, R. L., Devlin, M., Walsh, B. T., Hasin, D., Wing, R., Marcus, M., Stunkard, A., Wadden, T., Yanovski, S., Agras, S., Mitchell, J., & Nonas, C. (1992). Binge eating disorder: A multisite field trial of the diagnostic criteria. *International Journal of Eating Disorders*, *11*, 191–203.

Stern, S. (1986). The dynamics of clinical management in the treatment of anorexia nervosa and bulimia: An organizing theory. *International Journal of Eating Disorders*, *5*(2), 233–254.

Strober, M., & Humphrey, L. L. (1987). Familial contributions to the etiology and course of anorexia nervosa and bulimia. *Journal of Consulting and Clinical Psychology*, *55*, 654–659.

Strober, M., & Yager, J. (1985). A developmental perspective on the treatment of anorexia nervosa in adolescents. In D. M. Garner & P. E. Garfinkel (Eds.), *Handbook of psychotherapy for anorexia nervosa and bulimia* (pp. 363–390). New York: Guilford Press.

Theander, S. (1985). Outcome and prognosis in anorexia nervosa and bulimia: Some results of previous investigations, compared with those of a Swedish long-term study. *Journal of Psychiatric Research*, *19*, 493–508.

Tobin, D. L., & Johnson, C. L. (1991). The integration of psychodynamic and behavior therapy in the treatment of eating disorders: Clinical issues versus theoretical mystique. In C. L. Johnson (Ed.), *Psychodynamic treatment of anorexia nervosa and bulimia* (pp. 374–397). New York: The Guilford Press.

Tobin, D. L., Johnson, C., Steinberg, S., Staats, M., & Dennis, A. B. (1991). Multifactorial assessment of bulimia nervosa. *Journal of Abnormal Psychology*, *100*(1), 4–21.

Touyz, S. W., Beumont, P. J. V., Glaun, D., Phillips, T., & Cowie, J. (1984). A comparison of lenient and strict operant conditioning programmes in refeeding patients with anorexia nervosa. *British Journal of Psychiatry*, *144*, 512–520.

Vandereycken, W., & Meermann, R. (1984). *Anorexia nervosa: A clinician's guide to treatment*. New York: Walter de Gruyter.

Vandereycken, W., Kog, E., & Vanderlinden, J. (1989). *The family approach to eating disorders*. New York: PMA Publishing Corp.

Walsh, B. T., Hadigan, C. M., Devlin, M. J., Gladis, M., & Roose, S. P. (1991). Long-term outcome of antidepressant treatment for bulimia nervosa. *American Journal of Psychiatry*, *148*, 1206–1212.

Welch, G. W., Hall, A., & Renner, R. (1990). Patient subgrouping in anorexia nervosa using psychologically-based classification. *International Journal of Eating Disorders*, *9*, 311–322.

Wooley, S. C., & Wooley, O. W. (1985). Intensive outpatient and residential treatment for bulimia. In D. M. Garner & P. E. Garfinkel (Eds.), *Handbook of psychotherapy for anorexia nervosa and bulimia*. New York: Guilford Press.

24

Autism and Developmental Disorders

SANDRA L. HARRIS, DAVID CELIBERTI, and ERICA LILLELEHT

INTRODUCTION

The diagnosis and treatment of autistic disorder and related forms of pervasive developmental disorder have grown increasingly effective in the past several decades. After considerable study, autism has been differentiated from schizophrenia (Rumsey, Rapoport, & Scerry, 1985) and has been recognized as biological rather than psychogenic in origin (Schreibman, 1988), and as involving multiple etiologies (Reichler & Lee, 1987). Intensive behavioral interventions have been proved successful in bringing about important changes in persons with autism, although full recovery remains elusive for most patients (Schreibman, 1988).

Although recognized as a diagnostic entity for half a century (Kanner, 1943), autism did not become an official category of the American Psychiatric Association (APA) until 1980. With the publication of the latest edition of the *Diagnostic and Statistical Manual of Mental Disorders* (DSM-III-R; APA, 1987), this diagnosis appears firmly established, although detailed criteria are still being debated.

DSM-III-R CRITERIA

Autistic Disorder and Pervasive Developmental Disorder Not Otherwise Specified (PDDNOS) are the two diagnostic categories under the heading of Pervasive Developmental Disorders in the DSM-III-R. These diagnoses are made on Axis II rather than Axis I. When applied to a disorder of childhood origin, the use of Axis II indicates that the disorder involves major disturbances in the development of cognition, language, motor function, or social skills (APA, 1987). A second Axis II diagnosis of Mental Retardation often accompanies Autistic Disorder.

The DSM-III-R provides more explicit diagnostic criteria for Autistic Disorder than the DSM-III (APA, 1980), and greater attention is given to developmental changes in the expression of symptoms (Rapoport & Ismond, 1990). Sixteen specific criteria are listed under three broad

SANDRA L. HARRIS, DAVID CELIBERTI, and ERICA LILLELEHT • Rutgers, The State University of New Jersey, New Brunswick, New Jersey 08903.

Handbook of Behavior Therapy in the Psychiatric Setting, edited by Alan S. Bellack and Michel Hersen. Plenum Press, New York, 1993.

headings: (1) Qualitative Impairment in Reciprocal Social Interaction; (2) Qualitative Impairment in Verbal and Nonverbal Communication; and (3) Markedly Restricted Repertoire of Activities and Interests. The patient must exhibit at least 8 of the 16 criteria—at least 2 in the social domain, 1 in verbal and nonverbal communication, and 1 in restricted repertoire of activities and interests. A fourth criterion specifies that the onset of the disorder occurs during infancy or childhood.

According to the DSM-III-R criteria, a diagnosis of PDDNOS rather than Autistic Disorder is made when the patient exhibits impairments in social interaction and communication, but not at the level required for a diagnosis of Autistic Disorder. Thus, a person with PDDNOS may have fewer or milder symptoms. PDDNOS may or may not be accompanied by a markedly restricted repertoire of activities and interests. At present, this diagnosis is somewhat vague and may be applied inconsistently.

Social Interaction

In making decisions about impairment in social functioning, it is essential to consider the patient's level of cognitive development. Rapoport and Ismond (1990) argued that it is difficult, if not impossible, to make a differential diagnosis between autistic disorder and profound mental retardation in persons with an IQ lower than 35. The DSM-III-R does not establish such a cutoff, but the clinician must nonetheless be aware of the impact of profound mental retardation on social behavior, and she or he must be cautious in reaching judgments about whether social impairment should be attributed to the presence of autistic disorder at this level of cognitive functioning. Similarly, it is very difficult to make a reliable diagnosis in infancy.

For young children or older persons with marked degrees of intellectual dysfunction, one would diagnose impairment in reciprocal social interaction on the basis of a demonstrated lack of awareness of other people and their feelings. The very young child with autism may exhibit diminished signs of interest in her or his parents, particularly as manifested by the capacity to be sensitive to the affective response of others. Frith (1989) described as central in the expression of autism the inability of the person with autism to empathetically understand the perceptions of others.

According to the criteria of the DSM-III-R, children with autism may not seek comfort when hurt, fail to imitate on request and/or fail to show interest in modeling the behavior of adults, have limited if any interest in social play, and at the highest levels, may be impaired in the ability to form peer friendships. The criteria of social play and peer friendships are useful in evaluating children beyond the age of 3 (Rapoport & Ismond, 1990). These children may show a greater level of superficial social awareness and interest in their parents but may still be markedly deficient in the subtler skills needed to negotiate the social world of childhood or to respond empathetically to the needs of others.

Communication

Both the verbal and the nonverbal communication of people with autism may be impaired as well as their capacity for imagination. In the very young child, there may be little to no interactive babbling, use of facial expression or gesture to communicate, or spoken language. The impairment of nonverbal communication may include deficiencies in eye contact for communicative purposes and a failure to use gestures such as reaching to be picked up. Unlike normally developing children, the child with autism typically shows little, if any, capacity for fantasy or adult role play. Among those children who play with toys, the activities tend to be concrete, repetitive, and isolative.

For those persons with autistic disorder who speak, abnormalities in production such as in volume and intonation often exist. Their speech may, for example, be in a monotone, very soft, or high-pitched. When present, speech is usually abnormal in form or content, with immediate or delayed echolalia, as well as idiosyncratic, personalized use of language.

Even among persons with highly developed language, there is typically great difficulty in sustaining conversation. Thus, very high-functioning persons with autism may speak with grammatical accuracy and complexity about topics of narrow interest that do not hold the attention of the listener. At the same time, persons with autism may be unaware of the other person's lack of response. Their speech may also have a pedantic or formal aspect, further limiting the quality of sustained conversation.

As noted for the assessment of social responsiveness, it is essential that the patient's level of intellectual functioning be considered when determining whether dysfunction in communication is linked to the presence of autistic disorder or is the result of profound mental retardation.

Activities and Interests

Within the domain of "Markedly Restricted Repertoire of Activities and Interests," the authors of the DSM-III-R pointed to stereotyped body movements, such as rocking, hand waving, or head banging. This category also includes a persistent preoccupation with parts of objects, for example, turning a toy car over to spin the wheels, or grasping the wrist of every visitor to study his or her wristwatch while ignoring the person.

As the DSM-III-R notes, some people with autism show great distress over seemingly minor changes in the environment or over changes in routine. Parents may report that their child tantrums when they move a piece of furniture or take a left turn rather than a right turn on the way out of the driveway. Some children with autism may show a preoccupation with lining up objects in a set pattern, and higher functioning older persons may show a similar preoccupation with a narrow intellectual topic, such as facts about train schedules or brands of automobiles.

Onset during Infancy or Early Childhood

Consistent with the recognition that autism usually persists into adulthood, there has been a shift from the label *infantile autism* to the age-neutral term *autistic disorder*. Autistic disorder may be diagnosed at any age but must have its origins in infancy or early childhood. Childhood onset is noted if the symptoms first emerged after 36 months. According to the DSM-III-R, it is quite rare for the onset to occur after age 5 or 6, and alternative diagnoses must be carefully considered for such children. It is also noted that some children may show marked improvement in autistic symptoms at about age 5–6.

Although most persons with autism come to professional attention in early childhood, one is sometimes called on to make an initial diagnosis of autistic disorder in an older patient. The more advanced criteria listed under each of the major diagnostic categories in the DSM-III-R facilitate this decision making, as does a careful review of the developmental history. Unfortunately, developmental history is always viewed through the lens of life's experience, and it is difficult, if not impossible, for parents to be totally reliable reporters of their children's development.

PROTOTYPICAL ASSESSMENT

A meaningful assessment of the person with autism includes a detailed study of behavioral patterns, the functioning of the patient's family, and the community resources available to support one's treatment plans. Depending on the clinician's objectives, the assessment may include a diagnostic evaluation or may focus exclusively on an assessment of the client's behavioral excesses and deficits.

Differential Diagnosis

SANDRA L. HARRIS
et al.

The diagnosis of autistic disorder or PDDNOS requires that one discriminate these disorders from others that they may resemble. Additionally, within the category of autistic disorder, one must identify those persons whose autism is linked to a known biological disorder that has implications for treatment. Making these decisions often requires close multidisciplinary collaboration.

Among the diagnostic choices that may have to be ruled out in reaching a diagnosis of autistic disorder or PDDNOS are schizophrenia, hearing impairments, specific developmental language and speech disorders, schizoid and schizotypal personality disorders, tic disorders and stereotypy or habit disorder. Mental retardation may coexist with pervasive developmental disorder and should be included as a second Axis II diagnosis. Rapoport and Ismond (1990) described the criteria to be used in differentiating pervasive developmental disorders from other conditions.

A neurological assessment should be a part of every evaluation of a person who may have autism. Given autism's range of possible etiologies and the important implications of recognizing those biological factors that may be genetic, as in fragile-X (e.g., Watson, Leckman, Annex, Breg, Boles, Volkmar, Cohen, & Carter, 1984), or degenerative, as in Rett syndrome (e.g., Hagberg, Aicardi, Dias, & Ramos, 1983), it is essential that these factors be identified. Such an identification allows families to receive appropriate genetic counseling, and to make suitable plans for persons whose condition will inevitably deteriorate. Similarly, the diagnosis of a seizure disorder, present in about 25% of persons with autism (Rutter & Schopler, 1988), enables the use of appropriate anticonvulsant medication to minimize the impact of the seizures on the general treatment plan.

At our center, the diagnosis of autistic disorder is based on the criteria of the DSM-III-R. We also use the Childhood Autism Rating Scale (Schopler, Reichler, DeVellis, & Daly, 1980) to estimate the child's relative level of autistic involvement. Data for this evaluation are collected during an intake interview with the child's parents, direct observation of the child in structured and unstructured settings, and a review of the available medical records.

We routinely administer the fourth edition of the Stanford-Binet Intelligence Scale (Thorndike, Hagen, & Sattler, 1986), the Battelle Developmental Inventory (Newborg, Stock, Wnek, Guidubaldi, & Svinicki, 1984), the Peabody Picture Vocabulary Test (Dunn & Dunn, 1981), and the Preschool Language Scale (Zimmerman, Steiner, & Pond, 1979) to obtain normative data on the child's cognitive and language functioning. Data from cognitively oriented tests help determine the extent to which mental retardation may be a contributing factor.

Behavioral Assessment of the Individual

Although a diagnosis is important for many purposes, decisions about individual treatment planning are based far more on a behavioral assessment than on a diagnostic label. The behavioral assessment of the person with autism begins during the initial intake and continues throughout treatment. Over time, treatment is modulated according to feedback from programming data. One can divide the behavioral assessment into three somewhat arbitrary categories: behavioral excesses, behavioral deficits, and language deficits (Harris, 1984). It is typically the behavioral excesses that lead to inpatient hospitalization, that are often targeted for pharmacological interventions, and that may need to be resolved before discharge. Skill deficits and language deficits, although of great importance, can usually be treated on an outpatient basis.

Behavioral Excesses.   Persons with autism may exhibit a variety of troubling behavioral excesses, some of which may lead to hospitalization. Perhaps the most severe of these is self-injurious behavior, which sometimes reaches life-threatening proportions. Other behaviors that typically merit intensive intervention and may result in hospitalization include severe tantrums, aggression, and destruction of property. Self-stimulatory behavior, noncompliance, and some potentially dangerous behaviors such as running out of the house or classroom are more typically seen in an outpatient setting.

The clinician familiar with general strategies for the behavioral assessment of problems of childhood or of persons with mental retardation will have an understanding of the methods used in assessing the behavioral excesses of the person with autism. This assessment involves developing a clear definition of the target behavior and identifying the variables that appear to control the emission of the behavior (e.g., Kanfer & Saslow, 1969). Both naturalistic and analogue observation settings may be used in the collection of data; some analogue techniques allow for the rapid manipulation of potentially important controlling variables. Powers and Handleman (1984) provided an extended discussion of the behavioral assessment of persons with autism.

One particularly fruitful approach to the disruptive behaviors of persons with autism has been an assessment of the learning environment. For example, Carr, Newsom, and Binkoff (1980) documented that task complexity can be related to the presence of aberrant behavior. Edelson, Taubman, and Lovaas (1983) noted that, in some children, self-injurious behavior increases when staff members make demands on them. These observations have sensitized clinicians to examine the extent to which variables such as negative reinforcement may sustain unwanted behaviors.

Behavioral and Communication Deficits. Persons with autism typically exhibit a range of skill deficits that need to be addressed if overall functioning is to be enhanced. These include deficits in self-help; social, recreational, and cognitive skills; affective behavior; and communication skills. A rather extensive literature exists describing the assessment of these domains (e.g., Powers & Handleman, 1984; Schopler & Mesibov, 1985, 1986). The long-term nature of this assessment process makes it more appropriate to an educational setting than an inpatient hospital setting. Nonetheless, as part of a comprehensive treatment plan, consideration should be given to the patient's needs for adaptive skills.

Powers and Handleman (1984) noted the importance of discriminating between performance and skill deficits. Some patients may have the necessary skills to perform a task, but the specific stimulus conditions may not be sufficient to cue that performance. For example, if a child responds to requests from his teacher but fails to respond when the same command is given by his father, he is demonstrating a performance deficit as opposed to a skill deficit. Understanding the nature of the behavioral deficit in these terms has important implications for one's approach to treatment.

Assessment of the Family and the Community

Having a family member with a pervasive developmental disorder may have a significant impact on a family (Handleman & Harris, 1986; Harris, 1984, 1987). As part of a comprehensive evaluation, one needs to consider the family members' skills as behavior change agents, the psychological functioning of the individual members of the family, and the functioning of the family as a unit. This assessment should be sensitive to the developmental status of the child and the life cycle status of the family (Harris & Powers, 1984). In addition to evaluating the needs of the nuclear family, one may also need to consider members of the extended family. These family members may be a powerful source of support for the nuclear family, but their own lives may also be significantly affected by the presence of a family member with a disability (Harris, Handleman, & Palmer, 1985).

Just as the individual with autism does not function in a vacuum, so, too, the family responds to the wider context of the community. A full assessment requires that one consider the community resources available to support one's intervention plan. Who will execute the treatment program after the child is discharged from the hospital? Can the family implement the treatment program alone? Are respite services available to assist the family? Will a teacher in a regular class have to be trained to work with the child? Does this community rely on private schools, public schools, or some combination to provide services? What types of adult services are available? Is there a link between the educational system and the services provided to adults in the community?

There is good reason to believe that both the formal and the informal support services available to the family of a child with autism have an impact on family functioning (Bristol, 1984). One's assessment must therefore examine the informal support from friends and family as well as the formal services provided by the community. A thorough assessment should include a parental understanding of how to find the necessary assistance. Some families may need help in learning how to access these resources and support networks.

ACTUAL ASSESSMENT

Assessing the Benefits of Medication

Sudhir, a 12-year-old adolescent at the Douglass Developmental Disabilities Center, came to staff attention because of his increasing difficulty in school and at home. Over several months, he had engaged in a growing array of aggressive behaviors, including hitting, kicking, head banging, pinching, scratching, and biting. The severity, frequency, and duration of these behaviors led his teacher to request a case conference at which members of the professional staff reviewed the baseline data and records of behavioral interventions and then generated a set of potential treatment strategies. Because of the severity and dangerousness of the behavior, and because of Sudhir's lack of response to a variety of behavioral interventions and environmental manipulations, pharmacological alternatives were considered along with changes in educational programming.

Following this conference, Sudhir was referred to a major university medical center for a four-week evaluation of his potential response to medication. As a result of this assessment, the medical center staff suggested a trial with fenfluramine. The availability of our extended baseline data on Sudhir's behavior before the administration of fenfluramine made possible a rapid undertaking of this assessment.

During the three months before drug intervention, Sudhir had engaged in aggressive acts toward others an average of five times a day. With the exception of one day during which there were no aggressive episodes, the frequency of these acts ranged from 1 to 18 a day. For the three months following the introduction of fenfluramine, Sudhir engaged in aggressive behaviors toward others on only six occasions. On each of these six days, there was only a single episode of aggressive behavior. Changes in the intensity of these behaviors as a function of fenfluramine were also noted. In the three months preceding medication, there had been 12 instances in which his aggressive behavior was so severe that he had to be restrained to protect himself and others. By contrast, during the three months of fenfluramine administration, there were only two episodes that required such restraint. Additionally, the duration of Sudhir's aggressive outbursts decreased, and we also noted a modest decline in self-directed aggression during the fenfluramine trial.

A Behavioral Assessment: Tantrumming

Six-year-old Eric was a "model student" for his first six months at the Douglass Developmental Disabilities Center. He appeared happy, was attentive and compliant, followed directions well, and adapted to the routine of the classroom. Halfway through the year, however, a marked shift was noted in Eric's behavior. Although still attentive and eager to work, he began to tantrum. His teacher noted that this new behavior had begun just as Eric's communicative skills were showing considerable gains and as he became more aware of the people around him. The increasing frequency, intensity, and duration of these tantrums led his teacher to conduct a behavioral assessment to determine whether important antecedents or consequences might be maintaining Eric's disruptive behavior.

As the first step, his teacher assembled a behavior report form for the staff who worked with Eric. Based on Groden (1989), this single-page chart requires a staff member to describe the target behavior, the location of the incident, the immediate antecedents (e.g., the particular task being done), the distal antecedents (e.g., a poor night's sleep), and the environmental and program-oriented consequences. The day, date, and time are also noted.

For three weeks, daily data on Eric's tantrumming were recorded, and the individual reports were condensed on a summary form. These records revealed that he had had 18 tantrums in 13 days. The behavior appeared to be independent of the day of the week but to be linked to the time of day; tantrums were more prevalent in the early part of the school day, from 9:30 A.M. to 10:30 A.M. (8 episodes). Only 1 episode was recorded during the last hour of the school day, from 1:30 P.M. to 2:30 P.M. Although Eric's tantrums occurred in many settings, they were most often noted in his classroom (8 episodes). No other setting involved more than 1 or 2 episodes, and none occurred on the playground.

The most prominent immediate antecedent of the tantrums was instructional demands, which preceded 13 episodes. Social/interpersonal factors also seemed to be involved and served to clarify some of the reasons Eric tantrummed so much during individual work periods. Specifically, 5 episodes occurred when a staff member took a reinforcing item, such as a favorite toy, from Eric without asking him for it. When staff asked him to give up these items, 4 episodes occurred. When he requested an item but was asked to "wait" or to "work" for the toy, 4 episodes followed. Five episodes occurred after Eric was asked to follow an instruction. No tantrums were recorded during recreational periods.

Other antecedent variables that were related to tantrums were organismic-affective factors, including "upset" (6 episodes) and "tense" (3 episodes). Possible distal factors noted were previous tantrums that day (4 episodes), a poor night's sleep (4 episodes), a transition between classrooms (3 episodes), general noncompliance through the day (2 episodes), and excessive "silliness" throughout the day (1 episode).

Two types of program consequences occurred in response to Eric's tantrums. On 12 occasions, staff used response prevention, and on another 4 occasions, planned ignoring was implemented until he was calm. Two other environmental consequences were also noted. On 2 occasions, he received a requested reinforcer shortly after the onset of tantrumming, and on 5 occasions, additional staff had to come to the scene.

PROTOTYPICAL TREATMENT

It is convenient to consider the treatment of persons with autism under two broad headings: direct intervention with the client and intervention with the family. Both aspects of treatment are covered by extensive literatures. Our focus here is on some of the newer and more innovative approaches to these problems.

Treating the Person with Autism

Since the mid-1960s, there has been a rapid growth in the behavioral technology used to treat people with autism. Important early studies documenting the feasibility of using operant procedures with this population include the work of Ferster (1961), Hewett (1965), and Lovaas, Berberich, Perloff, and Schaeffer (1966). Since then, ongoing research has led to increasingly sophisticated techniques that treat the behavioral excesses and deficits that typically accompany autistic disorder. Examples of this technology include making reinforcements intrinsic to the response (e.g., Williams, Koegel, & Egel, 1981), using a variety of reinforcing events (Egel, 1981), and maintaining brief intertrial intervals (Koegel, Dunlap, & Dyer, 1980). These methods have all been found to enhance response acquisition.

In order to address the social deficits that are so prominent in persons with autism, attempts have been made to arrange the environment to enhance the awareness of social cues. For example, normal peers are used as models of appropriate behavior for young children with autism (e.g., Harris, Handleman, Kristoff, Bass, & Gordon, 1990; Odom, Hoyson, Jamieson, & Strain, 1985). Similarly, research has addressed the problems of enhancing the spontaneous language of persons with autism by arranging the natural environment so that they will be attracted to activities that provide occasions to learn functional language (e.g., McGee, Krantz, & McClannahan, 1985).

In the area of reduction of behavioral excesses it has been reported that teaching clients to engage in new, more adaptive alternative responses decreases self-stimulation (Eason, White, & Newsom, 1982) and self-injury (e.g., Favell, McGimsey, & Schell, 1982). Relatively mild punishment procedures, such as overcorrection (Azrin, Gottlieb, Hughart, Weslowski, & Rahn, 1975; Harris & Romanczyk, 1976) and physical exercise (e.g., Gordon, Handleman, & Harris, 1986; Luce, Delquadri, & Hall, 1980) have similarly been found useful in the suppression of disruptive behaviors.

For many persons with autism, medication may be an important component of treatment, especially on an inpatient unit. The effective use of medication for patients with autism requires a familiarity with the most current research. Many medications that appear effective for patients with psychiatric disorders have little apparent benefit for the person with a pervasive developmental disorder. It is therefore essential that one be conversant with this literature before recommending a specific medication.

Self-injurious and aggressive behaviors may be the most frequent behavioral complaints for which medication is considered. A full range of medications has been tested to treat these behaviors in people with autism, and some medications appear to hold more promise than others. Campbell, Anderson, Meier, Cohen, Small, Samit, and Sachar (1978) reported that, for children with autism, haloperidol may reduce symptom intensity and enhance learning. She cautioned, however, that chronic use of haloperidol is associated with tardive and withdrawal dyskinesias (Spencer & Campbell, 1990). These side effects, of course, limit the clinical utility of the drug.

Lithium carbonate has been reported useful in the control of aggressive behavior in some children with autism (Campbell, Schulman, & Rapoport, 1978). However, at present, we have few data about the long-term effects of this drug on children (Spencer & Campbell, 1990). Spencer and Campbell described carbamazepine as potentially useful for controlling aggressive and self-injurious behavior in some clients with autism. Beta-blockers and some of the opiate antagonists such as naloxone and naltrexone have similar potential value, although none of these drugs has given extensive empirical proof of efficacy at this time.

Working with the Family

Most families that include a person with autism require training in behavioral procedures. There is a large literature documenting that parents can master behavior modification techniques and use them skillfully with their own child (Harris, 1989; Harris, Alessandri, & Gill, 1991). These data indicate that parents, whether trained individual or in groups, improve in their ability to present instructions, use prompts, reinforce correctly, and so forth (e.g., Harris, Wolchik, & Weitz, 1981; Howlin, 1981; Koegel, Schreibman, Britten, Burke, & O'Neill, 1982).

Siblings may also be effective behavior-change agents (e.g., Colletti & Harris, 1977; Schreibman, O'Neill, & Koegel, 1983), although one must take particular care with children to avoid burdening them with excessive responsibility. Teaching siblings how to play with their brother or sister with autism is probably more appropriate than involving them in the acquisition of self-help skills or management of maladaptive behavior. We believe younger children should not be taught to use punishment procedures and may often function best as models rather than as teachers.

Didactically oriented training in behavioral techniques may not be sufficient for every family that includes a child with autism. Many families also need emotional support as they come to terms with the meaning of both their child's special needs for the future and their own. Our own clinical experience indicates that ignoring these needs in the family may undermine efforts to help the family members become behavior change agents.

Parents who feel sad, angry, or guilty about their child's handicapping condition are likely to have difficulty focusing their efforts on their child's instructional needs. Although we have worked with many families whose distress was reduced by didactic training and informal support, other families have required more formal intervention before they could mobilize themselves on their child's behalf.

It is also important to recognize that the role of the parents of an autistic child changes over time. It may be unrealistic to expect the parents of an adolescent to devote many hours a day to the instruction of their child, whereas the parents of a preschool child will be eager to spend that time in a teaching role. Parents of adolescents and adults may prefer to focus on advocacy for the young person. Such advocacy may include identifying group-home placements and vocational training resources. Understanding the developmental and lifelong needs of the family, as well as those of the person with autistic disorder, enables the clinician to set realistic treatment goals.

ACTUAL TREATMENT

Parents as Agents of Change

Four-year-old Randy M. was newly enrolled at the Douglass Developmental Disabilities Center when his parents approached the staff for help in toilet-training their son. Although Mr. and Mrs. M, like many parents, did not wish to rush Randy beyond his developmental limits, they found the endless round of wet clothing and bed sheets a particular burden. As he was growing older, the process of changing diapers was becoming increasingly disagreeable. Thus, toilet-training Randy was a high priority for the family. It also provided the center's staff with a useful context in which to provide home-based training to Randy's family. We used this opportunity to introduce them to a number of concepts, such as data collection, defining target behaviors, reinforcing desirable behavior, shaping a new skill, and ignoring undesirable responses.

The first step in creating a home program was a discussion between Randy's teacher and Mr. and Mrs. M. to explore how they dealt with his enuresis, to agree on the definitions to be used in the home program, and to design baseline procedures to determine how often Randy was wet and whether there was a temporal pattern to his wetness. Mr. and Mrs. M. had been responding to Randy's wetting by taking him to the toilet after an accident. Neither parent had punished him for accidents, but both had voiced their frustration over his lack of bladder control. For purposes of the baseline, it was agreed that an "accident" would be defined as Randy's underwear's being wet when he was checked at regular half-hour intervals from waking to bedtime.

A week of baseline data revealed that Randy was wet an average of six to seven times a day, and that no apparent temporal pattern was evident. Based on these data and her own work with him in the classroom, Randy's teacher suggested that the family adopt a procedure of asking him every 30 minutes whether he had to use the toilet. If Randy agreed (either verbally or with a sign), he would be taken to the bathroom. If Randy voided, he would be praised and allowed to jump on his trampoline or would be given tickles. Randy's not indicating a need to use the toilet or having an accident would be treated neutrally. A daily data sheet was maintained indicating whether he was wet or dry on the half hour and whether he voided in the toilet.

In the ensuing two weeks, Randy's number of toileting accidents decreased from the baseline 6 or 7 to 1 or 2 a day. He had 8 to 9 successful episodes of voiding in the toilet. At the end of the second two-week period, his mean daily accident rate was 1.3, and his mean success rate was 10.8. Over the following three two-week periods, this pattern continued, and in the final two-week period, Randy had a daily success rate of 14.95 and a daily accident rate of .8. This high rate of success included not only successful voiding at routine checks, but the times when Randy spontaneously initiated using the toilet. His time between toileting checks was increased from 30 minutes to 50 minutes.

Reducing the Frequency of Self-Stimulation

Five-year-old Jimmy exhibited high levels of self-stimulatory behavior throughout his school day. A variety of simple interventions, including reinforcing him when he was not engaged in self-stimulation, voicing a firm reprimand, promptly returning his hands to his lap and holding them there for a few seconds, consistent ignoring of self-stimulation, and an overcorrection procedure, had all failed to suppress the behavior, which appeared to be highly reinforcing for Jimmy. However, his teacher's preliminary observations did suggest that, following his physical education period, Jimmy engaged in less self-stimulatory behavior than at any other time during the day.

Based on these observations, and with the approval of Jimmy's parents and physician, a program of noncontingent physical exercise was included in Jimmy's curriculum. Jimmy was taken twice a day for a six-minute run and twice for a slow walk. Data were kept on his self-stimulatory behavior during the ensuing 40 minutes after walking or running and after three 40-minute intervals not preceded by any form of physical activity.

The baseline rate of self-stimulation in the 40-minute intervals not connected with physical activity was a mean of 60%. Self-stimulation after walking showed no change from the baseline rate, with a mean of 61%. By contrast, after the six-minute run, the mean rate of self-stimulation was 41%. The beneficial effects of jogging were noted to deteriorate over the 40-minute interval, with a mean rate of 28% in the first 10 minutes as contrasted with 46% in the last 10 minutes. In addition to decreasing Jimmy's self-stimulatory behavior, the vigorous running also led to a decrement in his bouncing in his chair during lessons.

Although this intervention did not eliminate Jimmy's self-stimulatory behavior, it led to a significant reduction and also appeared to be a pleasurable, healthy activity for him. The next steps in the treatment program included increasing the frequency of exercise to maximize its effects, and taking advantage of the reduced rate of self-stimulation to reinforce other appropriate behaviors, and thus to strengthen the likelihood that incompatible behaviors would occur.

Learning to Play

Mr. and Mrs. E.'s 6-year-old son, Billie, was a student with autism at the Douglass Developmental Disabilities Center. The E. family was very committed to Billie's welfare, and everyone, including his 9-year-old brother, Kevin, and his 13-year-old sister, Jill, was eager to make him a full-fledged member of the family. However, for Kevin and Jill, this was not an easy task. Every effort to include Billie in play activities was thwarted by his poor attending behaviors, inappropriate use of toys, limited speech, and sometimes volatile mood. In spite of Billie's behavioral limits, Mr. and Mrs. E. were aware of his siblings' wish to have a way of interacting with their brother. They wondered if, at the center, we might be able to help them develop a home-based program that would enable Kevin and Jill to relate to Billie in a more satisfying way.

A data-based, in-home training program was developed for the E. family. This two-phase program consisted of teaching the siblings how to elicit physical play responses and play-related language. The three basic skills targeted for acquisition by Kevin and Jill were delivering effective commands, prompting physical and verbal responses when Billie did not respond to a request, and reinforcing his appropriate play behaviors.

Each 20-minute play session was broken into three parts. During the first 5 minutes, the trainer demonstrated the appropriate target skill while Kevin or Jill watched. For the next 5 minutes, the sibling practiced the new skill while the trainer gave feedback on her or his performance. The final 10 minutes were used for data collection, and the trainer made no comments during this period.

Striking differences were noted in the siblings' behaviors during the pretraining baseline and the posttraining follow-up. For example, at baseline, Kevin was reinforcing 45% of Billie's appropriate play; this proportion rose to 95% after training. Similarly, Jill's reinforcement rate was 26% before training and 100% at follow-up. The use of prompts to elicit appropriate play behavior showed similar gains, Kevin going from a 16% rate at baseline to 90% at follow-up, and Jill progressing from 0% at baseline to 100% at follow-up. These changes in the siblings' behaviors seem to have altered Billie's responsiveness as well. At baseline, he complied with only 17% of Kevin's requests for a physical response and with 20% of his requests for a verbal response; at follow-up, Billie was complying with 75% of Kevin's requests for physical responses and 88% of the requests for verbal responses. Similarly, Jill's ability to elicit play responses from her brother was markedly improved. At baseline, Billie complied with only 31% of her requests for physical responses and with 34% of her requests for language; at follow-up, Billie's compliance rate was 92% and 89% for physical and verbal responses, respectively.

Following this training, Mr. and Mrs. E. reported an increase in both the frequency and the duration of play between the older children and Billie. Furthermore, both siblings were applying their skills in untrained play settings and in other interactions such as at mealtime. Jill and Kevin both reported feeling more confident in their interactions with Billie.

SUMMARY

Since its recognition as an official diagnostic category by the American Psychiatric Association (1980, 1987), autistic disorder has been the focus of increased clinical interest and research. There are ongoing efforts to refine the diagnostic criteria for this disorder and to identify the subcategories that fall under the broader rubric of *autism*. It is likely that such efforts will continue for some time, at least until the biological antecedents of the conditions are identified and specific corresponding behavioral and/or biological markers are noted.

Although the specific causes of autism remain obscure, we have become increasingly sophisticated in assessing the behaviors that accompany this disorder and in developing behavioral and educational treatment programs to meet the needs of these patients. Competent implementation of these procedures has markedly changed the long-term outlook of many persons with autism, often enabling them to live in the community and participate in work and recreational activities. The potential for such gratifying outcomes makes it all the more essential that initial diagnostic work and inpatient intervention be well informed by the current research.

REFERENCES

American Psychiatric Association. (1980). *Diagnostic and statistical manual of mental disorders* (3rd ed.; DSM-III). Washington, DC: Author.

American Psychiatric Association. (1987). *Diagnostic and statistical manual of mental disorders* (3rd ed. rev.; DSM-III-R). Washington, DC: Author.

Azrin, N. H,. Gottlieb, L,. Hughart, L., Weslowski, M. D., & Rahn, T. (1975). Eliminating self injurious behavior by educative procedures. *Behaviour Research and Therapy*, *313*, 101–111.

Bristol, M. M. (1984). Family resources and successful adaptation to autistic children. In E. Schopler & G. B. Mesibov (Eds.), *The effects of autism on the family* (pp. 289–310). New York: Plenum Press.

Campbell, M., Anderson, L. T., Meier, M., Cohen, I. L., Small, A. M., Samit, C., & Sachar, E. J. (1978). A comparison of haloperidol, behavior therapy and their interaction in autistic children. *Journal of the American Academy of Child Psychiatry*, *17*, 640–655.

Campbell, M., Schulman, D., & Rapoport, J. L. (1978). The current status of lithium therapy in child and adolescent psychiatry. *Journal of the American Academy of Child Psychiatry*, *17*, 717–720.

Carr, E. G., Newsom, C. D., & Binkoff, J. A. (1980). Escape as a factor in the aggressive behavior of two retarded children. *Journal of Applied Behavior Analysis*, *13*, 101–117.

Colletti, G., & Harris, S. L. (1977). Behavior modification in the home: Siblings as behavior modifiers, parents as observers. *Journal of Abnormal Child Psychology*, *1*, 21–30.

Dunn, L. M., & Dunn, L. M. (1981). *Peabody Picture Vocabulary Test—Revised*. Circle Pines, MN: American Guidance Service.

Eason, L. J., White, M. J., & Newsom, C. (1982). Generalized reduction of self-stimulatory behavior: An effect of teaching appropriate play to autistic children. *Analysis and Intervention in Developmental Disabilities*, *2*, 157–169.

Edelson, S. M., Taubman, M. T., & Lovaas, O. I. (1983). Some social contexts of self-destructive behavior. *Journal of Abnormal Child Psychology*, *11*, 299–312.

Egel, A. L. (1981). Reinforcer variation: Implications for motivating developmentally disabled children. *Journal of Applied Behavior Analysis*, *14*, 345–350.

Favell, J. E., McGimsey, J. F., & Schell, R. M. (1982). Treatment of self-injury by providing alternative sensory activities. *Analysis and Intervention in Developmental Disabilities*, *2*, 83–104.

Ferster, C. B. (1961). Positive reinforcement and behavioral deficits of autistic children. *Child Development*, *32*, 437–456.

Frith, U. (1989). *Autism: Explaining the enigma*. Cambridge, MA: Basil Blackwell.

Gordon, R., Handleman, J. S., & Harris, S. L. (1986). The effects of contingent versus non-contingent running on the out-of-seat behavior of an autistic boy. *Child and Family Behavior Therapy*, *8*, 337–344.

Groden, G. (1989). A guide for conducting a comprehensive behavioral analysis of a target behavior. *Journal of Behavior Therapy and Experimental Psychiatry*, *20*, 163–170.

Hagberg, B., Aicardi, J., Dias, K., & Ramos, O. (1983). A progressive syndrome of autism, dementia, ataxia, and loss of purposeful hand use in girls: Rett's syndrome: Report of 35 cases. *Annals of Neurology*, *14*, 471–479.

Handleman, J. S., & Harris, S. L. (1986). *Educating the developmentally disabled: Meeting the needs of children and families*. San Diego: College Hill Press.

Harris, S. L. (1984). Intervention planning for the family of the autistic child: A multilevel assessment of the family system. *Journal of Marital and Family Therapy*, *10*, 157–166.

Harris, S. L. (1987). The family crisis: Diagnosis of a severely disabled child. *Marriage and Family Review*, *11/12*, 107–118.

Harris, S. L. (1989). Training parents of children with autism: An update on models. *The Behavior Therapist*, *12*, 219–221.

Harris, S. L., Wolchik, S. A., & Weitz, S. (1981). The acquisition of language skills by autistic children: Can parents do the job? *Journal of Autism and Developmental Disorders*, *11*, 373–384.

Harris, S. L., & Powers, M. D. (1984). Behavior therapists look at the impact of an autistic child on the family system. In E. Schopler & G. B. Mesibov (Eds.), *The effects of autism on the family* (pp. 207–224). New York: Plenum Press.

Harris, S. L., Handleman, J. S., & Palmer, C. (1985). Parents and grandparents view the autistic child. *Journal of Autism and Developmental Disorders*, *15*, 127–137.

Harris, S. L., Handleman, J. S., Kristoff, B., Bass, L., & Gordon, R. (1990). Changes in language development among autistic and peer children in segregated and integrated preschool settings. *Journal of Autism and Developmental Disorders*, *20*, 23–31.

Harris, S. L., Alessandri, M., & Gill, M. J. (1991). Training parents of developmentally disabled children. In J. L. Matson & J. A. Mulick (Eds.), *Handbook of mental retardation* (2nd ed., pp. 373–381). Elmsford, NY: Pergamon Press.

Hewett, F. M. (1965). Teaching speech to an autistic child through operant conditioning. *American Journal of Orthopsychiatry*, *35*, 927–936.

Howlin, P. A. (1981). The effectiveness of operant language training with autistic children. *Journal of Autism and Developmental Disorders, 11*, 89–105.

Kanfer, F. H., & Saslow, G. (1969). Behavior diagnosis. In C. M. Franks (Ed.), *Behavior therapy: Appraisal and status* (pp. 417–444). New York: McGraw-Hill.

Kanner, L. (1943). Autistic disturbances of affective contact. *Nervous Child, 2*, 217–240.

Koegel, R. L., Dunlap, G., & Dyer, K. (1980). Intertrial interval duration and learning in autistic children. *Journal of Applied Behavior Analysis, 13*, 91–99.

Koegel, R. L., Schreibman, L., Britten, K. R., Burke, J. C., & O'Neill, R. E. (1982). A comparison of parent training to direct child treatment. In R. L. Koegel, A. Rincover, & A. L. Egel (Eds.), *Educating and understanding autistic children* (pp. 260–279). San Diego: College Hill Press.

Lovaas, O. I., Berberich, J. P., Perloff, B. F., & Schaeffer, B. (1966). Acquisition of imitative speech by schizophrenic children. *Science, 151*, 705–707.

Luce, S. C., Delquadri, J., & Hall, R. V. (1980). Contingent exercise: A mild but powerful procedure for suppressing inappropriate verbal and aggressive behavior. *Journal of Applied Behavior Analysis, 13*, 583–594.

McGee, G. G., Krantz, P. J., & McClannahan, L. E. (1985). The facilitative effects of incidental teaching on preposition use by autistic children. *Journal of Applied Behavior Analysis, 18*, 17–31.

Newborg, J., Stock, J. R., Wnek, L., Guidubaldi, J., & Svinicki, J. (1984). *Battelle Developmental Inventory, Examiner's manual.* Allen, TX: DLM Teaching Resources.

Odom, S. L., Hoyson, M., Jamieson, B., & Strain, P. S. (1985). Increasing handicapped preschoolers' peer social interactions: Cross-setting and component analysis. *Journal of Applied Behavior Analysis, 18*, 3–16.

Powers, M. D., & Handleman, J. S. (1984). *Behavioral assessment of severe developmental disabilities.* Rockville, MD: Aspen Systems Corporation.

Rapoport, J. L., & Ismond, D. R. (1990). *DSM-III-R training guide for diagnosis of childhood disorders.* New York: Brunner/Mazel.

Reichler, R. J., & Lee, E. M. C. (1987). Overview of biomedical issues in autism. In E. Schopler & G. B. Mesibov (Eds.), *Neurobiological issues in autism* (pp. 13–41). New York: Plenum Press.

Rumsey, J. M., Rapoport, J. L., & Scerry, W. R. (1985). Autistic children as adults: Psychiatric, social, and behavioral outcomes. *Journal of the American Academy of Child Psychiatry, 24*, 465–473.

Rutter, M., & Schopler, E. (1988). Autism and pervasive developmental disorders. Concepts and diagnostic issues. In E. Schopler & G. B. Mesibov (Eds.), *Diagnosis and assessment in autism* (pp. 15–36). New York: Plenum Press.

Schopler, E., & Mesibov, G. B. (Eds.). (1985). *Communication problems in autism.* New York: Plenum Press.

Schopler, E., & Mesibov, G. B. (Eds.). (1986). *Social behavior in autism.* New York: Plenum Press.

Schopler, E., Reichler, R. J., DeVellis, R. F., & Daly, K. (1980). Toward objective classification of childhood autism: Childhood autism rating scale (CARS). *Journal of Autism and Developmental Disorders, 10*, 91–103.

Schreibman, L. (1988). *Autism.* Newbury Park, CA: Sage.

Schreibman, L., O'Neill, R. E., & Koegel, R. L. (1983). Behavioral training for siblings of autistic children. *Journal of Applied Behavior Analysis, 16*, 129–138.

Spencer, E. K., & Campbell, M. (1990). Aggressiveness directed against self and others: Psychopharmacologic intervention. In S. L. Harris & J. S. Handleman (Eds.), *Aversive and nonaversive interventions: Controlling life threatening behaviors of the developmentally disabled* (pp. 163–181). New York: Springer.

Thorndike, R. L., Hagen, E. R., & Sattler, J. M. (1986). *The Stanford-Binet Intelligence Scale* (4th ed.). Chicago: Riverside.

Watson, M. S., Leckman, J. F., Annex, B., Breg, W. R., Boles, D., Volkmar, F. R., Cohen, D. J., & Carter, C. (1984). Fragile X in a survey of 75 autistic males. *New England Journal of Medicine, 310*, 1462.

Williams, J. A., Koegel, R. L., & Egel, A. L. (1981). Response-reinforcer relationships and improved learning in autistic children. *Journal of Applied Behavior Analysis, 14*, 53–60.

Zimmerman, I. L., Steiner, V. G., & Pond, R. E. (1979). *Preschool Language Scale manual.* Columbus, OH: Merrill.

25

Attention-Deficit Hyperactivity Disorder

CHARLES E. CUNNINGHAM and MARIO CAPPELLI

INTRODUCTION

Attention-deficit hyperactivity disorder (ADHD) is one of the most frequently diagnosed childhood psychiatric disorders. The burden this diagnosis places on the child, the family, and the educational system is reflected in the relatively large proportion of ADHD children referred to outpatient psychiatric settings. Consecutive referral studies in our own center, for example, reveal that 67% of the 4- to 11-year old boys and 41.9% of the girls referred meet the diagnostic criteria for ADHD. These figures are consistent with those reported by other investigators (Kahn & Gardner, 1975; Marine & Cohen, 1975). This chapter begins with an overview of the problems experienced by this very challenging group of children; considers epidemiological evidence regarding its prevalence, etiology, and longitudinal course; describes an approach to behavioral assessment and treatment; and concludes with two case studies.

According to the diagnostic criteria in the revised third edition of the *Diagnostic and Statistical Manual* (DSM-III-R; American Psychiatric Association, 1987), the ADHD child presents developmentally inappropriate difficulties with sustained attention, impulse regulation, and activity level. Although these problems typically emerge before the age of 7, and many parents report difficulties during the preschool years (Palfrey, Levine, Walker, & Sullivan, 1985), it has been suggested that some children do not manifest symptoms until the social and academic demands of adolescence are encountered (Coleman & Levine, 1988). Although the DSM-III-R criteria require the presence of symptoms for a period of at least six months, Barkley (1990) argued for a more conservative interval of one year. A longer symptom duration appears to be particularly important among preschoolers, whose problems, in a significant number of cases, remit within six months (Campbell & Ewing, 1990). The term *undifferentiated attention deficit disorder* is reserved for children presenting with attentional difficulties who do not evidence significant difficulties with activity level. This subgroup, referred to in the third edition of the *Diagnostic and Statistical Manual* (DSM-III; American Psychiatric Association, 1980) as

---

CHARLES E. CUNNINGHAM and MARIO CAPPELLI • Chedoke-McMaster Hospitals and Department of Psychiatry, McMaster University, Hamilton, Ontario L8N 3Z5, Canada.

Handbook of Behavior Therapy in the Psychiatric Setting, edited by Alan S. Bellack and Michel Hersen. Plenum Press, New York, 1993.

"attention-deficit disorder without hyperactivity," appears to have a lower risk of emotional problems and aggression than children with hyperactivity (Barkley, DuPaul, & McMurray, 1990a).

Prevalence

Epidemiological studies suggest that 3%–5% of primary-school–aged children meet the diagnostic criteria for ADHD (Costello, 1989; Costello, Costello, Edelbrock, Burns, Dulcan, Brent, & Janiszewski, 1988; McGee, Silva, & Williams, 1984a; Szatmari, Offord, & Boyle, 1989b). Although the prevalence of ADHD is generally found to be higher among boys than among girls (Szatmari *et al.*, 1989b), simple attention deficits may be equally prevalent among boys and girls (McGee, Williams, & Silva, 1987).

Associated Impairments

Psychiatric Difficulties.   The probability of comorbid psychiatric disorders among ADHD children is high. Data from the Ontario Child Health Study (Szatmari, Offord, & Boyle, 1989a), for example, suggest that among 4- to 11-year-olds, approximately 53% of ADHD boys and 42% of ADHD girls meet the diagnostic criteria for at least one other disorder. The most frequently reported second diagnosis is conduct disorder (Hinshaw, 1987; Szatmari *et al.*, 1989b), with approximately 42.2% of 4- to 11-year-old ADHD boys and 36% percent of 4- to 11-year-old ADHD girls meeting the diagnostic criteria (Szatmari *et al.*, 1989b). Although the degree of overlap between ADHD and conduct problems has led some investigators to question their status as independent syndromes (Shaffer & Greenhill, 1979), epidemiological studies reveal a different pattern of correlates, ADHD being linked to developmental variables and conduct disorder being associated with social adversity (Szatmari, Offord, & Boyle, 1989a). Longitudinal studies, moreover, reveal a different course: conduct-disordered children are at substantially greater psychiatric and social risk than their ADHD peers (Hinshaw, 1987).

ADHD children also evidence a markedly increased risk for other psychiatric difficulties (Szatmari *et al.*, 1989b). Szatmari, Offord, and Boyle (1989c) found that 24.4% of ADHD boys and 50%–35% of ADHD girls experienced neurotic and somatic disorders. Biederman, Munir, Knee, Armentano, Autor, Waternaux, and Tsuang (1987) found that 32% of a clinic sample of 6- to 17-year-old ADHD children suffered from major affective disorders, and longitudinal studies reveal an increased risk of suicidal attempts and deaths (Weiss & Hechtman, 1986).

Impaired Social Relationships.   The ADHD child's difficulties with activity level, sustained attention, impulse control, and self-regulation adversely affect their social relationships with their parents (Barkley, Karlsson, & Pollard, 1985a; Cunningham & Barkley, 1979; Mash & Johnston, 1982), their siblings, their peers (Cunningham & Siegel, 1987), and their teachers (Campbell, Endman, & Bernfield, 1977; Whalen, Henker, & Dotemoto, 1980). During interactions with their parents, for example, ADHD children are more active, less cooperative, and less likely to sustain their attention to play or task-related activities (Cunningham & Barkley, 1979; Mash & Johnston, 1982). Parents report difficulties in daily routines such as dressing, mealtimes, and bedtime (Barkley & Edelbrock, 1987). Problems are also experienced in social activities when visitors are in the home, the parents are on the phone, or the family is on a community outing. The ADHD child's behavior elicits a more controlling, less responsive and rewarding approach to parenting (Barkley, Karlsson, Strzelecki, & Murphy, 1984; Cunningham & Barkley, 1979), which may ultimately compound and perpetuate the child's difficulties (Patterson, 1982).

ADHD children also evidence considerable difficulty with their peers (Cunningham & Siegel, 1987; Pelham & Milich, 1984). They seem to lack knowledge about strategies for sustaining relationships and resolving conflicts with other children (Grenell, Glass, & Katz,

1987), to have more difficulty adjusting their behavior to situational demands (Landau & Milich, 1988; Whalen, Henker, Collins, McAuliffe, & Vaux, 1979), and to engage in more controlling, negative, and aggressive interaction than normal peers (Clark, Cheyne, Cunningham, & Siegel, 1988; Cunningham & Siegel, 1987; Johnston, Pelham, & Murphy, 1985). Other children, as a result, judge ADHD children negatively (Johnston *et al.*, 1985; Milich & Landau, 1982) and interact with them in a more coercive manner (Cunningham & Siegel, 1987; Cunningham, Siegel, & Offord, 1985).

Academic Failures. In classroom settings, ADHD children spend more time off-task and out of their seats, complete less work, and engage in more disruptive behavior than their peers (Barkley, 1990; Whalen, Henker, Dotemoto, & Hinshaw, 1983). ADHD children score lower on standardized intellectual tests, have difficulty with visual-motor coordination (Barkley *et al.*, 1990a; Cunningham & Siegel, 1987), and have deficiencies in complex problem-solving skills (Barkley, 1990). Although epidemiological studies suggest that approximately 25%–30% of ADHD children evidence poor school performance (Szatmari *et al.*, 1989b), the proportion of children referred to clinical settings who experience academic difficulties is much higher (Barkley, 1990). Although the prevalence of developmental learning disorders is difficult to establish in the absence of epidemiological data, it is estimated that between 19% and 26% of ADHD children have either math, reading, or spelling disabilities (Barkley *et al.*, 1990a). Some school surveys have placed the incidence of reading disabilities as high as 39% (August & Garfinkel, 1990).

Personal Accidents. The ADHD child's active, inattentive, and impulsive behavior is associated with an increased risk of personal accidents. ADHD children were significantly more likely to fracture bones or poison themselves than non-ADHD controls (Szatmari *et al.*, 1989c). The ADHD child's vulnerability to accidents, coupled with the increased risk of abuse of this population, clearly indicates the need for careful medical examination (Barkley, 1990).

Longitudinal Course

Although a significant number of parents find their children difficult to manage during the preschool years, these problems subside in a considerable number of cases (Campbell & Ewing, 1990). Studies of school-aged children, in contrast, suggest that ADHD is a remarkably persistent disorder (Mendelson, Johnson, & Stewart, 1971). Barkley *et al.* (1990a), for example, found that 71.5% of a clinic sample identified as ADHD during the early school years continued to meet the diagnostic criteria for ADHD as adolescents. Moreover, a significant percentage of ADHD children experience related difficulties as adults (Weiss & Hechtman, 1986).

By adolescence, ADHD children scored lower on educational tests (Fischer, Barkley, Edelbrock, & Smallish, 1990), received more suspensions, and failed more grades than controls (Barkley, Fischer, Edelbrock, & Smallish, 1990b). Difficulties with social conduct may intensify during adolescence. Barkley *et al.* (1990), for example, found that 59.3% of an adolescent ADHD sample met the DSM-III-R diagnostic criteria for oppositional-defiant disorder, and that 43.5% met the criteria for conduct disorder. These data are consistent with epidemiologically selected community samples of adolescent ADHD children (Szatmari *et al.*, 1989b). Cross sectional studies suggest that, while prevalence of conduct disorders among ADHD boys remains relatively stable, conduct disorders increase sharply among adolescent ADHD girls (Szatmari *et al.*, 1989b).

Etiology

It is generally agreed that the problems presented by this heterogeneous group of children reflect the complex interplay of genetic, biological, social, and environmental variables (Barkley,

1990). Although the mechanisms of transmission are not known, there is growing evidence that genetic variables may predispose children to ADHD. From 20% to 30% of the first-degree relatives of ADHD children may themselves experience ADHD (Alberts-Corush, Firestone, & Goodman, 1986; Biederman, Munir, Knee, Habelow, Armentano, Autor, Hoge, & Watenaux, 1987). Moreover, in an epidemiologically selected sample, Goodman and Stevenson (1989) estimated that approximately 30%–50% of the variance in laboratory measures of attention and activity was attributable to genetic factors.

Although the increased consumption of alcohol and tobacco reported by mothers of ADHD children during their pregnancies is correlated with inattentiveness at age 4 (Streissguth, Martin, Barr, Sandman, Kirchner, & Darby, 1984), a causal relationship has not been established (Barkley, 1990). Moreover, epidemiological studies do not yield consistent links between measures of perinatal adversity and ADHD (Goodman & Stevenson, 1989; McGee, Williams, & Silva, 1984b; Minde, Webb, & Sykes, 1968).

Although it is generally agreed that a small number of children respond adversely when challenged with specific foods or additives (Conners, 1989), most reviewers conclude that dietary variables such as sugar (Gross, 1984; Milich & Pelham, 1986; Wolraich, Milich, Stumbo, & Schultz, 1985) and additives (Harley, Ray, Tomasi, Eichman, Matthew, Chun, Cleelund, & Traisman, 1981) do not play a significant role in the etiology of ADHD (Barkley, 1990). Nonetheless, studies suggesting that the effects of sugar on the behavior and performance of ADHD children vary as a function of the food ingested have led some investigators to contend that definitive studies on this question have not been completed (Conners, 1989).

The role of parenting and family variables in the emergence of ADHD has been a topic of speculation among generations of developmental theorists (Bell & Harper, 1977; Jacobvitz & Sroufe, 1987). Although parents of ADHD children evidence a more controlling, less responsive approach to child management (Barkley et al., 1985a; Cunningham & Barkley, 1979; Mash & Johnston, 1982), pharmacological trials suggest that this strategy may be a response to the ADHD child's active, poorly regulated, noncompliant behavior (Barkley & Cunningham, 1979; Barkley, Karlsson, Pollard, & Murphy, 1985b; Cunningham & Barkley, 1978a; Humphries, Kinsbourne, & Swanson, 1978). Indeed, the behavior of ADHD children appears to elicit a similar response from their teachers (Whalen et al., 1980).

In contrast to conduct problems that are linked to measures of social adversity such as marital conflict and family dysfunction, ADHD is more closely associated with other measures of developmental difficulty (McGee, Williams, & Silva, 1984b; Szatmari et al., 1989; Taylor, Schachar, Thorley, & Wieselberg, 1986). Such correlational evidence is supported by genetic studies finding less than 10% of the variance in laboratory measures of ADHD attributable to markers of social adversity (Goodman & Stevenson, 1989). Nonetheless, child management skills, parental psychopathology, and family variables appear to modulate the expression of a predisposition to ADHD, to influence the course of the disorder, and to affect longer term adjustment (Barkley, 1990; Campbell & Ewing, 1990; Earls & Jung, 1987; Weiss & Hechtman, 1986).

Some investigators question whether academic failures may contribute to the emergence of difficulties with activity level, sustained attention, and self-regulation (Cunningham & Barkley, 1978b; McGee & Share, 1988). According to this model, predisposing cognitive, memory, attentional, or social factors may contribute to academic failures, increase frustration, and exacerbate ADHD symptoms. Impulsive, inattentive, or overtly disruptive behavior that is elicited by academic difficulties, may, in turn, be reinforced and perpetuated by the avoidance of aversive academic activities or by differential attention from peers and teachers (Cunningham & Barkley, 1978b). This pattern of self-perpetuating failures may erode self-efficacy attributions, reduce effort, and compound educational and behavioral difficulties (Kistner, White, Haskett, & Robbins, 1985). Although prospective longitudinal studies of epidemiologically selected ADHD children confirm that learning difficulties often predate the emergence of ADHD (McGee & Share, 1988), the links between early academic failures and ADHD require more careful study.

Although early studies failed to yield consistent differences between normal and ADHD children on resting psychophysiological measures (Hastings & Barkley, 1978), there has been significant progress in efforts to identify neurological or neurochemical correlates of ADHD (Zametkin & Rapoport, 1978). Positron emission tomography (PET) studies, for example, show a reduction in global cerebral glucose metabolism and a more pronounced reduction in those prefrontal motor cortex and superior prefrontal cortex areas implicated in the control of attention and motor activity (Zametkin, Nordahl, Gross, King, Semple, Rumsey, Hamburger, & Cohen, 1990).

PROTOTYPICAL ASSESSMENT

In formulating an approach to the assessment of ADHD children, the reader should consult the many thoughtful articles addressing this topic (Barkley, 1987, 1990; Barkley, Fischer, Newby, Breen, 1988; Edelbrock & Rancurello, 1985). We begin our discussion of assessment with several qualifying assumptions.

1. As the prevalence of comorbid psychiatric disorders is high, specialized evaluations should be preceded by a comprehensive review and a differential diagnostic interview. Certain medical conditions occur comorbidly with ADHD, or present symptoms similar to those of ADHD. Moreover, some medical treatments may exacerbate ADHD symptoms (Barkley, 1990). This assessment, therefore, should be preceded by medical examinations, audiological evaluations, and other assessments as indicated.

2. Because many referrals to psychiatric settings request a diagnostic opinion, the battery described here is designed to determine whether the child meets the DSM-III-R diagnostic criteria for ADHD.

3. No test is sufficient to accurately identify ADHD children, and no single battery will provide the detail needed to assess this heterogeneous group of children (Barkley, 1990). Thus, although we begin with a standard battery, follow-up assessments should be selected according to the pattern of problems that emerges.

4. Observations conducted in clinical contexts often fail to detect problems in attention, activity level, and impulse regulation (Sleater & Ullman, 1981). Office evaluations and observations, therefore, need to be supported by either direct observations or data from informants, such as teachers who observe the child in those settings where the problems occur.

5. Given the situational nature of this disorder, no single informant will provide reliable observations. Indeed parents and teachers rarely agree on the diagnoses of ADHD children (Szatmari et al., 1989b). Interviews and standardized questionnaires, should therefore be used to gather information from individuals who have an extended opportunity to observe the child in the home and school contexts where the problems are most likely to occur.

6. Assessments that yield comprehensive interventions addressing difficulties in educational, family, and extracurricular activities should result in a better outcome (Boyle & Offord, 1990; Dulcan, 1985; Satterfield, Satterfield, & Cantwell, 1981).

7. Finally, although social service systems typically report heavy case loads and long waiting lists, many children with psychiatric disorders do not receive professional assistance (Szatmari et al., 1989c). In an era of economic restraint and limited professional resources, each component of the assessment battery needs to be examined for its incremental benefit to treatment planning and, ultimately, the child's longer term adjustment.

Assessment Overview

The approach to assessment presented here is designed to identify problems, provide a differential diagnosis, construct the formulations needed to generate a comprehensive intervention, and evaluate treatment outcome. To ensure a comprehensive assessment, we routinely address the child's cognitive abilities, academic performance, family and peer relationships, and extracurricular recreational activities.

Initial Parent Interview

The assessment of most ADHD children begins with an open-ended review of parental concerns (without the child present), an individual interview with the child, and a joint discussion of the planned assessment.

Parent Questionnaires

The information obtained in the initial parent interview is used to select questionnaires allowing key informants to provide a more comprehensive description of the child. The data gathered via questionnaires is explored in a more detailed follow-up interview. The preschool (ages 2–3) and school-aged (ages 6–18) Parent Report Forms of the Child Behavior Checklist (CBCL) provide an overview of the problems presented by ADHD children (Achenbach & Edelbrock, 1983). The CBCL includes a broadband Externalizing score and individual factor scores, such as hyperactivity, aggression, and delinquent behavior, and an Internalizing score with individual factors, such as uncommunicative behavior, anxiety, depression, obsessive-compulsive behaviors, and somatic complaints and questions regarding academic achievement, special class placements, and grade repetitions.

To obtain the situationally specific information needed for treatment planning, we ask fathers and mothers to complete the Home Situations Questionnaire (Barkley & Edelbrock, 1987). This measure yields norm-based information about behavior in 16 situations in which ADHD children frequently cause problems, allows situationally specific interviewing, and provides a simple measure that may be repeated to evaluate treatment effectiveness.

Parental Psychopathology. Interpretations of parent reports should recognize that perceptions of the severity of the child's difficulty may be biased by marital conflict, social isolation, or parental psychopathology (Christensen, Phillips, Glasgow, & Johnson, 1983; Estroff, Herrera, Gaines, Shaffer, Gould, & Green, 1984; Fergusson, Horwood, Gretton, & Shannon, 1985; Forehand, Wells, McMahon, Griest, & Rogers, 1982; Friedlander, Weiss, & Taylor, 1986; Griest, Wells, & Forehand, 1979; Panaccione & Wahler, 1986; Rickard, Forehand, Wells, Griest, & McMahon, 1981; Schaughency & Lahey, 1985; Webster-Stratton & Hammond, 1988). Indeed, many studies report increased incidence of alcohol abuse (Cunningham et al., 1988; Owing-West & Prinz, 1987), antisocial personality (Lahey, Piacentini, McBurnett, Stone, Hartdagen, & Hynd, 1988), depression (Cunningham et al., 1988), and other psychiatric disorders among the parents of ADHD children. Parental psychopathology appears to be highest among those ADHD children with conduct problems (Reeves, Werry, Elkind, & Zametkin, 1987; Szatmari et al., 1989a). Because psychopathology may negatively bias parental perceptions of the child's difficulties, impair effective child management (Bond & McMahon, 1984; Mash & Johnston, 1983), and limit participation in interventions (Firestone & Witt, 1982; Rickard et al., 1981), apparent difficulties in this area should be pursued.

Follow-Up Parent Interview

The completion of standardized background and behavioral questionnaires is followed by a more detailed discussion of selected situations from the Home Situations Questionnaire (Barkley & Edelbrock, 1987). We begin with situations that the parents agree are unusually challenging, proceed to situations in which the problems reported by the fathers and the mothers differ in severity, and conclude with situations that the parents manage successfully. This interview reveals differences in parental perceptions, identifies situational influences on the child's behavior, yields information about the strategies adopted by the mothers and the fathers, and presents a balanced view of parenting strengths and weaknesses. In addition, it provides parents with an opportunity to review the most promising strategies in their repertoire and to conclude the interview on a positive note.

Follow-up interviews (1) begin with open-ended questions regarding a specific problem on the Home Situations Questionnaire; (2) explore a specific example; (3) determine the frequency, duration, and intensity of the problem; and (4) consider factors associated with its development. Interviewers (1) explore the emotional response of the individual parents to situational problems; (2) examine their explanations regarding the problem; and (3) note attributions and expectations that may influence the parental response to the situation (Sobol, Ashbourne, Earn, & Cunningham, 1989). The interviewer questions each parent about the various strategies that he or she uses in an effort to manage the problem and determines the child's response to specific strategies.

Family Functioning. There is an emerging consensus that child behavior problems must be understood within a more systemic framework (Mash, 1989; Mash & Terdal, 1988). This is particularly important because of the general relationship between marital conflict and childhood behavior problems (Emery, 1982) and the more specific association between family dysfunction and conduct disorder among ADHD children (McGee, Williams, & Silva, 1985; Szatmari et al., 1989b). In addition to discussions of the strategies adopted by the parents, the dimensions of marital and family functioning influencing child behavior and parenting effectiveness should be assessed. Home Situations Questionnaire follow-up interviews, for example, explore the allocation of parenting roles by determining who manages the child's behavior in different situations, performs child care tasks, and relates to educational or mental health professionals. Problem-solving skills may be explored by asking *how* the parents arrived at the strategies used in each situation, what alternatives they have tried, and which of these is likely to yield the most promising short-term and longer term outcomes. A more formal assessment of problem-solving skills may be obtained by coding the response of the parents to a standard written measure of behavior problem analogues (Johnston, Cunningham, & Hardy, 1988).

Communication skills may be assessed by prompting parents to give one another feedback on how effectively specific situations are managed. More affective dimensions of communication can be evaluated at points where the interviewer labels emotional responses by asking the spouses whether they were aware of their husband's or wife's feelings, how these feelings are typically communicated, and how each spouse responds to the other's efforts to discuss affective issues.

When significant difficulties in marital or family functioning emerge, more detailed interviews or questionnaires should be used (Epstein, Baldwin, & Bishop, 1983; Locke & Wallace, 1959).

Social Networks. Personal social networks are an important source of direct assistance, child-rearing information, and personal support (Cochran & Brassard, 1979). Families of ADHD children, however, move frequently (Barkley et al., 1990b), have fewer contacts with extended-family members, and consider relationships with relatives disruptive (Cunningham et al., 1988). As social isolation adversely affects child management (Dumas, 1986) and limits the outcome of parenting interventions (Wahler, 1980), the family's contact with supportive peers and useful community resources should be explored via either interviews or questionnaires (Dunst, Trivette, & Deal, 1988).

Assessing Relationships with Peers. Because the type of peer rejection experienced by ADHD children (Cunningham & Siegel, 1987; Milich & Landau, 1982; Pelham & Bender, 1982) is linked to longer term adjustment difficulties (Parker & Asher, 1987), the ADHD child's relationships with other children should be assessed. Although the sociometric evaluations used by researchers studying ADHD children (Milich & Landau, 1982) are expensive and logistically difficult to administer in applied settings, parent and teacher reports represent a viable alternative (Landau, Milich, & Whitten, 1984). The Parent report form of the Child Behavior Checklist, for example, reviews friendships, weekly contacts with other children, and the quality of the child's relations with siblings and peers. In addition, specific questions on the Teacher's versions of the CBCL (Achenbach & Edelbrock, 1986) provide information on the extent to which the ADHD child disturbs other pupils (#24), does not get along with other pupils (#25), teases a lot (#94), threatens (#97) or physically attacks people (#57), gets into many fights (#37), gets teased a lot (#38), and is not liked by other pupils (#48). Teachers may provide a more detailed description of social skills via the Taxonomy of Social Situations for Children (Dodge, McClaskey, & Feldman, 1985), a measure providing information regarding the child's competence in six domains: (1) peer group entry; (2) response to provocation; (3) response to failure; (4) response to success; (5) social expectations; and (6) teacher expectations. The child's perspective on peer relationships may be obtained via either interview or formal self-concept measures, such as the Self Description Questionnaire (Marsh, 1988).

Cognitive and Academic Assessment

Individual tests or patterns of scores on cognitive measures do not provide reliable diagnostic markers of ADHD (Barkley, 1990; Ownby & Matthews, 1985). Nonetheless, cognitive and academic assessments allow the examiner to observe the child's approach to the solution of a variety of intellectually challenging tasks and are needed to advise parents and teachers regarding the child's abilities, to identify learning disabilities, to develop an individualized education plan, and to secure specialized educational resources.

Classroom Assessment

Teachers observe children in settings that require ADHD children to mobilize their efforts, resist distractions, regulate their behavior, and sustain their attention to cognitively demanding tasks in the presence of very little incentive. Children must establish both cooperative and competitive relationships with their peers, adjust to classrooms with different rules and expectations, and relate to adults with different personalities, management styles, educational philosophies, and positions within the academic hierarchy. Teacher reports should be considered an *essential* component in the evaluation of ADHD children.

Teacher Report. Although interviews allow teachers to express their concerns and observations flexibly, standardized questionnaires permit comprehensive information to be gathered efficiently from different educational informants. Whereas primary-grade teachers are familiar enough with the child to complete the Teachers Report form of the Child Behavior Checklist (Achenbach & Edelbrock, 1986), in the middle and high school years, it will be necessary to select teachers who have enough contact with the child to respond accurately. From an educational perspective, the CBCL Teacher Report provides norm-referenced information about academic performance, effort, and adjustment. Specific questions address tutorial assistance, special class placement, grade failures, and the results of educational and psychological assessments. The CBCL provides a broadband Externalizing scale with subscales reflecting inattention, aggressiveness, and nervousness/overactivity. The Internalizing scale and individual subscores reflect problems with social withdrawal, unpopularity, immaturity, anxiety, and depression.

In addition to an examination of the patterns of the broadband and individual factor scores on the Teacher CBCL, follow-up interviews should be conducted regarding certain individual questions. For example, in view of the association between ADHD and movement disorders such as Tourette's syndrome (Barkley, 1990) and the possibility that stimulant medications may exacerbate these, it is instructive to explore positive responses to question #46 (nervous movement or twitching).

The School Situations Questionnaire (Barkley & Edelbrock, 1987) provides information about the ADHD child's behavior in settings that contain potential problems such as individual desk work, small-group activities, recess, lunch, hallways, bathrooms, field trips, and buses. A shorter revised version of this questionnaire focuses specifically on problems with attention and concentration (DuPaul, 1990). Determining the types of situations in which problems occur allows the consultant to use interview time efficiently, to target situations requiring detailed assessment, and to select times that will yield more informative classroom observations.

Diagnostic Decisions

Because the item content of the CBCL does not correspond to the DSM-III-R criteria, several normed DSM-III-R rating scales are of diagnostic assistance (Barkley, 1990; Pelham, Gnagy, Greenslade, & Milich, 1992). The Disruptive Behavior Disorders Scale (Pelham *et al.*, 1992), for example, places DSM-III-R symptom descriptions for attention-deficit hyperactivity disorder, oppositional defiant disorder, and conduct disorder along a 4-point Likert scale (Not at all, Just a little, Pretty much, and Very much). Although diagnosis should not be based on a single questionnaire, this one allows diagnostic decisions to be made according to standard criteria, cutoff scores to be determined empirically, and local norms to be developed.

Although teachers are generally reliable informants regarding ADHD children (e.g., Sleator & Ullmann, 1981), their evaluations of sustained attention and activity level may be inflated by the classroom management problems presented by ADHD children who also have oppositional or conduct disorders (Schachar, Sandberg, & Rutter, 1986).

Direct Observations

Classroom Observations. Classroom observations are time-consuming for consultants employed in noneducational psychiatric settings. Although students and teachers may react in unpredictable ways to the presence of observers, direct observations generally yield valuable information regarding the child, his or her peer relationships, classroom management strategies, teaching strategies, and the school environment. Moreover, classroom observations increase the credibility of the consultant's assessment and foster the rapport with key school personnel that will be needed to formulate and implement solutions collaboratively.

As noted above, problems identified on the School Situations Questionnaire or discussions with teachers should be used to identify times when a school visit will yield the most useful observations. We begin school visits by interviewing teachers and principals, proceed to classroom observations, and conclude with a debriefing discussion to determine the representativeness of the observations. Although classroom observation codes are available (Barkley, 1990), less formal recording of the situational, personal, and motivational variables influencing key targets, such as work completion and social interaction, should prove instructive.

Clinic Observations. Although clinic observations lack the ecological richness of school- or home-based observations, analogues simulating the demands of classrooms (Cunningham & Siegel, 1987; Cunningham *et al.*, 1985), task-related parent-child interactions (Barkley *et al.*, 1984; Cunningham & Barkley, 1979; Mash & Johnston, 1982), or potentially difficult interactions with peers (Cunningham & Siegel, Landau & Milich, 1988) may be constructed.

Laboratory Measures. There have been a number of efforts to develop laboratory measures of attention, activity level, and impulse regulation (Barkley, 1989). The Gordon Diagnostic System (GDS; Gordon, 1983), for example, is a computerized continuous-performance task that has satisfactory test-retest reliability (Gordon & Mettelman, 1988) and modest correlations with laboratory measures of attention (Barkley, 1989). Although the GDS provides a relatively objective measure of primary symptoms and an excellent setting in which to observe the child's response to an attentionally demanding task, relatively high false-negative rates limit its use as a stand-alone diagnostic tool (Barkley, 1990).

Assessing Extracurricular Activities. Extracurricular activities allow children to establish friendships, improve social competence, and develop skills that may compensate for difficulties in other areas (Jones & Offord, 1989). Informal discussions with the parents and the child will yield useful information about extracurricular activities. Supplementary information may be obtained from the CBCL's Parent Report questions regarding the frequency and quality of the child's participation in sports, hobbies, games, and clubs. The child's evaluation of her or his athletic competence may be inferred in the case of children over the age of 7 years from responses on the physical abilities scale of the Self Description Questionnaire (Marsh, 1988).

Behavioral Formulation

The data gathered via interviews, questionnaires, and direct observations should be integrated into a working formulation describing the functional relationships between key variables and the child's behavior. The S-O-R-K-C model described by Kanfer and Phillips (1970), for example, guides the collection of information during the assessment phase; provides a framework for organizing the data obtained from interviews, questionnaires, direct observations, and formal testing; suggests follow-up questions, allows the construction of a working formulation about the variables influencing the behaviors of concern; provides an explanatory model for parents and teachers; and suggests treatment hypotheses.

S: Exploring Situational Influences. The questionnaires, interviews, and observations discussed above will reveal the ADHD child's situationally specific pattern of problems and will suggest the variables influencing the probability of target behaviors and functional alternatives. Stimuli should be categorized as *discriminative stimuli*, which increase the probability of behavior by signaling a shift in situational contingencies; *conditioned stimuli*, which elicit emotional responses; or *modeling stimuli*, which influence behavior through observational learning. Because the type of intervention needed to alter the influence of various types of stimuli differs, this step will aid in treatment planning.

O: Individual Influences. Formulations should consider the mediational influences of stable personal characteristics, transient states, and cognitions on the ADHD child's response to situational variables and motivational consequences. *Stable characteristics* include information gained from formal interviews, questionnaires, tests, and observations regarding activity level, attention deficits, self-regulatory skills, temperament, and interpersonal competence. Behavior may also be influenced by *emotional responses* to specific stimuli or emotional states linked to more distal events in the child's life. States also include the conditions of social, physical, or nutritional deprivation, which may potentiate emotional responses or motivate a child to seek particular reinforcers.

Cognitions are a particularly important component in formulations of the ADHD child's difficulties with impulsivity and self-regulation. Indeed, some investigators have argued that the ADHD child's difficulties may reflect a deficit in the ability to regulate behavior according to internal mediational strategies (Douglas, 1980). Assessments, therefore, should explore the child's knowledge of important rules, awareness of alternative strategies, and ability to anticipate short-term and longer term positive and negative consequences. Moreover, behavior, educational performance (Kistner *et al.*, 1985), and emotional adjustment (Leitenberg, Yost, Carroll-Wilson, 1986) are influenced by the child's *interpretation* of important events. Interviews should examine the child's explanations of the extent to which social and academic successes and failures are (1) due to internal or external causes; (2) a result of global or specific factors ("I'm dumb" versus "I have to work hard at math"); (3) controllable ("If I work hard at math, I'll do OK"); or (4) stable ("I'll never understand this"). The Family Beliefs Inventory (Robin &

Foster, 1989) provides a measure of unreasonable assumptions and expectations that may increase conflict between adolescent ADHD children and their parents (Barkley, Anastopoulos, Guevremont, & Fletcher, 1992a). Finally, it is often helpful to conduct a brief functional analysis of the role of cognitions by (1) recording baseline behavior; (2) teaching an alternative cognitive strategy; and (3) monitoring shifts in performance.

R: Identifying Target Behaviors. Formulation begins with the identification of a specific problem and, for behavior problems that are to be reduced in frequency, the identification of a more positive competing response. Defining targets operationally permits reliable reporting and the construction of accurate formulations.

K: Contingencies. Although ADHD children are thought to need frequent immediate consequences (Barkley, 1990), parents (and presumably some teachers) of ADHD children seem to deliver both positive and negative consequences in a less contingent manner than they do to normal children (Cunningham & Barkley, 1979). The K in S-O-R-K-C formulations examines two variables influencing the effectiveness of each consequence: (1) the delay between the response and the consequence and (2) the probability that a given consequence will follow a response.

C: Consequences. ADHD children have difficulty sustaining effort and attention when rewards are delayed or infrequent (Barkley, 1990; Haenlein & Caul, 1987). Interviews, observations, or questionnaires should survey the positive reinforcers, the negative reinforcers, and the punishers that follow both negative and positive alternative behavioral targets of the formulation. Because ADHD children often fail in social or academic settings, particular attention should be given to negatively reinforced behaviors that allow the child to avoid or escape aversive situations. This segment of the evaluation should include a review of the reinforcers that may be used to motivate change during subsequent interventions.

Building a Working Formulation

Once the data have been organized within an S-O-R-K-C framework, a working formulation of the ADHD child's problems should be constructed. This formulation begins by identifying the *variables* that are amenable to change and the *constants* that, for logistical, developmental, or biological reasons, will not change significantly. Next, the relative weights of each constant and variable are estimated via a set of logical and theoretical principles. Thus, whereas the situational variables controlling the occurrence of problems are weighted heavily, inconsistent, infrequent, low-magnitude consequences should exert a less significant impact on behavior. Finally, we connect the various components of the equation with arrows depicting directional and reciprocal influences.

A Systemic Framework. As the proximal contextual influences described in an S-O-R-K-C formulation are modulated by events and relationships within the child's family, school, and community, formulations should be embedded within a descriptive formulation of the larger family and community, describing key functional links between systemic and S-O-R-K-C variables.

Actual Assessment

Referral Problem

Greg, a 7-year-old boy, was referred jointly by his parents and his school because of restless, inattentive, disruptive behavior during class; difficulty following instructions; failure to complete assigned work; and deficits in reading and written language skills. His parents noted that Greg was often restless and unable to sit through television programs or Sunday school classes, had difficulty following instructions, and was easily frustrated by difficulties with fine-motor activities such as drawing or coloring. In kindergarten and Grade 1, his teachers had reported significant problems with sustained attention, the completion of assignments, self-control, fine-motor coordination, and early reading skills. Continued difficulties in Grade 2 prompted this referral.

Background Information

Pediatric assessments revealed no significant medical problems. Greg had been delivered via an uncomplicated full-term cesarean section and had an unremarkable postnatal history. No history of accidents, head injuries, or serious illnesses was reported. Greg walked at 1 year, used single words at 11 months, and used two-word combinations at 18 months. His toilet training was accomplished with some difficulty at age 3. Although some articulation difficulties were initially noted, his fluency improved during the preschool years. Audiological evaluations yielded normal pure-tone and speech-discrimination scores and placed performance on central-auditory processing measures within normal limits.

Although Greg's mother had had an early history of reading and spelling difficulties, she had ultimately obtained a college degree. His father reported no educational and behavioral difficulties, and neither parent reported a personal or extended- family history of ADHD. Both parents were employed in middle- to upper-middle-class occupations.

Psychological Assessment

Selected results of Greg's cognitive and academic testing are summarized in Table 1. The intellectual assessments placed his Verbal, Performance, and Full Scale IQ scores on the Weschler Intelligence Scale for Children (WISC) within the normal range. Academic tests, however, placed his reading and spelling skills at the 3rd and 1st percentiles, scores that are significantly low according to both discrepancy and absolute criteria (Barkley, 1990). On the Gordon Diagnostic System, Greg experienced significant difficulties on tasks requiring sustained attention and impulse regulation.

Parent Report

Table 2 indicates that the reports of both Greg's parents exceeded DSM-III-R cutoffs on the ADHD rating Scale (Barkley, 1990). Although his mother reported significantly high scores on the Home Situations Questionnaire, his father's scores were within normal limits. Following an overview of parental concerns and background factors, a more detailed discussion of selected problems from the Home Situations Questionnaire was conducted. Greg's parents approached the most difficult situations by attempting to "nudge" and reinforce effort and

Table 1.   Case 1: Prototypical Assessment:
Selected Cognitive and Academic Percentile Scores

Measure	Percentile score
WISC-R Verbal Score	70
WISC-R Performance Score	50
McCarthy Memory	13
Visual Motor Integration	25
Wide Range Achievement Test—Revised (WRAT-R) Math	42
WRAT-R Reading	3
WRAT-R Spelling	1

success while avoiding pressure, conflicts, and confrontations. Greg's mother found his failure to follow instructions and complete tasks especially frustrating and made a special effort to avoid unnecessary nagging. As Greg often failed to make eye contact or to listen carefully to instructions, his parents engaged his attention before commands, presented short instructions, and paused if his attention lapsed. Greg was allowed to earn money or privileges for agreed-on goals while losing 10 minutes of television for breaking rules. His parents felt that most of their child management solutions had been formulated via discussion and consensus. Although Greg's father reported fewer difficulties with his behavior, both parents felt that they approached management in a cooperative and supportive manner, a report substantiated by observations during the interview.

Teacher Report

Both of Greg's teachers reported scores on the ADHD rating scale (Barkley, 1990) exceeding the DSM-III-R cutoffs for ADHD. The criteria for oppositional-defiant or conduct disorders were not met. On the School Situations Questionnaire, Greg's morning classroom teacher reported significant difficulties with sustained attention and concentration during individual desk work, small-group activities, class lectures, free time, field trips, assemblies, films, and class discussions. By contrast, during Greg's afternoon French language arts program, few significant difficulties were noted.

Classroom Observations

Because the ADHD rating scales and the school situations questionnaires revealed the most difficulty during individual morning seat work and small-group activities, a 9:00 A.M. school observation was scheduled. The teachers confirmed their concerns about sustained attention and academic difficulties. They noted that Greg was easily frustrated, had difficulty sustaining effort, guessed impulsively, and gave up on tasks that he was capable of doing. They noted that his performance improved if he was encouraged to calm himself, slow down, and consider how to approach a task.

Greg was observed in his regular classroom during small-group and independent assignments. He sat at the rear of his small group, did not attend visually to instructions, and did not raise his hand in response to questions. Although he made an effort to comply with the instructions, he was the last member of his group to begin activities, failed to collect the requisite materials, and was the only student failing to finish the assigned project. Greg fiddled with non-task-related materials on his desk, hummed, sang, and repeatedly interrupted other students by borrowing materials and blurting out questions. During a listening-comprehension activity, Greg

Table 2. Case 1: Prototypical Assessment: Selected Diagnostic Measures

ADHD rating scale		Gordon Diagnostic System: Delay	
Father rating positive	Yes	Total efficiency ratio	Borderline
Mother rating positive	Yes	Total responses	Borderline
Teacher 1 rating positive	Yes	Total correct	Normal
Teacher 2 rating positive	Yes	Gordon Diagnostic System: Vigilance	
Home Situations Questionnaire		Total commissions	Abnormal
Mother positive	Yes	Total correct	Borderline
Father positive	No	Gordon Diagnostic System: Distractibility	
School Situations Questionnaire		Total commissions	Abnormal
Teacher 1 positive	No	Total correct	Borderline
Teacher 2 positive	No		

seated himself at the back of the group, looked about the room, talked to other students, failed to raise his hand in response to questions, and was unable to answer the question addressed to him. Although Greg's teacher gave him repeated reminders, she did not engage his attention before presenting the instructions or prompt him to repeat or review complex commands. Whereas Greg was reprimanded for disruptive behaviors on several occasions, instances of on-task behavior were not rewarded. A postobservation debriefing suggested that, although the inattention, off-task behavior, and disorganized approach to assignments observed were typical, this had been an unusually good morning.

Social Relationships

On the CBCL, Greg's parents noted one friend that Greg visited two or three times a week. His relationships with his siblings and peers were considered by his parents typical of boys his age. His teachers confirmed that, although Greg often disturbed other students in class, his relations with other children were not a problem. Although Greg noted that one peer teased him, he tried to prevent conflict by simply avoiding the child.

Extracurricular Activities

Greg was a member of a local hockey team, took piano lessons, enjoyed swimming, and shared a paper route with another child. Although his parents considered him an average hockey player, Greg thought that he was a very competent defenseman.

Comment

This case illustrates a mild case of ADHD uncomplicated by oppositional or conduct disorder. Diagnostic questionnaires revealed consistent reports by both his parents and his teachers of Greg's problems with sustained attention, impulse control, and activity level beginning well before the age of 7. Teacher and parent reports were supported by classroom observations and performance on the GDS. Despite average intellectual ability, Greg evidenced significant reading and spelling difficulties. In addition to educational assistance, school observations suggested that consultation concerning more effective classroom management strategies would be helpful. Although Greg's mother reported significant difficulties, his parents had adopted a collaborative approach to management that had led to behavioral improvements. Greg was involved in a variety of extracurricular activities that provided him with a sense of competence. Although his parents felt that his peer relationships were satisfactory, classroom observations revealed a pattern of disruptive behaviors that might ultimately alienate other children.

PROTOTYPICAL TREATMENT

Treatment-Planning Assumptions

In considering interventions for ADHD children, we make several assumptions:

1. Treatment plans should be derived from a formulation of those variables influencing developmentally significant target problems.

2. Because many interventions yield situationally and temporally specific outcomes (Forehand & Atkeson, 1977), programs may need to target problems at home, at school, and in extracurricular contexts. Moreover, as the effects of many interventions fail to generalize beyond the termination of active treatment (Pelham & Hinshaw, 1992), programs need to incorporate booster components designed to maintain the gains accomplished in each setting.

3. As the logistical burden of individualized educational programs often limits adherence in both regular and special educational settings, classwide programs should be considered (Greenwood, Delquadri, & Hall, 1989).

4. Given the prevalence of ADHD, limited resources, and evidence that a significant number of children do not receive treatment (Szatmari *et al.*, 1989b), cost-effective models that increase the availability of services need to be developed. Although the needs of individual children often appear to be unique, it is generally possible to deliver services such as parent training (Cunningham, Bremner, & Secord-Gilbert, 1990) or social-skills training (Cunningham *et al.*, 1989) within cost-effective groups.

5. Finally, programs such as self-control training that have a strong theoretical rationale (Douglas, 1980; Kendall & Braswell, 1985) but that do not consistently yield sustained gains in short-term trials (Abikoff, 1985) need to be integrated into the educational curriculum, taught within the framework of daily academic and social activities, sustained consistently over a period of years, and evaluated for their longer term impact.

Feedback

Parents, children, and, with parental permission, educational representatives should be given feedback about the diagnostic results of the assessment. As parents and teachers often have incorrect information and beliefs regarding the cause or treatment of this disorder (Sobol *et al.*, 1989), it is important to present an accurate explanatory model describing the link between the child's characteristics, contextual influences, and the problems of concern. Feedback should include a discussion of the probable course of the individual child's difficulties and a review of the treatment options that merit consideration. As some parents have difficulty accepting and adjusting to this diagnosis, follow-up discussions may be required (Barkley, 1990). Where it is indicated, parents should discuss pharmacological management with a consulting physician. Parents and teachers interested in additional reading on the topic of ADHD may wish to explore the texts (Goldstein & Goldstein, 1987, 1989; Gordon, 1991) and videotapes (Goldstein, 1989; Goldstein & Goldstein, 1990) available.

Planning an Intervention

We adopt a three-stage approach to behavioral treatment planning. First, the general situations (home, school, and extracurricular activities) in which interventions are indicated are identified. At this level, generic programs such as parent training, social skills groups, or educational consultation may be considered. Second, within these situations, specific problems may be targeted for an S-O-R-K-C assessment, a formulation, and a more systematic effort to the shift controlling variables via the application of behavioral, cognitive, systemic, or pharmacological interventions. In Stage 3, the results of Stage 1 and 2 interventions are evaluated to determine the need for more intensive intervention.

Formulations should identify the variables influencing the target behaviors and allow the effect size of the interventions influencing alternative combinations of variables to be estimated. Parents, teachers, and consultants should rank problems with respect to their longer term developmental, social, or educational significance. In general, formulations should target measures of social or academic achievement (e.g., the number of math problems completed successfully), rather than primary symptoms such as off-task behavior or fidgetiness (Cunningham & Barkley, 1978b). Problem solving should begin with targets that are soluble given the resources of the consultee. Success on simpler problems often improves rapport among the consultant, the teacher, the parent, and the child; yields the information needed to formulate solutions for more complex problems; and builds the skill and confidence needed to execute more challenging strategies.

Management in Educational Settings. Because many ADHD children experience significant academic difficulties (Barkley *et al.*, 1990b), individualized educational assistance may be required. Classroom interventions begin with problem-solving sessions in which the consultants, the teacher, and the parents consider variables in the S-O-R-K-C equation that may yield meaningful shifts in behavior. This type of formulation-based problem solving generally contributes to agreement about the nature of the child's difficulties, builds a consensus for the intervention, increases consistency in the administration of home and school strategies, and fosters the collaborative relationship needed to implement the strategies consistently.

Modifying Situational Influences (Stimuli). Typically, shifts in the situational components of the formulation are indicated. Although intervention can often be accomplished in the context of a regular classroom, placement in a setting with a lower pupil-teacher ratio that is specialized in the management of behavioral and education problems may be indicated. Within either setting, formulations typically suggest that teachers (1) reduce time in situations, activities, and peer groups that are linked to problem behavior; (2) increase time in situations associated with more positive behavior; and (3) seat the child in a position that reduces salient distractions, enhances eye contact, and attention to the teachers' instructions, and permits teachers to deliver private prompts and rewards. Because classroom rules often fail to exert regulatory control over the ADHD child's behavior (Barkley, 1990), strategies that enhance the child's attention, improve retention, or increase the salience of key rules and instructions should be explored. For example, instructions that ADHD children typically have difficulty following should be presented in a clear, simple step-by-step manner, paired with nonverbal cues and prompts to review strategically positioned visual reminders. Finally, S-O-R-K-C formulations may suggest ways in which the complexity, length, and format of tasks and the time of the day when particular tasks are presented to ADHD children may be adjusted to enhance success.

Managing Personal Influences. The *individual* component of most S-O-R-K-C formulations suggests the need to improve educational or social skills deficits, to modulate emotional arousal, to improve self-regulation, and to correct counterproductive attributions or self-statements. The academic difficulties experienced by many ADHD children may necessitate an individualized remedial program for improving skill deficits. Formal relaxation procedures, such as the turtle technique (Robin, Schneider, & Dolnick, 1976), may be helpful in modulating emotional arousal. There are a variety of programs designed to enhance self-regulatory skills (Kendall & Braswell, 1985). Moreover, classrooms designed specifically to improve self-control in ADHD children have demonstrated promising short-term results (Barkley, Copeland, & Sivage, 1980). Nonetheless, as generalization of the gains accomplished via cognitive interventions is often limited (Abikoff, 1985), there is a need to explore strategies for enhancing the effectiveness of this approach.

Managing Motivational Contingencies and Consequences. The consequence and contingency components of most S-O-R-K-C formulations suggest improvements in the motivational dimensions of the classroom. These typically involve simultaneous efforts to reduce positive and negative reinforcers for disruptive behavior while increasing rewards for more positive alternatives. These goals may be accomplished via an increase in verbal reward ratios (Pfiffner, Rosen, & O'Leary, 1985) or more formal contingency-contracting procedures (Robinson, Newby, & Ganzell, 1981), in which points earned for targeted successes are exchanged for items on either school- or home-based menus of optional rewards (Barkley, 1990). Response cost procedures, in which the child loses points for specified infractions, often enhance the effectiveness of contingency-contracting procedures (Rapport, Murphy, & Bailey, 1982). Quiet rather than publicly delivered reprimands coupled with time-out or loss of privileges seem to enhance the effectiveness (Pfiffner & O'Leary, 1990; Rosen, O'Leary, Joyce, Conway, & Pfiffner, 1984) and the temporal generalization (Sullivan & O'Leary, 1989) of positive reinforcement procedures.

Highly individualized behavioral interventions (Allyon, Layman, & Kandel, 1975; Robinson *et al.*, 1981) and classroom programs designed specifically for ADHD children (Barkley *et al.*, 1980) have been shown to enhance both behavior and performance. Generalization to regular class placements is, however, often limited (Barkley *et al.*, 1980). Although some larger scale programs executed by teachers trained in classroom management procedures have demonstrated significant behavioral improvements (O'Leary & Pelham, 1978; Pelham, Schnedler, Bologna, & Contreras, 1980), others have reported less promising results (Abikoff & Gittelman, 1984). Moreover, although there is great variation in the response of individual children to classroom behavioral interventions, most ADHD children continue to cause more problems than normal peers. Because behavioral interventions conducted in highly controlled settings yield more impressive improvements than those in normal educational contexts, it is important to explore the factors enhancing adherence (Meichenbaum & Turk, 1987).

Improving Parenting Skills

The persistence, complexity, and severity of the problems that many ADHD children present make parenting an unusually challenging task. The ADHD child's poorly regulated oppositional behavior (Cunningham & Barkley, 1979; Mash & Johnston, 1982) elicits a less positive, inconsistent, more controlling approach to parenting, which may compound and perpetuate the child's problems (Cunningham & Barkley, 1978a, 1979; Mash & Johnston, 1982). Over the course of the ADHD child's development, parents are confronted with a substantially greater number of problems than are the parents of normal children. Improving child management strategies and building the problem-solving skills needed to solve future problems should be components in comprehensive interventions for the parents of many ADHD children.

A variety of useful programs are designed specifically for the parents of preschool (Pisterman, McGrath, Firestone, Goodman, Webster, & Mallory, 1989), school-aged (Dubey, O'Leary, & Kaufman, 1983; Pollard, Ward, & Barkley, 1983), and adolescent (Barkley, Guevremont, Anastopoulos, & Fletcher, 1992b; Robin, 1990) ADHD children. Outcome studies suggest that, although a significant number of parents elect not to participate (Firestone & Witt, 1982), those completing training programs experience an increase in parenting skill and a reduction in child behavior problems (Barkley *et al.*, 1992; Dubey *et al.*, 1983; Pisterman *et al.*, 1989; Pollard *et al.*, 1983). Although these gains are typically maintained at short-term follow-ups (Barkley *et al.*, 1990; Pisterman *et al.*, 1989), the longer term effectiveness of these interventions merits study.

Our parenting program (Cunningham, 1989, 1990; Cunningham *et al.*, 1990) evolved from hospital-based individual models to large-group community courses conducted in schools and day care facilities throughout our area. Scheduling large-group courses in neighborhood schools increases accessibility and permits a significantly greater number of parents to participate. Parents attend 15 weekly two-hour sessions designed to improve their child management skills. In Session 1, the participants formulate a more effective approach to the solution of child management problems. In Session 2, attending strategies are developed for reinforcing quiet, constructive, cooperative behavior; for facilitating conversation; and for strengthening parent-child relationships. Session 3 explores strategies for balancing time and attention among siblings and for promoting prosocial skills. Because ADHD children seem to need more immediate, more frequent rewards (Barkley, 1990), Session 4 focuses on formal strategies for reinforcing positive behavior.

As low-level conflicts between ADHD children and their parents may escalate into serious confrontations or self-perpetuating coercive cycles (Patterson, 1982), Session 5 focuses on strategies for ignoring minor irritants, disengaging from potentially explosive episodes, and regulating anger. Presenting commands and using preparatory strategies to facilitate transitions between activities are discussed in Session 6. Session 7 explores the Premack principle, through which completion of less rewarding tasks is reinforced by access to more rewarding activities. Sessions 8 and 9 focus on strategies for prompting and rewarding planning, problem solving, and the application of self-regulatory skills. In advance of potentially problems, for example, parents prompt children to consider helpful strategies, develop reminders, and negotiate incentives. Parents prompt the child to review plans immediately before the target situation, and they reward successful performance. Session 10 develops time-out from positive reinforcement strategies as a backup for those occasions when children fail to comply with nonnegotiable commands or refuse to terminate unacceptable behaviors. Sessions 11 through 15 are designed to strengthen the skills established in Sessions 1 through 10, to encourage their application to new problems, and to address concerns of special interest.

In addition to parenting skills, this program is designed to strengthen dimensions of marital and family functioning that are essential to effective child management. The process of each session, therefore, is designed to enhance problem-solving skills, encourage a more balanced allocation of child management responsibilities, and increase supportive communication (Cunningham, 1990). As the parents of ADHD children find themselves isolated from the supportive personal contacts critical to the maintenance of the gains established in parent-training programs (Wahler, 1980), the large-group format provides an opportunity to encourage the formation of supportive networks of personal contacts and local community resources.

A variety of written and videotaped materials provide suggestions about the management of ADHD (Gordon, 1991; Goldstein & Goldstein, 1989), or of generally problem-causing children (Wyckoff & Unell, 1984). Many families appreciate the assistance provided by parent support groups, such as CHADD (Children with Attention Deficit Disorders), a national organization for parents and professionals.

Follow-Up. Although successful interventions may yield modest short-term gains, ADHD is an extremely persistent disorder. Most parents face an enormous number of new problems. It is important, therefore, that programs develop a cost-effective follow-up component. To support the gains established in our parenting programs, for example, graduates are encouraged to attend monthly booster groups providing an opportunity to review successful strategies, solve new problems, explore community resources, and renew supportive personal contacts (Cunningham, 1990).

Improving Social Competence

As ADHD children experience significant difficulty with their peers (Cunningham & Siegel, 1987; Milich & Landau, 1982; Pelham & Bender, 1982), improving social competence is an important component of a comprehensive intervention. Although there are some promising approaches to building social competence in this population (Cunningham et al., 1989; Hinshaw, Henker, & Whalen, 1984; Kendall & Braswell, 1984), skills acquired in social training programs may not generalize to educational and social contexts (Berler, Gross, & Drabman, 1982). Moreover, the reputation of socially unpopular children may negatively bias the response of their peers to improvements in the children's behavior (Hymel, Wagner, & Butler, 1992). Thus, although our parent training program includes a 15-session children's group designed to improve social competence (Cunningham, 1990), we attempt to improve the social relationships of ADHD children by integrating social-skill-building activities into existing educational and extracurricular contexts. Cunningham et al. (1989), for example, conducted a morning social-skills-training program for ADHD and learning-disabled students enrolled in a summer computer camp. The students observed adult models role-playing common interactional errors, identified the errors and discussed their consequences, formulated alternative strategies and discussed their advantages, rehearsed new skills, and established personal goals for applying the strategy during their morning class. Continuous daily classroom observations showed a marked increase in prosocial interactions and a corresponding improvement in sociometric relationships. However, although social-skill-building exercises increased positive interactions, negative interactions did not decline until an in-class differential reinforcement of other behaviors (DRO) contingency was introduced. These data are consistent with those of other investigators who found that in-class contingencies are effective in reducing aggressive behavior (Abikoff & Gittelman, 1984).

531

MANAGING ADHD

Extracurricular Activities

Jones and Offord (1989) demonstrated that extracurricular programs designed to enhance the skills of children living in publicly funded housing complexes enhanced self-esteem and lowered rates of antisocial behavior. Moreover, the expense of mounting this program was offset by a reduction in police, fire-department, and vandalism costs. These effects did not generalize to educational performance, and they rebounded when the program was terminated. These findings are consistent with those of other investigators, showing that the beneficial effects of many interventions are situationally and temporally specific. Nonetheless, they suggest that well-organized activities that engage children in constructive alternative activities during high-risk times build the skills needed to continue participating in organized activities, strengthen social skills, and enhance self-confidence and may also reduce the opportunity to engage in antisocial behavior. A well-planned program of extracurricular activities, therefore, should be of benefit to ADHD children who are at high risk for conduct problems.

Combining Behavioral and Pharmacological Interventions

There is growing evidence that pharmacological interventions represent a useful adjunct to behavioral interventions for ADHD children. The positive effects of stimulants may enhance the effects of behavioral interventions, provide an alternative when well-executed behavioral interventions fail, afford an option when parents or teachers do not adhere to recommendations, or reduce the severity of the child's problems to a level that will permit teachers and parents to use newly acquired skills more successfully. Stimulants have been shown to enhance a variety of behavioral interventions including parent training (Firestone, Kelly, Goodman, & Davey, 1981; Pollard *et al.*, 1983; Speltz, Varley, Peterson, & Beilke, 1988), reinforced self-evaluation in playgrounds settings (Hinshaw, Henker, & Whalen, 1984), spelling performance (Pelham, Milich, & Walker, 1986), and classroom behavior therapy (Gittelman, Abikoff, Pollack, Klein, Katz, & Mattes, 1980). Although the effects of stimulants on long-term academic achievement are unclear (Barkley & Cunningham, 1979), short-term studies suggest that stimulants may improve cognitive and academic performance (Douglas, Barr, O'Neill, & Britton, 1988) and enhance the outcome of remedial educational interventions (Richardson, Kupietz, Winsberg, Maitinsky, & Mendell, 1988). Finally, stimulant medications that reduce conflict (Cunningham *et al.*, 1985, 1991), enhance social status (Whalen, Henker, Buhrmester, Hinshaw, Huber, & Laski, 1989), and improve attention during athletic activities (Pelham, McBurnett, Harper, Murphy, Milich, Clinton, & Thiele, 1990) may support training programs designed to improve social skills and extracurricular competence.

ACTUAL TREATMENT

Background Summary

Jason, age 6, was referred to the ADHD program by the family's pediatrician. Although his developmental milestones were within normal limits, Jason presented with a history of overactive, irritable behavior dating to early infancy. His school reports indicated difficulties with sustained attention, overactivity, impulsivity, and disruptive, noncompliant behavior. Jason was described as a stubborn, moody, argumentative child prone to temper tantrums and aggressive behavior. His parents confirmed similar difficulties at home. The psychological assessment summarized in Table 3 placed Jason's verbal abilities in the average range and his nonverbal abilities in the high-average range. Difficulties were noted on measures of short-term memory, auditory and verbal memory, and visual-motor coordination. Formal academic testing suggested emerging difficulties in reading skills but normal quantitative skills. The diagnostic battery described above confirmed a diagnosis of ADHD with oppositional-defiant disorder.

Treatment Plan

As Jason presented significant problems both at home and at school, this intervention included components designed to strengthen parenting skills, enhance classroom management, and improve academic performance.

Parent Training. Jason's parents enrolled in a 15-week parent-training course (Cunningham, 1990). The parents attended reliably and completed homework projects. Over the course of the program, they showed very significant improvements in their child management skills, a more effective approach to problem solving, a more balanced distribution of child management responsibilities, and more mutual support and reinforcement. At the completion of the course, the couple joined a monthly booster group designed to encourage continued application of the skills acquired in the parent-training program and to solve new problems.

School Consultation. Jason's pediatrician, therapist, parents, and teachers met on several occasions to review the results of his psychological testing, to discuss the diagnosis of ADHD, and to formulate collaborative solutions to Jason's academic and behavioral difficulties. The school management plan included (1) actively engaging Jason's attention; (2) presenting short instructions; (3) prompting his repetition of instructions; (4) giving him praise for follow-through; (5) instituting a three-way contract among Jason, his teachers, and his parents in which points earned for successfully completed work were exchanged for rewards at home (Barkley, 1990), and (6) setting aside two brief periods daily during which the teacher prompted Jason to formulate and review strategies for situations that were apt to cause him problems. Academically, Jason received daily individualized assistance in areas of difficulty.

Stimulant Medication. Given the severity of Jason's problems at home and school, his parents and his pediatrician elected to combine parent training and classroom consultations with a trial of the stimulant medication, Cylert (pemoline sulfate). As he responded favorably, this medication was continued.

Outcome. The preprogram, postprogram, and two-year follow-up scores presented in Table 4 show a very substantial decline in Jason's Internalizing and Externalizing scores on the Child Behavior Checklists completed by his mother and father. Both parents reported a significant reduction in management difficulties on the Home Situations Questionnaire. Jason's postprogram diagnostic scores for both ADHD and oppositional disorder were within normal

Table 3. Case 2: Selected Cognitive and Academic Scores Percentile Scores

Measure	Percentile score
WISC-R Verbal Score	37
WISC-R Performance Score	77
Visual motor integration	21
WRAT-R Reading	12
WRAT-R Spelling	19
WRAT-R Math	32

limits. The measures of marital satisfaction and depression, which were within normal limits at the outset of the program, did not shift significantly.

Follow-Up. Follow-up reviews conducted two years after the completion of this intervention revealed that Jason remained on Cylert, and his parents continued to use the strategies developed during the parent-training program. Follow-up scores on the Home Situations Questionnaire and the Child Behavior Checklist suggested that gains evident at posttest had been maintained; all scores were well within normal limits. Jason remained in a regular classroom placement with daily assistance from a learning-resource teacher in reading and language-related academic skills.

Comment. The very substantial sustained improvements evident here, in our opinion, reflect several factors. First, a situationally comprehensive intervention accomplished significant shifts in the management strategies adopted by both Jason's parents and his teachers. Second, adherence was enhanced with an approach in which the parents, the teachers, and the child collaborated in the formulation and implementation of the solutions. In contrast to didactic approaches that may increase resistance (Patterson & Forgatch, 1985), the participants are more committed to solutions that they have actively formulated (Meichenbaum & Turk, 1987). Third, the parent training was designed to strengthen the dimensions of family functioning needed to cope effectively with a chronically difficult child. Fourth, the interventions at school included strategies designed to enhance Jason's educational performance, strengthen his self-regulatory skills, and improve his behavior. The conjoint collaborative structure of the program made the approach to management by his parents and his teachers consistent. Moreover, his parents and his teachers facilitated transfer and generalization by prompting and reinforcing Jason to apply newly acquired social and self-regulatory skills. Fifth, the impact of the educational and behavioral interventions was enhanced by the stimulant medication Cylert. Finally, this program included monthly booster sessions and preventively scheduled school contacts to enhance longer term maintenance.

Table 4. Case 2: Pre-Post and Two-Year Follow-Up Parent-Training Program Scores Reported by Mother and Father

	Pre	Post	2-year follow-up
DSM-III-R mother report			
ADHD	Yes (11/14)	No (1/14)	No (4/14)
ODD	Yes (8/9)	No (0/9)	No (0/9)
CD	No (1/12)	No (0/12)	No (1/12)
DSM-II-R father report			
ADHD	Yes (8/14)	No (1/14)	No (5/14)
ODD	Yes (8/9)	No (0/9)	No (0/9)
CD	No (0/12)	No (0/12)	No (1/12)
CBCL Externalizing Z score			
Mother	2.7	.3	.9
Father	2.6	.5	—
CBCL Internalizing Z score			
Mother	2.4	−.4	−.4
Father	2.2	−.4	—
Home Situations Questionnaire severity Z score			
Mother	3.7	−.7	−.6
Father	2.6	.0	−.6

aFollow-up CBCL completed collaboratively by the parents.

CHARLES E.
CUNNINGHAM and
MARIO CAPPELLI

SUMMARY

ADHD is a persistent disorder that poses significant difficulties in school, home, and extracurricular social contexts. When it is complicated with conduct disorder, the risk of longer term social and emotional difficulties increases markedly. Successful management requires careful assessment and, in many cases, a sustained, situationally comprehensive focus on parenting skills, classroom management, academic skills, peer relationships, and extracurricular activities. Stimulant medication represents a useful adjunct in selected cases. Finally, an effective communitywide approach requires a consideration of the high prevalence of the disorder, an effective use of the limited professional resources, and the need for prevention and early intervention. Although behavioral interventions have proved useful, future studies need to address the incremental effectiveness of different combinations of interventions, the factors influencing adherence, and the long-term effects of various combinations of interventions.

REFERENCES

Abikoff, H. (1985). Efficacy of cognitive training interventions in hyperactive children: A critical review. *Clinical Psychology Review, 5*, 479–512.

Abikoff, H., & Gittelman, R. (1984). Does behavior therapy normalize the classroom behavior of hyperactive children? *Archives of General Psychiatry, 41*, 449–454.

Achenbach, T. M., & Edelbrock, C. (1983). *Manual for the Child Behavior Checklist and Revised Child Behavior Profile*. Burlington: University of Vermont, Department of Psychiatry.

Achenbach, T. M., & Edelbrock, C. (1986). *Manual for the Teacher Report Form and the Child Behavior Profile*. Burlington: University of Vermont, Department of Psychiatry.

Alberts-Corush, J., Firestone, P., & Goodman, J. T. (1986). Attention and impulsivity characteristics of the biological and adoptive parents of hyperactive and normal control children. *American Journal of Orthopsychiatry, 56*, 413–423.

Allyon, T., Layman, D., & Kandel, H. (1975). A behavioral-educational alternative to drug control of hyperactive children. *Journal of Applied Behavior Analysis, 8*, 137–146.

American Psychiatric Association. (1980). *Diagnostic and statistical manual of mental disorders* (3rd ed.; DSM-III). Washington, DC: Author.

American Psychiatric Association. (1987). *Diagnostic and statistical manual of mental disorders* (3rd ed. rev.; DSM-III-R). Washington, DC: Author.

Anderson, J. C., Williams, S., McGee, R., & Silva, P. A. (1987). DSM-III disorders in preadolescent children: Prevalence in a large sample from the general population. *Archives of General Psychiatry, 44*, 69–76.

August, G. J., & Garfinkel, B. D. (1990). Comorbidity of ADHD and reading disability among clinic referred children. *Journal of Abnormal Child Psychology, 18*, 29–45.

Barkley, R. A. (1987). The assessment of attention deficit-hyperactivity disorder. *Behavioral Assessment, 9*, 207–233.

Barkley, R. A. (1989). The ecological validity of laboratory and analogue assessments of ADHD symptoms. In J. Sargeant & A. Kalverboer (Eds.), *Proceedings of the Second International Symposium on ADHD*. Oxford, England: Pergamon Press.

Barkley, R. A. (1990). *Attention deficit hyperactivity disorder: A handbook for diagnosis and treatment*. New York: Guilford Press.

Barkley, R. A., & Cunningham, C. E. (1979). The effects of methylphenidate on the mother-child interactions of hyperactive children. *Archives of General Psychiatry, 36*, 201–208.

Barkley, R. A., & Edelbrock, C. S. (1987). Assessing situational variation in children's behavior problems: The Home and School Situations Questionnaires. In R. Prinz (Ed.), *Advances in behavioral assessment of children and families* (Vol. 3, pp. 157–176). Greenwich, CT: JAI Press.

Barkley, R. A., Copeland, A. P., & Sivage, C. (1980). A self-control classroom for hyperactive children. *Journal of Autism and Developmental Disorders, 10*, 75–89.

Barkley, R. A., Karlsson, J., Strzelecki, E., & Murphy, J. (1984). Effects of age and Ritalin dosage on the mother-child interactions of hyperactive children. *Journal of Consulting and Clinical Psychology, 52*, 750–758.

Barkley, R. A., Karlsson, J., & Pollard, S. (1985a). Effects of age on the mother-child interactions of hyperactive children. *Journal of Abnormal Child Psychology, 132*, 631–638.

Barkley, R. A., Karlsson, T., Pollard, S., & Murphy, J. (1985b). Developmental changes in mother-child interactions of hyperactive boys. Effects of two doses of Ritalin. *Journal of Child Psychology and Psychiatry, 24*, 705–715.

Barkley, R. A., Fischer, M., Newby, R., & Breen, M. (1988). Development of a multimethod clinical protocol for assessing stimulant drug responses in ADHD children. *Journal of Clinical Child Psychology, 17*, 14–24.

Barkley, R. A., DuPaul, G. J., & McMurray, M. B. (1990a). Comprehensive evaluation of attention deficit disorder with or without hyperactivity as defined by research criteria. *Journal of Consulting and Clinical Psychology, 58*, 775–789.

Barkley, R. A., Fischer, M., Edelbrock, C. S., & Smallish, L. (1990b). The adolescent outcome of hyperactive children diagnosed by research criteria: 1. An 8-year prospective follow-up study. *Journal of the American Academy of Child and Adolescent Psychiatry, 29*, 546–557.

Barkley, R. A., Anastopoulos, A., Guevremont, D., & Fletcher, K. (1992a). Attention deficit disorder in adolescence: Mother-adolescent interactions, family beliefs and conflicts, and maternal psychopathology. *Journal of Abnormal Child Psychology, 20*, 263–288.

Barkley, R. A., Guevremont, D. C., Anastopoulos, A. D., & Fletcher, K. E. (1992b). A comparison of three family therapy programs for treating family conflicts in adolescents with attention deficit hyperactivity disorder. *Journal of Consulting and Clinical Psychology, 60*, 450–462.

Bell, R. Q., & Harper, L. (1977). *Child effects on adults*. New York: Wiley.

Berler, E. S., Gross, A. M., & Drabman, R. S. (1982). Social skills training with children: Proceed with caution. *Journal of Applied Behavior Analysis, 15*, 41–53.

Biederman, J., Munir, K., Knee, D., Armentano, M., Autor, S., Waternaux, C., & Tsuang, M. (1987). High rate of affective disorders in probands with attention deficit disorder and in their relatives: A controlled family study. *American Journal of Psychiatry, 144*, 330–333.

Bond, C., & McMahon, R. J. (1984). Relationships between marital distress and child behavior problems, maternal personal adjustment, maternal personality, and maternal parenting behavior. *Journal of Abnormal Psychology, 93*, 348–351.

Boyle, M. H., & Offord, D. R. (1990). Primary prevention of conduct disorder: Issues and prospects. *Journal of the American Academy of Child and Adolescent Psychiatry, 29*, 227–233.

Campbell, S. B., & Ewing, L. J. (1990). Follow-up of hard to manage preschoolers: Adjustment at age 9 and predictors of continuing symptoms. *Journal of Child Psychology and Psychiatry, 31*, 871–890.

Campbell, S. B., Endman, M., & Bernfield, G. (1977). A three year follow-up of hyperactive preschoolers into elementary school. *Journal of Child Psychology and Psychiatry, 18*, 239–249.

Christensen, A., Phillips, S., Glasgow, R. E., & Johnson, S. M. (1983). Parental characteristics and interactional dysfunction in families with child behavior problems: A preliminary investigation. *Journal of Abnormal Child Psychology, 11*, 153–166.

Clark, M. L., Cheyne, J. A., Cunningham, C. E., & Siegel, L. S. (1988). Dyadic peer interaction and task orientation in attention-deficit-disordered children. *Journal of Abnormal Child Psychology, 16*, 1–15.

Cochran, M., & Brassard, J. A. (1979). Child development and personal social networks. *Child Development, 50*, 601–615.

Coleman, W., & Levine, M. (1988). Attention deficits in adolescence: Description, evaluation, and management. *Pediatrics in Review, 9*, 287–299.

Conners, C. K. (1989). *Feeding the brain: How foods affect children*. New York: Plenum Press.

Costello, E. J. (1989). Child psychiatric disorders and their correlates: A primary care pediatric sample. *Journal of the American Academy of Child and Adolescent Psychiatry, 28*, 851–855.

Costello, E. J., Costello, A. J., Edelbrock, C., Burns, B. J., Dulcan, M., Brent, D., & Janiszewski, S. (1988). Psychiatric disorders in pediatric primary care. *Archives of General Psychiatry, 45*, 1107–1116.

Cunningham, C. E., & Barkley, R. A. (1978a). The effects of Ritalin on the mother-child interactions of hyperactive identical twins. *Developmental Medicine and Child Neurology, 20*, 634–642.

Cunningham, C. E., & Barkley, R. A. (1978b). The role of academic failure in hyperactive behavior. *Journal of Learning Disabilities, 11*, 15–21.

Cunningham, C. E. (1989). A family-system-oriented training program for parents of language delayed children with behavior problems. In C. E. Schaefer & J. M. Breismeister (Eds.), *Handbook of parent training: Parents as cotherapists for children's behavior problems* (pp. 133–176). New York: Wiley.

Cunningham, C. E. (1990). A family systems approach to parent training. In R. A. Barkley (Ed.), *Attention deficit hyperactivity disorder: A handbook for diagnosis and treatment* (pp. 432–461). New York: Guilford Press.

Cunningham, C. E., & Barkley, R. A. (1979). The interactions of hyperactive and normal children with their mothers during free play and structured tasks. *Child Development, 50*, 217–224.

Cunningham, C. E., & Siegel, L. S. (1987). Peer interactions of normal and attention-deficit disordered boys during free-play, cooperative task, and simulated classroom situations. *Journal of Abnormal Child Psychology*, *15*, 247–268.

Cunningham, C. E., Siegel, C. S., & Offord, D. R. (1985). A developmental dose response analysis of the efforts of methylphenidate on the peer interactions of attention deficit disordered boys. *Journal of Child Psychology and Psychiatry*, *26*, 955–971.

Cunningham, C. E., Benness, B. B., & Siegel, L. S. (1988). Family functioning, time allocation, and parental depression in the families of normal and ADDH children. *Journal of Clinical Child Psychology*, *17*, 169–177.

Cunningham, C. E., Clark, M. C., Heaven, R. K., Dumant, J., & Cunningham, L. J. (1989). The effects of coping-modelling problem solving and contingency management procedures on the positive and negative interactions of learning disabled and attention deficit disordered children with an autistic peer. *Child and Family Behavior Therapy*, *11*, 89–106.

Cunningham, C. E., Bremner, B., & Secord-Gilbert, M. (1990). A family and community-systems-oriented course for parents of ADHD children. *Chadder*, *4*, 10–11, 26.

Dodge, K. A., McClaskey, C. L., & Feldman, E. (1985). A situational approach to the assessment of social competence in children. *Journal of Consulting and Clinical Psychology*, *53*, 344–353.

Douglas, V. I. (1980). Higher mental processes in hyperactive children. In R. M. Knights & D. J. Bakker (Eds.), *Treatment of hyperactive and learning disordered children* (pp. 65–92). Baltimore: University Park Press.

Douglas, V. I., Barr, R. G., O'Neill, M. E., & Britton, B. G. (1988). Dosage effects and individual responsivity to methylphenidate in attention deficit disorder. *Journal of Child Psychology and Psychiatry*, *29*, 453–475.

Dubey, D. R., O'Leary, S., & Kaufman, K. F. (1983). Training parents of hyperactive children in child management: A comparative outcome study. *Journal of Abnormal Child Psychology*, *11*, 229–246.

Dulcan, M. K. (1985). Attention deficit disorder: Evaluation and treatment. *Pediatric Annals*, *14*, 383–400.

Dumas, J. E. (1986). In direct influence of maternal social contacts on mother-child interactions: A setting event analysis. *Journal of Abnormal Child Psychology*, *14*, 205–216.

Dunst, C., Trivette, C., & Deal, A. (1988). *Enabling and empowering families: Principles and guidelines for practice*. Cambridge MA: Brookline Books.

DuPaul, G. J. (1990). *The Home and School Situations Questionnaires—Revised: Normative data, reliability, and validity*. Unpublished manuscript, University of Massachusetts Medical Center, Worcester.

Earls, F., & Jung, K. G. (1987). Temperament and home environment characteristics as causal factors in the early development of childhood psychopathology. *Journal of the American Academy of Child and Adolescent Psychiatry*, *26*, 491–498.

Edelbrock, C. S., & Rancurello, M. D. (1985). Childhood hyperactivity: An overview of rating scales and their applications. *Clinical Psychology Review*, *5*, 429–445.

Emery, R. E. (1982). Interparental conflict and the children of discord and divorce. *Psychological Bulletin*, *92*, 310–330.

Epstein, N. B., Baldwin, L. M., & Bishop, D. S. (1983). The McMaster Family Assessment Device. *Journal of Marital and Family Therapy*, *9*, 171–180.

Estroff, T. W., Herrera, C., Gaines, R., Shaffer, D., Gould, M., & Green, A. H. (1984). Maternal psychopathology and perception of child behavior in psychiatrically referred and child maltreatment families. *Journal of the American Academy of Child Psychiatry*, *23*, 649–652.

Fergusson, D. M., Horwood, L. J., Grettorn, M. E., & Shannon, F. T. (1985). Family Life events, maternal depression, and maternal and teacher descriptions of child behavior. *Pediatrics*, *75*, 30–35.

Firestone, P., & Witt, J. E. (1982). Characteristics of families completing and prematurely discontinuing a behavioral parent-training program. *Journal of Pediatric Psychology*, *7*, 209–222.

Firestone, P., Kelly, M. J., Goodman, J., & Davey, J. (1981). Differential effects of parent training and stimulant medication with hyperactive children. *Journal of the American Academy of Child Psychiatry*, *20*, 135–147.

Fischer, M., Barkley, R. A., Edelbrock, C. S., & Smallish, L. (1990). The adolescent outcome of hyperactive children diagnosed by research criteria: 2. Academic, attentional, and neuropsychological status. *Journal of Consulting and Clinical Psychology*, *58*, 580–588.

Forehand, R., & Atkeson, B. M. (1977). Generality of treatment effects with parents as therapists: A review of assessment and implementation procedures. *Behavior Therapy*, *8*, 575–593.

Forehand, R., Wells, K. C., McMahon, R. J., Griest, D., & Rogers, T. (1982). Maternal perceptions of maladjustment in clinic-referred children: An extension of earlier research. *Journal of Behavioral Assessment*, *4*, 145–151.

Friedlander, S., Weiss, D. S., & Taylor, J. (1986). Assessing the influence of maternal depression on the validity of the child behavior checklist. *Journal of Abnormal Child Psychology*, *14*, 123–133.

Gittelman, R., Abikoff, H., Pollack, E., Klein, D. F., Katz, S., & Mattes, J. (1980). A controlled trial of behavior modification and methylphenidate in hyperactive children. In C. K. Whalen & B. Henker (Eds.), *Hyperactive children: The social ecology of identification and treatment* (pp. 221–243). New York: Academic Press.

Goldstein, S. (1989). *Why won't my child pay attention? A video guide for parents of hyperactive and inattentive children.* Salt Lake City: Neurology, Learning & Behavior Center.

Goldstein, S., & Goldstein, M. (1987). *A teacher's guide: Attention-deficit hyperactivity disorder in children.* Salt Lake City: Neurology, Learning & Behavior Center.

Goldstein, S., & Goldstein, M. (1989). *A teacher's guide: Attention-deficit hyperactivity disorder in children.* Salt Lake City: Neurology, Learning & Behavior Center.

Goldstein, S., & Goldstein, M. (1990). *Educating inattentive children: A guide for the classroom.* Salt Lake City: Neurology, Learning & Behavior Center.

Goodman, R., & Stevenson, J. (1989). A twin study of hyperactivity: 2. The aetiological role of genes, family relationships and perinatal adversity. *Journal of Child Psychology and Psychiatry, 30,* 691–709.

Gordon, M. (1983). *The Gordon diagnostic system.* Boulder, CO: Clinical Diagnostic Systems.

Gordon, M. (1991). *ADHD/Hyperactivity: A consumer's guide for parents and teachers.* DeWitt: GSI Publications.

Gordon, M., & Mettelman, R. B. (1988). The assessment of attention: 1. Standardization and reliability of a behavior based measure. *Journal of Clinical Psychology, 44,* 682–690.

Greenwood, C. R., Delquadri, J. C., & Hall, R. V. (1989). Longitudinal effects of classwide peer tutoring. *Journal of Educational Psychology, 81,* 371–383.

Grenell, M. M., Glass, C. R., & Katz, K. S. (1987). Hyperactive children and peer interaction: Knowledge and performance of social skills. *Journal of Abnormal Child Psychology, 15,* 1–13.

Griest, D. L., Wells, K. C., & Forehand, R. (1979). An examination of predictors of maternal perceptions of maladjustment in clinic-referred children. *Journal of Abnormal Psychology, 88,* 277–281.

Gross, M. D. (1984). Effect of sucrose on hyperkinetic children. *Pediatrics, 74,* 876–878.

Haenlein, M., & Caul, W. F. (1987). Attention deficit disorder with hyperactivity: A specific hypothesis of reward dysfunction. *Journal of the American Academy of Child and Adolescent Psychiatry, 26,* 356–362.

Harley, J. P., Ray, R. S., Tomasi, L., Eichman, P. L., Matthews, C. G., Chun, R., Cleelund, C. S., & Traisman, E. (1981). Hyperkineses and food additives: Testing the Feingold hypothesis. *Pediatrics, 61,* 818–823.

Hastings, J. E., & Barkley, R. A. (1978). A review of psychophysiological research with hyperactive children. *Journal of Abnormal Child Psychology, 7,* 413–447.

Hinshaw, S. P., Henker, B., & Whalen, C. K. (1984). Cognitive-behavioral and pharmacologic interventions for hyperactive boys: Comparative and combined effects. *Journal of Consulting and Clinical Psychology, 52,* 739–749.

Hinshaw, S. P. (1987). On the distinction between attentional deficit/hyperactivity and conduct problems/aggression in child psychopathology. *Psychological Review, 101,* 443–463.

Humphries, T., Kinsbourne, N., & Swanson, J. (1978). Stimulant effects on cooperation and social interaction between hyperactive children and their mothers. *Journal of Child Psychology and Psychiatry, 19,* 13–22.

Hymel, S., Wagner, E., & Butler, L. J. (1992). Reputational bias: View from the peer group. In S. R. Asher & J. D. Coie (Eds.), *Peer rejection in childhood.* Cambridge: Cambridge University Press.

Jacobvitz, D., Sroufe, L. A. (1987). The early caregiver-child relationship and attention deficit disorder with hyperactivity in kindergarten: A prospective study. *Child Development, 58,* 1488–1495.

Johnston, C., Cunningham, C. E., & Hardy, C. L. (1988). A couples' parenting measure. Poster presented at the annual meeting of the Association for Advancement of Behavior Therapy.

Johnston, C., Pelham, W. E., & Murphy, H. (1985). Peer relationships in ADHD and normal children: A developmental analysis of peer and teacher ratings. *Journal of Abnormal Child Psychology, 13,* 89–100.

Jones, M. B., & Offord, D. R. (1989). Reduction of antisocial behavior in poor children by non-school skill development. *Journal of Child Psychology and Psychiatry, 30,* 737–750.

Kahn, D., & Gardner, G. (1975). Hyperactivity: Predominant diagnosis in child upheavals. *Frontiers of Psychiatry, 5,* 3.

Kanfer, F. J., & Phillips, J. S. (1970). *Learning foundations of behavior therapy.* New York: Wiley.

Kendall, P. C., & Braswell, L. (1985). *Cognitive-behavioral therapy for impulsive children.* New York: Guilford Press.

Kistner, J., White, K., Haskett, M., & Robbins, F. (1985). Development of learning-disabled and normally achieving children's causal attributions. *Journal of Abnormal Child Psychology, 13,* 639–347.

Lahey, B. B., Piacentini, J. C., McBurnett, K., Stone, P., Hartdagen, S., & Hynd, G. (1988). Psychopathology in the parents of children with conduct disorder and hyperactivity. *Journal of the American Academy of Child and Adolescent Psychiatry, 27,* 163–170.

Landau, S., & Milich, R. (1988). Social communication patterns of attention-deficit-disordered boys. *Journal of Abnormal Child Psychology, 16,* 69–81.

Landau, S., Milich, R., & Whitten, P. (1984). A comparison of teacher and peer assessment of social status. *Journal of Clinical Child Psychology, 13*, 44–49.

Leitenberg, H., Yost, L., & Carroll-Wilson, M. (1986). Negative cognitive errors in children: Questionnaire development, normative data, and comparisons between children with and without self-reported symptoms of depression, low self-esteem, and evaluation anxiety. *Journal of Consulting and Clinical Psychology, 54*, 328–536.

Locke, H. J., & Wallace, K. M. (1959). Short marital adjustment and prediction tests: Their reliability and validity. *Journal of Marriage and Family Living, 21*, 251–255.

Marine, E., & Cohen, R. (1975). The impact of a community mental health centre program on the operation of a university child guidance center. *Journal of the American Academy of Child Psychiatry, 14*, 49–65.

Marsh, H. E. (1988). *Self-description questionnaire: Vol. 1. Manual.* New York: The Psychological Corporation, Harcourt Brace Jovanovich.

Mash, E. J. (1989). Treatment of child and family disturbance: A behavioral-systems perspective. In E. J. Mash & R. A. Barkley (Eds.), *Treatment of childhood disorders* (pp. 3–36). New York: Guilford Press.

Mash, E. J., & Johnston, C. (1982). A comparison of the mother-child interactions of younger and older hyperactive and normal children. *Child Development, 53*, 1371–1381.

Mash, E. J., & Johnston, C. (1983). The prediction of mother's behavior with their hyperactive children during play and task situations. *Child and Family Behavior Therapy, 5*, 1–14.

Mash, E. J., & Terdal, L. G. (1988). *Behavioral assessment of childhood disorders* (2nd ed.). New York: Guilford Press.

McGee, R., & Share, D. L. (1988). Attention deficit disorder-hyperactivity and academic failure: Which comes first and what should be treated? *Journal of the American Academy of Child and Adolescent Psychiatry, 27*, 318–325.

McGee, R., Silva, P. A., & Williams, S. (1984a). Behaviour problems in a population of seven-year-old children: Prevalence, stability and types of disorder—A research report. *Journal of Child Psychology and Psychiatry, 25*, 251–259.

McGee, R., Williams, S., & Silva, P. A. (1984b). Background characteristics of aggressive, hyperactive, and aggressive-hyperactive boys. *Journal of the American Academy of Child Psychiatry, 23*, 280–284.

McGee, R., Williams, S., & Silva, P. A. (1985). Factor structure and correlates of ratings of inattention, hyperactivity, and antisocial behavior in a large sample of 9-year-old children from the general population. *Journal of Consulting and Clinical Psychology, 53*, 480–490.

McGee, R., Williams, S., & Silva, P. A. (1987). A comparison of girls and boys with teacher identified problems of attention. *Journal of the American Academy of Child and Adolescent Psychiatry, 26*, 711–717.

Meichenbaum, D., & Turk, D. C. (1987). *Facilitating treatment adherence: A practitioner's handbook.* New York: Plenum Press.

Mendelson, W., Johnson, N., & Stewart, M. A. (1971). Hyperactive children as teenagers: A follow-up study. *Journal of Nervous and Mental Disease, 153*, 273–279.

Milich, R., & Landau, S. (1982). Socialization and peer relations in hyperactive children. In K. D. Gadow & I. Bialer (Eds.), *Advances in learning and behavioral disabilities* (Vol. 1, pp. 283–339). Greenwich, CT: JAI Press.

Milich, R. S., & Pelham, W. E. (1986). Effects of sugar ingestion on the classroom and playgroup behavior of attention deficit disordered boys. *Journal of Consulting and Clinical Psychology, 54*, 714–718.

Minde, K., Webb, G., & Sykes, D. (1968). Studies on the hyperactive child: 6. Prenatal and perinatal factors associated with hyperactivity. *Developmental Medicine and Child Neurology, 10*, 355–363.

O'Leary, S. G., & Pelham, W. E. (1978). Behavior therapy and withdrawal of stimulant reduction with hyperactive children. *Pediatrics, 61*, 211–217.

Owing-West, N., & Prinz, R. J. (1987). Parental alcoholism and childhood psychopathology. *Psychological Bulletin, 102*, 204–218.

Ownby, R. L., & Matthews, C. G. (1985). On the meaning of the WISC-R third factor: Relations to selected neuropsychological measures. *Journal of Consulting and Clinical Psychology, 53*, 531–534.

Palfrey, J. S., Levine, M. D., Walker, D. K., & Sullivan, M. (1985). The emergence of attention deficits in early childhood: A prospective study. *Developmental and Behavioral Pediatrics, 6*, 339–348.

Panaccione, V. F., & Wahler, R. G. (1986). Child behavior, maternal depression, and social coercion as factors in the quality of child care. *Journal of Abnormal Child Psychology, 14*, 263–278.

Parker, J. G., & Asher, S. R. (1987). Peer relations and later personal adjustment: Are low-accepted children at risk? *Psychological Bulletin, 102*, 357–389.

Patterson, G. R. (1982). *Coercive family process.* Eugene, OR: Castalia.

Patterson, G. R., & Forgatch, M. S. (1985). Therapist behavior as a determinant for client noncompliance: A paradox for behavior modification. *Journal of Consulting and Clinical Psychology, 53*, 846–851.

Pelham, W. E., & Bender, M. E. (1982). Peer relationships in hyperactive children: Description and treatment. In K. D. Gadow & I. Bialer (Eds.), *Advances in learning and behavioral disabilities* (Vol. 1, pp., 365–436). Greenwich, CT: JAI Press.

Pelham, W. E., & Hinshaw, S. P. (1992). Behavioral intervention for attention deficit-hyperactivity disorder. In S. Turner, K. Calhoun, & H. Adams (Eds.), *Handbook of clinical behavior therapy*. New York: Wiley.

Pelham, W. E., & Milich, R. (1984). Peer relations in children with hyperactivity/attention deficit disorder. *Journal of Learning Disabilities, 17*, 560–567.

Pelham, W. E., Schnedler, R. W., Bologna, N., & Contreras, A. (1980). Behavioral and stimulant treatment of hyperactive children: A therapy study with methylphenidate probes in a within-subject design. *Journal of Applied Behavior Analysis, 13*, 221–236.

Pelham, W. E., Milich, R., & Walker, J. (1986). The effects on continuous and partial reinforcement and methylphenidate on learning in children with attention deficit disorder. *Journal of Abnormal Psychology, 95*, 319–325.

Pelham, W. E., McBurnett, K., Harper, G. W., Murphy, D. A., Milich, R., Clinton, J., & Thiele, C. (1990). Methylphenidate and baseball playing in ADD children: Who's on first? *Journal of Consulting and Clinical Psychology, 58*, 130–133.

Pelham, B., Gnagy, E. M., Greenslade, K. E., & Milich, R. (1992). Teacher rated DSM-III-R symptoms of the disruptive behavior disorders. *Journal of the American Academy of Child Psychiatry, 31*, 210–218.

Pfiffner, L. J., & O'Leary, S. G. (1990). Educational placement and classroom management. In R. A. Backley (Ed.), *Attention deficit hyperactivity disorder: A handbook for diagnosis and treatment* (pp. 498–539). New York: Guilford Press.

Pfiffner, L. J., Rosen, L. A., & O'Leary, S. G. (1985). The efficacy of an all-positive approach to classroom management. *Journal of Applied Behavior Analysis, 18*, 257–261.

Pisterman, S., McGrath, P. J., Firestone, P., Goodman, J. T., Webster, I., & Mallory, R. (1989). Outcome of parent-mediated treatment of preschoolers with attention deficit disorder with hyperactivity. *Journal of Consulting and Clinical Psychology, 57*, 628–635.

Pollard, S., Ward, E. M., & Barkley, R. A. (1983). The effects of parent training and Ritalin on the parent-child interactions of hyperactive boys. *Child and Family Therapy, 5*, 51–69.

Rapport, M. D., Murphy, H. A., & Bailey, J. S. (1982). Ritalin vs. response cost in the control of hyperactive children: A within-subject comparison. *Journal of Applied Behavior Analysis, 15*, 205–216.

Reeves, J. C., Werry, J., Elkind, G. J., & Zametkin, A. (1987). Attention deficit, conduct, oppositional, and anxiety disorders in children: 2. Clinical characteristics. *Journal of the American Academy of Child and Adolescent Psychiatry, 26*, 133–143.

Richardson, E., Kupietz, S. S., Winsberg, B. G., Maitinsky, S., & Mendell, N. (1988). Effects of methylphenidate dosage in hyperactive reading disabled children: 2. Reading achievement. *Journal of American Academy of Child and Adolescent Psychiatry, 27*, 78–87.

Rickard, K. M., Forehand, R., Wells, K. C., Griest, D. L., & McMahon, R. J. (1981). Factors in the referral of children for behavioral treatment: A comparison of mothers of clinic-referred deviant, clinic-referred non-deviant, and nonclinic children. *Behavior Research and Therapy, 19*, 201–205, 132.

Robin, A. L. (1990). Training families of ADHD adolescents. In R. A. Barkley (Ed.), *Attention deficit hyperactivity disorder: A handbook for diagnosis and treatment* (pp. 462–497). New York: Guilford.

Robin, A. L., Schneider, M., & Dolnick, J. (1976). The turtle technique: An extensive case study of self-control in the classroom. *Psychology in the Schools, 1*, 449–459.

Robinson, P. W., Newby, T. J., & Ganzell, S. L. (1981). A token system for a class of underachieving children. *Journal of Applied Behavior Analysis, 14*, 307–335.

Rosen, L. A., O'Leary, S. G., Joyce, S. A., Conway, G., & Pfiffner, L. J. (1984). The importance of prudent negative consequences for maintaining the appropriate behavior of hyperactive students. *Journal of Abnormal Child Psychology, 12*, 581–604.

Satterfield, J. H., Satterfield, B. T., & Cantwell, D. P. (1981). Three-year multimodality treatment study of 100 hyperactive boys. *Journal of Pediatrics, 98*, 650–655.

Schacher, R., Sandberg, S., & Rutter, M. (1986). Agreement between teachers' ratings and observations of hyperactivity, inattentiveness and defiance. *Journal of Abnormal Child Psychology, 14*, 331–345.

Schaughency, E. A., & Lahey, B. B. (1985). Mothers' and fathers' perceptions of child deviance: Roles of child behavior, parental depression, and marital satisfaction. *Journal of Consulting and Clinical Psychology, 53*, 718–723.

Shaffer, D., & Greenhill, L. (1979). A critical note on the predictive validity of "the hyperkinetic syndrome." *Journal of Child Psychology and Psychiatry*, *20*, 61–72.

Sleator, E. K., & Ullmann, R. K. (1981). Can the physician diagnose hyperactivity in the office? *Pediatrics*, *67*, 13–17.

Sobol, M. P., Ashbourne, D. T., Earn, B. M., & Cunningham, C. E. (1989). Parents' attributions for achieving compliance for attention-deficit disordered children. *Journal of Abnormal Child Psychology*, *17*, 359–369.

Speltz, M. L., Varley, C. K., Peterson, K., & Beilke, R. L. (1988). Effect of dextroamphetamine and contingency management on a preschooler with ADHD and oppositional deficient disorder. *Journal of American Academy of Child and Adolescent Psychiatry*, *27*, 175–178.

Streissguth, A. P., Martin, D. C., Barr, H. M., Sandman, B. M., Kirchner, G. L., & Darby, B. L. (1984). Intrauterine alcohol and nicotine exposure: Attention and reaction time in 4-year old children. *Developmental Psychology*, *20*, 533–541.

Sullivan, M. A., & O'Leary, S. G. (1989). Differential maintenance following reward and cost token programs with children. *Behavior Therapy*, *21*, 139–151.

Szatmari, P., Boyle, M., & Offord, D. R. (1989a). ADDH and conduct disorder: Degree of diagnostic overlap and differences among correlates. *Journal of the American Academy of Child and Adolescent Psychiatry*, *28*, 865–872.

Szatmari, P., Offord, D. R., & Boyle, M. H. (1989b). Ontario child health study: Prevalence of attention deficit disorder with hyperactivity. *Journal of Child Psychology and Psychiatry*, *30*, 219–230.

Szatmari, P., Offord, D. R., & Boyle, M. H. (1989c). Correlates, associated impairments and patterns of service utilization of children with attention deficit disorder: Findings from the Ontario child health study. *Journal of Child Psychology and Psychiatry*, *30*, 205–217.

Taylor, E., Schachar, R., Thorley, G., & Wieselberg, M. (1986). Conduct disorder and hyperactivity: separation of hyperactivity and anti-social conduct in British child psychiatric patients. *British Journal of Psychiatry*, *149*, 760–764.

Wahler, R. G. (1980). The insular mother: Her problems in parent-child treatment. *Journal of Applied Behavior Analysis*, *13*, 207–219.

Webster-Stratton, C., & Hammond, M. (1988). Material depression and its relationship to life stress, perceptions of child behavior problems, parenting behaviors, and child conduct problems. *Journal of Abnormal Child Psychology*, *16*, 299–315.

Weiss, G., & Hechtman, L. T. (1986). *Hyperactive children grown up: Empirical findings and theoretical considerations*. New York: Guilford Press.

Whalen, C. K., Henker, B., Collins, B. E., McAuliffe, S., & Vaux, A. (1979). Peer interaction in structured communication task: Comparisons of normal and hyperactive boys and of methylphenidate (Ritalin) and placebo effects. *Child Development*, *50*, 388–401.

Whalen, C. K., Henker, B., & Dotemoto, S. (1980). Methylphenidate and hyperactivity: Effects on teacher behaviors. *Science*, *208*, 1280–1282.

Whalen, C. K., Henker, B., Dotemoto, S., & Hinshaw, S. P. (1983). Child and adolescent perceptions of normal and atypical peers. *Child Development*, *54*, 1588–1598.

Whalen, C. K., Henker, B., Buhrmester, D., Hinshaw, S. P., Huber, A., & Laski, K. (1989). Does stimulant medication improve the peer status of hyperactive children? *Journal of Consulting and Clinical Psychology*, *57*, 545–549.

Wolraich, M., Milich, R., Stumbo, P., & Schultz, F. (1985). The effects of sucrose ingestion on the behavior of hyperactive boys. *Pediatrics*, *106*, 675–682.

Wyckoff, J., & Unell, B. C. (1984). *Discipline without shouting or spanking: Practical solutions to the most common preschool behavior problems*. Deephaven, MN: Meadowbrook.

Zametkin, A. L., & Rapoport, J. L. (1987). Neurobiology of attention deficit disorder with hyperactivity: Where have we come in 50 years? *Journal of the American Academy of Child and Adolescent Psychiatry*, *26*, 676–686.

Zametkin, A. L., Nordahl, T. E., Gross, M., King, C., Semple, W. E., Rumsey, J., Hamburger, S., & Cohen, R. M. (1990). Cerebral glucose metabolism in adults with hyperactivity of childhood onset. *The New England Journal of Medicine*, *323*, 1361–1366.

26

Conduct and Oppositional Disorders

MARC S. ATKINS and MARY L. OSBORNE

INTRODUCTION

Childhood antisocial behavior is a common problem with no single etiology or treatment. Estimates of prevalence rates range from 4% to 10%, and one third to one half of child and adolescent referrals to outpatient clinics include primary symptoms of antisocial, disruptive, or aggressive behaviors (Reeves, Werry, Elkind, & Zametkin, 1987; Rutter, Tizard, & Whitmore, 1970). Surveys of adolescent youth indicate that approximately 50% admit to theft, 35% admit to assault, 45% admit to property destruction, and as many as 60% admit to engaging in multiple antisocial acts (Kazdin, 1987a). Epidemiological studies indicate that antisocial behavior is stable over time and across generations and has a poor long-term prognosis (Huesmann, Eron, Lefkowitz, & Walder, 1984; Magnusson, Statlin, & Duner, 1983).

However, there is considerable evidence that conduct-problem children represent a heterogeneous group. Numerous factors contribute to the pervasiveness and intractability of childhood conduct problems. The most important of these are related psychiatric comorbidity, family history and family functioning, peer relations, and response topography.

Psychiatric Comorbidity

The most prominent concurrent diagnosis with conduct problems is Attention-Deficit Hyperactivity Disorder. Diagnostic overlap ranges from 30% to 60% depending on age, sex, and primary symptoms (Szatmari, Boyle, & Offord, 1989). Loney and colleagues (Loney, 1987; Loney & Milich, 1982) were the first to recognize the independent contributions of hyperactivity and aggression to etiology and course of treatment. There is considerable evidence that hyperactive children with concurrent aggression represent a distinct subgroup of behavior-disordered children (Hinshaw, 1987). For example, boys with co-occurring hyperactivity and

---

MARC S. ATKINS and MARY L. OSBORNE • University of Pennsylvania School of Medicine and Department of Pediatric Psychology, Children's Hospital of Philadelphia and Children's Seashore House, Philadelphia, Pennsylvania 19104.

Handbook of Behavior Therapy in the Psychiatric Setting, edited by Alan S. Bellack and Michel Hersen. Plenum Press, New York, 1993.

delinquency had greater family dysfunction, lower intelligence, and worse school performance than pure groups of hyperactive or delinquent boys (Moffitt, 1990). In addition, social competency may represent a core deficit for hyperactive-aggressive boys, as evidenced by higher rates of social-information-processing biases and a greater risk for future peer problems than boys who are hyperactive only (Johnston & Pelham, 1986; Milich & Dodge, 1984).

A second factor affecting the course and severity of conduct problems is learning problems and cognitive deficits. Longitudinal investigations revealed that delinquent adolescents had significantly lower IQs in early childhood than nondelinquents (Moffitt & Silva, 1988; White, Moffitt, & Silva, 1989). In addition, high IQ protected boys from the development of delinquency, even those who were at risk by virtue of parental history of antisocial behavior (White et al., 1989). The protection provided by IQ may be related to long-term prospects for school success (Feshbach & Price, 1984). For example, current academic dysfunction appeared to be more highly related to conduct problems than was low IQ (Kandel, Mednick, Kirkegaard-Sorensen, Hutchings, Knop, Rosenberg, & Schulsinger, 1988). Similarly, academic skill deficits were found to be the strongest covariate of adolescent antisocial behavior when they were evaluated in combination with interpersonal and work skills (Dishion, Loeber, Stouthamer-Loeber, & Patterson, 1984).

A third comorbid factor in conduct problems is depression. Conduct-disordered youth high in self-reported depression also reported higher rates of conduct problems and personality problems than conduct-disordered youth low in depression (Nieminen & Matson, 1989). Surveys of assaultive youth indicate a more than fourfold increase in suicide incidence in this population than in the general population (Cairns, Peterson, & Neckerman, 1988). As expected, aggressive youth who were suicidal were significantly more depressed than aggressive youth who were nonsuicidal (Pfeffer, Plutchik, & Mizruchi, 1983).

Family History and Family Functioning

Family factors that are related to the occurrence of delinquency in adolescence are the level of family support, marital adjustment, and social stress (Loeber & Dishion, 1983; Olweus, 1980; Tolan, 1988; Webster-Stratton & Hammond, 1990). However, when parental antisocial behavior and family functioning are considered concurrently, parental antisocial behavior is a stronger predictor of conduct problems in offspring than are divorce or marital satisfaction (Frick, Lahey, Hartdagen, & Hynd, 1989; Lahey, Hartdagen, Frick, McBurnett, Connor, & Hynd, 1988).

Another way in which parental antisocial behavior interacts with family functioning is through parenting skills. Parenting practice is among the most well-established factors influencing childhood conduct problems. Specifically, harsh and inconsistent parenting is highly predictive of aggressiveness in children, as is physical abuse or neglect (Dodge, Bates, & Pettit, 1990a; Gardner, 1989; Henggeler, McKee, & Borduin, 1989; Patterson, 1986).

Peer Relations

Social competency has been proposed as a core deficit of many aggressive children (Coie, Belding, & Underwood, 1988). Compared to nonaggressive children, socially rejected, aggressive children perceive more hostile intentions from others in ambiguous situations, minimize their perceptions of their own aggressiveness, and exaggerate the aggressiveness of their peers (Dodge, Pettit, McClaskey, & Brown, 1986; Lochman, 1987). These social-information-processing deficits form the basis of a subtyping model that distinguishes proactive aggression (e.g., bullying) from reactive aggression (e.g., overreaction to provocation); the latter presumably involves the most severe social cognitive deficits (Dodge & Coie, 1987). In a recent evaluation of this model in a population of juvenile offenders, reactive aggression was associated with aggression toward persons and violent antisocial acts, mediated by deficits in social problem solving (hostile attributional biases). In contrast, proactive aggression was related more to nonviolent crimes and socialized aggression (Dodge, Price, Bachorowski, & Newman, 1990b).

Peer relations are also implicated in the distinction between socialized and undersocialized aggression, which was originally derived from early factor-analytic studies of parent and teacher ratings (Quay, 1986). Socialized aggression involves delinquent activities pursued within the confines of the peer group. Theoretically, such youths do not have poor social skills *per se*; rather, the deficit is poor judgment. Conversely, undersocialized aggression occurs without significant peer support and presumably is often associated with social skill deficits.

Response Topography

Loeber and colleagues have identified two extremes of childhood antisocial behavior: covert antisocial behaviors that occur outside the supervision of adults (e.g., lying, stealing, and drug and alcohol use) and overt antisocial behaviors that occur in confrontation with adults or peers (e.g., assault and temper tantrums). These bipolar dimensions were identified in a meta-analysis of studies evaluating antisocial behavior in children (Loeber & Schmaling, 1985b), and in an empirical evaluation of 195 boys aged 10–17 (Loeber & Schmaling, 1985a). In the latter study, three relatively distinct subgroups of antisocial behavior were identified: the exclusive fighter group (overt antisocial behaviors), the exclusive theft group (covert antisocial behaviors), and the versatile antisocial group (both overt and covert antisocial behaviors).

Important differences are associated with the subtypes. The early onset of aggressive symptoms, though associated with the severity of the symptoms (Tolan, 1987), is not highly predictive of long-term outcome. In contrast, early covert activity is strongly associated with a worse prognosis (Loeber, 1985). In addition, as expected, the versatile antisocial group had the poorest long-term prognosis of the three groups (Loeber & Schmaling, 1985b).

DIAGNOSIS OF CONDUCT AND OPPOSITIONAL DISORDERS

Significant advances have evolved from the two latest revisions of the *Diagnostic and Statistical Manual of Mental Disorders* (DSM), the standard for psychiatric diagnoses in the United States (American Psychiatric Association, 1980, 1987). The revised third edition (DSM-III-R; APA, 1987) subsumes antisocial behavior under the general rubric of Disruptive Behavior Disorders. Specific criteria differentiate noncompliance and defiance toward authorities (Oppositional Defiant Disorders or ODD) and behavior that violates the rights of others, especially peers (Conduct Disorders or CD). CD is further subtyped according to whether these behaviors occur alone (Solitary Aggressive type), in the presence of peers (Group type), or both (Undifferentiated type).

A diagnosis of CD is made when a youth has displayed a disturbance of conduct for at least six months and meets 3 of 13 criteria. These criteria represent a wide range of behaviors in terms of symptomatology and severity (e.g., lying, physical cruelty, and using a weapon). ODD is viewed as being less severe than CD and is not considered if a diagnosis of CD is made. The ODD diagnosis is made when a disturbance of conduct has been present for at least six months and five of nine criteria are met (e.g., loses temper, swearing, and argues).

Although both the CD and the ODD criteria are more specific than past diagnostic criteria for these disorders, several problems remain. For one, the criteria were rationally, rather than empirically, derived. For example, overt and covert acts are combined in CD despite evidence that they have unique developmental pathways (Loeber, 1985). Second, ODD appears more closely related to Attention-Deficit Hyperactivity Disorder than to CD, so that the ODD and CD diagnoses may not be mutually exclusive (Reeves *et al.*, 1987).

Other problems with the diagnostic criteria are low interrater reliability, ambiguous wording of many core symptoms, and covariation among items both within and across categories (Kazdin, 1987a; Werry, Methven, Fitzpatrick, & Dixon, 1983). In addition, the criteria are specific but not operationalized. For example, it is not clear how to determine symptom presence or how to resolve differences across sources (e.g., parents and teachers). Especially important in its omission is the lack of specific measurement strategies and cutoff scores for diagnoses. Almost universally, the development of empirically derived, standardized, and explicit diagnostic criteria for childhood antisocial behavior has been advocated for both research and clinical practice (e.g., Achenbach, 1985; Kazdin, 1987a; Loney, 1987; McMahon, 1987; Quay, Routh, & Shapiro, 1987).

Prototypical Assessment

The heterogeneity associated with samples of conduct-problem children gives further evidence of the inadequacy of current psychiatric classification (Kazdin, 1987b). However, in part, this heterogeneity is also due to the difficulty of obtaining information that accurately reflects the complexity of antisocial behavior in the natural environment. Given the multitude of factors that have demonstrated relevance to the onset and maintenance of childhood conduct problems, assessment is a difficult and often ambiguous task. Multiple assessment strategies are often recommended, including direct observations and ratings by parents, teachers, and peers (e.g., Fergusson & Horwood, 1987; Loney & Milich, 1982; McMahon, 1987). However, there is currently no standard procedure for using these measures concurrently to yield an accurate assessment (Kazdin, 1987a).

One approach that illustrates the utility of multiple measurement strategies is the multiple gating technique for the large-scale screening of conduct problems (Loeber, Dishion, & Patterson, 1984). This approach consists of three increasingly intensive assessments. The first "gate" involves standardized ratings on a global instrument of externalizing disorder. We have used an 11-item scale for teachers developed specifically for this purpose. Several alternative scales are available, each well developed in regard to psychometric properties (e.g., Achenbach & Edelbrock, 1986; Burns & Owen, 1990; Gresham & Elliott, 1990; Pelham, Milich, Murphy, & Murphy, 1989; Quay & Peterson, 1987). In addition, peer ratings have also been used for large-scale conduct-problem screening (e.g., Coie, Rabiner, & Lochman, 1989).

The second "gate" consists of a telephone interview that asks the parent to assess conduct problems at home for those children identified as above the cutoff for conduct problems. The most extensive, and expensive, screening measure is reserved for the third "gate." An interview with the child and the parents about family-management practices is reserved for those children identified at the second screening as exhibiting conduct problems at school and at home.

On completion of the multiple gating procedure, a child identified as exhibiting sufficient conduct problems to warrant intervention requires further assessment. In this phase, the goal of assessment is to gather a wide breadth of information relevant to developing an individualized treatment (Hayes, Nelson, & Jarrett, 1987). As noted, multiple measures are often recommended for this purpose to offset the limitations of any single measure or source. For example, rating scales are an efficient and cost-effective means of providing standardized impressions of the type and frequency of conduct problems across multiple sources of information, such as parent and teacher reports and self-reports. However, because the ratings are subjective, they are liable to show possible bias (Schachar, Sandberg, & Rutter, 1986). In contrast to ratings, behavioral observations provide specific information about target behaviors using clearly defined measures with low inference on the part of the observers. However, direct observations are more expensive and more time-consuming than ratings. In addition, direct observations are not appropriate for low-rate but persistent aggression or covert delinquent activities (Atkins, Pelham, & Licht, 1988; Patterson & Bank, 1986). These shortcomings are especially prominent in outpatient settings. In inpatient settings, direct observations may be more feasible as part of an ongoing multivariate assessment that identifies the situational factors that influence the target behaviors (Charlebois, Tremblay, Gagnon, Larivee, & Laurent, 1989; Kolko, Loar, & Sturnick, 1990).

ACTUAL ASSESSMENT

John was a 14-year-old male with a 9-year history of behavior problems. He was referred for treatment because of school truancy and academic underachievement. Referral for treatment was solicited by his parents when he was suspended from parochial school.

Response Topography

The primary symptoms of antisocial and aggressive behavior were assessed through interviews and standardized rating scales. The Child Behavior Checklist (CBCL; Achenbach & Edelbrock, 1983) was completed by the parents, and self-report version, the Youth Self-Report Scale, was completed by John. The CBCL was selected as it is a well-validated broad-band scale for identifying externalizing and internalizing behaviors. John's homeroom teacher completed the Teacher Report Form of the Child Behavior Checklist (Achenbach & Edelbrock, 1986), a teacher scale that parallels the CBCL. In addition, open-ended interviews were conducted with all of the informants (i.e., John, his parents, and his teacher).

The results of the rating scales and the open-ended interviews revealed a very strong weighting on the covert dimension as evidenced by truancy, stealing without confrontation, lying, alcohol abuse, and elopement. On the overt dimension, John was infrequently exhibiting mildly assaultive behaviors.

Psychiatric Comorbidity

CBCL Internalizing factors were elevated on items indicating depression based on parent and teacher report. This diagnosis was later confirmed by an independent interview during a psychiatric hospitalization. During this hospitalization, psychoeducational testing was also conducted, which revealed significant learning deficits despite superior intellectual capability. John was identified by all sources as inattentive and impulsive. Thus, in addition to a DSM-III-R diagnosis of Conduct Disorder, Group Type, John met the additional criteria for Major Depression, Attention-Deficit Hyperactivity Disorder (ADHD), and Learning Disabilities.

Family Functioning

Family functioning was assessed through clinical interviews with John and his parents. The family was intact but quite distressed by John's behavior and what appeared to be clear defiance of parental authority. However, in other respects, the family appeared to be functioning reasonably well, despite John's troubles. This finding suggested potential resources for change once his antisocial activities had been controlled. John's parents were both working, had many friends, and were without significant marital conflict. Our assessment also revealed two important risk factors that required intervention: (1) John was essentially unmonitored during and after school, and (2) his parents were increasingly giving harsh and inconsistent discipline, which, at times, became physically abusive.

Peer Relations

John's peer relations were assessed through interviews with John, his teacher, his school counselor, and his parents. All of the interviews revealed that John had many friends but that he was eager to be accepted by high-status peers. On entering high school, he had joined a group of peers who, by the school counselor's report, were engaged in drug and alcohol abuse. It was apparent that John's antisocial activities were largely maintained by peer attention.

In addition, an assessment of John's social relations gave little evidence of a primary social skills deficit. Rather, John was using poor judgment in his choice of friends and activities. Based on interviews with him, it became clear that the choice point for truancy and drug use occurred in the morning on his way to school. In short, he was unable to resist peer pressure to conform to the group's norms, despite escalating parental punishment and anger. This point highlights the importance of situational factors in the assessment and treatment of peer relation difficulties (Coie & Koeppl, 1990; Dodge, McClaskey, & Feldman, 1985).

PROTOTYPICAL TREATMENT

The complexity and variety of conduct problems typically require a multimodal treatment. However, without question, the most well-documented treatment for childhood conduct problems is training the parents. Parent-training programs have been developed for a wide array of target problems, consistent with the variety of problems labeled as conduct disorders. Generally, the goals of parent-training programs are to increase positive attention, reduce harsh punishment, increase consistency, and improve communication (Forehand & Long, 1988; Patterson, 1986; Sayger, Horne, Walker, & Passmore, 1988).

However, parent training is often a necessary but insufficient treatment. Another treatment component administered concurrently with psychosocial interventions is psychostimulant medication (Pelham & Murphy, 1986). In evaluations of CD children with ADHD, stimulant medication yielded positive effects on aggression as well as on inattention and impulsivity (Gadow, Nolan, Sverd, Sprafkin, & Paolicelli, 1990; Kaplan, Busner, Kupietz, Wassermann, & Segal, 1990; Klorman, Brumaghin, Salzman, Strauss, Borgstedt, McBride, & Loeb, 1988). However, positive effects on conduct problems when symptoms of ADHD are not present have not been evaluated. For explosive forms of aggression, one report found lithium to be the drug of choice (Campbell, Small, Green, Jennings, Perry, Bennett, & Anderson, 1984).

Another common component of the successful treatment of conduct problems is a school-based intervention that remediates academic deficits (e.g., Coie & Krehbiel, 1984). A recent study, which is especially relevant to training in academic skills, documented the benefits of a reward-based intervention that targeted the attentional capacities of delinquents (Scerbo, Raine, O'Brien, Chan, Rhee, & Smiley, 1990). For elementary-school children who are aggressive, contingency management procedures, such as response cost, are often necessary adjuncts to treatment (e.g., Forman, 1980).

Inpatient or residential treatment is often needed in the management of severe-conduct-problem children and adolescents. Most settings use either a structured milieu or a token or level system and also incorporate individual, group, and family psychotherapy (Drabman, Jarvie, & Hammer, 1978). Most, if not all, also include some form of time-out procedure. With the more severely behaviorally disordered, a seclusion room may be necessary to manage escalating acting-out behavior (Antoinette, Iyengar, & Puig-Antich, 1990).

It is important to highlight the distinction between time-out and seclusion, as the two terms are often used interchangeably. Seclusion is a punishment procedure or a means of minimizing injury when a patient is acutely assaultive. Time-out, in contrast, is an extinction procedure in which all reinforcement is removed for a specified amount of time immediately following a target behavior (Lochman, White, Curry, & Rumer, 1992).

A recent report from a large state hospital for children and adolescents highlights the distinction between time-out and locked-door seclusion. Whereas guidelines for time-out rarely exceed durations of 30 minutes for adolescents (e.g., Drabman *et al.*, 1978), in this state hospital the average length of seclusion was over five hours (Atkins & Ricciuti, in press). Furthermore, about 15% of the patients accounted for over 70% of all the episodes leading to seclusion and almost 90% of the time spent in seclusion. Not surprisingly, the children and adolescents secluded at the highest rate were also most likely to have a diagnosis of Conduct Disorder or Oppositional Defiant Disorder with concurrent Attention-Deficit Hyperactivity Disorder.

In both inpatient and outpatient settings, cognitive behavioral therapies (CBT) have been implemented to modify specific behaviors or patterns of behavior in antisocial or aggressive youth. A common goal of CBT programs for conduct-problem youth is to change the cognitive processing of frustrating and provocative situations (Lochman *et al.*, 1992). A strength of CBT is its flexibility in targeting functional deficits in heterogeneous groups. CBT incorporates a wide variety of behavioral and cognitive techniques, such as social perspective taking, social problem solving, and training in specific social skills (Michelson, 1987). The effectiveness of CBT in inpatient settings has been evaluated in several controlled clinical trials (Kazdin, Bass, Siegel, & Thomas, 1989; Kazdin, Esveldt-Dawson, French, & Unis, 1987a, b; Kolko *et al.*, 1990). The results were promising in demonstrating significant reductions in maladaptive and aggressive behaviors. However, as these authors have noted, the findings have not been replicated consistently, nor have behaviors been modified into the normal range. Thus, at best, CBT is one component of a successful treatment but is not itself a sufficient treatment.

A variation on the CBT framework that includes both cognitive behavioral strategies and social skills training is aggression replacement training for delinquents (Glick & Goldstein, 1987). The focus of this approach is anger control training. Again, these authors found a reduction in staff ratings of acting-out behavior. However, the findings were not replicated in a second facility. This failure of replication may indicate that the treatment is less robust than first thought or may reflect the heterogeneity of patient groups across settings.

ACTUAL TREATMENT

Initially, John was seen individually and with his family in outpatient treatment. In addition, separate sessions with John's parents focused on establishing a consistent and positive approach to discipline, decreasing the emphasis on punishers, and encouraging problem solving in place of harsh discipline (Sayger *et al.*, 1988). Arrangements were made for John's parents to contact his school guidance counselor weekly to monitor his attendance as a way to increase their supervision of John's activities throughout the day. Weekly rewards in the form of weekend privileges were established for daily attendance.

Individual sessions with John involved supportive counseling, as well as social-problem-solving skills-training focused on teaching him to identify and avoid deviant peer-group pressure. Family meetings were held throughout the treatment as a way to share information among the family members and to foster improved communication. In addition to these sessions, a concurrent evaluation of stimulant medication was recommended to assess the possible additive effects of a behavioral and a pharmacological treatment (Atkins, Pelham, & White, 1990; Pelham & Murphy, 1986).

Initially, John's treatment progressed well. The school reported that he was attending class consistently, and he reported that a low dose of Ritalin (5 mg) improved his concentration. Weekly phone contact was maintained with the school counselor. John's parents were pleased by his progress but remained skeptical. After several months, John noted in his individual sessions that he had resumed school truancy by reporting to homeroom and leaving school shortly afterward. This admission came after he was suspected of stealing money from his parents. He seemed dejected and frightened. He had discontinued his medication, which, of course, served no useful purpose if he was not in school. At the height of his own and his parents' frustration and despair, psychiatric hospitalization was recommended to counter escalating truancy and alcohol abuse and to minimize the negative influence of his peer group.

Over the summer, John was admitted to a private psychiatric hospital for a 28-day inpatient stay on their adolescent drug and alcohol unit. The primary treatment modalities were group and individual psychotherapy, family therapy, and a school program. During his admission, John also attended an educational program for drug and alcohol abusers that incorporated the abstinence principles of Alcoholics Anonymous (AA).

John's initial response to his inpatient hospitalization was very favorable. He faithfully attended follow-up weekly group-therapy sessions in addition to his weekly outpatient sessions. Also, he became very active in AA and attended those meetings two or three times a week. When school began, he had renewed enthusiasm, and despite being in remedial classes because of past school failure, he expressed optimism that he would be able to attend class and perhaps advance to classes at his own grade level. At home, tensions were reduced, privileges were restored, and communication had improved. For example, John and his mother scheduled time to talk when not in crisis, and he and his father participated in several work-related father–son activities. Medicine was not reinstituted because of a concern about possible substance abuse.

During the next several months, John's individual sessions changed focus from peer-group issues to strategies that would enhance his attentional skills and self-control (e.g., Lochman, Burch, Curry, & Lampron, 1985). Sessions also focused on the prevention of relapse, not only to alcohol abuse but also to school truancy (cf. Marlatt, 1985). John took a part-time job after school with the goal of saving money for his first car. Nevertheless, despite these efforts, John was unable to overcome his boredom with school and to resist peer pressure to skip classes. His truancy triggered parental anger, which, in turn, led John to greater alienation. On a positive note, he focused his energy not on alcohol abuse and deviant peer interactions, but on earning more money by working overtime. It became clear that the school placement was not meeting his academic needs, and the goal for treatment was focused on identifying an alternative educational setting.

John had severed the link with his maladaptive peer group, and this progress was facilitated further by a school change. The new school was especially suited to John, as it included an accelerated program that allowed him to complete his high school degree in less than two years. Given his history of school failure, he appeared especially responsive to this increased motivation. Furthermore, he was able to establish relationships in a new peer group both in and out of school. In addition, family communication and support remained important assets for John, despite the significant family discord that was associated with his escalating behavior problems. It is unlikely, however, that they would have remained supportive without considerable efforts in parent-training sessions.

SUMMARY

Conduct problems in children and adolescents represent, in most cases, a chronic disorder with implications throughout the person's lifetime. Factors that influence the type and course of treatment have been summarized as relating to comorbidity, family functioning, peer relations, and symptomatology. Research is beginning to pinpoint effective strategies for specific conduct problems, but there is, as yet, no empirically validated systematic approach to all of the components of conduct problems (Kazdin, 1987b).

The case example was selected because it illustrates several important aspects of the treatment of childhood conduct problems. First, the importance of family support and peer-group influence was especially clear in this example. Second, the difficulty of monitoring and modifying covert activities hindered treatment for more than a year. Third, as is axiomatic in behavioral writings, multimodal assessment and treatment were clearly indicated. The complex interplay of learning problems, attentional deficits, and depression established the need for a multifocused treatment requiring considerable collaboration of the family, the school, and the inpatient and outpatient treatment teams. Medication played only a minor role in John's treatment, given the greater importance of elements in John's setting, such as parenting practices and peer-group influences.

The variable course of treatment, with intermittent periods of apparent success and failure, highlights the importance of long-term follow-up and the critical role of community-based interventions. In addition, this case illustrates the wide scope of conduct problems and the importance of refining the existing subtyping models to facilitate differential diagnosis and treatment efficacy.

REFERENCES

Achenbach, T. M. (1985). *Assessment and taxonomy of child and adolescent psychopathology*. Beverly Hills, CA: Sage.

Achenbach, T. M. & Edelbrock, C. S. (1983). *Manual for the Child Behavior Checklist*. Burlington: University of Vermont.

Achenbach, T. M. & Edelbrock, C. S. (1986). *Manual for the Teacher's Report Form and Teacher Version of the Child Behavior Profile*. Burlington: Department of Psychiatry, University of Vermont.

American Psychiatric Association. (1980). *Diagnostic and statistical manual of mental disorders* (3rd ed.; DSM-III). Washington, DC: Author.

American Psychiatric Association. (1987). *Diagnostic and statistical manual of mental disorders* (3rd ed., rev.; DSM-III-R). Washington, DC: Author.

Antoinette, T., Iyengar, S., & Puig-Antich, J. (1990). Is locked door seclusion necessary for children under the age of 14? *American Journal of Psychiatry, 147*, 1283–1289.

Atkins, M. S. & Ricciuti, A. (in press). *Characteristics of locked door seclusion in a children's psychiatric hospital, Residential Treatment for Children and Youth*.

Atkins, M. S., Pelham, W. E., & Licht, M. H. (1988). The development and validation of objective classroom measures for conduct and attention deficit disorders. In R. J. Prinz (Ed.), *Advances in behavioral assessment of children and families* (Vol. 4, pp. 3–31). Greenwich, CT: JAI Press.

Atkins, M. S., Pelham, W. E., & White, K. J. (1990). Hyperactivity and attention deficit disorders. In M. Hersen & V. B. Van Hasselt (Eds.), *Psychological aspects of developmental and physical disabilities: A casebook* (pp. 137–156). Newbury Park, CA: Sage.

Burns, G. L. & Owen, S. M. (1990). Disruptive behaviors in the classroom: Initial standardization data on a new teacher rating scale. *Journal of Abnormal Child Psychology, 18*, 515–525.

Cairns, R. B., Peterson, G., & Neckerman, H. J. (1988). Suicidal behavior in aggressive adolescents. *Journal of Clinical Child Psychology, 17*, 298–309.

Campbell, M., Small, A. M., Green, W. H., Jennings, S. J., Perry, R., Bennett, W. G., & Anderson, L. (1984). Behavioral efficacy of haloperidol and lithium carbonate: A comparison in hospitalized aggressive children with conduct disorder. *Archives of General Psychiatry, 41*, 650–656.

Charlebois, P., Tremblay, R. E., Gagnon, C., Larivee, S., & Laurent, D. (1989). Situational consistency in behavioral patterns of aggressive boys: Methodological considerations on observational measures. *Journal of Psychopathology and Behavioral Assessment, 11*, 15–27.

Coie, J. D. & Koeppl, G. K. (1990). Adapting intervention to the problems of aggressive and disruptive rejected children. In S. R. Asher & J. D. Coie (Eds.), *Peer rejection in childhood* (pp. 309–337). New York: Cambridge University Press.

Coie, J. D. & Krehbiel, G. (1984). Effects of academic tutoring on the social status of low achieving, socially rejected children. *Child Development, 55*, 1465–1478.

Coie, J. D., Belding, M., & Underwood, M. (1988). Aggression and peer rejection in childhood. In B. B. Lahey & A. E. Kazdin (Eds.), *Advances in clinical child psychology* (Vol. 11, pp. 125–158). New York: Plenum Press.

Coie, J. D., Rabiner, D. L., & Lochman, J. E. (1989). Promoting peer relations in a school setting. In L. A. Bond and B. E. Compas (Eds.), *Primary prevention and promotion in schools* (pp. 207–234). Newbury Park, CA: Sage.

Dishion, T. J., Loeber, R., Stouthamer-Loeber, M., & Patterson, G. R. (1984). Skill deficits and male adolescent delinquency. *Journal of Abnormal Child Psychology, 12*, 37–54.

Dodge, K. A. & Coie, J. D. (1987). Social information processing factors in reactive and proactive aggression in children's peer groups. *Journal of Personality and Social Psychology*, *53*, 1146–1158.

Dodge, K. A., McClaskey, C. L., & Feldman, E. (1985). Situational approach to the assessment of social competence in children. *Journal of Consulting and Clinical Psychology*, *53*, 344–353.

Dodge, K. A., Pettit, G. S., McClaskey, C. L., & Brown, M. M. (1986). Social competence in children. *Monographs of the Society for Research in Child Development*, *51* (2, Serial No. 213).

Dodge, K. A., Bates, J. E., & Pettit, G. S. (1990a). Mechanisms in the cycle of violence. *Science*, *250*, 1678–1683.

Dodge, K. A., Price, J. M., Bachorowski, J., & Newman, J. P. (1990b). Hostile attributional biases in severely aggressive adolescents. *Journal of Abnormal Psychology*, *99*, 385–392.

Drabman, R. S., Jarvie, G. J., & Hammer, D. (1978). Residential child treatment. In M. Hersen & A. S. Bellack (Eds.), *Behavior therapy in the psychiatric setting* (pp. 219–255). Baltimore: Williams & Wilkins.

Fergusson, D. M. & Horwood, L. J. (1987). The trait and method components of ratings of conduct disorder: I. Maternal and teacher evaluations of conduct disorder in young children. *Journal of Child Psychology and Psychiatry*, *28*, 249–260.

Feshbach, S. & Price, J. (1984). Cognitive competencies and aggressive behavior: A developmental study. *Aggressive Behavior*, *10* 185–200.

Forehand, R. & Long, N. (1988). Outpatient treatment of the acting out child: Procedures, long term follow-up data, and clinical problems. *Advances in Behavioral Research and Therapy*, *10*, 129–177.

Forman, S. G. (1980). A comparison of cognitive training and response cost procedures in modifying aggressive behavior of elementary school children. *Behavior Therapy*, *11*, 594–600.

Frick, P. J., Lahey, B. B., Hartdagen, S., & Hynd, G. W. (1989). Conduct problems in boys: Relations to maternal personality, marital satisfaction, and socioeconomic status. *Journal of Clinical Child Psychology*, *18*, 114–120.

Gadow, K. D., Nolan, E. E., Sverd, J., Sprafkin, J., Paolicelli, L. (1990). Methylphenidate in aggressive-hyperactive boys: 1. Effects on peer aggression in public school settings. *Journal of the American Academy of Child and Adolescent Psychiatry*, *29*, 710–718.

Gardner, F. E. (1989). Inconsistent parenting: Is there evidence for a link with children's conduct problems? *Journal of Abnormal Child Psychology*, *17*, 223–233.

Glick, B., & Goldstein, A. P. (1987). Aggression replacement training. *Journal of Counseling and Development*, *65*, 356–362.

Gresham, F. M. & Elliott, S. N. (1990). *Social Skills Rating System manual*. Circle Pines, MN: American Guidance Service.

Hayes, S. C., Nelson, R. O., & Jarrett, R. B. (1987). The treatment utility of assessment: A functional approach to evaluating assessment quality. *American Psychologist*, *42*, 963–974.

Henggeler, S. W., McKee, E., & Borduin, C. M. (1989). Is there a link between maternal neglect and adolescent delinquency? *Journal of Clinical Child Psychology*, *18*, 242–246.

Hinshaw, S. P. (1987). On the distinction between attentional deficits/hyperactivity and conduct problems/aggression in child psychopathology. *Psychological Bulletin*, *101*, 443–463.

Huesmann, L. R., Eron, L. D., Lefkowitz, M. M., & Walder, L. O. (1984). Stability of aggression over time and generations. *Developmental Psychology*, *20*, 1120–1134.

Johnston, C. & Pelham, W. E. (1986). Teacher ratings predict peer ratings of aggression at 3-year follow-up in boys with attention deficit disorder with hyperactivity. *Journal of Consulting and Clinical Psychology*, *54*, 571–572.

Kandel, E., Mednick, S., Kirkegaard-Sorensen, L., Hutchings, B., Knop, J., Rosenberg, R., & Schulsinger, F. (1988). IQ as a protective factor for subjects at high risk for antisocial behavior. *Journal of Consulting and Clinical Psychology*, *56*, 224–226.

Kaplan, S. L., Busner, J., Kupietz, S., Wassermann, E., & Segal, B. (1990). Effects of methylphenidate on adolescents with aggressive conduct disorder and ADDH: A preliminary report. *Journal of the American Academy of Child and Adolescent Psychiatry*, *29*, 719–723.

Kazdin, A. E. (1987a). *Conduct disorders in childhood and adolescence*. Newbury Park, CA: Sage.

Kazdin, A. E. (1987b). Treatment of antisocial behavior in children: Current status and future directions. *Psychological Bulletin*, *102*, 187–203.

Kazdin, A. E., Esveldt-Dawson, K., French, N. H., & Unis, A. S. (1987a). Effects of parent management training and problem-solving skills training combined in the treatment of antisocial child behavior. *Journal of the American Academy of Child and Adolescent Psychiatry*, *26*, 416–424.

Kazdin, A. E., Esveldt-Dawson, K., French, N. H., & Unis, A. S. (1987b). Problem-solving skills training and relationship therapy in the treatment of antisocial child behavior. *Journal of Consulting and Clinical Psychology*, *55*, 76–85.

Kazdin, A. E., Bass, D., Siegel, T., & Thomas, C. (1989). Cognitive-behavioral therapy and relationship therapy in the treatment of children referred for antisocial behavior. *Journal of Consulting and Clinical Psychology*, *57*, 522–535.

Klorman, R., Brumaghim, J. T., Salzman, L. F., Strauss, J., Borgstedt, A. D., McBride, M. C., & Loeb, S. (1988). Effects of methylphenidate on attention-deficit hyperactivity disorder with and without aggressive/noncompliant features. *Journal of Abnormal Psychology*, *97*, 413–422.

Kolko, D. J., Loar, L. L., & Sturnick, D. (1990). Inpatient social-cognitive skills training groups with conduct disordered and attention deficit disordered children. *Journal of Child Psychology and Psychiatry*, *31*, 737–748.

Lahey, B. B., Hartdagen, S. E., Frick, P. J., McBurnett, K., Connor, R., & Hynd, G. W. (1988). Conduct disorder: Parsing the confounded relation to parental divorce and antisocial personality. *Journal of Abnormal Psychology*, *97*, 334–337.

Lochman, J. E. (1987). Self and peer perceptions and attributional biases of aggressive and nonaggressive boys in dyadic interaction. *Journal of Consulting and Clinical Psychology*, *55*, 404–410.

Lochman, J. E., Burch, P. R., Curry, J. F., & Lampron, L. B. (1985). Treatment and generalization effects of cognitive-behavioral and goal-setting interventions with aggressive boys. *Journal of Consulting and Clinical Psychology*, *52*, 915–916.

Lochman, J. E., White, K. J., Curry, J. F., & Rumer, R. R. (1992). Antisocial behavior. In R. G. Slaby & D. J. Kolko (Eds.), *Inpatient behavior therapy with children and adolescents* (pp. 277–312). New York: Plenum Press.

Loeber, R. (1985). Patterns and development of antisocial child behavior. In G. J. Whitehurst (Ed.), *Annals of child development* (Vol. 2). New York: JAI Press.

Loeber, R. & Dishion, T. (1983). Early predictors of male delinquency: A review. *Psychological Bulletin*, *94*, 68–99.

Loeber, R. & Schmaling, K. B. (1985a). Empirical evidence for overt and covert patterns of antisocial conduct problems: A metaanalysis. *Journal of Abnormal Child Psychology*, *13*, 337–353.

Loeber, R. & Schmaling, K. B. (1985b). The utility of differentiating between mixed and pure forms of antisocial child behavior. *Journal of Abnormal Child Psychology*, *13*, 315–335.

Loeber, R., Dishion, T. J., & Patterson, G. R. (1984). Multiple gating: A multistage assessment procedure for identifying youths at risk for delinquency. *Journal of Research in Crime and Delinquency*, *21*, 7–32.

Loney, J. (1987). Hyperactivity and aggression in the diagnosis of attention deficit disorder. In B. B. Lahey & A. E. Kazdin (Eds.), *Advances in clinical child psychology* (Vol. 10, pp. 99–135). New York: Plenum Press.

Loney, J. & Milich, R. (1982). Hyperactivity, inattention, and aggression in clinical practice. In M. Wolraich & C. K. Routh (Eds.), *Advances in behavioral pediatrics* (Vol. 2, pp. 113–147). Greenwich, CN: JAI Press.

Magnusson, D., Statlin, H., & Duner, A. (1983). Aggression and criminality in a longitudinal perspective. In K. T. Van Dusen & S. A. Mednick (Eds.), *Prospective studies of crime and delinquency* (pp. 277–301). Boston: Kluwer-Nijhoff.

Marlatt, G. A. (1985). Relapse prevention: Theoretical rationale and overview of the model. In G. A. Marlatt & J. R. Gordon (Eds.), *Relapse prevention* (pp. 3–70). New York: Guilford Press.

McMahon, R. J. (1987). Some current issues in the behavioral assessment of conduct disordered children and their families. *Behavioral Assessment*, *9*, 235–252.

Michelson, L. (1987). Cognitive-behavioral strategies in the prevention and treatment of antisocial disorders in children and adolescents. In J. Burchard & S. Burchard (Eds.), *Prevention of delinquent behavior* (Vol. 10, pp. 275–310). Newbury Park, CA: Sage.

Milich, R. & Dodge, K. A. (1984). Social information processing in child psychiatric populations. *Journal of Abnormal Child Psychology*, *12*, 471–490.

Moffitt, T. E. (1990). Juvenile delinquency and attention deficit disorder: Boys' developmental trajectories from age 3 to age 15. *Child Development*, *61*, 893–910.

Moffitt, T. E. & Silva, P. A. (1988). IQ and delinquency: A direct test of the differential detection hypothesis. *Journal of Abnormal Psychology*, *97*, 330–333.

Nieminen, G. S. & Matson, J. L. (1989). Depressive problems in conduct-disordered adolescents. *Journal of School Psychology*, *27*, 175–188.

Olweus, D. (1980). Familial and temperamental determinants of aggressive behavior in adolescent boys: A causal analysis. *Developmental Psychology*, *16*, 644–660.

Patterson, G. R. (1986). Performance models for antisocial boys. *American Psychologist*, *41*, 432–444.

Patterson, G. R. & Bank, L. (1986). Bootstrapping your way in the nomological thicket. *Behavioral Assessment*, *8*, 49–73.

Pelham, W. E. & Murphy, H. A. (1986). Behavioral and pharmacological treatment of attention deficit and conduct disorders. In M. Hersen (Ed.), *Pharmacological and behavioral treatment: An integrative approach*. New York: Wiley.

Pelham, W. E., Milich, R., Murphy, D. A., & Murphy, H. A. (1989). Normative data on the IOWA Conners Teacher Rating Scale. *Journal of Clinical Child Psychology, 18*, 259–262.

Pfeffer, C. R., Plutchik, R., & Mizruchi, M. S. (1983). Suicidal and assaultive behavior in children: Classification, measurement, and interrelations. *American Journal of Psychiatry, 140*, 154–157.

Quay, H. C. (1986). Conduct disorders. In H. C. Quay & J. S. Werry (Eds.), *Psychopathological disorders of childhood* (3rd ed., pp. 35–72). New York: Wiley.

Quay, H. C. & Peterson, D. R. (1987). *Manual for the Revised Behavior Problem Checklist*. Coral Gables, FL: University of Miami.

Quay, H. C., Routh, D. K., & Shapiro, S. K. (1987). Psychopathology of childhood: From description to validation. *Annual Review of Psychology, 38*, 491–532.

Reeves, J. C., Werry, J. S., Elkind, G. S., & Zametkin, A. (1987). Attention deficit, conduct, oppositional, and anxiety disorders in children: 2. Clinical characteristics. *Journal of the American Academy of Child and Adolescent Psychiatry, 26*, 144–155.

Rutter, M., Tizard, J., & Whitmore, K. (1970). *Education, health and behaviour*. London: Longmans.

Sayger, T. V., Horne, A. M., Walker, J. M., & Passmore, J. L. (1988). Social learning family therapy with aggressive children: Treatment outcome and maintenance. *Journal of Family Psychology, 1*, 261–285.

Scerbo, A., Raine, A., O'Brien, M., Chan, C. J., Rhee, C., & Smiley, N. (1990). Reward dominance and passive avoidance learning in adolescent psychopaths. *Journal of Abnormal Child Psychology, 18*, 451–463.

Schachar, R., Sandberg, S., & Rutter, M. (1986). Agreement between teachers' ratings and observations of hyperactivity, inattentiveness, and defiance. *Journal of Abnormal Child Psychology, 14*, 331–345.

Szatmari, P., Boyle, M., & Offord, D. R. (1989). ADDH and conduct disorder: Degree of diagnostic overlap and differences among correlates. *Journal of the American Academy of Child and Adolescent Psychiatry, 28*, 865–872.

Tolan, P. H. (1987). Implications of age of onset for delinquency risk. *Journal of Abnormal Child Psychology, 15*, 47–65.

Tolan, P. H. (1988). Socioeconomic, family, and social stress correlates of adolescent antisocial and delinquent behavior. *Journal of Abnormal Psychology, 16*, 317–331.

Webster-Stratton, C. & Hammond, M. (1990). Predictors of treatment outcome in parent training for families with conduct problem children. *Behavior Therapy, 21*, 319–337.

Werry, J. S., Methven, R. J., Fitzpatrick, J., & Dixon, H. (1983). The interrater reliability of DSM-III in children. *Journal of Abnormal Child Psychology, 11*, 341–354.

White, J. L., Moffitt, T. E., & Silva, P. A. (1989). A prospective replication of the protective effects of IQ in subjects at high risk for juvenile delinquency. *Journal of Consulting and Clinical Psychology, 57*, 719–724.

IV

FAMILY PROBLEMS

27

Parent Training

LORI A. SISSON and JILL C. TAYLOR

INTRODUCTION

Since the mid-1960s, the work on behavioral parent training has burgeoned from a few single-case studies to a massive body of literature reporting the successful treatment of thousands of children with a wide variety of problems. Beginning in the late 1950s, behavior modification had its first impact on children diagnosed as autistic, schizophrenic, and mentally retarded (e.g., Lovaas, Freitag, Gold, & Kassorla, 1965). Once this approach had been demonstrated to be effective, it was applied to youngsters exhibiting other disorders, such as hyperactivity, school phobia, and enuresis (e.g., Ayllon, Layman, & Kendel, 1975; Azrin, Sneed, & Foxx, 1974). As clinicians began to consider the questions about the efficient delivery of services and the maintenance and generalization of behavioral improvements, increased attention was focused on training the child's parents to be the agents of change (O'Dell, 1974). Using parents as therapists had the potential of extending interventions to greater numbers of children in need of services and to those environments in which problem behaviors and/or skills deficits were evidenced. No longer viewed as an experimental technology, this mode of treatment has become an increasingly effective, accepted, and popular strategy.

There are several theoretical and practical arguments in support of the development and use of behavioral parent training. This intervention is based on an empirical methodology and specific principles drawn from the field of social learning theory. Extensive research with laboratory animals has demonstrated unequivocally that a wide range of behavior is functionally related to environmental events. The application of the principles and procedures of this body of knowledge to children suggests that many of their behaviors are shaped and maintained by events in the natural environment and therefore can best be changed by the modification of these events. Thus, parents are trained in the effective use of such techniques as reinforcement and punishment to increase or decrease specific child responses. The basic principles are relatively simple and can be learned and applied by comparatively unsophisticated and uneducated persons (Feldman, Case, Rincover, Towns, & Betel, 1989), can be imparted to many individuals at once in group instruction (Adesso & Lipson, 1981), can be acquired in a short training period

LORI A. SISSON • Western Pennsylvania School for Blind Children, Pittsburgh, Pennsylvania 15213.
JILL C. TAYLOR • Institute for Clinical Training and Research, The Devereux Foundation, Devon, Pennsylvania 19333.

Handbook of Behavior Therapy in the Psychiatric Setting, edited by Alan S. Bellack and Michel Hersen. Plenum Press, New York, 1993.

(Cava, 1991), and can be adapted to many of the behavior problems for which children are referred (O'Dell, 1974).

As noted above, behavioral parent training has become a standard tool of practitioners whose focus is on childhood disorders. Whether as a prevention strategy, a primary treatment, or an ancillary service, this approach has been applied to a number of childhood problems. These may be broadly categorized into four areas. First, medical-somatic complaints, such as seizures (Gardner, 1967), feeding problems (Lamm & Greer, 1988), enuresis (Houts & Mellon, 1989), toilet training (Foxx & Azrin, 1973), and asthma (Neisworth & Moore, 1972) have been shown to respond to parent-training interventions.

Second, in the area of developmental disabilities, teaching parents to facilitate self-help or preacademic skills (Moran & Whitman, 1991), communication (Laski, Charlop, & Schreibman, 1988), and behavior control (Van Hasselt, Sisson, & Aach, 1987) in their children with single and multiple handicaps appears to be an important component of effective treatments for this population.

Third, research and clinical practice recommends parents as therapists for internalizing disorders, including fears (Dolgin, Phipps, Harrow, & Zelter, 1990), phobias (Yule, 1989), and depression (Blechman, Tryon, Ruff, & McEnroe, 1989).

Finally, externalizing disorders—particularly conduct disorders and hyperactivity, with their associated negativistic, noncompliant, oppositional, and aggressive behaviors—constitute the class of behavior that has drawn the most attention and effort from behavior therapists who incorporate parent training into treatment (e.g., Anastopoulos & Barkley, 1989; McMahon & Forehand, 1984). In addition, it should be noted that parents referred because of abusive behavior toward their children (Campbell, O'Brien, Bickett, & Lutzker, 1983) and parents of children at risk for medical and developmental complications (Bruder, 1986) frequently receive parent training as part of their therapy. Although the primary focus in this chapter is on parent-training interventions to remediate disruptive child responding, much of the information presented also relates, either directly or indirectly, to a variety of referral problems.

Despite the diversity of the child populations treated with behavioral parent training, virtually all programs attempt to decrease children's disruptive or otherwise unwanted responses and/or to increase their adaptive or prosocial behaviors. Initial reports documented the efficacy of parent training for the remediation of relatively simple, discrete behavior problems (e.g., tantrumming; Williams, 1959). However, as the technology became more sophisticated, it was quickly applied to a variety of responses simultaneously, for example, aggression, enuresis, and crying (Patterson & Brosky, 1966) and self-help, motor, communication, and cognitive skills (Sandler, Coren, & Thurman, 1983). Further, in addition to affecting child behavior, parent training also should influence how parents teach and discipline their offspring. Relevant parent behaviors that have been changed include the strategies they use for instruction (Laski *et al.*, 1988; Moran & Whitman, 1991), the types of commands they give (Peed, Roberts, & Forehand, 1977), when and how they reinforce responses (Wahler, Winkel, Peterson, & Morrison, 1965), and when and how they deliver punishing consequences (Budd, Green, & Baer, 1976).

PROTOTYPICAL ASSESSMENT

It is not the type of child behavior problem that is addressed that distinguishes behavioral parent training from other approaches to treatment. Instead, one of the defining characteristics of this intervention is the fact that it is based on an initial and continuing assessment of what are perceived to be the relevant variables. Traditionally, direct observation has been used to examine child behaviors within the context of the social environment (McMahon, 1987). The parent-training strategy derived from this model focuses on teaching parents more appropriate parenting skills (e.g., differential reinforcement and time-out) to reduce their children's acting-out behavior and to foster prosocial responses. Although these assessment and treatment procedures have proved to be quite useful and effective for many families (O'Dell, 1974), both research findings and clinical experience have indicated that they have not worked well for others (Forehand & Atkeson, 1977; Griest & Wells, 1983). As a result, recent recommendations (e.g., Breiner, 1989; DuPaul, Guevremont, & Barkley, 1991; McMahon, 1987) specifically promote a broader and more comprehensive approach to assessment (as well as to any associated interventions) in order to maximize clinical efficacy with resistant populations. In this section, we provide an overview of the strategies and issues associated with what we believe to be prototypical assessment for behavioral parent training. The increased focus on evaluating possible functional relationships between child behavior and a wide range of environmental events will be apparent.

Problem Identification

The initial task in assessment is to engage in problem identification, which consists of pinpointing the presenting problems; obtaining a history of the disorder; determining the frequency, duration, and intensity of the maladaptive responses; and selecting tentative targets for modification. Typically, this stage begins with the therapist conducting a behavioral clinical interview with the child's parents, as well as with the child himself or herself (Gross & Wixted, 1988; Luiselli, 1991). Although criticized for their subjectivity, parent and child reports provide ecologically valid information, as the perceptions of these parties directly influence the nature of the referral and the likelihood of adherence to treatment recommendations (Wahler & Cormier, 1970).

Several structured interviews, comprising a prearranged set of questions to be asked in a sequential order, have been developed to assist the practitioner in isolating specific problems. Presumably, such standardized interviews increase the likelihood of obtaining reliable and valid information, yet adequate psychometric evaluation is still pending for most. Of those that are available to child therapists, the focus is on eliciting symptom history and severity that is sufficient to evoke a diagnosis based on the criteria in the revised third edition of the *Diagnostic and Statistical Manual* (DSM-III-R; American Psychiatric Association, 1987). These include the children's version of the Schedule for Affective Disorders and Schizophrenia (K-SADS; Chambers, Puig-Antich, Hirsch, Paez, Ambrosini, Tabrizi, & Davies, 1985), the Diagnostic Interview for Children and Adolescents (DICA; Herjanic, 1980), and the Diagnostic Interview Schedule for Children (DISC; Costello, Edelbrock, Kalas, Kessler, & Klaric, 1982).

To supplement information derived from the clinical interview, many therapists ask parents to complete a behavioral rating scale immediately before or after the first meeting. A typical rating scale includes a listing of child-behavior-specific statements, such as "Argues with other children" or "Disturbs others." The respondents are required to complete each statement by making one of several categories that refer to occurrence or nonoccurrence and degree of severity (e.g., "Does not occur," "Occurs seldom," "Occurs frequently"). Scores are derived from the completed scale, and these data constitute a profile of the child's behavior which is compared to that of a normative sample. A very large number of rating scales are available for evaluating a child's behavior. Some of the most popular are the Revised Behavior Problem Checklist (RBPC; Quay, 1983) and the Child Behavior Problem Checklist (CBCL; Achenbach & Edelbrock, 1983), which assess a wide range of adaptive and maladaptive responses, and the Conners Parent and Teacher Rating Scales (Conners, 1969, 1970), which target hyperactivity.

Finally, direct observation and quantification of the child's behavior in natural (home) or analogue (clinic) situations are often undertaken (Gross & Wixted, 1988). Historically, behavior therapists have found this type of assessment to be the most useful in providing information regarding response characteristics. It involves a far lower level of inference in interpreting findings and uses categories or dimensions of behavior that more closely approximate the concerns of parents than do other assessment strategies (DuPaul *et al.*, 1991). Typically, several targeted behaviors are isolated via interviews and rating scales and then measured by the practitioner and/or the parent by means of interval, frequency, or duration recording formats (e.g., Breiner, 1989). As an alternative to this time-consuming and expensive approach, Patterson and his associates (Chamberlain & Reid, 1987; Patterson, Reid, Jones, & Conger, 1975) have used the Parent Daily Report (PDR), a measure usually administered in a brief telephone interview, in which the parent is asked to note whether a variety of child symptoms have occurred over the past 24 hours.

It is clear that important information necessary to specify and monitor problem behaviors is gained through the use of these assessment procedures. Further, the responses to be targeted for treatment can be selected based on how disruptive or dangerous they are or how much their presence or absence interferes with adaptive functioning. Until recently, discrete responses have been emphasized in behavioral assessment (Voeltz & Evans, 1982). However, there has been a growing recognition that child disorders covary with one another (e.g., Milich, Landau, Kilby, & Whitten, 1982; Wells & Forehand, 1985); that is, they are related, so that a change in one affects the other. For example, Wahler and his colleagues (Kara & Wahler, 1977; Wahler, 1975; Wahler & Fox, 1980) have shown that the behaviors of children and youth with conduct disorders or autism are organized into clusters that covary both directly and inversely. The use of multiple assessment procedures has the potential to identify the range of behaviors that may be so related. Within that range, it is possible that behaviors that provide access to, or are maintained by, the same reinforcers will covary (Kazdin, 1982). Compliance with adult requests and disruptive behavior may both be effective in obtaining adult attention; therefore, reducing or increasing one may have the opposite effect on the other. In fact, using single-subject research methodology; Parrish, Cataldo, Kolko, Neef, and Egel (1986) established this inverse relationship between compliance and a variety of inappropriate activities displayed by four children by applying and withdrawing interventions. Knowledge of response covariation permits the selection of target behaviors whose modification is most likely to facilitate positive changes in multiple responses while minimizing negative side effects, thus improving the economy of the treatment (Voeltz & Evans, 1982).

Behaviors may also be related temporally and sequentially, as in behavioral chains. In this arrangement, each response serves as a discriminative (or eliciting) stimulus of the next behavior and as a secondary reinforcer of the preceding behavior (Kelleher, 1966). Specifying these behavioral chains is important in the selection of target behaviors because individual responses may exert more control over one another than any environmental events (Voeltz & Evans, 1982). Identifying and targeting a behavior that occurs early in a chain (e.g., teasing) may also prevent the occurrence of a more noxious terminal behavior (e.g., physical aggression) without waiting for the more severe behavior to occur and then applying treatment. Further, the initial behavior may occur more frequently, allowing more intervention opportunities and thus facilitating quicker results.

Functional Assessment of Problem Behavior

Once the target behaviors have been defined, a functional assessment should be conducted. The term *functional assessment* denotes an identification of the antecedent and consequent events that are temporally contiguous to the target response, and that occasion and maintain it. Presumably, an understanding of the controlling variables, achieved through a functional assessment of the aberrant behavior, will lead to the selection of more effective treatments. For example, a functional assessment may identify the reinforcing consequences of the target response, so that the practitioner is led to eliminate their occurrence following the response (e.g., Cooper, Wacker, Sasso, Reimers, & Donn, 1990). Alternatively, a functional assessment may pinpoint antecedent conditions that evoke the target behavior. By either removing these conditions or altering their characteristics, one can prevent the response (e.g., Roberts,

McMahon, Forehand, & Humphreys, 1978). Finally, information obtained from a functional assessment may aid the practitioner in identifying more appropriate but functionally equivalent alternatives (i.e., those that result in the same reinforcing consequences) to the target behavior. Then, these adaptive responses are trained in an effort to decrease disruptive responding (Carr & Durand, 1985). Although isolating the antecedents and consequences of problem behavior was advocated by the founders of applied behavior analysis (Baer, Wolf, & Risley, 1968; Kanfer & Saslow, 1969), this kind of evaluation has often been neglected (Axelrod, 1987; Durand, 1987).

Several methods of conducting a functional assessment of challenging behavior in applied settings have been described. The least rigorous procedure is the behavioral clinical interview, described earlier, which may incorporate questions about the antecedent and consequent events associated with the target behavior (e.g., Barkley, 1981). Durand and Crimmins (1988) presented the Motivational Assessment Scale (MAS) as an instrument to be used in conjunction with the interview to identify the contextual determinants of self-injurious and other disruptive responses exhibited by persons with developmental disabilities. The MAS consists of 16 questions that provide data useful in determining whether the problem behavior is reinforced by attention, tangibles, escape or avoidance, or sensory stimulation. A similar questionnaire has been developed for use with children who exhibit school refusal (Kearney & Silverman, 1990).

Direct observations conducted by the practitioner and/or the parents also highlight the relationships between the target behavior and various environmental events. In one approach, an observer or parent records those events that set the stage for the problem behavior, a description of the action that the child performs, and finally, those events that immediately follow the child's response. This narrative is then analyzed for antecedent-behavior-consequence (A-B-C) sequences. Over time, these data may reflect a correlational relationship leading to hypotheses about potentially important maintaining events (Cooper, Heron, & Heward, 1987). Alternatively, several formal observational coding schemes have been used to measure behavioral interactions in families with children who present conduct problems. For example, the Family Interaction Coding System (FICS; Jones, Reid, & Patterson, 1975) consists of 29 behavioral codes, including common problem behaviors (e.g., noncompliance and crying) and positive and negative parental responses (e.g., approval and ignoring). In a typical use of the FICS, an observer enters the home and targets each member of the family for at least five minutes of observation. During each six-second interval within that period, the observer codes the behavior of the targeted individual and the subsequent response(s) of the other family members. Similarly, Forehand and his colleagues (e.g., Forehand & McMahon, 1981) described a scoring system that focuses not only on child problem behavior and parental consequences, but also on parental antecedents, such as questions, clearly stated requests (alpha commands), and non-specific requests (beta commands). The sequential data obtained through the Patterson and Forehand codes should suggest the functional relationships among antecedents, problem behaviors, and consequences.

The final method for conducting a functional assessment involves the experimental manipulation of the controlling variables (Axelrod, 1987). By recording behavioral changes associated with the systematic introduction and withdrawal of various antecedent and consequent events, one can determine precisely the variables that are functionally related to the target behavior. Such control of maintaining variables is difficult to attain in the natural environment and often requires that the practitioner arrange an analogue situation in which the contingencies are essentially contrived. Once the controlling variables are identified in the analogue situation, functionally similar contingencies found in the natural environment can be altered in an effort to decrease the problem behavior.

Much of the research and clinical work involving experimental functional assessment has focused on self-injurious or aggressive behavior displayed in inpatient or school settings by persons with severe handicaps and has been conducted by therapists who are professionals well trained in behavior analysis techniques (e.g., Carr & Durand, 1985; Iwata *et al.*, 1982). However,

LORI A. SISSON and
JILL C. TAYLOR

Cooper *et al.* (1990) recently demonstrated the efficacy of using a 90-minute procedure, carried out by the parents of children of normal intelligence with conduct disorders, in an outpatient clinic. The parents varied their task demands (antecedents) and their attention (consequences) within a homework situation according to a multielement design, and the treatment recommendations were based on the assessment results. Because it is only through such experimental manipulations that controlling variables can be identified unequivocally (Axelrod, 1987), and because previous authors have demonstrated that functional assessments can provide the necessary bridge between assessment and treatment (Carr & Durand, 1985; Carr, Newsom, & Binkoff, 1980; Cooper *et al.*, 1990; Mace, Page, Ivancic, & O'Brien, 1986; Slifer, Ivancic, Parrish, Page, & Burgio, 1986), it is encouraging that efficient and user-friendly means of conducting these procedures are being developed and tested.

It must be noted that in most conceptualizations, child behavior is presumed to be controlled by adult-mediated antecedents and consequences. When these are found, the analysis is considered complete. Typically, it is not extended to determine the child-mediated events controlling the adult behavior that occurs within the context of maladaptive adult-child interaction (Emery, Binkoff, Houts, & Carr, 1983). Yet several hypotheses suggest that a child's behavior can promote environmental conditions that create or exacerbate problem responding (Lytton, 1990; Patterson, 1977; Stevens-Long, 1973; Wahler, 1975). For example, studies of the family interactions of conduct problem boys (Patterson, 1977) have revealed the following pattern: The child initiates noxious behavior (e.g., a temper tantrum) and ceases it contingent on adult acquiescence to a demand. In this type of interaction, the behavior of both parties is reinforced. The child receives positive reinforcement for the inappropriate behavior (i.e., the parent complies with the demand), and the adult receives negative reinforcement for giving in (i.e., the child ceases the noxious behavior). Each member of the dyad reciprocally reinforces the other's behavior, thus ensuring that the tantrums and the acquiescence to demands will recur. A strategy that recognizes these reciprocal influences includes both a functional assessment of the child's maladaptive behavior and the adult behavior that surrounds it. Such an analysis has been referred to as a *systems-functional analysis* (Emery *et al.*, 1983, p. 402). A systems-functional analysis may lead to the efficient targeting of both child and adult responses for treatment. In addition, a sensitivity to the effects of a child's behavior on the specific behavior of his or her parents may lead to the selection of treatment targets so that the changes will be most reinforcing to the referring party and therefore will be more likely to be maintained (Emery *et al.*, 1983). Responses related to independence, compliance, and affection are likely to be rewarding to parents.

Assessment of Setting Events

As discussed in the preceding sections, the assessment of children's problem behavior has focused on specifying the response and, less frequently, investigating the relationship between the target response and the events immediately preceding or following it. More recently, however, some researchers and clinicians have broadened the study of behavior-environment relationships to include an evaluation of the effects of temporally distinct antecedent conditions on maladaptive responding. These are commonly referred to as *setting events* (Bijou & Baer, 1978; Wahler & Graves, 1983). It is assumed that setting events do not have a direct effect on problem behavior (Durand & Crimmins, 1988). Instead, they influence the salience or valence of discrete stimuli, which, in turn, affect responding.

Setting events affect both children's problem behavior and parenting skills. A small literature (which is quite distinct from the parent-training literature) has identified a number of conditions that negatively influence child behavior, including illness and other abnormal biological conditions (Cataldo & Harris, 1982), agitation (Steen & Zuriff, 1977), high activity level (Krantz & Risley, 1977), social interactions with particular individuals (Gardner, Cole,

Davidson, & Karan, 1986), and aspects of the physical environment, such as crowding and noise level (Brackbill, Adams, Crowell, & Gray, 1966; Hutt & Vaizey, 1966). Within the parent-training literature, there has been ongoing interest in the relationship between various setting events and parents' perceptions of the child's adjustment, parent-child negative interactions, and the outcome of treatments. For example, maternal depression (McMahon Forehand, Griest, & Wells, 1981), marital problems (Reisinger, Frangia, & Hoffman, 1976), stressful life events (Patterson, 1983), and maternal social isolation (Wahler, 1980) have been shown to increase the likelihood of referral for treatment, to evoke child-directed aversive behavior, and/or to interfere with the maintenance of skills taught in therapy. Thus, if such conditions are not identified and ameliorated, it is unlikely that parent-training interventions will be effective in improving child or parent behavior.

Despite the importance of setting events, few guidelines exist for their assessment. Identifying setting events is a complex process that is poorly understood at this time. Three problems exist: (1) when setting events should be considered; (2) what conditions should be measured; and (3) how they should be assessed. Regarding the first, many authors have implied that the clinician should be prepared to incorporate multimethod assessment strategies into the initial evaluation in order to identify what factors are operating as the setting events for a child's problem behavior (Luiselli, 1991; McMahon, 1987). In this way, important treatment foci can be established, including environmental conditions (e.g., noise level), internal conditions (e.g., illness), familial conditions (e.g., depression), and extrafamilial conditions (e.g., insularity). Certainly, setting events must be measured when experimental analyses indicate that the behavior of interest is not largely controlled by temporally close stimulus associations, that is, when manipulations of routinely considered variables reveal unstable changes in the target behavior (Wahler, 1980).

Regarding the problem of what to assess, several authors have identified specific aversive situations that increase coercive parent-child interactions; these were listed above. However, it seems that there are individual differences in the type of aversive stimuli that produces these effects in particular families. Support for an idiographic analysis of setting events was provided by Furey and Forehand (1984), who found that for one mother, daily ratings of health and child behavior were associated with satisfaction with her child; for another subject, marital satisfaction and child behavior ratings were better predictors of satisfaction; and in a subsequent study (Furey & Forehand, 1986), negative child behavior and negative maternal activities were the strongest predictors of mothers' satisfaction with their children.

Finally, the existing models for measuring setting events include experimental manipulation of the presumed controlling variables, as in an experimental functional assessment, described earlier (e.g., Krantz & Risley, 1977), and administering questionnaires designed to uncover relevant stimulus conditions (see McMahon, 1987, for review). The instruments most frequently used to assess factors such as parental depression, marital adjustment, stressful events, and insularity in families are, respectively, the Beck Depression Inventory (Beck, Rush, Shaw, & Emery, 1979), the Marital Adjustment Test (Locke & Wallace, 1959), the Parenting Stress Index (Loyd & Abidin, 1985), and the Community Interaction Checklist (Wahler, Leske, & Rogers, 1979).

Actual Assessment

While acknowledging the importance of a broad-based, functional assessment of the child and his or her family to maximize the likelihood of a successful intervention, it is necessary to consider the cost-effectiveness of such an approach in terms of the monetary and time demands placed on the therapist and the family. Indeed, conducting such an extensive evaluation for each child who is referred would be prohibitively expensive. Therefore, actual clinical practice rarely incorporates all the components of the prototypical assessment procedures described above.

What is commonly used is an unstructured interview, often with the primary purpose of eliciting a symptom picture that suggests a diagnosis. Yet the application of diagnostic systems generally ignores the situational variables and family characteristics that influence problem behavior (Kendall, 1987). Sometimes, the clinical interview is supplemented with behavioral rating scales, and/or informal observations of parent and child interactions in a clinic play or task situation. However, responses to questionnaires do not necessarily mirror truly the behavior at home (e.g., Foster, 1987), and the relationship between the behaviors observed in naturalistic and those observed in analogue environments has not been investigated adequately (Hughes & Haynes, 1978).

One possible strategy for dealing with the problem of administering practical assessments of child and parent functioning in typical clinical settings is called *multiple gating* (Loeber, Dishion, & Patterson, 1984; McMahon, 1987; Reynolds, 1986). In this approach, less costly assessment procedures, such as brief interviews, behavioral rating scales, and clinic observations, are used to screen all children who are referred. More detailed and often more expensive procedures, such as structured interviews, behavior rating in the home, and experimental functional assessments, are used only for the subgroup of children for whom the screening techniques have indicated the desirability of further evaluation. Alternatively, these procedures may be used when a brief treatment trial is unsuccessful or when additional problems are uncovered as treatment progresses. A similar sequential strategy is recommended in the consideration of other child characteristics, environmental stimulus, and familial and extra-familial factors that may affect a child's problem behavior. Relatively low-cost methods, such as interview questions (e.g., concerning the child's and the parent's adjustment) and/or brief self-report measures (e.g., the Beck Depression Inventory) can be used as screening measures. If additional evaluation in these areas appears to be warranted, then a more thorough assessment is arranged. In this process, the procedures that yield the most relevant information are identified for use in a periodic, ongoing evaluation of the treatment's effectiveness.

PROTOTYPICAL TREATMENT

Training programs in child behavior management differ somewhat in their content, ranging from those that emphasize teaching parents the theory and concepts of operant behavior to those that focus on specific techniques designed to modify particular target responses. Notwithstanding these differences, it is typical for parents to be taught to (1) select and then define target child behaviors so that they are objectively measurable; (2) observe and record specific instances of the child's prosocial and antisocial behavior; and (3) respond contingently and consistently to this behavior with the help of social learning techniques. Originally, parent-training programs attempted to alter the types of consequences that parents provided for appropriate and inappropriate child responses (e.g., Forehand & King, 1977; Wahler, 1969). First, they were taught to ignore undesirable actions and to attend positively to independent play, compliance, and other desirable responses. Next, they received instruction in applying time-out from reinforcement for noncompliance. In addition, Forehand and his colleagues had parents alter the instructions they gave to their children, either by decreasing the number of commands given (Forehand & King, 1977) or by changing the verbal content so that the commands were more direct and concise (Roberts *et al.*, 1978). Although highly successful in a large number of families, these techniques fell short of the expectations held for behavioral parent training in that treatment failures remained. As noted previously, these failures led to the consideration of an expanded range of variables for assessment and intervention. More recently, because of the successful use of empirical functional-analytic procedures in the management of severe problem behavior displayed by individuals with developmental disabilities, closer attention has been given to assessment-derived treatments (see particularly Cooper *et al.*, 1990). These two trends are elaborated on in the following discussion of the procedures and issues associated with proto-typical treatment in behavioral parent training.

Treatment Issues Related to Problem Identification

A multifaceted assessment process should reveal not only a child's problem behavior but also those responses that are related in some way, such as those that covary with the problem behavior and those that are associated in response chains. Some implications of these behavior-behavior relationships for treatment have already been mentioned but are important enough to repeat here.

First, identifying responses that covary with the behavior that prompted referral pro-motes an identification of the pivotal responses (i.e., those whose alteration would have the most far-reaching positive effects and the fewest side effects), and these merit early intervention. Selecting a behavior that occurs early in a response chain may have similar broad effects. Consider a case in which whining is followed by crying, and crying leads to tantrumming. If whining is treated successfully, it is likely that instances of crying and tantrumming will be reduced as well. If tantrumming is targeted, however, it is possible that whining and crying will remain. Broad behavior change is most noticed by and acceptable to clients in behavior therapy (Voeltz & Evans, 1982). Further, countertherapeutic effects appear to contribute significantly to low ratings of treatment acceptability (Kazdin, 1981). Therefore, intervening in pivotal behaviors or responses occurring early in behavior chains should enhance the social validity of the intervention. This enhancement, in turn, should increase the probability that parents will apply the necessary behavior management procedures over time, thus maintaining the behavioral improvements exhibited by their children.

Second, knowledge of behaviors that covary with inappropriate target responses may promote the use of reinforcement-based interventions over punishment-based ones. For exam-ple, Wahler and Fox (1980) noted that, in several subjects, solitary toy play was inversely related to noncompliance. Rather than intervening directly in noncompliance, Wahler and Fox suc-cessfully reduced it by increasing solitary toy play through reinforcement procedures. Similarly, the modification of a less innocuous behavior that occurs early in a behavior chain may require a less intrusive treatment than changing the terminal response. It has been demonstrated that positive interventions are more acceptable to parents than negative ones (Reimers, Wacker, & Cooper, 1991; Singh, Watson, & Winton, 1987), and therefore, parents' willingness to follow treatment recommendations may be enhanced by their use.

Finally, precursor behaviors are probably seen more frequently than problem behavior that occurs at the end of response chains, as these initial behaviors may appear in isolation (as when response chains are interrupted naturally) or in conjunction with the more severe behavior. As a result, there are more opportunities to treat behaviors that occur early in response chains, thus hastening the intervention effects. Because the efficiency of a treatment is considered another important factor in its overall acceptability (Lennox & Miltenberger, 1990), therapists' efforts to increase efficiency, including applying intervention procedures to responses that reliably precede the problem behavior, should be encouraged.

Functionally Based Treatments

As previously elaborated, functional assessment has widespread implications for the treatment of children's problem behavior. When devising intervention strategies for parents to implement with their children, it is crucial to understand and address both the antecedent stimuli and the reinforcement processes controlling the target response. As one example, escape behavior maintained by negative reinforcement (Carr & Durand, 1985; Iwata, 1987; Patterson,

1982) is discussed here. Suppose a child is presented with a stimulus that is aversive, such as a request to eat vegetables. The child responds by exhibiting problem behavior (i.e., a tantrum). In desperation, the parent terminates the aversive stimulus by removing the vegetables from the child's plate. At this point, the child immediately stops tantrumming. In this situation, the responses of the child and the parent are negatively reinforced. The child's tantrum is reinforced by the termination of the aversive stimulus (in this case, the removal of the vegetables), and the parent's withdrawal of the request to eat vegetables is reinforced by the termination of the tantrums. Other examples of escape behavior include disruptive actions that follow the presentation of difficult academic tasks (Carr & Durand, 1985; Center, Deitz, & Kaufman, 1982); aggressive responses to teasing, yelling, and other negative verbalizations (Patterson, 1982); and misbehavior elicited by noninstructional parental commands (Forehand & McMahon, 1981).

A typical behavior-management strategy for noncompliance and aggression includes the implementation of differential attention and time-out, in which parents (1) ignore inappropriate behavior; (2) reward cooperative responses; and (3) remove the child from the situation to a time-out chair or room following the target action (Barkley, 1981; Forehand & McMahon, 1981; Patterson, 1976, 1982; Patterson et al., 1975). However, for escape behaviors, such as the ones listed above, time-out is not an effective procedure. In these cases, time-out delivered contingent on disruption would enable the child to escape from, or at least delay, the aversive stimulus (e.g., eating vegetables or completing a task), thereby negatively reinforcing disruption and increasing its frequency. Several studies have indicated that, if an individual who exhibits escape behavior is removed from the aversive situation when the problem behavior occurs, this behavior increases (Carr et al., 1980; Iwata et al., 1982). Further, there have been reports of time-out-related exacerbation of problem behavior. Plummer, Baer, and LeBlanc (1977) used time-out with two autistic children who exhibited a variety of disruptive behaviors in a task situation. The effect was to provide a marked and systematic increase in their disruptive behavior. In another study, Solnick, Rincover, and Peterson (1977) applied time-out for the self-injurious and aggressive behavior of two children with developmental disabilities. The result was heightened levels of both problem behaviors. It is possible that time-out failed as an intervention because the problem behaviors of the children in these studies were evoked by aversive task stimuli and maintained by negative reinforcement. This is not known, however, as the authors did not analyze the variables that controlled the problem behavior.

It appears that time-out is not a useful behavior-management technique to use with escape behavior. However, alternative strategies do address the function of such responses, although most have not been used in parent-training intervention. In particular, procedures that reduce the aversiveness of the antecedent stimuli may be successful. Parents might be instructed to divide the activity into smaller component skills that the child is able to accomplish successfully (Etzel & LeBlanc, 1979), such as taking one bite of vegetables or picking up one toy. Alternatively, parents can be taught how to give appropriate commands, that is, being specific and direct, giving one command at a time, and giving the child time to do the task before presenting other commands (Forehand & McMahon, 1981). Another antecedent-based approach involves the use of interspersed requests (Horner, Day, Sprague, O'Brien, & Heathfield, 1991; Mace, Hock, Lalli, West, Belfiore, Pinter, & Brown, 1988). This procedure requires the adult to present two to five short, easy requests immediately before delivering one that has been identified as difficult or likely to result in undesirable behaviors. The pattern of cooperative responding established with the easy requests appears to increase the likelihood of compliance with commands that might otherwise have provoked disruptive behavior. Recent research with persons who are developmentally disabled suggests that allowing choice-making between two or more responses or activities reduces challenging behavior (Dyer, Dunlap, & Winterling, 1990). Offering children the opportunity to choose between acceptable alternative behaviors (such as eating peas or carrots, picking up toys or doing the dishes) is a strategy that may easily be incorporated into parenting repertoires.

Finally, a new approach that might be an important component of a parent-training program involves teaching the child a functionally equivalent prosocial behavior to replace the target maladaptive response (Carr & Durand, 1985; Durand & Carr, 1987). In other words, the child would be provided with an appropriate means of escaping an aversive situation. For example, the child could request to skip the vegetables and forfeit dessert, take a short break from a cleanup task, and so on. Parental involvement in such a program would include determining acceptable alternative responses and providing reinforcement when they occurred (i.e., by honoring appropriate requests).

The strategies discussed above for dealing with escape behavior can be contrasted with those that would be appropriate for attention-seeking behavior that is maintained by positive reinforcement (Day, Rea, Schussler, Larsen, & Johnson, 1988; Taylor, Sisson, McKelvey, & Trefelner, in press). Consider a situation in which a parent is talking on the telephone while the child is playing alone nearby. After a brief period, the child calls to the parent, who continues the telephone conversation. Soon after, the child begins to throw and destroy toys. In exasperation, the parent hangs up the phone and then approaches and reprimands the youngster. The child stops throwing the toys at once. In this sequence, the child's disruptive behavior is positively reinforced by the parent's attention (the reprimands), and the parent's reprimands are negatively reinforced by the cessation of the child's disruptive behavior. Several empirical reports have demonstrated that, if a child who exhibits attention-seeking behavior receives adult attention (usually admonishments) following the target response, the problem worsens (Iwata *et al.*, 1982; Taylor *et al.*, in press). Further, in certain instances, reprimands have appeared to increase the frequency of problem behavior. Martin and Foxx (1973) found that, when they delivered warnings and comments (e.g., "Don't do that again!") contingent on the aggression of two children, the children's aggression increased. Similarly, Carr and McDowell (1980) discovered the same phenomenon with a boy who had scratched sores all over his body. During the periods of time when his parents asked him to stop scratching, his scratching increased to high levels. One explanation for these findings is that the individuals in these studies were engaging in problem behaviors that were evoked by low levels of adult attention and that were maintained through positive reinforcement. Unfortunately, the authors of these studies did not conduct functional assessments to determine the variables that controlled the problem behavior.

In the case of attention-seeking behavior, typical approaches to parent training are likely to be effective. Two prominent research groups begin treatment by developing more effective attending skills in parents (Barkley, 1981; Forehand & McMahon, 1981). Time is set aside each day during which the parents and the children interact in positive ways. During this period, the parents practice attending to prosocial behaviors differentially while ignoring negative actions. One outcome of this protocol should be to increase the amount and quality of parental attention to the child, thus ameliorating the antecedent conditions of low levels of attention that set the stage for the attention-seeking behavior. Further, removing adult attention following this type of problem behavior should reduce its frequency (e.g., Allen & Harris, 1966; Budd *et al.*, 1976). Similarly, the signaled withdrawal of attention contingent on problem behavior, as in time-out, should also be effective. The efficacy of time-out has been demonstrated repeatedly with many child populations and a variety of disturbing behaviors (Barkley, 1981; Forehand & McMahon, 1981; Patterson, 1982; White, Nielson, & Johnson, 1972; Zeilberger, Sampsen, & Sloane, 1968).

One additional procedure that has reduced the attention-seeking behavior of persons with severe disabilities deserves mention. This strategy involves teaching children alternative, appropriate methods of obtaining adult attention (Carr & Durand, 1985; Durand & Carr, 1987). In this procedure, children are taught phrases such as "Can you play with me now?", "Will you help?", or "Am I doing good work?" Research has shown that children use the most efficient response to obtain a reinforcer (i.e., adult attention) (Horner, Sprague, O'Brien, & Heathfield,

1990). Therefore, parents must consistently and promptly respond to such appropriate bids for attention; otherwise, the maladaptive responding will be resumed.

The above discussion highlights the treatment implications of a functional assessment of children's problem behavior. When such an evaluation is extended to determining a child's effects on adult behavior, additional intervention considerations are suggested. As noted in a prior section, when clinicians understand reciprocal reinforcement, they can be careful to select target behaviors so that the changes will be maximally reinforcing to the referring adult (Emery *et al.*, 1983). The more parents are reinforced by the child's behavior change, the more likely they will be to maintain their treatment efforts. Another approach resulting from the notion of reciprocal influences is the idea of using children, rather than parents, as behavior change agents (Emery *et al.*, 1983). Several early studies capitalized on child effects by teaching students to praise their teachers for attention and help (e.g., Sherman & Cormier, 1974; Stokes, Fowler, & Baer, 1978). The results were that positive teacher-student contacts increased and negative teacher-student interactions decreased. In the only study dealing with behavior problems at home, Fedoravicius (1973) taught a boy to modify his parents' behavior after they failed to implement a behavior change program. The child was taught to attend to and reinforce parental praise for his appropriate behavior and to remain silent when they criticized him. In response to this treatment, the boy reported improved family interactions and increased freedom from parental constraints. In addition, his parents, who had been unaware of the nature of the intervention, reported that their son had become more cooperative and friendly. As Emery *et al.* (1983) noted, "While this alternative may not always be the most appropriate, it may offer the advantages of empowering children who typically have little power, promoting attributions of internal control in children, and serving as a step in the direction toward behavioral family therapy" (p. 406).

Altering Setting Events

Although typical parent-training protocols focus almost exclusively on the remediation of parenting-skills deficits, other areas for modification are highlighted through the assessment of potential setting events for a child's problem behavior and/or parenting responses. In fact, in some cases, addressing the setting events may be the treatment of choice or, at least, should be done as a prerequisite to more traditional training in behavior management techniques. For example, inadequate sleep may result in child irritability manifested in noncompliance with adult commands. With careful intervention in sleeping habits, irritability and the associated noncompliance may be eliminated. If a youngster exhibits severe aggression in the presence of one family member but is cooperative when with another, the initial treatment recommendations may include increasing the time the child spends with the preferred individual. And when siblings distract each other during homework times, moving to separate study areas may result in better work behavior. There are several advantages in manipulating such setting events for problem behavior (Carr, Robinson, Taylor, & Carlson, 1990). First, challenging responses can be prevented or, at least, reduced significantly. Second, the effects are usually immediate. Third, changing many of the environmental conditions that serve as setting events is much easier than dealing with severe problem behavior when it occurs. Finally, these interventions are extremely cost-effective because, usually, neither the adult nor the child requires training. The therapist needs only to ensure that certain environmental manipulations will be conducted. Then, the parents and the children can be taught additional skills to facilitate the treatment gains. For these reasons, it is essential that a heightened awareness of the impact of setting events on problem behavior be promoted among clinicians and researchers who work with children and their families. To date, there has been a paucity of research in the parent-training literature evaluating the effect of such stimuli on children's responses.

Setting events that affect parents are receiving more attention (Dumas, 1989; Griest & Wells, 1983). However, this interest is reflected primarily in evaluations of the impact of various conditions (e.g., maternal depression, stress, and insularity) on parent-training outcome rather than in investigations of the effects of treatments specifically designed to alter these variables (e.g., McMahon *et al.*, 1981; Patterson, 1983; Wahler, 1980; Webster-Stratton & Hammond, 1990). In a few empirical reports, the combined use of traditional parent training and adjunctive treatments such as parent enhancement therapy (Griest, Forehand, Rogers, Breiner, Furey, & Williams, 1982), partner-support training (Dadds, Schwartz, & Sanders, 1987), problem-solving-skills intervention (Pfiffner, Jouriles, Brown, Etscheidt, & Kelly, 1990), and social skills approaches (Intagliata & Doyle, 1984) has been shown to have the potential to produce greater improvements in child behavior and family interactions than parent training alone. These gains have been especially pronounced at follow-up, a finding suggesting that the most significant result of a broad-based treatment approach may be to enhance the maintenance of newly acquired parenting skills.

ACTUAL TREATMENT

As noted previously, routine clinical assessments of children's problem behavior typically do not take into account the many variables that may be in operation and are not individualized and functional. It follows that actual parent training may be characterized by the application of a fairly standard intervention package. Without the benefit of comprehensive assessment, parent-training approaches typically focus on compliance and noncompliance as target behaviors. The decision to treat these responses is based on a sound empirical rationale. Loeber and Patterson (1981) clearly demonstrated that noncompliance was a core problem in all subgroups of children referred to child therapy centers for treatment of maladaptive responding. It leads to the majority of negative parent-child interactions, which in turn maintain tension in the family. Furthermore, noncompliance is the earliest link in the developmental progression of behavior disorders. Therefore, it makes sense to begin intervention by targeting noncompliance in most cases.

Typical parent-training programs teach techniques for both accelerating desirable behaviors and decelerating undesirable ones, to be used in conjunction with each other. Acceleration procedures are usually introduced first; they involve increasing the frequency and range of the reinforcers, especially the social reinforcers, used by parents. This approach may include helping parents to identify potential reinforcers (Rinn, Vernon, & Wise, 1975), establishing nondirective playtime to improve the parent-child relationship and enhance the value of parental social reinforcement (Barkley, 1981; Forehand & McMahon, 1981), and teaching parents to attend to positive behaviors while ignoring negative ones (Barkley, 1981; Forehand & McMahon, 1981; Patterson, 1982). Parents also are given specific techniques for increasing the effectiveness of their commands in eliciting compliance (e.g., using clear statements and establishing eye contact) (Forehand & McMahon, 1981; Neville & Jenson, 1984). In addition to providing parents with strategies for increasing the frequency of the desirable behaviors that already exist in their child's repertoire, this training often includes methods for developing new prosocial responses. These include shaping, modeling, and prompting. For example, parents can use a shaping procedure to encourage children to play independently when the parents are busy and cannot be interrupted. The parents are taught to give periodic positive attention to a child's independent play in order to gradually increase its duration (Barkley, 1981).

The most commonly taught behavior deceleration technique is time-out from positive reinforcement. Time-out may consist of removing the opportunity to gain praise or tangible rewards (Spitalnik & Drabman, 1976), withdrawing stimulus materials (Barton, Guess, Garcia, & Baer, 1970), or isolating the child in an area devoid of reinforcing persons and objects (Barkley, 1981; Forehand & McMahon, 1981; Patterson, 1982). It is recommended that the duration of time-out not exceed five minutes (Kendall, Nay, & Jeffers, 1976) or ten minutes (Patterson, 1982), that release from time-out be contingent on calm behavior plus an agreement to comply with the original directive (Hobbs & Forehand, 1975), and that parents give a warning before implementing time-out (Roberts, 1982). The efficacy of time-out in decreasing children's problem behavior has been well documented.

Finally, some parent-training programs have reported successfully teaching parents fairly complex and sophisticated methods of achieving behavior change by using token reinforcement (Christophersen, Arnold, Hill, & Quilitch, 1972) and contingency contracting (Patterson, 1982). In these programs, points or chips are earned for the performance of adaptive behaviors and lost for maladaptive actions. Typically, token programs are put into place once differential attention and time-out procedures are under way.

It is recognized widely that certain child populations require modifications in this standard parent-training program. For example, when children are developmentally delayed, parents may need to use simple procedures over longer time periods (Breiner, 1989), and when adolescents are referred for treatment, special interventions for improving family communication and negotiation skills are warranted (Patterson & Fogatch, 1987). Similarly, for treatment-resistant families, it has been recommended that a more individualized, assessment-based approach be used (Dumas, 1989; Griest & Wells, 1983). In fact, like the multiple-gating assessment strategy described earlier, a practical intervention program might start with the application of the standard parent-training protocol. Cost efficiency may be enhanced through the use of group training (Adesso & Lipson, 1981), written materials (Ferber, Keeley, & Shemberg, 1974), and videotaped demonstrations (Nay, 1975). When the initial assessment reveals that there are special needs, or when standard treatment fails, more individually tailored procedures are used.

SUMMARY

Our knowledge of the multiple factors influencing the development, manifestation, and maintenance of children's problem behavior has grown since the inception of parent training in the mid-1960s. Over this period, it has become apparent that a proper assessment of problem responding must make use of multiple methods (unstructured and structured interviews, rating scales and questionnaires, and direct observation) to identify the target child behavior. In addition, related child responses (i.e., those that covary with and/or lead up to the target behavior), as well as the variables controlling them, should be evaluated. These controlling events may include parental actions and reactions and more removed environmental, internal, familial, and extrafamilial conditions. With such a comprehensive functional assessment, an efficacious treatment approach can be designed. Further, the ongoing use of key assessment procedures will document the progress in treatment, pointing to the need for modifications in the intervention strategies and highlighting improvements that signal the time to terminate the therapy.

This type of assessment of children's problem behavior points to conditions that suggest interventions other than differential attention and time-out, which are fairly standard in parent-training protocols. These new treatments include stimulus-based procedures, such as requiring the completion of small components of a task, interspersing difficult requests and easy ones, and offering choices. Teaching behaviors that are functionally equivalent to maladaptive responses also represents a promising approach to behavior management in many child populations. In addition, teaching the child to be the behavior change agent in the family is underused as an intervention strategy. Finally, altering setting events may be the most cost-efficient and long-lasting approach of all. These procedures have been developed and tested in school or institutional settings, often with clients who have developmental disabilities. Thus, they have heuristic value for use by the parents of children with and without handicaps in their own homes. If the current model of parent training is expanded to include some or all of the factors discussed above, it appears that both the clinical and the theoretical gains will be substantial.

REFERENCES

Achenbach, T. M., & Edelbrock, C. (1983). *Manual for the Child Behavior Checklist and Revised Child Behavior Profile*. Burlington, VT: Thomas Achenbach.

Adesso, V. J., & Lipson, J. W. (1981). Group training of parents as therapists for their children. *Behavior Therapy*, *12*, 625–633.

Allen, K. E., & Harris, F. R. (1966). Elimination of a child's excessive scratching by training the mother in reinforcement procedures. *Behavior Research and Therapy*, *4*, 70–84.

American Psychiatric Association. (1987). *Diagnostic and statistical manual of mental disorders* (3rd ed., rev.; DSM-III-R). Washington, DC: Author.

Anastopoulos, A. D., & Barkley, R. A. (1989). A training program for parents of children with attention deficit-hyperactivity disorder. In C. E. Shaffer & J. M. Briesmeister (Eds.), *Handbook of parent training: Parents as cotherapists for children's behavior problems* (pp. 83–104). New York: Wiley.

Axelrod, S. (1987). Functional and structural analyses of behavior: Approaches leading to reduced use of punishment procedures? *Research in Developmental Disabilities*, *8*, 165–178.

Ayllon, T., Layman, D., & Kendel, H. J. (1975). A behavioral-educational alternative to drug control of hyperactive children. *Journal of Applied Behavior Analysis*, *8*, 137–146.

Azrin, N. H., Sneed, T. J., & Foxx, R. M. (1974). Dry-bed training: Rapid elimination of childhood enuresis. *Behaviour Research and Therapy*, *10*, 14–19.

Baer, D. M., Wolf, M. M., & Risley, T. R. (1968). Some current dimensions of applied behavior analysis. *Journal of Applied Behavior Analysis*, *1*, 91–97.

Barkley, R. A. (1981). *Hyperactive children: A handbook for diagnosis and treatment*. New York: Guilford Press.

Barton, E. S., Guess, D., Garcia, E., & Baer, D. M. (1970). Improvements of retardates' mealtime behaviors by timeout procedures using multiple baseline techniques. *Journal of Applied Behavior Analysis*, *3*, 77–84.

Beck, A. T., Rush, A. J., Shaw, B. F., & Emery, G. (1979). *Cognitive therapy of depression*. New York: Guilford Press.

Bijou, S. W., & Baer, D. M. (1978). *Behavior analysis of child development*. Englewood Cliffs, NJ: Prentice-Hall.

Blechman, E. A., Tryon, A. S., Ruff, M. H., & McEnroe, M. J. (1989). Family skills training and childhood depression. In C. E. Shaffer & J. M. Briesmeister (Eds.), *Handbook of parent training: Parents as cotherapists for children's behavior problems* (pp. 203–222). New York: Wiley.

Brackbill, Y., Adams, G., Crowell, D. H., & Gray, M. L. (1966). Arousal level in neonates and preschool children under continuous auditory stimulation. *Journal of Experimental Child Psychology*, *4*, 178–188.

Breiner, J. (1989). Training parents as change agents for their developmentally disabled children. In C. E. Shaffer & J. M. Briesmeister (Eds.), *Handbook of parent training: Parents as cotherapists for children's behavior problems* (pp. 269–304). New York: Wiley.

Bruder, M. B. (1986). Acquisition and generalization of teaching techniques: A study with parents of toddlers. *Behavior Modification*, *10*, 391–414.

Budd, K. S., Green, D. R., & Baer, D. M. (1976). An analysis of multiple misplaced parental social contingencies. *Journal of Applied Behavior Analysis*, *9*, 459–470.

Campbell, R. V., O'Brien, S., Bickett, A. D., & Lutzker, J. R. (1983). In-home parent training, treatment of migraine headaches, and marital counseling as an ecobehavioral approach to prevent child abuse. *Journal of Behavior Therapy and Experimental Psychiatry*, *14*, 147–154.

Carr, E. G., & Durand, V. M. (1985). Reducing behavior problems through functional communication training. *Journal of Applied Behavior Analysis*, *18*, 111–126.

Carr, E. G., & McDowell, J. J. (1980). Social control of self-injurious behavior of organic etiology. *Behavior Therapy*, *11*, 402–409.

Carr, E. G., Newsom, C. D., & Binkoff, J. A. (1980). Escape as a factor in the aggressive behavior of two retarded children. *Journal of Applied Behavior Analysis*, *13*, 393–409.

Carr, E. G., Robinson, S., Taylor, J. C., & Carlson, J. I. (1990). Positive approaches to the treatment of severe behavior problems in persons with developmental disabilities: A review and analysis of reinforcement and stimulus-based procedures. *Monograph of the Association for Persons with severe Handicaps*, *4*, 1–40.

Cataldo, M. G., & Harris, J. (1982). The biological basis for self-injury in the mentally retarded. *Analysis and Intervention in Developmental Disabilities*, *2*, 21–39.

Cava, E. L. (1991). Training parents in behavior modification during a single interview. *The Behavior Therapist,* *14,* 11–12.

Center, D. B., Deitz, S. M., & Kaufman, M. E. (1982). Student ability, task difficulty, and inappropriate classroom behavior. *Behavior Modification, 6,* 355–374.

Chamberlain, P., & Reid, J. B. (1987). Parent observation and report of child symptoms. *Behavioral Assessment, 9,* 97–109.

Chambers, W. J., Puig-Antich, J., Hirsch, M., Paez, P., Ambrosini, P. J., Tabrizi, M. A., & Davies, M. (1985). The assessment of affective disorders in children and adolescents by semi-structured interview: Test-retest reliability. *Archives of General Psychiatry, 42,* 696–702.

Christophersen, E. R., Arnold, C. M., Hill, D. W., & Quilitch, H. R. (1972). The home point system: Token reinforcement procedures for application by parents of children with behavior problems. *Journal of Applied Behavior Analysis, 5,* 485–497.

Conners, C. K. (1969). A teacher rating scale for use in drug studies with children. *American Journal of Psychiatry, 126,* 152–156.

Conners, C. K. (1970). Symptom patterns in hyperactive, neurotic and normal children. *Child Development, 41,* 667–682.

Cooper, J. O., Heron, T. E., & Heward, W. L. (1987). *Applied behavior analysis.* Columbus, OH: Merrill.

Cooper, L. J., Wacker, D. P., Sasso, G. M., Reimers, T. M., & Donn, L. K. (1990). Using parents as therapists to evaluate appropriate behavior of their children: Application to a tertiary diagnostic clinic. *Journal of Applied Behavior Analysis, 23,* 285–296.

Costello, A., Edelbrock, C., Kalas, R., Kessler, M., & Klaric, S. (1982). *The NIMH Diagnostic Interview Schedule for Children (DISC).* Pittsburgh: Author.

Dadds, M. R., Schwartz, S., & Sanders, M. R. (1987). Marital discord and treatment outcome in behavioral treatment of child conduct disorders. *Journal of Consulting and Clinical Psychology, 35,* 396–403.

Day, R. M., Rea, J. A., Schussler, N. G., Larsen, S. E., & Johnson, W. L. (1988). A functionally based approach to the treatment of self-injurious behavior. *Behavior Modification, 2,* 565–589.

Dolgin, M. J., Phipps, S., Harrow, E., & Zeltzer, L. K. (1990). Parental management of fear in chronically ill and healthy children. *Journal of Pediatric Psychology, 15,* 733–744.

Dumas, J. E. (1989). Treating antisocial behavior in children: Child and family approaches. *Clinical Psychology Review, 9,* 197–222.

DuPaul, G. J., Guevremont, D. C., & Barkley, R. A. (1991). Attention deficit-hyperactivity disorder in adolescents: Critical assessment parameters. *Clinical Psychology Review, 11,* 231–245.

Durand, V. M. (1987). "Look Homeward Angel": A call to return to our (functional) roots. *Behavior Analyst, 10,* 299–302.

Durand, V. M., & Carr, E. G. (1987). Social influences on "self-stimulatory" behavior: Analysis and treatment application. *Journal of Applied Behavior Analysis, 20,* 119–132.

Durand, V. M., & Crimmins, D. M. (1988). Identifying the variables maintaining self-injurious behaviors. *Journal of Autism and Developmental Disorders, 18,* 99–117.

Dyer, K., Dunlap, G., & Winterling, V. (1990). The effects of choice-making on the problem behavior of students with severe handicaps. *Journal of Applied Behavior Analysis, 23,* 515–524.

Emery, R. E., Binkoff, J. A., Houts, A. C., & Carr, E. G. (1983). Children as independent variables: Some clinical implications of child-effects. *Behavior Therapy, 14,* 398–412.

Etzel, B., & LeBlanc, J. (1979). The simplest treatment alternative: The law of parsimony applied to choosing appropriate instructional control and errorless-learning procedures for the difficult to teach child. *Journal of Autism and Developmental Disorders, 9,* 361–382.

Fedoravicius, A. S. (1973). The patient as shaper of required parental behavior: A case study. *Journal of Behavior Therapy and Experimental Psychiatry, 4,* 395–396.

Feldman, M. A., Case, L., Rincover, A., Towns, F., & Betel, J. (1989). Parent Education Project III: Increasing affection and responsivity in developmentally handicapped mothers: Component analysis, generalization, and effects on child language. *Journal of Applied Behavior Analysis, 22,* 211–222.

Ferber, H., Keeley, S. M., & Shemberg, K. M. (1974). Training parents in behavior modification: Outcome and problems encountered in a program after Patterson's work. *Behavior Therapy, 5,* 415–419.

Forehand, R., & Atkeson, B. M. (1977). Generality of treatment effects with parents as therapists: A review of assessment and implementation procedures. *Behavior Therapy, 8,* 575–593.

Forehand, R., & King, H. E. (1977). Noncompliant children: Effects of parent training on behavior and attitude change. *Behavior Modification, 1,* 93–108.

Forehand, R., & McMahon, R. J. (1981). *Helping the noncompliant child: A clinician's guide to effective parent training.* New York: Guilford Press.

Foster, S. L. (1987). Issues in behavioral assessment of parent-adolescent conflict. *Behavioral Assessment, 9,* 253–269.

Foxx, R. M., & Azrin, N. H. (1973). Dry pants: A rapid method of toilet training children. *Behavior Research and Therapy, 11,* 435–442.

Furey, W., & Forehand, R. (1984). Maternal satisfaction with clinic-referred children: Assessment by use of a single-subject methodology. *Journal of Behavioral Assessment, 5,* 345–355.

Furey, W., & Forehand, R. (1986). What factors are associated with mothers' evaluations of their clinic-referred children? *Child and Family Behavior Therapy, 8,* 21–42.

Gardner, W. I. (1967). Behavior therapy treatment approach to a psychogenic seizure case. *Journal of Consulting Psychology, 3,* 209–212.

Gardner, W. I., Cole, C. L., Davidson, D. P., & Karan, O. C. (1986). Reducing aggression in individuals with developmental disabilities: An expanded stimulus control, assessment, and intervention model. *Education and Training in Mental Retardation, 21,* 3–12.

Graziano, A. M. (1977). Parents as behavior therapists. In M. Hersen, R. M. Eisler, & P. M. Miller (Eds.), *Progress in behavior modification* (Vol. 4, pp. 251-298). New York: Academic Press.

Griest, D. L., & Wells, K. C. (1983). Behavioral family therapy with conduct disorders in children. *Behavior Therapy, 14,* 37–53.

Griest, D. L., Forehand, R., Rogers, T., Breiner, J., Furey, W., & Williams, C. A. (1982). Effects of parent enhancement therapy on the treatment outcome and generalization of a parent training program. *Behavior Research and Therapy, 20,* 429–436.

Gross, A. M., & Wixted, J. T. (1988). Assessment of child behavior problems. In A. S. Bellack & M. Hersen (Eds.), *Behavioral assessment: A practical handbook.* New York: Pergamon Press.

Herjanic, B. (1980). *Washington University Diagnostic Interview for Children and Adolescents (DICA).* St. Louis: Washington University School of Medicine.

Hobbs, S. M., & Forehand, R. (1975). Effects of differential release from time-out on children's behavior. *Journal of Behavior Therapy and Experimental Psychiatry, 6,* 256–257.

Hobbs, S. A., & Forehand, R. (1977). Important parameters in the use of timeout with children: A reexamination. *Journal of Behavior Therapy and Experimental Psychiatry, 8,* 365–370.

Horner, R. H., Sprague, J. R., O'Brien, M., & Heathfield, L. T. (1990). The role of response efficiency in the reduction of problem behaviors through functional equivalence training: A case study. *Journal of the Association of Persons with Severe Handicaps, 15,* 91–97.

Horner, R. J., Day, M., Sprague, J. R., O'Brien, M., & Heathfield, L. T. (1991). Interspersed requests: A nonaversive procedure for decreasing aggression and self-injury during instruction. *Journal of Applied Behavior Analysis, 24,* 265–278.

Houts, A. D., & Mellon, M. W. (1989). Home-based treatment for primary enuresis. In C. E. Shaffer & J. M. Briesmeister (Eds.), *Handbook of parent training: Parents as cotherapists for children's behavior problems* (pp. 60–80). New York: Wiley.

Hughes, H. M., & Haynes, S. N. (1978). Structured laboratory observation in the behavioral assessment of parent-child interactions: A methodological critique. *Behavior Therapy, 9,* 428–447.

Hutt, C., & Vaizey, M. J. (1966). Differential effects of group density on social behavior. *Nature, 209,* 1371–1372.

Intagliata, J., & Doyle, N. (1984). Enhancing social support for parents of developmentally disabled children: Training in interpersonal problem solving skills. *Mental Retardation, 22,* 4–11.

Iwata, B. A. (1987). Negative reinforcement in applied behavior analysis: An emerging technology. *Journal of Applied Behavior Analysis, 20,* 361–378.

Iwata, B. A., Dorsey, M. F., Slifer, K. J., Bauman, K. E., & Richman, G. S. (1982). Toward a functional analysis of self-injury. *Analysis and Intervention in Developmental Disabilities, 2,* 3–20.

Jones, R. R., Reid, J. B., & Patterson, G. R. (1975). Naturalistic observation in clinical assessment. In P. McReynolds (Ed.), *Advances in psychological assessment* (Vol. 3, pp. 42–95). San Francisco: Jossey-Bass.

Kanfer, F. H., & Saslow, G. (1969). Behavioral diagnosis. In C. M. Franks (Ed.), *Behavior therapy: Appraisal and status* (pp. 417–444). New York: McGraw-Hill.

Kara, A., & Wahler, R. G. (1977). Organizational features of a young child's behavior. *Journal of Experimental Child Psychology, 24,* 24–39.

Kazdin, A. E. (1981). Acceptability of child treatment techniques: The influence of treatment efficacy and adverse side effects. *Behavior Therapy, 12,* 493–506.

Kazdin, A. E. (1982). Symptom substitution, generalization, and response covariation: Implications for psychotherapy outcome. *Psychological Bulletin, 91,* 349–365.

Kearney, C. A., & Silverman, W. K. (1990). A preliminary analysis of a functional model of assessment and treatment for school refusal behavior. *Behavior Modification, 14,* 340–366.

Kelleher, R. T. (1966). Chaining and conditioned reinforcement. In W. K. Honig (Ed.), *Operant behavior: Areas of research and application* (pp. 160–212). New York: Meredith.

Kendall, P. C. (1987). Ahead to basics: Assessments with children and families. *Behavioral Assessment, 9,* 321–332.

Kendall, P. C., Nay, W. R., & Jeffers, J. (1976). Timeout duration and contrast effects: An evaluation of a successive treatment design. *Behavior Therapy, 7,* 609–615.

Krantz, P. J., & Risley, T. R. (1977). Behavioral ecology in the classroom. In S. G. O'Leary & K. D. O'Leary (Eds.), *Classroom management: The successful use of behavior modification* (pp. 222–240). New York: Pergamon Press.

Lamm, N., & Greer, R. D. (1988). Induction and maintenance of swallowing responses in infants with dysphagia. *Journal of Applied Behavior Analysis, 21,* 143–156.

Laski, K. E., Charlop, M. H., & Schreibman, L. (1988). Training parents to use the natural language paradigm to increase their autistic children's speech. *Journal of Applied Behavior Analysis, 21,* 391–400.

Lennox, D. B., & Miltenberger, R. G. (1990). On the conceptualization of treatment acceptability. *Education and Training in Mental Retardation, 25,* 211–224.

Locke, H. J., & Wallace, K. M. (1959). Short marital-adjustment and prediction tests: Their reliability and validity. *Marriage and Family Living, 21,* 251–255.

Loeber, R., & Patterson, G. R. (1981). The aggressive child: A concomitant of a coercive system. In J. P. Vincent (Ed.), *Advances in family intervention, assessment and theory: An annual compilation of research* (pp. 47–87). Greenwich, CT: JAI Press.

Loeber, R., Dishion, T. J., & Patterson, G. (1984). Multiple gating: A multi-stage assessment procedure for identifying youths at risk for delinquency. *Journal of Research in Crime and Delinquency, 21,* 7–32.

Lovaas, O. I., Freitag, G., Gold, V. J., & Kassorla, I. C. (1965). Recording apparatus and procedure for observation of behaviors of children in free play settings. *Journal of Experimental Child Psychology, 2,* 108–120.

Loyd, G. J., & Abidin, R. R. (1985). Revision of the Parenting Stress Index. *Journal of Pediatric Psychology, 10,* 169–177.

Luiselli, J. K. (1991). Assessment-derived treatment of children's disruptive behavior disorders. *Behavior Modification, 15,* 294–309.

Lytton, H. (1990). Child and parent effects in boys' conduct disorder: A reinterpretation. *Developmental Psychology, 26,* 683–697.

Mace, F. C., Page, T. J., Ivancic, M. T., & O'Brien, S. (1986). Analysis of environmental determinants of aggression and disruption in mentally retarded children. *Applied Research in Mental Retardation, 7,* 203–221.

Mace, F. C., Hock, M. L., Lalli, J. S., West, B. J., Belfiore, P., Pinter, E., & Brown, D. K. (1988). Behavioral momentum in the treatment of noncompliance. *Journal of Applied Behavior Analysis, 21,* 123–141.

Martin, P. L., & Foxx, R. M. (1973). Victim control of the aggression of an institutionalized retardate. *Journal of Behavior Therapy and Experimental Psychiatry, 4,* 161–165.

McMahon, R. J. (1987). Some current issues in the behavioral assessment of conduct disordered children and their families. *Behavioral Assessment, 9,* 235–252.

McMahon, R. J., & Forehand, R. (1984). Parent training for the noncompliant child: Treatment outcome, generalization, and adjunctive therapy procedures. In R. F. Dangel & A. Polster (Eds.), *Parent training: Foundations of research and practice* (pp. 298–323). New York: Guilford Press,

McMahon, R. J., Forehand, R., Greist, D. L., & Wells, K. C. (1981). Who drops out of treatment during parent behavioral training? *Behavioral Counseling Quarterly, 1,* 79–85.

Milich, R., Landau, S., Kilby, G., & Whitten, P. (1982). Preschool peer perceptions of the behavior of hyperactive and aggressive children. *Journal of Abnormal Child Psychology, 12,* 471–490.

Moran, D. R., & Whitman, T. L. (1991). Developing generalized teaching skills in mothers of autistic children. *Child and Family Behavior Therapy, 13,* 13–37.

Nay, W. R. (1975). A systematic comparison of instructional techniques for parents. *Behavior Therapy, 6,* 14–21.

Neisworth, J. T., & Moore, F. (1972). Operant treatment of asthmatic responding with the parent as therapist. *Behavior Therapy, 3,* 95–99.

Neville, M. H., & Jenson, W. R. (1984). Precision commands and the "Sure I will" program: A quick and efficient compliance training sequence. *Child and Family Behavior Therapy, 6,* 61–65.

O'Dell, S. (1974). Training parents in behavior modification: A review. *Psychological Bulletin, 81,* 418–433.

Parrish, J. M., Cataldo, M. F., Kolko, D. J., Neef, N. A., & Egel, A. L. (1986). Experimental analysis of response covariations among compliant and inappropriate behaviors. *Journal of Applied Behavior Analysis, 19,* 241–254.

Patterson, G. R. (1976). *Living with children: New methods for parents and teachers*. Champaign, IL: Research Press.

Patterson, G. R. (1977). Accelerating stimuli for two classes of coercive behavior. *Journal of Abnormal Child Psychology*, *5*, 335–350.

Patterson, G. R. (1982). *A social learning approach to family intervention: Vol. 3. Coercive family process*. Eugene, OR: Castalia.

Patterson, G. R. (1983). Stress: A change agent for family process. In N. Garmezy & M. Rutter (Eds.), *Stress, coping and development in children* (pp. 235–262). New York: McGraw-Hill.

Patterson, G. R., & Brosky, M. (1966). Behavior modification for a child with multiple problem behaviors. *Journal of Child Psychology and Psychiatry*, *7*, 277–295.

Patterson, G. R., & Fogatch, M. S. (1987). *Parents and adolescents living together: Part 1. The basics*. Eugene, OR: Castalia.

Patterson, G. R., Reid, J. B., Jones, R. R., & Conger, R. E. (1975). *A social learning approach to family intervention: Families with aggressive children* (Vol. 1). Eugene, OR: Castalia.

Peed, S., Roberts, M., & Forehand, R. (1977). Evaluation of the effectiveness of a standardized parent training program in altering the interaction of mothers and their noncompliant children. *Behavior Modification*, *1*, 323–349.

Pfiffner, L. J., Jouriles, E. N., Brown, M. M., Etscheidt, M. A., Kelly, J. A. (1990). Effects of problem-solving therapy on outcomes of parent training for single-parent families. *Child and Family Behavior Therapy*, *12*, 1–11.

Plummer, S., Baer, D. M., & LeBlanc, J. M. (1977). Functional considerations in the use of procedural timeout and an effective alternative. *Journal of Applied Behavior Analysis*, *10*, 689–705.

Puig-Antich, J., & Chambers, W. (1978). *Schedule for Affective Disorders and Schizophrenia for School-Aged Children (6–16 years)—Kiddie-SADS*. New York: New York State Psychiatric Institute.

Quay, H. C. (1983). A dimensional approach to children's behavior disorder: The Revised Behavior Problem Checklist. *School Psychology Review*, *12*, 244–249.

Reimers, T. M., Wacker, D. P., & Cooper, L. J. (1991). Evaluation of the acceptability of treatments for children's behavioral difficulties: Ratings by parents receiving services in an outpatient clinic. *Child and Family Behavior Therapy*, *13*, 53–71.

Reisinger, J. J., Frangia, G. W., & Hoffman, E. H. (1976). toddler management training: Generalization and marital status. *Journal of Behavior Therapy and Experimental Psychology*, *7*, 335–340.

Reynolds, W. M. (1986). A model for the screening and identification of depressed children and adolescents in school settings. *Professional School Psychology*, *1*, 117–129.

Rinn, R. C., Vernon, J. C., & Wise, M. J. (1975). Training parents of behavior-disordered children in groups: A three years' program evaluation. *Behavior Therapy*, *6*, 378–387.

Roberts, M. W. (1982). The effects of warned versus unwarned time-out procedures on child noncompliance. *Child and Family Behavior Therapy*, *4*, 37–53.

Roberts, M. W., McMahon, R. J., Forehand, R., & Humphreys, L. (1978). The effect of parental instruction-giving on child compliance. *Behavior Therapy*, *9*, 793–798.

Sandler, A., Coren, A., & Thurman, S. K. (1983). A training program for parents of handicapped preschool children: Effects upon mother, father, and child. *Exceptional Children*, *49*, 355–359.

Sherman, T. M., & Cormier, W. H. (1974). An investigation of the influence of student behavior on teacher behavior. *Journal of Applied Behavior Analysis*, *7*, 11–21.

Singh, N. N., Watson, J. E., & Winton, A. S. W. (1987). Parents' acceptability ratings of alternative treatments for use with mentally retarded children. *Behavior Modification*, *11*, 17–26.

Slifer, K. J., Ivancic, M. T., Parrish, J. M., Page, T. J., & Burgio, L. D. (1986). Assessment and treatment of multiple behavior problems exhibited by a profoundly retarded adolescent. *Journal of Behavior Therapy and Experimental Psychiatry*, *17*, 203–213.

Solnick, J. V., Rincover, A., & Peterson, C. R. (1977). Some determinants of the reinforcing and punishing effects of timeout. *Journal of Applied Behavior Analysis*, *10*, 415–424.

Spitalnik, R., & Drabman, R. (1976). A classroom timeout procedure for retarded children. *Journal of Behavior Therapy and Experimental Psychiatry*, *7*, 17–21.

Steen, P. L., & Zuriff, G. E. (1977). The use of relaxation in the treatment of self-injurious behavior. *Journal of Behavior Therapy and Experimental Psychiatry*, *8*, 447–448.

Stevens-Long, J. (1973). The effect of behavioral context on some aspects of adult disciplinary practice and affect. *Child Development*, *44*, 476–484.

Stokes, T. F., Fowler, S. A., & Baer, D. M. (1978). Training preschool children to recruit natural communities of reinforcement. *Journal of Applied Behavior Analysis*, *11*, 285–303.

Taylor, J. C., Sisson, L. A., McKelvey, J. L., & Trefelner, M. F. (in press). Situation specificity in attention seeking problem behavior: A case study. *Behavior Modification*.

Van Hasselt, V. B., Sisson, L. A., & Aach, S. R. (1987). Parent training to increase compliance in a young multihandicapped child. *Journal of Behavior Therapy and Experimental Psychiatry, 18*, 275–283.

Voeltz, L. M., & Evans, I. M. (1982). The assessment of behavioral interrelationships in child behavior therapy. *Behavioral Assessment, 4*, 131–165.

Wahler, R. G. (1969). Oppositional children: A quest for parental reinforcement control. *Journal of Applied Behavior Analysis, 2*, 159–170.

Wahler, R. G. (1965). Some structural aspects of deviant child behavior. *Journal of Applied Behavior Analysis, 8*, 27–42.

Wahler, R. G. (1980). The insular mother: Her problems in parent-child treatment. *Journal of Applied Behavior Analysis, 13*, 207–219.

Wahler, R. G., & Cormier, W. H. (1970). The ecological interview: A first step in outpatient child behavior therapy. *Journal of Behavior Therapy and Experimental Psychiatry, 1*, 279–289.

Wahler, R. G., & Fox, J. J. (1980). Solitary toy play and time out: A family treatment package for children with aggressive and oppositional behavior. *Journal of Applied Behavior Analysis, 13*, 23–39.

Wahler, R. G., & Graves, M. G. (1983). Setting events in social networks: Ally or enemy in child behavior therapy? *Behavior Therapy, 14*, 19–36.

Wahler, R. G., Winkel, G. H., Peterson, R. F., & Morrison, D. C. (1965). Mothers as behavior therapists for their own children. *Behavior Research and Therapy, 3*, 113–124.

Wahler, R. G., Leske, G., & Rogers, E. S. (1979). The insular family: A deviance support system for oppositional children. In L. A. Hamerlynck (Ed.), *Behavioral systems for the developmentally disabled: Vol. 1 School and family environments* (pp. 102–127). New York: Brunner/Mazel.

Webster-Stratton, C., & Hammond, M. (1990). Predictors of treatment outcome in parent training for families with conduct problem children. *Behavior Therapy, 21*, 319–337.

Wells, K. C., & Forehand, R. (1985). Conduct and oppositional disorder. In P. H. Bornstein & A. E. Kazdin (Eds.), *Handbook of clinical behavior therapy with children* (pp. 218–265). Homewood, IL: Dorsey.

White, G. D., Nielson, G., & Johnson, S. M. (1972). Timeout duration and the suppression of deviant behavior in children. *Journal of Applied Behavior Analysis, 5*, 111–120.

Williams, C. G. (1959). The elimination of tantrum behavior by extinction procedures. *Journal of Abnormal and Social Psychology, 59*, 269.

Yule, W. (1989). Parent involvement in the treatment of the school phobic child. In C. E. Shaffer & J. M. Briesmeister (Eds.), *Handbook of parent training: Parents as cotherapists for children's behavior problems* (pp. 223–244). New York: Wiley.

Zeilberger, J., Sampsen, S. E., & Sloane, H. N. (1968). Modification of a child's behavior problems in the home with the mother as therapist. *Journal of Applied Behavior Analysis, 1*, 47–53.

28

Marital Distress

STEVEN L. SAYERS, DONALD H. BAUCOM, and LYNN RANKIN

INTRODUCTION

Most clinicians have contact with individuals or couples who are experiencing marital conflict. Indeed, marital distress is quite common. At least half of all first marriages and half of all remarriages eventually fail (Glick, 1984, 1989a,b). Twenty percent of married couples at any particular time are likely to be distressed (Beach, Arias, & O'Leary, 1987a). Often marital issues must be addressed because of the interrelationship between marital problems and the psychological functioning of the individual. In some couples, marital conflict may precipitate or exacerbate the psychiatric symptoms of one of the spouses; in other couples, an existing psychiatric disorder may lead to the disruption of the marital relationship. Given these circumstances, it is encouraging that, since the late 1960s, an increasing number of investigations have shown behavioral marital therapy to be an effective treatment for marital distress (Baucom & Hoffman, 1986). Additionally, marital therapy shows promise in the treatment of concomitant psychiatric disorders such as depression. Before we elucidate these developments, it is necessary to describe marital distress from a behavioral perspective.

DESCRIPTION OF THE SYNDROME

Specific, observable patterns in distressed spouses' communication differentiate them from nondistressed spouses. As might be expected, distressed spouses exhibit predictably higher rates of negative behavior and lower rates of positive behavior than nondistressed spouses. The negative behavior characteristic of distressed couples during the discussion of problems includes criticism, putdowns, statements reflecting hostility or displeasure, excuses, complaints, and negative nonverbal behavior. They are less likely than nondistressed spouses to agree, to propose solutions, and to show empathy, humor, and positive affect (for reviews, see Baucom, Notarius, Burnett, & Haefner, 1990c; Weiss & Heyman, 1990).

Investigators have also examined the *sequential* patterns of communication behavior exhibited by distressed couples. Spouses in distressed relationships are more likely than those

STEVEN L. SAYERS • Medical College of Pennsylvania at EPPI, Philadelphia, Pennsylvania 19129. DONALD H. BAUCOM and LYNN RANKIN • Department of Psychology, University of North Carolina at Chapel Hill, Chapel Hill, North Carolina 27599.

Handbook of Behavior Therapy in the Psychiatric Setting, edited by Alan S. Bellack and Michel Hersen. Plenum Press, New York, 1993.

in nondistressed couples to respond to their partner's negative behavior with negative behavior (Hooley & Hahlweg, 1989; Margolin & Wampold, 1981). The immediate tendency to reciprocate the partner's negative behavior is termed *negative reciprocity*. Clinical observation suggests that this type of interaction quickly escalates into destructive verbal and physical conflict. Other, more specific "distressed" sequences include complaints followed by complaints, complaints followed by defensive remarks (and vice versa) (Ting-Toomey, 1983), and the husband's withdrawal followed by the wife's hostility (Roberts & Krokoff, 1990).

Recent studies suggest that behavior associated with conflict engagement, rather than conflict avoidance, may lead to improvements in marital satisfaction. Preliminary evidence indicates that there are specific kinds of negatively valenced behavior that facilitate increased satisfaction in the future, even though they are characteristic of current dissatisfaction (Gottman & Krokoff, 1989; Roberts & Krokoff, 1990; Sayers, Baucom, Sher, Weiss, & Heyman, 1991). Hopefully, future research will clarify what specific behavior helps maritally distressed couples improve the functioning of their relationship.

Distressed spouses also display dysfunctional patterns of cognitions about their relationship and relationship problems. Distinct kinds of *attributions*, or explanations of marital events, are exhibited by distressed couples. Unhappy spouses tend to attribute their relationship conflicts to faults in their partners and to feel that these faults are enduring, negative characteristics that affect many areas of the relationship (see Bradbury & Fincham, 1990). Distressed spouses may also perceive their partners' behavior more negatively than nondistressed partners and may feel that the negative behavior is meant to hurt them.

Other types of cognitions may also be associated with marital distress. For example, distressed spouses are likely to have inappropriate or unrealistic *standards* for relationships ("My partner should meet all my emotional needs") and *assumptions* ("My wife is typical in that she is domineering, monopolizes the children, and is not interested in being romantic with me") (Baucom & Epstein, 1990). Although a great deal of research is still needed in this area, clinicians should attend to evidence that these kinds of thoughts and beliefs contribute to the marital discord.

PROTOTYPICAL ASSESSMENT

A detailed discussion of how to assess marital discord from a cognitive behavioral perspective is beyond the scope of this chapter (for an in-depth discussion of this topic, see Baucom & Epstein, 1990; O'Leary, 1987); however, the major representative assessment strategies are discussed. For heuristic purposes, it is useful to differentiate among the couple's behavior, cognitions, and affect as the major domains relevant to the assessment of marital discord.

Assessing Behavior

A couple's behavior constitutes a broad class of activities, but two classes of behavior are of significance: *communication* and *noncommunication*. Communication concerns are the most frequent presenting complaints of married couples requesting assistance with their relationship (Geiss & O'Leary, 1981). Two very useful self-report measures that provide a global index of a couple's communication are the Marital Communication Inventory (MCI; Bienvenu, 1970) and the Primary Communication Inventory (PCI; Navran, 1967). To enhance the clinical utility of these inventories, the clinician can discuss with the spouses their responses to individual items in order to clarify the communication difficulties. Furthermore, Snyder (1981) developed two subscales from the Marital Satisfaction Inventory (MSI) to assess problem-solving communication and affective communication. These scales can help to narrow the nature of the concerns to more specific areas that the clinician can assess through behavioral observation, as described below.

Behavioral observation is particularly useful in assessing a couple's ability to solve problems because it is not subject to the spouses' reporting biases. The couple is asked to resolve a problem of moderate importance during a 10-minute conversation that the therapist observes. To allow for the possibility that the interaction may be influenced by the particular problem discussed (Weider & Weiss, 1980), it is best for the couple to discuss at least two problems during the assessment session.

The clinician must then evaluate the communication that has occurred. Several detailed, microanalytic coding systems have been developed for research purposes, including the Marital Interaction Coding System (MICS; Weiss & Summers, 1983; Weiss, 1990), the Couples Interaction Scoring System (CISS; Notarius, Markman, & Gottman, 1983), and the Kategoriensystem für Partnerschaftliche Interaktion (KPI; Hahlweg, Reisner, Kohli, Vollmer, Schindler, & Revenstorf, 1984). Whereas a systematic application of these coding systems is far beyond the resources available in most clinical contexts, familiarity with one or more of these systems allows the clinician an informal assessment of the communication. Alternatively, the clinician may use one of the global rating scales that have been developed for the assessment of problem-solving communication. These systems include the Marital Interaction Coding System—Global (MICS-G; Weiss & Tolman, 1990), the Global Rapid Couples Interaction Scoring System (RCISS; Krokoff, Gottman, & Haas, 1989), and the Interactional Dimensions Coding System (IDCS; Julien, Markman, & Lindahl, 1989). Furthermore, the clinician may opt to assess the couple's problem-solving communication skills by using the list in Table 1. The table can be used as a checklist by the clinician, who notes the frequency of each behavior during the problem-solving-assessment exercises. This list includes clinically established problem-solving guidelines and is based, in part, on studies differentiating the problem-solving behavior of nondistressed couples and the interactions of their distressed counterparts.

The couple's ability to express their thoughts and feelings to each other and to be effective listeners should also be evaluated through observation. To provide the context for this interaction, a variant of Guerney's Verbal Interaction Task (1977) may be used. One spouse is told to spend four minutes sharing his or her feelings and thoughts about something the speaker likes or appreciates about the partner. The partner is told that his or her role is to *help* the speaker to

Table 1. Communication Behaviors for Problem Solving

Functional communication behaviors
  Maintaining good eye contact
  Stating the problem in *behavioral* terms rather than in terms of negative traits of the partner
    Example: "We haven't been keeping up the maintenance on the car" (behavioral description).
               "We have to deal with your laziness" (negative trait description).
  Staying solution-oriented:
    Describe the problem.
    Propose solutions.
    Discuss the merits of the solutions.
  Presenting one's solutions only one or two times
  Summarizing the partner's viewpoint when possible to clarify his or her position
  Seeking solutions that meet both partners' needs and compromising when possible
Dysfunctional communication behaviors
  Blaming one's partner for the conflict
  Stating one's perceptions as facts rather than opinions or feelings
  Getting sidetracked onto other problems
  Dwelling on the past
  Interrupting the partner

STEVEN L. SAYERS
et al.

express the feelings. After four minutes, the two partners switch roles. The clinician repeats this format to assess the expression of negative feelings. Thus, each spouse is observed expressing both positive and negative feelings about the partner, and the partner's listening skills are also observed. Guerney (1977) and his colleagues have developed rating scales that assist in evaluating the extent to which spouses express feelings adaptively and the extent to which partners are effective listeners; again, informal application of this more time-consuming rating procedure is sufficient for most clinical purposes. The primary skills to be assessed in this exercise are listed in Table 2.

Because spouses interact with each other in numerous ways other than through direct communication (e.g., engaging in leisure activities or household tasks), noncommunication behavior should also be assessed. The behaviors that partners engage in or avoid may have a major impact on the happiness of the marriage (Christensen & Nies, 1980; Jacobson, Follette, & McDonald, 1982). Clarifying the behavioral excesses and deficits in the marriage becomes a major task of the marital assessment. Often, spouses have rather global perceptions of their problems, simply stating that they argue frequently or spend little time together. To give a more detailed picture of their behavior, self-report measures that focus on specific aspects of marital functioning are helpful. For example, the Areas-of-Change Questionnaire (Weiss & Perry, 1983) lists 34 specific areas of marital functioning (e.g., finances, leisure time, and sex) and asks the respondent to clarify the degree of change by the partner desired in each area. This information is discussed within the sessions to clarify each partner's specific behavioral concerns.

Assessing Cognitions

In recent years, behaviorally oriented therapists have gained greater appreciation that spouses' cognitions about the relationship are important determinants of relationship happiness. There are at least five cognitive factors to take into account when assessing a couple's relationship (Baucom, Epstein, Sayers, & Sher, 1989a). First, spouses may *selectively attend*

Table 2. Communication Behaviors for Empathic Listening and Expressing Feelings

Empathic listening
Functional communication behaviors
  Restating or summarizing the partner's message, emphasizing his or her feelings
  Maintaining good eye contact to express acceptance
  Tactfully indicating to the partner if she or he is telling you too much at one time
Dysfunctional communication behaviors
  Interrupting the partner
  Stating one's own interpretation of the partner's feelings
  Trying to solve the problem
Expressing feelings
Functional communication behaviors
  Using a "subjective" voice, combined with a behavioral description of the event
    Example: "I feel angry when you change the TV channel repeatedly without talking to me about it."
  Balancing a negative message with its positive aspects
    Example: "I usually enjoy watching TV with you, but I get angry when you change the channels quickly without asking me."
  Maintaining good eye contact
  Talking in short "paragraphs" to help the partner remember all that is said
Dysfunctional communication behaviors
  Blaming the partner for one's feelings
  Negative "mindreading," or assuming that the partner is thinking negatively.

to what events are occurring in the relationship; thus, if a husband increases his rate of affectionate behavior but the wife does not notice, his behavior change is unlikely to increase his wife's happiness. Second, once spouses do recognize that some behavior has occurred, they make *attributions* for the partner's behavior. For example, if a husband attributes his wife's working late to her commitment to providing for the family, her working late may have a positive effect on the relationship. Alternatively, if her behavior is viewed as an attempt to avoid him, her late hours may have a negative effect. Third, not only do spouses interpret events that have already occurred, they also have *expectancies* or make predictions about what behaviors are likely to occur in the future. Therefore, if a wife believes that her husband's increased affection is only temporary, she may not enjoy his behavior even while it is occurring. Fourth, spouses have *assumptions* about the basic nature of men, women, and relationships. For example, a husband may believe that women are not rational and that there is no reason to attempt to discuss problems with his wife. Such assumptions are dysfunctional and limit the spouses' efforts to change. Fifth, spouses have *standards* concerning relationships and how each partner should behave. Thus, one spouse may believe that marital partners should spend all of their free time together and that any violation of this standard is a clear indication of a lack of love.

At present, there are several strategies for assessing these cognitions in a clinical setting. First, couples often spontaneously offer information relevant to these cognitions during initial clinical interviews. While discussing a current concern, the spouses may offer their attributions or explanations for the existence of the problem. Similarly, spouses frequently provide standards concerning how they believe their partner should behave in a given area of the marriage. The clinician's task is to make an assessment of the extent to which the cognitions are distorted or extreme and thus require intervention. The mere fact that a partner has negative cognitions about the marriage does not mean that the cognitions are distorted. Therefore, if a husband believes that a wife stays at work late because she does not want to spend time with him and she confirms his attribution, a cognitive procedure is not the intervention of choice. Instead, it may be necessary to change the couple's interaction patterns in order to make them more enjoyable for the wife.

As therapy progresses, in-session events also provide the therapist with abundant cognitions. When a spouse's affect or behavior changes abruptly, the therapist solicits that spouse's cognitions. This approach is most effective after the spouses have become more accustomed to the process of scrutinizing their thoughts; otherwise, they may feel challenged by the therapist. Another possible source of cognitions is the couple's report of past upsetting events, as spouses often reveal their *interpretations* of events when reporting them. In addition to the information about the spouses' cognitions obtained from interviews, cognitive self-monitoring forms, such as the Daily Record of Dysfunctional Thoughts (Beck, Rush, Shaw, & Emery, 1979), may be helpful. This form helps the spouses collect examples of distressing events and the spouses' cognitions and emotional responses.

Standardized self-report measures focusing on couples' cognitions are currently being developed, although they are in only the initial stages of validation. The greatest attention has been given to the assessment of attributions by means of self-report measures (see Bradbury & Fincham, 1990, for a recent review). For example, Baucom, Sayers, and Duhe (1989b) developed the Dyadic Attribution Inventory, a 24-item measure that assesses a partner's attributions for both positive and negative relationship events. Alternatively, Baucom, Epstein, Rankin, and Burnett (1990b) developed the Inventory of Specific Relationship Standards to assess a broad range of relationship standards.

Assessing Affect

There are many factors to consider in assessing the emotional life of married couples, although we have space here for only a cursory look at these issues (see Baucom & Epstein,

1990). The most important of these factors are (1) a spouse's awareness of the specific emotion that he or she is experiencing; (2) a spouse's ability to relate this emotion to his or her own cognitions or to external events; (3) and a spouse's ability to express affect adaptively. When spouses experience emotions only on a global, diffuse, "positive-negative" level, it is difficult for them to understand the specifics of how their feelings are related to their thoughts or behaviors. These factors may be assessed by asking a spouse to report on his or her emotions concerning a past event. Alternatively, the therapist may query the spouse when he or she *appears* to be experiencing an affective response. The assessment of skills relating to the communication of emotions was discussed earlier.

In addition to short-lived affective responses in a particular situation, one or both partners may have a more enduring emotion that interferes with relationship functioning. In many maritally distressed couples, one partner is clinically depressed. Similarly, one spouse may frequently experience high levels of anxiety that interfere with social interaction or various aspects of relationship functioning (e.g., sexual interaction). The presence of these affective disturbances must be assessed. Numerous sources discuss the assessment of various disorders (e.g., see Chapters 11–18 of this book). As noted below, it is important to determine the existence of concomitant disorders because of the broader treatment implications.

ACTUAL ASSESSMENT

An assessment of the interrelated domains of behavior, cognitions, and emotions is structured around the clinical interview. Before the initial interview, the spouses are asked to complete a battery of self-report measures that assess the areas described above. This strategy directs the clinician to the areas that should be assessed with the couple in more detail. The actual clinical interview is divided into three segments: (1) a marital history; (2) a discussion of current relationship problems and strengths; and (3) an observation of the couple communicating. A discussion of the history of the relationship provides the clinician with a context for understanding the current concerns. Within such a context, many of the current problems form a relationship pattern rather than occurring as isolated behaviors or cognitions. Following the relationship history, the clinician asks each spouse to clarify his or her current concerns about the relationship. This phase of the interview may be structured around items from the Areas-of-Change Questionnaire or similar instruments. In order to maintain a proper perspective on the relationship, the clinician should also include a discussion of the relationship's strengths. Finally, the spouses are observed while they communicate with each other in different ways, including problem solving in areas of conflict and sharing positive and negative feelings with each other.

During this data-gathering process, the therapist often becomes aware that one or both of the spouses may have a psychiatric disorder. Alternatively, only one of the spouses may have originally presented for the treatment of individual distress, and it becomes apparent that he or she is experiencing considerable marital conflict. Given either situation, both spouses should be involved so that the clinician can conduct an assessment of individual psychopathology and of the marriage. In addition, the relationship between any existing disorders and the marital conflict must be fully explored.

Following a fairly standard set of procedures that one would use to assess individual psychopathology, the clinician turns to the question of the interrelationship between the marital conflicts and individual problems. It is not particularly difficult for the marital therapist to obtain information about the role of an individual disorder; however, obtaining it in a way that does not alienate one partner or encourage one spouse to blame the other is more difficult (i.e., one spouse says, "If you were not depressed all the time, our marriage would be fine"). Therefore, the clinician should tactfully make it clear that the notion of a single cause of any behavioral problem is almost always an oversimplification and that the couple's task will be to try to understand the multiple factors that contribute to both areas of concern. The temporal ordering of the marital discord and the disorder of one of the spouses should also be assessed through interview. Again, there is no certainty that such evaluations represent the true temporal or causal relationship of these complex areas of concern.

The therapist also focuses on the extent to which the couple is responding successfully to the individual's problems. The clinician should ask how the individual problems are manifested in the family context and how the partner responds to those problems. Furthermore, the communication samples may provide some information regarding the patterns of reinforcement for psychiatric symptoms by the nonaffected spouse.

Case Conceptualization and Treatment Planning

The therapist may increase his or her success with the strategies discussed above by using the findings of the assessment to construct a conceptualization of the couple's problems and by planning the treatment accordingly. The therapist should consider several questions in this conceptualization. Does the couple fight frequently and find fighting aversive? Are there discernible patterns in these transactions, judging by the couple's reports of arguments at home and the problem-solving assessments in the initial interviews? Do the spouses exhibit a skill *deficit* in problem-solving discussions, or do they simply choose ineffective skills when dealing with one another? The spouses' report of interactions with others, as well as interactions with the therapist, will aid the therapist in answering this question. Regarding cognitions, do the spouses hold beliefs about their relationship that inhibit them from changing? Are their expectations of themselves and each other reasonable? Do they track each other's behavior, waiting for the partner to act negatively? Furthermore, what seems to have been responsible for the development of the couple's current dissatisfaction? Does one of the spouses seem to be experiencing a disorder, such as major depression?

The conceptualization should be an integration of the findings from all of the domains of the couple's functioning. For instance, how do the spouses' beliefs about relationships, combined with their level of problem-solving skill, influence their day-to-day interactions? How do their patterns of avoidance prevent them from dealing effectively with the current stresses in their lives? Answering these questions will help the therapist to target his or her interventions to the areas most responsible for relationship dissatisfaction.

Given the array of interventions available, the clinician must decide which to use first. Immediate concerns cited by the couple may provide a guide to the selection of the initial intervention. If the couple has a number of specific problems to solve (e.g., the division of household chores and the discipline of the children), training in problem solving and communication is a logical choice. However, if the couple exhibits a great deal of negative reciprocity, it may be wiser to begin with skills training in expressing emotions. Reducing the intensity of these exchanges may do much to prepare the couple for the collaborative work of problem solving. Further, the spouses may also be closely tracking the partner's negative behavior. Such behavior indicates that techniques that affect spouses' selective attention to negative behavior should be used early in therapy.

Generally speaking, it may be better to delay the use of cognitive interventions until later in treatment. Even if it is apparent that one or both of the spouses have dysfunctional cognitions that contribute to their distress, they may not easily integrate the idea that how they think about their problems may be as important as the problems themselves. Further, it is not always easy to determine quickly what thoughts and beliefs contribute most to negative feelings and a lack of collaborative spirit in the marriage.

In some cases, the person with a specific disorder has received individual therapy before beginning marital therapy. In other instances, the marital therapist recommends individual therapy. In order for the marital therapist to develop a successful treatment plan for the marriage and also be of benefit to the individual, it is critical that there be a close collaboration between the marital therapist and any individual therapists involved. A mutual plan is necessary for dealing with the individual problems and the relationship. Thus, if the marital therapist believes that it is important that a wife not provide extensive reassurance to a husband who has obsessional fears of contamination, the individual therapist must concur and support this shift in her behavior.

PROTOTYPICAL TREATMENT

In its earliest form, behavioral marital therapy (BMT) was designed to effect *behavioral* changes in spouses' marital interactions as a way to increase their satisfaction. Based on the idea that couples' dissatisfaction is a result of disturbances in the spouses' rates of exchange of pleasing behaviors, Stuart (1969) helped couples negotiate changes in these behaviors. This approach formed the foundation of later techniques, which became more oriented toward how spouses communicate and negotiate their feelings, needs, wants, and desires. More recent developments in BMT include cognitive interventions that focus on helping spouses perceive and think about their partner and their relationship most appropriately. Precisely which areas of the relationship's functioning should be attended to greatly depends on the outcome of the assessment phase described above.

Skills-Training Techniques

Most BMT outcome studies and clinical descriptions feature *problem-solving/communication training (PST)* as the basic technique for the treatment of marital discord (e.g., Baucom & Epstein, 1990; Jacobson & Margolin, 1979; Weiss, 1980). The goal of PST is to teach couples *how* to solve problems, rather than to solve only the problems they are currently bringing to treatment.

The introduction of problem solving involves several aspects. The therapist first presents the steps to be followed in problem solving: (1) a definition of the problem and an agreement by both spouses to work on the problem; (2) the generation of solutions; (3) an evaluation of the solutions, the selection of the preferred solution, and a specification of the trial period; and (4) an evaluation of the success of the solution following the trial period. An important aspect of helping couples to follow these steps is to encourage them to use a *behaviorally defined* description at the problem definition stage. A vague or generally stated problem description often becomes a sweeping critical commentary about the partner. For example, the statement that "Amy is uncomfortable with the number of nights that she and Charles eat at the dinner table per week" is much more appropriate than "Charles doesn't care about the family enough to sit down to dinner."

The specific communication guidelines that accompany PST parallel those assessed in the problem-solving samples at the beginning of treatment (see Table 1). The therapist guides the spouses through the steps detailed previously and provides periodic encouragement, as well as feedback on how to communicate more effectively by using these principles. In general, the expression of highly negative affect is discouraged because it dampens creative problem-solving attempts. The key feature of PST is that it helps the couple negotiate changes in behavior in the relationship in a task-oriented way.

Another important procedure used in BMT is termed *emotional expressiveness training* (EET). It was pioneered by Guerney (1977) as a technique for relationship enhancement. Its purpose is to help encourage emotional intimacy by teaching couples reflective listening skills. It contrasts PST in that it emphasizes the affiliative aspects of the relationship. If the therapist helps the spouses to concentrate on *accepting* rather than *agreeing with* their partner's position, they may feel freer to be more empathic.

EET involves two roles for each spouse: listener and expresser. The spouses alternate roles so that each is able to express his or her feelings as the speaker. The guidelines associated with each role are detailed in Table 2. Initially, couples have the most difficulty with the empathic listening role. Spouses must often be coached to *listen* to their partners, rather than to formulate a challenging rebuttal. Other spouses immediately try to remedy the situation by offering solutions to the problem being presented to them. Because the spouse expressing his or her feelings may want only to feel heard and supported, the offer of a solution may be perceived as a lack of acceptance or understanding.

The strategies presented above are ways of helping spouses learn more constructive means of meeting their relationship goals (e.g., solving conflicts and feeling understood). They are the primary techniques for reducing the couple's overall level of negativity as well as their tendency to exhibit negative reciprocity. Further, the communication exercises improve spouses' ability to *self-monitor*, which is essential when these skills are being practiced outside the sessions. As discussed in a later section, the communication practice sessions also provide a structure for intervening in the cognitions that are frequently revealed in couples' communication.

Techniques for Increasing Positive Behavior

Spouses who become distressed have typically lost much of their ability to experience enjoyment and pleasure with one another. Often, the reason is simple neglect. The spouses may feel that, if their relationship were going better, positive events would simply "happen." In other couples, one spouse is angry at the partner and does not behave positively toward him or her until the partner yields to all demands for change. The therapist should discuss the idea of behavior exchange and suggest that exhibiting positive behavior may be the most effective way of improving the emotional climate and encouraging greater collaboration with the partner.

Several procedures are available that increase positive behavior in a relationship. "Love days" (Weiss, Hops, & Patterson, 1973) or "caring days" (Stuart, 1980) help the spouses identify their partners' pleasing behaviors. The therapist directs each spouse to perform certain behaviors on one or more days during the week. The behaviors identified should not require great effort or be too difficult to maintain. Examples of appropriate behaviors for love days may include a spouse's devoting at least 15 minutes to a discussion of the partner's day, going out to dinner during the week, or spending time in some pleasurable activity requested by the partner (e.g., a walk). Depending on the couple, the activity should not necessarily require *more* time together; for example, one spouse may desire more quiet time alone to read without being responsible for the care of the children.

One final procedure for increasing positivity in distressed marriages involves coaching the couple to *schedule* positive events with one another. Often, couples begin to avoid shared events, such as going out to eat or to the movies without their children, to minimize the arguments they have come to expect. It helps, however, to instruct them to select a simple, enjoyable activity and to consciously avoid a discussion of major areas of contention during the activity. The discussion of these conflicts may be reserved for problem-solving sessions at home or for therapy sessions. Suitable positive activities include taking a walk, working on a household project together, attending a lecture, or listening to music (see Baucom & Epstein, 1990, for a lengthier list).

In order to facilitate success in these techniques, the therapist should discuss how tempting it is to see the withholding of positive behavior as a way of motivating a partner to make some desired change. Spouses may be unwilling to engage in pleasing behavior voluntarily if they see it as "giving in" to their partner's resistance to change. Thus, more appropriate ways of communicating about negative relationship events, such as problem solving or emotional expressiveness, should be taught to couples to replace withholding maneuvers. Spouses also need to be reminded that behaving positively toward the partner *enhances* the ability to solve problems by increasing the sense of closeness to and cooperation with each other.

Cognitive Techniques

Dysfunctional cognitions often play a key role in marital difficulties, making it necessary to address spouses' thoughts and beliefs directly. As in individual cognitive therapy, the therapist's first task is to orient the couple to the cognitive approach and to educate them about it. Generally speaking, the therapist does this by describing the cognitive model and teaching the spouses how to monitor their thoughts. Later, they are taught to evaluate their thoughts and to change them to more functional and reasonable cognitions.

The therapist adopts a didactic style in the presentation of the cognitive marital model, which is largely consistent with the cognitive model described in Beck *et al.* (1979) and Ellis (1962, 1986). The major ideas to convey to couples are the following. First, all of us have ideas and beliefs about the world that help us understand and respond to our experiences. Second, these perceptions occur to us automatically, and we seldom expend much effort to make them explicit or to evaluate whether they are reasonable, accurate, or supported by objective evidence. Third, in distressed relationships, these cognitions may be quite dysfunctional because they lead the spouses to feel bad, to feel poorly motivated to improve the relationship, and to behave in ways that prevent relationship improvement. The therapist may also give a list of types of distorted cognitions drawn from those described by Beck *et al.* (1979) and Baucom and Epstein (1990). Although it is not wise to discuss initially all of the types of dysfunctional cognitions defined by Baucom and Epstein (1990), a sampling of the most relevant types may be selected for discussion.

One of the most straightforward cognitive techniques addresses a frequent problem: spouses' *selective attention* to negative events, to the exclusion of positive events. The spouses are asked to record on paper at least one positive behavior per day that the other spouse engaged in, no matter how small or seemingly inconsequential. During each subsequent session, the therapist reviews the lists, praising the spouses' efforts and discussing the natural tendency of maritally distressed individuals to overlook the positive behavior of the partner. The therapist gradually increases the recording "requirement" from one positive behavior to several behaviors per day. To help solidify these changes, the therapist asks each spouse to acknowledge the partner verbally for this positive behavior each time it occurs.

The therapist also addresses distorted cognitions recorded on the Daily Record of Dysfunctional Thoughts. Spouses are instructed to record their thoughts at home on an ongoing basis. It is useful to inform the spouses that important cognitions often occur when their own affect or behavior changes abruptly. For example, one wife noticed that she felt very angry and hopeless (an affective change) when her husband left the dinner table and began reading the newspaper soon after eating. She also noted that she left the dinner dishes on the table and sat in the bedroom in the dark (a behavioral change). She was able to record the following thoughts on the Daily Record of Dysfunctional Thoughts: "He never helps me clean up the dishes," "Who does he think he is?", "He doesn't care about talking to me," "I have to carry the work load for the two of us," and "I shouldn't have to ask him to help me clean up; he would help if he cared about my feelings." The next step is to help the wife identify the thoughts that may be inaccurate or unreasonable. For example, the last recorded thought reveals that she has expected her husband to know how she feels about cleaning the dinner dishes. This thought may be unwarranted if she has never fully discussed the issue with him.

In this case, the therapist is advised to keep the husband's contributions to the discussion to a minimum, especially early in therapy. It would be tempting for him to argue that his wife is to blame because she has misperceived the situation, when the goal is to help the wife feel less upset in preparing for more appropriate communication about the problem. The couple may subsequently use problem-solving procedures to negotiate a possible change in how the chore of cleaning the dinner dishes is handled. In addition, the husband may have recorded his own thoughts about the event, and these, in turn, may deserve attention.

One use of the large number of cognitions that may result from the procedures just described is the construction of underlying relationship themes. The therapist helps the spouses use this material to examine these themes for unrealistic or dysfunctional standards and/or assumptions. For example, one husband reported being upset with his wife for maintaining a negative mood after he had apologized for "snapping" at her. After the husband reported his thoughts about the incident, two general themes were pieced together. First, he seemed to hold the relationship standard "She should be able to control her moods as well as I do." Second, he operated under the relationship assumption "I can make her feel happier at all times if I try hard enough." The husband was coached to attack these dysfunctional beliefs on the grounds that they put him and his wife in unrealistic roles. Subsequently, both spouses felt liberated to develop new ways of responding to one another in similar situations.

There are two other techniques for altering dysfunctional cognitions: the *behavioral experiment* and *listing the pros and cons*. The behavioral experiment is a well-known cognitive technique useful in cases in which cognitions are interfering with behavioral change. For example, one husband believed that he would lose the ability to have any influence over the couple's decisions if he shared his feelings. He was encouraged to test this belief by actually sharing some of his feelings and evaluating their effects on the relationship. The technique of listing the "pros and cons" of a belief is another procedure borrowed from individual cognitive therapy. True to its name, the technique requires one to evaluate the value of a belief by actually listing its merits and liabilities.

ACTUAL TREATMENT

Many circumstances may hinder the clinician from carrying through even the most straightforward interventions. These circumstances can be organized in the following categories: compliance problems in communication training and homework assignments, the appropriateness of the timing of intervention shifts, the therapist's response to crises, and complications due to the presence of a concomitant psychiatric disorder.

Compliance Problems

There are minimal conditions for facilitating compliance with both communication training and homework assignments (Liberman, 1981). As in any therapy, it is important that the spouses have an opportunity to air their concerns before a structured intervention is begun. The therapist must demonstrate understanding and acceptance of each of the spouses. In particular, the therapist *must* be sensitive to the attributions that the spouses make for their marital difficulties. It is important to acknowledge the spouses' perceptions and integrate them into the rationale for the procedures suggested by the therapist.

Obviously, a rationale for the behavioral approach should be presented convincingly; otherwise, the couple may question the relevance of a procedure such as behavioral rehearsal in communication training. The ideas surrounding behavioral rehearsal are sufficiently alien so that it takes time for these ideas to sink in. It is often useful to discuss the differences between BMT and other types of marital treatment. Sometimes, it is necessary to ask the spouses to behave "as if" the conceptualization and the procedures feel natural and correct to them. Using a new communication style is nearly always associated with some discomfort, which can be expected to decrease after initial practice.

Noncompliance sometimes occurs when the communication guidelines presented by the therapist are too detailed, too numerous, or, alternatively, too vague. From among the large number of communication guidelines that a therapist may convey to a couple, they will remember and follow only a few. Thus, the therapist should mentally prioritize the guidelines based on his or her conceptualization of the case and should prepare to emphasize the most important of them.

Several other simple procedures facilitate better compliance with behavioral rehearsal in sessions. The participation in behavioral rehearsal may be shaped in small steps (Liberman, 1981). When asking a spouse about an interaction occurring at home, the therapist may say, "After she did that, you said what? Can you illustrate it to me here, as if I were her?" Also, spouses are asked to repeat the communication behavior modeled by the therapist, who says, "Now, try saying it to your partner that way."

Homework presents a special difficulty in compliance because it occurs outside the direct influence of the therapist. Therapists should realize that homework is crucial to the generalization of communication skills; unfortunately, the homework compliance of almost all couples will fall short of the expectations of the therapist. *Any* compliance with homework assignments should be treated with great excitement and interest, and the therapist should refrain from expressing disapproval or annoyance in response to noncompliance. After assigning homework, the therapist should take a troubleshooting approach and ask some of the following questions: (1) What interfered with last week's assignment? (2) When are the best three or four times for completing this week's assignment? (3) Who will initiate the homework session? (4) What might get in the way of these homework times? (5) Are all of the directions clear? (6) What kind of cues can be left around the house that will lead to homework completion? Furthermore, homework is discussed at the beginning of each session as part of the review of the couple's week. These procedures will build a belief that homework is important to the treatment and will be supported by the therapist.

Intervention Shifts

BMT is sometimes viewed as a form of marital treatment that should be the same for all couples. On the contrary, each case involves special needs and unexpected events that may cause the therapist to consider changing directions and attempting a different intervention. Indeed, there is evidence that a clinically flexible version of BMT leads to a superior maintenance of improvements, when compared to a structured, protocol format (Jacobson, Schmaling, Holtzworth-Munroe, Katt, Wood, & Follette, 1989b). When are the appropriate times to shift interventions?

Clearly, one situation that would call for a shift in direction is when additional information leads to a new conceptualization of the couple's difficulties. For example, after beginning EET, it was learned that one couple's major conflicts occurred around the discipline of the wife's children from a previous marriage. Thus, switching from EET to PST to solve the problem was necessary to remove that stumbling block in their relationship.

Another situation that might prompt an intervention shift occurs in PST when one or both spouses are too angry to be "solution-oriented" or to behave collaboratively. At this point, the therapist may have the couple set aside their goal of solving the problem in order to spend some time sharing their feelings about the conflict by using the EET guidelines. In a similar circumstance, the spouses may have cognitions that keep them from being flexible in PST, so that a shift to a cognitive intervention may be advisable. For example, a conflict about the dishwashing chores was reconceptualized for one couple as a clash of standards about relationship roles. The husband was persuaded to abandon the relationship standard that he should "never be expected to help with the dishes" in favor of the standard that "there may be some situations when it is desirable to help out with the dishes." This cognitive intervention allowed the spouses to return to problem solving to negotiate when, how often, and in what way the husband was to help with the dishes.

Intervention shifts should not occur reflexively when a couple is being resistant to a skills-training intervention. A therapist may be unknowingly reinforcing the couple's avoidance of the task. Instead, the therapist should inquire about their understanding of what is expected in the procedure. Further, a cognitive intervention such as a behavioral experiment might be useful in challenging cognitions that are leading to the resistance. The discussion of compliance, above, also is relevant to this issue.

Therapist Response to Crises

A special situation that sometimes precipitates an intervention shift is the emergence of a crisis. Crises come in various forms: reports of a large argument, threats to leave the relationship, threats to terminate therapy, or the announcement of an extramarital affair. Distressed spouses tend to experience their relationship with great uncertainty and emotional turmoil and often convey these feelings to the therapist. Under this pressure, it is easy for a beginning therapist to shift the direction of treatment in response to each crisis as it appears. There are two reasons for the therapist to resist these forces and to continue in the same direction. First, it is important to remember that behavioral treatment of marital discord involves learning new behaviors or increasing the frequency of specific, constructive behaviors. This task is undermined when skills training is abandoned in favor of attending to crises. If this happens often, the therapist will begin to feel that he or she is simply "putting out fires." Second, the presentation of crises may reflect an avoidance of skills-training exercises and may become a disruption to the session. In extreme cases, it is literally a battle for control of the session. Presented below are several methods of dealing with the occurrence of crises.

It is helpful for the therapist to understand the difference between the content of a session and the process of the intervention. *Process* refers to the communication guidelines, the problem-solving steps, or other "style" factors in the spouse's communication. The *content* of the problem is the conflict the couple defines: the fight over the dishes, the issue of disciplining the children, and conflicts about the practice of religion. To circumvent a control struggle, the therapist should concentrate on the process of the interventions, whereas the content should be defined by the couple. During the initial phases of PST, it is wise for the therapist to *guide* the couple in the selection of a specific problem to ensure that they will not tackle the largest problem first. However, the set of problems from which the couple chooses is nearly always generated by the couple. Thus, the therapist can deal with a crisis as a "new" content matter, and the intervention continues as planned.

If the direction is changed because of a crisis, it is often most appropriate to shift to EET. As noted above, when spouses become too preoccupied with or overwhelmed by affect to be productive, emotional expressiveness training may serve as a fall back intervention to help the spouses process the event and feel heard by each other. The added structure of the empathic listening format reduces the risk of the spouses' escalating with anger.

At other times, PST may be used to help the couple move through the crisis. One couple presented with a monetary crisis that had resulted from the husband's spending while he was in a manic episode. Recent negotiations with a credit card company had failed, and a financial adviser had presented the option of personal bankruptcy. The therapist in this case used problem solving in order to address this crisis and at the same time to reinforce the utility of the PST approach. In this type of situation, it is appropriate to be more directive in PST in order to steer the couple toward the most relevant problem-solving issues. This technique is called *traffic-copping* because the therapist takes more direct control of the process to make it more orderly. It should be used only sparingly, but it is a useful way to help couples resolve major disruptive crises.

STEVEN L. SAYERS
et al.

An important part of BMT is the therapist's commitment to the psychological well-being of each of the couple (Baucom, Burnett, Rankin, & Sher, 1990a). Individual pathology is an important area of concern in and of itself and may be intimately linked to ongoing marital problems. As discussed earlier, a thorough assessment of each spouse is often necessary when there is any reason to suspect the presence of individual psychopathology.

The role of marital interventions in the context of other pathology is potentially quite variable. In some cases, it is more clear than in others that the psychiatric symptoms are either maintained or exacerbated by marital conflict, and a larger role for BMT is suggested. Additionally, whether or not discord is identified as a problem often determines how successful a marital approach may be. Empirical evidence that a marital approach will be effective in solving the identified problem should be a key determinant in the decision to use BMT. Below, we discuss some of the most common disorders addressed with BMT.

Depression.   There is evidence that as many as 50% of women experiencing marital discord are also clinically depressed (Beach, Jouriles, & O'Leary, 1987b). Little is known about the direction of causality of depression and marital conflict; however, some research suggests that marital conflict may play a role in the etiology and maintenance of depression (see Beach, Sandeen, & O'Leary, 1990, for a review). At the very least, depression causes many problems in a relationship. The behavior of depressed individuals may be sufficiently aversive to inspire rejection and devaluation by others (Biglan, Rothlind, Hops, & Sherman, 1989). Furthermore, studies suggest that depressed spouses and their partners use their depressive and hostile behavior *coercively* (Biglan, Hops, & Sherman, 1988). For example, a depressed wife may escalate her depressive complaints to inhibit her husband's hostility; his cessation of hostility *negatively reinforces* her use of these complaints. Although models of this type need much further examination, the existing data suggest that conjoint therapy may be more desirable than individual therapy for some depressed spouses.

There are two primary models of spouse involvement in the conjoint treatment of major depression (Baucom & Epstein, 1990; Beach *et al.*, 1990; Schmaling & Jacobson, 1990). The first model places the nondepressed spouse in the role of an adjunctive therapist and is applicable to couples not reporting marital distress. Because these couples do not seem to have the same characteristics as discordant couples (Biglan, Hops, Sherman, Friedman, Arthur, & Osteen, 1985; Hooley, 1986; Schmaling & Jacobson, 1990), a limited, supportive role for the partner is appropriate. In this treatment model, early individual sessions with the depressed spouse are focused on standard cognitive-behavioral-therapy techniques (e.g., Beck *et al.*, 1979). Conjoint sessions are introduced slowly, and the emphasis is on procedures that increase positivity in the relationship (e.g., caring days). Conjoint sessions are used as an environment in which the depressed spouse can test his or her beliefs about the relationship or about the partner. For example, the depressed spouse may personalize the partner's behavior, taking the blame for any negativity expressed in the relationship. With the aid of the nondepressed spouse, the depressed spouse is helped to acknowledge other, more benign influences on both spouses' behavior. Other types of distorted cognitions also needing attention include the magnification of problems, negative or distorted expectations, and inaccurate beliefs about the spouse's ability or willingness to change. Furthermore, problem solving may be helpful in increasing the depressed spouse's role demands. Through the structure of PST, the therapist requires more participation from the depressed spouse, thus decreasing his or her dependency. Last, the maintenance of treatment gains is strengthened through the discussion of interpersonal and personal events that may precipitate a relapse. See Dobson, Jacobson, and Victor (1989) for a detailed description of this treatment.

The second model of conjoint treatment addresses both spouses' marital satisfaction as well as the depression. In contrast to the treatment model just described, the nondepressed spouse is a fully involved participant in this treatment. Several important characteristics may make a case suitable for BMT as the sole treatment intervention (Baucom & Epstein, 1990; Beach *et al.*, 1990; Jacobson, 1984; Jacobson, Holtzworth-Munroe, & Schmaling, 1989a). First, both spouses should be acknowledging marital discord in addition to the depression and should be willing to address relationship issues in treatment. Second, there should be evidence that (1) marital conflict plays an etiological or maintenance role in the depressive symptoms, and (2) the depression is a source of stress on the relationship. Obtaining a detailed history of the depressive episodes and the marital conflict is helpful in this regard. Third, suicide risk should be low because it is difficult to maintain a dyadic focus when one spouse is seriously suicidal. Last, hidden agendas and low commitment to the relationship should be assessed and ruled out.

The early phase of this treatment used conjoint sessions to increase positivity in the relationship. Compared to therapy with couples of whom one spouse is a depressed spouse but in which there is no concomitant marital discord, greater efforts are necessary to decrease mutual criticism. Again, "caring days" can be used to increase the positivity in the relationship, followed by EET to increase the spouses' cohesion and their sense of feeling understood. When one spouse is depressed, maritally distressed couples may be particularly likely to use hostile and dysphoric statements coercively. Thus, PST can be used to decrease these coercive patterns and provide a structure through which relationship problems can be resolved in a less emotionally charged atmosphere. Cognitive interventions may be necessary to address both spouses' dysfunctional beliefs about change, particularly to the extent to which they depend on biological explanations for depressive symptoms. Special attention should be given to helping the spouses anticipate potential future relationship stressors. In both treatment models, an allowance for depressive venting is often necessary; the therapist should not rigidly maintain a focused agenda but should provide support and encouragement for gains made by the depressed spouse.

Bipolar Disorder. Bipolar disorder is widely regarded as having a substantial biological component. However, even since the advent of lithium treatment, an estimated two thirds to three fourths of all bipolar patients are expected to relapse and require hospitalization at least once in their lifetime (Goodwin & Jamison, 1984). Recent evidence suggests that the risk of relapse is increased by patients' exposure to stressful interactions with family members (Miklowitz, Goldstein, Nuechterlein, Snyder, & Mintz, 1988). Thus, a marital intervention that includes communication training has great potential to improve the long-term functioning of married individuals with bipolar disorder.

Conjoint meetings that begin while the patient is still hospitalized may have a positive impact on the patient's overall social functioning and medication compliance (Clarkin, Haas, & Glick, 1989). The initial sessions should use a psychoeducational approach, including information about the diagnosis, the medications, their side effects, and relapses. Also, the clinician should assess the role of psychosocial stressors in any relapse, the family environment, and the couple's problem-solving skills. During these early sessions, however, it is not wise to explore in depth the conflict surrounding the present hospitalization because these issues are usually too emotionally laden.

The goals of reducing marital conflict and the risk of relapse are often sufficient enough to engage patients and their spouses in continued marital treatment following discharge. Assuming that the bipolar spouse is adequately stabilized, EET can be used in initial outpatient sessions to address any residual anger surrounding the recent hospitalization. Because patients with residual or hypomanic symptoms tend to increase their overall level of interactional activity (McKnight, Nelson-Gray, & Gullick, 1989), it is much safer to ask the couple initially to confine their planned discussion of negative topics to the marital sessions. When the affective climate in the relationship is improved, PST can be used to address the relationship conflicts identified by the spouses. After problem solving has been used for several weeks, relapse prevention is discussed again in order to identify potential future stressors that may place the patient at greater risk of relapse.

Agoraphobia. Traditionally, family and marital approaches to agoraphobia have emphasized the interdependency of the behavior of agoraphobic women and their husbands (Goldstein & Chambliss, 1978; Hafner, 1986). The husbands are thought to reinforce their wives' dependency and to assume dominant, independent roles in the family. However, methodological difficulties in the existing studies preclude this conclusion (Jacobson *et al.*, 1989a). Furthermore, there is not adequate evidence that the marriages of agoraphobics are more likely than average to be distressed. Despite these shortcomings in the literature, several studies have reported improved responses to exposure-based treatments when the spouse is involved in a supportive role (Barlow, Mavissakalin, & Hay, 1981; Barlow, O'Brien, & Last, 1984; Cerny, Barlow, Craske, & Himaldi, 1988).

There is also evidence that a communication-oriented marital treatment enhances the effectiveness of an exposure treatment for agoraphobia (Arnow, Taylor, Agras, & Telch, 1985). However, as noted by Jacobson *et al.* (1989a), one should not straightforwardly conclude that improved communication has mediated the improvement. Future research focusing on these mediators should clarify this question. Given the present evidence, however, it is prudent to involve the nonagoraphobic spouse when he or she is willing, and to use EET and PST, especially in cases where the couple clearly acknowledges marital discord.

Alcoholism. Recent studies of the marital interactions of alcoholics and their spouses have led to contradictory findings concerning Steinglass's proposition (1981) that intoxication serves a stabilizing and adaptive function in the family (Jacobson *et al.*, 1989a). However, this confusing picture was clarified somewhat by Jacob and Leonard (1988), who compared the marital interactions of steady, in-home drinkers to those of episodic, out-of-home drinkers. While intoxicated, the steady drinkers exhibited greater problem-oriented behavior during a problem discussion, a finding suggesting that alcohol temporarily served a facilitative effect. Under the same conditions, episodic drinkers exhibited more negativity and poorer problem-solving skills. Future research will be needed to clarify the role of marital therapy in these groups, but current studies suggest that BMT should focus on conflict resolution for the episodic, out-of-home drinkers and increasing positivity for the steady, in-home drinkers.

Several treatment packages have been developed that include love days, PST, and EET as an adjunct to standard outpatient alcohol treatment using an Antabuse contract (e.g., O'Farrell & Cutter, 1984). The evidence to date indicates that this type of treatment helps alcoholics decrease their drinking, improve their marital satisfaction through the resolution of conflicts, and delay their return to drinking (e.g., McCrady, Noel, Abrams, Stout, Nelson, & Hay, 1986; O'Farrell, Cutter, & Floyd, 1985). Furthermore, these studies suggest that the communication training should focus on broader relationship conflicts and that a sole focus on drinking issues may result in an increase in both marital discord and alcohol use. The preliminary evidence is encouraging and indicates that BMT can help spouses learn to resolve relationship conflicts that have typically been responded to by drinking.

SUMMARY

Marital discord is an important but sometimes overlooked source of personal distress in the psychiatric setting. We have used a broadly defined behavioral model of marital distress that has behavioral, cognitive, and affective components. Each of these domains must be assessed and integrated into a conceptualization that describes the current functioning of the couple. Whether or not marital unhappiness is the focus of the presenting complaint, clinicians must consider engaging both of the spouses in an assessment of the relationship. There are important clinical implications in the treatment of depression, for example, when it occurs in the context of marital discord.

As we have described, there is a large number of techniques for addressing the various components of marital discord. Communication training forms the foundation of BMT, although recent innovations in BMT include cognitive interventions drawn from individual cognitive therapy. This review represents a brief clinical guide to the selection of interventions for specific clinical situations. Unfortunately, we do not have the benefit of years of research findings to support these suggestions. However, we are cautiously optimistic that the importance of these issues will move the field in this direction.

BMT also has shown promise in the treatment of couples when one spouse suffers from major depression, agoraphobia, bipolar disorder, or alcoholism. The role of BMT in these circumstances varies; for example, BMT is an adjunctive treatment for alcoholism, whereas it is often the primary treatment for major depression. These exciting clinical innovations are relatively new; thus, future studies will be necessary before each approach achieves its fullest potential and the reasons for its effectiveness are understood. Given the impact of marriage on people's lives and the high rates of marital discord, it is likely that behavioral interventions for relationship conflict will continue to be highly useful.

REFERENCES

Arnow, B. A., Taylor, D. B., Agras, W. S., & Telch, M. J. (1985). Enhancing agoraphobia treatment outcome by changing couple communication patterns. *Behavior Therapy, 16,* 452–467.

Barlow, D. H., Mavissakalin, M., & Hay, L. R. (1981). Couples treatment of agoraphobia: Changes in marital satisfaction. *Behaviour Research and Therapy, 19,* 245–256.

Barlow, D. H., O'Brien, G. T., & Last, C. G. (1984). Couples treatment of agoraphobia. *Behavior Therapy, 15,* 41–58.

Baucom, D. H., & Epstein, N. (1990). *Cognitive-behavioral marital therapy.* New York: Brunner/Mazel.

Baucom, D. H., & Hoffman, J. A. (1986). The effectiveness of marital therapy: Current status and application the clinical setting. In N. S. Jacobson & A. S. Gurman (Eds.), *Clinical handbook of marital therapy.* New York: Guilford Press.

Baucom, D. H., Epstein, N., Sayers, S., & Sher, T. G. (1989a). The role of cognitions in marital relationships: Definitional, methodological, and conceptual issues. *Journal of Consulting and Clinical Psychology, 57,* 31–38.

Baucom, D. H., Sayers, S. L., & Duhe, A. (1989b). Marital attributions: Issues concerning attributional pattern and attributional style. *Journal of Personality and Social Psychology, 56,* 596–607.

Baucom, D. H., Burnett, C. K., Rankin, L., & Sher, T. G. (1990a, November). *Cognitive/behavior marital therapy outcome research: What is success?* Paper presented at the 24th Annual Convention of the Association for the Advancement of Behavior Therapy, San Francisco.

Baucom, D. H., Epstein, N., Rankin, L. A., & Burnett, C. K. (1990b). *New measures for assessing couples' standards.* Paper presented at the 24th Annual Convention of the Association for the Advancement of Behavior Therapy, San Francisco.

Baucom, D. H., Notarius, C. I., Burnett, C. K., & Haefner, P. (1990c). Gender differences and sex-role identity in marriage. In F. D. Fincham & T. N. Bradbury (Eds.), *The psychology of marriage.* New York: Guilford Press.

Beach, S. R. H., Arias, I., & O'Leary, K. D. (1987a). The relationship of social support to depressive symptomatology. *Journal of Psychopathology and Behavioral Assessment, 8,* 305–316.

Beach, S. R. H., Jouriles, E. N., & O'Leary, K. D. (1987b). Extramarital sex: Impact on depression and commitment in couples seeking marital therapy. *Journal of Sex and Marital Therapy, 11,* 99–108.

Beach, S. R. H., Sandeen, E. E., & O'Leary, K. D. (1990). *Depression in marriage: A model for etiology and treatment.* New York: Guilford Press.

Beck, A. T., Rush, A. J., Shaw, B. F., & Emery, G. (1979). *Cognitive therapy of depression.* New York: Guilford Press.

Bienvenu, J. J. (1970). Measurement of marital communication. *The Family Coordinator, 19,* 26–31.

Biglan, A., Hops, H., Sherman, L., Friedman, L. S., Arthur, J., & Osteen, V. (1985). Problem solving interactions of depressed women and their husbands. *Behavior Therapy, 16,* 431–451.

Biglan, A., Hops, H., & Sherman, L. (1988). Coercive family processes and maternal depression. In R. D. Peters & R. J. McMahon (Eds.), *Social learning and systems approaches to marriage and the family.* New York: Brunner/Mazel.

Biglan, A., Rothlind, J., Hops, H., & Sherman, L. (1989). Impact of distressed and aggressive behavior. *Journal of Abnormal Psychology, 98,* 218–228.

Bradbury, T. N., & Fincham, F. D. (1990). Attributions in marriage: Review and critique. *Psychological Bulletin, 107,* 3–33.

Cerny, J. A., Barlow, D. H., Craske, M. G., & Himaldi, W. G. (1988). Couples treatment of agoraphobia: A two year follow-up. *Behavior Therapy, 18,* 401–416.

Christensen, A., & Nies, D. C. (1980). The Spouse Observation Checklist: Empirical analysis and critique. *American Journal of Family Therapy, 8,* 69–79.

Clarkin, J. F., Haas, G. L., & Glick, I. D. (1989). Inpatient family intervention. In J. F. Clarkin, G. L. Haas, & I. D. Glick (Eds.), *Affective disorders and the family: Assessment and treatment.* New York: Guilford Press.

Dobson, K. S., Jacobson, N. S., & Victor, J. (1989). Integration of cognitive therapy and behavioral marital therapy. In J. F. Clarkin, G. L. Haas, & I. D. Glick (Eds.), *Affective disorders and the family: Assessment and treatment.* New York: Guilford Press.

Ellis, A. (1962). *Reason and emotion in psychotherapy.* New York: Lyle Stuart.

Ellis, A. (1986). Rational-emotive therapy applied to relationship therapy. *Journal of Rational-Emotive Therapy, 4,* 4–21.

Fincham, F. D., & Bradbury, R. N. (1990). *The psychology of marriage.* New York: Guilford Press.

Geiss, S. K., & O'Leary, K. D. (1981). Therapist ratings of frequency and severity of marital problems: Implications for research. *Journal of Marital and Family Therapy, 7,* 515–520.

Glick, P. C. (1984). How American families are changing. *American Demographics, 6,* 20–27.

Glick, P. C. (1989a). The family life cycle and social change. *Family Relations, 38,* 123–129.

Glick, P. C. (1989b). Remarried families, stepfamilies and stepchildren: A brief demographic profile. *Family Relations, 38,* 24–27.

Goldstein, A., & Chambliss, D. (1978). A reanalysis of agoraphobia. *Behavior Therapy, 9,* 47–59.

Goodwin, F. K., & Jamison, K. R. (1984). The natural course of manic-depressive illness. In R. M. Post & J. C. Ballenger (Eds.), *Neurobiology of mood disorders* (pp. 20–37). Baltimore: Williams and Wilkins.

Gottman, J. M., & Krokoff, L. J. (1989). Marital interaction and satisfaction: A longitudinal view. *Journal of Consulting and Clinical Psychology, 57,* 47–52.

Guerney, B. G. (1977). *Relationship enhancement.* San Francisco: Jossey-Bass.

Hafner, R. J. (1986). *Marriage and mental illness.* New York: Guilford Press.

Hahlweg, K., Reisner, L., Kohli, G., Vollmer, M., Schindler, L., & Revenstorf, D. (1984). Development and validity of a new system to analyze interpersonal communication: Kategoriensystem für Partnerschaftliche Interaktion. In K. Hahlweg & N. S. Jacobson (Eds.), *Marital interaction: Analysis and modification.* New York: Guilford Press.

Hooley, J. M. (1986). Expressed emotion and depression: Interactions between patients and high- vs. low-expressed emotion spouses. *Journal of Abnormal Psychology, 95,* 237–246.

Hooley, J. M., & Hahlweg, K. (1989). Marital satisfaction and marital communication in German and English couples. *Behavioral Assessment, 11,* 119–134.

Jacob, T., & Leonard, K. (1988). Alcoholic-spouse interaction as a function of drinking style and drinking setting. *Journal of Abnormal Psychology, 97,* 231–237.

Jacobson, N. S. (1984). Marital therapy and the cognitive-behavioral treatment of depression. *Behavior Therapist, 7,* 143–147.

Jacobson, N. S., & Margolin, G. (1979). *Marital therapy: Strategies based on social learning and behavior exchange principles.* New York: Brunner/Mazel.

Jacobson, N. S., Follette, W. C., & McDonald, D. W. (1982). Reactivity to positive and negative behavior in distressed and nondistressed married couples. *Journal of Consulting and Clinical Psychology, 50,* 706–714.

Jacobson, N. S., Holtzworth-Munroe, A., & Schmaling, K. B. (1989a). Marital therapy and spouse involvement in the treatment of depression, agoraphobia, and alcoholism. *Journal of Consulting and Clinical Psychology, 57,* 5–10.

Jacobson, N. S., Schmaling, K. B., Holtzworth-Munroe, A., Katt, J. L., Wood, L. F., & Follette, V. M. (1989b). Research-structured vs. clinically flexible versions of social learning-based marital therapy. *Behaviour Research and Therapy, 27,* 173–180.

Julien, D., Markman, H. J., & Lindahl, K. M. (1989). A comparison of a global and a microanalytic coding system: Implications for future trends in studying interactions. *Behavioral Assessment, 11,* 81–100.

Krokoff, L. J., Gottman, J. M., & Haas, S. D. (1989). Validation of a global rapid couples interaction scoring system. *Behavioral Assessment, 11,* 65–80.

Liberman, R. P. (1981). Managing resistance to behavioral family therapy. In A. S. Gurman (Ed.), *Questions and answers in the practice of family therapy.* New York: Brunner/Mazel.

Margolin, G., & Wampold, B. E. (1981). Sequential analysis of conflict and accord in distressed and nondistressed marital partners. *Journal of Consulting and Clinical Psychology, 49,* 554–567.

McCrady, B. S., Noel, N. E., Abrams, D. B., Stout, R. L., Nelson, H. F., & Hay, W. N. (1986). Comparative effectiveness of three types of spouse involvement in outpatient behavioral alcoholism treatment. *Journal of Studies on Alcohol, 47*, 459–467.

McKnight, D. L., Nelson-Gray, R. O., & Gullick, E. (1989). Interaction patterns of bipolar patients and their spouses. *Journal of Psychopathology and Behavioral Assessment, 11*, 269–289.

Miklowitz, D. J., Goldstein, M. J., Nuechterlein, K. H., Snyder, K. S., & Mintz, J. (1988). Family factors and the course of bipolar affective disorder. *Archives of General Psychiatry, 45*, 225–231.

Navran, L. (1967). Communication and adjustment in marriage. *Family Process, 6*, 173–184.

Notarius, C. I., Markman, H. J., & Gottman, J. M. (1983). The Couples Interaction Scoring System: Clinical implications. In E. E. Filsinger (Ed.), *Marriage and family assessment: A sourcebook for family therapy.* Beverly Hills, CA: Sage.

O'Farrell, T. J., & Cutter, H. S. G. (1984). Behavioral marital therapy for male alcoholics: Clinical procedures from a treatment outcome study in progress. *The American Journal of Family Therapy, 12*, 33–46.

O'Farrell, T. J., Cutter, H. S. G., & Floyd, F. J. (1985). Evaluating behavioral marital therapy for male alcoholics: Effects on marital adjustment and communication from before to after treatment. *Behavior Therapy, 16*, 147–167.

O'Leary, K. D. (1987). *Assessment of marital discord: An integration for research and clinical practice.* Hillsdale, NJ: Erlbaum.

Roberts, L. J., & Krokoff, L. J. (1990). A time-series analysis of withdrawal hostility, and displeasure in satisfied and dissatisfied marriages. *Journal of Marriage and the Family, 52*, 95–105.

Sayers, S. L., Baucom, D. H., Sher, T. G., Weiss, R. L., & Heyman, R. E. (1991). Constructive engagement, behavioral marital therapy and changes in marital satisfaction. *Behavioral Assessment, 13*, 25–49.

Schmaling, K. B., & Jacobson, N, S. (1990). Marital interaction and depression. *Journal of Abnormal Psychology, 99*, 229–236.

Steinglass, P. (1981). The alcoholic family at home: Patterns of interaction in dry, wet and transitional stages of alcoholism. *Archives of General Psychiatry, 8*, 441–470.

Stuart, R. B. (1969). Operant interpersonal treatment for marital discord. *Journal of Consulting and Clinical Psychology, 33*, 675–682.

Stuart, R. B. (1980). *Helping couples change: A social learning approach to marital therapy.* New York: Guilford Press.

Snyder, D. K. (1981). *Marital Satisfaction Inventory (MSI) manual.* Los Angeles: Western Psychological Services.

Ting-Toomey, S. (1983). An analysis of verbal communication patterns in high and low marital adjustment groups. *Human Communication Research, 9*, 306–319.

Weider, G. B., & Weiss, R. L. (1980). Generalizability theory and the coding of marital interactions. *Journal of Consulting and Clinical Psychology, 48*, 469–477.

Weiss, R. L. (1980). Strategic behavioral marital therapy: Toward a model for assessment and intervention. In J. P. Vincent (Ed.), *Advances in family intervention, assessment and theory* (Vol. 1). Greenwich, CT: JAI Press.

Weiss, R. L. (1990). *MICS-IV: Marital Interaction Coding System.* Unpublished manual.

Weiss, R. L., & Heyman, R. E. (1990). Observation of marital interaction. In F. D. Fincham & T. N. Bradbury (Eds.), *The psychology of marriage.* New York: Guilford Press.

Weiss, R. L., & Perry, B. A. (1983). The Spouse Observation Checklist: Development and clinical applications. In E. E. Filsinger (Ed.), *Marriage and family assessment: A sourcebook for family therapy* (pp. 65–84). Beverly Hills, CA: Sage.

Weiss, R. L., & Summers, K. J. (1983). Marital interaction coding system—III. In E. E. Filsinger (Ed.), *Marriage and family assessment: A sourcebook for family therapy* (pp. 85–115). Beverly Hills, CA: Sage.

Weiss, R. L., & Tolman, A. O. (1990). The marital interaction coding system—global (MICS-G): A global companion to the MICS. *Behavior Assessment, 12*, 271–294.

Weiss, R. L., Hops, H., & Patterson, G. R. (1973). A framework for conceptualizing marital conflict, a technology for altering it, some data for evaluating it. In L. A. Hamerlynck, L. C. Handy, & E. J. Mash (Eds.), *Behavior change: Methodology, concepts and practice* (pp. 309–342). Champaign, IL: Research Press.

29

Behavioral Family Therapy for Schizophrenic and Affective Disorders

IAN R. H. FALLOON

INTRODUCTION

Vulnerability Stress: A Model for Intervention

The behavioral approach to family interventions with schizophrenic and affective disorders is based on the vulnerability-stress model of major mental disorder. This model postulates that the impairment of mental disorders is most likely to become manifest at times when the combination of vulnerability and stress factors overwhelms an individual's biopsychosocial adjustment capacity and triggers the biobehavioral responses that characterize that person's disorder.

Vulnerability refers to factors that predispose a person to develop a particular syndrome at any time. Among these factors is genetic predisposition. The preexistence of a mental disorder in a first-degree relative tends to increase the risk of developing a similar mental disorder significantly above that of a person who does not have a family history of that disorder. However, in most cases, the increased risk is not substantial, and the patterns of genetic transmission remain unclear.

It may be presumed that genetic vulnerability is mediated through some abnormalities in brain metabolism, and that it is this weakness that contributes to the development of the disorder under certain conditions. Biomedical research has implicated a large number of possible abnormalities in persons with established mental disorders. For example, the metabolism of dopamine has been associated with schizophrenic disorders, and abnormalities of thyroid and adrenal hormones have been associated with affective disorders.

Current research suggests that biochemical changes are not always sufficient to cause mental disorders on their own and may require the interaction of psychological or social factors. Psychological traits that determine individuals' cognitive appraisal patterns may determine

IAN R. H. FALLOON • Department of Psychiatry and Behavioral Science, University of Auckland, New Zealand.

Handbook of Behavior Therapy in the Psychiatric Setting, edited by Alan S. Bellack and Michel Hersen. Plenum Press, New York, 1993.

whether a biochemical change is experienced positively, negatively, or neutrally, and results in further escalation of the mood disturbance or is passed off as a merely discomforting sensation. The physiological changes in the female hormones during the menstrual cycle, throughout pregnancy and childbirth, and at the menopause lead to a wide range of response patterns that contribute to the varying vulnerability associated with such changes.

Preexisting brain dysfunction, such as that associated with birth injury, viral encephalitis, or epilepsy, appears to be another factor that increases vulnerability to major mental disorders, including schizophrenia (Lewis & Murray, 1987).

Environmental stress is postulated as playing a role in triggering episodes of impairment in persons who are otherwise predisposed to a specific disorder. The risk of experiencing an episode appears to be increased where stress exceeds an individual's stress threshold. The level of this threshold is determined by a person's overall vulnerability at any one time. Exceeding this threshold will result in stress responses and is associated with a high risk of impaired health. Two types of stressor have been researched: ambient and life-event stress.

Ambient stress is the stress experienced in dealing with the day-to-day hassles of life in the community. It is an accumulation of stresses in the household, in social and leisure pursuits, and in the work environment. Such a wide range of stresses is extremely difficult to quantify. However, household stress has been measured by indices such as "expressed emotion" (Vaughn & Leff, 1976) and "family burden" (Grad & Sainsbury, 1963). Work-related stress and stress in social relationships, including the stresses associated with homemaking, child care, unemployment, and interpersonal relationships, have been less readily measured yet are undoubtedly as important as family relationships as sources of ambient stress. Indices of household stress have predicted the risk of recurrent episodes of schizophrenic and affective disorders (Leff & Vaughn, 1985; Miklowitz, Goldstein, Nuechterlein, Snyder, & Mintz, 1988). Persisting high levels of ambient stress in the environment have similarly predicted the development of depressive disorders (Brown & Harris, 1978).

Life event is the term used to define more discrete stresses, such as the loss of a job, the death of a close associate, or the breakup of an intimate relationship. Life events that lead to long-term ambient stress have been associated with the onset of major episodes of depressive (Brown & Harris, 1978), schizophrenic (Brown & Birley, 1968), and manic (Ambelas, 1987) disorders. It is evident that the subjective appraisal of the highly threatening quality of the event and the individual's perceived ability to cope with the associated stress are most closely associated with the onset of episodes of mental disorders. It is postulated that such cognitive awareness of stress is often associated with a physiological change in vulnerable biological pathways, thereby contributing to episodes of impairment. Relatively little research has been conducted to support this hypothesis, but there is some evidence that increased physiological arousal is associated with environmental stress in schizophrenia (Tarrier, Vaughn, Lader, & Leff, 1979).

Figure 1: Stress Flowchart

It has been noted that there is a substantial variation in the patterns of physiological change (including biochemical responses) observed in individual cases, even within a group of people experiencing the same mental disorder. Similar variation in the cognitive and behavioral responses to stresses have been found. It is likely that a person's response to stress is multidetermined, with biogenetic factors determining physiological response patterns, and psychological factors, such as personality, conditioning to past experiences, coping skills, and being prepared for an expected occurrence, all determining the individual's actions in response to the specific stress (see Figure 1).

Stress does not interact directly with vulnerability to produce the specific impairments that characterize specific mental disorders. It appears that stress responses may lead to a range of impairments in any individual. Although the possibilities are extensive, most persons have a

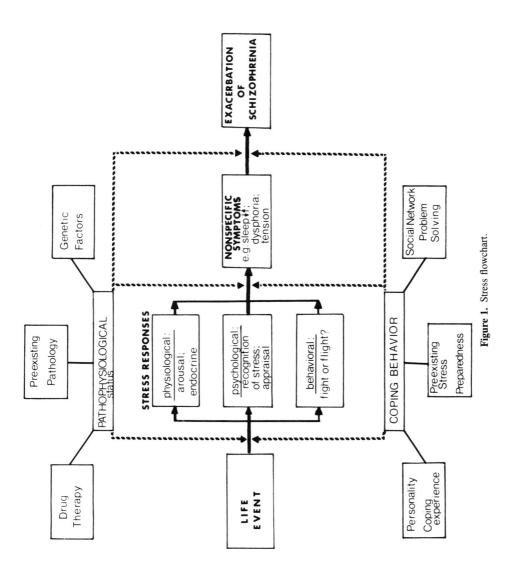

Figure 1. Stress flowchart.

more restricted range of nonspecific impairments that are characteristic stress responses for them. These impairments result from the excessive physiological changes that stress induces in that particular person. For example, one person experiences an increase in muscular tone that may lead to tension headaches or backache; another may have a stress-induced increase in gastric acid leading to reduced appetite and indigestion; another may have an increase in adrenergic activity leading to difficulty relaxing and disturbed sleep patterns. In persons vulnerable to specific mental disorders, these impairments may precede the onset of the specific features of the disorders to which they are especially prone, such as perceptual disturbances, mood changes, or behavioral abnormalities. The ability to recognize the prodromal nature of specific effects of stress may assist the person to seek early intervention and help in modifying the course of major episodes of mental disorder. The definition of these nonspecific early-warning signs may facilitate efficient crisis intervention aimed at buffering and subsequently resolving persisting stress, as well as countering the physiological responses with drugs or other agents to alter the biological patterns; these interventions may include hormonal adjustment to reduce premenstrual vulnerability or relaxation to modify muscle tension.

The indirect mediation of stress responses usually means that there is a delay between the onset of an overwhelming stressor and the development of an episode of a mental disorder. This delay may be a matter of hours in the case of persons with preexisting impairments (i.e., persisting subacute symptoms of a mental disorder) or may extend over several months in the case of some depressive episodes (Brown & Harris, 1978). For most schizophrenic, anxiety, and manic disorders, the lag period between the onset of stress and the development of a major episode is several days. During this time, prodromal signs are evident, and crisis intervention may avert a major episode or at least modify its severity.

Implications for Therapeutic Intervention

Several principles for the delivery of mental health services may be derived from the vulnerability-stress model:

1. The need to screen people who have high levels of vulnerability to mental disorders, and to ensure that they receive competent early mental-health assessment when they show early signs of major mental disorders.
2. A longitudinal perspective for persons who develop mental disorders that ensures that any reversible vulnerability factors will be treated and that clinical management will be continuous, with efforts directed at efficient stress management by optimal combinations of biological, psychological, and social procedures that vary according to the specific needs of each individual at each phase of the disorder.
3. A teamwork approach to case management that integrates medical, nursing, psychological, occupational, and social assessments and effective treatment strategies with the long-term goal of full recovery of community functioning, and that above all, ensures that the stress associated with the clinical management of mental disorders will be minimized at all times.
4. The people who care for those who are disabled by mental disorders are themselves often placed under considerable stress by their caregiving roles. In addition, they often have increased vulnerability to mental disorders as a result of shared genetic factors or assortative pairing (e.g., disabled persons sharing a household or marrying). Thus, clinical management should encompass both the index patient and the caregivers throughout.
5. The need to extend stress management beyond the immediate household environment so that highly vulnerable people can learn to manage a full range of stresses in areas such as occupation, recreation, and intimate relations in a wider social network.

It is increasingly evident that family-based interventions can play a critical role in the clinical management of major mental disorders. Evidence is accumulating that, where patients return to supportive households after recovering from acute episodes of schizophrenia, depression, or mania (Falloon & McGill, 1985; Hooley, Orley, & Teasdale, 1986; Miklowitz, Strachan, Goldstein, Doane, Snyder, Hogarty, & Falloon, 1986), the outcome is substantially improved. Furthermore, Brown and Harris (1978) identified the value of supportive confiding relationships as a major factor that protects women from depressive disorders associated with major life stresses. Thus, a family approach that focuses on enhancing the communication of important needs as well as on developing efficient problem solving to assist with stress management may be expected to reduce the long-term risk of recurrent episodes of mental disorders.

Behavioral Analysis of Mental Disorder in the Family

The baseline assessment of family functioning and the continual review that is a part of every session are the framework within which behavioral intervention strategies are constructed. The initial behavioral analysis may involve several hours of painstaking individual and conjoint interviews as well as systematic observation. Where one family member is vulnerable to a major mental disorder, a range of stressful problems are often evident. Each of these problems, including those associated with the key symptoms of the index patient, is explored in the assessment process. The therapist attempts to obtain:

1. *A therapeutic alliance with all family members*. The presenting problems are used as a starting point for the analysis of the functioning of the family as a problem-solving unit. Each component of the system (individual, dyad, triad, etc.) is explored for its strengths and weaknesses in relationship to those specific issues. At its most straightforward level, this exploration consists of defining the specific contingencies that surround a specific problem behavior. For example, what precedes a family row or increases agitated behavior, and what are the usual consequences of that behavior? By interviewing each family member individually, the therapist gains a broader picture of the setting of the presenting problem than the consensus view provided by a family group. Generalizations tend to be avoided. However, reports of problem behavior are often distorted by the search for simple causal relationships, so that, at this stage, the therapist can derive only a series of hypotheses to be confirmed in subsequent observation of the actual behavioral sequences.

2. *Detailed information about each family member's observations, thoughts, and feelings about the presenting problems*. This information includes the level of understanding of the nature and treatment of the index patient's disorder.

3. *Information about each family member's interaction within the family system*; this includes his or her attitudes, feelings, and behavior toward the other family members and his or her support of efforts to resolve the presenting problems.

4. *Information about each family member's functioning in settings outside the family unit*; this includes his or her personal assets and deficits that may be relevant to problem resolution.

Ideally, observations of the family's functioning are conducted in the circumstances where the presenting problems arise, usually at home. Such naturalistic observations are invaluable, but they may be too costly for routine practice. Alternatives include tape recordings of family interactions at targeted times, time sampling of recordings with automated time switches, reenactment of problem situations by family members, or family discussions of "hot issues." Nevertheless, at least one home visit is an essential part of the behavioral assessment and usually provides the therapist with an abundance of valuable information seldom accessible in clinic-based assessments.

The behavioral family therapist is interested not merely in pinpointing the setting in which problem behavior is most likely to arise, but also in the family's past and current efforts to cope with the behavior. It usually emerges that any problem is present only a small proportion of the time and arises only on a proportion of the occasions when it might be expected. Even the most depressed person has extensive periods when his or her main symptoms are not observed. From another viewpoint, most behavior observed in families is positive or neutral (i.e., nonproblem), and for the most part, families have already learned strategies to cope with the major problems. Thus, the therapist is interested in uncovering the contingencies that exist when the problem is quiescent, as well as those that exist when the problem is present but results in minimal distress. It is assumed that the family has generally developed patterns to cope with the problem, but that these coping behaviors are only partially effective, often because family members are inconsistent in their application or do not persist to derive the full benefits from these coping efforts. Where such effective strategies can be pinpointed, the therapist is left with the relatively straightforward task of assisting the family to enhance the efficacy of their preexisting interaction patterns. Such a targeted intervention may take a mere session or two, but the behavioral analysis that precedes it may be a much longer process.

Major mental disorders play havoc with the everyday routine of family living. A survey of the current activities of each family member is contrasted with his or her desired activity patterns. Each family is invited to describe his or her most frequent activities, as well as the people, places, and objects that he or she spends most time in contact with. Discrepancies between current and expected activity levels help the therapist pinpoint key areas of dissatisfaction that may assist in defining specific goals related to each family member's quality of life.

In addition to listing activities that induce pleasing responses, aversive situations are discussed. Unpleasant situations that tend to be avoided may vary from simple phobias to various family interactions, such as arguments or discussions about finances or sexual concerns. Feelings of rejection, isolation, frustration, coercion, lack of support, mistrust, and intrusiveness may be discussed in this context. Family members are asked to provide clear examples of interactions in which they experience these negative feelings.

This survey of reinforcing and aversive situations often provides a fascinating picture of the manner in which everyday activities intertwine with patterns of mutual reinforcement, positively in happy families, and negatively in distressed families, where marked avoidance of intimacy, confrontation, or coercion may predominate. Interviews about daily activities are notoriously unreliable, particularly those with patients during episodes of major affective disorders. To obtain a more precise assessment of family activity, it may be necessary to invite the family members to complete daily activity schedules.

A final use of the reinforcement survey involves the selection of positive reinforcers that may be used to promote specific behavior change during the intervention phase. Activities, places, people, and objects that are deemed highly desirable may be used to mediate change; they are used as specific rewards for the performance of the targeted behaviors.

At the completion of the behavioral analysis, the therapist will be able to specify the short-term personal goals of each family member, and the conflicts and problems that may need to be resolved to achieve these goals. These may include symptoms of the mental disorder, as well as relationship difficulties that appear to impede problem resolution within the family unit.

Functional Analysis: A Behavioral System

The behavioral analysis provides a clear basis for identifying a list of potential intervention targets. However, such a list does not tell us where to begin. The behavioral family therapist aims to pinpoint the key deficits within the family group that, once resolved, will lead to maximal change. It is assumed that the patterns of family behavior that are observed at any point represent the optimal response of every family member to the resolution of the existing problem. Even when chaotic, distressing responses are observed, it should be assumed that every family member is attempting to resolve the problem (or to achieve the goal) in the manner that he or she considers most rewarding (or least distressing), given all the constraints imposed by the biopsychosocial system at that time.

Rather than attempt to impose his or her own optimal solutions to the problem, the behavioral family therapist aims to use minimal intervention that will build on existing family assets. For example, where one family member is observed to be able to get a depressed person to assist with household chores, the therapist examines that person's behavior closely and pinpoints the specific effective strategies that that person uses. A note is made that effective strategies are already present within the family unit and that the skilled member may be used to train others in the intervention plan.

The functional analysis involves the exploration of the family system from a behavioral perspective so that a long list of potential targets for intervention can be reduced to one or two specific deficits that can be addressed straightforwardly. These issues are not restricted to purely psychosocial parameters; they may include biological variables such as changes in hormonal systems that may trigger or maintain affective disturbance, as well as the specific benefits of drug therapies. If the latter are observed to produce efficient and significant relief of specific symptoms, they are strongly advocated, despite evidence that family patterns of behavior may appear to have contributed to the onset or maintenance of the episode.

Thus, a purely pragmatic approach is used that endeavors to facilitate the most efficient and effective problem resolution and goal achievement for every family member. Of course, this approach includes efforts to ensure that similar problems will not recur in the future. In most cases of major disorders, interventions are aimed at multiple systems: drugs to correct biological deficiencies, psychological interventions to correct cognitive-behavioral disabilities, family interventions to enhance family problem solving functions, and social interventions to deal with financial, work, and friendship stresses.

These varied biomedical and psychosocial strategies can be subsumed in a problem-solving paradigm. Maximizing the efficiency of the mutual problem-solving functions of patients and their family members enables them to become actively involved in all aspects of clinical management. The final assessment of family functioning involves observation of the family group attempting to resolve a problem that is a current hot issue for them. Behavioral observation focuses on the strengths and weaknesses of interpersonal communication, such as clear expression of unpleasant feelings and active listening, as well as specific components of problem solving, such as defining the problem, choosing solutions, and planning.

An example of this behavioral assessment of a family system involved Jane, a depressed woman, who had recently resigned from her job as a social worker after the threat of an assault by a client's husband. Her problem was made worse by an exacerbation of her long-standing fear of crowds, which caused her to become housebound, to withdraw from social activities she found very rewarding, and to place increasing demands on her husband for friendship. The accidental death of their daughter five years earlier had not been discussed with her husband. This avoidance had created persistent tension between them that limited the emotional support he could give his wife at this time. He tended to take over her role as homemaker, leaving her with limited rewarding daily activities. In addition, she was experiencing the effects of the hormonal changes associated with menopause. Her family doctor had given her a course of antidepressants that she had not completed because of their unpleasant side effects. Observation of this couple's problem solving revealed major interpersonal communication deficits, with neither partner making eye contact, and a lack of structure in their problem-solving efforts.

The behavioral family therapist postulated that the key reason that Jane had become persistently depressed was not a biological, psychological, or social problem—despite the presence of abundant problems in these areas—but believed that the most likely explanation was the breakdown in her intimate communication with her husband, which had effectively precluded her obtaining support to resolve the stressors she had experienced at work and at home, as well as her symptoms of anxiety. A treatment plan was devised, the first step of which was reestablishing the intimate communication of feelings, needs, and wishes between husband and wife, initially directed toward the specific problem of Jane's anxiety symptoms, and then to facilitate open discussion about their daughter's death.

At the completion of a functional analysis, the behavioral family therapist is able to draw up an initial intervention program with one or two clearly defined therapy goals and a systematic treatment plan aimed at these goals. A time frame is defined, and a contract of a specific number of sessions agreed on with the family. Continuous measures of progress toward the goal are defined to guide the therapist from session-to-session, and a date is set for a detailed review at the end of the contracted sessions. After this review, the goals and intervention plans may be modified or changed, and a further contract for therapy may be developed.

Deviations from Assessment Procedures

Although it is rare that these semistructured assessment procedures cannot be completed in the manner outlined, some conditions impair the assessor's efficiency. Among these problems are the presence of severe and persistent cognitive impairment associated with thought interference, delusions, hallucinations, persistent worrying, and distractibility. In such circumstances, the assessor may be constrained to conduct inquiries in a series of brief interactions, and to settle for a limited initial data base that may be enriched throughout the course of the treatment. Similar impairment of attention and concentration, although seldom severe, may be found in family members who are experiencing severe stress and burden. This impairment is most evident in people who have had little previous opportunity to discuss their stresses with professionals, and who have an overwhelming desire to tell the assessor every detail of their unpleasant experiences and emotional traumas. It is essential that the assessor allow such people to express these emotional outpourings but at the same time set limits so that all key aspects of the assessment can be completed.

Many people find it difficult to define their short-term life goals, particularly at times when they have experienced considerable stress associated with a period of ill health in the family. It is often necessary to invite people to go away and think about their personal goals and to conduct further discussion at the next session.

It is evident that an assessment of a large household may take several hours and may extend over several weeks. Therapists and family may be eager to begin treatment sessions. However, a thorough assessment invariably saves time overall and is often highly therapeutic in its own right. Families are encouraged to begin to convene their own problem-solving sessions, and to continue their efforts to resolve any current problems. When a major crisis emerges during the assessment phase, the therapist is expected to provide crisis intervention with minimal delay.

Quite often, the therapist will not be able to persuade all household members to participate in the assessment. Where the members appear to play a limited role in the everyday affairs of the household, such members may be excused from regular participation. However, the family may wish to engage them in its family meetings, and to develop a clear contract concerning their increased involvement in household affairs. Strategies to engage reluctant participants may be planned with the family and may continue until all key people are actively involved in the therapeutic process.

Behavioral Family Intervention Strategies

It is still fairly common for acute episodes of major mental disorders to be treated in the hospital. The role of family caregiving is transferred to nursing and medical staff on a hospital ward. However, trends toward community care of mental disorders have tended to expect families to provide more extensive care at home. The family management of severe acute episodes involve training family members in many of the skills used by excellent nurses (Falloon, 1975). At all times, the management plan is based on the behavioral assessment of family functioning, although it is usually necessary to begin the initial intervention strategies before comprehensive family assessment has been conducted. However, when the therapist is able to operate from a community-based service, cases tend to be detected before the episode is fully developed, so that a more extensive assessment may be feasible.

The key intervention strategies used in behavioral family therapy for major mental disorders are

1. Education about the disorder and its clinical management.
2. Communication skills training.
3. Problem-solving training.
4. Specific cognitive-behavioral strategies.

Education about Mental Disorders. The initial sessions are usually devoted to providing the patient and the family with a straightforward explanation of the nature of the disorder and its treatment. Handouts are provided, and the index patient is invited to describe his or her experiences of the disorder and its treatment. The vulnerability-stress theory is outlined as a framework for integrating the benefits of combining biomedical and psychosocial interventions to reduce morbidity. Throughout the treatment, revision of this education is conducted whenever indicated, for example, when patients display reluctance to continue taking the recommended drug regimen, or when major stresses threaten to overwhelm the coping resources of the family. The early-warning signs of imminent episodes of the index patient's disorder are clearly delineated so that patients and family members can take immediate action to avert major episodes.

The educational strategies outlined above are remarkably free of major difficulties, although therapists who are unfamiliar with discussing the nature of disorders with patients and their caregivers may express considerable anxiety about the kinds of problems they may encounter. Traditionally, behavior therapists have eschewed the value of diagnostic classification and have favored a problem-oriented approach. A diagnosis *per se* is of limited value and may contribute to the stigmatized labeling of an individual and his or her behaviors. However, there are substantial gains from the cognitive restructuring of experiences in terms of pathophysiological processes, and from an enhanced awareness of the strategies that may facilitate recovery from distressing states. Such cognitive strategies have been widely used in the behavioral treatment of anxiety and depressive states and obsessive-compulsive disorder (OCD).

Educational strategies used in a cognitive-behavioral framework must focus on the specific strengths and weaknesses of each family. In particular, it is crucial to tailor teaching to the information-processing abilities of each participant. Where participants are experiencing deficits, such as those experienced during the florid episodes of a major mental disorder, it may be necessary to simplify information dissemination, to repeat key points, to take breaks every 5–10 minutes, and to make sure that the disabled family members have processed the information accurately. Although this approach may prolong the education process and may be a little tedious for the nondisabled participants, these techniques will help demonstrate to them that effective communication is possible even with people who seem to lack insight and who are apparently not aware of what is going on around them. Additionally, relatives' groups may provide family caregivers with further support and further understanding of the disorders that their disabled members are experiencing, but these groups are not an alternative to education that includes the index patients.

One common problem encountered in practice is the confusion between stress management and stress reduction. When participants are told that high level so stress may trigger episodes of a disorder, they frequently conclude that people who are vulnerable in this way should endeavor to minimize stress in their lives. Whereas such a strategy may prove beneficial during acute episodes, it is likely to prove detrimental to a person's quality of life when adopted as a lifestyle. Stress *management* on the other hand is an approach that encourages people to maximize their functioning while becoming increasingly efficient at coping with stress, so that they can lead increasingly active lives without being overwhelmed.

Training individuals to report the earliest signs they experience of major episodes of manic, schizophrenic, or depressive disorders may lead to increased presentations for crisis management, some of which will not be associated with the prodromes of these episodes. Although such false-positive reporting may lead to some additional strain on mental health resources, the benefits usually outweigh the costs. Unfortunately, a few patients tend to take advantage of the ready availability of therapists and present a problem when they seek attention inappropriately. Such cases require assertive limit setting by the therapy team.

Communication Skills Training. The goal of communication training in behavioral family therapy (BFT) is to facilitate family problem-solving discussions. The ability to define problems or goals in a highly specific fashion, to reinforce progress toward objectives in small steps, to prompt behavior change without coercion, and to listen with empathy enables problems and goals of all kinds to be dealt with optimally. Most families can improve their interpersonal communication substantially and benefit from several sessions of communication training. The skills are trained through repeated practice among family members, with instructions, coaching, and reinforcement of progress in a manner identical to that used in social skills training. Homework practice is a key component that ensures that the skills will not be restricted to practice within the therapy sessions but will generalize to everyday interaction.

The multistep structure of communication training with families is often difficult to follow rigidly. However, experienced therapists tend to be less distracted from the structure than novices. The main source of deviation results from concerns about the issues that are communicated by the participants, particularly when they are expressing unpleasant feelings of anger and frustration. Therapists may feel that these issues require immediate problem resolution and attempt to resolve the conflicts there and then. Such hot issues can often be avoided when the therapist has uncovered such animosity during the assessment process and steers the communication to more everyday concerns. However, in highly distressed families, even seemingly innocuous issues may lead to major emotional flare-ups. In such cases, the therapist may consider delaying training in expressing unpleasant feelings until after the family has received a few sessions of training in problem solving and goal achievement. When hostile outbursts do occur, it is crucial that the therapist stop the discussion immediately and take time out before reconvening the discussion in a problem-oriented framework.

Distressed families may complain that they cannot find any positive behaviors about which to express their pleasurable feelings. Such individuals are encouraged to reduce their expectations and to search for minor everyday events that trigger only slight feelings of pleasure. Once again, where hostility is running very high, it may be necessary to begin training with the problem-solving approach before refining the interpersonal communication skills of distressed individuals. However, the cognitive change that is associated with the ability to recognize and acknowledge small but significant pleasure generated by the behaviors of a person who is considered overwhelmingly negative may be considerable, and these benefits should not be underestimated by the therapist who is faced with hostile family conflicts.

Problem-Solving Training. The six-step method used in this approach resembles that used in several other BFT methods (D'Zurilla & Goldfried, 1971). However, unlike in some BFT approaches, the therapist's aim is to teach the family to convene their own structured sessions of problem solving, rather than to assist them in their problem solving in the sessions. The therapy sessions are merely used as workshops where the family learns the skills that they apply later in their own problem-solving discussions. Only at times when stresses threaten to overwhelm the family problem-solving capacity, and when the early signs of an impending major episode are detected, does the therapist consider becoming an active participant in the family problem-solving effort. The six steps are

1. *Defining the problem or goal.* The exact issue that is to be addressed is pinpointed.
2. *Listing five or six possible alternative solutions* by brainstorming.
3. *Evaluating the consequences of the proposed solutions.* A brief review highlights the main strengths and weaknesses of each alternative solution.
4. *Choosing the optimal solution.* The participants choose the solution that best suits the current resources and skills of the family.
5. *Planning.* A detailed plan is drawn up to define the specific steps that will ensure efficient implementation of the optimal solution.
6. *Reviewing the implementation.* The efforts of the participants in attempting to implement the agreed-on plan are reviewed in a constructive manner that facilitates continued efforts until resolution has been achieved.

Families are assisted to convene a regular family meeting, at least weekly, with a chairperson and a secretary to administer the meeting, and to report back on their efforts at each therapy session. A guide sheet, which outlines the six-step method, is used to record family discussions and assists the therapist in his or her review. Skills training is provided where family members are deficient in the use of one or more steps of the method. The therapist avoids getting personally involved in suggesting or choosing solutions, leaving that to the family.

The main difficulties that most therapists experience in the application of the six-step problem-solving approach concern the process of handing over the structuring of the session to the family chairperson. Most therapists take the role of co-chair of the problem-solving discussions and become increasingly enmeshed in the content of the issues, while failing to train the family members to convene their own discussions. The therapist is expected to conduct problem-solving training by using the identical procedures that he or she used in training communication skills. This training entails requesting the family to choose their own chairperson and secretary, who make sure that the six-step structure is followed according to the instructions outlined on the guide sheets. The therapist then hands over the discussion to the family and observes from well outside the family group. He or she interrupts the discussion from time to time to provide feedback and coaching. Whenever a therapist demonstration of specific steps is indicated, the therapist exchanges roles with the chairperson or the secretary to model the skills explicitly. Once the brief demonstration has been completed, the family members are restored to their roles and attempt to emulate the key skills demonstrated by the therapist, who provides praise for their efforts and excuses herself or himself from the family circle to return to the observing role once more. This approach ensures that the family will use the sessions to practice the structured problem-solving approach rather than to employ the therapist as an expert problem solver to sort out their problems for them.

BFT therapists are expected to contribute actively to resolving major family crises when it is evident that there is a large discrepancy between the problem-solving capacity of the family unit and the specific issue that they are attempting to resolve. The decision to join the problem-solving process requires considerable judgment, particularly in work with deprived, multiproblem families. The novice therapist tends to view the problem besetting a family from her or his own experience and to feel overwhelmed by issues, such as drug taking, poverty, and violence, that may be commonplace to such families and thus may not prove as distressing to them as to other families. Nevertheless, careful session-to-session assessment provides the therapist with cues to the levels of stress experienced by each family member and helps to establish a balance between training families in the problem-solving skills and actively supporting their problem resolution plans.

Another common difficulty encountered in the application of this approach is the tendency of families that are under stress to focus on the problems associated with the index patient.

Paradoxically, such efforts to provide extra assistance to a disabled family member may be perceived as very stressful by the person who is the exclusive focus of family aspirations, however well intentioned. On such occasions, the therapist may intervene to suggest that the family seek to address problems that are preventing other members' achieving their personal goals. Overinvolved families may find this focus extremely difficult. They will attempt to refer their own lack of progress back to the problems associated with the disabled persons in their care. The therapist may need to insist that at least half the issues addressed during the training sessions be independent of the index person. Of course, the therapist has little control over the topics addressed in day-to-day problem solving in the home.

Specific Cognitive-Behavioral Strategies. Once participants have learned to use the problem-solving approach, there are relatively few occasions on which families are unable to devise effective strategies for resolving their problems or achieving their goals. However, when a family appears to be struggling to come up with an effective strategy, and there is a well-validated procedure for the management of that particular issue, the therapist may offer that procedure to the family as one possible solution. Common examples are the use of operant reinforcement procedures to enhance motivation to perform tasks that are not inherently reinforcing, such as household chores and work activities; desensitization procedures for specific anxiety-provoking situations; cognitive strategies for eliminating persistent negative thoughts; social skills training for coping with difficult interpersonal situations; coping strategies for persistent hallucinations or delusions; strategies for alleviating sexual dysfunction; and relaxation strategies for relieving muscle tension and insomnia. Although the six-step method is preserved, the therapist outlines the strategy in detail for the family and assists them in its implementation.

Drug treatment may be targeted in a similar fashion to specific problems: tranquilizers for overactivity and psychotic perceptual distortions; lithium for mood swings especially elation; and tricyclics for generalized anxiety, retardation, appetite reduction, and late insomnia.

A second occasion when the therapist may become involved directly in the problem solving is when a major crisis impedes the family's ability to conduct its own problem solving calmly and constructively. On these occasions, the therapist may choose to chair the problem-solving discussion in order to facilitate rapid stress reduction and thereby prevent symptomatic exacerbation.

Finally, when family members fail to adhere to the recommended treatment program, thereby producing strong negative feelings in the therapist, the therapist may choose to express his or her feelings directly to the family, and to chair a problem-solving discussion whose aim is to relieve his or her distress. Failure to complete homework tasks, missing sessions, and not adhering to prescribed drug regimens are among the issues that engender high levels of therapist distress.

Wherever possible the specific effects of each intervention are assessed by introducing them one at a time and measuring specific change on the targeted problem behavior in a multiple-baseline design. This process assists in the continuing functional analysis of the disorder. For example, where generalized improvement occurs after the introduction of an antidepressant drug directed primarily at severe anorexia, it may be postulated that a primary disorder of biological systems existed. When a cognitive-behavioral strategy produces similar changes, this effect tends to support the existence of a predominantly psychosocial deficit. However, the conclusions of such a speculation should be viewed with caution in the light of our very limited understanding of the origins of mental disorders.

The severity of the disorder in the index patient and the management skills of the family members will determine the level of input by the therapy team. This will vary from once-weekly sessions to work with the patient and family two or three times daily. Wherever possible, these sessions are conducted in the family home, so that the generalization of skills is maximized. Each session involves practical training in specific skills, with instructions, demonstrations, guided practice, and supportive coaching. Emphasis is placed on shaping the preexisting skills of the family members and self-help strategies for the patients. Session-by-session review is conducted to evaluate patients' and family members' progress toward their personal goals, their acquisition of efficient problem-solving functions, and reductions in specified problem behaviors.

Deviations from the standardized applications of specific cognitive-behavioral strategies are common when they are applied within the BFT framework. *In vivo* sessions that are conducted by family members tend to be less structured than traditional therapist-led sessions. This is particularly evident in the timing of the sessions. Family life may provide a wealth of opportunity for real-life practice, but careful planning is necessary to ensure that these opportunities will be designed to maximize their therapeutic potential. For example, a trip to the market for a person with agoraphobic symptoms must be planned so that the person will be exposed to his or her feared situations for sufficient time to have the fear build up and then begin to abate, and to ensure that the accompanying persons are adequate prepared to assist with panic attacks and to cope with other potential problems that may arise. Such advanced planning is not commonplace in families, but its importance must be stressed if the family's resources are to be harnessed. Clear guidelines and rehearsal by all the relevant participants during the therapy sessions are essential to ensure that the strategies will be carried out in a way that is likely to prove therapeutic. Where deficits remain, it may be more efficient to contract additional therapist-led sessions rather than risk the harm caused by a poor application of effective strategies. This may include individual or group sessions as a supplement to the BFT.

Efficacy of BFT in Major Mental Disorders

The first question for the behavior therapist is whether the specific goals of the therapy were achieved in a specific way. The main goal of BFT in major mental disorders is to enhance the problem-solving efficiency of the family unit. In a controlled study that compared BFT with individual supportive therapy (IST) of similar intensity in the long-term management of schizophrenia (Falloon, 1985), measures of family problem solving indicated that, after the intensive first three-month phase, the quantity of problem-solving statements in the BFT condition had trebled, whereas no significant change in the number of family problem-solving statements were noted after three months of IST (Doane, Goldstein, Miklowitz, & Falloon, 1986). Perhaps more significantly, the quality of family problem solving that was observed by independent assessors who interviewed the families about everyday stressful events showed a significant linear improvement over the first nine months of treatment in families receiving BFT. No benefits were noted in IST families. Similar levels of stress were encountered by the families in each condition. Thus, it is reasonable to conclude that BFT may be associated with specific improvements in family problem-solving functions and consequent stress management.

It has been hypothesized that specific changes in the ability of families to cope with a wide range of stressful life situations is associated with clinical benefits. The supporting evidence is impressive (Falloon, 1985). First, BFT patients experienced fewer major episodes of schizophrenia during the two-year period. Three BFT patients (17%) experienced a total of seven major episodes, whereas 83% of IST patients experienced 41 major episodes of schizophrenia and 11 major depressive episodes (compared with 5 major depressive episodes in the BFT patients). These clinicians' observations were supported by blind ratings of psychopathology that indicated not only that the florid symptoms of schizophrenia were more stable in BFT patients, but that there was a sustained improvement from baseline levels, suggesting that BFT may have promoted further symptom remission (Falloon, Boyd, McGill, Gilderman, Williamson, & Simpson, 1985). A trend (almost reaching statistical significance at the 5% level) was noted on the BPRS withdrawal factor, which suggested that the BFT was associated with a reduction in negative symptoms of schizophrenia. At the end of two years, one half of the BFT patients showed no evidence of any mental disorder on blind Present State Examination interviews. By contrast, 83% of the IST patients still showed evidence of schizophrenic symptoms at two years, although they, too, showed a trend toward remission, although on a much slower trajectory. Thus, the benefits of BFT appear to be genuine, and not to be attributable to a comparative deterioration of the IST group. Nor were these benefits associated with differences in the drug treatment received by the patients in the two conditions. Indeed, the BFT patients tended to have lower doses of neuroleptics than the IST patients, and although the latter had more difficulty maintaining adequate compliance, this was remedied through the use of intramuscular preparations and other compliance strategies.

The achievement of clinical stability and remission is an important goal in the rehabilitation of a patient with a chronic disorder. However, a more crucial goal from the patient's perspective is the restoration of social functioning. We should never forget that clinical stability is readily achieved by removing schizophrenia sufferers from community living into less stressful settings (Lamb & Goertzel, 1971). BFT, with its emphasis on achieving functional goals for patients, was associated with social benefits (Falloon, McGill, Boyd, & Pederson, 1987). BFT patients doubled the time they spent in constructive work activities compared with the two years before the study. Blind ratings of measures of social performance showed significant improvements over the two-year study period as well as significantly greater benefits than those achieved by IST patients. The greatest comparative benefits for BFT were in the areas of work activity, household tasks and friendships outside the family.

The family members of persons suffering from chronic disorders tend to lead impoverished lives and to experience considerable distress themselves (Hatfield, 1978). An effective management approach should reduce the level of the burdens on caregivers. BFT was associated with increased satisfaction for relatives as well as patients, even when the benefits to individual patients were limited (Falloon & Pederson, 1985). The burden associated with the care of the patients was reduced over the two years so that 17% of family members reported moderate or severe levels of burden at this time. On the other hand, almost two thirds of families who received IST continued to complain of moderate or severe burden at two years. Together with the earlier evidence of enhanced management of a wide range of family stresses, this finding suggests that the benefits of BFT extended beyond those for the index patients and were experienced by the family as a whole.

Although the number of subjects in this study was too small to allow a detailed multivariate analysis, the data supported the conclusion that the specific changes in family problem-solving behavior that were induced by behavioral family therapy were associated with the clinical and social benefits (Doane & Falloon, 1985).

Furthermore, increasingly efficient family problem-solving behavior generalized to a wide range of family stresses and appeared to have an impact on major life events. BFT families appeared to use their problem-solving behavior to reduce the stressful impact of life events (Hardesty, Falloon, & Shirin, 1985). In the course of the first 12 months in the study, the 18 families suffered only three life events that were associated with high levels of long-term threat, as defined by Brown and Harris (1978). Thus, the benefits of the behavioral family therapy appeared to derive from a reduction both in the stress of everyday household difficulties and in the stress associated with major life events. This combined effect appeared to be sustained throughout the less intensive second year of the study, although the data were incomplete and a comprehensive analysis was not conducted. It is probable that the continued benefits in both clinical and social morbidity were achieved as a result of continued use of the structured problem-solving approach in the management of stress and the promotion of social functioning.

Later Studies

The third generation of behavioral family therapy studies is now well under way. These studies are of two types: first, studies that attempt to use the BFT methods with different clinical and social populations and, second, studies that analyze the relative contributions of the major components of the approach. Studies are in progress in Munich, Los Angeles (three studies, one with Hispanic families), Providence, Naples, Athens, Manchester, Birmingham, Southampton, Sydney, and Bonn, as well as a multicenter collaborative study in five U.S. cities. Publication of the results of these studies is awaited. The preliminary results suggest that most will replicate the major findings of the University of Southern California (USC) project (Falloon, 1985). One major study that has been completed in Salford, England, found similar benefits of a behavioral problem-solving approach for families (Tarrier, Barrowclough, Vaughn, Bamrah, Porceddu, Watts, & Freeman, 1989). Unfortunately, no specific benefits in social functioning appeared to be associated with this rather less intensive approach in the more chronically disabled population studied. Additional field trials have shown that similar results can be obtained when the approach is applied within everyday clinical practice (Brooker, Tarrier, Barrowclough, Butterworth, & Goldberg, 1992; Curran, Faraone, & Graves, 1988; Whitfield, Taylor, & Virgo, 1988).

The large number of controlled and uncontrolled studies of the use of BFT with schizophrenic disorders is contrasted with the few attempts to evaluate its effectiveness with affective disorders. Apart from the Seattle study of depressive disorders (Jacobson, 1988), the only other study in progress is a comparison of the effects of adding BFT to lithium in the long-term management of bipolar disorders (Miklowitz, Goldstein, Nuechterlein, Snyder, & Mintz, 1988).

The National Institute of Mental Health (NIMH) Treatment Strategies in Schizophrenia Collaborative Study is attempting to examine the interaction between neuroleptic drugs and family interventions in the aftercare of schizophrenics. Five centers have participated in the study: Payne-Whitney Clinic, Hillside Hospital (Long Island), Emery/Grady University, San Francisco General Hospital, and the Medical College of Pennsylvania (EPPI). Therapists at each center were trained to stabilize patients who have experienced a recent episode of schizophrenia with optimal doses of neuroleptic drugs before randomly allocating them to double-blind fluphenazine decanoate in one of three dosages:

1. Continued optimal dose.
2. One-fifth the optimal dose.
3. Targeted doses of fluphenazine associated with periods when early-warning signs of an impending episode are detected.

Random allocation to BFT or a supportive family intervention is made independently. All families are invited to participate in an educational workshop and a monthly educational support group, and they receive crisis support when needed. The BFT is similar to that used in the USC study (Falloon, 1985), with one significant modification: The therapists are not behavior therapists and have not been trained to apply sophisticated behavioral programs, such as depression or anxiety management, social skills training, or token economies, within the family problem-solving framework. Thus, the method concentrates almost entirely on enhancing the general problem-solving functions of the family units.

In this study, BFT is provided for at least 12 months after stabilization and continues throughout episodes of florid schizophrenia or hospital admissions, in a manner similar to that used in the USC study. The main hypothesis being tested is that BFT, with its effectiveness in enhancing stress management, may reduce the need for higher doses of neuroleptic medication and hence reduce the detrimental effects associated with these drugs. However, the large number of cases entering the study will enable a wide range of secondary issues to be explored: the association of therapist competency and therapeutic outcome; the association of problem-solving skills and outcome; the specific benefits of more intensive, targeted family therapy; the cost-effectiveness of these approaches; and predictors of therapeutic efficacy.

The Buckingham Early Intervention Project (Falloon, 1992; Falloon, Shanahan, & Laporta, 1992) was based on the assumption that if BFT is effective in reducing the frequency of major schizophrenic and depressive episodes in established cases of schizophrenia, a similar approach will reduce the morbidity associated with the initial episodes of schizophrenic and major affective disorders. An attempt was made to detect cases during the prodromal phases of these disorders, when major episodes appeared imminent. The current absence of clear biological measures of vulnerability limited the early-detection strategies to a recognition of the clinical features through screening by primary-carer physicians, who worked in close collaboration with highly trained mental-health professionals. The detection of a suspected prodromal state led to immediate intervention with BFT and targeted low-dose neuroleptics or antidepressants when appropriate. The BFT focused on stress management and on educating the index patient and the caregivers to recognize the main symptoms of these mental disorders. The drugs were discontinued as soon as the prodromal features had remitted.

Early results support the feasibility of this approach, over 100 cases having been successfully managed in this way. A 10-fold reduction in the expected incidence of schizophrenic and major affective disorders has been observed. Further efforts are being made to conduct a controlled evaluation of this approach.

SUMMARY

It is concluded that BFT is a promising adjunct to the biomedical management of schizophrenic and major affective disorders. Whereas a substantial body of research supports its utility and cost-effectiveness in the long-term management of schizophrenia, further work is needed to establish the relative merits of its use with affective disorders. The relative ease of training professional staff to administer this approach is contrasted with the more extensive training needed to apply other forms of family therapy. The problem-solving approach allows considerable flexibility in the application of all strategies so that deviations from the prototypical intervention tend to be planned within the overall scheme outlined in the assessment and treatment manuals.

REFERENCES

Ambelas, A. (1987). Life events and mania: A special relationship? *British Journal of Psychiatry*, *150*, 235–240.

Brooker, C., Tarrier, N., Barrowclough, C., Butterworth, C., & Goldberg, D. (1992). Training community psychiatric nurses to undertake psychosocial intervention: Report of a pilot study. *British Journal of Psychiatry*.

Brown, G. W., & Birley, J. L. T. (1968). Crises and life changes and the onset of schizophrenia. *Journal of Health and Social Behaviour*, *9*, 203–14.

Brown, G. W., & Harris, T. O. (1978). *Social origins of depression*. London: Tavistock Press.

Curran, J. P., Faraone, S. V., & Graves, D. J. (1988). Behavioral family therapy in an acute inpatient setting. In I. R. H. Falloon (Ed.), *Handbook of behavioral family therapy*. New York: Guilford Press.

Doane, J. A., Goldstein, M. J., Miklowitz, D. J., & Falloon, I. R. H. (1986). The impact of individual and family treatment on the affective climate of families of schizophrenics. *British Journal of Psychiatry*, *148*, 279.

Doane, J. A., & Falloon, I. R. H. (1985). Assessing change in family interaction: Methodology and findings. In I. R. H. Falloon (Ed.), *Family management of schizophrenia*. Baltimore: Johns Hopkins University Press.

D'Zurilla, T. J., & Goldfried, M. R. (1971). Problem solving and behavior modification. *Journal of Abnormal Psychology*, *78*, 107.

Falloon, I. R. H. (1975). The therapy of depression: A behavioural approach. *Psychotherapy and Psychosomatics*, *25*, 69–75.

Falloon, I. R. H. (1985). *Family management of schizophrenia: A study of clinical, social, family and economic benefits*. Baltimore: Johns Hopkins University Press.

Falloon, I. R. H. (1992). Early intervention for first episodes of schizophrenia: A preliminary exploration. *Psychiatry*, *55*, 1–12.

Falloon, I. R. H., & McGill, C. W. (1985). Family stress and the course of schizophrenia: a review. In I. R. H. Falloon (Ed.), *Family management of schizophrenia*. Baltimore: Johns Hopkins University Press.

Falloon, I. R. H., & Pederson, J. (1985). Family management in the prevention of morbidity of schizophrenia: Adjustment of the family unit. *British Journal of Psychiatry*, *147*, 156–163.

Falloon, I. R. H., Boyd, J. L., McGill, C. W., Gilderman, A., Williamson, M., & Simpson, G. M. (1985). Family management in the prevention of morbidity of schizophrenia: 1. Clinical outcome of a two-year longitudinal study. *Archives of General Psychiatry, 42,* 887.

Falloon, I. R. H., McGill, C. W., Boyd, J. L., & Pederson, J. (1987). Family management in the prevention of morbidity of schizophrenia: Social outcome of a two-year longitudinal study. *Psychological Medicine, 17,* 59.

Falloon, I. R. H., Shanahan, W., & Laporta, M. (1992). Prevention of major depressive episodes: Early intervention with family-based stress management. *Journal of Mental Health, 1,* 53–60.

Grad, J., & Sainsbury, P. (1963). Mental illness and the family. *Lancet, 11,* 544–547.

Hardesty, J. P., Falloon, I. R . H., & Shirin, K. (1985). The impact of life events, stress, and coping on the morbidity of schizophrenia. In I. R. H. Falloon (Ed.), *Family management of schizophrenia: A study of clinical, social, family and economic benefits.* Baltimore: Johns Hopkins University Press.

Hatfield, A. B. (1978). Psychological costs of schizophrenia to the family. *Social Work, 24,* 355.

Hooley, J. M., Orley, J., & Teasdale, J. (1986). Levels of expressed emotion and relapse in depressed patients. *British Journal of Psychiatry, 148,* 642–647.

Lamb, H. R., & Goertzel, V. (1971). Discharged mental patients—Are they really in the community? *Archives of General Psychiatry, 24,* 29.

Leff, J. P., & Vaughn, C. E. (1985). *Expressed emotion in families.* New York: Guilford Press.

Lewis, S. W., & Murray, R. M. (1987). Obstetric complications, neurodevelopmental deviance, and schizophrenia. *Journal of Psychiatric Research, 21,* 413–421.

Miklowitz, D. J., Strachan, A. M., Goldstein, M. J., Doane, J. A., Snyder, K. S., Hogarty, G. E., & Falloon, I. R. H. (1986). Expressed emotion and communication deviance in the families of schizophrenics. *Journal of Abnormal Psychology, 95,* 60–66.

Miklowitz, D. J., Goldstein, M. J., Nuechterlein, K. H., Snyder, K. S., & Mintz, J. (1988). Family factors and the course of bipolar affective disorder. *Archives of General Psychiatry, 45,* 225–231.

Tarrier, N., Vaughn, C. E., Lader, M. H., & Leff, J. P. (1979). Bodily reactions to people and events in schizophrenia. *Archives of General Psychiatry, 36,* 311–315.

Tarrier, N., Barrowclough, C., Vaughn, C., Bamrah, J. S., Porceddu, K., Watts, S., & Freeman, H. (1989). The community management of schizophrenia: A controlled trial of a behavioural intervention with families to reduce relapse. *British Journal of Psychiatry, 153,* 532.

Vaughn, C. E., & Leff, J. P. (1976). The influence of family and social factors on the course of psychiatric illness: A comparison of schizophrenic and depressed neurotic patients. *British Journal of Psychiatry, 129,* 125.

Whitfield, W., Taylor, C., & Virgo, N. (1988). Family care of schizophrenia. *Journal of the Royal Society of Health. 1,* 4–5.

30

Family Therapy with Adolescents

DIANE HOLDER

INTRODUCTION

There has been a dramatic increase in the number of adolescents admitted to psychiatric facilities since the early 1980s (AAPPH, 1980–1985). The prevalence of depression, attempted suicide, aggressive behavior, and drug and alcohol abuse among adolescents, as well as the breakdown of traditional family and community supports, appears to be contributing to this disturbing phenomenon. At the time of admission, most adolescents are accompanied to the hospital by their families, many of whom are in crisis and overwhelmed. Even though the vast majority of adolescents return home after brief inpatient treatment, relatively little attention has been paid to family therapy approaches within the psychiatric setting, and treatment in many adolescent units continues to be oriented primarily toward the individual patient (Anderson, 1977; Hanrahan, 1986; Singh, 1987).

The long-standing theoretical and political schism between family systems approaches and traditional psychiatric models has resulted in competing theories of causality and minimal integration of family interventions into inpatient settings (Walsh & Anderson, 1987). However, two major facts underscore why attention to the family is important. The first is that the majority of adolescents who are admitted to psychiatric inpatient units suffer from disorders that have been associated with significant rates of family risk factors, including parental psychiatric disorders, family and marital conflict, family violence, physical and sexual abuse, and economic hardship (Rosenstock, 1985; Rutter, Tuma, & Lann, 1988). The second is that these are highly stressed families; the events surrounding hospitalization have outstripped their emotional resources, and interventions that will reduce anxiety and increase coping skills are needed.

Incorporating family interventions into the hospital setting requires integrating diagnostic criteria and biological models with interactional paradigms. The theoretical framework for this approach is best captured by the biopsychosocial model of Engel (1977) and enriched by the concepts of risk and protective factors delineated by Rutter (1985; 1987) and Garmezy and Rutter

DIANE HOLDER • Department of Psychiatry, University of Pittsburgh, 3811 O'Hara Street, Pittsburgh, Pennsylvania 15213.

Handbook of Behavior Therapy in the Psychiatric Setting, edited by Alan S. Bellack and Michel Hersen. Plenum Press, New York, 1993.

(1983). This model hypothesizes that biological vulnerability may be expressed only when resistance is lowered because of psychological or social stressors such as marital discord or coercive parenting practices (Patterson, 1977; Rutter & Quinton, 1977). On the other hand, protective influences, such as a supportive and cohesive family milieu, an external social support system, and personality features in the child or adolescent, will enhance adaptive functioning (Garmezy, 1985).

In keeping with this perspective, the family therapy approach described in this chapter emphasizes interventions that alter the family environment so as to reduce risk factors and enhance protective influences. This approach includes reducing negative behaviors, such as coercion, discord, and parental inconsistency, and increasing protective forces, such as positive communication, effective problem solving, and social support.

OVERVIEW OF THE MODEL

Background

Systemic behavioral family therapy was developed as an outpatient model to treat depressed adolescents who had attempted suicide (Holder, Feinberg-Steinberg, Miller, & Madonia, 1990). The approach targets problem family processes and structure in order to aid in recovery from depression and alter future episodes. It draws heavily on the behavioral-systems model of Robin and Foster (1989), which was developed for use with high-conflict adolescents and their families, and the functional family therapy (FFT) model of Alexander and Parsons (1982), which has been used to treat juvenile offenders and their families. The approach is short-term and stems from the integration of two major perspective in the family therapy literature: *family systems theory*, which emphasizes constructs such as circular patterns of interaction, family structure, and adaption, and *behavioral family theory*, which emphasizes social learning, contingency contracting, and behavior exchange (Alexander & Parsons, 1982; Robin & Foster, 1989). In keeping with a behavioral tradition, systemic behavioral family therapy stresses the importance of both empirical validation and generalizability. It relies on the direct observation of family interaction for the assessment of factors that maintain behaviors (Robin & Foster, 1989).

Theoretical Assumptions

There are several basic assumptions in this approach. The first is that the *adolescent's symptoms are influenced by the interpersonal context in which they occur*. Although school and peer influences become increasingly strong at this developmental stage, the family continues to serve as the adolescent's basic social environment and remains a powerful source of comfort or stress, depending on the quality of the relationships of the family members. The tasks for the individual and the family are different from those in earlier stages of childhood, but the basic themes remain. Adolescents continue to need affection, affiliation, limits, appropriate autonomy, and a sense of hope, optimism, and predictability. The physiological changes, the increased capacity for abstract thinking, and greater exposure to social stimulation typically lead to shifts in the power and intimacy balance between teenagers and their parents, resulting in a challenge to the family's usual patterns or homeostatic balance (Martin, 1987; McGoldrick & Carter, 1988). Although most families experience some increased conflict with the adolescent, highly stressed families or families with poor problem-solving skills, poor communication, negative reinforcement patterns, rigid boundaries, or inflexible patterns and hierarchies are more likely to experience excessive conflict with their adolescent, to foster other types of symptomatic behavior patterns, or to be less able to cope with a teenager who has special vulnerabilities.

The second assumption is that *thoughts, feelings, and behavior are interactive* (Izard & Schwartz, 1986). In line with this perspective, positive and negative emotions are viewed as being mediated by cognitions, including beliefs, attributions, and expectations, which in turn influence behavior. Moreover, the family problem-solving behavior is significantly hampered by negative emotional patterns (Forgatch, 1989). In other words, if I think my adolescent put a dent in my car because she is a careless person, I may be more angry and more likely to withhold privileges unfairly than if I believe that she is inexperienced and the poor road conditions contributed to the accident. Consequently, interventions target negative expectations and attributions that family members have about each other's behavior in order to reduce negative emotions and increase positive thoughts and feelings. Reducing negativity creates what has been called a *positive set* (Maier, 1937). This positive set readies the family for collaborative and successful problem-solving attempts (Morris, Alexander, & Waldron, 1988; Trautman & Rotheram-Borus, 1988).

Third, the model assumes that *specific skill-building interventions are needed to enhance positive communication and increase problem-solving abilities*. These improved skills are expected to provide an ongoing resource that will reduce family stress and enhance family support and that will thus have an effect on the amelioration and prevention of symptoms (Pearlin & Schooler, 1978; Turner, 1983).

PHASES OF TREATMENT

There are three basic tasks for the therapist in the systemic behavioral approach: (1) to engage the family in treatment; (2) to assess the family functioning and family resources; and (3) to provide therapeutic interventions that facilitate behavior change.

Changing behavior, one's own or somebody else's, is not a simple task (Alexander & Parsons, 1982; Anderson & Stewart, 1983; Meichenbaum & Turk, 1987). This model assumes that family members are hesitant to change their behavior unless they are sufficiently motivated to do so. Consequently, following in the tradition of the functional family therapy model, this approach has two broad phases: motivation/assessment and behavior change.

In Phase 1, the therapist assesses family functioning and uses interventions specifically designed to increase people's motivation to make behavioral change. Motivation for change is linked to family members' perception of what causes the problems as well as to their affective state. In Phase 2, the therapist assists the family to make behavioral changes that include improved communication and problem-solving skills, as well as changes related to problem family structures or functions. In the following section, each phase of the model is delineated and clinical examples highlight the theoretical issues.

Phase 1: Assessment/Motivation

The therapist has several tasks: to engage the family in treatment; to assess the family's functioning; and to attempt to shift attitudes, expectations, and beliefs. In very brief inpatient stays, Phase 1 occurs during hospitalization, and Phase 2 occurs during outpatient follow-up. In longer hospitalizations, it is possible to begin Phase 2 as well. This chapter focuses primarily on the assessment/motivation phase and gives a brief overview of the behavior change phase.

Goal 1: Engaging the Family in Treatment. The first task is to engage the family in treatment and to create an alliance with the family. As in most types of psychotherapy, the alliance is critical and is associated with positive therapy outcomes (Hartley, 1985). Most adolescents can be treated in outpatient settings; consequently, it is only when severe symptoms arise that threaten health or safety that inpatient treatment is recommended. The immediate needs of the family at the time of admission will depend largely on the reasons for the adolescent's admission, including the type and severity of the symptoms as well as the extent of the family crisis.

The inpatient setting requires intensifying the treatment and involving families *rapidly*. Parents and siblings may be experiencing severe symptoms of their own and may require immediate intervention to address suicidal or aggressive impulses or severe family conflict. A crisis intervention mode with elongated sessions spaced closely together is a useful framework (Budman, 1981). The basic goals are to assess the problem, defuse the current crisis, reduce the adolescent's acute symptoms, identify resources, and prime the patient and family for outpatient therapy.

The initial family session is a critical point in the therapeutic process and ideally occurs during the admission itself. Often, hospitalization can be avoided; however, in the process of deciding to use the inpatient service, a family and their adolescent can be empowered to take some control and responsibility and to help to determine which goals can be accomplished. An increased sense of control and hope can be provided in several ways:

1. In situations in which the adolescent is psychotic, has made a suicide attempt, or is severely depressed, the symptoms are often confusing or frightening to the patient and the family. Information about the disorder and the treatment options may be a powerful intervention that helps reduce anxiety and helps the family to handle the crisis more effectively (Anderson, Hogarty, & Reiss, 1980).

2. Hospital settings with complex rules and procedures may make a family feel excluded or intimidated. Introducing members of the treatment team, providing flexible visitation policies, and offering multiple therapy contacts, including parent and family groups within the milieu, may help to reduce tension between staff and family. This approach will help families join with the larger system and reduce the tendency of the staff to become aligned with the patient against the family (Anderson & Stewart, 1983; Lefley & Johnson, 1990).

3. It is important that the therapist convey a sense of understanding and concern about the dilemmas the family faces. Minuchin (1974) described this process as "joining" with the family and stressed the need for the therapist to "accept the family's organization and style and blend with them" (p. 123). This process involves rapport-building skills, including warmth, positivity, concern, humor, and nonblaming language.

Not all families are motivated to be involved in treatment. Common reasons for such resistance include a fear of being blamed, a poor understanding of why attendance is needed, anger at the patient, minimal hope that change is possible, a fear of reprisals outside the session, previous negative experiences with mental health settings or conditions such as substance abuse problems or depression, which may interfere with the family's interest in becoming involved or ability to become involved (Anderson & Stewart, 1983).

In some cases, the family is opposed to the hospitalization and the courts have facilitated the admission. In these cases, it is helpful to align with the parents in their goal of getting the child home quickly, if that is a realistic plan. In these cases, the family usually views the hospital as an arm of the court and is anxious about how information will be shared. The therapist should be clear about the confidentiality laws and provide the family and the patient with an accurate description of how information will be used. In some situations the hospital serves as an advocate for the adolescent if physical or sexual abuse makes returning home immediately a poor idea. In these situations, the therapist works with protective-service agencies and the family to find a safe environment for the adolescent while further evaluation and treatment occur.

Goal 2: Modifying Negative Beliefs, Attributions, and Expectations. Parent-child conflict and marital discord have been associated with a wide range of disorders (Jacob, 1987). The highly discordant family has well-rehearsed patterns of blaming and negativity that are exacerbated during a crisis. The stress preceding most hospitalizations increases the potential for the initial family sessions to stimulate angry, defensive, and blaming behavior. The therapist must quickly intervene to reduce negativity or the session will deteriorate.

Morris *et al*. (1988) suggested that attribution theory helps to explain the regulation of negative blaming behaviors. According to this view, people have a need to explain their world and provide meaning to events, particularly those events that affect their own lives. Very often, the causal interpretation is reduced to "trait" explanations. In discordant families, negative traits such as "laziness," "selfishness," and "irresponsibility" are often used to account for "bad" behavior. For example, Mary fails in school because she is a "lazy" person. These cognitions stimulate negative feelings and may lead to negative actions. In some families, one member may be viewed from a globally negative perspective (scapegoated), in which case any new behaviors are seen through the "trait" labels, which automatically lead to a negative emotional response. Very often, it is not the behavior *per se* but the expectations or attributions or meaning ascribed to the behavior that determines how a parent or teen reacts (Morris *et al.*, 1988).

Many parents have minimal knowledge of normative behavior. In addition, beliefs or basic assumptions about how parents and children should interact also influence behavior. Robin and Foster (1989) identified several cross-situational attributions and expectations that may lead to increased negativity between parents and teens:

1. *Perfectionism*: "My son should be the star."
2. *Ruination*: "If she wears lipstick, she'll become sexually active."
3. *Fairness*: "My parents should treat my brother exactly the way they treat me."
4. *Obedience*: "Good kids never talk back; good kids always do what they are told; good kids don't need to be 'paid' to do their chores."
5. *Malicious intent*: "He is failing in order to get even with me."
6. *Self-blame*: "He's failing math; I must be a bad mother."

These beliefs may lead to disappointment or anger when the teen or the parent cannot fulfill the requirement.

Interventions are needed to modify negative cognitions. Systemic behavioral therapy proposes that the shifting of attributions, attitudes, expectations, and beliefs can be effected through reframing, modeling, positive reinforcement, the provision of information, and a goal-oriented focus. The therapist counters negativity by structuring the session and actively searching for positive feelings and positive statements. While learning about the presenting problems, the therapist gradually shifts the family's focus toward goals and solutions. Reframing interventions are useful in helping to provide this shift. Reframing is a technique that provides an alternative explanation for a problem behavior by changing the class membership of an event. It provides a new interpretation for the reason the behavior occurs (Morris *et al.*, 1988). The reframings confuse the family and startle them into slowing down their automatic reactions. Reframing is based on common patterns as well as those that reflect the dynamic of the particular family. For example, oppositional behavior may be reframed as wanting more from a parent, either increased attention or its opposite, increase autonomy. An angry teen may be reframed as "hiding sadness."

A particularly useful type of reframing intervention is separating the actual behavior from the intention motivating the behavior (Morris *et al.*, 1988). In this approach, negative behaviors are not defined as other than negative, but the motivation for the behavior is ascribed a more benign meaning. For example, if a mother believes that her teenager has temper outbursts because he hates her, it is important to offer a different motive for the misbehavior. Or if a teen has attempted suicide and the father views the suicide attempt as a way to retaliate against him following an argument, the therapist offers an alternative explanation or "relational reframing" (Alexander & Parsons, 1982) for the teen's behavior, such as "It sounds as if, to you, Dad, Bill's overdose felt as if he was trying to hurt you or get back at you. But for you, Bill, it was your way of saying 'help me'." A series of reframings emphasizing more benign intentions may make family members less upset with each other and often allows the "offending party" to be less defensive. If family members begin to view each other's behavior as less malicious or intentionally hurtful, they may be more willing to compromise.

One of the most critical reframings to begin to build during Phase 1 is that parents can be one of the most influential forces in a teenager's life. Parents can become change agents to establish the conditions under which a teen will be more likely to function adaptively. Parenting methods and problem-solving abilities are framed as skills that anyone can learn but that few are taught. The goal is to help parents feel more competent and hopeful. Other common reframings include reframing malicious intent into positive intent, symptoms into attempted solutions, overly controlling behavior into a form of protection, oppositional behavior as an attempt at mastery, and crises as opportunities.

It is critical that the reframing not be completely out of line with the family's worldview and that it be delivered respectfully and thoughtfully. If the family disputes the reframing, it may be that the therapist has hypothesized incorrectly about what is motivating the behavior, that the reframing is too unbelievable, or that the therapist's delivery was mismanaged.

Goal 3: Family Assessment. Adolescents who are treated in inpatient settings have a complex set of problems, and a multidisciplinary team will assess the problems and provide a comprehensive evaluation that includes a family evaluation. An integrated treatment plan will address the problems identified in the various areas. The family assessment and treatment are conceptually distinct, but in the practice of this model, the two are intimately connected. From the point of initial contact, the therapist is assessing the critical domains of family functioning and family resources, and simultaneously engaging the family in the treatment process. The outcome of the assessment is a mutually negotiated initial contract.

The following case example will serve as an illustration of the key elements in the family assessment process:

> The parents of John, age 13, reported that he was "immature" and "violent" and "failing every subject." He frequently broke household objects in the midst of temper tantrums, which occurred on an average of two to three times a week. In the midst of one episode, he swallowed a large amount of aspirin, stating that he planned to kill himself. The father was particularly angry with the boy and was threatening to hurt him physically if he continued to provoke.
>
> In the recounting of a recent episode the following scene was described: The father and John were in a department store. John asked for new pants, which he said his mother had agreed to buy, and the father said no. John continued to ask and began yelling at his father, who in turn became very angry and left the store. John complained all the way home and, when he got home, told his mother who criticized the father for not buying the pants, which were on sale. The father and mother got into an argument, and the father told the mother to take John shopping herself, which she did that afternoon and purchased the pants. After dinner, John asked his father for a ride to the shopping mall, and the father refused. John went into the bathroom and destroyed the shower curtain and several bottles of toiletries. The father and the mother both yelled at John, who began complaining about missing his friends at the mall and accusing his father of wanting him to lose all his friends and become "a loser" just like him. An argument started between the parents, in which the mother accused the father of never being willing to "do anything" for the boy. Eventually, the father left the house, and the mother and John watched television for the rest of the evening.

Assessment Instruments

The family assessment is completed with a behavioral interview, which includes a family task and is supplemented by family questionnaires. There are numerous self-report instruments that may be of value. Some that are considered theoretically and psychometrically sound are the Areas of Change Questionnaire (ACQ; Jacob & Seilhamer, 1985), the Parent–Adolescent Relationship Questionnaire (PARQ; Robin & Foster, 1989), the Family Environment Scale (FES; Moos & Moos, 1981), the Family Adaptability and Cohesion Scales (FACES; Olson & Portner, 1983), and the Family Assessment Measure (FAM; Skinner, Steinhauer, & Santa-Barbara, 1983). (See Jacob & Tennenbaum, [1988], for a review of family assessment methods for children and adolescents.)

The family task is a 10-minute discussion, during which the therapist observes the family interaction in the room or through a one-way mirror. The task asks the family to talk about issues identified on the self-reports. Or it may use non–problem-focused hypothetical situations, such as planning a way to spend $200 or planning a family vacation (Watzlawick, 1966). The task provides an opportunity to observe the communication process in the family and to obtain an initial understanding of family structure. Immediately following the task, the therapist should provide positive feedback to the family about any communication or problem-solving strength observed.

The Contextual Model

The systemic behavioral approach uses a contextual assessment model that focuses primarily on the current functioning of the family. Although there is an interest in obtaining information about the duration of the current problems and significant life events, it is assumed that, for the purposes of establishing behavioral change, the influence of the past is manifested in the current feelings, attitudes, and behaviors displayed in the session. The therapist asks content- and process-focused questions and uses observational skills to evaluate the family's interaction. This process may be supplemented by family self-reports, which assess the family members' perceptions of their relationships and functioning.

The initial focus of the assessment begins with the current presenting problems and goals. Usually, families describe behaviors as discrete events and have a minimal recognition of the antecedents and consequences that provide the context and the rationale for understanding the behavior. It is useful for the therapist to conceptualize antecedents and consequences as a broad range of behaviors that include thoughts, feelings, and actions. These behaviors may precede or follow events immediately or may have less temporal proximity but form a part of a larger sequence or change of behaviors that affect the target event (Arrington, Sullaway, & Christensen, 1988).

The therapist should assess behavior patterns in the family, asking, "What is the behavioral payoff of this repeated sequence in the family interaction?" Patterns of positive and negative reinforcement, punishment, avoidance, reciprocity, and coercion are identified. Particular attention is paid to "social reinforcers," which are very powerful. Functional family therapy hypothesizes three interpersonal reinforcers for family interactions: closeness, distance, and regulation. The therapist identifies family members' behavioral responses to specific symptomatic behaviors in order to ascertain which behaviors may be reinforced by other family members' providing more or less contact. In families with symptomatic adolescents, the motivation of the behavior is sometimes to draw the parents in closer so as to obtain more connection. In other instances, the symptoms represent a method of "escaping" from an overly close or overly controlling parent. In our case example:

> Contextual assessment looks at how John's behavior is maintained by the mother's intermittent reinforcement of his complaining as well as the potential role of the parents' marital conflicts in preventing them from agreeing on privileges and consequences for John. The father's leaving may be negatively reinforcing to both the son's and wife's complaining, as they both prefer evenings together with the father out of the house. The contextual assessment should evaluate repeated patterns that involve all the relevant family members. The subsystems in the family include the individuals, the marital dyad, and the interlocking triads within larger family systems.

Communication and Problem Solving

Positive, effective communication processes facilitate family problem solving and reduce stress. During the family task and the initial sessions, the family demonstrate how they communicate their thoughts and feelings to each other. Falloon, Boyd, and McGill (1984) identified several important components of the communication process that the therapist evaluates: the degree of expressiveness, the positiveness or negativity of the tone, the degree of verbal ability, and the clarity of the messages. In addition, the therapist notes the degree of reciprocity among family members, which includes the similarities in nonverbal cues such as posture, eye contact, gestures, and expressions; the congruity between verbal and nonverbal messages; the extent of pseudomutuality; the level of disagreement; and tolerance and respect of versus intrusiveness into or invalidation of others' thoughts or feelings. In addition, it is also important to identify the patterns in which family members talk to each other, support each other's position, or disagree with each other. These provide clues to the family structure. In John's case:

> The father was exceedingly angry and stated repeatedly that John was "destroying" the family. John and his father engaged in mutual name calling and threats. John's mother announced with flat affect that John was "impossible" but defended him when the father attacked him.

Family Structure

The therapist uses the initial sessions to identify any problems in the family structure that may contribute to the adolescent's difficulties. These problems fall into two broad areas: cohesion problems and alignment problems (Robin & Foster, 1989).

Family cohesion is the amount of emotional bonding that is present between individuals in the family as well as the amount or extent of individual autonomy available in the family system. Cohesion is conceptualized on a continuum, ranging disengagement to enmeshment (Olson, Sprenkle, & Russell, 1979). Disengaged families do not provide adequate structure or support, often prematurely ejecting a teen into the adult world, where the adolescent experiences a lack of nurturance and support. Enmeshed families do not encourage independence, mastery, or differentiation. Adolescents in these types of families are often hesitant to speak up and do not overtly disagree with other family members. For example, Minuchin described the families of anorexics as enmeshed; the one way to rebel and assert autonomy was self-starvation (Minuchin, Rosman, & Baker, 1978).

Alignment is joining someone in the family who is involved in a task or function. In some families, members scapegoat, joining together at the expense of one person who is repeatedly blamed or ridiculed. In other cases, a parent and a child align against the other parent in order to secure increased power and thereby undermine an appropriate parent–child hierarchy and boundaries. In families with marital distress, a parent may seek a teen to inappropriately meet his or her emotional needs, or the adolescent may become triangulated, or caught in parental conflict. Adolescents who have parents experiencing marital conflict have been found to have more trouble separating from home or making a smooth transition into early adulthood (Haley, 1980; Martin, 1987). In the case example:

> John was triangulated in his parents' long-standing marital conflict. The mother had left twice, and according to the parents, John had "talked them into getting back together." John had more power to influence his mother than did his father, and the mother and John typically aligned together.

Adaptability

During the course of a family's history together, the family tasks and needs vary, depending on the stage of the marriage, the age of the children, the health and functioning of the individuals, the demands exerted by extended-family members, the requirements of the work place, and the pressures from the larger social-cultural environment. As described by the circumflex model of family systems (Olson *et al.*, 1979), this ability of a family to adjust to the needs of its members in response to situational and developmental stress is the measure of the family adaptability, which ranges from rigid to structured to flexible to chaotic.

Families that are at the rigid extreme are characterized by parenting styles that are autocratic, and it is more difficult for an adolescent to negotiate increased amounts of personal power and influence. Lack of autonomy and assertiveness has been identified as significant in adolescents who attempt suicide (Trautman & Rotheram-Borus, 1988). In extremely dysfunctional families, inappropriate power may take the form of physical and sexual abuse and isolation of the children from external supports.

Households with chaotic structures are characterized by minimal consistency, poor predictability, and erratic contingencies. Families whose children present with conduct problems are often at the chaotic end of the continuum and require help with basic parenting skills and household management. Parental inconsistency has been repeatedly demonstrated to be a critical factor in the development of conduct problems (Patterson, 1977). In the example of John's family:

> Rules were unclear and unpredictable. Chores and responsibilities were not delineated; privileges were vague, and consequences were erratic.

Reinforcement Patterns

In addition to family reinforcers, it is important to assess who and what else reinforces the adolescent's behavior. In highly disengaged families, the parents may no longer control significant reinforcers. In these cases, contingency contracting between the parent and the adolescent is insufficient. Integrating the family, the school, and sometimes the juvenile court authority is necessary in order to influence the adolescent.

Acute and Chronic Stress

In addition to the family process, structure, communication, and reinforcement patterns, it is important to assess the family's recent or chronic stressors, including physical and psychiatric illness, and financial, housing, or employment concerns. Poverty is a significant risk factor for the development of a disorder. Severe economic stress has a devastating impact on families and is associated with inadequate nutrition and housing (Segal & Yahraes, 1978) and adverse child-rearing and parenting practices (Schorr, 1988). Family therapists can facilitate family problem-solving skills to help families try to advocate for needed resources. If a family is dominated by stress related to basic necessities, such as food and shelter, it is very difficult to focus on meeting the children's emotional needs and providing them the basic assistance needed to develop adequately.

Family Strengths

In each area of family functioning there are strengths as well as deficits. The therapist should identify the ways in which the family functions well and demonstrates competency. It is useful for the therapist to provide feedback to the family about the skills and areas of resiliency that exist, as families in the early phase of therapy may feel pessimistic and incompetent.

It is extremely important for the therapist to determine the resources available to the family. The therapist then attempts to help the family mobilize its strengths to reduce the current crisis. These resources can be broadly defined as economic, social, intellectual, and emotional (Dunst, Trivette, & Deal, 1988). The strength of the social support system is correlated with adaptive functioning. Social support is a function of what is available in the environment and also reflects the abilities of the person to elicit or attract that support (Cohen & Syme, 1985).

Interventions should focus on helping families problem-solve regarding how to reconnect or build an adequate support system that emphasizes the role of the extended family, friends, and community organizations.

Conducting the Assessment

The therapist interviews the entire family and also interviews the parents and the adolescent individually. Most hospitalized adolescents are able to attend the initial family session, although some are reluctant because of the family conflicts that preceded the admission. The initial family sessions of these families can be expected to be tumultuous, and the therapist should be prepared to set very clear limits and to intervene rapidly to prevent escalating conflict. One method of containing conflict is for the therapist to remain highly active throughout the session, to interrupt negative exchanges, and to reframe perceptions quickly. The timing of including psychotic adolescents in family sessions should follow the psychoeducational model, which advises slow integration of the patient into the process (Anderson, Reiss, & Hogarty, 1986).

Although the therapist uses the assessment to identify family problems, the session is conducted in a way that also identifies family strengths. The following dialogue is an example from the first session of a family with a 16-year-old girl, Janet, who was seriously depressed. The therapist began with the adolescent and moved to the parent, with the goal of eliciting the goals for treatment, understanding the context, and reinforcing and modeling positive behavior.

Therapist: Can you tell me your top two concerns right now? Things that you want to fix in order to leave the hospital?

Janet: I want to stop feeling depressed, and I want everyone to quit bugging me.

Therapist: Thanks. That's terrific. You were able to be very clear about what you want. Can you tell me a little more about whom specifically you want to "quit bugging you"?

Janet: My mom mostly.

Therapist: My guess is that, if yours is like most families, there are times that do not go well and there are other times that do go well. I'd like to hear about both. Can you give me a specific example of some time this week when things went ok between the two of you.

Janet: Never.

Therapist: How about a time that was so-so.

Janet (*after a pause*): When we went to Donna's house, we didn't have a fight.

Therapist: Good. That was difficult, but you were able to come up with an example.

The therapist then tracked the specific behaviors and tried to highlight positive interactions to serve as a counterpoint to the problems readily listed. Below are examples of content- and process-focused questions that allow an evaluation of various areas of functioning:

Questions Related to Attributions. It is helpful to understand the family's history of causality.

1. How do each of you understand (John's) attempt to hurt himself?
2. What would need to be changed for (John) to stop running away?

Questions Related to Affective Expressions. In some families, there is minimal permission to express much emotion; in others, high levels of expressiveness are encouraged. Impaired expressiveness or high levels of negative emotionality reduce the family's ability to provide emotional support and reduce effective problem solving (Forgatch, 1989).

1. What are the clues that (mom, dad, sister, etc.) are disappointed (sad, angry, happy, etc.)?
2. How do you know when your mother (son, father, husband, etc.) likes something you did?

3. Whose feelings are the easiest to "read" in your family? Whose are the hardest to "read"?

Questions that Link Behavior, Thoughts, and Feelings. Trautman and Rotheram-Borum (1988) suggested teaching families to use a "feeling thermometer," which is a tool for identifying and communicating feelings to one another. Feelings are described as ranging from zero degrees to 100 degrees, with zero indicating positive, calm internal states and 100 indicating the worst feeling states:

1. Can you tell me a situation this week in which you were feeling in a good range? What was happening, and who was there? What were you thinking about? What was your temperature?
2. Everyone seems tense right now. What is your temperature? (The therapist checks with each person in the room and also tells the family her or his own stress level.)

Questions that Identify Interpersonal Reinforcers. The therapist asks questions that track a complete sequence:

1. If (John) is mad at his mother, who will be the first person in the family to know? How will others find out? How will each person react? How does the tension end?
2. Tell me about a time that went well in the last month at home. Who were involved and what were they doing?

Questions Related to Problem-Solving and Coercive Communications and Behaviors. Families with symptomatic children often have problems with clear expectations, inconsistent and harsh limit setting, and poor conflict resolution skills:

1. What are the most important rules in your family? What happens when people go along with the rules? What happens if they don't?
2. How are the rules or expectations different for each child? How are they the same?
3. What decisions are totally up to the adolescent? What decisions are totally up to the parents?
4. If I were in your house during the last disagreement, what would I have seen? How does the discussion usually end?
5. How do you keep from getting into disagreements?

Initial Contract

If successful, the assessment/motivation phase results in engaging the family in a therapy process and contracting for specific goals that the family wants to achieve. There is less negative emotionality, and there are more positive exchanges among the group. Moreover, there is a broader definition of the problems and goals for the family, which include a beginning understanding of the role that antecedents and consequences play in maintaining problem behaviors. In brief admissions, the initial contract focuses on problems relating to the acute crisis, and the adolescent and family agree to participate in outpatient treatment. If the family has a better understanding of the problems, more hope that change is possible, a less negative or blaming attitude toward each other, and a better understanding of how family involvement can be helpful, there is a greater likelihood that follow-through will occur. In the best circumstances, the family therapist remains the same. If this is not possible, it is necessary either to have the outpatient therapist join the discharge session or, at a minimum, to arrange an appointment time before discharge. Family members can be very helpful in keeping adolescents in therapy if the family has had a positive experience during the inpatient care.

Phase 2: Behavior Change

Behavior changes begin in either the inpatient or the outpatient setting, depending on the length of hospitalization. There are two components in the behavior change phase: (1) skill training in parenting, problem solving, and communication, and (2) functional or structural interventions to alleviate problems. The assessment indicates which of the skill areas must be targeted first. In some cases, basic parenting skills must be addressed. In other cases, the family can begin with problem-solving and communication skills, which involves learning a structured method for approaching the various problems they confront.

Parenting Skills. Problem-solving and communication skills are vital to effective family functioning, but in many cases other basic parenting skills must be strengthened first. Many parents define problems with their children using trait labels such as "lazy" or "irresponsible." Parents may need help learning to be behaviorally specific. They often need help with clarifying their expectations, rules, consequences, and rewards. Parents often need to learn to monitor their teenager's behavior to identify the rate at which positive and negative actions are occurring. Additionally, they need help to set appropriate limits. Problem-solving and communication skills are easier for families that have a basic understanding of reinforcement principles. Patterson and Forgatch (1987) provided an overview of parenting skills for early and mid-adolescents.

Problem-Solving Skills

Problem-solving is a structured approach that was first described by Spivack, Platt, and Shure (1976) and was adapted by others, including Falloon *et al.* (1984) and Robin and Foster (1989). This type of intervention can be provided in individual family sessions as well as in parent and adolescent groups and workshops. The latter may be very effective in helping parents to recognize common parenting problems and to get support. There are six steps in problem solving:

Defining the Problem. Blaming, global, and vague problem definitions defeat problem solving. Problems that are defined as "character pathology," such as "He's a manipulative liar," or vaguely, such as "We don't communicate" or "I want him to behave," will set up a failure experience for the family. An adequate problem definition is specific and can be turned into a goal statement, such as "I don't get to go out as often as my friends, and I feel as if I'm missing out on things." Goal: "I want to spend more time with my friends." If the speaker has not created an adequate problem definition, the therapist helps her or him to do so by prompting or modeling. As much as possible, the therapist provides positive feedback to each family member and the group at large; attaining an appropriate and workable problem definition may take many attempts. Often, it is helpful to start with a hypothetical problem in order to outline the general approach before moving into the actual issues. In general, the family should tackle the less severe problems first in order to experience some success with the approach.

Generating Alternative Solutions. After defining the problem and goals, the family needs to generate a range of alternatives, even absurd ideas. Occasionally, the therapist may add additional ideas when a family is stuck in order to positively reinforce creative thinking. Family members are taught not to evaluate ideas at this point, because evaluation leads to fewer suggestions. Everyone gives ideas, and the therapist interrupts criticism of any suggestions, using humor to deflect tension. For example, a 16-year-old has a nightly curfew of 10 o'clock and continues to break the rule and stays out late. The teenager wants to renegotiate the rule. Alternative solutions may be that there is no curfew; the curfew is the same or earlier; a younger sibling decides the curfew; there is one curfew for week nights and a different curfew for weekends; adherence to the curfew during the week earns extra time on the weekends; the curfew is related to the event; the curfew is fixed every night; the curfew is fixed regardless of the event; or the teen calls at 10 to obtain additional time. Usually, 8–10 solutions should be generated before the alternatives are evaluated.

Evaluating the Solutions.   Each suggestion is evaluated independently by each person and is rated on a 5-point scale.

Decision Making.   At this point, the pros and cons of each idea are discussed by the family. Negative stories about past events may emerge, and the therapist redirects the family to a future-tense orientation. As the family attempts to choose one alternative or a combination of alternatives, the therapist monitors the discussion to reinforce positively any efforts toward compromise, flexibility, and creativity.

Planning the Implementation.   In order to implement the negotiated solution, the family must be specific about the who, what, where, when, and how of the plan. Usually, several steps must be taken to achieve the goal, and the family should identify possible impediments and brainstorm about solutions to those difficulties. The agreed-upon alternative should be implemented on a trial basis, usually for no more than one week. The therapist helps the family anticipate actions that may increase the likelihood of success. For example, if the agreed-upon solution to the curfew problem is that the adolescent will earn extra time on the weekend if he comes home promptly on school nights, the therapist will help the parents and the teen to set up a monitoring system for weeknights, to agree on exactly how much time can be earned, and to negotiate what percentage of compliance that must be achieved during the week for the reward to be earned. (Expecting 100% compliance is strongly discouraged.)

Reviewing the Implementation.   At the next session, the plan and the implementation are reviewed for positive and negative outcomes. Positive reinforcement is provided for positive results or for approximation and effort. If necessary, the solution is renegotiated after a careful discussion of where the problems occurred. Renegotiation is needed on a fairly regular basis. (See Robin & Foster, 1989, for detailed information regarding problem-solving strategies.)

The therapist uses a variety of in-session tasks and techniques to facilitate the problem solving, including modeling, role playing, rehearsal, and feedback. Although problem solving is a very structured activity, attempts should be made not to create a classroom atmosphere, or adults and adolescents alike will balk. The therapist continues to reframe and give positive connotations to efforts and ideas. The therapist should also remind the family periodically of the connection between the problem solving skills, the communication skills, and the treatment goals.

Each problem that the family brings up can be addressed sequentially. As the family develops improved skills, the therapist becomes less directive and lets the negotiations proceed. If the family members are bogged down, the therapist asks them to review the process and try to figure out what has gone wrong. The therapist uses prompting and provides information if the family gets stuck.

Communication Skills

Problem solving relies on basic communication skills (Falloon *et al.*, 1984). In families where affect is constricted, the members are often likely to communicate indirectly, and conflict may be covert. Eye contact, the ability to identify feeling states, and verbal expressiveness are often inadequate. Conflict is frequently covert and not openly acknowledged. Helping the family members to express their respective thoughts and feelings at a pace that does not overwhelm them is useful. Discouraging the need to "walk on eggshells" may be helpful.

In families with more expressed emotion, conflict is usually greater, and the communication deficits may include blaming, interrupting, criticizing, commanding, or catastrophizing. Conflict may be frequent, but resolution is rare. Teaching family members anger management skills, assertiveness skills, and supportive communication is useful.

Problem communications fall into the nonverbal and verbal categories. Emotions are often conveyed nonverbally, and people with a paucity of nonverbal skills may give inadequate clues to their needs. Body posture, facial expressions, and reciprocity provide opportunities to send and read messages. Family members are taught to read and send these messages more clearly.

Verbal skills include sending messages—clearly, directly, briefly, and positively. In addition, families are encouraged to speak for themselves; to accept alternative points of view; to listen attentively; to eliminate overgeneralizations, such as "You always do that"; to eliminate "psychologizing" and "mind reading"; to cease dwelling on the past; and to minimize interrupting and changing the topic before the discussion is finished (Gottman *et al.*, 1976).

It is helpful to have family members identify who is proficient in which skills and to experiment as a group with one or two behaviors at a time. The therapist continues to model and reinforce appropriate types of communication.

Structural and Functional Family Problems

During the course of problem-solving and communication training, more serious family problems often emerge. During inpatient treatment these can be clarified and identified as issues for the family to continue to address in the outpatient treatment phase. Structural and functional therapy interventions are useful; however, it is beyond the scope of this chapter to discuss these methods in depth. A few of the more common difficulties are highlighted here. (For a more in-depth discussion of these interventions, see Alexander & Parsons, 1982; Minuchin, 1974; Robin & Foster, 1989).

One of the more frequent problems to emerge in family treatment is to boundary issues. When an adolescent's behavior problems are exacerbated by a lack of parental limit setting, there is often an inadequate parental coalition. In two-parent families, marital problems may be part of the issue, and the adolescent may be inappropriately empowered by a cross-generational alliance with one parent against the other. The therapist works to strengthen the parental bond and may need to obtain a contract with the couple for marital work. In some cases, marital issues are identified, but the couple is not interested in addressing them. Attempts are then made to solve the parenting and the marital issues separately. The severity of the marital problems may continue to interfere seriously with parenting practices, and as a consequence, minimal change may occur. In such cases, the teenager can be supported to recognize how he or she becomes triangulated in the battles and can be encouraged to stay out of the middle.

In other cases, the adolescent lacks a supportive and structured environment because of parental absence and neglect. The causes may be various, such as parental psychiatric impairment, drug abuse, or intellectual deficits. When parents are unable to cope, a referral for their own treatment is needed. In other cases, the lack of appropriate monitoring and nurturance is related to the parent's being overwhelmed by life stressors. Single parents with limited resources may find themselves too stressed to provide supervision and support. Helping the parent obtain additional resources should be targeted in treatment. (See Dunst *et al.*, [1988], for an overview of a resource-building model that is useful for highly stressed families.)

In some situations, the therapist hypothesizes that the symptoms are ineffective methods of regulating the interpersonal distance between the adolescent and one or more family members (*i.e.*, the symptoms are a method of drawing others in closer for more contact, driving people further away, or a combination of the two). The therapist attempts to provide an alternative, less symptomatic way of getting contact and distance needs met without changing the actual amount of intensity in the current arrangement (Alexander & Parsons, 1982). For example, a father who is not very involved with his children, except occasionally to punish them, would be asked to positively reinforce certain behaviors; he would not be involved in the family more intensely, but the children would have an alternative way of obtaining the same amount of contact.

A final problem of note occurs when acting-out behavior is directed against an overly rigid set of rules and a lack of family flexibility. In such cases, the therapist attempts to challenge the family rules by education, exploring the parents' catastrophic fears, and highlighting the relationship between excessive controls and acting out behavior. Cultural and religious influences as well as gender roles are highly influential in creating family expectations. It is useful for the therapist to help the parents differentiate between the content of the rules and the process through which they attempt to enforce them. For example, the parents may insist that their 17-year-old attend church, but they may choose to insist either coercively or more positively.

Summary

This chapter has attempted to demonstrate that the factors that affect the adolescent's ability to learn, to develop attachments and social relationships, and to cope effectively with the demands of family and community roles are broad-ranging and require a holistic perspective (Reiss, Plomin, & Hetherington, 1991). The family treatment outlined attempts to recognize the confluence of the psychosocial, psychological, and biological factors that shape symptom development, and it focuses on interventions that provide families with specific skills to reduce negativity and enhance support.

References

AAPPH (1981–1985). *Annual Survey*. Washington DC: American Association of Private Psychiatric Hospitals.

Alexander, J., & Parsons, B. (1982). *Functional family therapy*. Monterey, CA: Brooks/Cole.

Anderson, C. M. (1977). Family intervention with severely disturbed inpatients. *Archives of General Psychiatry*, *34*, 697–702.

Anderson, C. M., & Stewart, S. (1983). *Mastering resistance: A practical guide to family therapy*. New York: Guilford Press.

Anderson, C. M., Hogarty, G. E., & Reiss, D. J. (1980). Family treatment of adult schizophrenic patients: A psychoeducational approach. *Schizophrenia Bulletin*, *6*, 490–505.

Anderson, C. M., Reiss, D. J., & Hogarty, G. E. (1986). *Schizophrenia and the family*. New York: Guilford Press.

Arrington, A., Sullaway, M., & Christensen, A. (1988). Behavioral family assessment. In I. A. R. Falloon (Ed.), *Handbook of behavioral family therapy* (pp. 78–106). New York: Guilford Press.

Budman, S. H. (1981). *Forms of brief therapy*. New York, London: Guilford Press.

Cohen, S., & Syme, L. S. (Eds.). (1985). *Social support and health*. New York: Academic Press.

Dunst, C., Trivette, C., & Deal, A. (1988). *Enabling and empowering families*. Cambridge, MA: Brookline Books.

Engel, G. L. (1977). The need for a new medical model: A challenge for biomedicine. *Science*, *196*, 129–136.

Falloon, I. R. H., Boyd, J. L., & McGill, C. W., (1984). *Family care of schizophrenia*. New York: Guilford Press.

Forgatch, M. S. (1989). Patterns and outcome in family problem solving: The disrupting effect of negative emotion. *Journal of Marriage and the Family*, *51*, 115–124.

Garmezy, N., & Rutter, M. (1983). *Stress, coping and development in children*. New York: McGraw-Hill.

Gottman, J., Notarius, C., Gonso, J., Markman, H. (1976). *A couple's guide to communication*. Champaign, IL: Research Press.

Haley, J. (1980). *Leaving home*. New York: McGraw-Hill.

Hanrahan, G. (1986). Beginning work with families of hospitalized adolescents. *Family Process*, *25*, 391–405.

Holder, D., Feinberg-Steinberg, T., Miller, A., & Madonia, M. (1990). *Systematic behavioral family therapy—A problem-solving approach*. Unpublished treatment manual.

Jacob, T. (1987). *Family interaction and psychopathology*. New York: Plenum Press.

Jacob, T., & Seilhamer, R. A. (1985). Adaption of the areas of change questionnaire for parent-child relationship assessment. *The American Journal of Family Therapy*, *13*, 28–38.

Jacob, T., & Tennenbaum, D. L. (1988). Family assessment methods. In M. Rutter, A. H. Tuma, & I. S. Lann (Eds.), *Assessment and diagnosis in child psychopathology* (pp. 196–231). New York: Guilford Press.

Lefley, P., & Johnson, D. L. (1990). *Families as allies in treatment of the mentally ill: New directions for mental health professionals*. Washington, DC: American Psychiatric Press.

Maier, N. R. F. (1937). Reasoning in rats and human beings. *Psychological Review*, *44*, 365–378.

Martin, B. (1987). Developmental perspectives on family theory and psychopathology. In T. Jacob (Ed.), *Family interaction and psychopathology* (pp. 163–195). New York: Plenum Press.

McGoldrick, M. & Carter, B. (1988). Forming a remarried family. In B. Carter & M. McGoldrick (Eds.), *The changing family life cycle* (pp. 399–429). New York: Gardner Press.

Meichenbaum, D. & Turk, D. (1987). *Facilitating treatment adherence: A practitioner's guidebook*. New York: Plenum Press.

Minuchin, S. (1974). *Families and family therapy*. Cambridge: Harvard University Press.

Minuchin, S., Rosman, B. L., & Baker, L. (1978). *Psychosomatic families*. Cambridge: Harvard University Press.

Moos, R., & Moos, B. S. (1981). *Family environment scale: Manual*. Palo Alto, CA: Consulting Psychologists Press.

Morris, S. B., Alexander, J. F., & Waldron, H. (1988). Functional family therapy. In I. R. Falloon (Ed.), *Handbook of behavioral family therapy* (pp. 107–127). New York: Guilford Press.

Olson, D. H., & Portner, J. (1983). Family adaptability and cohesion evaluation scales. In E. E. Filsinger (Ed.), *Marriage and family assessment* (pp. 299–315). Beverly Hills, CA: Sage.

Olson, D. H., Sprenkle, D. H., & Russell, C. S. (1979). Circumplex model of marital and family systems: 1. Cohesion and adaptability dimensions, family types, and clinical applications. *Family Process, 18*, 3–28.

Patterson, G. R. (1977). The aggressive child: Victim and architect of a coercive system. In E. J. Nash, L. A. Hamerlynck, & L. C. Handy (Eds.), *Behavior modification and families: Vol. 1. Theory and research* (pp. 267–316). New York: Brunner/Mazel.

Patterson, G. R., & Forgatch, M. S. (1987). *Parents and adolescents living together: Part 1: The basics*. Eugene, OR: Castalia.

Pearlin, L. I., & Schooler, C. (1978). The structure of coping. *Journal of Health and Social Behavior, 22*, 368–378.

Reiss, D., Plomin, R., & Hetherington, E. M. (1991). Genetics and psychiatry: An unheralded window on the environment. *American Journal of Psychiatry, 148*, 283–291.

Robin, A. L., & Foster, S. L. (1989). *Negotiating parent adolescent conflict*. New York: Guilford Press.

Rosenstock, H. A. (1985). The first 900: A nine-year longitudinal analysis of consecutive adolescent inpatients. *Adolescence, 20*, 959–973.

Rutter, M. (1985). Resilience in the face of adversity: Protective factors and resistance to psychiatric disorders. *British Journal of Psychiatry, 147*, 598–611.

Rutter, M. (1987). Parental mental disorder as a psychiatric risk factor. In R. Hales & A. Frances (Eds.), *American Psychiatric Association annual review (Vol. 6)*, (pp. 647–663). Washington, DC: American Psychiatric Press.

Rutter, M., & Quinton, D. (1977). Psychiatric disorder: Ecological factors and concepts of causation. In H. McGurk (Ed.), *Ecological factors in human development* (pp. 173–187). North Holland: Amsterdam.

Rutter, M., Tizard, J., Yule, W., Graham, P., & Whitmore, K. (1976). Research report: Isle of Wight studies, 1964–1974. *Psychological Medicine, 6*, 313–332.

Rutter, M., Tuma, A. H., & Lann, I. S. (Eds.). (1988). *Assessment and diagnosis in child psychopathology*. New York: Guilford Press.

Schorr, L. B. (1988). *Within our reach: Breaking the cycle of disadvantage*. New York: Doubleday.

Segal, J., & Yahraes, H. (1978). *A child's journey: Forces that shape the lives of our young*. New York: McGraw-Hill.

Singh, N. (1987). A perspective on therapeutic work with in-patient adolescents. *Journal of Adolescence, 10*, 119–131.

Skinner, H. A., Steinhauer, P. D., & Santa-Barbara, J. (1983). The family assessment measure. *Canadian Journal of Community Mental Health, 2*, 91–105.

Spivack, G., Platt, J. J., & Shure, M. D. (1976). *The problem-solving approach to adjustment*. San Francisco: Jossey-Bass.

Trautman, P. D., & Rotheram-Borus, M. J. (1988). Cognitive behavior therapy with children and adolescents. In J. Rush & F. Allen (Eds.), *Review of psychiatry (Vol. 1)* (pp. (584–607). Washington, DC: American Psychiatric Association.

Turner, R. J. (1983). Direct, indirect, and moderating effects of social support on psychological distress and associated conditions. In H. Kaplan (Ed.), *Psychosocial stress: Trends in theory and research* (pp. 105–155). New York: Academic Press.

Walsh, F. & Anderson, C. (Eds.). (1987, Fall). "Severe and chronic disorders and the family." Special issue of *The Journal of Psychotherapy and the Family, 3* (3).

Watzlawick, P. (1986). A structured family interview. *Family Process, 5*, 256–271.

31

Child Abuse and Neglect

ROBERT T. AMMERMAN and ERIC F. WAGNER

INTRODUCTION

The Problem of Definition

Few social phenomena are as elusive as child abuse and neglect. From the beginning, the field has struggled to arrive at a clear operational definition of child maltreatment. Unfortunately, no satisfactory consensus has been achieved, beyond the broad view that abuse comprises the commission of acts that are or may be detrimental to the child's health, development, or well-being, and neglect consists of the omission of care that may result in equally negative outcomes. Pinning down the specific elements of maltreatment, however, has been virtually impossible.

One of the reasons for this problem is that maltreatment is a private event, unavailable to public scrutiny. Frequently, maltreatment is inferred from its consequences (e.g., physical injury or sudden change in behavior). Unclear reports by parents and children are common. Under these circumstances, researchers have had a difficult time isolating specific parameters of maltreatment that will lead to clearer definitions. Perhaps of even grater importance, however, child abuse and neglect are intricately tied to societal views of adequate child care, which in turn are in a continual state of flux (see Garbarino, 1990). Even within one society, there are vast differences between what is viewed as maltreatment among different cultural groups and professions. In the face of such shifting beliefs and values, it is unlikely that a universally accepted definition of maltreatment will be developed in the near future.

The focus of this chapter is child physical abuse and neglect. These forms of child maltreatment, however, often occur in conjunction with other forms of family violence or inadequate care, as well as with additional negative influences on the child and the family. Examples of such additional deleterious factors are sexual abuse, the child's witnessing of spouse battering, psychological abuse, parental substance abuse, neighborhood violence and crime, chronic poverty, overcrowding, poor educational opportunities, and racism. The unique contributions of maltreatment and the above complicating influences to child and family functioning

ROBERT T. AMMERMAN • Western Pennsylvania School for Blind Children, Pittsburgh, Pennsylvania 15213.   ERIC F. WAGNER • Emma Pendleton Bradley Hospital, Department of Psychiatry and Human Behavior, Brown University School of Medicine, East Providence, Rhode Island 02915.

Handbook of Behavior Therapy in the Psychiatric Setting, edited by Alan S. Bellack and Michel Hersen. Plenum Press, New York, 1993.

are unknown. Therefore, child abuse and neglect are best understood within the context of numerous ecological influences on the child and the family.

Epidemiology

Not surprisingly, the lack of a consensual definition of child abuse and neglect has impeded efforts to determine accurately the incidence and prevalence rates of maltreatment. As a result, epidemiological data have been gathered by means of several different methodologies. Official reports of maltreatment to child protective service agencies (reporting practices of which vary considerably between states) were filed on 1,335,000 families in 1986 (American Association for Protecting Children, 1988). Of the cases in which maltreatment was indicated, over 80% involved physical abuse and/or neglect. These data must be interpreted with caution, however, because it is estimated that almost half of maltreatment cases are never reported to protective service agencies.

In an incidence survey of professionals involved with maltreated children, the National Center on Child Abuse and Neglect (1988) estimated that approximately 1.5 million children were maltreated in 1986. Of these, 43% were physically abused, and 63% were neglected. Once again, methodological limitations probably render these data an underestimate of the actual figures (see Starr, Dubowitz, & Bush, 1990).

Telephone surveys of the general public have also revealed the extent of violence toward children. For example, Gelles and Straus (1987) estimated that, in 1985, 750,000 children were targets of potentially abusive violence.

PROTOTYPICAL ASSESSMENT

An essential component of the treatment of child physical abuse and neglect is the assessment of maltreating parents and their children. *Assessment* in this context refers to the methods used by clinicians to validate the presence of abuse, to identify target areas in need of intervention, and/or to monitor the progress of treatment (Hansen & Warner, 1992). Typically, assessment involves the use of instruments designed specifically to evaluate abuse (e.g., the Child Abuse Potential Inventory; Milner, 1986), as well as more general measures of domains related to maltreatment (e.g., the Novaco Provocation Inventory; Novaco, 1975). Such techniques run the gamut from self-report to interview to observational approaches. The perpetrator and the victim are the individuals most involved in evaluation. However, it is often desirable to include in the assessment additional family members and/or significant others outside the family system (e.g., teachers).

Unique Aspects of Maltreating Families

When evaluating maltreating families, it is important to consider the unique aspects of this population that may directly influence assessment (Wolfe, 1988). First, their participation in services may be involuntary. As a result, noncompliance, resistance, or even open hostility may be encountered by the evaluator. Second, the target behavior or abuse cannot be readily observed. The evaluating clinician must typically rely on indirect (i.e., error-prone) methods (e.g., self-report inventories and parent–child interaction analogues) to obtain information concerning abuse.

A third important aspect of maltreating families is that they are a varied and multiproblem group. No single marker can be used to identify abusing families, nor is there a specific stressor or condition that commonly precipitates abuse. Although there is good evidence that child abuse and neglect are associated with a number of variables, such as increased stress, parental modeling of violent approaches to conflict resolution, and a past history of maltreatment, attempts to isolate specific causal factors have failed. Currently, a constellation of factors has been identified that appears to increase the risk of maltreatment. These variables are best viewed as correlates of abuse and neglect because, among them, it has yet to be conclusively demonstrated which are antecedents, concomitants, and consequences of maltreatment.

Abused and neglected children and their families are a heterogeneous group. Maltreated children have been found to show (1) perceptual-motor deficits; (2) lower scores on measures of intelligence; (3) lower scores on measures of academic achievement; (4) internalizing problems, including depression, hopelessness, and low self-worth; (5) externalizing problems, particularly hyperactivity; (6) impaired interpersonal relations, characterized by aggression, resistance, and avoidance; (7) health-related problems, including prematurity, chronic illness, and physical handicaps; and (8) mental retardation (see review by Ammerman, Cassisi, Van Hasselt, & Hersen, 1986). Maltreating parents often demonstrate (1) low frustration tolerance and inappropriate expression of anger; (2) isolation and social incompetence; (3) impaired parenting skills; (4) a tendency to view themselves as inadequate parents; (5) unrealistic expectations of their children's behavior; (6) the perception that their children's behavior causes stress; (7) mild to moderate emotional distress; (8) a history of abuse themselves; (9) more negative interaction with other family members; (10) a tendency to respond reciprocally to their child's aversive behavior; and (11) a tendency to react negatively even when their child engages in prosocial behavior (see review by Wolfe, 1985). Moreover, the demographic and family correlates of maltreatment suggest that (1) neglect is more likely to occur among African Americans than abuse, whereas Caucasians are more likely to engage in physical abuse or physical abuse *and* neglect; (2) fathers are more likely to be reported for abuse, and mothers are more likely to be reported for neglect; (3) abusive parents tend to be younger than average when their first child is born; (4) mothers are more likely to be abusive and neglectful than fathers; (5) families with more than three children are more likely than smaller families to be maltreating; and (6) families from lower socioeconomic strata are more likely than other families to be abusive or neglectful (see Wolfe, 1987).

Cautionary Note on Biases among Professionals

An additional consideration when conducting an evaluation concerns the biases that sometimes influence professionals' judgment in cases of suspected abuse. In a study of mental health and social service workers' perceptions of child maltreatment, Howe, Herzberger, and Tennen (1988) found that discipline by mothers is viewed by professionals as being less severe and its effects as being more temporary than the same behavior exhibited by fathers. This bias exists despite data indicating that mothers are more likely to be abusive and neglectful than fathers by a ratio of 3:2. Further, Howe *et al.* found that discipline directed at daughters is judged as less severe and more appropriate than the same actions toward sons. This perception persists even though girls and boys are more-or-less equally likely to be abused and neglected. Other biases were documented by Howe *et al.*: Professionals with a personal history of abuse judge abusive behavior as more severe and its effects as being of greater magnitude than professionals without an abuse history, and female clinicians rate disciplinary actions by parents as being more severe and as having a greater negative impact than do male clinicians.

Assessment Procedures

The impediments to a straightforward and unbiased assessment of child abuse make the task especially challenging to clinicians. Fortunately, these obstacles are not insurmountable and can be overcome by professionals who are well informed, well prepared, and clinically skilled. Such individuals must be deliberate and goal-oriented in their assessment efforts and must be able to anticipate and cope with the problems that are likely to arise.

The ideal assessment approach is a multicomponent evaluation strategy that addresses the broad range of etiological and maintaining factors related to child abuse and neglect. This type of approach has the advantages of offering multiple data sources so that conclusions can be built on converging evidence, specific areas in need of intervention can be identified, and the progress of treatment can be monitored. Furthermore, whenever possible, the assessment of maltreatment should be multidisciplinary. A truly comprehensive evaluation can be achieved only when input from the various disciplines of pediatrics, psychiatry, psychology, social work, and nursing are integrated in a team approach.

Because abuse and neglect are symptomatic of a general disturbance in parenting and family adjustment (Wolfe, 1987), the scope of maltreatment assessment consists of (1) the child abuse potential of parents; (2) parental psychopathology; (3) family stress; (4) parental social support; (5) child behavior problems; (6) parent–child relations; (7) parental child-management skills; (8) parental problem-solving and coping skills; (9) parental anger management; (10) home safety and cleanliness; and (11) marital relations. The following section provides examples of the most common or promising approaches to each of these areas. Given our space limitations, only brief presentations are given. Data concerning the psychometric properties of each instrument are omitted, although an attempt has been made to include only those instruments for which there is empirical support. For greater detail, the reader is referred to other reviews of the assessment of child abuse and neglect (e.g., Ammerman, 1989; Hansen & MacMillan, 1990; Hansen & Warner, 1992) and the specific source materials cited with each method described.

Several instruments have been developed that are specifically designed to evaluate the maltreatment potential of parents. These typically use an interview format and provide an excellent foundation for the assessment of child abuse and neglect. The Child Abuse and Neglect Interview Schedule (CANIS; Ammerman, Hersen, & Van Hasselt, 1988a), for example, is an extensive semistructured interview that assesses the presence of maltreatment and factors related to abuse and neglect. The Childhood Level of Living Scale (CLLS; Hally, Polansky, & Polansky, 1980) evaluates essential elements of child care and neglect. A third widely used measure is the Child Abuse Potential Inventory (CAPI; Milner, 1986), which functions best as a screening measure for the detection of parents at high risk of engaging in abuse.

Psychopathology may interfere with a parent's ability to care for a child in a number of ways, and thus it is an essential area of functioning to assess. Objective measures such as the Minnesota Multiphasic Personality Inventory-2 (MMPI-2; Butcher, Dahlstrom, Graham, Tellegen, & Kaemmer, 1989), the Hopkins Symptom Checklist (SCL-90; Derogatis, 1983), and the Beck Depression Inventory (BDI; Beck, Ward, Mendelsohn, Mock, & Erbaugh, 1961) are useful in this regard. Particular attention should be devoted to evaluating for the presence of substance abuse, major depression, and psychosis, as these disorders correlate positively with child maltreatment.

Family stress may contribute to child abuse and neglect because of the demands placed on both parents and children. The Life Experiences Survey (Sarason, Johnson, & Siegel, 1978), which assesses major life events, and the Hassles Scale (Kanner, Coyne, Schaefer, & Lazarus, 1981), which assesses daily stressors, are two measures that may be used to evaluate the occurrence and impact of stress. The Parenting Stress Index (PSI; Abidin, 1986), which is designed to assess stresses specifically associated with parenting, is a third measure that often proves valuable in the assessment of child maltreatment.

Social support can act as buffer for family stress. Thus, the role of stress in a given case of child maltreatment cannot be completely understood unless the degree to which social support is available and fulfilling is measured. The Interpersonal Support Evaluation List (ISEL; Cohen, Mermelstein, Karmarck, & Hoberman, 1985) is a self-report questionnaire that evaluates the availability of support across a number of functional domains, including tangible support, appraisal support, self-esteem support, and belonging support. The Social Provisions Scale (Russell & Cutrona, 1984) provides a quick self-report assessment of the adequacy of an individual's social support network for satisfying needs in the areas of attachment, reassurance of worth, reliable alliance, and guidance. A somewhat different approach to measuring social support is the Community Interaction Checklist (CIC; Wahler, Leske, & Rogers, 1979), a semistructured interview that examines the frequency and nature of social contacts.

Measures of child misbehavior are important in identifying specific areas of child functioning that are a problem. The Child Behavior Checklist (CBCL; Achenbach & Edelbrock, 1983) is a comprehensive age- and gender-normed questionnaire completed by parents or teachers. The CBCL generates a variety of scale scores reflecting internalizing and externalizing disorders. The Revised Behavior Problem Checklist (Quay & Peterson, 1987) is a similar but shorter measure on which ratings of deviant child behavior yield scale scores for acting out and internalizing problems. The Eyberg Child Behavior Inventory (ECBI; Eyberg & Ross, 1978) is a comparable instrument, on which parents rate the frequency and difficulty of several different behavior problems.

An assessment of parent–child relations is crucial to any child abuse evaluation (Hansen & Warner, 1992). Most typically, this involves direct observation of parent–child interactions and a subsequent evaluation of the quality and content of their exchanges. In some cases, the ways in which a parent and a child relate are so obviously unusual that a simple narrative of the interaction may capture its dysfunctional quality. In most cases, however, the difficulties are more subtle and thus are better documented by systematic means. To this end, several direct-observation coding methods have been developed for assessing parent–child interactions. Three of the better known approaches are the Dyadic Parent-Child Interaction Coding System (DPICS; Eyberg & Robinson, 1981), the Family Interaction Coding System (FICS; Reid, 1978), and the Behavioral Coding System (Forehand & McMahon, 1981). It should be noted, however, that each of these procedures may be extremely labor- and time-intensive.

A related area is parental child management skills, which are important to assess because physical abuse, when it arises, usually occurs during disciplinary attempts. Because direct observation of parents' performance in a discipline context is often difficult for legal, ethical, or pragmatic reasons (Hansen & MacMillan, 1990), the preferred assessment strategies include analogue and self-report techniques. The Home Situation Assessment (MacMillan, Olson, & Hansen, 1991) is an example of a role-play procedure that uses an adult actor to present deviant child behavior across several different scenarios. A second type of analogue procedure requires parents to detect deviant child behavior in written or video stimuli (Holleran, Littman, Freund, & Schmaling, 1982; Wood-Shuman & Cone, 1986). Examples of self-report measures of child management skills include the Knowledge of Behavioral Principles as Applied to Children (KBPAC; O'Dell, Tarler-Benlolo, & Flynn, 1979), the Michigan Screening Profile of Parenting (Helfer, Schneider, & Hoffmeister, 1977), and the Parent Opinion Questionnaire (Twentyman, Plotkin, Dodge, & Rohrbeck, 1981).

An assessment of parental problem-solving and coping skills is also integral to understanding specific parenting deficits that may lead to abuse. The Parental Problem-Solving Measure (PPSM; Hansen, Pallotta, Tishelman, Conaway, & MacMillan, 1989; Pallotta, Conaway, Christopher, & Hansen, 1989) uses parents' verbal report to assess problem-solving skills in the areas of child behavior and child management, anger and stress control, finances, child care resources, and interpersonal problems. The Parental Locus of Control Scale (PLOC; Campis, Lyman, & Prentice-Dunn, 1986) is a self-report scale that yields an overall perceived control score as well as subscale scores for parental efficacy, parental responsibility, child control of parents, parental belief in fate or chance, and parental control of the child's behavior. Other self-report measures that provide a more general evaluation of parents' coping competence are the Social Problem-Solving Inventory (SPSI; D'Zurilla & Nezu, 1988) and the Ways of Coping Checklist—Revised (WOC-R; Folkman & Lazarus, 1985).

As noted by Hansen and Warner (1992), anger related to child behavior should be an assessment priority with abusive parents. The MacMillan-Olson-Hansen Anger Control Scale (MOHAC; MacMillan, Olson, & Hansen, 1988) is a self-report measure that examines distress

ROBERT T.
AMMERMAN and
ERIC F. WAGNER

and anger in response to several child-related situations. A similar self-report instrument is the Issues Checklist (IC; Robin & Foster, 1989), which evaluates parent–adolescent conflict. The High-Deviance Home Simulation Assessment (MacMillan *et al.*, 1991) is a high-demand version of the Home Situation Assessment (MacMillan *et al.*, 1991) described above. The role plays include higher levels of child demand or deviance and are rated for parental stress, anger, and anxiousness. Finally, a more general self-report measure that often proves helpful in assessing anger responsivity is the Novaco Provocation Inventory (Novaco, 1975).

The home physical environment of a neglected child is often deficient in ways that contribute to and/or reflect maltreatment. The Checklist for Living Environments to Assess Neglect (CLEAN; Watson-Perczel, Lutzker, Greene, & McGimpsey, 1988) is an observational rating system for identifying and monitoring home cleanliness across the three dimensions of the presence of dirt or organic matter, the number of clothes or linens in contact with a target area (e.g., a sink or counter), and the number of nonclothing items or other organic matter in contact with a target area. A companion measure, the Home Accident Prevention Inventory (HAPI; Tertinger, Greene, & Lutzker, 1984), is devoted to assessing home safety across five categories: fire and electrical, suffocation by ingested objects, suffocation by mechanical objects, firearms, and solid and liquid poisons. The Home Observation for Measurement of the Environment (HOME; Bradley & Caldwell, 1984) uses data from both observation and parental report to measure the quantity and quality of social, emotional, and cognitive support available to a child.

Marital problems are often associated with child maltreatment and may play a causal role in the perpetuation of abuse. The Marital Adjustment Scale (MAS; Locke & Wallace, 1959) and the Dyadic Adjustment Scale (DAS; Spanier, 1976) are two similar self-report measures commonly used to assess marital relations. The Conflict Tactics Scales (CTS; Straus, 1979) evaluate dyadic conflict resolution skills and use of violence, can be administered as an interview or questionnaire, and involve the respondents' reporting on their own as well as their significant other's behavior. The Spouse Observation Checklist (SOC; Weiss & Perry, 1983) is an extensive questionnaire on which spouses rate their satisfaction with daily joint activities. Additionally, as in the assessment of parent–child relations, direct-observation coding procedures are available. Two popular systems are the Marital Interaction Coding System—III (MICS-III; Weiss & Summers, 1983) and the Couples Interaction Scoring System (CISS; Gottman, 1979), both of which are comprehensive but time-consuming.

ACTUAL ASSESSMENT

As noted above, the ideal assessment is cross-disciplinary and has multiple components. Areas ranging from parental psychopathology to marital relations are evaluated, and an unbiased and comprehensive understanding of a given case of maltreatment is achieved. In actual practice, however, obstacles to ideal assessment are frequently encountered. The following sections describe some of the most common of these difficulties and suggest ways to deal with problems when they arise.

Acceptability of Assessment Procedures

An often neglected issue in the assessment of maltreating parents is the acceptability of the assessment procedures (Hansen & MacMillan, 1990). If not explained thoroughly and appropriately, such procedures may be interpreted inaccurately by a parent who is being evaluated. As an example, Hansen and MacMillan suggested that the videotaping of parent–child play behavior may be misconstrued as an attempt to demonstrate that the child does not like the parent. Such a misperception, if allowed to persist, can serve only to undermine a clinician's efforts to accurately assess parent–child relations. Thus, assessors must be careful to ensure that parents understand a given assessment procedure and the rationale behind it. At minimum, clinicians should provide an accurate and nontechnical verbal description of the assessment procedures to be used. This should be done before administering any tests. Written materials may also prove helpful but should not serve as a substitute for a verbal discussion of the procedures.

Perpetrator's Biases

When performing an abuse assessment, the clinician must take into account biases on the perpetrator's part that may affect the accuracy of the evaluation. First, because of the social undesirability associated with child maltreatment, abusive parents may minimize the extent to which abuse took place. The possibility that acts of maltreatment have been underreported must be considered. Second, abusive parents have been found to overreport negative behavior in their children (Reid, Kavanaugh, & Baldwin, 1987). When parental reports indicate child behavior problems, it is important to seek data from other sources (e.g., teachers' reports and clinical observations) before making a decision about the existence of child behavior difficulties. Third, in some cases, particularly when neglect rather than abuse is involved, ignorance may have led to maltreatment. In such cases, unusual candor about incidents of abuse may be expected. Thus, what may at first glance appear to be an intractable pattern of extreme insensitivity and abuse is better understood as behavior that results from relatively correctable deficits in parenting knowledge and skills.

Legal Concerns

Mental health professionals who work in the area of child maltreatment will inevitably have interactions with the legal system. As noted by Hansen and Warner (1992), there are two general areas of legal involvement in cases of abuse and neglect. The first concerns the protection of children, which typically consists of the mandated reporting of suspected child maltreatment to the appropriate authorities by professionals. Clinicians who work with children should be thoroughly versed in the current laws and practices in their state regarding child abuse and neglect, as well as the reporting procedures and requirements. The second area concerns the criminal prosecution of the child abuser when the abuse is severe. In these cases, clinicians may be asked to participate in procedures including report taking, screening, investigation, initial risk assessment, crisis intervention, and/or report disposition. Involvement often culminates in participation in courtroom proceedings, which may include providing expert testimony or preparing children for testimony.

When mental health professionals become involved in the investigatory and adjudicative phases of child maltreatment cases, ethical problems are often encountered. Melton and Limber (1989) outlined the most common of these and offered guidelines for clinicians' involvement, based on ethical and legal considerations. First, defendants must have an opportunity to consult with legal counsel before participation in assessment procedures. Second, assessors must be thoroughly familiar with the instruments that they use, including the psychometric characteristics, to guard against challenges to professional credibility. Third, clinicians must ensure that assessment instruments and their results will not be used in ways that exceed the limits of these procedures. It is important to remember that there is no test that "proves" child abuse. Thus, clinicians must do their utmost to prevent legal and social service authorities from substantiating abuse allegations merely on the basis of such tests. Fourth, defendants should be made clearly aware when material from an interview or a testing session may be admitted into evidence in court or may be used by a prosecutor in making a decision about whether to pursue criminal charges. Finally, whenever possible, mental health professionals should limit their role to one of the following: investigator, evaluator, or therapist. Thus, they will avoid misunderstandings about role expectations for clinicians, defendants, and legal authorities alike.

Practical Limitations

Time, resources, and/or other clinical limitations may preclude implementation of the full range of assessment approaches described earlier. An economical solution in the face of such constraints is to rely on data from self-report inventories. The benefits of using self-report measures are well-known, and include (1) the relative ease and brevity with which they can be administered and scored and (2) the ability to make comparisons between the respondent and the normative sample used to develop the measure. The primary drawback of self-report assessments, however, is that they are open to distortion and fabrication and thus should be interpreted cautiously.

A second solution is to concentrate on the measures that are most related to the construct of interest. For example, if the identification of maladaptive interactive patterns that may contribute to the occurrence of maltreatment is the primary concern, observation and coding of family interactions is important. Although such procedures are time- and labor-intensive and may result in decreased attention to other areas, the information obtained may prove invaluable to an understanding of the interactional factors that contribute to the abuse.

A third solution is to use a combination of general and specific measures. As noted by Hansen and Warner (1992), a good interview is essential to identifying the circumstances surrounding maltreatment and to assessing risk. A comprehensive interview may first be used to obtain a broad sense of the presence of and the factors related to abuse and neglect. More precise measures may subsequently be administered to obtain detailed information about the areas of concern raised during the interview. Such an approach has the advantage of being both extensive and practical.

PROTOTYPICAL TREATMENT

The word *prototypical* as applied to the treatment of abuse and neglect is something of a misnomer. The complexities of child maltreatment, combined with the deterioration evident in multiple areas of family functioning, ensure significant impediments to intervention in virtually every case. Indeed, child abuse and neglect are indicative of family disorganization, stress, loss of control, being overwhelmed, and general family dysfunction. The smooth carrying out of treatment in this context is very much the exception rather than the rule.

The psychiatric setting is also infrequently the primary site of treatment for abusive and neglectful families. First of all, it is likely that maltreatment will be uncovered elsewhere: at school, in a physician's office, or at home via a neighbor's report. Child protective services are mandated to provide preliminary interventions, and services in the community (e.g., Parents Anonymous) are thus the most likely locations of intervention. With its emphasis on remedial treatment, however, the psychiatric setting (and other mental health clinics) is a critical component in the acute response to child maltreatment, and to its prevention.

As is evident from previous sections of this chapter, behavior therapy for abuse and neglect is conducted against a background of powerful and shifting influences on the family. Poverty, crowding, neighborhood violence, low parental IQ, parental past history of mistreatment, lack of social support, and preexisting psychiatric disorders are only a few of the factors that contribute negatively to family functioning and that often play a role in bringing about maltreatment. Moreover, some of these influences are stable and relatively immutable (e.g., parental IQ and a parental history of abuse and neglect), whereas others are transient and fluctuating (e.g., death of a loved one). The success or failure of a behavioral intervention may depend, in part, on these factors and their impact, even though many of them will not be the direct targets of treatment. Behavior therapy, then, should be part of a comprehensive intervention effort incorporating other needed social services and medical treatment.

A Cognitive Behavioral Formulation within an Ecological Context

Behavior therapy in child abuse and neglect is driven primarily by social learning theory (Ammerman, 1990; O'Leary, 1988). Such an approach emphasizes skills deficits and the modeling of inadequate care behavior as central to an etiological model of maltreatment, and it views these areas as targets of intervention. More recently, misattributions of child behavior and cognitive deficits in problem solving have been integrated within the social learning model of abuse and neglect (Azar & Siegel, 1990; Hansen *et al.*, 1989). Although the cognitive behavioral conceptualization of child abuse and neglect provides a useful heuristic for guiding treatment, it is critical to note that "child maltreatment has proven to be so complex that it defies a single theoretical explanation" (Ammerman, 1990, p. 246). Treatment must be conducted with a full awareness of the varied additional negative influences on individual and family functioning, such as substance abuse, chronic unemployment, and neighborhood violence.

Before we discuss specific treatment approaches, we present the characteristics of abusive and neglectful families that are important in considerations of treatment planning. This presentation will set the stage for treatment and its targets. It must be recognized, however, that the empirical studies on maltreating families have been conducted almost exclusively on abusive low-income mothers (Fantuzzo & Twentyman, 1986). Neglect alone has received scant research attention. Similarly, abusive fathers, although responsible for almost half the mistreatment (and most of the serious injury stemming from abuse), rarely participate in research. (Discussions of the difficulties of conducting research in this area are found in Fantuzzo & Twentyman, 1986, and Herrenkohl, 1990.)

Child Characteristics. According to officially reported cases of maltreatment, abused and neglected children are younger (mean age = 7.2 years) than the general population (mean age = 8.6) (American Association for Protecting Children, 1988). Boys are slightly more likely to be maltreated than girls. African-American children are overrepresented in the reported cases (the reasons are most likely due to socioeconomic status; see Wolfe, 1987). Maltreated children are likely to insecurely attached to their caregiver (see Youngblade & Belsky, 1990), to be behaviorally difficult to manage (Reid, Taplin, & Loeber, 1981), and to display long-term deficits in social, emotional, and cognitive functioning. Also, children who were of low birth weight, who were born prematurely, or who exhibit disabilities are found disproportionately in some samples of abused and neglected children (see Ammerman, Van Hasselt, & Hersen, 1988b).

Parent Characteristics. It is widely acknowledged that there is no set of characteristics, or "syndrome," uniquely associated with the maltreating parent. However, abusive and neglectful mothers have been differentiated from their nonmaltreating counterparts in a number of areas. Abusive mothers, for example, report higher levels of unhappiness and dissatisfaction (see Wolfe, 1985). They often begin their families at an early age and are likely to be single-parent heads of households. They report greater perceived life stress and are more apt to be socially isolated (Salzinger, Kaplan, & Artemyeff, 1983). Abusive mothers often have excessive expectations about their child's capabilities (Azar & Rohrbeck, 1986), and they tend to view their children as more behaviorally disruptive (Reid, Kavanagh, & Baldwin, 1987). They have low frustration tolerance (Frodi & Lamb, 1980) and are inconsistent in their discipline. On the whole, they have a disproportionate amount of negative to positive interactions with their children and other family members (Reid *et al.*, 1981). They may, themselves, have been abused as children; approximately 35% of abused children grow up to abuse their own children (see Kaufman & Zigler, 1987). Their parenting styles are rigid and authoritarian (see Wolfe, 1987).

Considerably less information is available on parents who engage in neglect. Polansky and his associates (e.g., Polansky, Chalmers, Williams, & Buttenweiser, 1981), however, have found such parents to be lonely, disattached, socially isolated, hopeless about the future, and apathetic.

Family Characteristics.   A majority of families involved in maltreatment come from lower socioeconomic groups. Although this is probably partly an artifact of reporting procedures and practices, poverty often brings with it many of the stressors and disruptive influences (e.g., crowding and financial pressures) that contribute to the development of maltreatment. Abusive families are also likely to display coercive interactional styles (Reid *et al.*, 1981). These are characterized by reciprocal negative interactions between parent and child that escalate conflict to the point of violence.

In sum, abusive parents have been shown to have poor parenting skills, inadequate coping mechanisms, poor problem-solving abilities, misattributions and unrealistic expectations regarding their child's behavior and development, poor impulse control, and deficits in social skills. Maltreated children may exhibit a variety of deficits in psychosocial functioning. All of these are embedded in an environment that more often than not impinges on individual and family adaptation, and that contributes to instability and further deterioration.

Treatment Approaches

The multidetermined and heterogeneous nature of child maltreatment necessitates a broad, comprehensive, and flexible intervention approach. The goals of behavioral treatments are to remediate deficits in parenting, social, and problem-solving skills, with the intention of lowering the probability of recurrent maltreatment, improving the quality of family interactions, and maximizing the child's developmental potential over the long run. Although the perpetrator is the primary focus of intervention, it is essential that the child (and other family members) participate in treatment in one form or another.

Parent training is typically provided for maltreating parents (see Kelly, 1983). The objective here is to teach parents alternative child management techniques and to provide effective alternatives to physical punishment. Positive reinforcement approaches, implemented in order to increase appropriate behavior and thus prevent behavior problems and potential conflict, form the crux of parent training. Also important is the consistent application of appropriate rules and limitations on the child's behavior. Indeed, abusive mothers typically are inconsistent in their disciplining, often intervening well into the child's carrying out of a transgression (unlike more effective parents), at which point the likelihood of conflict and frustration is heightened. Parent training also teaches parents to monitor their children more closely, and to be more responsive and sensitive to their needs. Integral to the approach is learning about child development and appropriate expectations for child capabilities and behavior. Finally, by its very nature, parent training teaches parents problem-solving skills in that they are called on to respond to their child's behavior in creative ways, using previously learned principles and guidelines.

Problem-solving skills can also be trained directly. This protocol emphasizes following several steps in solving parenting problems. Included are clearly identifying the problem, speculating about its possible causes, generating possible solutions, implementing and evaluating the chosen solutions, and selecting another solution of the first one is unsuccessful. Parents are asked to practice problem-solving by using hypothetical examples, and then to move on to real-life situations.

Impulse (or anger) control training is a useful adjunct to treatment. The purpose of impulse control training is to teach parents how to defuse potentially explosive situations and gain control over their overexpression of anger (see Novaco, 1975; Walker, Bonner, & Kaufman, 1988). Parents are trained to recognize physiological cues indicative of anger; to identify and alter cognitions that facilitate an impulsive, angry outburst; and to engage in behaviors alternative to violence (e.g., to leave the room). Impulse control training may be a necessary first step to bring impulsive physical abuse under some control. However, it is used in conjunction with other interventions designed to prevent situations that may contribute to an abusive response in the first place.

Restoring stability is a critical aspect of the behavioral treatment of abuse and neglect. Household organization is an "umbrella" term encompassing interventions designed to provide structure, reduce chaos, and provide a safe and stimulating environment for the child and the family. Illustrative are programs developed by Lutzker and his colleagues (e.g., Barone, Greene, & Lutzker, 1986) to promote home safety and consistent health care. In their ongoing investigation of behavioral treatments for the maltreating parents of children with disabilities, Ammerman, Hersen, and Lubetsky (1991) emphasized providing the child with a regular eating and bedtime schedule, "child-proofing" the home to prevent accidents, and incorporating time for family leisure activities to reduce stress and permit opportunities for positive family interactions.

An innovative behavioral approach to abuse and neglect is Project 12-Ways (Lutzker, Frame, & Rice, 1982) and its more recent offshoot, Project Ecosystems (Lutzker, 1991). Project 12-Ways uses an ecobehavioral approach in which treatment stems directly from a comprehensive functional analysis. Based on such an assessment, needed interventions are selected from up to 14 programs (e.g., self-control training and job finding training). Project 12-Ways acknowledges that each family is different in its needs and presentation, and that no one intervention will satisfactorily address the concerns of all families. Ammerman *et al.*'s approach (1991) is to give families a 16-session intervention in which they are offered up to three treatment components selected from a "menu" of seven interventions, depending on the family's needs.

Empirical Support for Behavioral Interventions

The evidence supporting at least the short-term effectiveness of behavior therapy for abuse and neglect is compelling (see Ammerman, 1989; Azar & Siegel, 1990; Schilling, 1990). With the use of well-controlled experimental designs, incorporating both single-case and group methodologies, the short-term effectiveness of behavior therapy has been documented with moderately to severely abusive and neglectful parents (see more extensive reviews by Ammerman, 1989; Azar & Siegel, 1990). For example, Wolfe and his colleagues (e.g., Wolfe, Edwards, Manion, & Koverola, 1988) have used parent training to treat abusive mothers. In one study (Wolfe *et al.*, 1988), mothers of young children were given a comprehensive parent-training package that resulted in decreases in child abuse potential, depressive symptomatology, and child behavior problems, as well as lower risk for future maltreatment (as judged by the caseworker) up to three months following treatment.

Demonstrating the ecobehavioral approach of Project 12-Ways, Campbell, O'Brien, Bickett, and Lutzker (1983) successfully used stress reduction training, parent training, and marital counseling in treating a high-risk mother complaining of marital dissatisfaction and migraine headaches. In another study, Barone *et al.* (1986) intervened with a neglectful parent by using a psychoeducational home-safety program. Frequent feedback was provided, and a multiple-baseline design across safety domains revealed a decrease in the hazards existing in the home.

Future Directions in Treatment

Although the empirical literature on behavior therapy and child maltreatment has grown substantially since the early 1980s, much work remains to be done. For example, what are the broad effects of behavioral treatment? With a few exceptions, most studies use relatively circumscribed assessment approaches, overlooking the possible secondary effects of the treatment. Also, the long-term impact of behavior therapy is largely unexplored. The prospects here are discouraging. Recidivism rates are very high in maltreatment, even when comprehensive behavioral treatment is provided (Lutzker & Rice, 1987). It is likely that intermittent contact with the family over a long period (perhaps years) may be necessary to maintain gains and promote continued improvement. "Booster" sessions may encourage generalization across settings and as the child develops. Finally, continued efforts are needed to match families with the appropriate intervention. Individually tailored treatment, with the long-term impact in mind, is the *sine qua non* for this population.

ACTUAL TREATMENT

Ideally, behavior therapy is carried out with cooperative, highly motivated parents who are fully compliant with the therapist's directives. Similarly, external stressors or potentially disruptive factors are absent or under control, so that parental compliance is facilitated and the benefits of treatment are maximized. In actuality, numerous impediments interfere with the behavioral treatment of abuse and neglect. Many obstacles must be overcome, and several are seemingly insurmountable on the level of individual therapy.

Child maltreatment does not occur in isolation. Individual, family, neighborhood, and societal factors interfere with family functioning and negatively influence therapeutic efforts. Alcoholism and drug abuse, for example, are often evident concurrently with child maltreatment. The perpetrators may require detoxification and drug and alcohol treatment before interventions can be focused on child abuse and neglect. Or the perpetrators may live in households in which another family member is a substance abuser who adds to family stress and confounds parental attempts to regain stability. Chronic unemployment ensures constant financial pressures and contributes to low self-esteem and demoralization. Violence may be endemic in the community, as is illustrated by the alarming rise in drug-related crime in inner-city neighborhoods. All of these factors may disrupt treatment. Moreover, they underscore the need for a variety of social services (e.g., job counseling) in addition to behavior therapy if clinically meaningful and lasting change in the family are to be realized.

Irregular attendance for clinic-based interventions is a frequent problem in the treatment of child abuse and neglect. There are several reasons for this. First, most parents do not enter treatment voluntarily. Child-protective services are often involved, and there is a threat of removing the child from the home if the parents do not seek help. The involvement of child-protective services is (understandably) perceived by the parents as intrusive. Under these circumstances, parental resentment and anger may lead to lack of cooperation in the form of infrequent attendance at sessions. Indeed, establishing a therapeutic alliance under these circumstances is a critical first step in the treatment process (Wolfe, 1991). Practical limitations are a second impediment to regular attendance. Transportation from home to the clinic may be difficult or prohibitively expensive. Parents with other children may have difficulty arranging for baby-sitting. Some communities offer transportation or day-care services that circumvent these problems. However, such services are not always available. A third reason for erratic attendance is that the disorganized and often chaotic lives led by families implicated in abuse and neglect make regular attendance extremely difficult. Indeed, restoring stability and enhancing household organization are often important goals of treatment.

More and more, treatment providers are conducting treatment in the home to bypass the aforementioned attendance problems, as well as to ensure a more ecologically valid intervention. This is a recent development (and its utility relative to other intervention formats is questionable, see Barth, 1991). In the past, most treatment was conducted in clinic settings, often in a group format. Project 12-Ways (Lutzker *et al.*, 1982) is a notable exception, having always stressed the importance of in-home services. Individual treatment rather than group interventions is also gaining favor. Although group formats are more cost-effective, individually tailored interventions address the most salient issues for each parent and family, and these may be lost in a group intervention. For example, child-management-skills training is useful for parents who lack such skills. Some parents, however, are inconsistent and ineffective in child management not because they lack the skills, but because other factors (e.g., marital distress and external stressors) interfere with the full implementation of appropriate management techniques. Individualized in-home interventions are becoming the treatment formats of choice for child maltreatment.

It is evident that booster sessions and long-term follow-ups and contacts are essential to maintain the gains in the families involved in maltreatment. Unfortunately, follow-up is often difficult to carry out. Families may move frequently, and contact may be lost. Also, movements outside catchment areas may result in a transfer of treatment providers from one agency to another that interferes with continuity of care. Intermittent phone contact following termination improves the likelihood of maintaining contact with the family. Similarly, coordination of services promotes continuity of care.

SUMMARY

The etiology of child maltreatment is complex and multifactorial. Although a number of variables that increase the risk of child abuse and neglect have been identified, there does not appear to be a specific factor or set of factors that result in either child abuse or neglect. Each family in which maltreatment occurs is different, and clinicians who assess and treat these families need to take this difference into account.

Assessment approaches should be multicomponent and multidisciplinary. Although obstacles are often encountered during attempts to provide an unbiased and comprehensive evaluation of maltreatment, clinicians who are careful and patient can overcome most impediments. Similarly, the treatment approaches that are most effective are comprehensive and flexible and should be specifically tailored to meet the needs of each family.

ACKNOWLEDGMENTS. Preparation of this chapter was facilitated in part by grant No. H133G10008 from The National Institute on Disabilities and Rehabilitation Research, U.S. Department of Education, and a grant from the Vira I. Heinz Endowment (to the first author). However, the opinions reflected herein do not necessarily reflect the position of policy of the U.S. Department of Education or the Vira I. Heinz Endowment and no official endorsement should be inferred.

REFERENCES

Abidin, R. R. (1986). *Parenting Stress Index* (2nd ed.). Charlottesville, VA: Pediatric Psychology Press.

Achenbach, T. M., & Edelbrock, C. (1983). *Manual for the Child Behavior Checklist and Revised Child Behavior Profile*. Burlington, VT: Thomas M. Achenbach.

American Association for Protecting Children. (1988). *Highlights of official child neglect and abuse reporting 1986*. Denver: American Humane Association.

Ammerman, R. T. (1989). Child abuse and neglect. In M. Hersen (Ed.), *Innovations in child behavior therapy* (pp. 353–394). New York: Springer.

Ammerman, R. T. (1990). Etiological models of child maltreatment: A behavioral perspective. *Behavior Modification, 14*, 230–254.

Ammerman, R. T., Cassisi, J. E., Hersen, M., & Van Hasselt, V. B. (1986). Consequences of physical abuse and neglect in children. *Clinical Psychology Review, 6*, 291–310.

Ammerman, R. T., Hersen, M., & Van Hasselt, V. B. (1988a). *The Child Abuse and Neglect Interview Schedule (CANIS)*. Unpublished instrument, Western Pennsylvania School for Blind Children, Pittsburgh.

Ammerman, R. T., Van Hasselt, V. B., & Hersen, M. (1988b). Maltreatment of handicapped children: A critical review. *Journal of Family Violence, 3*, 53–72.

Ammerman, R. T., Hersen, M., & Lubetsky, M. J. (1991). *Treatment of physical abuse and neglect in families of handicapped and multihandicapped children: A comparison of two interventions*. Funded grant application (H133G10008), National Institute on Disabilities and Rehabilitation Research, U.S. Department of Education, Washington, DC.

Azar, S. T., & Rohrbeck, C. A. (1986). Child abuse and unrealistic expectations: Further validation of the Parent Opinion Questionnaire. *Journal of Consulting and Clinical Psychology, 54,* 867–868.

Azar, S. T., & Siegel, B. R. (1990). Behavioral treatment of child abuse: A developmental perspective. *Behavior Modification, 14,* 279–300.

Barone, V. J., Green, B. F., & Lutzker, J. R. (1986). Home safety with families being treated for child abuse and neglect. *Behavior Modification, 10,* 93–114.

Barth, R. P. (1991). An experimental evaluation of in-home child abuse prevention services. *Child Abuse and Neglect, 15,* 363–376.

Beck, A. T., Ward, C. H., Mendelsohn, M., Mock, J., & Erbaugh, J. (1961). An inventory for measuring depression. *Archives of General Psychiatry, 4,* 561–571.

Bradley, R. H., & Caldwell, B. M. (1984). 174 children: A study of the relationship between home environment and cognitive development during the first 5 years. In A. W. Gottfried (Ed.), *Home environment and early cognitive development: Longitudinal research.* New York: Academic Press.

Butcher, J. N., Dahlstrom, W. G., Graham, J. R., Tellegen, A., & Kaemmer, B. (1989). *Minnesota Multiphasic Personality Inventory-2 (MMPI-2): Manual for administration and scoring.* Minneapolis: University of Minnesota Press.

Campbell, R., O'Brien, S., Bickett, A., & Lutzker, J. R. (1983). In-home parent training, treatment of migraine headaches, and marital counseling as an ecobehavioral approach to prevent child abuse. *Journal of Behavior Therapy and Experimental Psychiatry, 14,* 147–154.

Campis, L. K., Lyman, R. D., & Prentice-Dunn, S. (1986). The Parental Locus of Control Scale: Development and validation. *Journal of Clinical Child Psychology, 15,* 260–267.

Cohen, S., Mermelstein, R., Kamarck, T., & Hoberman, H. M. (1985). Measuring the functional components of social support. In I. G. Sarason & B. R. Sarason (Eds.), *Social support: Theory, research, and applications.* The Hague: Martinus Nijhoff.

Derogatis, L. R. (1983). *SCL-90-R: Administration, scoring, and procedures manual-II.* Towson, MD: Clinical Psychometric Research.

D'Zurilla, T. J., & Nezu, A. M. (1988, November). *Developmental and preliminary evaluation of the Social Problem-Solving Inventory.* Paper presented at the Association for the Advancement of Behavior Therapy Convention, New York.

Eyberg, S. M., & Robinson, E. A. (1981). *Dyadic Parent-Child Interaction Coding System: A manual.* Unpublished manuscript, Oregon Health Sciences University, Eugene, OR.

Eyberg, S. M., & Ross, A. W. (1978). Assessment of child behavior problems: The validation of a new inventory. *Journal of Clinical Child Psychology, 7,* 113–116.

Fantuzzo, J. W., & Twentyman, C. T. (1986). Child abuse and psychotherapy research: Merging social concerns and empirical investigation. *Professional Psychology: Research and Practice, 17,* 375–380.

Folkman, S., & Lazarus, R. S. (1985). If it changes it must be a precess: Study of emotions and coping during three stages of a college examination. *Journal of Personality and Social Psychology, 48,* 150–170.

Forehand, R. L., & MacMahon, R. J. (1981). *Helping the noncompliant child: A clinician's guide to parent training.* New York: Guilford Press.

Frodi, A. M., & Lamb, M. E. (1980). Child abusers' responses to infant smiles and cries. *Child Development, 51,* 238–241.

Garbarino, J. (1990). Future directions. In R. T. Ammerman & M. Hersen (Eds.), *Children at risk: An evaluation of factors contributing to child abuse and neglect* (pp. 291–298). New York: Plenum Press.

Gelles, R. J., & Straus, M. A. (1987). Is violence toward children increasing? A comparison of 1975 and 1985 national survey rates. *Journal of Interpersonal Violence, 2,* 212–222.

Gottman, J. M. (1979). *Marital interaction: Experimental investigations.* New York: Academic Press.

Hally, C., Polansky, N. F., & Polansky, N. A. (1980). *Child Neglect: Mobilizing services* (DHHS Publication No. OHDS 80-30257). Washington, DC: U.S. Government Printing Office.

Hansen, D. J., & MacMillan, V. M. (1990). Behavioral assessment of child-abusive and neglectful families: Recent developments and current issues. *Behavior Modification, 14,* 255–278.

Hansen, D. J., & Warner, J. E. (1992). Assessment of child physical abuse and neglect. In R. T. Ammerman & M. Hersen (Eds.), *Assessment of family violence: A clinical and legal sourcebook* (pp. 123–147). New York: Wiley.

Hansen, D. J., Pallota, G. M., Tishelman, A. C., Conaway, L. P., & MacMillan, V. M. (1989). Parental problem-solving skills and child behavior problems: A comparison of physically abusive, neglectful, clinic, and community families. *Journal of Family Violence, 4,* 353–368.

Helfer, R., Schneider, C., & Hoffmeister, J. (1977). *Manual for the use of the Michigan Screening Profile of Parenting.* East Lansing, MI: Department of Human Development, Michigan State University.

Herrenkohl, R. C. (1990). Research directions related to child abuse and neglect. In R. T. Ammerman & M. Hersen (Eds.), *Children at risk: An evaluation of factors contributing to child abuse and neglect* (pp. 85–108). New York: Plenum Press.

Holleran, P. A., Littman, D. C., Freund, R. D., & Schmaling, K. B. (1982). A signal detection approach to social perception: Identification of negative and positive behaviors by parents of normal and problem children. *Journal of Abnormal Child Psychology, 4*, 547–558.

Howe, A. C., Herzberger, S., & Tennen, H. (1988). The influence of personal history of abuse and gender on clinicians' judgments of child abuse. *Journal of Family Violence, 3*, 105–119.

Kanner, A. D., Coyne, J., Schaefer, C., & Lazarus, R. S. (1981). Comparison of two modes of stress measurement: Daily hassles and uplifts versus major events. *Journal of Behavioral Medicine, 4*, 1–39.

Kaufman, J., & Zigler, E. (1987). Do abusive children become abusive parents? *American Journal of Orthopsychiatry, 57*, 186–192.

Kelly, J. A. (1983). *Treating child abusive families: Intervention based on skills-training principles.* New York: Plenum Press.

Locke, H. J., & Wallace, K. M. (1959). Short marital adjustment and prediction tests: Their reliability and validity. *Journal of Marriage and Family Living, 21*, 251–255.

Lutzker, J. R. (1991, August). *Project ecosystems: Ecobehavioral prevention of child abuse in developmental disabilities.* Symposium presented at the American Psychological Association, San Francisco.

Lutzker, J. R., & Rice, J. M. (1987). Using recidivism data to evaluate Project 12-Ways: An ecobehavioral approach to the treatment and prevention of child abuse and neglect. *Journal of Family Violence, 2*, 283–290.

Lutzker, J. R., Frame, R. E., & Rice, J. M. (1982). Project 12-Ways: An ecobehavioral approach to treatment and prevention of child abuse and neglect. *Education and Treatment of Children, 5*, 141–155.

MacMillan, V. M., Olson, R. L., & Hansen, D. J. (1988, November). *The development of an anger inventory for use with maltreating parents.* Paper presented at the Association of the Advancement of Behavior Therapy Convention, New York.

MacMillan, V. M., Olson, R. L., & Hansen, D. J. (1991). *Low and high stress analogue assessment of parent training/stress minimization package with physically abusive parents.* Manuscript submitted for publication.

Melton, G. B., & Limber, S. (1989). Psychologists' involvement in cases of child maltreatment. *American Psychologist, 44*, 1225–1233.

Milner, J. C. (1986). *The Child Abuse Potential Inventory.* Webster, NC: Psytec.

National Center on Child Abuse and Neglect. (1988). *Study findings: Study of national incidence and prevalence of child abuse and neglect: 1988.* Washington, DC: U.S. Department of Health and Human Services.

Novaco, R. W. (1975). *Anger control: The development and evaluation of an experimental treatment.* Lexington, MA: Health.

O'Dell, S. L., Tarler-Benlolo, L., & Flynn, J. M. (1979). An instrument to measure knowledge of behavioral principles as applied to children. *Journal of Behavior Therapy and Experimental Psychiatry, 10*, 29–34.

O'Leary, K. D. (1988). Physical aggression between spouses: A social learning theory perspective. In V. B. Van Hasselt, R. L. Morrison, A. S. Bellack, & M. Hersen (Eds.), *Handbook of family violence* (pp. 31–55). New York: Plenum Press.

Pallotta, G. M., Conaway, L. P., Christopher, J. S., & Hansen, D. J. (1989, November). *The Parental Problem-Solving Measure: Evaluation with maltreating, clinic, and community parents.* Paper presented at the Association for the Advancement of Behavior Therapy Convention, Washington, DC.

Polansky, N. A., Chalmers, M. A., Williams, D. P., & Buttenweiser, E. W. (1981). *Damaged parents: An anatomy of child neglect.* Chicago: University of Chicago Press.

Quay, H. C., & Peterson, D. R. (1987). *Manual for the Revised Behavior Problem Checklist.* Miami, FL: University of Miami.

Reid, J. B. (1978). *A social learning approach to family intervention: Vol. 2. Observation in home settings.* Eugene, OR: Castralia.

Reid, J. B., Taplin, P., & Loeber, R. (1981). A social interactional approach to the treatment of abusive families. In R. B. Stuart (Ed.), *Violent behavior: Social learning approaches to predicting, management, and treatment.* New York: Brunner/Mazel.

Reid, J. B., Kavanagh, K., & Baldwin, D. V. (1987). Abusive parents' perceptions of child problem behaviors: An example of parental bias. *Journal of Abnormal Child Psychology, 15*, 457–466.

Robin, A. L., & Foster, S. L. (1989). *Negotiating parent-adolescent conflict: A behavioral-family systems approach.* New York: Guilford Press.

Russell, D., & Cutrona, C. E. (1984). *The Social Provisions Scale.* Unpublished manuscript, University of Iowa, College of Medicine, Iowa City.

ROBERT T.
AMMERMAN and
ERIC F. WAGNER

Salzinger, S., Kaplan, S., & Artemyeff, C. (1983). Mothers' personal social networks and child maltreatment. *Journal of Abnormal Psychology*, *92*, 68–76.

Sarason, I. G., Johnson, J. H., & Siegel, J. M. (1978). Assessing the impact of life change: Development of the Life Experiences Survey. *Journal of Consulting and Clinical Psychology*, *46*, 932–946.

Schilling, R. F. (1990). Perpetrators of child physical abuse. In R. T. Ammerman & M. Hersen (Eds.), *Treatment of family violence: A sourcebook* (pp. 243–265). New York: Wiley.

Spanier, G. B. (1976). Measuring dyadic adjustment: New scales for assessing the quality of marriage and similar dyads. *Journal of Marriage and the Family*, *38*, 15–28.

Starr, R. H., Jr., Dubowitz, H., & Bush, B. A. (1990). The epidemiology of child maltreatment. In R. T. Ammerman & M. Hersen (Eds.), *Children at risk: Evaluation of factors contributing to child abuse and neglect*. New York: Plenum Press.

Straus, M. A. (1979). Measuring intrafamily conflict and violence: The Conflict Tactics (CT) Scales. *Journal of Marriage and the Family*, *41*, 75–88.

Tertinger, D. A., Greene, B. F., & Lutzker, J. R. (1984). Home safety: Development and validation of one component of an ecobehavioral treatment program for abused and neglected children. *Journal of Applied Behavior Analysis*, *17*, 159–174.

Twentyman, C. T., Plotkin, R., Dodge, D., & Rohrbeck, C. A. (1981, November). *Inappropriate expectations of parents who maltreat their children: Initial descriptive survey and cross-validation*. Paper presented at the Association for the Advancement of Behavior Therapy, Toronto.

Wahler, R. G., Leske, G., & Rogers, E. S. (1979). The insular family: A deviance support system of oppositional children. In L. A. Hamerlynck (Ed.), *Behavioral systems for the developmentally disabled: Vol. 1. School and family environments*. New York: Brunner/Mazel.

Walker, C. E., Bonner, B. L., & Kaufman, K. L. (1988). *The physically and sexually abused child: Evaluation and treatment*. New York: Pergamon Press.

Watson-Perczel, M., Lutzker, J. R., Greene, B. F., & McGimpsey, B. J. (1988). Assessment and modification of home cleanliness among families adjudicated for child neglect. *Behavior Modification*, *12*, 57–81.

Weiss, R. L., & Perry, B. A. (1983). The Spouse Observation Checklist: Development and clinical applications. In E. E. Filsinger (Ed.), *Marriage and family assessment: A Sourcebook for family therapy*. Beverly Hills, CA: Sage.

Weiss, R. L., & Summers, K. J. (1983). Marital Interaction Coding System—III. In E. E. Filsinger (Ed.), *Marriage and family assessment: A sourcebook for family therapy*. Beverly Hills, CA: Sage.

Wolfe, D. A. (1985). Child abusive parents: An empirical review and analysis. *Psychological Bulletin*, *97*, 462–482.

Wolfe, D. A. (1987). *Child abuse: Implications for child development and psychopathology*. Newbury Park, CA: Sage.

Wolfe, D. A. (1988). Child abuse and neglect. In E. J. Mash & L. G. Terdal (Eds.), *Behavioral assessment of childhood disorders* (2nd ed.). New York: Guilford Press.

Wolfe, D. A. (1991). *Preventing physical and emotional abuse of children*. New York: Guilford Press.

Wolfe, D. A., Edwards, B., Manion, I., & Koverola, C. (1988). Early intervention for parents at risk of child abuse and neglect A preliminary investigation. *Journal of Consulting and Clinical Psychology*, *56*, 40–47.

Wood-Shuman, S., & Cone, J. D. (1986). Differences in abusive, at-risk for abuse, and control mothers' descriptions of normal child behavior. *Child Abuse and Neglect*, *10*, 397–405.

Youngblade, L. M., & Belsky, J. (1990). Social and emotional consequences of child maltreatment. In R. T. Ammerman & M. Hersen (Eds.), *Children at risk: An evaluation of factors contributing to child abuse and neglect* (pp. 109–146). New York: Plenum Press.

Index